Oncology Clinical Trials

Oncology Clinical Trials
Successful Design, Conduct, and Analysis

Second Edition

Editors

William Kevin Kelly, DO

Professor
Department of Medical Oncology and Urology;
Director
Division of Solid Tumor Oncology
Thomas Jefferson University;
Associate Director of Clinical Research
Sidney Kimmel Cancer Center
Philadelphia, Pennsylvania

Susan Halabi, PhD

Professor
Department of Biostatistics & Bioinformatics
Duke University
Durham, North Carolina

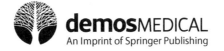

demosMEDICAL
An Imprint of Springer Publishing

Visit our website at www.springerpub.com

ISBN: 9780826168726
ebook ISBN: 9780826168733

Acquisitions Editor: David D'Addona
Compositor: Exeter Premedia Services Private Ltd.

Medicine is an ever-changing science. Research and clinical experience are continually expanding our knowledge, in particular our understanding of proper treatment and drug therapy. The authors, editors, and publisher have made every effort to ensure that all information in this book is in accordance with the state of knowledge at the time of production of the book. Nevertheless, the authors, editors, and publisher are not responsible for errors or omissions or for any consequences from application of the information in this book and make no warranty, expressed or implied, with respect to the contents of the publication. Every reader should examine carefully the package inserts accompanying each drug and should carefully check whether the dosage schedules mentioned therein or the contraindications stated by the manufacturer differ from the statements made in this book. Such examination is particularly important with drugs that are either rarely used or have been newly released on the market.

Library of Congress Cataloging-in-Publication Data

Names: Kelly, Wm. Kevin (William Kevin), editor. | Halabi, Susan, editor.
Title: Oncology clinical trials : successful design, conduct, and analysis /
  editors, William Kevin Kelly, Susan Halabi.
Description: Second edition. | New York : Demos Medical Publishing, [2018] |
  Includes bibliographical references and index.
Identifiers: LCCN 2017046144| ISBN 9780826168726 | ISBN 9780826168733 (ebook)
Subjects: | MESH: Neoplasms—drug therapy | Clinical Trials as Topic
Classification: LCC RC267 | NLM QZ 267 | DDC 362.196/994061—dc23
LC record available at https://lccn.loc.gov/2017046144

Printed in the United States of America.
18 19 20 21 22 / 5 4 3 2 1

We dedicate this book to the mentors, collaborators, researchers, and, most importantly, those patients who participate in clinical trials. These patients are not only scientific collaborators but, in many ways, are the ones who make the greatest contribution to the advancement of our collective quest to conquer cancer.

All royalties from this book have been donated to the American Society of Clinical Oncology to support the next generation of cancer researchers to ensure we continue our fight against cancer.

Contents

Contributors   *xi*
Foreword   Clifford A. Hudis, MD and Richard L. Schilsky, MD   *xxi*
Preface   *xxiii*

PART I. BACKGROUND AND INTRODUCTION TO ONCOLOGY CLINICAL TRIALS

1. The Changing Landscape of Clinical Research and Trials   *2*
    Susan Halabi and William Kevin Kelly

2. Historical Perspectives of Oncology Clinical Trials   *7*
    Ada H. Braun and David M. Reese

3. Ethical Principles Guiding Clinical Research   *13*
    Jackson Bruce Smith

4. Industry Collaboration When Developing Novel Agents in Oncology   *24*
    Hong Xie

5. The Trials and Tribulations of Writing and Conducting an Investigator Initiated Trial   *33*
    Jake Vinson, Josh Buddle, Julie Filipenko, Christine Tran, Kristofer Prepelica, and Sarah Wise

6. Writing a Consent Form   *40*
    Christine Grady

7. Why Do Clinical Trials Fail?   *48*
    Laurence Collette, Jan Bogaerts, and Xavier Paoletti

PART II. DESIGNING ONCOLOGY CLINICAL TRIALS

8. Choice of Endpoints in Cancer Clinical Trials   *64*
    Mei-Yin Polley, Wenting Wu, and Daniel J. Sargent

9. Design, Testing, and Estimation in Clinical Trials   *72*
    Barry Kurt Moser

10. Innovative Phase I Clinical Trials   *85*
    Nolan A. Wages

11. Pharmacokinetics in Clinical Oncology   *98*
    Jill M. Kolesar

12. Dose Finding Using the Continual Reassessment Method   *108*
    Mark R. Conaway

13. Design of Phase II Trials   *113*
    Hongkun Wang and Gina R. Petroni

14. Biomarkers in Confirmatory Clinical Trials   *122*
   Thomas Gwise

15. Bayesian Designs in Clinical Trials   *131*
   Gary L. Rosner, B. Nebiyou Bekele, and Yuan Ji

16. Selection Designs   *143*
   Suzanne E. Dahlberg

17. Phase III Oncology Clinical Trials   *148*
   Antje Hoering and John Crowley

18. Design of Noninferiority Trials in Oncology   *159*
   Lei Nie and Zhiwei Zhang

19. Design of Quality of Life Studies   *165*
   Amylou C. Dueck and Katie L. Kunze

20. Adaptive Designs   *176*
   Tze L. Lai, Ying Lu, and Ka Wai Tsang

PART III. CONDUCTING ONCOLOGY CLINICAL TRIALS

21. Randomization   *188*
   Susan Groshen

22. Case Report Form Development   *198*
   Susan Barry

23. Monitoring, Assessing, and Reporting Adverse Events   *207*
   Amy Callahan, Elizabeth Ness, and Helen Chen

24. Dose Modification and Use of Ancillary Treatments in Investigational Studies in
   Clinical Trials   *221*
   Yoshihito David Saito, Pamela Harris, Ming Poi, and Robert Wesolowski

25. Assessment of Patient-Reported Outcomes in Industry-Sponsored
   Clinical Trials   *233*
   Ari Gnanasakthy and Ethan Basch

26. Recruitment of Research Participants   *247*
   Christopher Gantz

27. Barriers to Oncology Clinical Trials   *251*
   Chethan Ramamurthy and Yu-Ning Wong

28. The Role of Novel Imaging Techniques in Clinical Trials   *258*
   Binsheng Zhao and Lawrence H. Schwartz

29. Practical Issues With Correlative Studies   *270*
   David McConkey and Woonyoung Choi

30. The Development of Companion Diagnostics in Oncology Clinical Trials   *277*
   Zixuan Wang and Stephen C. Peiper

PART IV. ANALYZING RESULTS OF ONCOLOGY CLINICAL TRIALS

31. Interim Analysis and Data Monitoring   *290*
   Scott R. Evans and William T. Barry

32. Reporting of Results: Data Analysis and Interpretation   *303*
   Donna Niedzwiecki

33. Statistical Considerations for Developing and Validating Prognostic Models of
   Clinical Outcomes   *313*
   Susan Halabi and Lira Pi

34. Statistical Evaluation of Surrogate Endpoints in Cancer Clinical Trials   *323*
    Marc Buyse, Geert Molenberghs, Xavier Paoletti, Koji Oba, Ariel Alonso,
    Wim Van der Elst, and Tomasz Burzykowski

35. Development and Validation of Genomic Signatures   *336*
    Stefan Michiels, Nils Ternès, and Federico Rotolo

36. Competing Risks Analysis in Clinical Trials   *346*
    Solange Bassale, Jeong Youn Lim, and Motomi Mori

37. Systematic Reviews and Meta-Analysis   *354*
    Claire Vale, Sarah Burdett, David Fisher, Larysa Rydzewska, and Jayne Tierney

38. Statistical Methods for Genomics-Driven Clinical Studies   *369*
    Richard Simon

39. Handling Missing Data in Oncology Clinical Trials   *375*
    Xiaoyun (Nicole) Li, Cong Chen, and Xiaoyin (Frank) Fan

PART V. SPECIAL CONSIDERATIONS IN ONCOLOGY CLINICAL TRIALS

40. Health-Related Quality of Life Studies in International Randomized Controlled
    Oncology Clinical Trials   *386*
    Andrew Bottomley, Corneel Coens, Murielle Mauer, Madeline Pe,
    and Francesca Martinelli

41. The Economics of Oncology Clinical Trials   *393*
    Michaela A. Dinan and Shelby D. Reed

42. Special Considerations in Immunotherapy Trials   *399*
    Claire F. Friedman, Katherine S. Panageas, and Jedd D. Wolchok

43. Special Considerations in Radiation Therapy Trials   *410*
    Amanda J. Walker, Hyun Kim, Paul G. Kluetz, Julia A. Beaver, Gideon
    Blumenthal, and Richard Pazdur

44. Clinical Trials in Hematologic Malignancies   *419*
    Neil Palmisiano, Bradley M. Haverkos, Sameh Gaballa, Joanne Filicko-O'Hara,
    Pierluigi Porcu, and Margaret Kasner

45. Issues in Recruiting Elderly, Underserved, Minority, and Rural Populations
    (and Solutions)   *428*
    Cecilia R. DeGraffinreid, Jill Oliveri, Chasity Washington, Cathy Tatum, and
    Electra D. Paskett

46. Telemedicine and Clinical Trials   *441*
    Ana Maria Lopez

PART VI. COOPERATIVE GROUPS, REGULATORY AND GOVERNING BODIES

47. Cooperative Groups and Global Clinical Trials in the Future   *452*
    Cooperative Groups: An American and Canadian Perspective   *452*
    Joseph A. Sparano, Judith Manola, and Robert L. Comis

    Cooperative Groups: A Japanese Perspective   *463*
    Kenichi Nakamura, Haruhiko Fukuda, and Yasuo Ohashi

    Cooperative Groups: The Australian Perspective   *476*
    Prudence A. Francis, Katrin Sjoquist, and Linda Mileshkin

    Cooperative Groups: A Latin American Perspective   *483*
    Gustavo Werutsky

48. The Evolution of the Drug Evaluation Process in Oncology: Regulatory
    Perspective   *489*

    The Evolution of Oncology Drug Evaluation at the FDA   *489*
    *Steven J. Lemery, Gideon Blumenthal, Paul G. Kluetz, Patricia Keegan, Amy
    McKee, and Richard Pazdur*

    The Evolution of the Drug Evaluation Process in the EU   *499*
    Francesco Pignatti, Emmanuelle Kempf, and Pierre Demolis

    The Evolution of the Drug Evaluation Process in Japan   *507*
    Hiroyuki Sato, Tomohiro Yamaguchi, Yuki Ando, and Takahiro Nonaka

49. Clinical Trials in the Year 2025   *516*
    Apostolia M. Tsimberidou, Peter Müller, and Richard L. Schilsky

Index   *527*

Contributors

Ariel Alonso, PhD
Professor of Biostatistics
Interuniversity Institute for Biostatistics and Statistical
   Bioinformatics (I-BioStat)
KU Leuven
Leuven, Belgium

Yuki Ando, PhD
Senior Scientist for Biostatistics
Pharmaceuticals and Medical Devices Agency
Tokyo, Japan

Susan Barry, BS
Senior Project Manager
Office of Clinical Research
Dana-Farber Cancer Institute
Boston, Massachusetts

William T. Barry, PhD
Assistant Professor of Medicine
Department of Biostatistics and Computation Biology
Dana-Farber Cancer Institute
Boston, Massachusetts

Ethan Basch, MD, MSc
Professor of Medicine
Lineberger Comprehensive Cancer Center
University of North Carolina
Chapel Hill, North Carolina

Solange Bassale, MS
Senior Biostatistician
Biostatistics Shared Resource
Knight Cancer Institute
Oregon Health & Science University
Portland, Oregon

Julia A. Beaver, MD
Acting Division Director
Division of Oncology Products 1
Office of Hematology and Oncology Products
Center for Drug Evaluation and Research
United States Food and Drug Administration
Silver Spring, Maryland

B. Nebiyou Bekele, PhD
Vice President
Biostatistics & Statistical Programming
Gilead Sciences, Inc.
Foster City, California

Gideon Blumenthal, MD
Acting Deputy Office Director
Office of Hematology and Oncology Products
Center for Drug Evaluation and Research
United States Food and Drug Administration
Silver Spring, Maryland

Jan Bogaerts, MSc, PhD
Scientific Director
European Organisation for Research and Treatment of
   Cancer (EORTC)
Brussels, Belgium

Andrew Bottomley, PhD
Assistant Director and Head of Quality of Life
   Department
EORTC
Brussels, Belgium

Ada H. Braun, MD, PhD
Executive Director, Regulatory Affairs
Pharmacyclics
Sunnyvale, California

Josh Buddle
Clinical Research Manager
The Prostate Cancer Clinical Trials Consortium
New York, New York

Sarah Burdett, MSc
Senior Research Scientist
Medical Research Council Clinical Trials Unit at
   UCL
London, UK

Tomasz Burzykowski, PhD
Professor of Biostatistics (Hasselt University)
Vice-President of Research (IDDI)
Interuniversity Institute for Biostatistics and Statistical
    Bioinformatics (I-BioStat)
Hasselt University
Hasselt, Belgium;
International Drug Development Institute (IDDI)
Louvain-la-Neuve, Belgium

Marc Buyse, ScD
Chief Scientific Officer (IDDI)
Associate Professor of Biostatistics (Hasselt University)
International Drug Development Institute (IDDI)
San Francisco, California;
Interuniversity Institute for Biostatistics and Statistical
    Bioinformatics (I-BioStat)
Hasselt University
Hasselt, Belgium

Amy Callahan, DNP, APRN, RN, AOCNS
Nurse Manager
Telemetry and Oncology
Paoli Hospital
Mainline Health
Paoli, Pennsylvania

Cong Chen, PhD
Director
Biostatistics and Research Decision Sciences
Merck & Co., Inc.
Kenilworth, New Jersey

Helen Chen, MD
Associate Chief, Investigational Drug Branch
Cancer Therapy Evaluation Program
National Cancer Institute
Rockville, Maryland

Woonyoung Choi, PhD
Assistant Professor
Department of Urology
Johns Hopkins Greenberg Bladder Cancer Institute
Brady Urological Institute
Baltimore, Maryland

Corneel Coens, MSc
Biostatistician
EORTC
Brussels, Belgium

Laurence Collette, PhD, MSc
Head of Statistics
Statistics Department
European Organisation for Research and Treatment of
    Cancer (EORTC)
Brussels, Belgium

Robert L. Comis, MD†
Co-Chair
ECOG-ACRIN Research Group
Philadelphia, Pennsylvania

Mark R. Conaway, PhD
Professor
Division of Translational Research and Applied
    Statistics
Department of Public Health Sciences
University of Virginia School of Medicine
Charlottesville, Virginia

John Crowley, PhD
Founder and Chief of Strategic Alliances
Cancer Research and Biostatistics
Seattle, Washington

Suzanne E. Dahlberg, PhD
Senior Research Scientist
Department of Biostatistics and Computational Biology
Dana-Farber Cancer Institute
Harvard T. H. Chan School of Public Health
Boston, Massachusetts

Cecilia R. DeGraffinreid, MHS, RHIA
Program Director
Department of Population Sciences
The Ohio State University Comprehensive Cancer
    Center
Columbus, Ohio

Pierre Demolis, MD, PhD
Chairman
Oncology Working Party of the Committee for
    Medicinal Products for Human Use, European
    Medicines Agency;
Director
Oncology and Haematology Division
French Medicines Agency (ANSM)
London, UK

Michaela A. Dinan, PhD
Assistant Professor
Division of Medical Oncology
Duke Cancer Institute
Duke Clinical Research Institute
Duke University
Durham, North Carolina

Amylou C. Dueck, PhD
Associate Professor of Biostatistics
Department of Health Sciences Research
Mayo Clinic
Scottsdale, Arizona

---

†Deceased.

Scott R. Evans, PhD, MS
Director, Biostatistics Center
Professor, Department of Epidemiology and
    Biostatistics
George Washington University
Rockville, Maryland

Xiaoyin (Frank) Fan, PhD
Director
Clinical Development & Analytics
Early Development Biostatistics
Novartis Global Drug Development (US)
Cambridge, Massachusetts

Joanne Filicko-O'Hara, MD
Associate Professor
Division of Hematologic Malignancies and
    Hematopoietic Stem Cell Transplantation
Department of Medical Oncology, and Sidney Kimmel
    Cancer Center
Thomas Jefferson University
Philadelphia, Pennsylvania

Julie Filipenko
Director
Clinical Data Management and Informatics
The Prostate Cancer Clinical Trials Consortium
New York, New York

David Fisher, MSc
Statistician
Medical Research Council Clinical Trials Unit at UCL
London, UK

Prudence A. Francis, MD, MBBS, BMedSc
Medical Oncology Department
Peter MacCallum Cancer Centre
St. Vincent's Hospital
The University of Melbourne
Victoria, Australia;
Australia and New Zealand Breast Cancer Trials
    Group
University of Newcastle
New South Wales, Australia

Claire F. Friedman, MD
Assistant Attending
Gynecologic Medical Oncology Service
Department of Medicine
Memorial Sloan Kettering Cancer Center
Weill Cornell Medical College
New York, New York

Haruhiko Fukuda, MD
Director
JCOG Data Center
National Cancer Center
Tokyo, Japan

Sameh Gaballa, MD
Assistant Professor
Division of Hematologic Malignancies and
    Hematopoietic Stem Cell Transplantation
Department of Medical Oncology, and Sidney
    Kimmel Cancer Center
Thomas Jefferson University
Philadelphia, Pennsylvania

Christopher Gantz, MBA
Program Manager
Clinical Research Support Office
Recruitment Enhancement Core
The Children's Hospital of Philadelphia
Philadelphia, Pennsylvania

Ari Gnanasakthy, MSc, MBA
Principal Scientist
Patient-Centered Outcomes Assessment
RTI Health Solutions
Research Triangle Park, North Carolina

Christine Grady, RN, PhD
Chair
Department of Bioethics
National Institutes of Health Clinical Center
Bethesda, Maryland

Susan Groshen, PhD
Professor
Department of Preventive Medicine
University of Southern California/Keck School of
    Medicine
USC/Norris Comprehensive Cancer Center
Los Angeles, California

Thomas Gwise, PhD
Deputy Director
Division of Biometrics V, FDA/CDER
Silver Spring, Maryland

Susan Halabi, PhD
Professor
Department of Biostatistics & Bioinformatics
Duke University
Durham, North Carolina

Pamela Harris, MD
Medical Officer
National Cancer Institute
Rockville, Maryland

Bradley M. Haverkos, MD, MPH
Assistant Professor
Division of Hematology
University of Colorado
Denver, Colorado

Antje Hoering, PhD
President and Chief Executive Officer
Cancer Research and Biostatistics
Seattle, Washington

Yuan Ji, PhD
Assistant Vice President
Director
Program for Computational Genomics & Medicine
NorthShore University HealthSystem
Evanston, Illinois;
Professor (part time, Biostatistics)
Department of Public Health Sciences
The University of Chicago
Chicago, Illinois

Margaret Kasner, MD, MSCE
Associate Professor of Medical Oncology
Clinical Director, Acute Leukemia Program
Division of Hematologic Malignancies and
    Hematopoietic Stem Cell Transplantation
Sidney Kimmel Cancer Center
Thomas Jefferson University
Philadelphia, Pennsylvania

Patricia Keegan, MD
Division Director
Office of Hematology and Oncology Products
Center for Drug Evaluation and Research
United States Food and Drug Administration
Silver Spring, Maryland

William Kevin Kelly, DO
Professor
Department of Medical Oncology and Urology;
Director
Division of Solid Tumor Oncology
Thomas Jefferson University;
Associate Director of Clinical Research
Sidney Kimmel Cancer Center
Philadelphia, Pennsylvania

Emmanuelle Kempf, MD, MSc
Department of Medical Oncology
Henri Mondor Teaching Hospital
Creteil, France

Hyun Kim, MD
Assistant Professor
Department of Radiation Oncology
Washington University School of Medicine
St. Louis, Missouri

Paul G. Kluetz, MD
Associate Director for Clinical Science
Office of Hematology and Oncology Products
Center for Drug Evaluation and Research;
Acting Associate Director of Patient Outcomes
Oncology Center of Excellence
United States Food and Drug Administration
Silver Spring, Maryland

Jill M. Kolesar, PharmD
Professor
College of Pharmacy
University of Kentucky
Lexington, Kentucky

Katie L. Kunze, PhD
Biostatistician
Department of Health Sciences Research
Mayo Clinic
Scottsdale, Arizona

Tze L. Lai, PhD
Professor
Department of Statistics
Stanford University
Palo Alto, California

Steven J. Lemery, MD, MHS
Lead Medical Officer (Team Leader)
Office of Hematology and Oncology Products
Center for Drug Evaluation and Research
United States Food and Drug Administration
Silver Spring, Maryland

Xiaoyun (Nicole) Li, PhD
Principal Scientist
Biostatistics and Research Decision Sciences
Merck & Co., Inc.
Kenilworth, New Jersey

Jeong Youn Lim, PhD
Assistant Staff Scientist
Biostatistics Shared Resource
Knight Cancer Institute
Oregon Health & Science University
Portland, Oregon

Ana Maria Lopez, MD, MPH, FACP
Associate Vice President for Health Equity and Inclusion
University of Utah Health Sciences;
Associate Director
Collaboration and Engagement
Utah Center for Clinical and Translational
    Science;
Director of Cancer Health Equity
Huntsman Cancer Institute;
Professor of Medicine
Department of Internal Medicine
University of Utah School of Medicine
Salt Lake City, Utah

Ying Lu, PhD
Professor
Department of Biomedical Data Science
Stanford University
Palo Alto, California

Judith Manola, MSc
Assistant Director of Operations
ECOG-ACRIN Boston Biostatistics Center
Boston, Massachusetts

Francesca Martinelli, MSc
Specialist in Quality of Life
European Organisation for Research and Treatment of
    Cancer (EORTC)
Brussels, Belgium

Murielle Mauer, PhD
Biostatistician
European Organisation for Research and Treatment of
    Cancer (EORTC)
Brussels, Belgium

David McConkey, PhD
Director and Professor
Department of Urology
Johns Hopkins Greenberg Bladder Cancer Institute
Brady Urological Institute
Baltimore, Maryland

Amy McKee, MD
Deputy Director (Acting)
Office of Hematology and Oncology Products
Center for Drug Evaluation and Research
United States Food and Drug Administration
Silver Spring, Maryland

Stefan Michiels, PhD
Gustave Roussy
Service de Biostatistique et d'Epidémiologie;
Université Paris-Saclay
Université Paris-Sud
Villejuif, France

Linda Mileshkin, MD, MBBS, MBioeth (Mon)
Medical Oncology Department
Peter MacCallum Cancer Centre
Sir Peter MacCallum Department of Oncology
The University of Melbourne
Victoria, Australia;
Australia New Zealand Gynaecological Oncology Group
Camperdown
New South Wales, Australia

Geert Molenberghs, PhD
Professor and Director
Interuniversity Institute for Biostatistics and Statistical
    Bioinformatics (I-BioStat)
Hasselt University
Hasselt, Belgium;
Interuniversity Institute for Biostatistics and Statistical
    Bioinformatics (I-BioStat)
KU Leuven
Leuven, Belgium

Motomi Mori, PhD
Professor of Biostatistics
Knight Cancer Institute
Oregon Health & Science University
Portland, Oregon

Barry Kurt Moser, PhD
Research Professor
Department of Biostatistics and Bioinformatics
Duke University Medical Center
Durham, North Carolina

Peter Müller, PhD
Professor
Department of Mathematics
The University of Texas at Austin
Austin, Texas

Kenichi Nakamura, MD, PhD
Director
JCOG Operations Office
National Cancer Center
Tokyo, Japan

Elizabeth Ness, MS, BSN, RN
Director
Office of Education and Compliance
Center for Cancer Research
National Cancer Institute
Bethesda, Maryland

Lei Nie, PhD
Division of Biometrics V
OB/OTS/CDER/FDA
Silver Spring, Maryland

Donna Niedzwiecki, PhD
Associate Professor of Biostatistics and Bioinformatics
Duke University
Durham, North Carolina

Takahiro Nonaka, PhD
Review Director
Office of New Drug V
Pharmaceuticals and Medical Devices Agency
Tokyo, Japan

Koji Oba, PhD
Associate Professor
Department of Biostatistics
School of Public Health
The University of Tokyo
Tokyo, Japan

Yasuo Ohashi, PhD
Professor
Department of Integrated Science and Engineering for
    Sustainable Society
Chuo University
Tokyo, Japan

Jill Oliveri, DrPH
Program Director
Department of Population Sciences
The Ohio State University Comprehensive Cancer
    Center
Columbus, Ohio

Neil Palmisiano, MD
Assistant Professor
Division of Hematologic Malignancies and
    Hematopoietic Stem Cell Transplantation
Department of Medical Oncology and Sidney Kimmel
    Cancer Center
Thomas Jefferson University
Philadelphia, Pennsylvania

Katherine S. Panageas, PhD
Associate Attending
Department of Epidemiology and Biostatistics
Memorial Sloan Kettering Cancer Center
New York, New York

Xavier Paoletti, PhD
Research Statistician
Department of Biostatistics and Epidemiology
Institut Gustave Roussy;
Service de Biostatistiques et Epidemiologie and
    INSERM CESP-OncoStat
Gustave Roussy Cancer Center
Villejuif, France

Electra D. Paskett, PhD
Marion N. Rowley Professor of Cancer Research and
    Director
Division of Cancer Prevention and Control
Associate Director for Population Sciences
The Ohio State University Comprehensive Cancer
    Center
Columbus, Ohio

Richard Pazdur, MD
Office Director
Office of Hematology and Oncology Products
Center for Drug Evaluation and Research
United States Food and Drug Administration
Silver Spring, Maryland

Madeline Pe, PhD
Specialist in Quality of Life
European Organisation for Research and Treatment of
    Cancer (EORTC)
Brussels, Belgium

Stephen C. Peiper, MD
Peter A. Herbut Professor and Chair
Department of Pathology, Anatomy and Cell Biology
Sidney Kimmel Medical College, Thomas Jefferson
    University
Philadelphia, Pennsylvania

Gina R. Petroni, PhD
Professor
Division of Translational Research and Applied Statistics
Department of Public Health Sciences
University of Virginia School of Medicine
Charlottesville, Virginia

Lira Pi, PhD
Postdoctoral Fellow
Department of Biostatistics and Bioinformatics
Duke University
Durham, North Carolina

Francesco Pignatti, MD
Head
Oncology, Haematology and Diagnostics Office
European Medicines Agency
London, UK

Ming Poi, PharmD, PhD
Assistant Professor
Department of Investigational Drug Service
Ohio State University Comprehensive Cancer Center
Columbus, Ohio

Mei-Yin Polley, PhD
Associate Professor of Biostatistics
Division of Biomedical Statistics and Informatics
Department of Health Sciences Research
Mayo Clinic
Rochester, Minnesota

Pierluigi Porcu, MD
Professor
Division of Hematologic Malignancies and
    Hematopoietic Stem Cell Transplantation
Department of Medical Oncology and Sidney Kimmel
    Cancer Center
Thomas Jefferson University
Philadelphia, Pennsylvania

Kristofer Prepelica, PhD
Medical Research Writing Manager
The Prostate Cancer Clinical Trials Consortium
New York, New York

Chethan Ramamurthy, MD
Institutional Affiliations Fellow
Hematology and Oncology Fox Chase Cancer Center
Temple University Health System
Philadelphia, Pennsylvania

Shelby D. Reed, PhD, RPh
Professor
Department of Medicine
Duke Clinical Research Institute
Duke University
Durham, North Carolina

David M. Reese, MD
Senior Vice President of Translational Sciences
Amgen Inc.
Thousand Oaks, California

Gary L. Rosner, ScD
E. K. Marshall, Jr. Professor of Oncology and Head
Division of Biostatistics and Bioinformatics
Department of Oncology
Johns Hopkins School of Medicine
Baltimore, Maryland

Federico Rotolo, PhD
Gustave Roussy
Service de Biostatistique et d'Epidémiologie;
Université Paris-Saclay
Université Paris-Sud
Villejuif, France

Larysa Rydzewska, BSc
Research Scientist
Medical Research Council Clinical Trials Unit
    at UCL
London, UK

Yoshihito David Saito, MD, MS
Hematology and Medical Oncology Fellow
Department of Internal Medicine/Division of Medical
    Oncology
Ohio State University Comprehensive Cancer
    Center
Columbus, Ohio

Daniel J. Sargent, PhD†
Ralph S. and Beverley E. Caulkins Professor of Cancer
    Research
Chair of the Division of Biomedical Statistics and
    Informatics
Department of Health Sciences Research
Mayo Clinic
Rochester, Minnesota

Hiroyuki Sato, PhD
Biostatistics Reviewer
Office of New Drug V
Pharmaceuticals and Medical Devices Agency
Tokyo, Japan

†Deceased.

Richard L. Schilsky, MD, FACP, FASCO
Senior Vice President and Chief Medical
    Officer
American Society of Clinical Oncology
Alexandria, Virginia

Lawrence H. Schwartz, MD
James Picker Professor and Chairman
Department of Radiology
Columbia University Medical Center
New York, New York

Richard Simon, DSc
Division of Cancer Treatment and Diagnosis
Director, Biometric Research Program
Chief, Computational & Systems Biology Branch
National Cancer Institute, National Institutes of
    Health
Rockville, Maryland

Katrin Sjoquist, BSc (Med), MBBS, MClinT(R)
Australasian Gastro-Intestinal Trials Group
Australia New Zealand Gynaecological Oncology
    Group
National Health & Medical Research Council
    (NHMRC) Clinical Trials Centre
The University of Sydney
New South Wales, Australia

Jackson Bruce Smith, MD
Emeritus Professor of Medicine
Thomas Jefferson University
Sidney Kimmel College of Medicine
Philadelphia, Pennsylvania

Joseph A. Sparano, MD
Associate Chairman
Department of Oncology
Montefiore Medical Center
Albert Einstein College of Medicine
Bronx, New York

Cathy Tatum, MA
Program Director
Department of Population Sciences
The Ohio State University Comprehensive Cancer
    Center
Columbus, Ohio

Nils Ternès, PhD
Gustave Roussy
Service de Biostatistique et d'Epidémiologie;
Université Paris-Saclay
Université Paris-Sud
Villejuif, France

Jayne Tierney, PhD
Reader in Evidence Synthesis
Medical Research Council Clinical Trials Unit at UCL
London, UK

Christine Tran, MS, CCRP
Jefferson Innovation
Center for Digital Innovation & Consumer
    Experience
Clinical Trials Office, Sidney Kimmel Cancer Center at
    Thomas Jefferson University
Philadelphia, Pennsylvania

Ka Wai Tsang, PhD, MS, MPhil
Assistant Professor
School of Science and Engineering
The Chinese University of Hong Kong, Shenzhen
Shenzhen, China

Apostolia M. Tsimberidou, MD, PhD
Professor
Department of Investigational Cancer Therapeutics
Phase I Clinical Trials Program
The University of Texas MD Anderson Cancer Center
Houston, Texas

Claire Vale, PhD
Senior Research Scientist
Medical Research Council Clinical Trials Unit at UCL
London, UK

Wim Van der Elst, PhD
Senior Statistician
Quantitative Sciences
The Janssen Pharmaceutical Companies of Johnson &
    Johnson
Beerse, Belgium

Jake Vinson, MHA
CEO
The Prostate Cancer Clinical Trials Consortium
New York, New York

Nolan A. Wages, PhD
Associate Professor
Department of Public Health Sciences
Division of Translational Research & Applied
    Statistics
University of Virginia
Public Health Sciences
Charlottesville, Virginia

Amanda J. Walker, MD
Acting Associate Director of Radiation Oncology
Oncology Center of Excellence;
Medical Officer
Division of Oncology Products 1
Office of Hematology and Oncology Products
Center for Drug Evaluation and Research
United States Food and Drug Administration
Silver Spring, Maryland

Hongkun Wang, PhD
Associate Professor
Department of Biostatistics, Bioinformatics &
    Biomathematics
Georgetown University
Washington, DC

Zixuan Wang, PhD
Associate Professor
Departments of Surgery and Pathology, Anatomy and
    Cell Biology
Sidney Kimmel Medical College, Thomas Jefferson
    University
Philadelphia, Pennsylvania

Chasity Washington, MPH
Director
Center for Cancer Health Equity
The Ohio State University James Cancer Hospital and
    Solove Research Institute
Columbus, Ohio

Gustavo Werutsky, MD
Latin American Cooperative Oncology Group
Porto Alegre, Brazil

Robert Wesolowski, MD
Assistant Professor
Department of Internal Medicine/Division of Medical
    Oncology
Ohio State University Comprehensive Cancer Center
Columbus, Ohio

Sarah Wise, MS
Regulatory and Quality Manager
The Prostate Cancer Clinical Trials Consortium
New York, New York

Jedd D. Wolchok, MD, PhD
Lloyd J. Old/Virginia and Daniel K. Ludwig Chair in
    Clinical Investigation
Chief, Melanoma & Immunotherapeutics Service
Department of Medicine
Memorial Sloan Kettering Cancer Center
Weill Cornell Medical College
New York, New York

Yu-Ning Wong, MD, MSCE
Associate Professor
Hematology and Oncology Fox Chase Cancer
    Center
Temple University Health System
Philadelphia, Pennsylvania

Wenting Wu, PhD
Statistical Science Director
Department of Oncology
AstraZeneca
Gaithersburg, Maryland

Hong Xie, MD, MSc, MBA
Senior Director
Oncology Early Development
Janssen Pharmaceutical Research and
    Development, LLC
Spring House, Pennsylvania

Tomohiro Yamaguchi, MD, PhD
Medical Reviewer
Office of New Drug V
Pharmaceuticals and Medical Devices Agency
Tokyo, Japan

Zhiwei Zhang, PhD
Associate Professor, Director of Statistical
    Collaboratory
Department of Statistics
University of California
Riverside, California

Binsheng Zhao, DSc
Professor
Department of Radiology
Columbia University Medical Center
New York, New York

Foreword

Clinical trials are the engine of progress in the development of new drugs, procedures, and devices for the detection, monitoring, prevention, and treatment of cancer. A well-conceived, carefully designed, and efficiently conducted clinical trial can produce results that change clinical practice; deliver new oncology drugs, interventions, and diagnostics to the marketplace; and expand our understanding of cancer biology. A poorly done trial does little to advance the field or guide clinical practice, consumes precious clinical and financial resources, and challenges the validity of the ethical contract between investigators and the volunteers who willingly give their time and effort to benefit future patients.

In the first edition of their book, *Oncology Clinical Trials: Successful Design, Conduct, and Analysis*, Kelly and Halabi delivered an outstanding primer that addressed the fundamentals of clinical trial design, execution, analysis, and reporting in easily consumed chapters written by experts in the field. Since publication of the first edition in 2009, much has changed in our approach to cancer treatment and, of necessity, in the methods used to evaluate new agents and devices. The understanding of the cancer genome has led to the recognition that most common tumors are collections of rare molecular subtypes that may have similar histology but can harbor unique molecular drivers, display distinct natural histories, and require targeted treatment approaches. The field of precision medicine has blossomed with the development of molecular diagnostic tests that are increasingly used to interrogate the cancer genome and guide therapy selection as well as trial eligibility. But with these new opportunities have come new challenges in clinical trial design and execution. Simply finding enough patients with rare tumor genotypes to participate in clinical trials is often difficult and expensive. It can require that thousands of patients be screened to find the few with the requisite genotype. The clinical research community has responded with new clinical trial designs aimed at increasing the efficiency of molecularly driven studies and a new lexicon of clinical trial terminology. "Basket" trials, "umbrella" trials, "platform" trials, some using Bayesian or "adaptive" designs that incorporate dynamic randomization, early

futility assessment, or "seamless" transition to expanded cohorts have now become commonplace. The execution of these trials is complex and requires unique design elements; near real-time monitoring; rapid data collection; and clear communication among sponsors, investigators, regulators, and study participants about trial modifications over time.

The rapid recent growth of immunotherapy for cancer has already produced long-term remissions in some patients despite their having far-advanced and refractory disease. The rise of immuno-oncology has revealed new patterns of tumor response and progression not well characterized by conventional response criteria and produced new toxicities not well described by standard toxicity grading scales. Thus, new treatment endpoints have begun to emerge that impact the design and execution of clinical trials, and new outcome measures, such as patient-reported outcomes, have become an important source of information about treatment tolerability.

As the investigator community has been challenged to respond to the opportunities and challenges presented by precision medicine and immuno-oncology, so has the global regulatory community been challenged in its assessment of the risks and benefits of these new therapeutic options. In some jurisdictions, new regulatory pathways have been introduced, such as Breakthrough Therapy in the United States and Adaptive Pathways piloted by the European Medicines Agency. In both cases, the goal is to introduce new cancer drugs into clinical use as quickly as possible, particularly in populations with high unmet medical need. Yet doing so may allow drugs into widespread clinical use based on limited data sets from clinical trials performed in highly selected populations. Thus, learning from the use of new agents in the real-world setting is increasingly important to optimize dosing, clarify labeling, and identify patients most or least likely to benefit or at highest risk of severe toxicity. Real-world evidence thus becomes a necessary and important complement to clinical trial data in drug development and evaluation, and we anticipate a deepening of our understanding of its utility and limitations in the next few years.

It is gratifying to see that Kelly and Halabi have produced a second edition of *Oncology Clinical Trials* that has kept pace with the rapid evolution of cancer treatment approaches. The increased focus on biomarker-driven trials, adaptive trial designs, companion diagnostics, patient-reported outcomes, immunotherapy, rare populations, and the perspective of regulatory agencies are all welcome additions that enhance the fundamental approaches to clinical trial design and execution emphasized in the first edition.

Today's cancer clinical trials are more complex, more expensive, and subject to more regulatory oversight than ever before. Current and future trainees in clinical research are challenged by enormous clinical demands, a highly competitive funding climate, and an administrative bureaucracy that can delay activation and then conclusion of a research study for months and sometimes years while the science moves on. More than ever, trainees in cancer clinical research need a concise yet comprehensive primer to guide them through the scientific, technical, ethical, and regulatory aspects of performing clinical trials. With this edition, Drs. Kelly and Halabi have again assembled an outstanding group of authors who are uniquely qualified to address the many complexities of cancer clinical trials. Historically, it has taken 10 to 15 years and cost hundreds of millions of dollars to bring a new cancer drug to the market, with only 5% to 8% of drugs that enter clinical testing emerging as marketed products. Hundreds of potential new cancer drugs now flood industry pipelines and, given relatively low rates of trial participation—especially among adults with solid tumors—there simply are not enough patients, dollars, or time to test them all using conventional clinical trial paradigms. As clinical investigators, we have both the opportunity and the responsibility to design trials that are efficient, informative, and robust. In short, we must learn as much as possible from each and every study participant. This book will help investigators achieve these goals and will also stimulate continued innovation in clinical trial design.

As with the first edition, the editors and publisher of this volume have agreed to provide the royalties from the book sales to the Conquer Cancer Foundation of the American Society of Clinical Oncology. Since the inception of the Young Investigator Awards and Career Development Awards programs in 1984, the Conquer Cancer Foundation has provided more than $83 million in support of clinical and translational research undertaken by oncology fellows and junior faculty. Many of the contributors to this book have served as mentors for applicants to these programs, acted as reviewers of submitted applications, or have themselves been grantees. The authors have all contributed in many ways to the education of young clinical researchers and it is fitting that through this work and the proceeds it generates, they will continue to mentor and support the next generation. For that, we should all be most grateful.

Clifford A. Hudis, MD
Richard L. Schilsky, MD
American Society of Clinical Oncology
Alexandria, Virginia

Preface

More than a decade ago, the concept of preserving the experience of many of those researchers that shaped modern oncology came to life in the first edition of *Oncology Clinical Trials: Successful Design, Conduct, and Analysis*. The book was a collaborative effort and brought the knowledge and expertise of leading oncologists, statisticians, and all clinical trial professionals from academia, industry, and government together to share their experience in designing, conducting, analyzing, and reporting clinical trials in cancer. This allowed these seasoned investigators to pass on their knowledge to those who are entering the field and those already engaged in research to expand their knowledge base. In so doing, our mission was to enhance the successful design, development, management, and analysis of oncology clinical trials for the next generation and beyond.

Since the book was published eight years ago, there has been an exponential growth in our understanding in the biology that underlies the growth of malignancies that has accelerated the number of novel agents entering into the clinic. This has increased the complexities of clinical trials, requiring innovative trial designs and more sophisticated methods to screen, enroll, treat, collect, and analyze the data. These new therapies also taught us how we need to monitor patient safety and gauge the effectiveness of a therapy differently than in the past. This has been paralleled by a tremendous effort from the regulatory agencies to streamline the new drug approval process which not only ensures safety for patients but also provides breakthrough therapies to patients quicker. Results have been astonishing: more drugs that treat and prevent the suffering of cancer have been approved for patients in the past 8 years than in the preceding 20 years.

While this book focuses on oncology clinical trials, the fundamental concepts and basic principles are applicable to all trials in many medical disciplines. We hope that this work will aid the junior investigator's academic, industry, or government career in order to improve the quality of clinical trials. In so doing, their discoveries can be quickly and efficiently translated into improved patient outcomes and future care.

The views expressed in the book are solely those of the contributors and do not represent those of the organizations or of the universities that the authors are affiliated with. In addition, the authors accept all responsibility for any errors or omissions in this work.

William Kevin Kelly, DO
Susan Halabi, PhD

Background and Introduction to Oncology Clinical Trials

The Changing Landscape of Clinical Research and Trials

Susan Halabi and William Kevin Kelly

"Learn from yesterday, live for today, hope for tomorrow.
The important thing is not to stop questioning."
—Albert Einstein, 1879–1955

The number of cancer cases diagnosed daily continues to increase around the world, and we urgently need to develop more effective therapies for this disease. Although there are a plethora of new agents that have shown promise in preclinical cancer models, clinical trials in patients remain the hallmark for clinical research in oncology and the key to developing more effective therapies for patients with cancer. We define clinical trials as scientific investigations that evaluate the safety and\or particular outcome(s) of a therapeutic or nontherapeutic intervention in a defined group of patients.

According to ClinicalTrials.gov, "a clinical trial is a research study to answer specific questions about vaccines or new therapies or new ways of using known treatments." Clinical trials are used to determine whether new drugs or treatments are both safe and effective; and they comprise the main conduit the Food and Drug Administration (FDA) uses to approve agents for use in humans. Over the past several decades, clinical trial methodology has evolved from simple, small, prospective studies to large, sophisticated studies that incorporate many correlative-science and quality-of-life objectives. Although studies have become more complex, they still can be broken down broadly into four categories or phases:

> phase I tests a new drug or treatment in a small group to evaluate dose and safety; phase II expands the study to a larger group of similar patients with a defined treatment or intervention; phase III expands the study to an even larger group of people; and phase IV takes place after the drug or treatment has been licensed and marketed (1).

Phase III clinical trials are usually the definitive trials providing evidence for or against a new experimental therapy, and they have become the gold standard in assessing the efficacy of a new experimental arm or a device (2,3). In the past this has been accomplished in a sequential manner. However, this paradigm has been more recently challenged with more fluid phase I trials that expand into large multi-arm trials in selected cohorts pending on tolerability and early indicators of clinical activity. However, well-conducted phase III studies remain the cornerstone for drug approval.

Friedman et al. define a phase III clinical trial as "a prospective controlled evaluation of an intervention for some disease or condition in human beings" (2). There are generally three purposes of randomized phase III trials: (i) to determine the efficacy of a new treatment compared to an observation/placebo arm, (ii) to determine the efficacy of a new treatment versus a standard therapy, or (iii) to test whether a new treatment is more effective relative to a standard therapy, but is associated with less morbidity (3). The main objectives of a clinical trial are to obtain reliable answers to important clinical questions and, more importantly, to change medical practice. Results from a single phase III trial are not sufficient for the intervention to be considered definitive or to change medical practice. When considering the strength of evidence of data, investigators should interpret data from other sources including other phase III trials and results from epidemiologic and other meta-analyses. As presented in Figure 1.1, Green and Byar argued that confirmed randomized controlled phase III trials form the strongest evidence of support for an intervention (4). The basic principles of design are to minimize bias and increase precision in the estimation of the treatment effect, which will improve the delivery of treatment and eventually improve care for oncology patients.

1. Anecdotal case reports
2. Case series without controls
3. Series with literature controls
4. Analyses using computer databases
5. "Case-control" observational studies
6. Series based on historical control groups
7. Single randomized controlled clinical trials
8. Confirmed randomized controlled clinical trials

FIGURE 1.1 Hierarchy of strength of evidence.

Source: Green & Bayer, Using observational data from registries to compare treatments: The fallacy of omnimetrices. *Statistics in Medicine*, 1984;3(4):361–370. Used by permission of John Wiley and Sons, Inc.

MOTIVATION

Clinical trials are expensive and time-consuming, and a lot of thought goes into their planning, execution, and reporting. The time involved from concept development to study activation varies, depending on the phase of the trial and whether it is a single or multi-institutional study. In recent reports, Dilts et al. indicated that there were 296 processes from concept inception to study activation in phase III trials sponsored by the Cancer Therapy Evaluation Program (CTEP), and the median time that the trials were activated was 602 days (interquartile range, 454–861 days) (5–7). This shows the complexity of clinical trials and highlights the fact that there are many areas where insufficiency and errors can occur if one does not have the experience, the guidance, or the appropriate personnel to aid in trial development and execution.

The development and conduct of a trial require a multidisciplinary approach that involves physicians, scientists, biostatisticians, research nurses, experts in regulatory affairs and contract negotiations, data coordinators, and research technicians, who are all critical for the success of the study (8). In particular, statisticians play a central role in clinical trials, and collaborating with biostatisticians in the early design stage ensures that the trial will yield valid and interpretable results. Close collaboration with statisticians results in trials with clearly defined objectives, study designs well-suited to address the hypotheses being posited, and appropriate analyses. This book is unique because it has contributions from a broad range of members of the multidisciplinary team, who provide their experience and expertise to guide investigators to a successful study.

SCOPE

The landscape of conducting clinical trials in oncology is quickly changing, and many investigators are now exposed to clinical trials without a deep appreciation for or understanding of the basic principles and practical issues of conducting clinical research. Although

historically this knowledge has been passed down from mentor to student, that practice is increasingly not the case in today's educational environment.

The goal of the second edition of this book is to provide an understanding of and a sound foundation for clinical trials and to pass on the decades of experience from seasoned investigators concerning a wide range of topics that are critical to formulate, write, conduct, and report clinical trials. This book is intended for investigators with some experience in clinical trials in oncology, who are interested in pursuing a career in academia or industry. In this sense, it seeks to be a guide, if not a mentor. In addition, this book provides a comprehensive, integrated presentation of principles and methodologies for clinical trials to enable readers to become active, competent investigators.

Altman describes the general sequence of steps in a research project as follows: planning, design, execution (data collection), data processing, data analysis, presentation, interpretation, and publication (9). The second edition of this book is arranged in a similar order, and it focuses on studies in humans, with emphasis on safety consideration in trial design. Furthermore, the second edition of *Oncology Clinical Trials* has been updated and now includes new chapters to address the latest designs and methods of planning, conducting, and analyzing clinical trials in the era of precision medicine and immunotherapy. The book is divided into six different parts that cover the general principles of clinical research, design, conduct, analysis of clinical trials, special considerations in clinical trials, cooperative groups, and the rapidly evolving regulatory and governing science that surrounds clinical trials. In Part I, the chapters discuss historical perspectives, along with ethical issues that have been raised with oncology clinical trials, which give one a basis for understanding the evolution that has occurred over the past several decades. Braun et al. provide an overview of the historical perspective of clinical trials and Smith discusses the ethical principles that guide clinical research. Xie describes how an investigator should interact with industry. In the past, there were few standards for writing a protocol, but through immense work from CTEP and other agencies, writing a protocol has been greatly simplified by the use of standardized templates. Although these templates have simplified the writing of a study, there is an art to writing a study, and there are many obstacles that investigators need to consider. Vinson et al. take you through the writing of an investigator-initiated study, and Grady et al. provide a clear summary on how to write a consent form while the pitfalls of conducting a clinical trial are elucidated by Collette et al.

Input from statisticians is important and critical at each stage of the process of protocol development, and Part II focuses on the design that a new investigator needs to consider for phase I through III trials. Throughout these chapters, the authors provide their extensive experience in trial design and provide actual examples to demonstrate their points. Once agents are chosen, defining the questions, objectives, and endpoints of the trial is crucial, and these aspects of planning must receive the critical consideration they deserve. Polley et al. highlight important issues on the choice on endpoint for a clinical trial, while Moser provides detailed discussion on the basic statistical concepts, such as estimation and hypothesis testing, and how to apply these principles to clinical trials. Innovative topics on clinical trial designs have been added to this part. In lieu of the 3 + 3 design, Conaway and Wages each provides discussion on innovative designs in the phase I setting and Koelsar et al. show the importance of pharmacokinetics in clinical trials. The chapter by Gwise et al. gives firsthand experience from the FDA on the role of biomarkers in confirmatory clinical trials. Dahlberg discusses selection designs, where they are useful for go/no-go decisions. Hoering et al. describe the design of phase III trials, the gold standard design in clinical trials. This part covers advanced topics such as noninferiority trials, Bayesian designs, and adaptive design. Bekele et al. discuss Bayesian design, while Nie et al. discuss important principles in the design of noninferiority trials. Dueck describes the design of quality-of-life studies, which are becoming more critical in trials. This part concludes with a discussion of adaptive designs by Lai et al., which have become critical in recent years.

Once the study is under way, the emphasis is on the conduct of the trial as outlined in Part III. This part starts with randomization as described by Groshen. A critical part of any study is to collect the appropriate data so that the results can be analyzed and Barry walks us through the development of study case report forms. Callahan, drawing on years of experience with clinical research patients, guides us through the monitoring, assessing, and reporting of adverse events encountered during a trial and Saito et al. review how dose modifications and use of ancillary treatments will ensure the safety of the patient. Historically, adverse events and overall tolerance for a treatment were accessed by an observer; however, Gnansakthy and Basch outline the importance of patient-reported outcomes and how this may become the standard in clinical trials in the future. After hours of planning and writing a clinical trial, having poor accrual and not completing a trial is a tribulation all clinical researchers face. Gantz describes practical issues on how to recruit participants into a study while Ramamurthy and Wong enlighten us on some of the unforeseen barriers of clinical trials. Most modern clinical trials have integrated imaging and other blood-based correlative studies embedded within the study. Zhoa reviews the role of novel imaging techniques while McConkey and Choi review the practical issues with using correlative studies. Especially in the era of precision medicine, many of these embedded correlative studies are looking to develop a companion diagnostic to aid in the selection of patients for a targeted therapy. Wang and Peiper eloquently review the complexities of developing a companion diagnostic test.

Studies need to be monitored continuously from the first patient to the last patient enrolled in the trial and Evans and Barry discuss the role of interim analysis and data monitoring during this journey (Part IV). Once the study has been completed, there are many pitfalls that can be encountered in conducting and interpreting a clinical trial, which is well illustrated by Niedzwiecki; and Halabi et al. discuss the importance of assessing prognostic factors and developing and validating prognostic models in cancer studies. In the past decade, there has been increased emphasis in decreasing the time for a new drug to be approved. Thus, biomarkers and surrogate endpoints are examined by Buyse et al. The development and validation of genomic signature has been incorporated into investigational studies to help move the development of drugs along. Michiels et al. provide an in-depth discussion on this topic, while Simon describes statistical methods for genomics-driven trials. Bassale and colleagues identify scenarios where competing risk analysis should be implemented. At times a single trial may not give enough information to produce a conclusive result. With their in-depth expertise in meta-analysis, Vale et al. discuss the importance of meta-analysis. Missing data is ubiquitous in clinical trials and Li et al. provide an outline on how to remedy missing data in trials.

As clinical trials have become more sophisticated over the past decade, investigators found that there are unique issues to consider, such as those described by Bottomley et al. that highlight practical and other analytic issues in health-related studies (Part V). The economics of clinical trials is often a limiting factor, and Dinan and colleagues offer some practical solutions to deal with these issues. As the field of oncology moves forward, researchers introduce more sophisticated and novel treatments, which are making significant differences in patients. Immunotherapy has redefined the landscape of oncology; however, this was not without its trials and tribulations as described by Freidman et al. The same holds true for designing and conducting clinical trials with radiotherapy; Walker and her colleagues outline these challenges. Doing studies in patient populations that have compromised hematologic status or are immune-competent raises significant issues as described by Palmisiano and colleagues. In addition, the frail, elderly, underserved, and rural patients have unique barriers to clinical trials, which are reviewed by DeGraffinreid et al., and Lopez suggests that telemedicine may help us with some of these barriers and enable these vulnerable populations to enroll on trials.

Historically, clinical trials on cancer in the United States were first sponsored by the National Cancer Institute. Part VI is dedicated to the cooperative groups in the United States working globally, as we have seen trials being conducted globally (Chapter 47). We now have global overviews from cooperative groups including those working in Australia, Canada, Japan, and Latin America.

Part VI also focusses on regulatory and governing bodies not only in the United States but also in Europe and Japan (Chapter 48). The material highlights some of the more practical issues that novice investigators encounter, but for which they cannot always get straight answers. Chapter 48 describes the requirements of regulatory affairs in studies and how the regulatory bodies review and approve new agents. Developing an understanding of all these issues is imperative for successful clinical trialists. Finally, Tsimberidou et al. (Chapter 49) outline their thoughts on where we should be in the next decade and how clinical trials will evolve further.

RESOURCES

Several books that have been written on clinical trials have focused on randomized phase III trials (10–14). The available books emphasize statistical or clinical principles and concepts, whereas in this book we present a balanced perspective on clinical trials. Our intention is to enhance statistical thinking and understanding among a wider professional audience. Unlike other books that focus only on randomized phase III clinical trials, we include topics that emerge earlier in the traditional paradigm, design of phase I trials, and selection design and phase II trials.

There are many resources dedicated to clinical trials. These include web-based resources for clinical trials. The list is not inclusive but we present some valuable links in Table 1.1. In addition, the Society of Clinical Trials (www.sctweb.org) is an organization dedicated to the study, design, and analysis of clinical trials, with a peer-reviewed journal (*Controlled Trials*).

There are other educational resources, including workshops, offered to junior faculty members in academic centers, such as the American Society of Clinical Oncology (ASCO) workshops, with the purpose of training junior faculty members in North America, Australia, and Europe.

SUMMARY

There is an ever-increasing need for educational resources and this book will serve as a road map for the next generation of clinical trialists in oncology. The objective is to enable the reader to understand the different stages involved in the design, conduct, and analysis of clinical trials. In addition, this book can be used as an aid in teaching clinical fellows in training programs complemented by lectures and discussion. This book may be of interest to public health students and public health workers and for contract research organizations and departments of medicine, where people are involved with clinical trials. Our hope is that the reader will find this book valuable, especially the practical issues we have encountered in conducting clinical trials, which are exemplified by citing real life examples of clinical trial failures and successes.

Rigorous clinical trials can address important questions relevant to a patient population in which one can make valid inferences about the therapy being tested. Such studies should be designed starting with a hypothesis, an explicit definition of endpoints, appropriate identification and selection of the patient population, and a sufficiently large sample size with high power to detect small to moderate clinical effect sizes. In addition, these studies should be monitored for terminating a trial early so that patients can benefit from a promising treatment or are spared from a harmful regimen.

TABLE 1.1 Web-based resources

https://www.asco.org/
http://www.cancer.gov/
www.clinicaltrials.gov
http://www.ema.europa.eu/ema/
http://eng.sfda.gov.cn/WS03/CL0755/
http://www.esmo.org/
https://www.fda.gov/
http://www.foodstandards.gov.au/Pages/default.aspx
https://latampharmara.com/mexico/cofepris-the-mexican-health-authority/
https://www.ncbi.nlm.nih.gov/pubmedhealth/PMHT0029908/
https://www.pmda.go.jp/english/
http://journals.sagepub.com/home/ctj
http://www.sctweb.org/public/home.cfm
https://seer.cancer.gov/
https://stattools.crab.org/

REFERENCES

1. U.S. National Library of Medicine. ClinicalTrials.gov. www.clinicaltrials.gov
2. Friedman LM, Furberg CD, DeMets DL, et al. *Fundamentals of Clinical Trials*. 5th ed. New York, NY: Springer-Verlag; 2015.
3. Simon RS. Design and conduct of clinical trials. In DeVita VT, Hellman S, Rosenberg SA, eds. *Cancer: Principles and Practice of Oncology*. Philadelphia, PA: J.B. Lippincott; 1993:418–440.
4. Green SB, Byar DP. Using observational data from registries to compare treatments: The fallacy of omnimetrics (with discussion). *Stat Med*. 1984;3:361–373.
5. Dilts DM, Sandler A, Cheng S, et al. Development of clinical trials in a cooperative group setting: the eastern cooperative oncology group. *Clin Cancer Res*. 2008;14:3427–3433.
6. Dilts DM, Sandler A, Cheng S, et al. Processes to activate phase III clinical trials in a cooperative oncology group: the case of cancer and leukemia group B. *J Clin Oncol*. 2006;24:4553–4557.
7. Dilts DM, Sandler AB, Cheng SK, et al. Steps and time to process clinical trials at the Cancer Therapy Evaluation Program. *J Clin Oncol*. 2009;27:1761–1766.

8. Kelly WK, Halabi S. *Oncology Clinical Trials: Successful Design, Conduct and Analysis*. 1st ed. New York, NY: Springer Publishing; 2009.
9. Altman, DG. *Practical Statistics for Medical Research*. 1st ed. London; New York, NY: Chapman and Hall; 1991:1–9.
10. Everitt BS, Pickles A. *Statistical Aspects of the Design and Analysis of Clinical Trials*. 2nd ed. London, UK: Imperial College Press; 2004.
11. Green S, Benedetti J, Crowley J. *Clinical Trials in Oncology*. 3rd ed. New York, NY: Chapman and Hall; 2016.
12. Crowley J, Hoering A. *Handbook of Statistics in Clinical Oncology*. 3rd ed. New York, NY: Chapman and Hall/CRC; 2017.
13. Piantadosi S. Clinical Trials. *A Methodologic Perspective*. 3rd ed. New York, NY: John Wiley & Sons; 2017.
14. Spiegelhalter DJ, Abrams KR, Myles JP. *Bayesian Approaches to Clinical Trials and Health-Care Evaluation*. New York, NY: Wiley & Sons; 2004.

Historical Perspectives of Oncology Clinical Trials

Ada H. Braun and David M. Reese

ORIGINS OF ONCOLOGY: ANTIQUITY, GREECE, AND ROME

Cancer is older than human life, and in fact it is intrinsic to terrestrial biology. The first evidence of tumors was found in bones from dinosaurs of the Jurassic period that lived some 200 million years ago (1). All vertebrate and many invertebrate species can develop cancer (2). Early human evidence of neoplasia includes both primary tumors and metastatic lesions; this evidence spans over 5,000 years, from predynastic Egyptian mummies to early Christian times, and over multiple continents, from the Far East to South America (3–5). The Babylonian "Code of Hammurabi" (1750 BCE), Chinese folklore ("Rites of the Zhou Dynasty"; 1100–400 BCE), as well as medical documents from India ("Ramayana"; 500 BCE) and Egypt, attest to the early recognition of cancer. Perhaps most famously, the George Ebers and Edwin Smith papyri (Egypt, ca. 1550 and 1600 BCE) describe several tumor ailments and their treatment. The Ebers papyrus, which may be considered the oldest textbook of medicine, recommends operations for certain accessible tumors and outlines palliative treatment for inoperable disease, including topical applications (6). The Smith papyrus provides more prosaic case reports. Describing what is likely a tumor of the breast, the scribe annotates, "there is no treatment" (7).

Although these ancient documents describe what we now recognize as malignant tumors, for millennia there was no attempt to study cancer systematically, until Greek physicians founded what we consider Western medicine. These doctors regarded all diseases—cancer included—as having natural (as opposed to supernatural) causes. Traditionally, Hippocrates (ca. 460–377 BCE) first described cancer as a biological process, a disease entity with both local and distant consequences. Based on observation of the growth patterns of tumors directly visualizable, such as breast cancers, he coined the term *karkinoma,* from the Greek word for crab; the term was later Latinized to the familiar carcinoma. According to legend, Galen of Pergamon (ca. 129–200 CE) thought the disease was "so called because it appears at length with turgid veins shooting out from it, so as to resemble the figure of a crab; or as others say, because like a crab, where it has once got, it is scarce possible to drive it away" (8).

If Hippocratic physicians laid the foundation of empiric medicine by replacing supernatural concepts of disease with meticulous observation and logical inference, Galen has been recognized as the founder of experimental science. The last prominent physician of the Greco-Roman school, he combined results of animal dissections, experiments in physiology, and clinical observation to construct models of human physiology and disease, which he recorded and taught systematically (9).

Following the Hippocratic physicians, Galen asserted that cancer originated in an imbalance of the four humors: specifically, an excess of *melan chole* (black bile) over yellow bile, phlegm, and blood was thought to drive the formation of malignant tumors. Because excess black bile was the cause of cancer, efforts to remove black bile were the logical treatment. Bloodletting, purgatives, and emetics thus entered the armamentarium of physicians attempting to treat the disease. No one as yet, however, thought to systematically record the results of treatment in a group of patients, or to directly compare one cancer treatment (or no treatment at all) with another. These astute observers did understand that most of their therapies were ineffective, though, and one teaching summarized a view dating to the time of Hippocrates: superficial tumors could sometimes be treated with surgery, but deep-seated tumors should be left alone, as patients often died more quickly with treatment compared with when they were left alone (8).

When he died, Galen left behind a formidable literary legacy comprising over 10,000 pages of authoritative treatises. These were a combination of science blended with Greek philosophy, and they profoundly influenced medicine for 1,500 years, cancer medicine included. The eminent Canadian doctor Sir William Osler (1849–1919) best described what followed: "fifteen centuries stopped thinking and slept, until awakened by the De Fabrica of Vesalius" (10). Cancer medicine slumbered with the rest of the profession.

THE DAWN OF CANCER SCIENCE: ADVANCES IN PATHOLOGY

In the 16th century, advances in anatomy heralded a new era of empiricism. Physicians such as Antonio Benivieni (1443–1502; Florence) pioneered the use of autopsy to understand the causes of death, correlating clinical conditions with postmortem findings. In 1543, based on hundreds of dissections, Andreas Vesalius of Brussels (1514–1564) published "De Humani Corporis Fabrica" (On the Fabric of the Human Body), a groundbreaking first complete depiction of human anatomy, lavishly illustrated with detailed drawings of the body. Within another century, Italy's Giovanni Battista Morgagni (1682–1771) inaugurated the field of pathological anatomy with his masterpiece "De Sedibus et Causis Morborum per Anatomen Indagatis" (The Seats and Causes of Diseases Investigated by Anatomy). Thereafter, a succession of investigators used increasingly specialized technology to localize disease with an ever-increasing clarity. Marie François Xavier Bichat (1771–1802; France) identified tissues underlying recognizable organ systems with the naked eye, thus laying the groundwork for histology. With the introduction of improved microscopes in the 1800s, Rudolf Virchow (1821–1902; Germany) honed in on the newly discovered building blocks of life: the cell.

Cell theory revolutionized the understanding of cancer, making possible for the first time the systematic study of the disease in the laboratory and the clinic. Virchow defined cancer as a disease of abnormal cells emanating from other cells through division. As he famously stated, "from every cell a cell" (*omnis cellula e cellula*) (11). Early in his career, Virchow described an abnormal proliferation of malignant white blood cells in a patient. Based on this case study, he coined the term "leukemia" ("white blood"; from Greek *leukos*, white, and *aima*, blood), shortly after Thomas Hodgkin (1798–1866; Great Britain) characterized the proliferation of malignant cells in lymph glands as "lymphoma" (12).

In 1863, the German pathologist Wilhelm von Waldeyer-Hartz (1836–1921) further outlined the fundamentals of malignant transformation and carcinogenesis. He postulated that cancer cells originate from normal cells, multiply by cell division, and metastasize (spread to distant sites; from Greek *methistanai,* to place away) through lymph or blood (13). Observing a nonrandom pattern of metastatic growth in hundreds of autopsy records, Stephen Paget (1855–1926) subsequently proposed that the predilection of cancer cells to metastasize to certain organs was "not a matter of chance." In 1889, the British surgeon articulated the groundbreaking "seed and soil" hypothesis that prevails to date: "when a plant [cancer] goes to seed, its seeds [the cancer cells] are carried in all directions; but they can live and grow only if they fall on congenial soil [a conducive organ microenvironment]" (14). Another 100 years passed before experimental evidence substantiated the theory. Indeed, though 19th-century pathology provided an increasingly accurate description of cancer, it offered little pathobiologic insight. The transition of oncology from a largely descriptive art to an experimental science finally occurred around the turn of the 20th century.

ONCOLOGY IN THE MODERN ERA: A VERY BRIEF OVERVIEW

The 20th century opens as the experimental era with the systematic study of tumors throughout the animal kingdom, and it . . . promises to widely separate many neoplastic diseases formerly held to be closely related. It may thereby prove to be the era of successful therapeutics and prophylaxis.
—*James Ewing (1919)*

The notion that cancer is not a single entity but rather hundreds of biologically distinct illnesses really dates to James Ewing's (1866–1943, United States) monumental textbook *Neoplastic Diseases,* in which he classified tumors according to the tissue they arose from or resembled (15). Ewing, who became the first director of what is now Memorial Sloan Kettering Cancer Center, tirelessly cataloged tumor cells according to their microscopic features, but he was more than a brilliant laboratory researcher. He recognized the substantial clinical implications his work could have, and he wrote in the preface to the third edition of his text,

Up to a very recent time the practical physician or surgeon has been content to regard all fibromas, sarcomas, or cancers [carcinomas] as equivalent conditions . . . and on this theory to treat the members of each class alike. Upon this theory it was also legitimate to conceive of a universal causative agent of malignant tumors and thus to subordinate many very obvious differences which clinical experience has established in the origin and behavior of different related tumors. (16)

Ewing's insight that different tumor types might arise from distinct sources and might require specific treatment approaches represented a breakthrough in thinking about cancer. In essence, it envisioned targeted treatment and precision medicine.

Ewing's achievement arose in an era of great excitement about the promise of scientific medicine. Claude Bernard (1813–1878; France) had propagated a stringent scientific method and, through intricate experiments in live animals (vivisection), achieved major advances in physiology (17). The fields of radiology and radiation therapy were born with the fortuitous discovery of x-rays by Wilhelm Conrad Röntgen in 1895, and the discovery of natural radioactivity by Henri Becquerel and Pierre and Marie Curie (18). Surgery matured, spurred by technical improvements and, foremost, by innovations in aseptic techniques and anesthesiology (19). Nursing became a skilled profession and a key component in the fight against disease (20). Alongside and contributing to these advances, hospitals were transformed from charitable asylums for the sick to medical institutions (21). All of these developments together helped lay the scientific groundwork for clinical research as we have come to practice it today.

THE ORIGINS OF ONCOLOGY CLINICAL TRIALS

Although there are references to what may be loosely considered clinical studies dating back at least to Biblical times, the first true medical trials depended on a specific breakthrough in medical thinking, namely the acceptance of quantitative methods as a fundamental component of clinical research.

The notion that simple counting could be a useful tool in medical research arose, as with so many other things, with the ancient Greeks. Epidemiology (from the Greek *epi demios,* among the people) began with Hippocrates and other Greek physicians, who made rudimentary generalizations about infectious epidemics, such as their seasonal nature. Understanding was limited, however, as the number of cases of specific diseases in defined populations was not collected. The birth of modern epidemiology can be traced to the haberdasher John Graunt (1620–1674; Great Britain), who among his varied pursuits studied patterns of death among residents of various London parishes, using numbers and causes reported in the parish clerks' weekly burial lists (22). By tracking outbreaks of fever and other common causes of death, Graunt demonstrated in stark terms the uses to which simple statistics could be put.

Quantitative observation was first introduced to experimental medicine by the groundbreaking work of William Harvey (1578–1657) in the 17th century, with the description of the circulation of blood on observational and mathematical grounds (23). One of the reasons Harvey's arguments carried such great weight—were ultimately irresistible—was because of simple calculations he made. Based on the anatomy of the heart

(the volume of the left ventricle) and the normal heart rate, Harvey estimated that the average person pumped approximately 540 pounds of blood in an hour. By simple inference, Galen's theory that the blood supply was replenished daily in the liver could not be true. What human could manufacture, in a 24-hour period, the staggering amount of blood required? A little bit of arithmetic put the lie to 1,500 years of dogma.

The first use of simple statistics in a clinical-trial setting occurred in the 18th century. Anecdotal reports dating to the 1600s had suggested that citrus fruits could prevent scurvy, which was extraordinarily common among sailors undertaking long ocean voyages. Drawing on his personal observations, the Scottish naval surgeon James Lind determined to test the hypothesis that citrus fruits were effective antiscorbutics. In 1747, on board the HMS *Salisbury,* he selected 12 patients with scurvy, and allocated them to six different treatment groups, including oil of vitriol, vinegar, sea water, oranges and lemons, cider, and a combination of garlic, radish, balsam, and myrrh. The two lucky sailors who received the fruit recovered within a week (24). Once the Navy adopted these findings and began issuing lemon juice to all its sailors, scurvy was essentially eliminated from the fleet.

Despite successes as pioneered by Lind, it was not until well into the 20th century that the randomized clinical trial—enshrined as the gold standard by which medical therapies are assessed—was formally introduced. The landmark study that launched the modern era of clinical trials evaluated the effectiveness of streptomycin as an antituberculosis agent, and owed its design and execution in large part to the efforts of a statistician who wanted to introduce physicians gently to the concepts of randomization and experimental design, as outlined by colleagues such as Fisher. Austin Bradford Hill, a professor at the London School of Tropical Medicine and Hygiene, was the primary driver behind the study and later the author of a landmark textbook of medical statistics.

At the time of the study, there was a limited amount of streptomycin available in Great Britain. This drug scarcity, coupled with the variable natural history of the disease, led Hill and his coinvestigators to believe that a randomized study in which half of the patients would not receive the experimental medication could be ethically justified. Anticipating our contemporary studies, the trial had strict eligibility criteria, including bilateral, progressive lung infiltrates, bacteriologically documented disease, and age between 15 and 30 years. Patients were randomly assigned to bed rest (standard therapy) or streptomycin. Standardized case reports were developed and used, and radiologists were blinded to treatment assignment–assessed serial chest x-rays. When the data were examined, the results could not have been more clear-cut. Substantially greater numbers of patients receiving streptomycin experienced radiographic improvement, and at the end of the 6-month observation period only 8% of those receiving the antibacterial had died, compared with 51% in the bed-rest arm of the study (25). The feasibility and practical utility of a randomized trial had been demonstrated beyond a shadow of a doubt.

Additional evidence for the utility of a statistical approach in medicine came from the field of cancer itself, with the publication in the 1950s of the landmark studies correlating smoking with the development of lung cancer. As early as 1761, a linkage between the development of cancer and exposure to an external agent (a carcinogen) was first postulated, when the London physician and polymath John Hill issued his pamphlet "Cautions Against the immoderate Use of Snuff: Founded on the known Qualities of the Tobacco Plant; and the Effects it must produce when this Way taken into the Body: and Enforced by Instances of Persons who have perished miserably of Diseases, occasioned, or rendered incurable by its Use." Hill associated heavy snuff use with nasal tumors and, bucking the tide of medical opinion, recommended against its use (26). It was not until the middle of the 20th century, however, with the development of sophisticated statistical techniques, that the causative relationship between tobacco and cancer became irrefutable. Commissioned by the British Medical Research Council in 1947, Austin Bradford Hill and Richard Doll analyzed potential causes for the dramatically rising mortality from lung cancer. Their comprehensive case–control study of over 2,400 patients identified unequivocally that "smoking is a factor, and an important factor, in the lung" (27). Ernst Wynder and Evarts Graham in the United States published a similar, large survey in over 1,200 patients the same year, again identifying "tobacco smoking as a possible etiologic factor in bronchiogenic carcinoma" (28). Finally, in the 1960s, the link between smoking and cancer was officially recognized.

The streptomycin trial, along with the lung cancer epidemiologic studies, powerfully established the value of a statistical approach to medical research. How was this new thinking incorporated into the just-developing field of oncology? In the remainder of this chapter we briefly review the rise of clinical studies in cancer medicine, with a particular emphasis on the development of chemotherapy as illustrative of the wholesale adoption of controlled trials.

The notion that chemicals might control cancer actually has an ancient history. Hippocratic doctors treated superficial tumors with ointments containing toxic copper compounds. Later, in the first century BCE, the physician and compounder Dioscorides, one of the patron saints of pharmacy, employed autumn crocus, which has as an active ingredient colchicine, later shown to be possessed of mild antitumor effects.

Arsenicals in particular enjoyed widespread use, mostly as topical applications, from ancient Egypt, through Galen and Falloppio, until the early 19th century (29). The first successful systemic cancer chemotherapy was published by Heinrich Lissauer, who reported remissions in two patients with leukemia using Fowler's solution, a then common cure-all based on arsenic (30). In spite of these anecdotal reports, though, and given a profound lack of evidence to support the use of drugs or chemicals, standard treatment for cancer in the early 20th century remained either surgery or radiation therapy.

The terminology and concept of modern chemotherapy, the use of chemicals to treat disease, was coined by Paul Ehrlich (1854–1915) in the early 1900s. Ehrlich introduced the use of laboratory animals to screen chemicals for their potency against diseases, leading to the development of arsenicals to treat syphilis and trypanosomiasis. He investigated aniline dyes and the first alkylating agents as potential drugs to treat cancer, and summarized his observations in what is known to be the first textbook of chemotherapy (31). In experimental oncology, in the first four decades of the 20th century, the development of adequate models for cancer drug screening then took center stage (32). A major breakthrough was achieved by George Clowes of Roswell Park Memorial Institute, who developed the first transplantable tumor systems in rodents, allowing for standardized testing of a larger number of drugs (33).

Initiation of clinical studies of modern chemotherapy can be traced to World Wars I and II. Use of mustard gas in World War I and an accidental spill of sulfur mustards (Bari Harbor, Italy) in World War II were observed to cause severe lymphoid hypoplasia and myelosuppression in exposed soldiers (34,35). In 1942, Alfred Gilman and Louis S. Goodman were commissioned by the U.S. State Department to examine the potential therapeutic use of toxic agents developed for chemical warfare (36). When they observed marked regression of lymphoid tumors in mice, they convinced their colleague, thoracic surgeon Gustav Lindskog, to treat a patient with non-Hodgkin's lymphoma (NHL) with a closely related compound, nitrogen mustard. Significant, albeit temporary, tumor remission was observed. The investigators and colleagues went on to treat several dozen more patients, with variable success. Although nitrogen mustard was clearly no magic bullet for hematologic malignancies, for the first time in history a systemic chemical agent had been shown, under controlled clinical conditions, to combat cancer cells. The principle was established that cancer cells may be more susceptible to certain toxins than are normal cells. In 1946, after wartime secrecy restrictions had been lifted, the clinical data were published, and the era of cancer chemotherapy had arrived (37,38).

In the two decades that followed, improved alkylating agents were developed (e.g., cyclophosphamide, chlorambucil) that became key components of leukemia and lymphoma treatment regimens. More chemotherapeutic approaches were to follow. Sydney Farber observed that folic acid, the vitamin deficient in megaloblastic anemia, stimulated proliferation of acute lymphoblastic leukemia (ALL) cells in children. In collaboration with industry, antifolates (aminopterin, amethopterin [methotrexate]) were synthesized and were the first drugs to induce remissions in children with ALL (39). Methotrexate displayed activity against a variety of other malignancies, including breast cancer, ovarian cancer, and head and neck cancer. Most remarkably, single-agent methotrexate was found to be the first chemotherapy agent to cure a solid tumor, choriocarcinoma, a germ cell malignancy originating in the placenta. Methotrexate was also the first agent to demonstrate benefit of adjuvant chemotherapy treatment—to prevent recurrence of osteosarcoma following surgery. Additional anticancer drugs entered clinical trials in the 1950s, including the inhibitor of adenine metabolism 6-mercaptopurine (6-MP), vinca alkaloids, and 5-fluorouracil, an inhibitor of DNA synthesis (32). Natural products such as taxanes (e.g., paclitaxel; 1964; from the bark of the Pacific Yew tree) or camptothecins (e.g., irinotecan; 1966; from a Chinese ornamental tree) were developed under the auspices of C. Gordon Zubrod at the National Cancer Institute (NCI) (40). Many more were to follow, including platinum compounds (e.g., cisplatin, carboplatin) or topoisomerase II inhibitors (e.g., anthracyclines or epipodophyllotoxins). In the development of all of these drugs, controlled clinical studies were essential to establish their effectiveness, and it can be argued that oncology has more systematically used the randomized study than any other field in medicine.

It has been only 150 years since cancer was recognized as a disease of cells, and a mere six decades since the introduction of the randomized clinical trial. Today, multimodality treatment, often incorporating molecular markers, targeted therapy, and, more recently, immunotherapy has become standard treatment for many malignancies. Our task for the future will be to retain the essential features of the randomized study, while developing new clinical trial methodologies that allow the most efficient investigation of novel therapeutics.

REFERENCES

1. Greaves MF. *Cancer: The Evolutionary Legacy*. Oxford, NY: Oxford University Press; 2000.
2. Huxley J. *Biological Aspects of Cancer*. London, UK: Allen & Unwin; 1958.
3. Urtega OB, Pack GT. On the antiquity of melanoma. *Cancer*. 1966;19:607–610.
4. Strouhal E. Tumors in the remains of ancient Egyptians. *Am J Physical Anthropol*. 1976;45:613–620.
5. Weiss L. Observations on the antiquity of cancer and metastasis. *Cancer*. 2000;19(3–4):193–204.
6. Bryan CP. *The Papyrus Ebers*. New York, NY: Appleton; 1931.
7. Breasted JH. *The Edwin Smith Surgical Papyrus*. Special ed. Chicago, IL: University of Chicago Press; 1930.
8. Kardinal CG, Yarbro JW. A conceptual history of cancer. *Sem Oncol*. 1979;6(4):396–408.
9. Siegel RE. *Galen's System of Physiology and Medicine*. Basel, NY: Karger; 1968.
10. Osler W, Camac CNB. *Counsels and Ideals from the Writings of William Osler*. Boston, MA: Houghton Mifflin; 1906.
11. Rather LJ. Rudolf Virchow's views on pathology, pathological anatomy, and cellular pathology. *Arch Pathol*. 1966;82:197–204.
12. Hodgkin T, Lister JJ. Notice of some microscopic observations of the blood and animal tissues. *Philos Mag*. 1827;2:130–138.
13. Triolo VA. Nineteenth century foundations of cancer research: advances in tumor pathology, nomenclature, and theories of oncogenesis. *Cancer Res*. 1965;25:75–106.
14. Paget S. The distribution of secondary growths in cancer of the breast. *Lancet*. 1889;133(3421):571–573.
15. Ewing J. *Neoplastic Diseases: A Treatise on Tumors*. Philadelphia, PA and London, UK: W.B. Saunders Company; 1919.
16. Ewing J, Raney RB. *Neoplastic Diseases: A Treatise on Tumors*. 3d ed. rev. and enl., with 546 illustrations. Philadelphia, PA and London, UK: W.B. Saunders; 1928.
17. Bernard C. *Introduction à l'étude de la médecine expérimentale*. Paris: Baillière; 1865.
18. Hayter CR. The clinic as laboratory: the case of radiation therapy, 1896–1920. *Bull Hist Med*. 1998;72(4):663–688.
19. Wangensteen OH, Wangensteen SD. *The Rise of Surgery: From Empiric Craft to Scientific Discipline*. Minneapolis, MN: University of Minnesota Press; 1978.
20. Maggs C. A General History of Nursing: 1800—1900. In: Bynum WF, Porter R, eds. *Companion Encyclopedia of the History of Medicine*. London, UK: Routledge; 1993:1300–1320.
21. Risley M. House of Healing: *The Story of the Hospital*. New York, NY: Doubleday, 1961.
22. Rothman KJ. Lessons from John Graunt. *Lancet*. 1996; 347(8993):37–39.
23. Harvey W. *An Anatomical Disputation Concerning the Movement of the Heart and Blood in Living Creatures*. Oxford: Blackwell Scientific; 1976.
24. Porter R. *The Greatest Benefit to Mankind: A Medical History of Humanity*. New York, NY: Norton; 1997.
25. Medical Research Council Investigation. Streptomycin treatment of tuberculosis. *Br Med J*. 1948;2:769–782.
26. Petrakis NL. Historic milestones in cancer epidemiology. *Sem Oncol*. 1979;6:433–444.
27. Doll R, Hill AB. Smoking and carcinoma of the lung: preliminary report. *Br Med J*. 1950;2:739–748.
28. Wynder EL, Graham EA. Tobacco smoking as a possible etiologic factor in bronchiogenic carcinoma: a study of 684 proved cases. *JAMA*. 1950;143:329–336.
29. Burchenal JH. The historical development of cancer chemotherapy. *Sem Oncol*. 1977;4:135–146.
30. Lissauer H. Zwei Fälle von Leucaemie. *Berl Klin Wochenschr*. 1865;2:403–405.
31. Ehrlich P. *Beiträge zur experimentellen Pathologie und Chemotherapie*. Leipzig: Akademischer Verlag; 1909.
32. DeVita VT, Jr., Chu E. A history of cancer chemotherapy. *Cancer Res*. 2008;68:8643–8653.
33. Clowes GHA. A study of the influence exerted by a variety of physical and chemical forces on the virulence of carcinoma in mice. *Br Med J*. 1906:1548–1554.
34. Krumbhaar EB, Krumbhaar HD. The blood and bone marrow in yellow cross gas poisoning. *J Med Res*. 1919;40:497–506.

35. Einhorn J. Nitrogen mustard: the origin of chemotherapy for cancer. *Int J Radiation Oncol Biol Physics*. 1985;11:1375–1378.
36. Gilman A. The initial clinical trial of nitrogen mustard. *American J Surg*. 1963;105:574–578.
37. Goodman LS, Wintrobe MM, Dameshek W, et al. Nitrogen mustard therapy. Use of methyl-bis(beta-chloroethyl)amine hydrochloride and tris (beta-chloroethyl)amine hydrochloride for Hodgkin's disease, lymphosarcoma, leukemia and certain allied and miscellaneous disorders. *JAMA*. 1946;132:126–132.
38. Gilman A, Philips FS. The biological actions and therapeutic applications of the B-chloroethyl amines and sulfides. *Science*. 1946;103:409–436.
39. Farber S, Diamond LK, Mercer RD, et al. Temporary remissions in acute leukemia in children produced by folic acid antagonist, 4-aminopteroyl-glutamic acid (aminopterin). *N Engl J Med*. 1948;238:787–793.
40. Chabner BA, Roberts TG. Chemotherapy and the War on Cancer. *Nature Rev Cancer*. 2005;5:65–72.

Ethical Principles Guiding Clinical Research

Jackson Bruce Smith

HISTORICAL PERSPECTIVES, REGULATIONS, AND ETHICAL PRINCIPLES

In the United States, research involving human subjects is overseen by local institutional review boards (IRBs), central cooperative IRBs (such as the National Cancer Institute Central Institutional Review Board [cIRB]), or independent (commercial) IRBs. All of these operate within the framework of regulations set forth in the Code of Federal Regulations (CFR) (1), also known as the "Common Rule" as it is followed by 17 federal departments that conduct human subjects research, and the ethical principles set forth in the Belmont Report (2). These principles are respect for persons, justice, and beneficence. Historically, the Belmont Report (2) was preceded by other sets of rules and regulations. These include the Nuremberg Code (3), the Declaration of Helsinki (4), and the U.S. National Research Act (5). The Nuremberg Code addressed voluntariness, informed consent (IC), and qualifications of researchers, among other things, and was a result of the Nuremberg Doctors Trial in which 23 defendants including 20 physicians were charged with murder, torture, and other atrocities for experiments conducted on concentration camp internees during World War II. The Declaration of Helsinki was written by the World Federation of Physicians. It incorporated the Nuremberg Code, clarified therapeutic versus nontherapeutic research, and allowed bona fide guardians to enroll subjects in research studies (Table 3.1). The main impetus for the National Research Act was the revelations of ethical lapses associated with the U.S. Public Health Service sponsored Tuskegee Study of Untreated Syphilis in the Negro Male (6) but also took into account other ethical infractions by researchers. Some of these along with the regulations resulting from those revelations are listed in Table 3.2. The National Research Act required review of human research by an IRB at any institution receiving federal funds and established the National Commission for the Protection of Human Subjects of Biomedical and

Behavioral Research (the "Commission") charged with developing guidelines for the conduct of human subjects research. The deliberations of the Commission resulted in modifications to 45 CFR 46 that added additional protections for vulnerable populations in research, The Belmont Report (2), in addition to expounding the three ethical principles noted previously, considered such concepts as differences between biomedical and behavioral research and standard clinical care, mechanisms for evaluating risks and benefits attending a research study, guidelines for selection of research subjects, and how IC is sought. The Commission's deliberations also established what is now known as the Office for Human Research Protections (OHRP), in the U.S. Department of Health and Human Services, which has regulatory oversight responsibilities for human subjects research sponsored by government agencies.

More recently, in 1995, the federal Advisory Committee on Human Radiation Experiments (ACHRE) (7) reviewed U.S. government sponsored clandestine research that occurred during the Cold War. Experiments involving release of radioactive materials into the environment and administering whole body radiation to terminal cancer patients, often without consent, resulted in establishing the National Bioethics Advisory Committee (8), which provides advice to the president and various government entities about research related to such topics as biobanking, stem cell research, and research subject privacy, and other public health issues in research.

The upshot of the history of ethical violations in human subjects research is that the regulatory environment surrounding human subjects research is vast and comprehensive including regulations at national, state, and local levels. Nationally, human subjects research is regulated by the OHRP via the Common Rule, 45 CFR 46, the Food and Drug Administration (FDA) via 21 CFR 50, Medicare for clinical trials billing, the Department of Health and Human Services for financial oversight of grants and contracts, and the Health

TABLE 3.1 Nuremberg Code and the Declaration of Helsinki

Nuremberg Code (1947)	Declaration Of Helsinki (1964)
Voluntary informed consent without coercion is essential	Incorporates the tenets of the Nuremberg Code
Human experiments should be based on prior animal experiments	Defines therapeutic versus nontherapeutic research
Anticipated results should justify the experiment	Allows enrollment of certain subjects in therapeutic research so they might benefit from important medical advances
Only qualified scientists should conduct the experiments	Allows legal guardians to enroll patients in therapeutic and nontherapeutic trials
Risks and benefits should be commensurate with the problem	
Physical and/or mental suffering is unacceptable	
There should be no expectation of death or disabling injury from the experiment	
Investigator must be prepared to stop the experiment if there is indication of danger	
Subjects should be able to withdraw without penalty	

Insurance Portability and Accountability Act (HIPAA) regarding privacy and protection of subject identity. State and federal regulations are generally congruent with federal regulations but where divergent, it is the responsibility of the researcher and the IRB to follow whichever regulations provide more stringent protections. At the local level, regulatory oversight is primarily the responsibility of on-site or contracted external IRBs, but conflict of interest (COI) committees, biosafety committees, and legal counsel also have important roles in administering regulatory and safety oversight of clinical researchers and their activities.

The regulatory environment is often perceived by researchers, clinical coordinators, and administrative personnel as overly burdensome and restrictive but the laws and regulations have served to largely prevent the types of research disasters listed in Table 3.2. While the regulations serve to protect individuals participating in clinical research studies, missteps and egregious harm still occur. It should not be assumed that researchers today are impervious to bias and the many temptations, both financial and prestige-related, in the world of clinical research. We must always be vigilant in order to prevent research abuses and protect research participants.

The primary responsibility of the IRB is to protect individuals in research studies from physical, psychological, social, or financial harm. This is best accomplished by establishing institutional systems to adhere to the Common Rule and being mindful of the ethical principles of *respect for persons*, *justice*, and *beneficence* as set forth in the Belmont Report.

Respect for Persons: Individuals should be treated as autonomous agents able to make their own informed decisions and those with diminished autonomy such as prisoners, the cognitively impaired, pregnant women and fetuses, students, and other vulnerable populations, should be afforded additional protections as needed. Table 3.3 provides a synopsis of federally defined vulnerable populations and additional considerations that may apply to oncology patients entering clinical trials. Such additional protections are determined by the investigative team in concert with the IRB and may include appointment of a subject advocate, an independent study monitor with experience or with knowledge of the vulnerable population, or employing surrogate consent (also discussed in the following in other contexts). Respecting an individual's autonomy also includes: (a) measures taken to protect identity, confidentiality, and privacy, (b) ensuring that the IC document and the process of IC meet all federally mandated disclosure requirements, and (c) sufficient time is given for the potential subject to consider the study and to discuss it with family and/or trusted friends. People considering joining a research study must be provided with all information necessary, both positive and negative, to allow them to make an informed decision regarding participation in the research.

Justice: When possible those willing to risk being in a research study should reap whatever benefits accrue either as individuals, or as members of groups of individuals or a community. Justice also requires that burdens of the research be spread as equally as possible through all strata of society. Thus, the investigator should exercise fairness in the selection of subjects and not recruit potential subjects simply on the basis of availability such as students, institutionalized individuals, prisoners, racial or ethnic minorities, or very ill patients unless the research targets such individuals or groups. Thus, justice overlaps in this case with respect for persons. While justice focuses more on groups or communities and respect for persons usually focuses on the individual, both individuals and communities may be vulnerable to coercion or disrespect and should be afforded additional protections.

TABLE 3.2 Regulatory Milestones in Human Subjects Research Protection

Year	Milestone	Impetus	Notes
1906	Pure Food and Drug Act	Publication of *The Jungle*–Upton Sinclair	Exposé of unsanitary conditions in the meatpacking industry in Chicago.
1938	Food, Drug and Cosmetic Act, Informed Consent	Sulfanilamide elixir	Distributed in doctors' offices for treatment of colds and coughs in children—107 cases of death from renal failure.
1947	Nuremberg Code	WWII Nazi research atrocities	Includes requirement for informed consent, voluntary participation (no coercion), sound science conducted by qualified investigators, risks commensurate with the problem being investigated, no expectation of injury or death, clear stopping rules, and subject able to withdraw without penalty.
1962	Kefauver–Harris amendment to Food, Drug and Cosmetic Act	Thalidomide	Drug for treating nausea of early pregnancy resulted in 30,000+ cases of phocomelia. Requirement for animal data, reproductive toxicity studies, and two human studies for approved use in humans.
1964	Declaration of Helsinki	Standardized international code of research ethics	Incorporated Nuremberg Code, allowed for enrollment of decisionally impaired patients into therapeutic and nontherapeutic trials.
1974	National Research Act	Tuskegee revelations	Study of the natural course of untreated syphilis in Negro males–act established the National Commission for the Protection of Human Subjects of Biomedical and Behavioral Research leading to the publication of the Belmont Report and the Common Rule.
1979	Belmont Report	Federally commissioned review of human research practices	Ethical principles of respect, justice, and beneficence, also addressed differences between standard medical care and research, risk assessment, selection of research subjects, and informed consent.
1991	Common Rule	National Research Act of 1974	Additional protections for vulnerable populations and eventual unification of CFR related to human research, adopted by 17 federal agencies that fund human subjects research–FDA remains separate (21 CFR 50).
1995	NBAC	U.S. government sponsored radiation experiments done during Cold War	Many U.S. government sponsored atmospheric radiation releases, total body irradiation of patients with terminal cancer to look at effects on normal cells. NBAC provides advice about public health issues to the president and other key government officials.

CFR, Code of Federal Regulations; FDA, Food and Drug Administration; NBAC, National Bioethics Advisory Committee; WWII, World War II.

Beneficence: This can be captured in the Hippocratic Oath, a main tenet of which is to not cause harm. Upon obtaining their degree physicians pledge to follow the Hippocratic Oath. The oath applies whether treating a disease process or running a research study. In both roles, there is a need to assess risks and benefits based on the severity of the condition being treated or investigated. Increased risk may be justified when treating or investigating a serious illness. Harm can affect an individual, a family, a class of individuals, special groups in society, or society at large.

Beneficence is also served by following research protocols that will likely result in useful or new data; why ask a research subject to take any risk at all by participating in a study that has no potential for meaningful results? Other key aspects of minimizing risk include strictly adhering to inclusion and exclusion criteria, reasonable stopping rules and, depending on risk level, appointment of an independent medical monitor or establishing a more comprehensive data safety monitoring plan. For all human research the Common Rule should be applied to the extent possible including the

TABLE 3.3 Vulnerable Subjects and Additional Considerations Concerning Oncology Trials

Federal Definition of Vulnerable Populations (45 CFR 46, Subparts B, C, and D)
Pregnant women, fetuses, and neonates
Prisoners
Children
Others Usually Considered Vulnerable
Aged or infirm
Cognitively impaired including comatose or traumatized individuals, Alzheimer's disease patients, or those with other brain conditions
Students
Individuals of very low educational or economic status
Homeless individuals/refugees
Additional Considerations Regarding Vulnerability of Oncology Patients
Advanced age-related decline
Pediatric oncology patients
Presence of brain metastases
Sequelae of cranial/brain radiation

subparts that add protections for research involving prisoners, children, and pregnant women and fetuses, whether or not these are specified in the Federalwide Assurance (FWA) agreed to and signed by the institution. The content of an FWA is provided in Box 3.1.

BOX 3.1 Federalwide Assurance Defined

Under the DHHS human subjects protection regulations (at 45 CFR 46.103), every institution engaged in human subjects research that is funded or conducted by DHHS must obtain an Assurance Of Compliance approved by the OHRP. This Assurance Of Compliance, when granted, is called a Federalwide Assurance. Both "awardee" institutions and collaborating "performance site" institutions must file assurances. The signed Federalwide Assurance obligates the institution to follow the ethical principles of the Belmont Report and to apply the federal regulations to **all** human subjects research being conducted at the institution.

DHHS, Department of Health and Human Services; OHRP, Office for Human Research Protections.

The ethical principles noted previously should be interpreted in a fluid way since our society has changed over time since they were first published. Consideration of the three principles should take into account the nature of society today with particular attention to cultural situations or an individual's privacy, ethnicity, race, or gender. For example, consideration of transgender individuals as a potentially vulnerable population would not have concerned most IRBs until recently.

INFORMED CONSENT

IC usually consists of a *document*, the informed consent form (ICF), and a consent *process*—the ongoing conversation about the research between the researcher and research staff and the research subject. The required and "optional" elements to be addressed in the consent to participate in research, whether written or oral, as specified in 45 CFR 46.116 are listed in Table 3.4. Ideally in greater than minimal risk studies the IC process should be initiated by the research physician or a coinvestigator who is totally familiar with the objectives and background of the study. While many times the initial IC interview is delegated to a research coordinator or coinvestigator, the principal investigator (PI) is ultimately responsible for the ethical conduct of the trial and should ensure that coinvestigators and designated research staff are appropriately trained to execute the IC interview. For high-risk studies the PI should be available in person or by phone to answer any questions potential subjects may have. In that regard, IC documents, while theoretically written in lay language understandable to someone with an eighth-grade reading level, are too often filled with medical jargon and legalese. If that is the case someone on the research team may have to review the document with the potential subject in order to ensure understanding. In the ICF and in ongoing discussions with subjects, terms suggesting improvement or cure should not be used. Also coercive, misleading, and exculpatory language should be avoided. Table 3.5 provides examples of appropriate and inappropriate consent language. Regarding ICFs written by "professionals" (e.g., in an industry-sponsored study or cooperative oncology group) do not assume that the form(s) is written in understandable and unambiguous language that addresses all federally mandated elements of IC plus any additional information appropriate to the study. It is critically important that the PI and research staff review all sponsor-proposed study-related documents with care prior to submitting for IRB review.

While the signed or oral consent (when can you use an oral consent?) usually provides the go-ahead signal from the patient (now subject), consent is an ongoing process throughout the entire study; from screening through some reasonable time period after study

TABLE 3.4 Elements of Informed Consent (45 CFR 46.116)

Required	Optional Depending on Study
Statement that the study involves research	Statement that there may be risks to subject, or embryo/fetus if subject is or may become pregnant, that are unforeseeable
The purpose of the research	Circumstances under which subject may be terminated from study by the investigator w/o subject's consent
Duration of the subject's participation	Any additional costs that may accrue to subject as a result of being in study
Description of procedures to be followed	Consequences of subject withdrawal from study and any procedures required for orderly termination
Identification of procedures that are experimental	Statement that any significant new findings that might be related to subject's willingness to continue in study will be revealed to subject and explained
Description of reasonably foreseeable risks or discomforts	The approximate number of subjects involved in the study
Description of any potential benefits to subjects or others	
Description of any reasonable alternative to being in study	
Statement describing the extent to which confidentiality will be protected	
Statement about compensation in case of research-related injury and how to obtain further information (greater than minimal risk studies)	
Contact information for questions about research, participants' rights, and in case of suspected research-related injury	
Statement that participation is voluntary, that participant can quit study for any reason without penalty, and that not participating will not affect any benefits to which subject is otherwise entitled	

TABLE 3.5 Consent Language

MISLEADING	NOT MISLEADING
The compound we are testing is *very similar to an FDA approved drug that is known to have a beneficial effect.*	The compound we are testing *may or may not have a beneficial effect. . .*
COERCIVE	**NOT COERCIVE**
The sponsor *will not* reimburse you for lost time from work if you experience a research-related injury.	The sponsor *has no plan to* reimburse you for lost time from work if you experience a research-related injury.
MISLEADING	**NOT MISLEADING**
The questionnaires are *simple and are easy to complete.*	The questionnaires *will take approximately 15 to 20 minutes to complete. You do not have to answer questions that make you feel uncomfortable.*

intervention is completed in order to inform subjects of trial results or late-occurring unanticipated risks.

In the context of respecting the potential research subject as an autonomous individual able to make informed decisions, the consent interview should not simply be a form signing exercise but rather an intelligent and intelligible discussion between the investigator/research staff and the potential subject. The ongoing discussion should include illumination of all required elements of consent as noted in Table 3.4 as well as any optional elements that are study-specific or related to risk. The researcher should be honest and forthcoming and not prone to minimizing the importance of rarely encountered risks. Risks should be presented in the consent form and in the consent discussion in clear and understandable lay language that includes any symptoms a subject may need to report to the study staff. Most patients/subjects do not understand medical jargon; therefore, providing a clinical context that includes a description of symptoms or signs to look for is important. An example would be "jaundice/yellow color of skin or eyes" to accompany a risk of "abnormal liver function tests." A statement that regularly obtained blood tests will be done to screen for possible adverse effects on body functions should be included as appropriate to the research.

Beyond the IC document, in order to help ensure that the IC process is adequate throughout the study, the PI or study staff should monitor a subject's willingness to continue in a study. This can be accomplished by determining at each visit, or at certain intervals depending on study design, that the subject still understands the study and the requirements of participation and is willing to continue study participation.

The PI is obligated to keep participants informed of new findings, positive or negative, during and after participation. The PI must also be willing to inform a subject that continuing in a study is not in his or her best interest. If it is determined that a subject following a research protocol requires medical intervention that is ex-protocol, then unless a formal waiver is approved by the IRB and sponsor the subject should be removed from the study and provided the appropriate treatment.

Physician investigators must be constantly aware of which "hat they are wearing" so that neither the researcher nor the subject becomes ensnared in what is commonly referred to as the "therapeutic misconception"; the subject may think he or she is following a protocol in the interest of improvement in a disease process but is mainly doing so in order for the researcher to collect sound data for evaluation of the experimental intervention (9). Improvement in a condition may be hoped for and may occur but it is not the primary reason for the conduct of the research. The therapeutic misconception can be particularly vexing when the researcher and the physician are the same individual enrolling his or her own patients as research subjects. IRBs and researchers need to be aware of the inherent conflict between these dual roles. Patients may join a study as a conscious or subconscious motive for gaining approval of the physician researcher, the misapprehension that they will receive more personalized care, or the perception that the physician would not ask them to join a study unless he or she as the physician thought there would be therapeutic benefit.

Special Consent Situations

In addition to the requirements of the CFR and added protections for vulnerable subjects, justice and autonomy require a nuanced and thoughtful approach when recruiting and enrolling individuals who may be subject to coercion.

Children

Studies involving children as subjects pose challenges regarding IC/assent. While parental permission is required prior to (usually) age 18, care must be taken to obtain assent from the child with respect being paid to the perceived degree of maturity of the child, or at least from age 6 and up. Assent, in this context, is the agreement of a minor to be in a research study once it has been explained to the minor in age-appropriate terms (often with an IRB approved script). Once assent has been obtained, parents or guardians should sign an IRB approved parent or guardian permission form that incorporates all federal and local requirements pertaining to the research. There should also be a plan in place to obtain formal consent when age of majority is reached.

Non-English Speaking

When recruiting and consenting non-English speaking individuals for a study being done in the United States one should employ a certified translated consent for studies that are expected to include more than an occasional non-English speaking subject. The short form consent may be used on an ad hoc basis if non-English speakers are expected only sporadically. The short form should be followed by a certified translated full consent as soon as possible and the subject reconsented. During the consent interview and in the ongoing consent process it is best to have an interpreter who is not related to the subject as a relative may have his or her own agenda regarding enrollment of the subject, for example, interpret in an upbeat or downbeat fashion to steer the subject one way or the other.

Cognitively Impaired

Cognitively impaired individuals are often not included in complex studies. However, in studies where there is reasonable potential for benefit regarding the target disease, one should consider enrolling them. When appropriate, consent should be obtained through a legally authorized representative (LAR). When there is not a court appointed LAR or a clearly defined surrogate named in an advanced directive for medical care there is usually a hierarchy of family members able to be surrogates by hospital or IRB policy (which are hopefully congruent). A caution is that family members may have a personal agenda for the subject that is not necessarily in the subject's best interest. Every attempt should be made to ensure that the subject, to the best of his or her ability, understands the study and its requirements. Assent should be obtained from the subject if at all possible. Also keep in mind that individuals with certain conditions may fluctuate between periods of impairment and lucidity and need to be reinforced regarding their participation depending on their clinical condition.

Emergency Use of a Drug or Biologic

Emergency use may be done when a human subject is in a life- or limb-threatening situation, there is no recourse to standard of care, and there is not sufficient time to obtain IRB approval. This type of *exemption* from prior review and approval by the IRB, which is not rare in the oncology clinical research setting, may not be used unless all of the conditions described in 21 CFR 56.102(d) exist. The requirements are as follows:

1. The subject is in a life- or limb-threatening situation necessitating the use of the test article.
2. IC cannot be obtained because of an inability to communicate with, or obtain legally effective consent from, the subject.
3. Time is not sufficient to obtain consent from the subject's legal representative.
4. No alternative method of approved or generally recognized therapy is available that provides an equal or greater likelihood of saving the subject's life.

Policy specifics may vary from institution to institution but usually the investigator provides a letter to the IRB describing the clinical situation of the patient along with a confirming letter from a physician not involved with the case. If, in the investigator's opinion, the preceding conditions are met and immediate use of the test article is required to preserve or extend the subject's life or limb, and there is not time to obtain an independent physician's determination, the clinical investigator may proceed with treatment and, within 5 working days after the use of the article, provide the IRB with the letter corroborating the necessity for emergency use. In general, one emergency use per test article is allowed and further use requires prospective IRB review, although a second use in a life-threatening situation is possible. If the judgment of the investigator is that additional patients may require similar emergency use of a particular drug or biologic, an emergency use protocol and consent should be submitted to the IRB along with an investigational new drug (IND) application for prospective review.

In the emergency use situation, IC is required but the consent form, which may be adapted from the IRB approved research ICF, must make it clear that the use of the test article is treatment and not research. Generally the FDA requires that a single patient IND application be submitted and approved in order for the test article to be shipped to the site.

EARLY-PHASE CLINICAL TRIALS

Phase I clinical trials are performed to study the pharmacokinetics and safety of a drug. The testing of therapeutic benefit is not a primary goal of these studies. Because phase I studies begin at a point of limited human data, they usually enroll only the number of individuals sufficient to collect the pharmacokinetic and initial safety data. Such trials usually start with a low dose of drug based on prior animal studies if no data on humans are available.

Nononcology phase I studies are generally done on healthy volunteers. Oncology phase I trials enroll cancer patients who have failed conventional (standard of care) treatment and for whom there are no known further treatment options. Healthy volunteers understand that enrolling in phase I research provides no benefit except perhaps a feeling of satisfaction related to helping to develop a new treatment. The primary reason healthy volunteers enroll in phase I studies is to receive study payments. However, for cancer or other patients with life-threatening conditions enrolling in phase I trials there is often an expectation of clinical benefit—the therapeutic misconception (9)—even though the consent form clearly indicates they may receive a dose too low to have clinical effect and that any positive clinical effect on a disease is unknown at this stage of drug development. Thus the onus is on the researcher to ensure the subject understands the nature and reasons for the research without dashing hope for a positive clinical result.

Phase II clinical trials may enroll up to several hundred individuals in order to get preliminary information on dose response, efficacy, and safety. In these trials there may be some expectation of benefit but the consent should make clear that benefit or degree of benefit compared to existing treatments remains unknown. Participants in some phase II trials may be randomized to an approved therapy or the new drug. However, placebo trials may be done if there is no known standard of care or if there is low risk to subjects and reasonable rescue criteria for worsening symptoms or disease. Placebos are appropriately used in clinical trials comparing standard treatment plus a placebo with standard treatment plus the new treatment. While the potential for benefit is higher than in phase I trials, the researcher needs to ensure the written consent and the ongoing consent process are clear about expectation of benefit.

TISSUE BANKING, GENETIC ANALYSIS, AND DATABANKS

The explosion of data and tissue banking over the past decade has led to concerns and controversy over how identity and confidentiality are protected. Tissue sample collection and pharmacogenetic/genomic testing examining genetic influences on drug metabolism are often integral to commercially sponsored clinical trials and consent forms generally address privacy and confidentiality issues appropriately. A larger concern is banking tissue or genetic information for future unspecified research. Subject wishes concerning future use of tissue and data should be respected through opt-in or opt-out provisions in the consent form and by discussing specific issues with the donor of the tissue or information (10,11). Some of the issues that should be addressed with the tissue donor are (a) designation of types of research that can be conducted, (b) recovery of tissue for use elsewhere, in another study, or if new diagnostic tests become available that would benefit the original donor of the tissue, and (c) the handling of valuable clinical information that would need to be linked to tissue for future studies. In addition, genetic information that is "de-identified" does not fall under the protection of the HIPAA regulations and it has been demonstrated that reidentification is possible (12).

Some protection of individuals whose genetic information is stored in gene banks is afforded by the federal Genetic Information Nondiscrimination Act (GINA). This was enacted in 2008 to protect individuals from discrimination by insurance companies or employers because they have a gene mutation that causes or increases the risk of an inherited disorder (13).

An additional concern with gene databases is to whom data should be released. There is little quarrel with releasing information to a subject if the genetic test provides important clinically actionable information. For example, a subject is found to have a pathogenic variant of BRCA1/2 genes that confer a high risk for developing ovarian or a second primary breast cancer (14).

Ownership of tissue has been partly addressed by the courts and decisions have generally been in favor of ownership by the entity employing the researcher who collected the tissue (15,16). However future lawsuits or decisions concerning tissue ownership are to be expected.

GENE THERAPY/TRANSFER STUDIES

Gene transfer means the treatment of disease by replacing, altering, or supplementing a gene that is absent, underexpressed, or abnormal and involved in a disease process. An example in oncology is transfer of a gene directly to tumor cells that enhances programmed cell death. The gene of interest is delivered to the target cell via a vector, usually a replication deficient virus such as adenovirus, adeno-associated virus, or a retrovirus.

Initiating a gene transfer study requires input and regulation at both federal and local levels. Federally or commercially sponsored gene transfer studies are reviewed by the National Institutes of Health (NIH) Recombinant DNA Advisory Committee (RAC), a panel of experts that provides recommendations to the NIH director regarding any study involving recombinant or synthetic nucleic acids. Recommendations are in part based on the information provided in Appendix M from the NIH Guidelines (17). Appendix M requires details about study design and procedures, information about the vector and the gene of interest and its expression, safety and risk to the participant, research staff, pharmacy personnel, local environment, and preclinical data. Appendix M also addresses reporting serious adverse events that are unexpected and possibly associated with the gene transfer product. These must be reported to the NIH Office of Biotechnology Activities and the FDA within 15 calendar days of sponsor notification, unless the event was life-threatening or fatal, in which case, it should be reported within 7 calendar days.

The FDA requires an IND application if the study is commercially sponsored. The IND is overseen by the FDA Center for Biologics Evaluation and Research (CBER). Somatic cell gene transfer is treated as a drug/biologic since its effects are finite. Currently there is a federal ban on germ-line cell gene transfer/therapy.

The reviewing IRB must ensure that all criteria of 45 CFR 46 for human subjects research are met along with any additional ethical considerations or protections specific to the study. Also, the site Institutional Biosafety Committee (IBC) reviews the recommendations of the RAC and the answers to questions in Appendix M along with any other local safety considerations. IBC determinations are shared with the IRB in order to ensure ability of the IRBs to thoroughly review safety issues as well as ethical considerations regarding the protocol, consent, and other documents.

Tremendously powerful techniques for gene editing have been discovered in the past few years and techniques such as clustered regularly interspaced short palindromic repeats (CRISPR) that can be used for gene insertion or deletion in both somatic and germ-line cells are clearly applicable to genetic manipulation in humans (18). Use of such new techniques for gene manipulation will undoubtedly pose new ethical and safety considerations that IRBs will have to address. Of note, an international group of scientists have called for a moratorium on the use of CRISPR-Cas9 where gene insertion or deletion would be used on germ-line cells (19).

IRB SUBMISSIONS

It behooves the PI to interact with IRB leadership and staff prior to submitting a study for IRB review. This can avoid tedious back-and-forth about the nature of the study and what is required for IRB approval. Most IRBs provide forms that when completed appropriately address all federal and local requirements for obtaining IRB approval to conduct a study. The IRB usually requires the study synopsis to be presented in lay language since many IRB members who will review the submission are not physicians or scientists.

Submissions for initial review by the IRB should include all study documents including the protocol, consent form, study synopsis, and Investigator's Brochure, if applicable. Advertisements or social media scripts along with a copy or script of any video should also be included.

Continuing review of research is required one year after initial approval and subsequently on a yearly basis unless the IRB has specified more frequent reviews. The initial continuing review represents the first chance for the IRB to reexamine the entire study with study-generated information not available or known at the time of initial review. Updated information on risks and side effects, efficacy, drug tolerance, or device issues should be provided for IRB review.

Amendments to the protocol, consent form, or other study documents should be provided in sufficient detail to allow the IRB to make informed decisions regarding any increased or decreased risk and should also address requirement or a plan for reconsent of subjects.

CONDUCTING A STUDY

No aspect of a study may be initiated, including screening, until written acknowledgment of IRB approval is in hand. However, certain generic information may be obtained prior to IRB approval. There is a provision in the HIPAA regulations for obtaining information that is preparatory to research. That information includes assessment of how many patients are available who fit a certain diagnostic code or certain other preliminary information but does not include obtaining contact information or specific test results. Approval for acquiring such information is generally obtained by following standardized institutional procedures to ensure patient confidentiality.

Checklists serve to keep a study on track regarding day-to-day study activities and regulatory compliance. Helpful checklists may include preenrollment information such as human subjects research and HIPAA training for investigators and research staff, COI disclosure for all personnel, IRB approval letter and other study documents on file, and date of IRB approval. Checklists are also helpful for the items related to the IC, and appropriate signatures, inclusion/exclusion criteria, and protocol requirements such as required lab or imaging tests and dates.

Following the protocol is paramount but there are certain protocol deviations/violations that are expected.

Violations and deviations are discussed here as having the same meaning although some IRBs define deviations as being minor infractions and violations as being more serious in nature. Expected deviations/violations include slightly out-of-window visits, missed lab tests, and other nonserious events. A record of these should be maintained but generally they are not reportable to the IRB unless they become repetitive and pose a risk. More serious deviations/violations that may involve risks should be reported as per your local IRB policy.

Reporting adverse events and unanticipated problems involving risks to subjects or others is often a challenge for investigators and IRB staff. The Common Rule and the FDA regulations are specific about what requires reporting but neither address reporting time frames. Most IRBs specify reporting requirements in their policies. Regarding unanticipated problems involving risk to subjects or others, the key word is risk. While many risks are easily deciphered, such as loss or theft of a computer with files containing protected health information (PHI), many require medical judgment. The latter may include the host of abnormal laboratory values encountered postoperatively in a surgical study. In that instance, a preemptive review of reportable items with the IRB may be helpful (Box 3.2).

Individuals participating in studies involving sensitive issues can be afforded additional protection under a Certificate of Confidentiality (COC) (20). COCs are used to protect against forced disclosure of information that may have adverse effects on a research subject's financial standing, employability, insurability, or reputation. Typical research areas where COC are useful include child health, reproductive health, mental health, substance and/or alcohol abuse, health issues of older adults, and cancer screening, diagnosis, and treatment. A COC allows a researcher to refuse to provide identifiable information in a civil, criminal, administrative, legislative, or other proceeding at any jurisdictional level. The consent form HIPAA section or addendum should contain information about the COC and include that the subject may voluntarily override

---

BOX 3.2 Some Examples of IRB-Reportable Unanticipated Problems Involving Potential Risk

Suspected noncompliance
For-cause audit
Trial suspension by sponsor
Incarceration of a research subject
New or increased risk
Adverse event requiring protocol/consent amendment
Breach of confidentiality
Exception to inclusion/exclusion criterion w/o IRB approval

the protection afforded by the COC. Certificates are issued by the NIH and applications are usually prepared by the research administration office. On occasion, a granting agency may require a COC to protect vulnerable populations.

CONFLICT OF INTEREST

The importance of financial COI in the clinical research arena, whether real or perceived, cannot be overemphasized. Passage of the Bayh–Dole Act in 1980 (21) encouraged cooperation between industry and academia by allowing inventions made with federal funding to be licensed to industry and, hopefully, provide a faster path to the marketplace for important drugs, treatments, or devices. The resultant comingling of the interests of researchers and industry or other sponsors has made COI disclosure more critical to maintaining public trust and ensuring objectivity in the design and conduct of human subjects research, and in the analysis and presentation of study-related data. The intent of COI regulations is to ensure that:

- Research is not biased by any financial or other interest of an investigator or key personnel.
- Public trust in the integrity of the researcher, the research, and the institution is not damaged by any apparent COI.
- Subjects in research studies are protected from harm.

A robust COI oversight program maintains public and institutional trust in the research enterprise. Institutions with federal funding are obligated to follow NIH guidelines for COI disclosure. However, federal funding notwithstanding, all investigators and research staff must be aware of their institutions' policies on COI.

COI regulations are not meant to be punitive but rather they should allow research subjects to make informed and rational decisions about joining a study and ensure that the research is consistent with the ethical tenets of the Belmont Report. In that context, respect for persons is satisfied by not allowing the COI to result in subtle coercion to join a study, beneficence is served by ensuring reporting of adverse events, and justice is satisfied by preventing a skewed subject selection process.

Reporting potential COI is of critical importance to research as the COI committee in concert with the investigator must devise a plan to manage or eliminate any potential conflict. COI management options include divesting the financial interest to reach an acceptable dollar figure, moving funds to an escrow account until an agreed upon time after study closure, appointing an independent study monitor to oversee conduct of the study, or not participating in the relevant research. When the conflicted investigator plays a crucial role in the study—such as being the only surgeon able to perform a technique or implant a particular device, the COI committee may allow continued participation as an investigator but would stipulate that the conflicted individual cannot be involved in subject selection, the consent process, or in recording or analyzing study data.

Whatever management plan is put into place a mechanism to monitor compliance with the management plan is required. Depending on the degree or nature of the conflict this could mean periodic monitoring by a department chair or business administrator, appointing an oversight committee, or enlisting services of a contract research organization (CRO). Monitor reports generally would be sent to the COI committee and the IRB.

NEW DIRECTIONS

In the interest of enhancing the transparency of clinical trial results and streamlining the IRB process in general, the U.S. Department of Health and Human Services has posted a number of modifications to the Common Rule to become effective January 2018 (22). These include:

- Shortening the IC document and online posting of IC documents for federally funded studies
- Eliminating continuing review requirements for some studies originally reviewed as expedited and for studies that have completed interventions and are open for data analysis only
- Eliminating the need for IRB review of some studies now requiring review for determination of exempt status, and
- The use of single IRBs for review of federally funded multisite studies.

CONCLUSIONS

Following the ethical principles of the Belmont Report and assiduously following the rules for conducting human subjects research as set forth in the CFR, state law, and local IRB policies helps to ensure but does not guarantee the safety of individuals who volunteer to take part in clinical research studies. An additional protection of great importance is the ongoing dialog between the research participant and the researcher and the research staff. While the rules and regulations governing human subjects research may seem onerous and at times excessive, they actually are not considering what is at stake for the volunteer. Recent initiatives by the OHRP in the Department of Health and Human Services will hopefully serve to ease the regulatory burden on IRBs and researchers.

ACKNOWLEDGMENTS

I am grateful to Walter K. Kraft, MD, Kyle Conner, MA, CIP, and Penny Prusa Smith for their helpful editorial review and thoughtful comments.

REFERENCES

1. Code of Federal Regulations. Title 45 Public Welfare Department of Health and Human Services; Part 46 Protection of Human Subjects. https://www.hhs.gov/ohrp/humansubjects/guidance/45cfr46.htm
2. The National Commission for the Protection of Human Subjects of Biomedical and Behavioral Research. The Belmont Report, Ethical Principles and Guidelines for the Protection of Human Subjects of Research; 1979. http://www.hhs.gov/ohrp/humansubjects/guidance/belmont.htm
3. Nuremberg Code. *Trials of War Criminals before the Nuremberg Military Tribunal under Control Council Law No. 10, Vol. 2.* Washington, DC: US Government Printing Office; 1949:181–182. http://www.hhs.gov/ohrp/references/nurcode.htm
4. World Medical Association. Declaration of Helsinki: Ethical Principles for Medical Research Involving Human Subjects. Adopted by the 18th WMA General Assembly, Helsinki, Finland, June 1964, and as revised by the 52nd WMA General Assembly, Edinburgh, Scotland, October 2000 with note of clarification on paragraph 29 added by the WMA General Assembly, Washington, DC; 2002. http://www.wma.net/e/policy/b3.htm
5. US National Research Act. https://history.nih.gov/research/downloads/PL93-348.pdf
6. Brandt AM. Racism and research: the case of the Tuskegee Syphilis Study. *Hastings Ctr Rep.* 1978;8:21–29.
7. Advisory Committee on Human Radiation experiments. *Final Report.* Washington DC: US Gov Pr Office; 1995
8. National Bioethics Advisory Commission Reports. https://ntrl.ntis.gov/NTRL
9. Lidz CW, Appelbaum PS. The therapeutic misconception problems and solutions. *Medical Care.* 2002;40:V55–V63.
10. Editorial, Genetic Privacy. *Nature.* 2013;493:451.
11. Future Genomics research. https://www.genome.gov/27026588/informed-consent-for-genomics-research
12. Gymrek M, Maguire AL, Golan D, et al. Identifying personal genomes by surname inference. *Science,* 2013;339:321–332.
13. Genetic Information Nondiscrimination Act Guidance. Guidance on the Genetic Information Nondiscrimination Act: Implications for Investigators and Institutional Review Boards; 2009. https://www.hhs.gov/ohrp
14. Eccles DM, Mitchell G, Montiero ANA, et al. BRCA1 and BRCA2 genetic testing–pitfalls and recommendations for managing variants of uncertain clinical significance. *Ann Oncol.* 2015;26:2057–2065.
15. Charo RA, Body of research-ownership and use of human tissue. *N Engl J Med.* 2006;355:1517–1519.
16. Allen, MJ, Powers MLE, Gronowski, et al. Human tissue ownership and use in research: what laboratorians and researches should know. *Clinchem.* 2010;56:1675–1682.
17. Lenzi RN, Altevogt BM, Gostin LO, et al, eds. Oversight and Review of Clinical Gene Transfer Protocols: Assessing the Role of the Recombinant DNA Advisory Committee. Washington (DC): National Academies Press (US); 2014. https://www.ncbi.nlm.nih.gov/books/NBK195894
18. Shalem O, Sanjana NE, Hartenian E, et al. Genome-Scale CRISPR-Cas9 knockout screening in human cells. *Science.* 2014;343;84–87.
19. Baltimore D, Berg P, Botchan M, et al. A prudent path forward for genomic engineering and germline gene modification. *Science.* 2015;348;36–38.
20. Certificates of Confidentiality–Privacy Protection for Research Subjects: OHRP Guidance; 2003. https://www.hhs.gov/ohrp/regulations-and-policy/guidance/certificates-of-confidentiality/index.html
21. Markel H. Patents, profits, and the American people: the Bayh–Dole Act of 1980. *N Engl J Med.* 2013:369;794–796.
22. Common rule changes. https://www.federalregister.gov/documents/2017/01/19/2017-01058/federal-policy-for-the-protection-of-human-subjects

4

Industry Collaboration When Developing Novel Agents in Oncology

Hong Xie

The relationship between academia and industry has shifted in recent years, particularly in the realm of oncology clinical studies. With the development and approval of rituximab, trastuzumab, and imatinib, a new era of targeted therapies has been ushered in. The pharmaceutical industry has since changed its oncology business paradigm with increased funding in the areas of discovery, translational research, and clinical development. As a result, there has been dramatic growth in the number of novel agents that enter late-phase clinical testing or have been approved in the fight against cancer. Included among these are immune-checkpoint inhibitors that have captured the attention of the field. These immune-checkpoint inhibitors are working their way into the backbone of cancer treatment in combination with chemotherapies or targeted agents. The field of immuno-oncology beyond checkpoint inhibitors has also experienced rapid growth in clinical development as exemplified by targeted antibody therapies, antibody drug conjugates, bispecifics, and T-cell-based therapies. With the discovery of new molecular entities that have moved from the bench to the clinic, as well as the progression of existing molecules into late or combination development, the number of oncology clinical trials sponsored by industry has risen markedly, providing more opportunities for academia–industry collaborations.

As the understanding of cancer biology deepens, new tools have emerged resulting in the development of new cell lines and humanized mouse models that more closely reflect the human disease. Sophisticated bioinformatics tools enable the analysis of vast amount of data generated from whole-genome and exome sequencing of tumor samples. These tools have generated a wealth of preclinical data to direct the path for clinical development of new anticancer agents.

Clinical evaluation of new agents remains the cornerstone of oncology drug development. In the pharmaceutical industry, each new agent is rigorously evaluated following a clinical development plan (CDP), which integrates the scientific, clinical, regulatory, and commercial considerations into a comprehensive clinical strategy. The first version of the CDP should be created at a new molecular entity (NME) declaration, when the new agent is determined to meet a group of preset criteria for a potential therapeutic. As new information becomes available, both clinical and preclinical, decisions are made that alter the CDP between major milestones. The CDP also details the clinical studies required of the company to reach drug approval. The CDP outlines the process, starting with the first-in-human (FIH) study through to the proof of concept (POC) and the initial and subsequent registration studies, with estimated timelines for each stage. The CDP is critical to the project because it serves as the roadmap for all necessary clinical activities and outlines each milestone from drug discovery to marketing authorization.

The CDP development begins with and is guided by the target product profile (TPP), which states the desired pharmaceutical attributes or properties for a given agent. The TPP is based on the Food and Drug Administration (FDA) Guidance for Industry and Review Staff Target Product Profile—A Strategic Development Process Tool (1). A TPP includes but is not limited to pharmacological, safety, and efficacy targets, with each aspect resembling the major sections of a drug label. The TPP provides a statement of the overall intent of the drug development program elaborating with emphasis on the position of the drug under study and how it will improve upon the current standard of care (SOC) as well as other drugs being developed in the same or similar space. The primary elements are the foundation of the future new drug application and product label, and include: Indication and Usage (including stipulation of patient populations), Dosage and Administration, Dosage Form and Strengths, Contraindications, Warnings and

Precautions, Adverse Reactions, Drug Interactions, Use in Specific Populations (e.g., pregnancy, nursing mothers, pediatric and geriatric uses), Drug Abuse and Dependence, Overdosage, Description, Clinical Pharmacology, Nonclinical Toxicology, Clinical Studies, How Supplied/Storage and Handling, Patient Counseling Information, and References.

The CDP addresses the clinical evaluations required to achieve the criteria set forth in the TPP and details the company vision for drug approval, and thus forms the basis for the upcoming planned clinical trials. Each CDP should include the elements in Table 4.1.

The development of TPP and CDP is a multidisciplinary process following a bench-to-bedside approach. These documents are dynamic and are revised when new information becomes available.

The selection of an indication is evidence-based. In the early stage before any experience in humans is

available (including clinical data in the public domain from other drugs or drug candidates in the same class with similar mechanisms of action [MoA]), the following critical factors are considered:

- Validation of drug targets (such as genomic alterations or overexpression of tumor-associated antigens)
- Understanding of the biological pathway
- Evaluation of tumor killing activities in diverse cell lines
- Examining tumor inhibition in animal models
- Assessing in more robust models of clinical diseases (e.g., patient-derived xenografts)
- Identification of tumor subtypes via screening biobanks
- Data mining in gene/protein expression databases

Analysis of these factors may result in the identification of a specific targeted indication, for example androgen receptor antagonists for the treatment of prostate cancer. For some compounds the indications can be histology independent, as long as the targeted pathway or overexpressed cell surface antigen is present. An example in this category is the Bruton's tyrosine kinase (BTK) inhibitor, ibrutinib, which is indicated for B-cell cancers chronic lymphocytic leukemia, mantle cell lymphoma, Waldenström's macroglobulinemia, and marginal zone lymphoma. Another example would be trastuzumab for HER2 receptor overexpressing breast cancer and metastatic gastric or gastroesophageal junction adenocarcinoma. Yet, for other agents such as immuno-oncology agents or epigenetic agents, the indications are less clearly defined as the activity may be dependent on the tumor microenvironment or may be too broad to provide a focal point.

Once clinical data become available, including reported clinical data on a competitor's agent in the same class, the clinical data take precedence over the preclinical data. While preclinical cell lines or animal models provide answers to some basic questions, these data are generated from highly contrived systems and cannot always translate into efficacy in humans. Similarly, toxicology findings in animals do not always translate into safety signals in humans. Early signals from humans in tumor response or disease control, analysis and validation of biomarkers in posttreatment samples, and safety profile direct the subsequent indication selections.

Currently, for the majority of NMEs, a molecular selection is also often considered upfront to enrich the possibility of efficacy detection in early-phase oncology clinical trials by utilizing the bioinformation analysis of diverse cell line screens and animal models. This has undergone several iterations throughout the past years including personalized medicine, precision medicine, and synthetic lethality. The ability to select patients for some clinical trials requires a companion diagnostic test, which must be developed unless there is an alternative

TABLE 4.1 Elements for a Clinical Development Plan

Required Elements	Optional Elements
• Listing of each indication for which clinical development is planned and regulatory approval is to be sought and the foreseen timelines, including sequence of indications • By planned indication, a description of clinical trials required to reach the next major decision point (e.g., POC for early development programs or registration submission for late development programs) • For compounds in later stages of development, a listing of planned clinical pharmacology and special population studies that may not be indication-specific, but are part of the planned registration package • Listing of completed, company-sponsored clinical trials with summary data	• Multiple development scenarios and decision criteria • Risks and key development challenges and the accompanying mitigation strategies • A list of the key deliverables/objectives for each clinical trial in the CDP • A discussion of how each trial addresses elements of the target product profile • A high-level overview of clinical trial operational considerations • A description of the regulatory strategy • A description of the biomarker and translational research strategies • Integration of clinical pharmacology, biostatistics, and model-based drug development, by decision points, to ensure appropriate decision making at the earliest time point in the most efficient manner

CDP, clinical development plan; POC, proof of concept.

regulatory-approved test readily available. The development of a companion diagnostic is a parallel, lengthy regulatory pathway. The molecular selection assay needs to be evaluated in patient samples to ensure it appropriately identifies the marker with the necessary sensitivity and accuracy. In addition, the utility of the diagnostic test needs to be validated in registration clinical trials. Hence the planning for the companion diagnostic must be initiated early.

The development of a companion diagnostic is a challenge for both the pharmaceutical company as well as the investigators involved in the clinical trial. Appropriate samples must be collected from the early studies to validate the diagnostic. This includes evaluation of samples from subjects who were negative for the biomarker and, thus, not eligible for the study. At times, additional samples may be required to confirm results even after a subject has discontinued study drug treatment. It takes close collaboration between industry and investigators to ensure an appropriate companion diagnostic test is available to select the patients who are most likely to respond to a specific agent.

Preclinical toxicology and pharmacology experiments must be conducted not only to fulfill the regulatory requirements to file for an investigational new drug (IND) in the United States and/or clinical trial agreement (CTA) in Europe, but also to gain invaluable in vivo data on pharmacokinetic and pharmacodynamic predictors. For FIH clinical trials, safety signals detected—or expected but undetected—from toxicology studies done in relevant animal species, provide first clues on the predicted therapeutic window, mechanism in vivo, and potential side effects to be monitored and mitigated in clinical trials. All these data are summarized in the Investigator's Brochure (IB).

Existing standard medical practice for the potential indication—both regional and global—will be surveyed and emerging new agents will be closely monitored. The approvals of novel oncological drug candidates are based on efficacy improvements over SOC and at least the same—if not better—safety profile is desired. Therefore, careful selection of SOC as the control arm for phase III randomized trials is of great importance in order for the results to be accepted by regulatory agencies for marketing authorization. Lately, the trend is on the rise for combining novel agents with SOC regimens. However, the CDP should also address the necessary clinical data to move beyond SOC, even if the first indication is as an add-on therapy. Combinations primarily need to be based on complimentary MoA to derive synergy in efficacy. If the rational selection for the combination therapy is a SOC regimen, the phase III study design is more straightforward. Otherwise, if neither partner in the combination regimen has obvious efficacy separately, the phase III study design may need multiple arms to tease out the contribution of each therapy to the safety and efficacy profile of the combination.

The regulatory environment is changing with accelerated regulatory review processes, including breakthrough therapy designation (BTD) in the United States and priority medicines (PRIME) in Europe. Historically, a three-phase drug development paradigm had been followed in oncology for more than five decades, and this paradigm of oncology drug development would take on average 10 years or longer from FIH studies to regulatory approval. However, driven by a sense of urgency to bring transformative therapies to patients, an increasing number of agents with promising anticancer activities have challenged the sequential three-phase paradigm.

• The initial accelerated approval of pembrolizumab illustrates a model of seamless drug development where an FIH study (ClinicalTrials.gov, NCT01295827) was amended a number of times based on promising response rates in specific tumor types that were observed early in the trial. Gradually, the focus of the study shifted to melanoma and non–small-cell-lung cancer (NSCLC). Additionally, the study design incorporated randomized substudies to compare multiple doses and schedules as well as to confirm efficacy. In total, more than 1,200 subjects were recruited. This creative approach to drug development resulted in data that ultimately supported the accelerated approval of pembrolizumab in melanoma and in NSCLC, as well as the approval of a companion diagnostic test. The conduct of this study showed how it is now possible to use phase I trial data to apply for accelerated approvals. Hence, the three distinct sequential phases of the past in drug development have become increasingly blurred (2,3).

For indications with the potential for orphan drug status, BTD, and accelerated approval, the regulatory strategy outlined in the CDP identifies the key milestones for interactions with the regulatory authorities, including requests for scientific advice.

Clinical planning is the centerpiece of the CDP that integrates all the aforementioned elements. Each clinical trial in the CDP serves a specific purpose and collects data around a particular set of questions. Collectively, the CDP assesses all attributes of a drug candidate so that a comprehensive data package can be prepared for a marketing authorization application (MAA). In addition to studies evaluating the safety and efficacy profile, various special studies, such as food effect, drug–drug interaction, thorough QT, and special population studies need to be deliberated and determined depending on the drug attributes. Planning for changes in formulation or route of administration should also be considered.

Gantt charts are often used in a CDP providing a visual display of the activities involved in a CDP. During CDP drafting, the very critical and often forgotten piece is the identification of potential issues and bottlenecks in the drug development process. For example, if a cell line for an antibody production needs to be subcloned or switched to a different cell line, the CDP must either use an existing trial to characterize the new cell line product or dedicate a new bridging study to prove the compatibility between the products produced in the new cell line and the old cell line.

The CDP enables disciplined assessments and executions of a drug development program. At critical points such as start of a trial, a planned interim analysis, or the end of a trial, success criteria need to be well defined in advance based on the desired attributes defined in the TPP. Each step is a trigger to move to the next phase of clinical activities. These are dubbed the go/no-go decision points and go/no-go criteria. For example, at the end of the phase I trial, if the risk/benefit ratio attained is acceptable to warrant further research, then a larger scale production of clinical grade drug material may be initiated. A phase II study may start to refine the dose regimen and explore efficacy in a more homogeneous population. If a promising efficacy signal is detected in the FIH trial, the sponsor needs to be prepared to accelerate the development plan. On the contrary, if the drug candidate does not improve on efficacy over existing treatment options or does not provide a better safety profile in phase II, the indication, if not the entire program, may be terminated.

The CDP does not exist in isolation. As expected and unexpected events occur within the clinical program as well as in the external environment, critical evaluation of the impact of these events on the CPD should be considered and the CDP should be revised to reflect the current environment.

Decades of cancer research have led to fundamental improvements in our understanding of tumor genesis and treatment. Academia has made significant contributions to tumor biology, target identification and validation, biomarker identification, diagnostic tests, and drug inventions. On the other hand, the pharmaceutical industry has modernized oncology development and brought many transformative therapies to patients with various types of cancer. These advances have demonstrated the strengths and aptitudes of both academia and industry. Both sides now have a greater desire to collaborate so that overall cancer drug development can be more effective and efficient. Ultimately, our patients are better served and societal resources are better utilized.

There are many modes of collaboration between academia and industry. Through collaborations, academic investigators can access investigational drug candidates created by pharmaceutical companies to facilitate the investigators' own laboratory research (4). There is often financial support from the industry towards external research directly related to targets of the company's interest that can represent supplemental funding for the investigator. Furthermore, on the clinical side, the investigator can gain exposure to drug candidates earlier in their development, and contribute to toxicity management and drug registration strategies, while evaluating the potential benefit of the drug candidate. Through these collaborations, pharmaceutical companies can gain access to translational and clinical expertise that they may lack, as well as access to patients who may be eligible for clinical trials. The following list includes some of the common collaborations during and around oncology clinical trials:

- Academic clinicians can participate in industry-sponsored clinical trials as clinical investigators. Industry-sponsored clinical trials, especially those conducted in the United States and European Union, follow International Council for Harmonisation Good Clinical Practice (ICH-GCP) guidelines, which are a set of standards for the design, conduct, performance, monitoring, auditing, recording, analyses, and reporting of clinical trials. ICH-GCP compliance ensures that the clinical data and derived conclusions are credible and accurate, and that the rights, integrity, and confidentiality of patients are protected.

  Communication between the clinical investigators and the industry sponsor is vital to the quality of clinical research, especially during phase I trials where safety signals emerge rapidly. The types of toxicity encountered for targeted or immune therapies are vastly different compared with those of classical chemotherapeutic agents, and it is recognized that preclinical toxicology studies conducted in animal species do not necessarily translate to humans and may not predict novel toxicities. For example, ocular toxicities, such as central serous retinopathy and retinal pigment epithelial detachments, were observed in the treatment with MEK inhibitors (5). The investigators of several clinical trials of MEK inhibitors described these new eye toxicities and proposed to the industry sponsors more stringent eye examinations and toxicity management guidelines for use with MEK inhibitors. In addition to safety monitoring and toxicity management, the clinical investigators are also encouraged to provide feedback on the objectives, endpoints, eligibility criteria, enrollment difficulties, and data analysis plan of the trial that they are part of. These examples highlight the important relationship between investigators and industry sponsors and the importance of continuous open communication.

  o Correlative studies (also called biomarker programs) conducted during oncology clinical trials are of great importance to the understanding of the proposed MoA of a drug candidate. As the convergence of basic discovery and development, correlative studies are increasingly incorporated into early-phase, even FIH trials, to assess pharmacodynamic changes based on MoA, aid selection of therapeutic doses, and monitor therapeutic resistance.

In the development of vemurafenib, paired biopsies were obtained from a subset of melanoma patients in the phase I trial. Through monitoring the activation of the BRAF pathway by measuring ERK phosphorylation (pERK), it was found that tumor regressions were only noted following 80% or more of pERK inhibition. It was also discovered in the phase I trial that although vemurafenib was very effective against BRAF mutant melanoma, it was ineffective against BRAF mutant colorectal cancer, presumably due to the activation of the EGFR pathway in colorectal cancer as a mechanism of inherent resistance. Furthermore, the work on the mechanism of resistance to BRAF inhibition led to the proposal of combining vemurafenib with an MEK inhibitor in melanoma to derive greater efficacy, as the combination would provide concomitant inhibition of two elements along the RAS–RAF–MEK–ERK pathway (6).

Correlative studies may also help refine the patient selection if a biomarker of predictive value can be identified and fits the proposed MoA. For example, crizotinib was first developed as a c-MET inhibitor, but was later found to have activity against ALK rearrangements. In early clinical development, there was a case report showing that crizotinib had significant antitumor activity in one patient with ROS1-positive NSCLC (7). Following the promising efficacy signal, the industry sponsor pursued this molecularly-defined indication by amending the crizotinib FIH study (PROFILE1001) to include a cohort of ROS1-positive tumors. As a result, the sponsor received FDA accelerated approval for ROS1-positive NSCLC based on results from 50 subjects.

Currently, technological advances enable many sophisticated assays such as flow cytometry on tumor samples or gene expression profiling to identify potentially druggable gene alterations. However, many of these technologies are limited to special bedside sample handling that is impossible to carry out by a multicenter study. Investigators may consider their own technological expertise and laboratory settings to pursue a subcorrelative study focusing on the patients they recruit at their own center for the industry-sponsored study, to augment the biomarker plan of the entire study. Given the added costs and logistics, as well as the potential risk to trial subjects associated with invasive procedures, it is critical that all correlative studies are scientifically justified, carefully designed, and well organized.

Agreement with the industry sponsor as well as institutional review boards (IRBs) must be obtained upfront, as well as the informed consent of the patient.

- Besides being clinical investigators, academicians and clinicians can serve other roles in industry-sponsored clinical trials such as:
  o Advisory board: A meeting in which distinguished clinicians and translational scientists are invited to help pharmaceutical companies craft and execute development strategies. These advisors provide their expertise on questions fundamental to the CDP in development continuum of a prospective approved compound. During the conduct of a clinical trial, or a number of trials with a drug candidate, advisory boards can be held periodically to enable companies to review emerging clinical data with experts, confirm or disapprove proposed MoA, raise and answer development-related questions, and adjust CDPs. Advisory boards fulfill a specific and critical business need of a pharmaceutical company by providing expert opinions and direction on the development of a compound.
  o Steering committee: A small group of experts, typically senior clinicians participating in the study, are selected by the pharmaceutical company to oversee a large phase II or phase III clinical study. Large-scale phase II or III studies are major endeavors for pharmaceutical companies due to the financial and resource costs. To the community and patients, commencement of large-scale trials signifies a commitment by the company to a drug candidate. As the name suggests, steering committees are tasked with steering one or more large-scale trials. They review the conceptual plans for a study to ensure its objectives and goals are scientifically sound. They are also directly involved in the full development of a trial protocol, including details regarding statistical design, proposed control arm, patient eligibility and exclusion criteria, procedures for assessing and reporting adverse events, management plans of side effects, and data analysis plans. When the trial is under way, they monitor recruitment strategy, data collection, and the overall safety of participants as a whole. After the trial is completed, they scrutinize and interpret the data collected and draw conclusions based on their experience and expertise. They are responsible for publication strategies as well. Their responsibilities and functions are usually defined in a formal charter before a trial starts.
  o Independent data monitoring committees (IDMC): these are committees of clinical and statistical experts not associated with a particular clinical trial, selected to independently

review trial-associated data. They are in charge of reviewing unblinded safety data while a trial is ongoing, and they may make recommendations based on prespecified statistical rules regarding prespecified changes to the trial conduct. The committee members are independent of the sponsor, which allows the investigators and company staff working on a specific trial to remain blinded to clinical data. In their role, the IDMC provides important oversight on the safety and overall quality control of the trial conduct, thus preventing potential bias that could be introduced by frequent interim analyses conducted by the trial team.

o Safety evaluation team (SET): In phase I trials, the SET is composed mainly of clinical investigators who monitor safety data at scheduled pauses (e.g., dose-limiting toxicity [DLT] observation period), determine dose escalation or de-escalation, add or close patient cohorts based on safety findings, potentially expand cohorts, and advise other participating investigators about emerging new toxicities and their management.

• Since the industry CDP is mainly focused on getting regulatory approval as opposed to general practice, there are many data gaps in the knowledge about the optimal usage of a drug in general medical practice. Clinical investigators with interest in clinical research of an exploratory nature can address many of the scientific or clinical questions left out by the drug manufacturer's CDP by proposing their own clinical trials. In an investigator-initiated study (IIS), the investigator is the trial sponsor with total responsibilities for the design and conduct of the trial. Usual practice is for the investigator to apply to the drug manufacturer for drug supplies, and often times for funds as well. Based on the merits of the proposed study with consideration to the CDP (i.e., a similar study that is already part of the drug candidate's CDP), pharmaceutical companies may grant these requests. There are responsibilities beyond funds and drug supplies on the part of the drug manufacturer in IIS collaborations. Oversight of pharmacovigilance is mandatory and these activities are coordinated between the drug manufacturer and the sponsor investigator.

Similar to IISs are trials run by various consortia. Some consortia are set up as companies while others are networks of medical centers or clinics. There are also government backed cooperative groups in the United States. These consortia, especially those that operate as contract research organizations (CRO), can sponsor or colead large-scale clinical trials. Their experience, sophisticated infrastructures, access to large numbers of participating centers, and wide access to patients make them attractive candidates for conducting clinical trials. They may

also propose clinical trials for consideration in the pharmaceutical company CDP, or clinical trials to address practice-related questions such as optimal dose administration, sequencing of therapies, and comparisons to a number of SOCs.

• In the past decades, many breakthrough discoveries have been made in academia. However, discoveries in academia rarely move through the drug development process or as far as the clinic. Among the main reasons are:

o Academic centers or individual investigators do not have the know-how and equipment to produce clinical grade drugs on the scale required for a clinical study.

o The funds required to support the regulation-mandated nonclinical toxicology studies and clinical trials are prohibitive to academic centers.

o They lack the experiences and resources to be compliant with the increasing complexity of regulations in drug development and/or diagnostic testing.

o Some of the necessary disciplines such as pharmacology, translational research, legal, regulatory, project management, and marketing to bring a therapeutic to a broad patient population are inadequate in an academic center.

o They lack operational teams for data management, data analysis, pharmacovigilance, drug supply chain management, and management of CROs.

Pharmaceutical companies recognize that some of the best ideas and innovations are within academia. Therefore, most large pharmaceutical companies have set up venture investment funds to invest in areas of strategic interest to the company portfolio. These venture investors have an interest in identifying and investing in compounds that have the potential to be developed into drugs to complement their company's own pipelines. Academicians and investigators with drug innovations can seek funding opportunities with these venture investments. Alternatively, they can work with the pharmaceutical companies directly via licensing agreements, in order to move their innovative drug candidate into the clinical stage and ultimately to marketing approval to benefit cancer patients.

Regardless of the mode of collaboration, a contract and budget must be agreed upon by both the pharmaceutical company and academic collaborator before any actual work starts. This allows for transparency related to the activities and fees for those activities. The contract should state the purpose of the collaboration, expected roles and responsibilities, deliverables, timelines, confidentialities, and rights to intellectual properties. The contract is usually negotiated by a contract specialist for each party involved. Attorneys are enlisted to review intellectual property clauses. These contract negotiations can be time- and effort-consuming. National Cancer Institute (NCI) and CEO Roundtable on Cancer have developed a set of standardized clauses for use in CTAs (8). The START (Standard Terms of Agreement for Research Trial) clauses were developed with an intent to simplify and accelerate the contracting process, as contract negotiation is viewed as one of the key barriers to timely initiation of clinical trials.

Separately, milestones and associated payments are covered by grant/budget negotiations. Budgets for academic collaborations must reflect the current fair market value (FMV) for similar amount and complexity of work to ensure compliance with industry legal requirements. For clinical trials, there are line items in the budget that are one-time payments, as these items are required independent of the number of patients to be enrolled. These items include those related to start-up activities such as institutional review board (IRB) or ethics committee (EC) submissions and trial-specific trainings. There are also items related to the procedures that are based on the number of subjects and subject visits. Non-standard-of-care tests and procedures (e.g., biopsies, PET scans, or extra ECGs), which are denied by third-party payers to reimburse, are also included in the trial budget.

The investigators should be actively involved in the contract and budget negotiations, although contracts and budgets are negotiated for the most part by special delegates who may not have the scientific or medical background and knowledge to clearly understand the technical terms and the impact to the proposed clinical study. This hindrance leads to project delays and potential legal or financial entanglements down the road, ultimately affecting the project timeline and the evaluation of the drug under study.

Many pharmaceutical companies have dedicated field-based medical science liaison (MSL) teams to build strategic relationships with academic investigators and research sites. MSLs have separate and unique areas of focus in contrast with commercial sales teams. They are highly educated in a life science field (e.g., PharmD, PhD, MD, and MSN) and are responsible for peer-to-peer scientific knowledge exchange. Their proximity to and constant interactions with academic and community research sites in their respective geographic location enable them to be able to provide two-way in-depth communications and knowledge exchanges regarding research interests, activities, and collaborations on both sides. Their facilitating skills ensure timely issue escalation and problem solving during all clinical research initiatives, both for company- and investigator-sponsored clinical trials. In one area that the MSL teams support: site selection for company-sponsored studies, awareness of research sites' areas of focus can be leveraged to estimate engagement for specific clinical trials. Some research sites may have an interest in early development while others may be more focused on phase III clinical

trials. Knowledge of a patient population at the site or competing clinical trials may inform anticipated accrual patterns from a specific site. The MSL's insights can help guide clinical trial operation teams and/or CROs in fostering a more focused and streamlined site feasibility and selection process. Additionally, the MSL can facilitate communication of investigators' clinical research focuses and ideas to the pharmaceutical company. Therefore, the sponsor MSL team represents a resource that can bridge academia and industry to increase the collaborations in oncology clinical trials.

One area in the academia–industry relationship that often draws severe criticism by the public is "publication bias," in which a large number of clinical trials with negative results unfavorable to the sponsor's drug or drug candidate are unpublished or downplayed, while positive trials confirming effectiveness and safety are readily published (9,10). A frequently criticized practice is ghostwriting, where manuscripts or books are produced by paid medical writers while the named authors may not have had any significant contributions to the conceptualization, conduct, or data reporting of a clinical trial. In 2001, the International Committee of Medical Journal Editors (ICMJE) (11), concerned about publication bias, revised the sections related to potential conflicts of interest in its policy "Uniform Requirements for Manuscripts Submitted to Biomedical Journals: Writing and Editing for Biomedical Publication." This ICMJE policy (the most recent update was from 2016 [(12)]) has been widely adopted by many peer-reviewed scientific journals as the basis for editorial policy. Many journals now routinely require each author to disclose his or her contributions to the manuscript and ask the responsible author to sign a statement indicating that he or she accepts full responsibility for the conduct of the trial, has had full access to the data, ensures the integrity of the data, and is willing to publish the data.

Later, Title VIII of the FDA Amendments Act of 2007 (FDAAA) expanded the legal mandate for sponsors of certain clinical trials with FDA-regulated drug products to register their studies and report summary results to ClinicalTrials.gov (13). The two major pharmaceutical trade associations—European Federation of Pharmaceutical Industries and Associations (EFPIA) and the Pharmaceutical Research and Manufacturers of America (PhRMA)—jointly developed and voluntarily implemented Principles for Responsible Clinical Trial Data Sharing beginning in January 2014 (14). Member companies belonging to these two associations pledge to publish aggregate results of every phase II and phase III clinical trial within 1 year of trial completion, regardless of whether the trial outcome is positive or negative. Certain companies even allow outside researchers who are not engaged in the clinical research collaboration to access clinical trial data, such as clinical study reports (CSRs) and de-identified participant level data (15).

Cancer patients participate in clinical trials with the hope of potential personal benefit from a new treatment but also for altruistic reasons. The ultimate goal of conducting clinical trials in humans is to collectively understand the complex disease process of cancer and the potential benefits of new cancer treatments. It is the combined responsibility of both academia and industry to ensure the full disclosure of clinical research findings to help investigators and practitioners make informed treatment decisions, and to advance generalizable knowledge of cancer and cancer treatment. Only through improved and expanded disclosure of clinical trial data can we address publication bias and improve accountability between industry and investigators.

In addition to the concern of publication bias, financial conflict over the academia–industry relationship is of interest to the public. Conflict of interest on the part of investigators can compromise the well-being of research subjects, introduce bias in the conduct of clinical trials, and distort conclusions of trial data. Therefore, perceived or real conflict of interest may undermine public trust in the results of clinical trials either sponsored by industry or an investigator. Both academia and industry need to take responsibilities for these negative perceptions and distrust. Academia and industry must do a better job in explaining why companies and healthcare professionals interact, how they interact, and how their interactions contribute to better understanding of the disease, novel technologies, new drug development, and ultimately improved patient care.

Financial relationships (such as consultancies, research grants, stock ownership, honoraria, patents, and employment) need to be fully disclosed at scientific conferences when clinical data are presented or exchanged. ICMJE policy mandates full financial disclosure from authors at the time they submit a manuscript. Authors are also warned by ICMJE to avoid entering into agreements that interfere with their access to all of the study data or that interfere with their ability to analyze and interpret the data. Authors need to prepare and publish manuscripts independently.

In the United States, the Physician Payments Sunshine Act, commonly known as the Sunshine Act or Open Payments, was enacted by Congress in 2010 as part of the Patient Protection and Affordable Care Act. The law requires Centers for Medicare and Medicaid Services (CMS) to collect and display information reported by pharmaceutical companies about the payments and other transfers of value made to healthcare professionals and teaching hospitals (16). Note, the federal Sunshine Act does not replace state marketing laws that require explicit financial disclosures as well. The EFPIA has also in June 2016 formally adopted a code of conduct on disclosure of transfers of value from pharmaceutical companies to healthcare professionals in an effort to promote transparency and further self-regulate. The individual healthcare professionals refer to all types of practitioners including but not limited to physicians, pharmacists, nurses, research staff, and administrators. Academic investigators belong to healthcare professions, and in certain countries government officials as well. A "reportable payment" can be fees for advice or service, travel, meals, or education cost. Companies are responsible for reporting payments associated with company-initiated activities and meetings, whether these are organized directly or by an agency. If a company provides sponsorship to an academic center or educational agency to hold its own educational meeting, these sponsorships will be separately reported. Reportable payments will be published on companies' websites by individual and by event.

The information presented here briefly describes the planning process (CDP), regulatory considerations, and collaborations between industry and academia on the road from drug discovery to health agency approval and beyond. The road from "bench to bedside" for cancer research is a long process involving significant financial and human resources, and impacts the patients who participate in the clinical trials. Although improvements have been made in cancer research in recent years, more is yet to be done to better the outcomes for cancer patients.

This shared goal brings academia and industry together so that each side can contribute their unique creativities, talents, and skills. Only through joining forces will we be able to advance cancer research and develop more precision medicines. Collaborations need to be conducted carefully to avoid real or perceived biases so that we can ensure public confidence in results from oncology clinical trials. These results need to be accurate and disclosed properly to the medical community in a timely and transparent fashion. It is the partnership between industry and academia that is truly critical to improving cancer care and transforming cancer treatment.

REFERENCES

1. Guidance for industry and review staff target product profile—a strategic development process tool. http://www.fda.gov/downloads/Drugs/GuidanceCompliance RegulatoryInformation/Guidances/ucm080593.pdf. Published 2007.
2. Bates SE, Berry DA, Balasubramaniam S, et al. Advancing clinical trials to streamline drug development. *Clin Cancer Res.* 2015;21(20):4527–4535.
3. Prowell TM, Theoret MR, Pazdur R. Seamless oncology-drug development. *N Engl J Med.* 2016;374:2001–2003.
4. Published Kinase Inhibitor Set. https://www.ebi.ac.uk/chembldb/extra/PKIS
5. McCannel TA, Chmielowski B, Finn RS, et al. Bilateral subfoveal neurosensory retinal detachment associated with MEK inhibitor use for metastatic cancer. *JAMA Ophthalmol.* 2014;132:1005–1009.
6. Bollag G, Tsai J, Zhang J, et al. Vemurafenib: the first drug approved for BRAF-mutant cancer. *Nat Rev Drug Discov.* 2012; 11:873–886.

7. Davies KD, Le AT, Theodoro MF, et al. Identifying and targeting ROS1 gene fusions in non-small cell lung cancer. *Clin Cancer Res*. 2012;18:4570–4579.

8. Proposed Standardized/Harmonized Clauses for Clinical Trial Agreements. https://www.cancer.gov/about-nci/organization/ccct/resources/start-clauses-info.pdf

9. Lexchin J. Those who have the gold make the evidence: how the pharmaceutical industry biases the outcomes of clinical trials of medications. *Sci Eng Ethics*. 2012;18:247–261.

10. Ross JS, Gross CP, Krumholz HM. Promoting transparency in pharmaceutical industry–sponsored research. *Am J Public Health*. 2012;102(1):72–80.

11. Davidoff F, DeAngelis CD, Drazen JM, et al: Sponsorship, authorship and accountability. *CMAJ*. 2001;165(6):786–788.

12. Recommendations for the conduct, reporting, editing, and publication of scholarly work in medical journals. http://www.icmje.org/icmje-recommendations.pdf. Updated 2016.

13. Zarin DA, Tse T, Williams RJ, et al. Trial reporting in ClinicalTrials.gov—the final rule. *N Engl J Med*. 2016;375:1998–2004.

14. EFPIA-PhRMA rules for clinical trial data sharing active [Press release]. http://www.phrma.org/press-release/joint-efpia-phrma-principles-for-responsible-clinical-trial-data-sharing-become-effective-today

15. How to request data. http://yoda.yale.edu/how-request-data

16. U.S. Centers for Medicare & Medicaid Services. How open payments works. https://www.cms.gov/OpenPayments/About/How-Open-Payments-Works.html

The Trials and Tribulations of Writing and Conducting an Investigator Initiated Trial

Jake Vinson, Josh Buddle, Julie Filipenko, Christine Tran, Kristofer Prepelica, and Sarah Wise

Clinical trials sponsored by pharmaceutical, biotech, medical device companies, or specialized groups can often be referred to as industry-sponsored trials. However, in cases where the principal investigator (PI) would like to serve as the sponsor for his or her own study, investigator initiated trials (IITs) can be conducted. While these types of trials can also be referred to as investigator initiated studies, investigator sponsored trials, third party studies, or medical school grants, it all calls attention to the PI taking on the role of both sponsor and investigator. According to the Code of Federal Regulations (CFR) (1) an investigator is "an individual who actually conducts a clinical investigation (i.e., under whose immediate direction the drug is administered or dispensed to a subject)," while a sponsor is a person who "takes responsibility for and initiates a clinical investigation. This can be an individual, academic institution, pharmaceutical company, government agency, private or nonprofit organization." As outlined in FDA 21 CFR Part 312 (1), the sponsor–investigator role in an IIT must plan, design, conduct, monitor, manage data, prepare reports, and oversee all regulatory and ethical matters, in addition to owning data and publication privileges. The benefit to patients, demand for efficiency in health care, gap in knowledge, a need for more cost-effective ways to advance research, or to spark innovation are just some reasons why IITs are needed. However, IITs are not without their trials and tribulations. As both an investigator and a sponsor, there are numerous aspects of planning, conducting, and completing a successful IIT to consider. This chapter provides principles of how to address scientific, legal, regulatory, data, budgetary, and oversight concerns throughout the life cycle of an IIT.

CONCEPT DEVELOPMENT AND THE REALITY OF WRITING AND REVIEWING AN IIT

IITs are primarily conceptualized by an investigator to test a specific hypothesis that may or may not be of primary interest to traditional "sponsors" (e.g., pharmaceutical companies). This unique circumstance allows the investigator significant flexibility to innovate a new concept (e.g., combining two Food and Drug Administration [FDA] approved drugs in an untested population), test a novel agent, and so on. A two- to three-page concept sheet, drafted by the investigator, which details the background, hypothesis, objectives, correlatives, study design, and statistical assumptions is critical in the early stages of an IIT. This concept sheet will be the snapshot that a potential supporting entity will use to vet the science and originality of the concept. A primary statistician and a seasoned clinical researcher (nurse, coordinator, manager, etc.) should review the concept sheet for scientific merit, programmatic fit, practicality, and resourcing (among other things). It is also important at the very early stages of concept design to have an experienced coordinator or research manager who will manage communication, review comments, versioning, and keep track of timelines. It is vital to understand the risks associated with an IIT, which can be as simple as competition among investigators testing similar or identical concepts and lack of originality, to managing complex scientific and operational communication, and so on. Two vitally important components to consider during the concept phase are (a) delineating between the possible and the impossible and (b) managing a concept/protocol timeline in a constantly evolving clinical and scientific landscape.

Conceptual Versus Practical

Many IITs are burdened with lofty hypotheses and outcome expectations that must be constantly checked at the development stage against the reality of clinical trial design, costs, and operational mechanics. The trial's coordinator needs to review the concept against institutional requirements; engaging relevant personnel such as research nurses and research operations staff who see clinical trial patients in this assessment helps determine feasibility to an even greater extent. The individual responsible for drafting the protocol must constantly ask if something is feasible and should strongly consider a real-world "dry-run" testing of procedures. For example, an investigator may have cardiac toxicity concerns and require 12-lead electrocardiograms at specific intervals and a supporting company may "require" completing them within 10-minute windows in triplicate pre- and post-therapy. However, this is most likely impractical, overly costly, and unlikely to succeed. Similar consideration should be given throughout the review of a concept.

Changing Clinical Landscape

IITs are often timeline-challenged. The typical resources in an industry-sponsored study are usually not available in an IIT, and this often results in a very lengthy development process. A new drug combination strategy may no longer be clinically relevant to the field if, for example, a large phase III study reports results that change the field. An innovative and forward-thinking trial design is important, as well as having a thorough understanding of the current research landscape. Understanding the greater clinical trials landscape, whether results from other ongoing trials will impact the scientific question(s) of one's IIT, is also critical. Communicating openly with colleagues and potential supporters is key.

The IIT is often one of the best ways to test a hypothesis in a phase I or phase II setting; careful attention to detail, maintaining strict timelines, and open communication are keys to success. The process is complicated and can be thought through as a timeline (Figure 5.1).

PROTOCOL DEVELOPMENT

Writing a good protocol is both a science and an art. It must represent an actionable plan that is readable, repeatable, nonduplicative, and include reasonable accommodations for subjects while maintaining scientific integrity and following all federal, state, and local regulations. The best way to take a concept to a full protocol is to start with a protocol template that has been accepted previously at the lead institution or is a commonly accepted format (e.g., National Cancer Institute [NCI]).

Protocol Templates; Version Control

Starting with a well-structured protocol template is the best way to ensure that the document has the correct flow of information and appropriately covers how to perform the study within the legal regulations. Many institutions and numerous federal regulatory agencies offer protocol templates including required language as a starting point. It is up to the investigator to take the concept and translate it into an actionable plan that describes the background of the study, objectives, clinical plan, correlative plan, and statistical assumptions. Pull the key information from the concept sheet to the protocol template and identify key individuals who can collaborate and/or write each section of the document.

It is highly likely that a protocol will go through 10 or more versions before a final document is ready for submission—version control is critical. Version control is best managed by the assigned research manager and this role has to be defined early in the process. Often, the most efficient methodology is to allow multiple reviewers to write, comment, and edit simultaneously, with the research manager ensuring that each set of changes and comments is included in a "master" version. After edits and comments have been incorporated into the master, a coordinating meeting among all stakeholders to address outlying questions and identify weaknesses is most efficient.

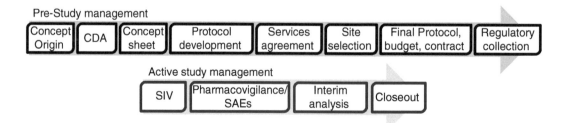

FIGURE 5.1 The study management process from concept origin to trial closeout.
CDA, confidential disclosure agreement; SAE, serious adverse event; SIV, site initiation visit.

There are several software platforms that can assist in this process by allowing multiple reviewers to annotate and comment on a developing protocol document simultaneously.

Regulatory Requirements

Conducting a clinical study with human research subjects requires significant regulatory oversight and understanding of which regulations apply to the clinical investigation. Generally, the investigation will include drugs, biologics, and/or devices. Depending on the drug and/or device being tested, specific regulatory language may need to be included in the protocol document and considered in the overall timeline. Further, the International Council for Harmonisation (ICH) has established ethical and scientific quality standards for clinical trials known as Good Clinical Practice (GCP) guidelines that are recommended for adoption to regulatory bodies of the European Union, Japan, and the United States. Many elements of GCP are incorporated into the U.S. CFR, but the ICH GCP E6 guideline itself is also an important reference when conducting an IIT.

Federal Regulatory Requirements

CFR Title 21 applies when research is being conducted to develop a medical product that will be licensed for sale in the United States. An IIT inherently infers that the sponsorship of the clinical study is with the investigator; the investigator must therefore understand and apply the federal regulatory requirements for an investigational new drug (IND; 21 CFR 312) (1) and/or investigational device exemption (21 CFR 812) (2).

21 CFR 312 details the regulations for human research done with investigational drugs. It also discusses regulations for applying to FDA to conduct research under an IND application (21 CFR 312 Subpart B), responsibilities of sponsors and investigators under an IND (21 CFR 312 Subpart D), and expanded access to investigational drugs (21 CFR 312 Subpart I). 21 CFR 812 outlines the regulations for human research with investigational devices. Conducting human subjects research with investigational devices is covered in 21 CFR 812 Subpart B, responsibilities of sponsors in 21 CFR 812 Subpart C, investigators in 21 CFR 812 Subpart E, and institutional review board (IRB) approval in 21 CFR 812 Subpart D.

There are additionally many less common regulatory oversight bodies such as the National Institutes of Health's Recombinant DNA Advisory Committee (RAC), and so on. It is important for the IIT to determine the regulatory pathway, including the regulatory bodies involved, determine who interacts with regulatory bodies, and plan the protocol activation steps and timeline accordingly. Typical industry sponsors have entire divisions of people with years of regulatory experience to navigate these complicated pathways. A PI leading an IIT needs to evaluate whether there are any institutional resources available to develop the regulatory document package and navigate communication with the regulatory bodies.

Institutional Review Process

Institutions have different requirements for institutional review, so an important first step in planning for an IIT is understanding specific institutional review requirements. Examples of review requirements or committees an institution may have include review for fit within a department's research portfolio and patient population and review of the scientific merit of the research. Depending on the type of trial, a trial may also require review of radiation safety or biosafety. Other groups/departments contributing to a trial may require their own review, such as a radiology department performing scans on the clinical trial participants or a biostatistics department contributing to the statistical design of the trial. There are often more review steps for an IIT than for other protocols, since there are often other groups involved in helping the investigator write the protocol. It is important to anticipate the institutional review requirements and associated timeline for each review, so that necessary reviews can be aligned with other necessary activities prior to opening a trial; such as obtaining drug/device supply, identifying staff resources, and so on.

IRB—Local and Central

IRB review is one step in the review process that is required for all research considered human subjects research, regardless of other institutional review requirements. There are some limited scenarios when research may be exempt from IRB review or a waiver of IRB review and approval may be obtained, but it is still essential to review the scenarios with an IRB to determine applicable regulations.

IRB review may be accomplished by a "local" IRB or a "central" IRB depending on the requirements of the investigator's institution. A local IRB is an IRB associated with the institution performing the research; a central IRB is independent of any specific institution performing research. When a local IRB is reviewing an IIT, the review may be more critical than when the IRB is reviewing other trials, since the institution is the sponsor of the trial and has greater accountability for the conduct of the trial. The obligation to review and ensure strict compliance with institutional guidelines is prioritized, and this mentality may be seen at all levels of review leading up to IRB review as well.

Institutions with a local IRB often require review by the local IRB and will not allow central IRB review of a protocol. However, central IRBs are often much more efficient than local IRBs. For IITs with multiple participating sites, a central IRB can save time and effort by performing protocol review one time for all sites, thus consolidating the review process. The efficiency of a central IRB has been acknowledged within the research community and regulations have been adapted to apply this efficiency more broadly. Revisions to the Common Rule (45 C.F.R. § 46) (3) require that all multicenter trials, whether IIT or not, utilize a single IRB for protocol review by 2020 (4).

Supporting Company Requirements

If an outside company is supporting the protocol (e.g., a pharmaceutical or biotechnology company), the company will likely have protocol requirements to include as well. These often come in the form of a protocol template, which will include background on a specific drug, required inclusion and/or exclusion criteria, safety reporting guidelines, and drug/manufacturing details. The investigator will need to work with the company to determine the review pathway, timeline, and requirements for the protocol. Often, a negotiation of protocol terms is required to meet both company and institutional requirements, which can be time consuming.

CONSENT DEVELOPMENT

As with writing a good protocol, writing a good consent form could also be considered a science and an art. Contrary to externally sponsored trials that often have an informed consent form (ICF) template, an investigator often has to start from scratch when writing the consent for an IIT. Some institutions have an institutional ICF template, but the protocol-specific content must be written by the investigator or a member of the investigator's team. When writing an ICF, the CFR provides a detailed list of required content. However, one of the most challenging elements of writing a good ICF is translating the complex scientific content of a protocol into a readable document for a potential clinical trial participant.

Consent Requirements Change

The potential for changes in the regulatory environment of clinical trials and changes in scientific information available related to the protocol require that consent documents are viewed as living documents that must be adjusted as needed. New risks emerge in the safety profile of a drug and disclosures of investigators affecting conflict of interest can change. The nature of genomic testing is constantly evolving, and evaluating how to share discoveries with patients is vital.

Managing consent changes is particularly complicated for multicenter IITs. While most institutions typically have a consistently used "consent template," every institution has a different template (sometimes drastically different). Ensuring that consenting terms are consistent becomes very challenging to manage across multiple institutions, which will be discussed in a later section on multicenter studies.

Next-Generation Sequencing; Future Use; Sharing Results

As with any protocol intending to collect samples for future use, an investigator conducting an IIT must communicate the plan to subjects during informed consent. While the specific testing to be performed may not be known, the informed consent should communicate to subjects how samples will be stored, the nature and purpose of the future research to be conducted, and whether results will be shared when the samples are analyzed in the future.

BUDGETS/CONTRACTS

Execution of an IIT can only be successful when adequately supported financially, which makes establishing a protocol-specific budget a necessary step prior to protocol activation. Depending on the funding source, and whether there are any vendors needed to execute the research, one or more contracts may be necessary as well. Aligning the budget and contract steps in the activation process with the protocol development will help ensure that a protocol is truly ready to be activated once institutional and regulatory approvals have been attained.

Budgets

A protocol budget should accurately reflect the costs associated with running the trial. This includes staff time and effort, institutional administrative fees, patient care services being performed for research, correlative studies, supplies, and any other protocol-specific expenses. While it can be tempting to make a protocol budget match the amount of whatever funding has been obtained, it is important to consider the true expenses of the trial in order to proactively identify secondary funding if needed. Underbudgeting and thus becoming unable to ultimately complete the protocol and/or the intended analyses does not benefit the patients or the scientific process.

Once a budget is established and adequate funding is secured, it is important to ensure proper financial management of the trial during the conduct. This includes managing payables and receivables according to the budget and forecasting fixed and variable costs associated with the life cycle of the project. If a protocol is amended, it is important to consider the financial implications of the amendment.

Contracts

If external funding is secured, a contract with the funding source will be needed. A contract may also be needed if a manufacturer has agreed to provide a drug or device for the trial, or if a lab or another external vendor will be involved in the execution of the clinical trial protocol. It is important to involve appropriate institutional legal groups in contract review, though negotiation can sometimes extend the protocol timeline. An institution may have a master agreement with a certain drug or device manufacturer or certain labs, which can help streamline contract negotiation but may not apply for an IIT. IITs may have more complex terms than other trials, particularly for intellectual property. If a drug or device manufacturer has agreed to provide its product for use in the trial, it will want intellectual property rights to any discoveries made during the trial relating to its product; however, as the sponsor of the IIT, it is important for the investigator and institution to maintain their intellectual property rights to discoveries made during the trial.

It is important to engage early with a skilled legal team or contracting group to ensure contract negotiation timelines are in line with the protocol activation timeline. In addition to legal review of a contract, it is important to reconcile the contract with the protocol to ensure consistency in terms such as safety reporting requirements or lab supplies and analyses.

STUDY ACTIVATION

Before activation, it is critical to ensure proper training for personnel who will work on the protocol and ensure a complete set of essential regulatory documentation, as defined in ICH E6 Section 8. The research manager who has helped the protocol reach this point now needs to champion the final collection of documents, ensure all regulatory and ethics approvals are in place, contracts are executed, budgets are agreed to, drugs/devices and so on have been resourced, and a date is picked to "activate." Organization of the final steps is critical.

SITE INITIATION VISIT

The site initiation visit (SIV) is the final opportunity to ensure that all protocol elements align and the study is ready to start enrolling subjects. The industry expectation of this alignment of multiple pieces is often impossible to match in an IIT. The SIV is a training exercise, but it is always best to have already worked out all of the details as this is the time to "get in the weeds" and explain the minutiae. "Pre-SIVs" can be informal meetings that take place with the study team, pharmacy team, and so on to ensure there is understanding of roles and responsibilities before the official kickoff of the protocol during the SIV.

ACTIVE STUDY MANAGEMENT

Clinical Data Management

Oncology trials pose many unique challenges to data management: numerous adverse events associated with treatments with concurrent comorbidities and medications to manage them, higher number of protocol violations due to complexity of study design, extended trial durations and follow-up for survival, frequent scheduled and unscheduled lab tests, complicated database setups to accommodate dose escalation, reduction, crossover to alternative treatment arms, overlapping treatment combinations, and complexity of external genetic and imaging data.

This leads to protocols collecting large amounts of data and time-consuming data cleaning, external data transfers, integration, and reconciliation, and many interim deliverables. The use of electronic data capture (EDC) technology is undoubtedly the best route for faster data collection and implementation of system edit check to validate it in real time. While researchers have a tendency toward collecting as much data as possible, collecting only what is necessary for analysis will reduce the effort of collecting and cleaning extraneous data and will have a direct impact on the budget.

Good Clinical Data Management Practices by Society of Clinical Data Management (5) should be used to promote current industry best procedures and practices. Clear case report form (CRF) completion guidelines, standard operating procedures (SOPs), and a data management plan will add tremendously to the quality of data.

The future of clinical data management is in leveraging technology, such as direct data feeds into EDC from, for example, electronic health records, without having sites to transcribe it, cloud solutions to manage huge volumes of data from different sources; using the Clinical Data Interchange Standard Consortium (CDISC) standards, and implementation of a risk-based approach to data processing (cleaning data with high risk levels such as efficacy and safety thoroughly).

Monitoring/Oversight

The sponsor of a trial has responsibility for proper monitoring and oversight of the trial as a whole. This includes monitoring and oversight for all sites if the trial is multicenter. The guideline for GCP found in ICH E6 (6) requires the sponsor to establish a means to manage quality throughout the trial. Quality assurance and quality control measures such as monitoring and auditing are often used to accomplish this responsibility. This applies to IIT sponsors as well, which may also fall under FDA requirements for sponsor monitoring found in 21 C.F.R. § 312 (1) and 21 C.F.R. § 812 (1), which apply when the trial is conducted under an IND or IDE (respectively).

Industry sponsors historically relied on the costly process of frequent on-site monitoring visits where source documents are verified for 100% of the data collected. The source documents represent the original documentation for relevant data (e.g., hospital records, office charts, laboratory reports, etc.). Particularly for an IIT sponsor who is often on a more limited budget, leveraging the principals of risk-based monitoring becomes especially important. The FDA and ICH have endorsed leveraging technology and using more centralized monitoring practices to establish quality in a more cost-efficient and effective manner.

Pharmacovigilance

As an IIT sponsor, the sponsor–investigator also has responsibility for safety oversight of the trial. Reporting requirements for serious adverse events (SAEs) or other events of clinical interest should be incorporated into the protocol based on relevant regulations. This includes requirements to report to an IRB/institutional ethics committee (IEC), and the FDA if the trial is conducted under an IND or investigational device exemption (IDE). The reporting requirements, in particular the reporting timeframe, require assessment of the relationship of the event to the study drug/device and assessment of whether the event was expected based on the data available in the Investigator's Brochure (IB) or other product information. If a drug or device is being provided for use in the study by the drug/device manufacturer, the manufacturer typically has its own reporting requirements to follow as well. In addition to reporting to the drug/device manufacturer, IRB/IEC, and FDA, the IIT sponsor also has an obligation to report relevant safety information to participating sites in a multicenter trial. As the safety of clinical trial participants is always a top priority, proper pharmacovigilance is an important part of any IIT.

MULTICENTER STUDIES

A multicenter trial is defined in ICH E6 as, "A clinical trial conducted according to a single protocol but at more than one site, and, therefore, carried out by more than one investigator." Pharmaceutical sponsored studies are almost universally multicenter as they often have the resources and expertise available to coordinate a study at multiple investigator sites. However, coordinating a single protocol at multiple sites is complicated, time-consuming, and expensive. In the pharmaceutical sponsored trial arena, often the oversight of coordinating a multicenter trial is facilitated by a contract research organization (CRO), defined by ICH E6 as "A person or an organization (commercial, academic, or other) contracted by the sponsor to perform one or more of a sponsor's trial-related duties and functions."

In an IIT, these obligations may be held by the sponsor–investigator, sometimes referred to as the coordinating investigator.

Selecting Sites/Investigators (1,6)

Selecting qualified and committed investigators to participate is one of the first obligations of the coordinating investigator. Usually, the protocol and an up-to-date IB should be provided and sufficient time given for the investigator/institution to review the protocol and the information provided. Selection of a site/investigator should be documented appropriately with the site agreeing to abide by the protocol.

Subsite Clinical Trial Agreements

The sponsor–investigator, having contracted with a supporting entity (pharma, biotech, etc.), which provides study drug and/or funds for the conduct of a clinical trial, may identify potential subsite medical institutions. The sponsor–investigator (or their institution) is responsible for negotiating, executing, and/or administering contracts with the subsite governing their conduct of the clinical trial subject to all terms and conditions of primary study contract, to the extent defined and passed through in the subsite agreement. The clinical trial would be of mutual interest and benefit to the subsite and the sponsor–investigator, furthering the institutional and research objectives of subsite as well as the conduct of the clinical trial by the sponsor–investigator.

Sponsor Obligations in Multicenter Trials

The sponsor–investigator must oversee the trial at all participating sites, including the following, as per ICH E6:

1. 5.23.1 All investigators conduct the trial in strict compliance with the protocol agreed to by the sponsor and, if required, by the regulatory authority(ies), and given approval/favorable opinion by the IRB/IEC.
2. 5.23.2 The CRFs are designed to capture the required data at all multicenter trial sites. For those investigators who are collecting additional data, supplemental CRFs should also be provided that are designed to capture the additional data.
3. 5.23.3 The responsibilities of the coordinating investigator(s) and the other participating investigators are documented prior to the start of the trial.
4. 5.23.4 All investigators are given instructions on following the protocol, on complying with a uniform set of standards for the assessment of clinical and laboratory findings, and on completing the CRFs.
5. 5.23.5 Communication between investigators is facilitated.

Maintaining Communication in Multicenter Studies

One of the most important factors in multicenter trial success is open and direct communication among all investigators and sites. Facilitating conference calls where real clinical trial data and information is shared with all investigators and research staff is critical. For high/medium risk phase I studies, these calls should occur weekly while a less frequent occurrence is reasonable for a lower risk phase I or phase II study. Minutes and actions from the calls should be recorded and filed with all sites.

CONCLUSION

IITs are an important component of drug development as they address critical research questions beyond the scope of an industry-sponsored trial's ultimate objective of regulatory approval. While an industry partner may still provide drug product or financial assistance to operate an IIT, it is left to the investigator to successfully manage the study's unique legal, regulatory, data, budgetary, oversight, and scientific needs. This requires considerable planning and organization and, importantly, teamwork. The CFR outlines procedures and requirements governing the use of INDs while local institutional SOPs further define best practices for planning, conducting, and completing IITs.

REFERENCES

1. Electronic Code of Federal Regulations. Title 21: Food and drugs. Part 312—Investigational new drug application. Food and Drug Administration 2017. https://www.ecfr.gov/cgi-bin/text-idx?SID=80e3d2c53a55113d58899e5a13ee36b8&mc=true&node=pt21.5.312&rgn=div5
2. Electronic Code of Federal Regulations. Title 21: Food and Drugs. Part 812—Investigational device exemptions. Food and drug administration 2017. https://www.ecfr.gov/cgi-bin/text-idx?SID=efbd1f0c3094d632f0775d3e120d2e01&mc=true&node=pt21.8.812&rgn=div5
3. Code of Federal Regulations. Title 45: Public welfare. Part 46—Protection of human subjects. Department of Health and Human Services 2017. https://www.hhs.gov/ohrp/regulations-and-policy/regulations/45-cfr-46/index.html
4. Final NIH Policy on the Use of a Single Institutional Review Board for Multi-Site Research: National Institutes of Health 2017. https://grants.nih.gov/grants/guide/notice-files/NOT-OD-16-094.html
5. Good Clinical Data Management Practices. Society for Clinical Data Management. October 2013. https://www.scdm.org/publications/gcdmp/
6. Guidance for Industry. E6 Good Clinical Practice: Consolidated Guidance. International Conference for Harmonisation. FDA. April 1996. https://www.fda.gov/downloads/drugs/guidances/ucm073122.pdf

6

Writing a Consent Form

Christine Grady

Informed consent is an important component of ethical clinical research. Planning for informed consent involves decisions about (a) what information to provide to potential participants or their legally authorized representatives (LARs), both in writing and in discussions; (b) how the information will be presented; (c) how participant capacity to consent and understanding will be considered; and (d) how to obtain the participant's signature.

PURPOSE AND RATIONALE FOR INFORMED CONSENT

Informed consent is a legal, regulatory, and ethical requirement for most clinical research and is widely accepted as an integral part of the ethical conduct of clinical research (1). Current requirements for informed consent owe much to the legal system, but the underlying values are deeply culturally embedded. Fundamentally, informed consent is based on the ethical principle of respect for persons (2). This principle recognizes and compels us to respect an individual's right and capacity to determine his or her own life goals and make autonomous choices consistent with those goals. Informed consent is integral to clinical practice, in that patients are given information about the nature, consequences, benefits, risks, and alternatives of a treatment to help them decide whether to accept the treatment (3). Similarly, informed consent in clinical research is a process by which we enable individuals considering research to exercise their right to autonomous choice about whether or not to participate or continue to participate in the research.

Existing research ethics guidelines (4–7), laws, and federal regulations governing clinical research, including the Food and Drug Administration (FDA) regulations and the Common Rule (8,9) emphasize the need

for the voluntary and informed consent of research participants. For example, the 2013 version of the World Medical Association's Declaration of Helsinki states:

> Participation by individuals capable of giving informed consent as subjects in medical research must be voluntary.
> . . . each potential subject must be adequately informed of the aims, methods, sources of funding, any possible conflicts of interest, institutional affiliations of the researcher, the anticipated benefits and potential risks of the study and the discomfort it may entail, post-study provisions and any other relevant aspects of the study. The potential subject must be informed of the right to refuse to participate in the study or to withdraw consent to participate at any time without reprisal. Special attention should be given to the specific information needs of individual potential subjects as well as to the methods used to deliver the information. . . . After ensuring that the potential subject has understood the information, the physician or another appropriately qualified individual must then seek the potential subject's freely-given informed consent, preferably in writing. (10)

The process of informed consent is generally understood to include: (a) **disclosure** of relevant information about the research to prospective participants who have the capacity to consent or to their LARs; (b) their **understanding** of the information and appreciation of what it means for them; (c) their **voluntary agreement to participate**; and (d) their **authorization** (11). By regulation, an institutional review board (IRB) or research ethics committee (REC) reviews and approves the proposed process for obtaining research informed consent as well as the written information to be given to prospective participants before participants are approached. The usual process of informed decision making by potential

The views expressed here are those of the author and do not necessarily reflect those of the Clinical Center, the National Institutes of Health, or the Department of Health and Human Services.

research participants about whether or not to enroll in a study follows discussion of relevant information about the research study with the principal investigator (PI) and other members of the research team, as well as reading and signing a written consent document. Participants should be given sufficient time to read the consent information and consider the decision and should be encouraged to ask questions before being asked to sign the consent document. After the consent form is signed, ongoing discussion and education of participants appropriate to the nature, type, and duration of the study should continue. The participant retains the right to change his or her mind and withdraw consent for participation at any time without penalty.

THE WRITTEN CONSENT DOCUMENT

Early in the research process and well before any potential participants are approached, the investigator prepares a written consent document for review and approval by the IRB(s). Advertisements, fliers, or brochures that are prepared to recruit and inform potential participants about a study are considered part of informed consent and also require review and approval by an IRB. Traditionally, informed consent documents have been paper, but in recent years there has been a growth in the use of electronic versions of consent (e-consent) (12).

The consent document (whether paper or electronic) aims to summarize information about the study that a reasonable person would want to know to make an informed decision about whether or not to participate in research, including that it is research, an explanation of the research procedures, related risks and possible benefits, alternatives to participation, and research participant rights. Federal regulations at 45 CFR 46.116 and 21 CFR 50.25 (listed in Table 6.1) (13-15) specify the informational elements that should be included in consent documents for clinical research (16,17). The consent document should clearly state that participation in research is voluntary and should not include any language waiving or appearing to waive participants' rights. Revisions to the Common Rule, effective in 2018, require that the informed consent document "...begin with a concise and focused presentation of the key information...organized in a way that facilitates prospective participant understanding of why one might or might not want to participate,".. and that is not "...merely lists of isolated facts" (45 CFR.46 (a)(5) (ii)).

Written consent information can be used to guide discussion between the potential participant and the investigator or research team. Participants may find the consent document helpful to their enrollment decisions by using the written information to understand what the study is about and what is required of them and by using it as a tool when discussing possible study participation decisions with their family, friends, or healthcare providers. Participants may also refer to the written consent information throughout their study participation. Regulations require participants under most circumstances to sign the consent form to indicate that they have agreed to participate in the study. Electronic signatures are also acceptable under FDA regulations (18). According to both the Common Rule and FDA regulations, "A copy shall be given to the person signing the form" (19,20).

Consent information for clinical research should be written clearly with the goal of promoting informed decision making by participants. Both the content and format of the consent document are important to making it readable and understandable. Plain language guidelines offer clear instructions for writing in an understandable manner (21). The National Cancer Institute (NCI) has convened several informed consent working groups who have developed guidance on plain writing (Table 6.2) (22,23), oncology trial consent templates, and sample consent language for investigators as they are preparing consent forms for their cancer studies (24).

To promote understanding, consent information should be written so that it could be understood by the proposed participant population and is consistent with their educational level, familiarity with research, language, and cultural views. Since most people are less familiar with scientific and cancer language than investigators are, investigators should strive to write consent documents in plain language, and ". . . as non-technical as practical" (25).

Consent documents should be clear and concise, and use active voice, short sentences, and uncomplicated words. Language should be simple and direct but not simplistic and patronizing (26). Straightforward descriptions of what participants need to know about a study and devoid of scientific jargon are important for potential participants who are already coping with the stresses of cancer and treatment decisions. U.S. guidelines suggest that documents be written at the eighth-grade reading level (27). Approximately 44% of U.S. adults read at the basic or below basic level (28). Online readability programs, such as Flesch–Kincaid, Flesch Index, Fog Index, and Smog Grading, among others are available to assess reading level (29). Yet, despite such recommendations, data show that research consent forms are often lengthy, complex, and written at or above the 12th-grade level (30). Substituting scientific or medical terms with words more familiar to the nonscientist can be very helpful. Using charts, pictures, flowcharts, or graphics in addition to text may further facilitate understanding (31).

Readability and understandability are also influenced by consent document format. Information should be arranged logically and should be easy to follow. Paper documents that use text in small font, single spaced text, or large chunks of text are difficult to read. Documents that balance words with graphics and white space are

TABLE 6.1   Information to Be Included in the Consent Document

1. A statement that the study involves research
2. An explanation of the purpose of the research, an invitation to participate and explanation of why the subject was selected, and the expected duration of the subject's participation
3. A description of procedures to be followed and identification of which procedures are investigational and which might be provided as standard care to the subject in another setting
4. Explanation of research methods such as randomization, placebo controls, dose escalation
5. A description of any foreseeable risks or discomforts to the subject, an estimate of their likelihood, and a description of what steps will be taken to prevent or minimize them; as well as acknowledgment of potentially unforeseeable risks
6. A description of any benefits to the subject or to others that may reasonably be expected from the research, and an estimate of their likelihood
7. A disclosure of any appropriate alternative procedures or courses of treatment that might be advantageous to the subject
8. A statement describing to what extent records will be kept confidential, including examples of who may have access to research records such as hospital personnel, the FDA, and drug sponsors
9. For research involving more than minimal risk, an explanation and description of any compensation and any medical treatments that are available if subjects are injured through participation; where further information can be obtained, and whom to contact in the event of research-related injury
10. An explanation of whom to contact for answers to questions about the research and the research subject's rights (including the name and phone number of the PI)
11. A statement that research is voluntary and that refusal to participate or a decision to withdraw at any time will involve no penalty or loss of benefits to which the subject is otherwise entitled
12. A statement indicating that the subject is making a decision whether or not to participate, and that his or her signature indicates that he or she has decided to participate having read and discussed the information presented
13. (effective January 2018). A statement for any research involving collection of identifiable private information or biospecimens, that identifiers will be removed and the information or biospecimens will be shared and used for future research OR that they will not be used for future research

When appropriate, or when required by the IRB, one or more of the following elements of information will also be included in the consent document:

1. If the subject is or may become pregnant, a statement that the particular treatment or procedure may involve risks, foreseeable or currently unforeseeable, to the subject, or to the embryo or fetus
2. A description of circumstances in which the subject's participation may be terminated by the investigator without the subject's consent
3. Any costs to the subject that may result from participation in the research
4. The possible consequences of a subject's decision to withdraw from the research and procedures for orderly termination of participation
5. A statement that the PI will notify subjects of any significant new findings developed during the course of the study that may affect them and influence their willingness to continue participation
6. The approximate number of subjects involved in the study
7. The plan for follow-up or access to an intervention proven effective through the research
8. (effective January 2018) A statement that biospecimens may be used for commercial profit, and whether subjects will or will not share in this profit
9. Statement whether clinically relevant research results, including individual research results, will be disclosed and under what conditions
10. Statement about whether research with biospecimens might include whole genome sequencing §__.116(c)(7)–(9)

FDA, Food and Drug Administration; IRB, institutional review board; PI, principal investigator.
Source: Adapted from 45 CFR 46.116; 21 CFR 50.25; ICH-GCP E6, 4.8.10.

more readable. Electronic documents are more likely to be read if they are short and engaging. The use of headings in the consent document can help investigators and the IRBs ensure that all the regulatory-required elements are included and communicated to the participants. Headings can also promote comprehension and readability. The NCI template uses questions for headings. In this format, the headings take a conversational tone, such as *Why is this research being done?* Headings can also be in the form of statements, such as *The purpose of this study* (32).

The written consent document and any other written information provided to participants should be updated when new information becomes available that might be relevant to the participant's consent or his or her willingness to continue in a study. An IRB/REC reviews and approves revisions to the written consent information before it is provided to research participants.

TABLE 6.2 Tips for Easy-to-Read Informed Consent Documents

Text
- Words familiar to the reader; clearly defined scientific, medical, or legal words
- No abbreviations and acronyms
- Consistent words and terminology throughout the document
- Short, simple, and direct sentences
- Short paragraphs that convey one idea per paragraph
- Active voice verbs, personal pronouns
- Clear and logically sequenced ideas
- Important points highlighted by underlining, bold, or separating into boxes
- Simple titles, subtitles, and other headers
- Balance of white space with words and graphics
- Left margins are justified; right margins are ragged
- Font of 12 points or higher, and use of both upper and lower case letters
- Readability analysis (should be ≤eighth-grade reading level)

Graphics
- Easy to understand to explain the text
- Meaningful to the audience, culturally appropriate
- Appropriately located
- Simple and uncluttered
- Visuals with one message and captions
- Cues, such as circles or arrows, to point out key information
- Appealing colors

Source: From Plain Language. Improving communication from the federal government to the public. http://www.plainlanguage.gov/howto/guidelines/FederalPLGuidelines/TOC.cfm; NCI Simplification of Informed Consent Documents, http://www.cancer.gov/clinicaltrials/understanding/simplification-of-informed-consent-docs/page1

Valid informed consent assumes that the participant has a substantial understanding of the nature of the study, the benefits, risks, and alternatives to participating, and the fact that participation is voluntary. Unfortunately, participants do not always understand information that might be relevant to an informed decision about participation. Although research has shown that the majority of research participants report satisfaction with the process of informed consent, understanding of important aspects of the studies in which they are participating is variable at best (33–37).

The National Cancer Institute Informed Consent Working Groups and Templates

Several groups, including the Association of American Medical Colleges, the NCI, and others, have introduced initiatives to improve research consent forms recognizing that consent documents for clinical research are long, complicated, and difficult to understand, and becoming longer, more difficult, more legalistic, and therefore less likely to be read or comprehended by potential research participants (37–40).

The NCI, in collaboration with the FDA and the U.S. Office of Human Research Protections, convened an informed consent working group of multidisciplinary experts in the late 1990s. The initial NCI group offered specific "Recommendations for the Development of Informed Consent Documents for Cancer Clinical Trials" (40), and released a consent form template for cancer treatment trials. Subsequent working groups have modified and expanded these templates. NCI informed consent templates include all the elements of consent required by the federal regulations, and ". . . recognize the significant differences between various types of trials and provide phase-specific examples of recommended consent form language" (see examples in Table 6.3). Templates include instructions about consent form length and format and advise that "In all cases, consent form authors should use simple language and be concise" (40). NCI templates offer sample language and recommend that the lay language and the format be followed as closely as possible when applying it to a specific study. These templates are available at the Cancer Therapy Evaluation Program (CTEP) website (40).

With respect to risks and side effects, for example, NCI recommendations suggest including language such as the following, and then tables of side effects categorized by severity and frequency.

The *(specify type of study intervention, such as surgery, radiation therapy, drugs, etc.)* used in this study may affect how different parts of your body work such as your liver, kidneys, heart, and blood. The study doctor will be testing your blood and will let you know if changes occur that may affect your health.

There is also a risk that you could have side effects from the study drug(s)/study approach.

Here are important points about side effects:

- The study doctors do not know who will or will not have side effects.
- Some side effects may go away soon, some may last a long time, or some may never go away.
- Some side effects may interfere with your ability to have children.
- Some side effects may be serious and may even result in death.

Here are important points about how you and the study doctor can make side effects less of a problem:

- Tell the study doctor if you notice or feel anything different so they can see if you are having a side effect.
- The study doctor may be able to treat some side effects.

TABLE 6.3 NCI Template Sample Consent Wording for Clinical Trials

---

Why is this study being done?

Text Example: Phase 2 or 3 Randomized Chemoprevention Studies

The purpose of this study is to compare the safety and effects of *(insert name of drug or agent)* with *(insert name of currently used drug or placebo)* on people and their risk of *(insert type)* cancer. In this study, you will get either *(insert name of drug/agent)* or placebo, a *(insert appropriate description for the placebo, e.g., pill/liquid)* that looks like the study drug but contains no medication. To be better, the study drug should increase life by 1 year or more compared to the usual approach. There will be about *(insert number)* people taking part in this study.

Text Example: Phase 1 Dose Escalation Studies

The purpose of this study is to test the safety of a study drug called *(insert name of research drug, e.g., TST1234)*. This drug has been tested in animals but not yet in people. This study tests different doses of the drug to see which dose is safer in people. There will be about *(insert number)* people taking part in this study.

Text Example: Phase 1 Novel Route/Combination Studies

This study uses a combination of drugs *(insert names of drugs, e.g., carboplatin and paclitaxel)* that have already been FDA-approved to be given by vein. The purpose of this study is to test whether giving one of the drugs *(insert name of drug, e.g., carboplatin)* through the belly along with the other drug *(insert name of drug, e.g., paclitaxel)* by vein is safe. There will be about *(insert number)* people taking part in this study.

Text Example: Phase 2 Nonrandomized Studies

The purpose of this study is to test any good and bad effects of the study drug called *(insert name of drug, e.g., bevacizumab)*. *(Insert name of drug(s) or investigational approach)* could shrink your cancer but it could also cause side effects. Researchers hope to learn if the study drug will shrink the cancer by at least one quarter compared to its present size. *(The following sentence should be included as appropriate). (Insert name of drug(s))* has already been FDA-approved to treat other cancers. *(The following sentence should be included only if the agent has not shown evidence of activity in humans).* It has not been tested in *(insert type of cancer, e.g., rectal)* cancer, but has shrunk several types of tumors in animals. There will be about *(insert number)* people taking part in this study.

Text Example: Phase 2 or 3 Randomized Studies

The purpose of this study is to compare any good and bad effects of using a *(specific drug, surgery, or radiation approach)* *along with* the usual *chemotherapy*, surgery, or radiation therapy to using the usual chemotherapy, surgery, or radiation approach alone. The addition of *(insert name of drug(s) or investigational approach)* to the usual *(chemotherapy, surgery, or radiation)* could shrink your cancer/prevent it from returning *(as appropriate)* but it could also cause side effects. This study will allow the researchers to know whether this different approach is better, the same, or worse than the usual approach. To be better, the study drug(s)/study approach should increase life by 6 months or more compared to the usual approach *(select other study primary endpoints as appropriate). (The following sentence should be included if appropriate).* This chemotherapy drug, *(insert name of drug, e.g., docetaxel)*, is already FDA-approved for use in *(insert type of cancer, e.g., prostate)* cancer but is usually not used until *(e.g., hormone drug)* stops working. There will be about *(insert number)* people taking part in this study.

- The study doctor may adjust the study drugs to try to reduce side effects.

The following tables show the most common and the most serious side effects that researchers know about. There might be other side effects that researchers do not yet know about. If important new side effects are found, the study doctor will discuss these with you. (40)

NCI recommends categorizing and describing in tables the study-related risks and side effects according to their likelihood and severity in the following categories: (a) Common, some may be serious; (b) Occasional, some may be serious; (c) Rare, and serious; (d) Serious; and (e) Possible, some may be serious. (Table 6.4). The

CTEP website also includes examples of tables that could be used for particular drugs or regimens (40).

Exceptions to the Requirement for Written Informed Consent

Written informed consent signed by the research participant is required by the FDA regulations and the International Council for Harmonisation Good Clinical Practice (ICH-GCP) Tripartite guide (41,42). Written informed consent is also required, with clearly defined exceptions, by the Common Rule ". . . informed consent shall be documented by the use of a written consent form approved by the IRB and signed by the subject or the subject's legally authorized representative" (43).

TABLE 6.4 NCI Template Instructions on Presenting Side Effects in Consent Forms

---

Notes to consent form authors on how to present possible side effects

1. Side effects of study group(s):
   a. For single-arm studies, list all possible side effects of the study drugs according to the recommendations given in 2 to 6 in the following.
   b. For multiple-arm studies with a control, the Table(s) of Possible Side Effects for the control arm should appear first and be followed by the Tables of Possible Side Effects for the drugs/agents used in the experimental arm(s).
   c. If the experimental arm consists of the usual treatment drugs/regimens (the control arm) plus experimental agent(s)/drug(s), the Table of Possible Side Effects for the usual treatment should not be repeated. The following statement should appear before the Table of Possible Side Effects for the investigational drugs/agents: "In addition to side effects outlined above for Group 1 and Group 2, people in this study who are in Group 2 may also experience the possible side effects of (insert name of research drug) listed below."
2. Side effects of procedures:
   a. When describing risks for procedures, describe risks only for procedures that are beyond what would be considered as occurring during the usual treatment approach. The determination of deeming a procedure as part or not part of the usual treatment approach is left to the discretion of the investigator.
   b. Examples of procedures that are not part of the usual treatment approach could include an unusually large amount of blood to be drawn for PK, central line placement to administer the investigational agent, research biopsy, etc.
3. Side effects of supportive drugs named in the consent form:
   a. Nonexperimental supportive drugs need not have their side effects listed unless the treatment they support is the research question tested in the study. For example, side effects of Bactrim need not be listed when transplant is part of a study unless transplant is the actual study question in the trial.
4. Side effects of classes of medications:
   a. If general classes of approved medications, such as a hormonal therapy or antiemetics—where no specific drug is named—are required by the protocol, these do not need to be listed, nor their possible side effects included, in the consent form.
5. Extremely specific possible side effects that are not perceived by the study participant, such as minor changes in lab values, should not be included in the consent form. Lab value changes that could be perceived by the study participant, or could be indicative of harm, should be listed, for example, the phrase "you could have liver damage," would be much more understandable to the study participant than "you could have elevated liver enzymes" or "you could have an elevation in (such-and-such lab value)."
6. Definitions of frequency categories:
   a. "Common, some may be serious"—There is no standard definition of the frequency of risks included in this category; however, as a guideline, "Common, some may be serious" can be viewed as occurring in greater than 20% and up to 100% of patients receiving the drug/agent.
   b. "Occasional, some may be serious"—There is no standard definition of the frequency of risks included in this category; however, as a guideline, "Occasional, some may be serious" can be viewed as occurring between 4% and 20% of patients.
   c. "Rare, and serious"—Side effects that occur in less than 3% of patients do not have to be listed unless they are serious, in which case they should appear in the "Rare, and serious" category. This categorization will need to be modified for prevention studies.
   d. "Serious" is defined as side effects that may require hospitalization or may be irreversible, long term, or life-threatening.
   e. "Possible, some may be serious"—This is a unique frequency category and may be used, when appropriate, for informing study participants of possible side effects related to IND agents for which the frequency of individual side effects has not yet been determined.

IND, investigational new drug; PK, pharmacokinetics.

The federal Common Rule, however, allows the IRB under certain specified circumstances to approve changes to some of the required elements of informed consent, or allow a waiver of informed consent or of the need to document consent. In order to waive or alter the requirement for, or some of, the elements of informed consent, the IRB must determine that (a) the research involves no more than minimal risk to participants, (b) waiving or changing the requirements will not adversely affect the rights and welfare of subjects, (c) the research could not practicably be carried out without the waiver, and (d) when appropriate, additional information will be given to participants at the conclusion of the study (44). The revised Common Rule added a 4th criteria for waiver of informed consent that says that for research involving identifiable private information or identifiable biospecimens, the research could not practicably be carried out without using them in an identifiable format. Importantly, FDA does not have a similar regulatory option for a waiver and requires written informed consent in all studies testing drugs, biologics, or devices under an investigational new drug (IND) or investigational device exemption (IDE). The FDA only allows a waiver of informed consent under a specific exception for emergency research (45).

Federal regulations usually require that investigators document informed consent using a written consent form that is approved by an IRB and signed by the participant or an LAR, except in limited circumstances delineated in the regulations. Both the Common Rule and the FDA regulations allow the use of a short written consent form that does not include all the detailed information usually found in a written consent form if complemented by oral presentation of relevant study information and approved by an IRB (46,47). According to the regulations, the IRB must approve a summary of what is to be included in the oral presentation, there must be a witness to the oral presentation, and the participant or LAR must sign the short form for the record (47). This process can be useful, for example, when a prospective participant cannot read or is blind or when the consent form is written in a language that the prospective participant cannot read. In the latter case, a qualified interpreter conversant in the language of the participant works with the investigator to explain information about the study to the participant and answer questions, and a short form is used to document that the participant consented. Some institutions, such as the intramural National Institutes of Health (NIH), have created short consent forms in multiple languages to be used along with a detailed explanation of the particulars of the study through an interpreter. When an investigator anticipates enrolling a non-English speaking population, consent information should be translated into the appropriate languages.

When the prospective research participant or LAR is unable to read, the ICH-GCP recommends a witnessed process of providing oral information to the participant, including reading and explaining to the participant the information in the written consent form or other written documents. The participant should then give an oral indication of agreement to participation, and, if capable, should sign and date the consent form. In these cases, a witness—who is independent of the participant and the research team—should also sign and date the consent form, attesting that the information in the written documents was accurately explained to the participant, and that informed consent was freely given (48).

The Common Rule also allows a waiver of the requirement for documentation by a signed consent form if the IRB determines that: (a) there is a risk from a breach of confidentiality and the only link between the subject and the research would be the consent document; (b) the research is minimal risk and involves no procedures that normally require written consent outside of research or, (c) if the subjects or LAR are members of a group or community in which signing is not a norm, the research is minimal risk, and there is an alternative method of documenting consent (49).

CONCLUSION

Informed consent, a central ethical requirement for most clinical research, is a process that includes disclosing study information to potential participants so that they can make informed and voluntary choices about participating or continuing to participate in a cancer research study. Study information is usually disclosed to participants both in written paper or electronic consent documents and through discussions with the investigator and research team. Investigators should strive to write consent information in a way that facilitates understanding among participants, that is, in simple language, with information relevant to participant decisions and required by regulations, and using a coherent and reader-friendly format. Simplifying writing, avoiding scientific jargon, using charts and graphics, and employing template language with appropriate study-specific modifications is likely to result in better consent documents and better informed research participants.

REFERENCES

1. Emanuel E, Wendler D, Grady C. What makes clinical research ethical? *J Am Med Assoc.* 2000;283(20):2701–2711.
2. National Commission for the Protection of Human Subjects of Biomedical and Behavioral Research. *The Belmont Report: Ethical Principles and Guidelines for the Protection of Human Subjects of Research.* Washington, DC, U.S. Government Printing Office; 1979.
3. Berg J, Appelbaum P, Lidz C, Parker L. *Informed Consent.* New York, NY: Oxford University Press; 2001.
4. The Nuremberg Code, 1949. http://wayback.archive-it .org/4657/20150930181802/http://www.hhs.gov/ohrp/ archive/nurcode.html
5. World Medical Association, Declaration of Helsinki, Ethical Principles for Medical Research Involving Human Subjects; October 2013. https://www.wma.net/policies-post/ wma-declaration-of-helsinki-ethical-principles-for-medical -research-involving-human-subjects/
6. Council for International Organizations of Medical Sciences. *International Ethical Guidelines for Biomedical Research Involving Human Subjects.* Geneva, CIOMS/WHO, 2002. Soon to be replaced by the 2016 *International Ethical Guidelines for Health-Related Research involving Human Subjects.* https://cioms.ch/wp-content/uploads/2017/01/WEB -CIOMS-EthicalGuidelines.pdf
7. International Conference for Harmonisation (ICH) Harmonised Tripartite Guideline, Guideline for Good Clinical Practice, E6 (R1) June 1996, and Integrated Addendum (R2) November 2016. http://www.ich.org/products/guidelines/ efficacy/article/efficacy-guidelines.html#6-2
8. U.S. Code of Federal Regulations Title 21, Part 50. (21CFR50) "Protection of Human Subjects." http://www.accessdata.fda .gov/scripts/cdrh/cfdocs/cfcfr/cfrsearch.cfm?fr=50.20
9. U.S. Code of Federal Regulations Title 45, Part 46. (45CFR.46). http://www.hhs.gov/ohrp/regulations-and-policy/regulations/ 45-cfr-46/index.html

10. World Medical Association, supra #5
11. Beauchamp T, Childress J. *Principles of Biomedical Ethics*, 5th ed. New York, NY: Oxford University Press; 2001.
12. U.S. Office of Human Research Protections and U.S. FDA. Use of Electronic Informed Consent: Questions and Answers Guidance for Institutional Review Boards, Investigators, and Sponsors, 2016. http://www.fda.gov/downloads/drugs/guidancecomplianceregulatoryinformation/guidances/ucm436811.pdf
13. 45CFR.46.116
14. 21CFR50.25
15. ICH-GCP E6, 4.8.10
16. 45CFR §46.117
17. 21CFR §50.25
18. US FDA Part 11, Electronic Records; Electronic Signatures—Scope and Application. http://www.fda.gov/regulatoryinformation/guidances/ucm125067.htm
19. 45CFR §46.117
20. 21CFR §50.25
21. Federal Plain language.gov http://www.plainlanguage.gov/howto/guidelines/FederalPLGuidelines/TOC.cfm
22. Plain Language. Improving communication from the federal government to the public. http://www.plainlanguage.gov/howto/guidelines/FederalPLGuidelines/TOC.cfm
23. NCI **Simplification of Informed Consent Documents**, http://www.cancer.gov/clinicaltrials/understanding/simplification-of-informed-consent-docs/page1>
24. Comprehensive Working Group on Informed Consent in Cancer Clinical Trials. Recommendations for the Development of informed consent documents for cancer clinical trials. National Cancer Institute. https://ctep.cancer.gov/protocolDevelopment/informed_consent.htm
25. ICH-GCP. http://www.ich.org/LOB/media/MEDIA482.pdf, item 4.86, page 21, supra #7.
26. Federal Plain language.gov. Clear writing and plain language. http://www.plainlanguage.gov/whatisPL/definitions/wright.cfm
27. Office of Human Subjects Research, National Institutes of Health. SOP #12 Requirements for Informed Consent. https://ohsr.od.nih.gov/ohsr/public/SOP_12_v4_3-8-16.pdf
28. National Center for Education Statistics. National Assessment of Adult Literacy. http://nces.ed.gov/naal/kf_demographics.asp
29. Online Readability tests. https://readability-score.com or http://www.readabilityformulas.com/free-readability-formula-tests.php
30. Paasche-Orlow M, Taylor H, Brancati F. Readability standards for informed consent forms as compared with actual readability. *N Engl J Med*. 2003;348:721–726.
31. Houts P, Doak C, Doak L, Loscalzo M. The role of pictures in improving health communications: a review of research on attention, comprehension, recall, and adherence. *Pat Ed Counseling*. 2006;61(2):173–190.
32. NCI, Supra note #19
33. Jefford M, Mileshkin L, Raunow H, et al. Satisfaction with the decision to participate in cancer clinical trials is high, but understanding is a problem *J Clin Oncol*. 2005;23(suppl 16):6067.
34. Joffe S, Cook E, Cleary P, et al. The quality of informed consent in cancer clinical trials: A cross sectional survey. *The Lancet*. 2001;358:1772–1777.
35. Sharp S. Consent documents for oncology trials: does anybody read these things? *Am J Clin Oncol*. 2004;27:570–575.
36. Mandava A, Pace C, Campbell B, et al. The quality of informed consent: mapping the landscape. A review of empirical data from developing and developed countries. *J Med Ethics*. 2012;38:356–365.
37. Beardsley E, Jefford M, Mileshkin L. Longer consent forms for clinical trials compromise patient understanding: so why are they lengthening? *J Clin Oncol*. 2007;25(9):e13–e14.
38. Jefford M, Moore R. Improvement of informed consent and the quality of consent documents. *Lancet Oncol*. 2008;9:485–493.
39. Association of American Medical Colleges. Universal Use of Short and Readable Informed Consent Documents: How do we get there? https://www.aamc.org/download/75282/data/hdicklermtgsumrpt53007.pdf
40. NCI Cancer Therapy Evaluation Program. Informed Consent. https://ctep.cancer.gov/protocoldevelopment/sideeffects/drugs.htm
41. International Conference on Harmonization- Good Clinical Practice Guidelines. http://www.ich.org/fileadmin/Public_Web_Site/ICH_Products/Guidelines/Efficacy/E6/E6_R1_Guideline.pdf
42. 21CFR §50.23
43. 45CFR §46.117(a)
44. 45CFR §46.116(d)
45. 21CFR §50.24
46. 45CFR §46.117 (b)
47. 21CFR §50.27(b).
48. Copernicus Group. The role of an impartial witness in informed consent. http://www.cgirb.com/irb-insights/the-role-and-use-of-impartial-witnesses-in-the-informed-consent-process
49. 45CFR §46.117(c).

7

Why Do Clinical Trials Fail?

Laurence Collette, Jan Bogaerts, and Xavier Paoletti

INTRODUCTION

Failure is a concept that will shift with perspective. For new pharmaceutical entities for which access to market is sought, failure has the connotation of "not making it." For trials studying important unanswered questions in the medical setting, failure could have a different meaning of "not answering the question to a satisfying degree." There are also other types of failure, with varying degrees of incurred damage. Trial failure may include features such as misleading the community, which is an especially nasty way of failing to answer the question, or failure by lack of quality. In this chapter, we discuss trial failure in various forms and propose some prevention measures to help avoid failure. First, however, we discuss how failure affects different interested stakeholders and what the costs of these types of failure are (Table 7.1).

Admittedly this table is a messy undertaking, but we feel it can be an interesting model to discuss the outcomes of various types of failure. To a large extent, the stakes of various parties (the patients in the study, population with the disease, medical community, public health system, and investors in the pharmaceutical industry) are the same. We all want safe and effective treatments to be available in as brief a time as possible to correctly selected patients for a reasonable price. What we have tried to highlight in the table are some of the differential outcomes of failure types with regards to stakeholder groups, magnifying them beyond the background of the common good. The reader may come up with their own interpretation of the entries in this table. We wanted to make it available as a model of thinking about failure.

The following examples illustrate our proposed use of the table:

- If a trial never enrolled any patients, this may mean the question was not applicable; the patient population did not sustain any effect from that failure, but the scientific community and the financers of that trial certainly lost from it. Even the patients indirectly suffered because the community set up to research the question was spending efforts on the wrong question.
- Erroneous conclusions from a trial may actually benefit the financial investor, while setting up patients with a suboptimal treatment, leading the scientific community astray, and not providing best value for money for the health system.
- Drawing conclusions too early from an ongoing trial (stopping the trial) may lead to vastly different outcomes, ranging from early acceptance of a good drug (where everybody benefits) to the whole community being stuck with inconclusive data, while being unable to repeat the experiment.
- Another failure type that deserves highlighting is the case where the research was good, but nothing happened with the conclusions. The world has experienced this in the past 65 years, with the very slow implementation of antismoking policies after the proof that smoking leads to lung cancer in 1950 (1).

The following sections further discuss several types of failure with illustrative examples and make recommendations to help avoid them.

FAILURE RESULTING FROM LACK OF RECRUITMENT

By far the most common reference to "trial failure" is when a trial cannot recruit the number of patients needed to test the hypothesis that it was designed to test. We detail in this section several circumstances that may lead to difficulties in completing accrual to (mostly randomized) studies.

Failure Because the Randomization is Too Challenging for the Patients

Trials that were designed to address clinical questions of extreme interest for the medical community

TABLE 7.1 Taxonomy of Trial Failure

Failure Type*	Cost of Failure by Stakeholder[†]			
	Patients (on and off trial)	Scientific Community	Payers/Health System	Industry/Investor
The trial is needed but is never done (or too late, leading to no enrollment)	May be very high	Missing information		
Wrong control arm or controversial control arm	Participation loses benefit Suboptimal treatment	Harder progress	Wrong information	May benefit or lose from this
Wrong end point(s)	Participation loses benefit	May be misled	May be misled or not be convinced	May benefit or lose from this
Wrong timing (too early or too late) Nonexistent or disappearing population (too late) Trial uses wrong assumptions (too early)	No effect Participation loses benefit	Loss of initiative Research field may suffer a lot	No effect Lack of information	Loss of investment Loss of market
Insufficient or misleading upfront biomarker science	Participation loses benefit	Waste of time/ resources	Wrong information	Potential loss of market
Failure to enroll	No effect for nonparticipants Population may lose benefit of learning	Loss of initiative Loss of coherence Failure to convince patients	No information	Loss of investment/ loss of market
Low recruitment but only trial of its kind	Decreased benefit	Can still be very successful	Uncertainty	Unlikely to lead to registration
Impossibility to reach number of events (lack of power)	May miss an effective drug	Some lack of information	Lack of information	May miss a market
Lack of quality (surgery, biomarker work)	Suboptimal treatment	Wrong learning	Lack of correct information	Can obstruct good development
The "negative trial"	No effect	Disappointment	No effect	Loss of investment
Failure to convince When "significant" data do not lead to significant change Phase I does not inform correctly the phase II dose	Can be huge Toxicity, lack of effect	Failure to learn Loss of time	Mission failure	Market failure Loss of time
Convincing—but wrong—conclusions, leading to erroneous development program	Can be huge	Huge loss of time and effort	Wrong information	Loss of time, investment
Poor interim decisions leading to disclosing significant results too early (e.g., on nonfinal end point)	Too optimistic messages, drug on the market may not be good	Wrong drug for use	Suboptimal drug	Highly variable from failure to register to full registration

(continued)

TABLE 7.1 Taxonomy of Trial Failure (*continued*)

Failure Type*	Cost of Failure by Stakeholder†			
	Patients (on and off trial)	Scientific Community	Payers/Health System	Industry/ Investor
Too many questions in one trial		Confusion – difficulty for next developments	Confused information	Loss of time, difficulty to have converging development

*This column is loosely ordered by the time of the failure, from concept to final interpretation.
†This table indicates some possibilities for the various stakeholders but is not exhaustive. The description is necessarily short and must be seen as one of many outcomes.

paradoxically seem to not be exempt of the risk of failure to recruit patients. A striking example is the yet impossible realization of a randomized controlled trial to compare radical prostatectomy with radical radiotherapy for localized prostate cancer. The two therapeutic approaches, which are well established in clinical practice, are regarded as bearing similar long-term oncologic outcome but are associated with different side-effect profiles. Yet the best available evidence to inform head-to-head comparison of these concurrent approaches relies on retrospective, matched case-control studies (2) and a few prospective population cohort studies (3).

Traditionally, studies that compared a same treatment started immediately or deferred to signs of disease progression proved difficult to conduct. One example is the randomized Eastern Cooperative Oncology Group study EST 3886 (4) that aimed to compare immediate versus deferred adjuvant hormonal therapy for patients with positive lymph nodes after radical prostatectomy and lymphadenectomy: 36 institutes in the United States altogether randomized only 98 patients in 1988–1993. The trial was then closed, but it so far remains the sole reliable comparison supporting the current treatment guidelines for this group of patients. Similarly, a European Organization for Research and Treatment of Cancer (EORTC) trial that tested the same questions for patients with positive lymph nodes for whom the radical prostatectomy was abandoned (5), recruited very slowly and was eventually closed after 12 years of recruitment and 234 patients randomized, not reaching its target sample size. Similarly, the intergroup study testing immediate versus deferred chemotherapy after radical cystectomy in patients with pT3–pT4 or N+ M0 urothelial carcinoma of the bladder recruited with difficulty, although it recruited across 12 European countries and Canada (6). In all these examples, lack of enthusiasm resided in good part on the side of the patients, who had strong preference for either being offered treatment shortly after diagnosis or being spared therapy and its side effects for as long as possible. This issue

highlights a particularly difficult area of clinical trial research, where the medical community is considering potential reduction of treatment or a drastic change in treatment a potentially viable option, but finding it difficult to implement the necessary research to obtain proof of the potential significant change in practice. Patients may find it impossible to accept randomization between being treated or not being treated (immediately) or between two different modes of treatment. Indeed, the medical community may not be optimally conducive to such research because of siloing, hospital processes, and habit.

Failure Because the Clinicians Have Conflicting Interests

However, clinician views may also strongly affect trial feasibility. In 2000, the EORTC genitourinary group launched a phase III trial (EORTC 30004) to evaluate if chemoresection with 4 weekly intravesical instillations of mitomycin-C could substitute for the existing practice of transurethral resection (TUR) followed by 1 single immediate instillation of mitomycin-C for solitary low noninvasive bladder cancer. The study aimed for 1,000 patients and was closed after 3 years and several attempts to facilitate recruitment, with only 58 patients recruited from 12 centers. Interestingly, the same group had recruited 512 patients over a period of just 3 years in their former trial in the same indication (7). The EORTC trial failed to recruit despite amendments and surveys at the centers that aimed to broaden entry criteria and facilitate patient access to the trial.

The true reason for the failure ironically is written in the study protocol itself. The introduction ends by the premonitory statement that "The philosophy of this trial, that is to question the value of TUR, will be difficult for urologists who are surgeons by education and profession. However, evidence based EORTC data, quality of life aspects and health economic reasons make this study a unique opportunity to investigate the rationale of ablative intravesical chemotherapy in low risk Ta, T1 bladder cancer." It seems that the perspective that this trial might change practice and reduce the amount of surgical procedures might have hampered the willingness to recruit patients in the study. A similar trial was attempted in the United Kingdom in the mid-2000s and failed the same way. Since then, the multidisciplinary approach made its way to the clinics. Interestingly enough, a new study, called CALIBER (8), was launched in the United Kingdom by the Institute of Cancer Research in January 2015 to address the very question. The study is a randomized, multicenter, phase II feasibility study that aims to recruit 174 patients from approximately 25 UK sites over 3 years. The study is currently open, and it is recruiting slower than expected but is likely to complete with some delay. Although all of the examples covered here relate to urologic oncology, the problem of recruiting patients in studies testing markedly different treatments is not unique to that specialty.

Experience shows that the risk of randomized trials failing increases as the difference in the types of treatment increases, and when this difference becomes too big, the trials are deemed to fail, irrespective of the relevance of the question (Figure 7.1). Everybody would want to know the result of such a trial, but no one is brave enough to do it.

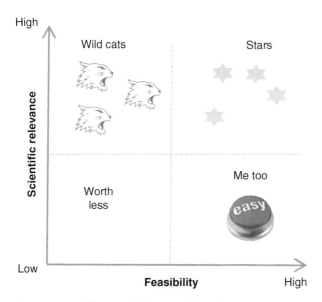

FIGURE 7.1 Clinical trials scientific relevance versus feasibility chart. Studies with great scientific relevance but too extreme difference between arms appear at high risk of failure. The "me too" type of study does not bring huge scientific advances but has low risk of failing due to lack of recruitment. Detailed assessment of trial acceptance to patients, interest of medical specialists involved, practical and financial feasibility in the center, prevalence of the disease of interest, and competing studies is needed to differentiate the "star" from the "wild cat" studies.

Failure Because of Insufficient Coordination Across Departments

A trial may also fail to recruit because of suboptimal coordination between the medical and specialist departments involved in the process of patient selection. Often, this happens because of failure to refer patients from the unit where the disease is diagnosed to that where the patient may be recruited and treated in the study. Restrictions to eligibility, relating to prior treatments, and time allowed after or documentation of diagnostic procedures (imaging, pathology) are likewise likely to hamper recruitment if communication between departments is not perfectly coordinated. Ideally, all departments should be aware of the study protocol and should support it. For example, if credentialing of a radiation technique via dummy run is required prior to activating a center, it is important that the radiation physics department be involved in the decision to contribute to the study so that they include this contribution in their workload. Failure to organize this coordination results in delays of site activation that directly affect study completion timelines.

FAILURE BY EXCESS OF COMPLEXITY

The ongoing study EORTC 22113-LungTech (9) launched by the EORTC radiation oncology group in November 2014 perfectly illustrates the challenges that complex site credentialing and prospective quality assurance represent and how these affect accrual. The study is a single-arm phase II testing image-guided stereotactic body radiotherapy (IG-SBRT) in patients who present with centrally located non–small cell lung tumor 7 cm or less in diameter and are unsuitable or unwilling to undergo surgery. The study is therefore testing a challenging technologically involved potentially curative approach for patients who would otherwise undergo palliative care. The primary measure of effectiveness will be freedom from local progression at 3 years after start of IG-SBRT as assessed by serial computed tomography (CT) scans. To secure patient safety, the protocol requires all centers to perform delineation and radiation treatment planning for benchmark cases and to present valid beam output audit in addition to completing a radiation facility questionnaire. Furthermore, the sites must also be credentialed for the use of their positron emission tomography (PET) scanner, four-dimensional CT, and intensity-modulated radiotherapy techniques via one or more phantoms (Figure 7.2). This is done by means of site visit during which the planning system on the phantom cases is checked.

Figure 7.3 shows the actual and planned recruitment in the study as of November 2016. The vertical blue bars in the figure show that these requirements severely delayed site activation, with less than half of the centers activated at 1 year after study start. In addition,

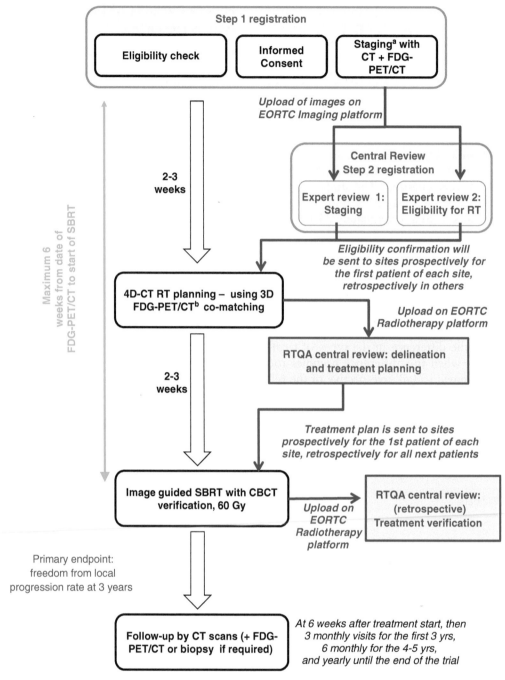

FIGURE 7.2 Trial 22113 LungTech study scheme. The scheme shows the various steps of central review and quality assurance required to recruit a patient in a center that is credentialed. After informed consent, initial radiologic staging and histologic confirmation, the diagnostic images are uploaded on the European Organization for Research and Treatment of Cancer (EORTC) central server. Two independent reviewers confirm patient eligibility. The radiation treatment planning is performed and uploaded on the EORTC central server for prospective radiotherapy (RT) quality assurance (RTQA). Once the plan adequacy is confirmed, the patient is treated. All radiotherapy images are then uploaded on the EORTC central server for retrospective quality assurance. The patient then proceeds to follow-up. CBCT, cone beam computed tomography; NSCLC, non–small cell lung cancer; SBRT, stereotactic body radiotherapy.

*Staging is based on two-dimensional or three-dimensional FDG-PET/CT.

†If the patient consented to participate to the optional translational research, four-dimensional FDG- PET/CT may be used as imaging coregistration.

Source: Modified from Adebahr S, Collette S, Shash E, et al. LungTech, an EORTC phase II trial of Stereotactic Body Radiotherapy for centrally located lung tumours—A clinical perspective. *Br J Radiol*; 88:2015.

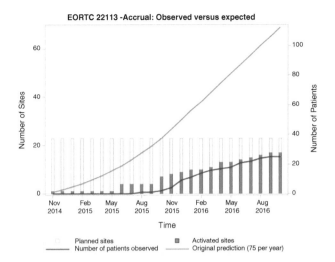

FIGURE 7.3 Site activation and patient recruitment in the European Organization for Research and Treatment of Cancer (EORTC) study LungTech from initiation in November 2014 until November 2016.

several review committees are involved before a patient may be treated (see Figure 7.2). A central review pathology panel confirms histology and a prospective quality assurance program necessitates that centers send their treatment plans for review by an expert committee prior to treating each patient. This results in extreme delay of patient recruitment as shown by the red curve in Figure 7.3. For this type of study, one may either challenge whether all credentialing, quality assurance, and central review procedures are critical to the study and if the tested approach can be translated to the clinical practice. If they are, one may consider adapting study timelines and trial financing.

Missing the Window of Opportunity

Studies may also be abandoned or fail to recruit because they do not come at the right time. For example, studies of ablative chemotherapy in bladder cancer against TUR discussed previously may have been launched too early. Conversely, some studies are launched too late. This may happen when the question addressed by the study becomes irrelevant while the trial is ongoing. An example of this may be when a patient population is redefined on the basis of new knowledge or new diagnostic method, so that the patient group targeted by the study protocol no longer exists as such, or because the study did not collect information about a biomarker that meanwhile has been discovered and strongly affects prognosis and/or response to treatment, such as human papillomavirus status for head and neck cancer. Another example is when the experimental intervention that the study tests is adopted in clinical practice without waiting for clinical trial results—thus in absence of level-1 evidence. Clearly, the likelihood that the study question becomes obsolete increases as the total time

the study takes to be initiated and to complete recruitment increases. Conversely, the recruitment rate usually sharply declines as the study relevance decreases.

The LungART study (10) sponsored by the Gustave Roussy Institute in Villejuif, France, offers an example of such circumstances. LungART is a phase III study that tests if postoperative conformal radiotherapy increases disease-free survival compared with no postoperative radiotherapy in patients with completely resected non–small cell lung cancer and mediastinal nodal (N2) involvement. The study needs 700 patients and was scheduled to take at least 10 years of recruitment when it started in February 2007. However, the study has only recruited 60% of its planned number as of November 2016 and despite intergroup collaboration across Europe, it is expected to complete recruitment only by 2021. Reasons for the slow recruitment are several:

1. A number of studies testing adjuvant immunotherapy for advanced non–small cell lung cancer patients have been launched (e.g., the intergroup study PEARLS in Europe [(11)] and the intergroup study BR31 in Canada [(12)], which are competing partially with the study).
2. A more thorough preoperative staging, including endobronchial ultrasound–guided biopsy and/or mediastinoscopy, reduces the frequency of intraoperative detection of unexpected N2 disease so that the patient population of interest diminishes.
3. Induction chemotherapy is not allowed by the study, thus making a number of patients ineligible.
4. Disappointed by the success rates of upfront surgery and induction chemotherapy with surgery, some centers have reverted to an approach of preoperative radiochemotherapy for their patients with non–small cell lung cancer, thus making them unsuitable for this study.
5. Patient acceptance of the randomization to no adjuvant therapy seems low.

All of these reasons explain why the study is poorly recruiting.

Sometimes, new treatments are adopted in the clinic without formal testing. In most instances, this phenomenon occurs when treatment novelty results from technologic advances, such as intensity-modulated irradiation laparoscopic surgery. Such technologic advances are often a priori regarded as progress. Their implementation requires investment in infrastructure and machines, which once made, results in adoption of the new technique without formal comparative testing.

Clinical interventions do not follow different pathways of diffusion from other innovations. Diffusion of innovation, as modeled by Everett Rogers (13), has five stages: the launch by the (1) innovators followed in successive stages by the (2) early adopters; (3) early majority; (4) late majority; and, finally, (5) laggards (Figure 7.4).

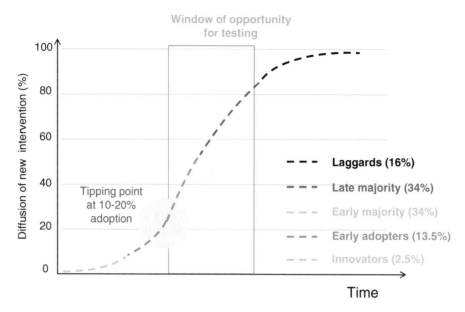

FIGURE 7.4 Adoption of new health interventions, the window of opportunity.

The speed of diffusion accelerates to a peak (the tipping point), which occurs on average at 20% adoption. Studies testing new interventions on a large scale (multicenter, multiregions) are best performed after the technology has been pioneered but before it has been widely adopted. If evaluated too early, the community feels that patient safety and learning curves are insufficiently documented to embark in wide-scale testing. However, once most physicians and centers have adopted the new approach, it is too late because the equipoise required for formal comparative assessment in randomized clinical trials is no longer present. Patients and/or physicians would refuse to enter the study at that time. An objective assessment of the timing of the study with regard to this model of innovation adoption may help launch studies at the right time and maximize success.

How to Make a Study That Completes Within Timelines

No sponsor surely wishes to invest in a trial that will never deliver, and a good share of the clinical trial costs are invested at the time of trial conception and implementation. Therefore, an extensive and objective assessment of the true feasibility of trial recruitment within timelines is essential. Besides evaluation of the relevance and appropriateness of the study design by an independent committee of experts, several steps can be taken prior to starting a clinical trial:

- The use of detailed feasibility questionnaires prior to trial launch is strongly recommended. Such questionnaires must address all aspects of the logistics and patient availability at the centers. Elements that feasibility questionnaires should address are listed

in Table 7.2 and guidance documents and checklists are available online (14).

- Acceptance of the study by patients is not an element to neglect. Success calls for involvement of patient representatives at every stage of a study development. Indeed, patients representatives are most knowledgeable by their experience, of the concerns of patients who will be proposed to participate in a clinical experiment. Their input provides critical highlights on the feasibility of recruitment. The use of patient survey questionnaires or feasibility of randomization studies is encouraged prior to launching the most challenging studies. It is important to highlight that in the setting of a randomized trial, and as part of informed consent, the investigator is tasked with communicating uncertainty to the patient they are treating. The way the logic of the trial is elaborated, preferably with the help of patients, can be very beneficial (or detrimental) to the ultimate success of the trial.

- Financial support to the centers contributing patients and to the various laboratories and committees involved in the study should be sufficient to cover both the real costs required by the study protocol (such as extra diagnostics or extra visits) and to support the time spent by staff to perform the study. This is usually easier for commercial sponsors who can offer financial compensation as well as data management and other administrative support to the centers. For academic sponsors, the impact of limited financial support must not be underestimated. In this case, it is strongly recommended that commitment to perform a study be obtained at the level of the hospital direction, rather than at the level of a hospital department or by an individual investigator, in order to avoid overoptimistic estimates of recruitment potential based on feasibility questionnaires.

TABLE 7.2 Elements to Consider in Assessing Trial Feasibility at the Recruitment Centers

Protocol	
Competing studies	In center or in referring centers.
Prior successful experience conducting studies in same indication	
Number of patients with indication seen in the department	Patient volume should be sufficient to balance hurdles of doing the study.
Practical Feasibility	
Deviation from standard practice	How much does the protocol deviate from standard practice (e.g., schedule of visits, frequency of visits, procedures or examinations)? Does the the protocol require specific organization in the department or center? If the study is blinded, does this affect feasibility?
Equipment required	Availability, adequacy, and cost.
Personnel required	Availability, willingness (e.g., does protocol require special organization after work, weekend work), coordination, and cost of supplementary work covered?
Other departments involved (for referring patients or else)	Do they support the trial? Is multidisciplinary team work in place?
Credentialing requirements (material)	Are credentialing procedures required (eg, radiation, radiation physics, laboratory, imaging) and departments involved informed and willing to perform? Is staffing sufficient to perform within protocol timelines? Are costs covered?
Requirements for central collection or review of samples	Are departments required to send material for central banking informed and willing to contribute? Are costs of the above covered?
Data management	Is it offered by the sponsor? If not, are resources available on site?
Administration	Does sponsor help with (1) regulatory and ethics submissions and (2) translations and other administrative tasks, or is there staff in place?
Training	Does the protocol require specific training? (for medical interventions, for protocol-specific systems [e.g., electronic case report forms]).
Patient Availability	
Acceptability of randomization to patients	Sponsor or site to assess with patients, equipoise, and procedures or frequency of visits or other protocol restrictions difficult for patients to accept.
Benefit-to-risk ratio	Is it balanced? Does risk require specific measures in the center (e.g., for management of side effects)? Are those measures in place?
Eligibility criteria	Do any criteria impede recruitment (constraints on time intervals, nonstandard exams, preexisting conditions)?
Source of patients	Are potential patients seen in the department? In another department (in which case is collaboration set up)? From registry? From screening tests? From general practice? Make sure referral channel is in place.
Estimates of effective numbers likely to enroll Total number that can be screened and screen failure ratio	Pessimistic rather than optimistic figures preferred. Test eligibility criteria on records of former patients. Consider feasibility of recruitment study. Keep screening logs during trial.

(*continued*)

TABLE 7.2 Elements to Consider in Assessing Trial Feasibility at the Recruitment Centers (*continued*)

Study Timelines	
Are study timelines for recruitment realistic?	Report if considered not realistic and why.
Is there support from the department for the whole duration of the study?	Commitment is for several years.
Funding	
Compensation to sites	Is compensation sufficient for the institution to support it? Are additional costs incurred by the site not covered that would jeopardize recruitment?
Additional Considerations	**Indicate any additional considerations that would increase complexity. Indicate any additional considerations of performing the study that would not have been listed previously.**

A study should be launched only if it is financially tenable for the participating institutions and if their commitment to perform the study is high, if patient availability and protocol acceptance to patients are high, and if both of these are sufficiently strong to sustain competition from other studies for the same population in the same institutions (Figure 7.5).

Once the study is ongoing, several measures may be envisaged in case of lack of recruitment.

First, the screening logs at the participating institutions must be carefully reviewed to identify any difficulties with the study. Often, delays imposed between diagnostic examinations and patient registration in a study or too-narrow conditions on some measurable parameters may result in exclusion of patients from the study. If patient safety allows, the study eligibility criteria should be relaxed as much as possible. Next, additional sites or intergroup participation must be envisaged, whenever the recruitment capacity of the centers has been overestimated, if the trial remains scientifically relevant. However, this often necessitates additional finances. Protocol procedures may also be simplified, whenever possible. Finally, an Independent Data Monitoring Committee (IDMC) may be called to review the current risk-benefit balance for patients entering the study. The committee may also confirm if the study scientific merit holds despite the delay. In randomized comparative trials, the implementation of formal interim analyses for futility should be discouraged, unless a substantial part of the planned sample

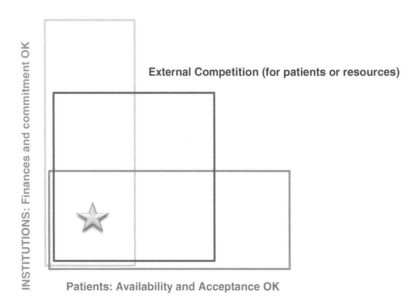

FIGURE 7.5 How to select trials that will not fail by lack of accrual.

is already recruited. Indeed, such interim analyses will further decrease the final study power. It is generally not recommended to conduct them early in the information time, when less than 40% of the planned events have been observed (15).

If the study recruitment remains poor, the trial may never recruit the planned number of patients. In that case, options to make the best use of the data that is already collected or that may become available from the patients already recruited in the study must be envisaged. If only very few patients were entered, a short communication about the data may be the only option. However, if a non-negligible number of patients are available, a revision of the statistical analysis plan may be envisaged in order to define new timelines for data analysis or reset achievable secondary objectives. With time-to-event end points, the number of events needed to test the original trial hypothesis at the desired power level may never be reached. In that case, a statistician, possibly with medical experts who have not seen any interim trial results, should propose a plan for data release. This plan may be for testing the original hypothesis at a reduced power (e.g., 70%). If the numbers are too small for any meaningful power level, then the plan may be based on length of follow-up. Further alternatives consist of redefining a noncomparative phase II–type of objective, either based on a secondary end point or on the primary, such as estimating the rate of the end point at a fixed time point. This way, the study may at least inform the design of future studies.

This approach was used in the intergroup study EORTC 40004-CLOCC (16). The study was launched in 2002 as a phase III study and was designed to compare overall survival (OS) in patients with nonresectable colorectal liver metastases randomly assigned to systemic treatment (the comparator arm) or systemic treatment plus radiofrequency ablation (RFA). The plan was to recruit 390 patients over 3 years and to conduct the analysis at year 6, when 317 patients would have died. In March 2005, it became clear that recruitment remained too low, as only 77 patients had been randomized. Because this was the only trial testing RFA in this setting, the study was formally amended to continue as a noncomparative randomized phase II trial. A Fleming one-stage design was implemented in the combination arm, with OS rate at 30 months as the primary end point. The target sample size was reduced to 142 patients so that another 75 patients were needed to be recruited over an additional 1.5 years. Eventually, the study was closed in June 2007, with only 119 patients recruited from 22 hospitals. The first results were published in 2012 (17) with 4.4 years of median follow-up. Despite the lower number of patients, the study met its primary objective with a 30-month OS rate of 61.7% (95% confidence interval [CI], 48.2–73.9) for the combined treatment group. However, results were in the same range for the systemic treatment group so that OS benefit remained uncertain at the time of that analysis. Follow-up of all patients continued, and an update of the study with 9.9 years of median follow-up was presented in 2015 (18). The data then indicated a significant long-term benefit of combined treatment using RFA over systemic treatment in an exploratory comparative assessment (hazard ratio [HR] = 0.58, 95% CI, 0.38-0.88, p = .010). These results raised enthusiasm in further testing this approach in new trials.

FAILURE IN LATE STAGE: THE PHASE II–TO–PHASE III TRANSITION

In this section we discuss the risky transition from (late) phase II to phase III.

Lack of Understanding of a Drug Mechanism of Action

A number of phase III studies in oncology have failed to meet their primary end point yet have demonstrated marked effects on important secondary end points in all or a subset of the patients. Such results most often lead to controversy in interpretation and as such, often fail to affect clinical practice.

In the mid-1990s, prostate-specific antigen (PSA) appeared to be a promising biomarker for detection and monitoring of progression of prostate cancer. Data also suggested that in patients whose disease no longer responded to hormonal manipulation (castration-resistant prostate cancer or CRPC; the hormone-insensitive refractory setting), a decrease of 50% of the PSA during treatment was associated with OS (19). From that time, phase II trials in this disease setting started using this definition of response as their primary end point. This approached worked well for chemotherapeutic agents. But when the end point was used in a study of 250 patients testing high-dose calcitriol and docetaxel to placebo and docetaxel in CRPC, the study showed no benefit for this end point, but there was a significant benefit in OS (20). It was later understood that this drug effect is not mediated through the same mechanisms as that of cytotoxic agents and that the drug does not lower PSA. The trial end point was thus inadequate to detect effects of this treatment.

Likewise, the first two studies that tested the immunotherapeutic agent sipuleucel-T against placebo in CRPC failed to meet their set primary end point of objective progression-free survival (PFS). In the first trial of 127 patients, the sipuleucel-T group had a significant reduction of the risk of death of 41%, as compared with those in the placebo group (p = .01) (21), whereas the benefit seen in the second study was not statistically significant (22). A further double-blind, placebo-controlled, multicenter trial, called the Immunotherapy for Prostate Adenocarcinoma Treatment (IMPACT) study, involving 512 men with metastatic CRPC, was then conducted. The initial protocol had PFS and OS as coprimary end points. However, learning from the results of the former two studies, it was amended prior to study unblinding, to set OS as the only primary end point. The results confirmed a survival advantage of 4 months with immunotherapy and there was again no effect on disease progression or PSA (23). The US Food and Drug Administration approved sipuleucel-T for the treatment of asymptomatic or minimally symptomatic patients with CRPC in April 2010, recognizing that questions about mechanism of action and combination and sequencing with other agents remained. We now know that immunotherapeutic agents may have delayed effects, the documentation of which require follow-up beyond progression. Lack of understanding of a drug mechanism of action is often the cause of unsuccessful drug development programs.

Some other drugs have demonstrated benefit on OS without gain in PFS (24–26). Whether the gains in survival in these studies are truly due to the drug or to problems in the measurement of disease progression, to posttreatment therapies, or to the play of chance is at present unknown (27). For these reasons, these studies have limited impact on clinical practice because their results remain controversial.

Excess of Optimism

Cancer vaccine development programs are challenging, as recently illustrated by the early termination for futility of the phase III study of the human epidermal growth factor receptor 2/new (ErbB-2)-positive/neu vaccine Neuvax (E75), which was meant to prevent recurrence in high-risk breast cancer. The phase III study was initiated after results of phase I and II studies in 195 patients showed borderline significant increase of the 24-month PFS rates from 86.8% for the controls to 94.3% for the vaccinated patients ($p = .08$) (28). However, the development team considered that because of trial design, 65% of patients received a lower-than-optimal vaccine dose and conducted subgroup analyses to refine the patient population likely to benefit. The authors concluded that a phase III trial targeting the specific population of patients with lymph node–positive, HER2 low-expressing tumors was warranted. In 2012, the company launched the phase IIb study PRESENT (29) of 300 patients with HER2 that is one- and two-node positive and high-risk node-negative patients to study NeuVax in combination with trastuzumab (Herceptin; Genentech/Roche). The end point is disease-free survival at 36 months. On June 2016, the IDMC met to review the efficacy and safety data available for the study. On June 26, 2016, it recommended that the trial should be stopped for futility as the results suggested NeuVax may have actually performed worse than the placebo in this

study (30). In this example, one could argue that the evidence available early on was sufficient to support the development of the larger program.

It is not uncommon that promising phase II results are followed by disappointing phase III results. Sometimes, the difference stems from different patient populations or different end points used, as in trials of gemcitabine and bevacizumab in patients with advanced pancreatic cancer. The phase II nonrandomized study conducted in 7 centers recruited 52 previously untreated patients with advanced (stage IV) disease. It showed a response rate of 21% and promising median PFS and OS of 5.4 months and 8.8 months, respectively (31). The subsequent phase III study was conducted by the Cancer and Leukemia Group B (CALGB) collaborative group and randomized 602 patients between gemcitabine and bevacizumab as in the phase II and gemcitabine and placebo. In the phase III study, the median OS was 5.8 months with bevacizumab and 5.9 months with placebo ($p = .95$); the median PFS was 3.8 and 2.9 months, respectively ($p = .07$); and overall response rates were 13% and 10%, respectively (32). Here the authors concluded that patient selection is likely the most important factor in the disparate results of the phase III CALGB study and the phase II trial that provided the study rationale. In retrospect, it is clear that the phase II accrued a more fit population. Although all of the patients had metastatic disease and 83% had liver metastases, both of which augur a poor prognosis, that trial also contained more patients with a performance status of 0, excluded patients with prior thrombosis, and had more patients who had received adjuvant therapy. When prognosis substantially varies within a same disease stage, a single-arm phase II trial design may not be optimal. A randomized phase II study would likely have showed no difference between groups, with similarly fitter patients in the 2 arms. More generally, the small number of patients tested in a phase II makes these studies more prone to selection bias. Furthermore, phase II studies are generally conducted in a smaller number of usually more selected centers, so that institution expertise may also play a role in achieving, on average, better outcomes than in a less selected phase III trial or in the clinic. These aspects should not be underestimated when making the decision to initiate a phase III study.

The development of the poly-ADP ribose polymerase, or PARP, inhibitor iniparib in combination with chemotherapy in metastatic triple-negative breast cancer offers another informative example of discrepant phase II and III results. The phase II study randomized 123 patients between the combination of gemcitabine and carboplatin with and without iniparib. The primary end point was the clinical benefit rate. PFS and OS were secondary end points. The phase II results published in 2011 (33) showed that iniparib not only significantly increased the clinical benefit rate from 21% to 34% but also significantly increased the median PFS time by 2 months. The median survival was significantly increased from 7.7 months to 12.3 months with iniparib. On that basis, the same team quickly launched a phase III study. The phase III results first presented in 2013 (34), disappointingly showing no benefit in the coprimary end points survival or in PFS in 519 randomized patients. The median OS was 11.8 months with iniparib and 11.1 months without, and the median PFS was 5.1 months with iniparib and 4.1 months without. The authors concluded that there were no obvious differences in the patient populations (although Breast Cancer 1 and 2 genes [BRCA1/2] status data were unavailable) or in trial designs in the phase II and III studies that could explain the discrepancies. Some have considered the possibility to crossover to iniparib for patients in the control arm as a possible explanation for the survival benefit in the phase II (35). They argued that the patients in the control arm who crossed over to treatment with iniparib were not offered optimal salvage and that this negatively impacted their overall survival. Others (36) argued that preclinical data and early development studies on iniparib did not sufficiently elucidate the mechanism of action of this agent before clinical trials were initiated. Randomized phase II trials have a significant rate of false positivity, so promising results should be interpreted cautiously until other confirmatory studies are reported.

FAILURE IN EARLY PHASES

Early-phase clinical trials (phase I or early phase II) raise specific concerns. They are designed to be short and should end by a go–no go decision for the next step. Early trials of personalized (or precision) medicine typically test delivering treatments selected according to an algorithm that matches a given treatment to a given molecular abnormality found in the patient tumour versus a standard of care approach. Such trials face numerous logistical challenges. In early-phase studies, however, a failure is not a so-called "negative" trial (i.e., one where the investigational agent has no effect). Rather, it is the inability to complete the trial in a short enough time to make their outcome useful to further developments.

Phase I Trials

Phase I clinical trials are often designed as biological experiments that require repeated biopsies (37), multiple samplings, and heavy imaging at various time points to elicit the mechanisms of action of the new agent. Although such trials usually benefit from top-level research laboratories, such requirements make trial logistics for imaging platforms, interventional radiology, tumor processing, and storage quite complex. They also deter from the quality of life of the patients who need to repeatedly visit the hospital or need to be hospitalized and undergo invasive investigations (38).

Patients may then become reluctant to participate in the trial (39) or withdraw approval. Investigators may participate less actively or propose the trial only to a subset of patients expected to comply with the extra burden of the research. The fair compromise between feasibility and collection of information useful for the research is needed to ensure trial success.

One major cause of the high attrition rate in oncology is probably the identification of an incorrect "optimal" dose (40). In oncology, the optimal dose is the maximum tolerated dose (MTD), and phase I trials should identify the MTD. The fraction of incorrect recommendations at the end of phase I trials is difficult to estimate. An accurate overview of the toxicity and efficiency of a new compound is typically derived from the large phase III trials. However, agents that are overdosed or underdosed are likely to be dropped after phase II because of lack of activity or excess of toxicity. This fact led David Von Hoff to declare that "there were no bad anticancer agents, only poor clinical trials" (41). A review of phase I trials in pediatric oncology showed that of the three agents that were tested twice in phase I trials, the phase I recommended completely different maximum doses for two (42), suggesting that there is a huge variability in the final estimates of the MTD. This finding is consistent with statistical work. Based on simulations, statisticians have estimated that a phase I trial has about a 50% chance of identifying the correct dose; hence, it has a 50% chance of recommending too high or too low a dose (43). The two causes of this high error rate are the small sample size and the questionable validity of the fundamental assumption that the higher the dose, the more active the treatment.

Can we improve on this? A method has been proposed to serve as a benchmark in simulation studies to quantify the best performance that can be obtained from a phase I, given a dose-toxicity relationship and a fixed sample size (44). This approach relies on a notion of "complete" information, as if a patient could be independently treated at each dose level. Thus, the method cannot be used in real trials (where a patient is exposed to a single dose), but it can serve in simulations. Using this method, the authors showed that in a large number of scenarios, the highest probability of selecting the right dose (without an informative prior) in a study of 25 patients was less than 60%. Any dose-finding method is limited by the variability induced by the use of a binary outcome (dose-limiting toxicity [DLT] or no DLT), which is not informative. It is regrettable that so little data are used for decision making in phase I trials, when so much more data (e.g., lower grade toxicities or laboratory values) are available. Future improvements in dose-finding designs will result from the incorporation of more information, rather than from refinement of the methods described.

Whether the MTD is the optimal dose is also the subject of heated debates. Recently, pembrolizumab, an immune checkpoint blocker, was tested in a dose-escalation phase I study (45). The highest dose, 10 mg/kg, was recommended for and tested in phase II and phase III trials. Two doses of pembrolizumab (2 vs. 10 mg/kg) were randomly compared in 173 patients with advanced melanoma (46). A total of 82% of the patients had drug-related adverse events at each dose (15% vs. 8% of grade 3/4). The overall response rate was also similar. As a consequence, the regulatory agencies requested that the lowest dose be included in the submission dossier, which raised difficulties because most data in phase III trials had been collected for the 10-mg dose. This illustrates the risk of extrapolating the hypotheses set up for cytotoxic agents to the field of monoclonal antibodies.

Window-of-Opportunity Trials

Window-of-opportunity trials take advantage of the time lapse between cancer diagnosis and surgery to test treatments preoperatively for a short time (usually 3–6 weeks) (47). The purpose is to investigate how the treatment affects biomarkers using measurements obtained on the diagnostic biopsy (pretreatment) and on the resected tumor sample (after treatment) using each patient as his or her own control. The surgeon in charge of the resection usually identifies the patients. The timing of the surgery is precisely defined. The medical oncologist informs and consents the patient and initiates the experimental treatment. Success of the studies lies in the collaboration between the surgery and the medical oncology departments. Lack of such collaboration is probably the reason why the RADHER study (48) that randomized everolimus plus Herceptin versus Herceptin alone before surgery was interrupted after 4 years with only 66% of the targeted sample size. That trial was exclusively steered by oncologists and pathologists. Surgeons were not strongly associated and the accrual was much lower than anticipated.

Trials of Personalized Medicine

Most new agents are designed to target molecular alterations involved in carcinogenesis. They are expected to produce antitumor activity only in the presence of the matching molecular alteration. The prevalence of the relevant molecular alteration is often low so that testing the treatment in each tumor type becomes virtually impossible. Therefore, several histologic-agnostic trials have been initiated to test several treatments directed against several molecular alterations across tumor types (49). The objective of such "personalized medicine" trials is then to investigate the added value of a treatment algorithm to select the best treatment based on molecular abnormalities.

Complexity is a major issue in trials assessing personalized medicine. The process needed to provide a standardized molecular profile is demanding (50). The tumor or metastasis material must be frozen rapidly after the biopsy, the DNA then needs to be extracted and processed on the sequencing or microarray platforms, and the data obtained from the processed sample requires normalization and bioinformatics processing. In turn, these data are interpreted by the biologists before one eventually applies an algorithm that matches a given drug with the molecular profile. Each step is associated with errors that may accumulate. Quality control must therefore be performed at each step of the process and traceability is required. In order not to delay the treatment administration, the entire process must be conducted within strict timelines.

Such trials involve a number of key specialists: physicians, radiologists, pathologists, biostatisticians, sequencing platforms managers, bioinformaticians, and biologists. Although the first 4 are accustomed to working together, the last 3 usually work in research laboratories and are not used to the time constraints related to patient care. Personalized medicine trials require that all these people coordinate their activities to ensure that treatment decisions are made in a timely manner. In the SHIVA trial, for example, the median duration of this multistep process was 4 weeks, with a maximum of less than 6 weeks (51). Such timelines are very challenging and may explain why several such trials struggle to accrue patients. The SHIVA trial accrued patients faster than anticipated but is an exception (52). It is worth noting that in this study even if a complete molecular profile was systematically investigated, results on only a part of the profile were deemed acceptable for entering a patient in the study. This most likely played a role in the success of the study.

To control for the histology, some trials such as the nonrandomized basked trial CUSTOM in advanced thoracic malignancies (53) have been designed as multicohort studies with stratification by histology. A total of 569 patients underwent successful molecular profiling. Although more than 280 profiles matched the target of one of the five investigational molecular targeted agents tested in the study, only 45 patients were eventually treated. Many were excluded because of clinical history, inclusion criteria required for treatment in a specific arm, or sudden worsening of their general status while the molecular analysis was being conducted. Furthermore, of the 280 eligible mutations identified, some such as the ErbB-2 or KIT/PDGFRA mutations/amplifications were present in only 5% and 3% of the cases, respectively. Further splitting those by histology resulted in several empty sets. The number of patients needed to screen to assess the activity in each subgroup rapidly increases as prevalence decreases, which severely limits the trial feasibility. Incorrect estimation of the prevalence of the rarer subgroups at the trial design stage has dramatic consequences on the study feasibility and on its costs. Careful monitoring as the trial goes is paramount. The right balance between homogeneous populations and feasibility of the trial is even more challenging than it is in untargeted populations.

CONCLUSIONS

From the authors' perspective as clinical trial professionals, the concept of considering a taxonomy for trial failure can be very thought provoking with regard to our role to the community and our own mission. On a daily basis, we evaluate trials on factors such as feasibility, scientific value, rigor, patient acceptance, financing, timing, and communication of results. We must ask ourselves what the cost of a failure on any of those points would be. Measures to prevent each type of failure would best be aligned with the cost of failure on each respective point. We hope that the readers, from their own perspective, find some value in a similar exercise.

It is important to us to highlight that the "negative trial" (i.e., one with statistically nonsignificant results) is but one case of a much broader group of research initiatives that do not lead to the desired outcome. In this perspective, it is very important to remind ourselves that science is not broken (54) but that it is a difficult undertaking. Part of the research we undertake will fail, and that is in fact desirable. When a trial "fails" because the tested treatment truly did not work, one has to embrace this as a learning experience. The goal should not be to set up research programs where you know you can win to avoid failure, but rather to fail if the tested approach does not work (55). If we never undertook initiatives that ultimately fail, we would indeed be erring on the side of caution, with little chance of making discoveries that change the outlook of cancer.

REFERENCES

1. Doll R, Hill A. Smoking and carcinoma of the lung; preliminary report. *Br Med J.* 1950;2(4682):739–748.
2. Nam RK, Cheung P, Herschorn S, et al. Incidence of complications other than urinary incontinence or erectile dysfunction after radical prostatectomy or radiotherapy for prostate cancer: a population-based cohort study. *Lancet Oncol.* 2014;15:223–231.
3. Resnick MJ, Koyama T, Fan KH, et al. Long-term functional outcomes after treatment for localized prostate cancer. *N Engl J Med.* 2013;368(5):436–445.
4. Messing EM, Manola J, Yao J, et al. Immediate versus deferred androgen deprivation treatment in patients with node-positive prostate cancer after radical prostatectomy and pelvic lymphadenectomy. *Lancet Oncol.* 2006;7(6): 472–479.
5. Schröder FH, Kurth KH, Fossa S, et al. Early versus delayed endocrine treatment of T2-T3 pN1-3 M0 prostate cancer without local treatment of the primary tumour: final results of European Organisation for the Research and Treatment of Cancer protocol 30846 after 13 years of follow-up (a randomised controlled trial). *Eur Urol.* 2009;55(1): 14–22.
6. Sternberg CN, Skoneczna I, Kerst JM, et al. Immediate versus deferred chemotherapy after radical cystectomy in patients with pT3-pT4 or N+ M0 urothelial carcinoma of the bladder (EORTC 30994): an intergroup, open-label, randomised phase 3 trial. *Lancet Oncol.* 2015;16(1):76–86.
7. Oosterlinck W, Kurth KH, Schröder F, et al. A prospective European Organization for Research and Treatment of Cancer Genitourinary Group randomized trial comparing transurethral resection followed by a single intravesical instillation of epirubicin or water in single stage Ta, T1 papillary carcinoma of the bladder. *J Urol.* 1993;149:749–752.
8. http://www.icr.ac.uk/our-research/our-research-centres/clinical-trials-and-statistics-unit/clinical-trials/caliber
9. Adebahr S, Collette S, Shash E, et al. LungTech, an EORTC Phase II trial of stereotactic body radiotherapy for centrally located lung tumours: a clinical perspective. *Br J Radiol.* 2015;88(1051):201–205.
10. https://clinicaltrials.gov/ct2/show/NCT00410683
11. https://clinicaltrials.gov/ct2/show/NCT02504372
12. https://clinicaltrials.gov/ct2/show/NCT02273375
13. Rogers EM. Diffusion of Innovations. 5th Edition. New York, NY: Free Press, a division of Simon and Schuster Inc.; 2003: 267–300.
14. http://hub.ucsf.edu/sites/hub.ucsf.edu/files/Clinical%20Trial%20Feasibility%20Checklist.pdf
15. Freidling B, Korn EL, Gray R. A general inefficacy interim monitoring rule for clinical trials. *Clin Trial.* 2010;7(3):197–208.
16. https://clinicaltrials.gov/ct2/show/NCT00043004
17. Ruers T, Punt C, Van Coevorden F, et al. Radiofrequency ablation combined with systemic treatment versus systemic treatment alone in patients with non-resectable colorectal liver metastases: a randomized EORTC Intergroup phase II study (EORTC 40004). *Ann Oncol.* 2012;23(10):2619–2626.
18. Theo Ruers, Cornelis J. A. Punt et al. Radiofrequency ablation (RFA) combined with chemotherapy for unresectable colorectal liver metastases (CRC LM): long-term survival results of a randomized phase II study of the EORTC-NCRI CCSG-ALM Intergroup 40004 (CLOCC). *J Clin Oncol.* 2015;3(suppl):abstr 3501.
19. Smith DC, Dunn RL, Strawderman MS, et al. Change in serum prostate-specific antigen as a marker of response to cytotoxic therapy for hormone-refractory prostate cancer. *J Clin Oncol.* 1998;16(5):1835–1843.
20. Beer TM, Ryan CW, Venner PM, et al. Double-blinded randomized study of high–dose calcitriol plus docetaxel compared with placebo plus docetaxel in androgen-independent prostate cancer: a report from the ASCENT investigators. *J Clin Oncol.* 2007;26(6):669–674.
21. Small EJ, Schellhammer PF, Higano CS, et al. Placebo-controlled phase III trial of immunologic therapy with sipuleucel-T (APC8015) in patients with metastatic, asymptomatic hormone refractory prostate cancer. *J Clin Oncol.* 2006;24:3089–3094.
22. Higano CS, Schellhammer PF, Small EJ, et al. Integrated data from 2 randomized double-blind, placebo-controlled, phase 3 trials of active cellular immunotherapy with sipuleucel-T in advanced prostate cancer. *Cancer.* 2009;115:3670–3679.
23. Kantoff PW, Higano CS, Shore ND, et al. Sipuleucel-T immunotherapy for castration-resistant prostate cancer. *N Engl J Med.* 2010;363:411–422.
24. Motzer RJ, Escudier B, Tomczak P, et al. Axitinib versus sorafenib as second-line treatment for advanced renal cell carcinoma: overall survival analysis and updated results from a randomised phase 3 trial. *Lancet Oncol.* 2013;14: 552–562.
25. Pirker R, Pereira JR, Szczesna A, et al. Cetuximab plus chemotherapy in patients with advanced non-small-cell lung cancer (FLEX): an open-label randomized phase III trial. *Lancet.* 2009;373:1525–1531.
26. Cortes J, O'Shaughnessy J, Loesch D, et al. Eribulin monotherapy versus treatment of physician's choice in patients with metastatic breast cancer (EMBRACE): a phase 3 open-label randomised study. *Lancet.* 2011;377:914–923.
27. Saad ED, Buyse M. Statistical controversies in clinical research: end points other than overall survival are vital for regulatory approval of anticancer agents. *Annals Oncol.* 2016;27:373–378.

28. Mittendorf EA, Clifton GT, Holmes JP, et al. Clinical trial results of the HER-2/neu (E75) vaccine to prevent breast cancer recurrence in high-risk patients: From US Military Cancer Institute Clinical Trials Group Study I-01 and I-02. *Cancer*. 2012;118(10):2594–2602.

29. https://clinicaltrials.gov/ct2/show/NCT01570036

30. https://globenewswire.com/news-release/2016/06/29/852251/0/en/Galena-Biopharma-Discontinues-NeuVax-nelipepimut-S-Phase-3-PRESENT-Interim-Analysis-based-on-Independent-Data-Monitoring-Committee-Recommendation.html

31. Kindler HL, Friberg G, Singh DA, et al. Phase II trial of bevacizumab plus gemcitabine in patients with advanced pancreatic cancer. *J Clin Oncol*. 2005;23(31):8033–8040.

32. Kindler HL, Niedzwiecki D, Hollis D, et al. Gemcitabine plus bevacizumab compared with gemcitabine plus placebo in patients with advanced pancreatic cancer: phase III trial of the Cancer and Leukemia Group B (CALGB 80303). *J Clin Oncol*. 2010;28(22):3617–3622.

33. O'Shaughnessy J, Osborne C, Pippen JE, et al. Iniparib plus chemotherapy in metastatic triple-negative breast cancer. *N Engl J Med*. 2011;364:205–214.

34. O'Shaughnessy J, Schwartzberg L, Danso MA, et al. Phase III study of iniparib plus gemcitabine and carboplatin versus gemcitabine and carboplatin in patients with metastatic triple-negative breast cancer. *J Clin Oncol*. 2014;32(34):3840–3847.

35. Fojo T, Amiri-Kordestani L, Bates SE. Potential pitfalls of crossover and thoughts on iniparib in triple-negative breast cancer . *J Natl Cancer Inst*. 2011;103:1738–1740.

36. Mateo J, Ong M, Tan DSP, et al. Appraising iniparib, the PARP inhibitor that never was—what must we learn? *Nat Rev Clin Oncol*. 2013;10:688–696.

37. Gomez-Roca CA, Lacroix L, Massard C, et al. Sequential research-related biopsies in phase I trials: acceptance, feasibility and safety. *Ann Oncol*. 2012;23(5):1301–1306.

38. Craft BS, Kurzrock R, Lei X, et al. The changing face of phase 1 cancer clinical trials: new challenges in study requirements. *Cancer*. 2009;115:1592–1597.

39. van der Biessen DA, Cranendonk MA, Schiavon G, et al. Evaluation of patient enrollment in oncology phase I clinical trials. *Oncologist*. 2013;18(3):323–329.

40. Kola I, Landis J. Can the pharmaceutical industry reduce attrition rates? *Nat Rev Drug Discov*. 2004;3(8):711–715.

41. Von Hoff DD. There are no bad anticancer agents, only bad clinical trial designs–twenty-first Richard and Hinda Rosenthal Foundation Award Lecture. *Clin Cancer Res*. 1998;4(5):1079–1086.

42. Paoletti X, Geoerger B, Doz F. A comparative analysis of paediatric dose-finding trials of molecularly targeted agent with adults' trials. *Eur J Cancer*. 2013;49(10):2392–2402.

43. Paoletti X, Kramar A. A comparison of model choices for the continual reassessment method in phase I cancer trials. *Stat Med*. 2009;28(24):3012–3028.

44. Paoletti X, O'Quigley J, Maccario J. Design efficiency in dose finding studies, 2004;45(2):197–214.

45. Patnaik A, Kang SP, Rasco D, et al. Phase I study of pembrolizumab (MK-3475; Anti-PD-1 Monoclonal Antibody) in patients with advanced solid tumors. *Clin Cancer Res*. 2015;21(19):4286–4293.

46. Robert C, Ribas A, Wolchok JD, et al. Anti-programmed-death-receptor-1 treatment with pembrolizumab in ipilimumab-refractory advanced melanoma: a randomised dose-comparison cohort of a phase 1 trial. *Lancet*. 2014;384(9948):1109–1117.

47. Ratain MJ. Bar the windows but open the door to randomization. *J Clin Oncol*. 2010;28(19):3104–3106.

48. Campone M, Treilleux I, Salleron J. Predictive value of intratumoral signaling and immune infiltrate for response to preoperative (PO) trastuzumab (T) vs trastuzumab + everolimus (T+E) in patients (pts) with primary breast cancer (PBC): UNICANCER RADHER trial results. *J Clin Oncol*. 2016;34 (suppl):abstr 606.

49. Le Tourneau C, Kamal M, Alt M, et al. The spectrum of clinical trials aiming at personalizing medicine. *Chin Clin Oncol*. 2014;3(2):13.

50. Servant N, Roméjon J, Gestraud P, et al. Bioinformatics for precision medicine in oncology: principles and application to the SHIVA clinical trial. *Front Genet*. 2014;30(5):152.

51. Le Tourneau C, Paoletti X, Servant N, et al. Randomised proof-of-concept phase II trial comparing targeted therapy based on tumour molecular profiling vs conventional therapy in patients with refractory cancer: results of the feasibility part of the SHIVA trial. *Br J Cancer*. 2014;111(1):17–24.

52. Le Tourneau C, Delord JP, Gonçalves A, et al. Molecularly targeted therapy based on tumour molecular profiling versus conventional therapy for advanced cancer (SHIVA): a multicentre, open-label, proof-of-concept, randomised, controlled phase 2 trial. *Lancet Oncol*. 2015;16(13):1324–1334.

53. Lopez-Chavez A, Thomas A, Rajan A, et al. Molecular profiling and targeted therapy for advanced thoracic malignancies: a biomarker-derived, multiarm, multihistology phase II basket trial. *J Clin Oncol*. 2015;33(9):1000–1007.

54. http://fivethirtyeight.com/features/science-isnt-broken

55. West HJ. 'Failing Fast' and moving forward: setting the right pace for clinical cancer research. *Medscape*. 2016.

Designing Oncology Clinical Trials

Choice of Endpoints in Cancer Clinical Trials

Mei-Yin Polley, Wenting Wu, and Daniel J. Sargent[†]

A critical element to the success of any clinical trial is the choice of the appropriate endpoint(s). In the context of a clinical trial, an endpoint is defined as a characteristic of a patient that is assessed by a protocol specified mechanism. Examples of endpoints commonly assessed in cancer clinical trials include adverse events, measures of tumor growth or shrinkage, or time-related endpoints such as overall survival (OS). The choice of the endpoint for any given trial depends primarily on the trial's objectives. In this chapter we first present general considerations related to the choice of an endpoint for a trial, and then focus on specific endpoints that may be appropriate for various trial types, specifically phase I, phase II, or phase III trials.

GENERAL CONSIDERATIONS

Each clinical trial should specify a single, primary endpoint. This endpoint is the patient characteristic that will most directly capture whether the therapy being tested is having the desired (or undesired, in the case of an adverse event) effect on the patient. The primary endpoint also typically determines the trial's sample size, through the process of specifying what effect on the primary endpoint is desired to be detected in the trial with a sufficiently high chance (study power). The primary endpoint must be appropriately justified, and typically should be a well-defined and commonly accepted endpoint in that cancer type and/or study phase.

Once a primary endpoint has been determined, typically multiple additional endpoints, known as secondary endpoints, are specified. Secondary endpoints should be variables that are of interest to study investigators, such that the examination of these endpoints will enhance the utility of the trial to address clinically or biologically relevant questions. Formally, statistical testing for treatment-related effects on these secondary endpoints should only

occur if there is a statistically significant effect on the primary endpoint so as to avoid inflating the study-wide type I error. In practice, however, these endpoints are typically examined regardless of the primary endpoint results.

When considering possible endpoints for a clinical trial, an important distinction exists between clinical and surrogate endpoints. A clinical endpoint is one with direct clinical and patient relevance, such as patient quality of life (QOL) or survival. In most cases, if possible and feasible, a clinical endpoint should be preferred for a protocol. However, in many cases, the optimal clinical endpoint may take very long to assess (such as patient survival), require a costly procedure (such as imaging), or be too invasive to be practical or ethical (such as requiring a patient biopsy). In such cases, a surrogate endpoint is often considered. A surrogate endpoint is defined as an endpoint obtained more quickly, at lower cost, or less invasively than the true clinical endpoint of interest (1). The practice of validating, or confirming the accuracy, of a surrogate endpoint is challenging, and there are many examples of endpoints that were considered promising surrogates only to be subsequently shown to have a poor or even negative association with the true endpoint of interest (2). The topic of surrogate endpoints is addressed in depth in Chapter 34 of this book (3); we do not consider this further here.

ENDPOINTS FOR PHASE I TRIALS

Historically, cancer therapies have been designed to act as cytotoxic, or cell killing, agents. The fundamental assumption regarding the dose-related activity of such agents is that there exists a monotone nondecreasing dose–response curve, meaning that as the dose increases, tumor shrinkage will also increase, which should translate into increasing clinical benefit. Under this assumption, both toxicity and the clinical benefit of the agent under study will increase with increasing dose. Since the monotone nondecreasing dose–response curve has been

---

[†]Deceased.

observed for most cytotoxic therapies, toxicity has historically been used as the primary endpoint to identify the dose that has an acceptable toxicity profile and has the greatest chance to be effective in subsequent testing.

Specifically, the typical goal for phase I clinical trials, for instance, by the cohort-of-3 design, has been to determine the highest dose level where one third of treated patients or fewer experience unacceptable dose-limiting toxicity (DLT). This highest dose level is referred to as the maximum tolerated dose (MTD). The use of toxicity as an endpoint and thus defining the MTD as the primary goal of a phase I trial has considerable appeal. This endpoint is clinically relevant, is straightforward to observe, is easy to explain, and has clear intuitive rationale and considerable historical precedent. With the advent of newer therapies in oncology, however, the use of toxicity as the primary endpoint poses increasing challenges in modern clinical trials.

A particular difficulty of using toxicity as a phase I endpoint is posed by noncytotoxic therapies. At the cell level, targets in cytoplasmic and cell-surface signaling molecules, processes of cell-cycle control and mutations, or lack of expression of suppressor genes have yielded many novel agents for evaluation. At the extracellular level, novel drugs designed to limit tumor penetration and metastasis or directly inhibit angiogenesis are being pursued. Vaccines to overcome immune tolerance of cancer are also being developed. These *cytostatic* or *targeted* therapies, many of which seem to be nontoxic at doses that achieve concentrations with desired biologic effects, have become more common. In these cases, a dose-escalation trial incorporating a biologic endpoint specific for the agent in addition to toxicity might be appropriate (4,5); these trials are sometimes referred to as phase Ib studies.

For cytostatic agents with a nontoxicity endpoint, the assumption that increasing dose will always lead to increasing biological activity may not be reasonable. In particular, the shape of the dose outcome curve could be monotone nondecreasing, quadratic, or increasing with a plateau. In a phase I trial with such an agent, an appropriate goal is to estimate the biologically optimal dose (BOD); that is, the dose that has maximal biological activity, with acceptable toxicity (6). As such, the trial must incorporate both toxicity and biological activity as endpoints while estimating the BOD. Several endpoints that could serve as endpoints for biological activity to supplement toxicity as the single endpoint for trials of cytostatic/targeted therapies are discussed in the following.

A possible endpoint for biological activity in this setting would be an endpoint that represents a measurement of the effect of the agent on the molecular target. The use of this kind of endpoint should have reproducible assays available, and optimally be shown to correlate with a clinical endpoint, such as tumor response, in human or at minimum animal models. In practice, several challenges exist for such an endpoint. These include that a reliable assay for measurement of the drug effect must be available, that the relevant tissue in which to measure target inhibition is readily available, that serial tumor sampling is usually invasive and associated with sampling error, and that at this early stage of a drug's development it may be difficult to define the appropriate measure of achieved target effects for a specific drug. The issue of ready availability of tissue may be addressed by restricting patient enrollment to those with accessible disease for assessment of the drug effect on the tumor, but this may severely restrict the number of patients eligible for the trial.

Other possible measurements for activity of an agent, and thus potential endpoints, include pharmacokinetic analysis, which would be appropriate if sufficient preclinical data exist demonstrating a convincing pharmacokinetic–pharmacodynamic relationship. More specifically, an endpoint of assessing whether the minimum effective blood concentration level of the agent has been attained could be considered. Again, such an endpoint would require preclinical data that have demonstrated that the target blood or serum level correlates with clinically relevant efficacy.

To date, few published phase I trials have used nontoxicity endpoints such as we have described, for both biologic and practical reasons. First, at this point in an agent's development, it may be difficult to define the desired target biological effect. Even if the target is known and an effect level known, it may be difficult to define and validate an appropriate measurement for that endpoint. Practical difficulties in measuring target levels once they have been defined include the lack of reliable, real-time assays and the difficulty in obtaining the required tumor specimens. The real-time nature of the assay is critical, as if dosing decisions are to be made based on the endpoint, turnaround must be rapid, and batch processing is not likely acceptable. Finally, statistical trial designs for identifying a dose that maximizes the biologic response would likely require more patients than are typically studied in phase I trials.

ENDPOINTS FOR PHASE II AND III TRIALS

Phase II and phase III clinical trials, as opposed to phase I trials, are designed to obtain a preliminary (phase II) or definitive (phase III) determination of a new agent's efficacy. As such, the endpoints for these trials tend to be clinical in nature, designed to directly assess the impact of a therapy on patient-relevant phenomena. The four endpoints most commonly used in phase II and phase III oncology trials are tumor response rate, patient progression-free survival (PFS; in the advanced disease setting)/disease-free survival (DFS; in the adjuvant setting), OS, and QOL. Historically, response rate has been the most common endpoint for phase II trials, and OS for phase III trials. However, in the past 10 to 20 years, both PFS/DFS and OS have been used increasingly as an endpoint in the phase II setting. Thus, in this section we discuss these endpoints, as they are relevant for both phase II and phase III trials.

Response Rate

Response rate has been the major primary endpoint for phase II trials in the past 40 years. The response rate in a trial is defined as the proportion of responders (complete or partial) among all eligible patients. The use of response rate as a primary endpoint has substantial biological plausibility: as tumors rarely shrink by themselves, a tumor response can be considered as a clear signal of activity of a new therapy. In addition, in most solid tumors with cytotoxic therapies, response occurs quickly after the initiation of therapy, most often within 3 months. As such, tumor response provides an endpoint that can be assessed rapidly, allowing a timely determination of whether an agent is sufficiently promising to warrant phase III testing.

Since the establishment of the Response Evaluation Criteria in Solid Tumors (RECIST) in 2000 (7), this standard has become widely accepted as the preferred method to assess tumor shrinkage. Under RECIST, all measurable lesions up to a maximum of 10 are identified as target lesions and the baseline measurements for these lesions are recorded. During treatment, for target lesions, complete response (CR) is defined as the disappearance of all target lesions, and partial response (PR) as a decrease of at least 30% in the sum of the longest diameter (LD) of target lesions, taking as reference the baseline sum of the LD. Progressive disease (PD) is defined as at least a 20% increase in the sum of the LD of target lesions, taking as reference the smallest sum LD recorded since the treatment started or the appearance of one or more new lesions. Stable disease (SD) is defined as neither sufficient shrinkage to qualify for PR nor sufficient increase to qualify for PD, taking as reference the smallest sum LD since the treatment started.

Lesions that are not measurable as per RECIST (typically due to poorly defined dimensions) are classified as nontarget lesions. For nontarget lesions, CR is defined as the disappearance of all nontarget lesions. Incomplete Response/SD is defined as the persistence of one or more nontarget lesions or/and maintenance of tumor marker level above the normal limits, with PD defined as appearance of one or more new lesions and/or unequivocal progression of existing nontarget lesions. To be assigned a status of PR or CR as per RECIST, changes in tumor measurements must be confirmed by repeat assessment performed no less than 4 weeks after the criteria for response are first met.

Since the publication of RECIST (version 1.0) in 2000, a number of issues and questions were raised, which led to the development of a revised RECIST guideline (version 1.1) (8). Major changes in RECIST v1.1 include the following: (a) the number of lesions required to assess tumor burden is reduced from a maximum of 10 to a maximum of 5 total (and from 5 to 2 lesions per organ maximum); (b) pathological lymph nodes are included in the sum of lesions in the calculation of tumor response. In particular, nodes with a short axis of ≥15 mm are considered measurable and assessed as target lesions. Nodes that shrink to <10 mm short axis are considered normal; (c) confirmation of response is only required for trials with response as primary endpoint but is no longer required in randomized studies; (d) in addition to the previous definition of PD in target disease of 20% increase in the sum of LD, the new guideline requires also a 5 mm absolute increase so as to guard against overcalling progression when the total disease burden is very small. Finally, the new guidelines offer further clarity on what constitutes "unequivocal progression" of nonmeasurable/nontarget disease and how to interpret fluorodeoxyglucose (FDG) PET scan assessment in the context of new lesion detections. Under RECIST v1.1, the best overall response at the patient level is the best response recorded from the start of the treatment until disease progression/recurrence, and it is evaluated as per Table 8.1.

In the past 10 to 15 years, the appropriateness of tumor response as a trial endpoint has been challenged (9–11). The RECIST criteria for response were designed primarily to assess cytotoxic agents. For drugs that might

TABLE 8.1 Patient Overall Response Based on Target Lesions, Nontarget Lesions, and New Lesions

Target Lesions	Nontarget Lesions	New Lesions	Overall Response
CR	CR	No	CR
CR	Non-CR/non-PD	No	PR
CR	Not evaluated	No	PR
PR	Non-PD or not all evaluated	No	PR
SD	Non-PD or not all evaluated	No	SD
Not all evaluated	Non-PD	No	NE
PD	Any	Yes or No	PD
Any	PD	Yes or No	PD
Any	Any	Yes	PD

CR, complete response; NE, inevaluable; PD, progressive disease; PR, partial response; SD, stable disease.

be active in slowing the cancer disease process, but without consistent achievement of tumor shrinkage, such as the epidermal growth factor tyrosine kinase inhibitors (gefitinib and erlotinib), or the multiple new agents targeting the vascular endothelial growth factor pathway (bevacizumab and sorafenib), the tumor response endpoint does not consider durable modest regressions or prolonged disease stability as activity, which we now know is an effect of those agents. For example, consider a randomized trial of bevacizumab, an antivascular endothelial growth factor antibody, in the setting of metastatic renal cancer (12). This randomized, double-blind, phase II trial was conducted comparing placebo with bevacizumab at doses of 3 and 10 mg/kg of body weight with time to disease progression and response rate as primary endpoints. In this trial, only 4 out of 116 patients demonstrated tumor response (all PRs), and all of them were in the high-dose arm. However, the time to progression (TTP) of disease in the high-dose group was significantly superior to that in the placebo group, with a median TTP of 4.8 versus 2.5 months, $p < .001$ by the log-rank test. The clinical benefit of bevacizumab in this trial was modest, only a few months extension of TTP, but the likelihood is high that this difference was due to true biologic activity, which might have been missed if response rate was the only endpoint considered.

In addition, the assessment of response rate may be complicated by factors other than the treatment intervention. For instance, in central nervous system (CNS) tumors, there are several factors that increase the potential for false-positive and false-negative responses. The blood–brain barrier and slow debris-clearing mechanisms in the brain make the brain tumor a special case. The use of steroids in CNS tumors may improve patient symptoms, maintain clinical improvement for extended periods of time even at low or reduced doses, and decrease the size of some malignant gliomas as assessed by CT scan. These benefits mimic treatment effects; thus a neurooncologist's assessment of the tumor's response to concurrent therapies could be a false positive. Further, distinguishing tumor shrinkage or growth from surgical changes and radiation effects is challenging. Delayed radiation effects may mimic tumor progression, and this pseudo tumor progression could confound interpretation of clinical trial results. Those effects may subside spontaneously over time without intervention. But at the present time, there is no demonstrated technology that can discern late radiation changes from tumor progression. Thus radiation effects may lead the investigator to conclude the intervention is either ineffective or effective when in reality the patient may not have experienced any impact of the intervention whatsoever. Other factors mimicking response, thus contributing to false-positive responses, include spontaneous resolution of postoperative or hemorrhage-related CT enhancement, spontaneous resolution of CT enhancing radiation effects,

and apparent CT improvement due to changes in scanning technique (13,14).

Recently, advancements in cancer immunotherapies have offered promising strategies for cancer treatment. Immune modulation refers to a range of treatments that aim at harnessing the patient's own immune system to achieve tumor control. Immuno-oncology therapies have been shown to provide anticancer benefits to patients. One such example is ipilimumab, the first-in-class fully human monoclonal antibody that blocks cytotoxic T-lymphocyte-associated protein 4 (CTLA-4). In studies with immunotherapeutic agents, clinical experience has shown that response may still be achieved after an initial increase in overall tumor burden. As such, the RECIST may not adequately characterize tumor response patterns as an early increase in tumor size or the appearance of new lesions would have been clarified as PD. Several other response criteria have been developed to overcome the limitations of RECIST with specific immunotherapeutic agents. In 2009, the Immune-Related Response Criteria (irRC) was developed to define patterns of tumor response that are observed in patients receiving immunotherapy and to identify successful treatment outcomes that would have been missed by the RECIST criteria (15). In contrast to RECIST, which uses unidimensional measurements, the irRC utilizes bidimensional tumor measurements of target lesions. At each follow-up assessment, both the sum of the products of the two longest perpendicular diameters of the target lesions and new measurable lesions are included in the calculation of the total tumor burden. This is in stark contrast with RECIST in that RECIST does not measure new lesions and the presence of a new lesion would be qualified as a progression. With irRC, patients are not assessed as having a progression in the presence of a new lesion as long as the tumor burden is not increased by 25% or more. Additionally, patients are considered to have PR or SD if the tumor burden meets the thresholds of response, even in the presence of a new lesion. Finally, irRC requires confirmation of progression by a second scan within 4 weeks after the initial progression determination to capture the late responding patterns of some patients. Generally, the irRC has the advantage of not calling a PD prematurely when the treatment effect may not yet have been fully apparent.

More recently, studies have shown that utilization of unidimensional measurements in irRC may be more reproducible than bidimensional measurements, have less measurement variabilities, and have lower misclassification rate when compared with bidimensional measurements (16). The Immune-Related Response Evaluation Criteria in Solid Tumors (irRECIST) was then developed to combine the advantages of both RECIST and irRC (17). Specifically, the irRECIST criteria utilize unidimensional measurements like the standard RECIST but include all detected lesions and at the same time avoid early declaration of PD like the irRC.

The irRECIST is expected to provide simpler and more reliable and reproducible assessment of response for targeted immunotherapeutic agents in oncology clinical trials.

Despite the aforementioned limitations of the response endpoint, many of which have been known for years, response rate has been considered as the primary endpoint of phase II trials primarily because tumor shrinkage was believed to be linked to the drug's biological activity, and drugs that induced tumor response were felt to be those most likely to lead to improved survival or decreased symptoms. However, some research has shown that an improved response rate may not always translate to a survival improvement. Significant association (or correlation) between response and progression (or survival) does not imply that response is a viable endpoint for chemotherapy trials in the current era. For example, in colorectal cancer, the meta-analysis conducted by Buyse et al. (10) showed that:

> an increase in tumor response rate translates into an increase in overall survival for patients with advanced colorectal cancer, but in the context of individual trials, knowledge that a treatment has benefits on tumor response does not allow accurate prediction of the ultimate benefit of survival.

At the present time, the use of response rate as a phase II endpoint is trial specific. For a trial with an agent thought to be cytotoxic, and a need for a rapid initial assessment of activity, tumor response may be an appropriate primary endpoint. However, as discussed in the next section, PFS allows a possibly more complete assessment of an agent's potential to improve patient outcome in a phase III trial. With the possible exception of tumors that are highly symptomatic, where tumor shrinkage results in meaningful patient symptomatic benefit, response rate is not appropriate as a primary endpoint for phase III trials, due to (a) inherent measurement issues, (b) unclear clinical relevance, and (c) poor prediction of ultimate survival benefit.

Progression-Free Survival/ Disease-Free Survival

Progression- and disease-free survival (PFS/DFS) are time-related endpoints that in principle measure the time from initiation of therapy to disease worsening. In a patient with existing disease (for example, with unresectable metastases), the event of interest for this endpoint is growth or progression of disease. Thus the term PFS is used in this setting to refer to the time to disease worsening in the advanced disease setting. In a patient with a complete surgical resection (as judged by standard surgical and pathological parameters), the event of interest is recurrence of disease. Thus in the adjuvant setting the term is DFS, measuring the time from surgery (or start of chemotherapy or randomization, depending on the study) to disease recurrence.

PFS/DFS, and OS, which will follow, are known as time-to-event endpoints. In a typical clinical trial, there is an accrual period plus an additional follow-up time prior to analysis of the data. At the time of the final analysis, some patients will have had the event of interest (a progression, for example), while some patients will remain event free. For those who remain event free, the total time of observations will vary, depending upon when in the accrual period the patient was registered to the trial. The actual event time for these patients is unknown, but it is known that they were event free at least from registration until the date of their last known contact. The event times for these patients whose events have not occurred at the time of analysis are referred to as being "censored." The Kaplan–Meier method (product-limit estimate) (18) is the most common method used to estimate time-to-event endpoints in clinical trials in the presence of censoring. For both endpoints of PFS and DFS, a death from any cause is considered an event, to remove any possible bias due to unknown disease status at death. Currently, PFS is increasingly being used as the primary endpoint for both phase II and phase III trials in advanced disease such as in renal and breast cancer, and DFS is increasingly being used as a primary endpoint in adjuvant phase III trials. Here we discuss advantages and challenges with these endpoints.

Because PFS requires a consistent definition as to what constitutes disease progression, similarly to response rate, this endpoint does depend on imaging techniques. However, the imaging subtleties for PFS are much less problematic than for the response endpoint, which requires agreement on definitions of what constitutes clinically important tumor shrinkage as well as what constitutes tumor progression. A more important advantage to PFS and DFS is that these endpoints are not affected by therapies administered subsequent to the therapy under study. In disease settings in which there are clearly beneficial therapies that may be administered subsequent to the interventional therapy, PFS/DFS provide an assessment that can isolate the effect of the specific intervention being tested. In contrast, OS is impacted by both the therapy in the specific trial as well as any therapies the patient may subsequently receive (19).

The use of PFS/DFS as an endpoint presents several practical and methodological challenges. First, if a patient is taken off protocol treatment (e.g., due to toxicity or refusal), other nonprotocol specified anticancer therapy may be initiated, which could impact the occurrence and timing of subsequent progression. To avoid ambiguity in the final analysis, specific rules as to whether PFS/DFS should include the subsequent progression as an event or censor at the time of the nonprotocol anticancer treatment is initiated should be prespecified in a protocol. Second, some patients stop treatment and/or follow-up due to symptomatic worsening, with no radiologic confirmation of progression. The method of analysis for such clinical progressions must also be prospectively specified. Additional items that must be considered when using a PFS or DFS endpoint include the necessity that the assessment frequency is identical between the treatment arms (20), and the possible need for confirmation of a tumor progression by an independent radiology review (21). Such an independent review might increase the confidence in a PFS endpoint, but may also complicate the statistical analysis due to informative censoring (22). These issues have potential major consequences; see Saltz et al. (23) for an example of analysis when seemingly subtle differences in censoring definitions or scan timings have had a major impact on trial conclusions. These and other examples demonstrate the need for careful sensitivity analyses when PFS or DFS is used as a primary endpoint. Finally, the clinical relevance of minor PFS differences remains questionable.

The clinical relevance of PFS/DFS as an endpoint for phase III studies has been the subject of debate. Indeed, detection of progression or recurrence is typically based on radiologic measurements, as opposed to increase in patient symptoms; thus it may not be considered directly relevant to patient well-being. However, based on current knowledge, progression or recurrence is clearly a signal of increasing disease burden at the patient level, and also results in substantial additional, most likely toxic, therapy. The Food and Drug Administration (FDA) has recently approved multiple agents (e.g., bevacizumab in breast cancer [(24)], sorafenib in renal cancer [(25)], and gemcitabine in second-line ovarian cancer [(26)]) based on an improvement in PFS in spite of no improvement in OS. In the setting of adjuvant colon cancer, the Oncologic Drugs Advisory Committee (ODAC) of the FDA voted unanimously that DFS was an endpoint of clinical relevance regardless of its surrogacy with OS (27).

Overall Survival

OS is defined as the time from study registration to time of death due to any cause. OS had historically been the primary outcome for most phase III trials, and some phase II trials. The virtues of OS as a clinical trial endpoint are clear. OS is simple to measure, unambiguous, and of unquestionable clinical relevance. It is the endpoint least susceptible to investigator bias. It is also very noninvasive and cost-effective to collect in a trial database (requiring no special scans), and often can be determined through searches of public databases even if a patient does not return to the trial institution.

In spite of these many advantages, modern phase III clinical trials are increasingly moving away from OS as a primary endpoint. Because mortality occurs after a relatively long time in many disease settings, statistically significant differences in OS require large numbers of patients and several years to reliably detect. For example, in a trial where women with metastatic breast cancer were randomized to receive bevacizumab or not in addition to first-line paclitaxel, the survival data for the trial population were not mature until nearly 8 years after the trial was opened—a full 2 years after initial results, based on a PFS endpoint, were made public (24).

For reasons discussed previously regarding the advantages of PFS/DFS as an endpoint, OS may also be insensitive to a true effect of a new therapy. For many new agents, patients assigned to the control arm are either allowed to cross over to the investigational agent, or receive the investigational agent off-study upon disease progression or recurrence. This strategy dilutes the difference between arms of an agent on OS, since patients in both arms will receive the new agent at some point. Although a prohibition of such crossover is scientifically appealing, ethical considerations, particularly if earlier trials have found the agent to be promising or the drug is approved in later line settings, often preclude it. For example, consider the case of two trials of similar drugs—cetuximab (28) and panitumumab (29)—in last-line colorectal cancer. In both trials, the agent under study provided a highly significant improvement in patient PFS. In the trial that allowed patients to cross over from best supportive care to active drug after disease progression, 75% did cross over, and no survival improvement was detected (29). In the other trial no crossover was allowed, and in that trial the PFS advantage translated into a significant survival advantage (28).

OS is also challenging as an endpoint because of the prolongation of OS as a result of many antineoplastic therapies now available. In the case of breast cancer, over the past few decades, OS has increased substantially for patients with metastatic disease. For example, in retrospective population-based analysis of patients with metastatic breast cancer treated in British Columbia, OS improved from approximately 14.5 months for those diagnosed in 1991 to approximately 22 months for women diagnosed in 2001 (30). As median survival continues to increase, the sample size necessary to conclusively identify the same absolute improvement in survival increases considerably, as the same 3-month absolute improvement results in a hazard ratio closer to unity as the control arm survival increases.

Additional challenges with OS as an endpoint are due to a long survival in some cancer patients. While OS is generally the most easily assessed endpoint, high uncertainty and/or bias can result when there are many patients for whom OS status is unknown. Patients on advanced disease studies may go elsewhere if they are not doing well; thus the survival estimate will be biased high if patients are lost to follow-up because they are beginning to fail. Patients on early-stage trials who remain disease free for many years may not return to the clinic for appointments; in this case, the survival estimate may be biased low. If most patients are still alive at the time of analysis, survival estimates can be highly variable, or not even defined. Finally, if many patients die of causes other than the cancer under the study, the interpretation of survival can be problematic, since the effect of treatment on the disease under study is of primary interest.

Despite these limitations, due to the simplicity and clear relevance of the OS endpoint, if feasible, OS should be the preferred endpoint for phase III trials. In addition, in phase II trials where death occurs quickly and imaging is problematic, OS may be an appropriate endpoint.

Quality of Life

QOL, typically measured through patient self-assessment, is an important outcome in the evaluation of the net benefit of antineoplastic therapies, particularly when the impact of treatment in terms of survival is expected to be small. QOL has mainly been included as a secondary endpoint in randomized phase III studies. QOL evaluations are not generally included in single-arm phase II trials primarily due to relatively small sample size and the absence of comparison groups. On the other hand, in randomized phase II studies that if successful will lead to a phase III trial where QOL will be regarded as an important outcome, QOL assessment should be included during the phase II study to assess feasibility, to possibly choose a most appropriate instrument, and to obtain a preliminary estimate of effect size. Extensive documentation on the use of QOL as an endpoint in cancer trials has recently been published (31). The topic of patient-related outcomes is covered in detail in Chapters 19 and 25 of this book.

NEW ENDPOINTS FOR EFFICACY

As the science of cancer research continues to rapidly expand, novel measurements may become increasingly relevant as endpoints for all phases of cancer trials. These endpoints include measures of the functional status of tumors by imaging (PET), measures of circulating tumor cells in blood, tumor-specific biomarkers such as prostate-specific antigen (PSA) for prostate cancer or CA-125 in ovarian cancer, or biological measures of target inhibition of a targeted therapy. While these endpoints are indeed promising, and offer the potential to speed clinical development of new agents, many issues remain with all of them prior to their appropriate use as primary endpoints. These include practical issues such as feasibility, accuracy issues such as test/retest variability, and surrogacy issues related to the ability of the endpoint to predict clinically relevant phenomena. Careful assessment of these endpoints, using the principles outlined in this chapter, should facilitate their evaluation regarding their optimal use as trial endpoints.

REFERENCES

1. Prentice RL. Surrogate endpoints in clinical trials: definition and operational criteria. *Stat Medicine*. 1989;8:431–440.
2. Fleming TR, DeMets DL. Surrogate end points in clinical trials: are we being misled? *Ann Intern Med*. 1996;125(7): 605–613.
3. Buyse, M. Statistical Evaluation of Surrogate Endpoints in Cancer Clinical Trials. *Oncology Clinical Trials: Successful Design, Conduct, and Analysis*.
4. Gelmon KA, Eisenhauer EA, Harris AL, et al. Anticancer agents targeting signaling molecules and cancer cell environment: challenges for drug development? *J Natl Cancer Inst*. 1999;91(15):1281–1287.
5. Korn EL, Arbuck SG, Pluda JM, et al. Clinical trial designs for cytostatic agents: are new approaches needed? *J Clin Oncol*. 2001;19:265–272.
6. Zhang W, Sargent DJ, Mandrekar S. An adaptive dose-finding design incorporating both toxicity and efficacy. *Stat Med*. 2006;25(14):2365–2383.
7. Therasse P, Arbuck SG, Eisenhauer EA, et al. New guidelines to evaluate the response to treatment in solid tumors. *J Natl Cancer Inst*. 2000;92(3):205–216.
8. Eisenhauer EA, Therasse P, Bogaert J, et al. New response evaluation criteria in solid tumors: revised RECIST guideline (version 1.1). *Eur J Cancer*. 2009; 45(2):228–247.
9. Ratain MJ. Phase II studies of modern drugs directed against new targets: if you are fazed, too, then resist RECIST. *J Clin Oncol*. 2004;22:4442–4445.
10. Buyse M, Thirion P, Carlson RW, et al. Relation between tumour response to first-line chemotherapy and survival in advanced colorectal cancer: a meta-analysis. *Lancet*. 2000;356:373–378.
11. Dowlati A, Fu P. Is response rate relevant to the Phase II trial design of targeted agents? *J Clin Oncol*. 2008;26:1204–1205.
12. Yang JC, Haworth L, Sherry RM, et al. A randomized trial of bevacizumab, an anti-vascular endothelial growth factor anti-body, for metastatic renal cancer. *N Engl J Med*. 2003;349:427–434.
13. Macdonald DR, Cascino TL, Schold SC Jr, Cairncross JG. Response criteria for Phase II studies of supratentorial malignant glioma. *J Clin Oncol*. 1990;8:1277–1280.
14. Rajan B, Ross G, Lim CC, et al. Survival in patients with recurrent gliomas as a measure of treatment efficacy: prognostic factors following nitrosourea chemotherapy. *Eur J Cancer*.1994;30A:1809–1815.
15. Wolchok JD, Hoos A, Bohnsack O, et.al., Guidelines for the evaluation of immune therapy activity in solid tumors: immune-related response criteria, *Clin Cancer Res*. 2009;15(23):7412–7420.
16. Nishino M, Giobbie-Hurder A, Gargano M, et al. Developing a common language for tumor response to immunotherapy: immune-related response criteria using unidimensional measurements. *Clin Cancer Res*. 2013;19(14):3936–3943.
17. Bohnsack O, Ludajic K, Hoos A. Adaptation of the immune-related response criteria: irRECIST. *ESMO*. 2014;(abstract 4958).
18. Kaplan EL, Meier P. Nonparametric estimation from incomplete observations. *J Am Stat Assoc*. 1958;53:457–481.
19. Sargent DJ, Hayes DF. Assessing the measure of a new drug: is survival the only thing that matters? *J Clin Oncol*. 2008;26(12):1922–1923.
20. Panageas KS, Ben-Porat L, Dickler MN, et al. When you look matters: the effect of assessment schedule on progression-free survival. *J Natl Cancer Inst*. 2007;99:428–432.
21. Food and Drug Administration. Guidance for industry: clinical trial endpoints for the approval of cancer drugs and biologics. 2007. http://www.fda.gov/downloads/Drugs/GuidanceComplianceRegulatoryInformation/Guidances/UCM071590.pdf

22. Dodd LE, Korn EL, Freidlin B, et al. Blinded independent central review of progression-free survival in Phase III clinical trials: important design element or unnecessary expense? *J Clin Oncol.* 2008;26(22):3791–3796.

23. Saltz LB, Clarke S, Diaz-Rubio E. Bevacizumab in combination with oxaliplatin-based chemotherapy as first-line therapy in metastatic colorectal cancer: a randomized Phase III study. *J Clin Oncol.* 2008; 26(12):2013–2019.

24. Miller K, Wang M, Gralow J, et al. Paclitaxel plus bevacizumab versus paclitaxel alone for metastatic breast cancer. *N Engl J Med.* 2007;357:2666–2676.

25. Escudier B, Eisen T, Stadler WM, et al. Sorafenib in advanced clear-cell renal-cell carcinoma. *N Engl J Med.* 2007;356:125–134.

26. Pfisterer J, Plante M, Vergote I, et al. Gemcitabine plus carboplatin compared with carboplatin in patients with platinum-sensitive recurrent ovarian cancer: an intergroup trial of the AGO-OVAR, the NCIC CTG, and the EORTC GCG. *J Clin Oncol.* 2006;24(29):4699–4707.

27. Department of Health and Human Services, Food and Drug Administration, Center for Drug Evaluation and Research. Oncologic drugs advisory committee. May 2004. http://www.fda.gov/ohrms/dockets/ac/04/transcripts/4037T2.htm

28. Jonker DJ, O'Callaghan CJ, Karapetis CS, et al. Cetuximab for the treatment of colorectal cancer. *N Engl J Med.* 2007;357:2040–2048.

29. Van Cutsem E, Peeters M, Siena S. Open-label Phase III trial of panitumumab plus best supportive care compared with best supportive care alone in patients with chemotherapy-refractory metastatic colorectal cancer. *J Clin Oncol.* 2007;25:1658–1664.

30. Chia SK, Speers CH, D'yachkova Y, et al. The impact of new chemotherapeutic and hormone agents on survival in a population-based cohort of women with metastatic breast cancer. *Cancer.* 2007;110(5):973–979.

31. Sloan JA, Halyard MY, Frost MH, et al. The Mayo Clinic manuscript series relative to the discussion, dissemination, and operationalization of the Food and Drug Administration guidance on patient-reported outcomes. *Value Health.* 2007;10(Suppl 2):S59–S63.

9

Design, Testing, and Estimation in Clinical Trials

Barry Kurt Moser

After a cancer clinical trial has been well designed, hypothesis testing and parameter estimation are the two most important statistical aspects of any study. Within this chapter several clinical trial design and test approaches are discussed including a one-stage binomial design to test the proportion of one population, Simon's (1) two-stage optimal design to test the proportion of one population, a design to test the difference in means from two correlated normally distributed populations, and optimal designs to test the differences in time-to-event survival functions from two independent populations (2,3). Commonly used estimation procedures are then highlighted and include: a Bayesian posterior distribution to estimate the mean of a binomial population; a Bayesian credible region on a population proportion (4); a maximum likelihood binomial estimate of a population proportion; a standard normal approximation of a $100(1 - a)\%$ confidence interval on a population proportion; mean difference, variance, and correlation estimates from two correlated normally distributed populations (5); a confidence interval on the mean difference from two correlated normally distributed populations; a log-rank test for comparing the survival curves from two independent populations (6); and confidence intervals on a survival function.

DESIGN, HYPOTHESIS TESTS, AND ESTIMATION PROCEDURES

The single most important aspect of a clinical trial is the design stage. If the trial is well designed to address the questions of interest the study has the best chance of producing interpretable and meaningful results. Note that the trial should be fully designed before any patients are registered to the trial and thus before any analysis is performed on observed data. The results of a poorly

designed trial are open to criticism due to such problems as bias, poorly defined hypotheses, sample size and power inadequacies, confounding, and other difficulties. A sound design promotes (a) well-chosen and worded objectives, (b) careful selection of endpoints, (c) hypotheses that directly address the objectives, (d) properly selected hypothesis testing and estimation procedures, (e) sample size calculations that provide sufficient power to successfully address a level hypothesis test decisions, and when needed (f) randomization schemes that help clearly answer the objectives.

In the following segments of this chapter, three phase II and two phase III cancer clinical studies are discussed. Appropriate trial designs are formulated, hypothesis tests are developed and illustrated, and estimation procedures are explained numerically.

Example 1: A Randomized Phase II Trial of Eicosanoid Pathway Modulators and Cytotoxic Chemotherapy in Advanced Non–Small-Cell Lung Cancer

Discussion
The primary objective of the trial was to evaluate the efficacy of carboplatin/gemcitabine with one or two modulators of eicosanoid metabolism (celecoxib, zileuton, or both) for the treatment of patients with advanced non–small-cell lung cancer (7). The primary endpoint was the proportion of patients alive without disease progression 9 months after treatment initiation (failure-free survival). Although patients in this trial were randomized to the three arms, the objective of the study is not to compare the three arms. Rather, each treatment was examined separately to see if it merits inclusion in a larger phase III trial.

Design and Hypothesis Test
Since the three treatment arms are analyzed separately the following discussion applies to any of them. If the

failure-free survival rate at 9 months was less than 30% there would be little interest in developing the treatment regimen further. However, if the failure-free survival rate at 9 months was 50% or greater then future treatment development would be of interest. Formally, this comparison can be written as the hypotheses: $H_0: p \leq p_0$ versus $H_1: p \geq p_1$, where p is the failure-free survival rate of the population at 9 months for any of the treatment arms, $p_0 = .30$ and $p_1 = .50$. The objective is to define a design (a test criterion and sample size) that produces a type I error rate less than or equal to a and a type II error rate less than or equal to β ($a = \beta = .10$ in this trial), where the type I error is calculated as the probability of incorrectly concluding that $p = .50$ when $p = .30$ and the type II error is calculated as the probability of incorrectly concluding that $p = .30$ when $p = .50$. The test criterion takes the form: if fewer than x^* of the n patients achieve failure-free survival at 9 months then the treatment regimen will not merit further study. But if x^* or more of the n patients achieve failure-free survival at 9 months then the treatment regimen will merit further study. Formally stated,

Reject $H_0: p \leq .30$ in favor of $H_1: p \geq .50$
if $X \geq x^*$, (Eq. 9-1)

where X is a random variable representing the number of failure-free survivors at 9 months in a sample of size n and x^* is the critical cutoff point. Note that H_0 is rejected in favor of H_1 and the treatment regimen is worthy of further study if the number of observed failure-free survivors X is large (larger than the critical value x^*). Formally, we seek the minimum value of n, where there exists a value of x^* such that:

Type I error requirement: $P(X \geq x^* \mid n, p = .3)$
$\leq = .1$ and (Eq. 9-2)

Type II error requirement: $P(X < x^* \mid n, p = .5)$
$\leq \beta = .1$.

Specifically, for increasing values of n the two probabilities in (Eq. 9-2) are calculated for increasing values of $0 \leq x^* \leq n$ until the first x^*, n pair meets the preceding type I and type II requirements. In this case, for $n = 39$ if $X \geq 16$ ($x^* = 16$ or more failure-free survivors out of 39 patients) then H_0 is rejected in favor of H_1 and the treatment regimen has sufficient merit to deserve further study. This test procedure produces type I and type II error rates equal to .094 and .099, respectively.

Testing, Estimation, and Confidence Intervals
We examine the results of the trial for the third arm where the regimen consists of carboplatin/gemcitabine with both modulators celecoxib and zileuton. Although the design called for 39 patients a total of 45 eligible patients were enrolled in the third arm. With 45 patients a test criterion: reject $H_0: p \leq .30$ in favor of $H_1: p \geq .50$

if $X \geq 18$ provides a type I error rate equal to .099 and a type II error rate equal to .068.

After $n = 45$ eligible patients were enrolled and observed for 9 months the number of failure-free survivors in the third arm was $x = 11$ (7). Since $x = 11 < 18$ the treatment regimen does not have sufficient merit to deserve further study.

Using a Bayesian approach, a $100(1 - a)\%$ credible region (8) on p can be constructed through the posterior distribution of binomial distribution using a noninformative uniform prior. Given the observed failure-free survivors x the parameter p has a Beta($x + 1, n - x + 1$) posterior distribution, whose functional form is given by:

$$f(p \mid x, n) = \frac{\Gamma(n + 2)}{\Gamma(x + 1)\Gamma(n - x + 1)} p^x (1 - p)^{n - x} \quad \text{(Eq. 9-3)}$$
for $0 \leq x \leq n, 0 \leq p \leq 1$.

The Bayesian estimator of p is provided by the posterior mean

$$\hat{p}_B = (x + 1) / (n + 2) \quad \text{(Eq. 9-4)}$$

For $n = 45$ and $x = 11$, $\hat{p}_B = 12 / 47$. A graph of the Beta ($x + 1, n - x + 1$) = Beta(12,35) distribution is provided in Figure 9.1.

The $100(1 - a)$ credible region is then the interval (p_L, p_U) such that:

$$1 - a = \int_{p_L}^{p_U} f(p \mid n, x) dp, \quad \text{(Eq. 9-5)}$$

where $f(p \mid n, x)$ is given in (Eq. 9-3). Using (Eq. 9-5) for $n = 45$, $x = 11$, and $a = .05$ a 95% credible region on p is given by $(p_L, p_U) = (.133, .377)$ and presented in Figure 9.1. These lower and upper bounds of the credible region are constructed so that they are equidistant from the posterior mean $\hat{p}_B$, where the area between the bounds under the posterior equals $(1 - a)$. Alternatively, $100(1 - a)\%$ credible region bounds can be constructed

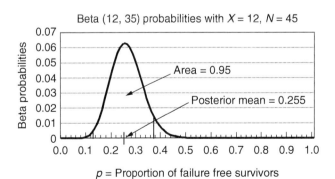

FIGURE 9.1 A credible region on the parameter p = the proportion of failure-free survivors from a Beta(12,35) distribution.

so that the areas under the posterior to the right of the lower bound and to the left of the upper bound each equal $a/2$.

For large samples another approach for constructing a $100(1 - a)\%$ confidence interval on p is to use the normal approximation to the binomial distribution. For the binomial distribution an unbiased estimate of p is given by:

$$\hat{p} = x / n. \qquad \text{(Eq. 9-6)}$$

A simple formula for the $100(1 - a)\%$ confidence interval is then provided by:

$$p_L = \hat{p} - z_{a/2}\sqrt{\hat{p}(1-\hat{p})/n}, \ p_U = \hat{p} + z_{a/2}\sqrt{\hat{p}(1-\hat{p})/n},$$
$$\text{(Eq. 9-7)}$$

where z_γ is the $100(1 - \gamma)$ percentile value of a standard normal distribution. Using the large sample normal approximation from (Eq. 9-6) and (Eq. 9-7) with $n = 45$, $\hat{p} = 11/45$, and $a = .05$, a 95% confidence interval on p is given by:

$$p_L = 11/45 - 1.96\sqrt{(11/45)[1-(11/45)]/45} = .119$$
$$\text{(Eq. 9-8)}$$

$$p_U = 11/45 + 1.96\sqrt{(11/45)[1-(11/45)]/45} = .370.$$

Example 2: A Nonrandomized Phase II Trial of Gemtuzumab Ozogamicin (Mylotarg) With High-Dose Cytarabine in Patients With Refractory or Relapsed Acute Myeloid Leukemia (AML)

Discussion

The primary objective of the trial was to determine the adequacy of the complete remission rate with complete platelet recovery (complete remission [CR]) or without complete platelet recovery (partial remission [CRp]) when gemtuzumab ozogamicin was administered in two weekly doses following a standard high-dose cytarabine course in patients with refractory or relapse AML. The primary endpoint was the CR + CRp rate.

Design and Hypothesis Test

If the complete remission rate with or without platelet recovery was less than 15% there would be little interest in developing the treatment regimen further. However, if the complete remission rate with or without platelet recovery was 35% or greater then future treatment development would be of interest. Formally, this comparison can be written as the hypotheses: $H_0: p \leq p_0$ versus $H_1: p \leq p_1$, where p is the complete remission rate with or without platelet recovery, $p_0 = .15$ and $p_1 = .35$. In Example 1, a test criterion was developed for a similar hypothesis using one sample of size n. That is, all n

patients had to be observed before an efficacy decision on the treatment could be made. However, historically, most drug regimens that are tested in a phase II setting fail to demonstrate sufficient efficacy to merit further study. For this reason, Simon (1) developed a two-stage phase II procedure whereby the trial can be terminated after the first stage if early results indicated that the treatment is not worthy of further study, thereby eliminating the need to administer ineffective treatment regimens to all n patients before making a conclusion. The two-stage test criterion takes the form:

1. Observe n_1 patients and terminate the trial if r_1 or fewer responses occur.
2. If more than r_1 of the first n_1 patients achieve a response, observe n_2 more patients ($n = n_1 + n_2$) and if r or fewer responses occur out of the total sample of n patients then the treatment regimen does not merit further study. But if more than r of the n patients sampled achieve a response then the treatment regimen merits further study.

The optimal design is chosen to minimize the expected sample size when the response rate equals p_0, for specified values of p_0, p_1, a, β. The probability of terminating the trial early (PET) given a response rate p is given by:

$$PET = \sum_{i=0}^{r_1} p^{r_1}(1-p)^{n_1 - r_1}. \qquad \text{(Eq. 9-9)}$$

Therefore, the expected sample size

$$EN = n_1 PET + (1 - PET)n. \qquad \text{(Eq. 9-10)}$$

For a given test criterion to calculate the expected sample size when the response equals p_0 simply replace p by p_0 in (Eq. 9-9) to calculate PET and then calculate EN as a function of PET, n_1, and n in (Eq. 9-10). Simon's optimal two-stage procedure cannot be developed through a closed-form equation but must be calculated iteratively through a computer program. A website that provides a program to calculate the optimal design as a function of a, β, p_0, p_1 is https://brb.nci.nih.gov/brb/samplesize/otsd.html. For Example 2 with $p_0 = .15$, $p_1 = .35$, $a = \beta = .1$ the optimal Simon two-stage procedure is:

1. Observe $n_1 = 19$ patients and terminate the trial if $r_1 = 3$ or fewer responses occur.
2. If more than $r_1 = 3$ of the first $n_1 = 19$ patients achieve responses, observe $n_2 = 14$ more patients ($n = 19 + 14 = 33$) and if $r = 7$ or fewer responses occur out of the total sample of $n = 33$ patients then the treatment regimen does not merit further study. But if more than $r = 7$ of the $n = 33$ patients sampled achieve a response then the treatment regimen merits further study.

With $r = 3$, $n_1 = 19$, and $p = p_0 = .15$ from (Eq. 9-9) and (Eq. 9-10) the probability of terminating the trial early and the expected sample size are given by: $PET = .684$ and $EN = 19 + (1 - .684)14 = 23.4$. The exact type I and type II error rates for this design are .096 and .096, respectively.

Simply for comparison purposes, a one-stage design to test $H_0: p \leq .15$ versus $H_1: p \geq .35$ with $a = \beta = .1$ requires a sample of $n = 32$ and if 7 or fewer responses occur out of the total sample of $n = 32$ patients then the treatment regimen does not merit further study. But if more than 8 of the $n = 32$ patients sampled achieve a response then the treatment regimen merits further study. The exact type I and type II error rates for this design are .096 and .082, respectively. Note that in this case the one-stage and two-stage designs require almost the exact total sample size $n = 32$ (and 32). The advantage of the one-stage design is that it provides slightly smaller type II error (i.e., slightly higher power) than the two-stage design. However, if H_0 is true then the two-stage design is more efficient than the one-stage design, stopping early and correctly concluding the treatment does not merit further study with probability .684, resulting in an expected sample size of 23.4 patients versus a required 32 patients in the one-stage design.

Testing, Estimation, and Confidence Intervals

During the course of the two-stage trial 6 of the first 19 eligible patients achieved CR or CRp. Therefore, the trial did continue and 14 more eligible patients were enrolled to the trial. Of those next 14 patients 4 achieved CR or CRp, for a total of 10 (= 6 + 4) out of 33 responders (9). Therefore, at least 8 of the first 33 patients were responders and according to the original test criteria the treatment regimen merits further study.

From (Eq. 9-4) a Bayesian estimate of the proportion of CR + CRp patients in the population is $\hat{p}_B = (x + 1)/(n + 2) = 11/35$. Then from (Eq. 9-5) for $n = 33$, $x = 10$, and $a = .05$, a 95% credible region on p is given by $(p_L, p_U) = (.164, .464)$.

Using the large sample normal approximation from (Eq. 9-7) with $\hat{p} = 10/33$ and $a = .05$, a 95% confidence interval on p is given by $(p_L, p_U) = (.146, .460)$.

Example 3: A Phase II Trial of Thalidomide for Patients With Relapsed or Refractory Low-Grade Non-Hodgkin's Lymphoma

Discussion

A secondary objective of the trial was to determine the effect of thalidomide on microvessel density. Antiangiogenesis effects were measured by the mean change in microvessel density between pre and posttreatment time points.

Design and Hypothesis Test

Antiangiogenesis effects were estimated by the mean observed change in microvessel density between pre and posttreatment (6 months) time points on $n = 45$ patients. Based on preliminary data a standard deviation of $\sigma = 17.5$ microvessels per mm^2 was anticipated. Since the microvessel data were observed at pre- and post-times on each patient it was assumed that these 45 pairs of pre- and postmeasurements were equally correlated with a correlation denoted by p. The population pre- and posttreatment microvessel density means are denoted by μ_1 and μ_2. Therefore, it was of interest to produce a two-sided a level test on the hypothesis that no detectable mean difference exists between the pre- and post-micro-vessel densities versus that a detectable difference does exist. Formally, this comparison can be written as the hypotheses: $H_0: \mu_1 - \mu_2 = 0$ versus $H_1: \mu_1 - \mu_2 \neq 0$. For any value of p, σ, n the two-sided a level test criterion takes the form:

Reject $H_0: \mu_1 - \mu_2 = 0$ in favor of $H_1: \mu_1 - \mu_2 \neq 0$
if $|\bar{y}_1 - \bar{y}_2| \geq z_{a/2} \, \hat{\sigma}\sqrt{2(1 - \hat{p})/n}$ (Eq. 9-11)

where $\bar{y}_1$ and $\bar{y}_2$ are the observed mean pre- and post-micro-vessel densities for the n patients. If it is of interest to provide a p value rather than an a level test criterion then the p value of the two-sided test is given by:

$$p \text{ value} = 2P\left[N(0,1) > \frac{|\bar{y}_1 - \bar{y}_2|}{\hat{\sigma}\sqrt{2(1 - \hat{p})/n}}\right] \quad (\text{Eq. 9-12})$$

or equivalently,

$$p \text{ value} = P\left[F_{1,n-1} > \frac{MS(\text{Pre/Post})}{MS(\text{Patient*Pre/Post})}\right],$$

where $MS(\text{Pre/Post})$ and $MS(\text{Patient*Pre/Post})$ are the analysis of variance (ANOVA) mean square due to the pre-/posteffect and the mean square due to interaction of patients by the pre-/posteffect, respectively. For any detectable absolute difference under the alternative hypothesis $|\mu_1 - \mu_2| = \delta > 0$ the power of the (Eq. 9-11) procedure is given by:

$$\text{power} = 1 - P\left[N(0,1) < z_{a/2} - \frac{\delta}{\sigma\sqrt{2(1 - p)/n}}\right].$$
$$(\text{Eq. 9-13})$$

Table 9.1 provides powers for various correlations p and mean detectable differences δ given $a = .05$, $n = .05$, and $\sigma = 17.5$.

The sample size of $n = 45$ for this trial was set to accommodate the power calculations of the primary objective of the study, not to accommodate the power calculations of the microvessel density analysis, which was a secondary objective. However, by solving (Eq. 9-13) for n it is possible to calculate the sample size

TABLE 9.1 Powers Associated With the Two-Sided σ Level Test Procedure (Eq. 9-11) for Various Mean Detectable Differences δ and Correlations p Given $a = 0.05$, $n = 45$, and $\sigma = 17.5$

Correlation p	Absolute Mean Detectable Difference δ			
	5	7	9	11
0	.273	.298	.483	.858
.1	.475	.516	.765	.989
.5	.684	.730	.932	>.999
.8	.847	.882	.988	>.999

required to attain a specified power for an a level two-sided test for the hypothesis $H_0: \mu_1 - \mu_2 = 0$ versus $H_1: \mu_1 - \mu_2 \neq 0$ for a specified correlation p. The resulting equation is:

$$n = \frac{2\sigma^2(1-p)(z_{a/2} + z_\beta)}{\delta^2}, \qquad \text{(Eq. 9-14)}$$

where the specified power equals $1 - \beta$. From (Eq. 9-14) for an $a = .05$ two-sided test of $H_0: \mu_1 - \mu_2 = 0$ versus $H_1: \mu_1 - \mu_2 \neq 0$ with $\sigma = 17.5$ the sample size required to achieve a power of .80 is provided in Table 9.2 for various absolute mean detectable differences δ and correlations p.

For a one-sided a level test where the alternative hypothesis is either $H_0: \mu_1 - \mu_2 > 0$ or $H_1: \mu_1 - \mu_2 < 0$ equations (Eq. 9-13) and (Eq. 9-14) still hold provided $a/2$ is replaced by a and δ continues to represent the absolute difference $|\mu_1 - \mu_2| = \delta > 0$ under the alternative hypothesis. Note that under a normal distribution assumption the test criterion (Eq. 9-11), the p value (Eq. 9-12), the power function (Eq. 9-13), and the sample size function (Eq. 9-14) can also be applied to two independent samples by setting $p = 0$.

Testing, Estimation, and Confidence Intervals
Although this trial closed due to poor accrual, Table 9.3 provides simulated pre- and post-micro-vessel density data for 45 patients.

The observed mean difference between the post- and pre-micro-vessel density averaged over the 45 patients was $\bar{y}_1 - \bar{y}_2 = 61.13 - 57.33 = 3.8$. The ANOVA mean square for the patients' effect with 44 degrees of freedom was 426.7, the ANOVA mean square due to the pre-/post-time effect with 1 degree of freedom was 324.9, and the ANOVA mean square due to the patient by pre-/post-time interaction effect with 44 degrees of freedom was 135.3. The mean square due to patients and the mean square due to the patient by pre-/post-time interaction are ANOVA estimates of $\sigma^2(1 + p)$ and $\sigma^2(1 - p)$, respectively. Setting the $\sigma^2(1 + p)$ equal to 426.7 and $\sigma^2(1 - p)$ equal to 135.3 and solving for σ^2, p we obtain $\hat{\sigma}^2 = 281.3 (\hat{\sigma} = 16.772)$ and $p = .519$. Therefore the p value of the test on $H_0: \mu_1 - \mu_2 = 0$ versus $H_1: \mu_1 - \mu_2 \neq 0$ equals:

$$p \text{ value} = 2P\left[N(0,1) > \frac{|3.8|}{16.772 \cdot \sqrt{2 \cdot (1 - .519)/45}}\right]$$
$$= 2P[N(0,1) > 1.56] = .12$$

$$\text{(Eq. 9-15)}$$

or equivalently

$$p \text{ value} = P\left[F_{1,n-1} > \frac{324.9}{135.3}\right] = P[F_{1,n-1} > 2.4] = .12.$$

TABLE 9.2 Sample Sizes (n) Required to Attain a Power of .80 Associated With the Two-Sided Hypothesis Test (Eq. 9-12) for Various Mean Detectable Differences δ and Correlations p Given $a = .05$ and $\sigma = 17.5$

Correlation p	Absolute Mean Detectable Difference δ			
	5	7	9	11
0	192	173	96	38
.1	98	88	49	20
.5	59	53	30	12
.8	40	36	20	8

TABLE 9.3 Pre- and Posttreatment Microvessel Density Simulated Data on 45 Patients

Patient	1	2	3	4	5	6	7	8	9	10	11	12	13	14	15
Pre	64	59	52	70	81	64	28	72	29	68	67	38	110	43	57
Post	36	67	72	78	64	56	42	75	56	50	66	46	68	62	39

Patient	16	17	18	19	20	21	22	23	24	25	26	27	28	29	30
Pre	47	53	60	54	56	72	83	70	67	40	27	71	70	40	89
Post	13	44	47	45	99	89	73	65	64	33	43	64	57	54	57

Patient	31	32	33	34	35	36	37	38	39	40	41	42	43	44	45
Pre	78	52	71	73	55	55	57	61	63	58	49	70	56	104	48
Post	75	53	64	71	46	45	47	54	56	64	53	44	40	91	53

An unbiased estimate of the mean difference $\mu_1 - \mu_2$ is provided by $\bar{y}_1 - \bar{y}_2 = 3.8$. Furthermore, a $100(1 - a)\%$ confidence interval on $\mu_1 - \mu_2$ is given by:

$$\bar{y}_1 - \bar{y}_2 \pm z_{a/2}\hat{\sigma}\sqrt{2(1 - \hat{\rho})/n}. \qquad \text{(Eq. 9-16)}$$

For this example using (Eq. 9-16) 95% confidence bounds on $\mu_1 - \mu_2$ are given by $(-1.01, 8.61)$.

Example 4: A Randomized Phase III Trial of Gemcitabine Plus Bevacizumab Versus Gemcitabine Plus Placebo in Patients With Advanced Pancreatic Cancer

Discussion

The primary objective of the trial was to determine if gemcitabine plus bevacizumab achieved superior overall survival compared to gemcitabine plus placebo in patients with advanced pancreatic cancer. As a secondary objective the toxicity rates between the two treatment arms were compared.

Design and Hypothesis Test

To address the primary objective of comparing the overall survival of the two treatments the patients were randomized with equal probability to the treatment gemcitabine plus bevacizumab or gemcitabine plus placebo. The assumed total enrollment rate was 20 patients per month. For an $a = .05$ two-sided test the trial was powered to distinguish a difference in the survival curves of the two treatments when the median survival of the gemcitabine plus bevacizumab arm was 6 months and the median survival of the gemcitabine plus placebo arm was 8.1 months, producing a 1.35 hazard ratio under an exponential event time assumption. Using results from George and Desu

(2) and Rubenstein et al. (3) (calculated by a computer program DSTPLAN downloaded from http://biostatistics.mdanderson.org/SoftwareDownload/SingleSoftware.aspx?Software_Id=41) an enrollment of $n = 528$ patients was required with a 26.4-month enrollment period (at 20 patients enrolled/month) and a 12-month follow-up period to attain a 90% power to detect a hazard rate of 1.35 using a two-sided log-rank test. During the enrollment and follow-up period 470 events were expected.

The secondary objective of the trial was to test whether the toxicity rates of the two treatment arms were equal or differed by Δ or more, assuming the toxicity rate of the gemcitabine plus placebo treatment was .10. Formally, this comparison can be written as the hypotheses: $H_0: p_1 - p_2 = 0$ versus $H_1: p_1 - p_2 = \Delta > 0$, where p_1, p_2 are the population toxicity rates of the gemcitabine plus bevacizumab and gemcitabine plus placebo treatment, respectively. Since the sample sizes in each treatment arm are large an approximate normal arcsin transformation procedure was used to test the hypothesis. Under this assumption, $\arcsin\left(\sqrt{\hat{p}_1}\right)$, $\arcsin\left(\sqrt{\hat{p}_2}\right)$ are independent normal random variables with means $\arcsin\left(\sqrt{p_1}\right)$, $\arcsin\left(\sqrt{p_2}\right)$, and variances $1/(4n_1)$, $1/(4n_2)$, respectively, where n_1, n_2 are the sample sizes and $\hat{p}_1$, $\hat{p}_2$ are the observed toxicity rates for the gemcitabine plus bevacizumab and gemcitabine plus placebo, respectively. The criterion to test this hypothesis is:

Reject $H_0: p_1 - p_2 = 0$ in favor of $H_1: p_1 - p_2 = \Delta > 0$ if

$$\arcsin\left(\sqrt{\hat{p}_1}\right) - \arcsin\left(\sqrt{\hat{p}_2}\right) \geq z_a\sqrt{1/(4n_1) + 1/(4n_2)}.$$

(Eq. 9-17)

If it is of interest to provide a p value rather than an a level test criterion then the p value of the one-sided test is given by:

$$p \text{ value} = P\left[N(0,1) > \frac{\arcsin\sqrt{\hat{p}_1} - \arcsin\sqrt{\hat{p}_2}}{\sqrt{\frac{1}{4n_1} + \frac{1}{4n_2}}}\right].$$

(Eq. 9-18)

For any values of p_1, p_2 under H_1: $p_1 - p_2 = \Delta > 0$ the power of the (Eq. 9-17) procedure is given by:

$$Power = 1 - P\left[N(0,1) < z_a - \frac{\arcsin\left(\sqrt{p_1}\right) - \arcsin\left(\sqrt{p_2}\right)}{\sqrt{1/(4n_1) + 1/(4n_2)}}\right].$$

(Eq. 9-19)

From (Eq. 9-19), Table 9.4 provides powers for combinations of p_1 = .10, .20, .30, .40, and Δ = .08, .10, .12 for a one-sided a = .05 test with $n_1 = n_2 = n/2 = 264$.

The sample size of n = 528 for this trial was set to accommodate the power calculations of the primary objective of the study, not to accommodate the power calculations of the toxicity rate comparison, which was a secondary objective. However, for equal allocation to each treatment (i.e., $n_1 = n_2 = n/2$) it is possible from (Eq. 9-19) to calculate the sample size n required to attain

a specified power for an a level one-sided test for the hypothesis H_0: $p_1 - p_2 = 0$ versus H_1: $p_1 - p_2 = \Delta > 0$. The resulting equation is:

$$n = \frac{(z_a + z_\beta)^2}{\left[\arcsin\left(\sqrt{p_1}\right) - \arcsin\left(\sqrt{p_2}\right)\right]^2}$$

(Eq. 9-20)

where the specified power equals $1 - \beta$. So from (Eq. 9-20) for an a = .05 one-sided test of H_0: $p_1 - p_2 = 0$ versus H_1: $p_1 - p_2 = \Delta > 0$ the sample size required to achieve a power of .80 is provided in Table 9.5 for combinations of p_1 = .10, .20, .30, .40 and Δ = .08, .10, .12.

For a two-sided a level test where the alternative hypothesis is H_1: $p_1 - p_2 \neq 0$ equations (Eq. 9-19) and (Eq. 9-20) still hold provided $a/2$ is replaced by a and in (Eq. 9-19) $\arcsin(p_1) - \arcsin(p_2)$ is replaced by $|\arcsin(p_1) - \arcsin(p_2)|$.

Testing, Estimation, and Confidence Intervals

Testing and estimation of the primary endpoint overall survival is not examined for this example since the log-rank and Kaplan–Meier analysis procedure is examined in detail in Example 5. Instead, in this example we use the secondary objective to examine the difference in grade 4 and 5 maximum hematologic toxicity rates between the two treatment arms.

The number of patients with grade 4 and 5 hematologic toxic events (9) was x_1 = 30 and x_2 = 21 from samples of size n_1 = 263 and n_2 = 277 in the bevacizumab

TABLE 9.4 Powers Associated With the One-Sided a Level Test Procedure (Eq. 9-17) for Various Combinations of p_1 and $\Delta = p_1 - p_2$ for a = .05 and $n_1 = n_2 = n/2 = 264$

p_1	p_2	Power
.18	.10	.848
.20	.10	.947
.22	.10	.985
.28	.20	.696
.30	.20	.846
.32	.20	.935
.38	.30	.617
.40	.30	.779
.42	.30	.892
.48	.40	.583
.50	.40	.748
.52	.40	.870

TABLE 9.5 Sample Size Required to Attain a Power of .80 Associated With the One-Sided Hypothesis Test (Eq. 9-17) for Various Values of p_1 and p_2 given a = .05

p_1	p_2	n
.18	.10	456
.20	.10	307
.22	.10	223
.28	.20	700
.30	.20	460
.32	.20	326
.38	.30	864
.40	.30	560
.42	.30	393
.48	.40	950
.50	.40	610
.52	.40	424

and placebo arms, respectively. Therefore, the observed toxicity rates for the bevacizumab and placebo arms were $\hat{p}_1 = 30/263 = .1141$ and $\hat{p}_2 = 21/277 = .0758$. From (Eq. 9-18) the p value to test the one-sided hypothesis $H_0: p_1 - p_2 = 0$ versus $H_1: p_1 - p_2 = \Delta > 0$ is given by:

$$p \text{ value} = P\left[N(0,1) > \frac{\arcsin\sqrt{.1141} - \arcsin\sqrt{.00758}}{\sqrt{\frac{1}{4(263)} + \frac{1}{4(277)}}} \right]$$

$$= .0639.$$

(Eq. 9-21)

Example 5: A Randomized Phase III Trial of Induction (Daunorubicin/Cytarabine) and Consolidation (High-Dose Cytarabine) Plus Midostaurin or Placebo in Newly Diagnosed FLT3 Mutated AML Patients

Discussion

The primary objective of the trial was to determine if the addition of midostaurin to daunorubicin/cytarabine induction, high-dose cytarabine consolidation, and continuation therapy improves overall survival in mutant FLT3 AML patients. A secondary objective was to determine if the addition of midostaurin to daunorubicin/cytarabine induction, high-dose cytarabine consolidation, and continuation therapy improves disease-free survival (DFS) in mutant FLT3 AML patients.

Design and Hypothesis Test

To address the primary objective of comparing the overall survival of the two treatments in newly diagnosed FLT3 mutated AML patients, the patients were randomized with equal probability to the two treatments: (a) induction (daunorubicin/cytarabine) and consolidation (high-dose cytarabine) plus midostaurin and (b) induction (daunorubicin/cytarabine) and consolidation (high-dose cytarabine) plus placebo. A formal one-sided hypothesis to compare whether the midostaurin arm improves overall survival is: $H_0: \lambda = 1$ versus $H_0: \lambda > 1$, where λ is the hazard ratio of the two survival curves. Assuming exponential event times, $\lambda = m_M/m_P$, where m_M, m_P are the median survival times of the midostaurin and placebo patient populations, respectively.

The assumed total enrollment rate was 25 patients per month. For an $a = .05$ one-sided test the trial was powered to distinguish a difference in the survival curves of the two treatments when the median survival of the daunorubicin/cytarabine plus midostaurin arm was 21 months and the median survival of the daunorubicin/cytarabine plus placebo arm was 15 months, producing a 1.4 hazard ratio under an exponential event time assumption. Using results from George and Desu (2) and Rubenstein et al. (3) an enrollment of $n = 514$ patients

was required with a 20.5-month enrollment period and a 24-month follow-up period to attain a 90% power to detect a hazard rate of 1.4 using a one-sided log-rank test. During the enrollment and follow-up period 374 survival events were expected.

The secondary objective of the trial was to compare the DFS between patients in the midostaurin and placebo arms. Among patients who achieved CR after the induction phase DFS time is the period from CR to relapse or death, whichever comes first. Seventy-nine percent of the FLT3 mutated patients were expected to achieve CR in each treatment arm after the induction phase, producing 406 patients (=.79*514) to investigate DFS. Assuming a median DFS time of 11 months in the placebo arm provides an 87% power (2,3) to detect an increase to 15.4 months in the midostaurin arm. During the postinduction enrollment period and the follow-up period 335 DFS events are expected.

The comparison of overall survival between the two treatment arms and the comparison between the DFS between the two treatment arms can both be performed through the log-rank test. Therefore the log-rank test is discussed relative to overall survival time and a comparable application can be made to the DFS time. An excellent discussion of the log-rank test is provided by Collett (6).

Suppose that there are r distinct death times occurring in either arm and let t_j represent the times when the deaths occurred for $j = 1, 2, \ldots, r$ and $t_1 < t_2 < \ldots < t_r$. Further suppose that d_{1j} and d_{2j} deaths occurred at time t_j in treatment arms 1 and 2, respectively with a total of $d_j = d_{1j} + d_{2j}$ deaths occurring at time t_j. Under $H_0: \lambda = 1$ (i.e., if no difference exists between the two survival curves) then the expected number of deaths in arm 1 at time t_j equals $e_{1j} = n_{1j}d_j/n_j$, where n_{1j} and n_{2j} are the patients who are at risk (have not died) in treatment arms 1 and 2, respectively, just prior to time t_j with the total number of patients at risk $n_j = n_{1j} + n_{2j}$. Then the a level log-rank one-sided test criterion takes the form:

Reject $H_0: \lambda = 1$ in favor of $H_1: \lambda > 1$ if $R_L > za$,

(Eq. 9-22)

where

$$R_L = \frac{U_L}{\sqrt{V_L}}$$

$$U_L = \sum_{j=1}^{r} (d_{1j} - e_{1j})$$

$$V_L = \sum_{j=1}^{r} v_{1j}$$

$$v_{1j} = \frac{n_{1j}n_{2j}d_j(n_j - d_j)}{n_j^2(n_j - 1)}.$$

The p value for the one-sided test is given by:

$$p \text{ value} = P[N(0, 1) > R_L]. \qquad \text{(Eq. 9-23)}$$

The a level log-rank two-sided test criterion to test the hypothesis H_0: $\lambda = 1$ versus H_0: $\lambda \neq 1$ takes the form:

$$\text{Reject } H_0: \lambda = 1 \text{ in favor of } H_0: \lambda \neq 1 \text{ if } R_L^2 > \chi_{1,a}^2(0),$$
$$\text{(Eq. 9-24)}$$

where $\chi_{v,a}^2(0)$ is the $100(1 - a)$ percentile of a central chi-square distribution with v degrees of freedom. The p value for the two-sided test is given by:

$$p\text{-value} = P\left[\chi_1^2(0) > R_L^2\right], \qquad \text{(Eq. 9-25)}$$

where $\chi_v^2(0)$ is a central chi-square random variable with v degrees of freedom.

An estimate of the survivor curve $S_i(t)$ in the ith arm can be generated through a Kaplan–Meier curve for $i = 1, 2$. The Kaplan–Meier survival curve estimate $\hat{S}_i(t)$ for any time t in the interval t_k to t_{k+1}, $k = 1, 2, \ldots r$, where t_{r+1} is defined to be ∞ is given by:

$$\hat{S}_i(t) = \prod_{j=1}^{k}\left(\frac{n_{ij} - d_{ij}}{n_j}\right) \qquad \text{(Eq. 9-26)}$$

for arms $i = 1, 2$. The standard error of the Kaplan–Meier estimate of the survival function is given by the Greenwood formula:

$$\text{s.e.}\left\{\hat{S}_i(t)\right\} \approx \left[\hat{S}_i(t)\right]\left\{\sum_{j=1}^{k}\frac{d_{ij}}{n_{ij}(n_{ij} - d_{ij})}\right\}^{1/2} \qquad \text{(Eq. 9-27)}$$

for $t_k \leq t < t_{k+1}$. Therefore, a $100(1 - a)\%$ confidence interval on the survival curve $S_i(t)$ at time $t_k \leq t < t_{k+1}$ for treatment $i = 1, 2$ is given by

$$\hat{S}_i(t) \pm z_{a/2}\text{s.e.}\left\{\hat{S}_i(t)\right\}. \qquad \text{(Eq. 9-28)}$$

However, confidence intervals (Eq. 9-28) are symmetric and therefore can produce confidence intervals outside the range $(0,1)$ for values of $\hat{S}_i(t)$ near 0 or 1. To correct this situation an alternative confidence interval on $S_i(t)$ produced through a logistic transformation on $S_i(t)$ is given by:

$$\left[\hat{S}_i(t)^{\exp\left[z_{a/2}\text{s.e.}\left\{\log\left[-\log\hat{S}_i(t)\right]\right\}\right]}, \hat{S}_i(t)^{\exp\left[-z_{a/2}\text{s.e.}\left\{\log\left[-\log\hat{S}_i(t)\right]\right\}\right]}\right].$$
$$\text{(Eq. 9-29)}$$

where

$$\text{var}\left\{\log\left[-\log\hat{S}_i(t)\right]\right\} = \frac{1}{\left[\log\hat{S}(t)\right]^2}\sum_{j=1}^{k}\frac{d_{ij}}{\left(n_{ij} - d_{ij}\right)}$$
$$\text{(Eq. 9-30)}$$

and s.e.$\left\{\log\left[-\log\hat{S}_i(t)\right]\right\} = \left\{\text{var}\left\{\log\left[-\log\hat{S}_i(t)\right]\right\}\right\}^{1/2}$.

Testing, Estimation, and Confidence Intervals

Although this trial was just opened to enrollment at the time of this writing, Table 9.6 provides representative death times t_j and values of d_{1j}, n_{1j}, d_{2j}, n_{2j}, d_j, n_j, e_{1j}, and v_{1j} for a total enrollment of 514 patients. The times are grouped in tenths of year increments, so there will be a manageable number of death times to demonstrate the numerical calculations.

From Table 9.6, $U_L = 38.2903$ and $V_L = 86.5266$. Therefore,

$$R_L = 38.5266 / \sqrt{86.5266} = 4.14 \qquad \text{(Eq. 9-31)}$$

and from (Eq. 9-23) the p value $< .0001$.

Since the follow-up time in this simulated data example is 2 years all censored observations have times greater than or equal to 2 years. Conversely, all patients who have event times less than 2 years are associated with deaths, not with censored events. This fact can be observed in Table 9.6 by noting that the number of deaths in either arm d_{1j}, d_{2j} at any time $t_j \leq 2$ equals the decrease in the number of patients at risk at the next time point t_{j+1}, that is, $d_{ij} = n_{i,j} - n_{i+j}$ or $n_{i+j} = n_{i,j} - d_{ij}$ for $i = 1, 2$, respectively.

For example, from Table 9.6 at time $t_j = .3$ years the number of deaths in treatment 1 is $d_{1j} = 16$ and the number at risk is $n_{1j} = 228$. Then since all patients in treatment 1 at time $t_j = .3$ years died (i.e., no censored observations) the number at risk at the next time $t_{j+1} = .4$ is $n_{i,j+1} = n_{i,j} - d_j = 228 - 16 = 212$. For times greater than 2 years some events are deaths and some events are censored. For example, at time $t_j = 2.7$ years the number of deaths in treatment 2 is $d_{2j} = 3$ and the number at risk is $n_{2j} = 72$. Then in treatment 2 at time $t_{j+1} = 2.8$ years the number at risk is $n_{1,j+1} = 64$ indicating a decrease in the number of patients at risk of $n_{2j} - n_{2,j+1} = 72 - 64 = 8$; $d_{2j} = 3$ are deaths and 5 are censored observations. The previous discussion is presented to explain how the difference in the number of patients at risk between times t_j and t_{j+1} is influenced by the number of deaths and censored observations at time t_j. Note that in actual trials not all patients are followed for the full follow-up period. Therefore, the event time is the period from the enrollment date to the last observed date. If the difference between the last observed date and the enrollment date is less than the follow-up period and no event has occurred then these censored observations have event times that are smaller than the follow-up time.

To develop a Kaplan–Meier survival function estimate and an estimate of the standard error of the Kaplan–Meier estimate (Eq. 9-26), (Eq. 9-27), and the values in Table 9.6 are used jointly. The required values $t_k \leq t < t_{k+1}, n_{ij}, d_{ij}, n_j$ are reproduced in the first six columns of Table 9.7 followed by the Kaplan–Meier

TABLE 9.6 Example Deaths and Associated Times for Two Treatment Arms

t_j^*	d_{1j}	n_{1j}	d_{2j}	n_{2j}	d_j	n_j	e_{1j}	$d_{1j} - e_{1j}$	v_{1j}
0.1	15	257	7	257	22	514	11.0000	4.00000	5.27485
0.2	14	242	9	250	23	492	11.3130	2.68699	5.49091
0.3	16	228	12	241	28	469	13.6119	2.38806	6.59109
0.4	13	212	11	229	24	441	11.5374	1.46259	5.67791
0.5	14	199	11	218	25	417	11.9305	2.06954	5.87720
0.6	10	185	7	207	17	392	8.0230	1.97704	4.06325
0.7	10	175	5	200	15	375	7.0000	3.00000	3.59358
0.8	7	165	6	195	13	360	5.9583	1.04167	3.11955
0.9	12	158	10	189	22	347	10.0173	1.98271	5.12495
1.0	7	146	9	179	16	325	7.1877	0.18769	3.77548
1.1	5	139	10	170	15	309	6.7476	1.74757	3.54352
1.2	6	134	7	160	13	294	5.9252	0.07483	3.09252
1.3	7	128	5	153	12	281	5.4662	1.53381	2.85933
1.4	4	121	4	148	8	269	3.5985	0.40149	1.92814
1.5	8	117	2	144	10	261	4.4828	3.51724	2.38763
1.6	9	109	3	142	12	251	5.2112	3.78884	2.81843
1.7	6	100	5	139	11	239	4.6025	1.39749	2.56430
1.8	4	94	6	134	10	228	4.1228	0.12281	2.32699
1.9	4	90	5	128	9	218	3.7156	0.28440	2.10121
2.0	7	86	1	123	8	209	3.2919	3.70813	1.87212
2.1	5	79	3	122	8	201	3.1443	1.85572	1.84167
2.2	2	71	3	109	5	180	1.9722	0.02778	1.16760
2.3	2	65	3	100	5	165	1.9697	0.03030	1.16464
2.4	4	59	2	88	6	147	2.4082	1.59184	1.39225
2.5	4	52	4	80	8	132	3.1515	0.84848	1.80795
2.6	4	46	0	75	4	121	1.5207	2.47934	0.91899
2.7	1	39	3	72	4	111	1.4054	0.40541	0.88675
2.8	0	34	1	64	1	98	0.3469	0.34694	0.22657
2.9	2	31	4	53	6	84	2.2143	-0.21429	1.31295
3.0	0	22	4	44	4	66	1.3333	-1.33333	0.84786
3.1	1	21	0	35	1	56	0.3750	0.62500	0.23438
3.2	0	18	0	30	0	48	0.0000	0.00000	0.00000
3.3	0	15	0	25	0	40	0.0000	0.00000	0.00000

(continued)

TABLE 9.6 Example Deaths and Associated Times for Two Treatment Arms (*continued*)

t_j^*	d_{1j}	n_{1j}	d_{2j}	n_{2j}	d_j	n_j	e_{1j}	$d_{1j} - e_{1j}$	v_{1j}
3.4	0	9	0	18	0	27	0.0000	0.00000	0.00000
3.5	1	9	2	15	3	24	1.1250	-0.12500	0.64198
3.6	0	4	0	7	0	11	0.0000	0.00000	0.00000
3.7	0	1	0	1	0	4	0.0000	0.00000	0.00000
Total	204	-	164	-	368	-	-	38.2903	86.5266

*Years.

t_j^*= associated times, d_{1j}= deaths in placebo, d_{2j}= deaths in midostaurin

TABLE 9.7 Kaplan–Meier Survival Function Estimates and Standard Errors

t	d_{1j}	n_{1j}	$\hat{S}_1(t)$	s.e. $\{\hat{S}_1(t)\}$	d_{2j}	n_{2j}	$\hat{S}_2(t)$	s.e. $\{\hat{S}_2(t)\}$
$0.1 \leq t < 0.2$	15	257	.942	.258	7	257	.973	.378
$0.2 \leq t < 0.3$	14	242	.887	.186	9	250	.938	.250
$0.3 \leq t < 0.4$	16	228	.825	.149	12	241	.891	.190
$0.4 \leq t < 0.5$	13	212	.7745	.132	11	229	.848	.160
$0.5 \leq t < 0.6$	14	199	.720	.118	11	218	.805	.142
$0.6 \leq t < 0.7$	10	185	.681	.111	7	207	.778	.133
$0.7 \leq t < 0.8$	10	175	.642	.105	5	200	.759	.127
$0.8 \leq t < 0.9$	7	165	.615	.101	6	195	.735	.122
$0.9 \leq t < 1.0$	12	158	.568	.096	10	189	.696	.114
$1.0 \leq t < 1.1$	7	146	.541	.094	9	179	.661	.108
$1.1 \leq t < 1.2$	5	139	.521	.092	10	170	.623	.102
$1.2 \leq t < 1.3$	6	134	.498	.090	7	160	.595	.099
$1.3 \leq t < 1.4$	7	128	.471	.088	5	153	.576	.097
$1.4 \leq t < 1.5$	4	121	.455	.087	4	148	.560	.095
$1.5 \leq t < 1.6$	8	117	.424	.085	2	144	.553	.095
$1.6 \leq t < 1.7$	9	109	.389	.083	3	142	.541	.094
$1.7 \leq t < 1.8$	6	100	.366	.082	5	139	.521	.092
$1.8 \leq t < 1.9$	4	94	.350	.081	6	134	.498	.090
$1.9 \leq t < 2.0$	4	90	.335	.080	5	128	.479	.088
$2.0 \leq t < 2.1$	7	86	.307	.079	1	123	.475	.088
$2.1 \leq t < 2.2$	5	79	.288	.079	3	122	.463	.087
$2.2 \leq t < 2.3$	2	71	.280	.079	3	109	.450	.087
$2.3 \leq t < 2.4$	2	65	.271	.079	3	100	.437	.086

(*continued*)

TABLE 9.7 Kaplan–Meier Survival Function Estimates and Standard Errors (*continued*)

t	d_{1j}	n_{1j}	$\hat{S}_1(t)$	s.e.$\{\hat{S}_1(t)\}$	d_{2j}	n_{2j}	$\hat{S}_2(t)$	s.e.$\{\hat{S}_2(t)\}$
$2.4 \le t < 2.5$	4	59	.253	.079	2	88	.427	.086
$2.5 \le t < 2.6$	4	52	.233	.080	4	80	.406	.086
$2.6 \le t < 2.7$	4	46	.213	.081	0	75	.406	.086
$2.7 \le t < 2.8$	1	39	.208	.081	3	72	.389	.086
$2.8 \le t < 2.9$	0	34	.208	.081	1	64	.383	.086
$2.9 \le t < 3.0$	2	31	.194	.083	4	53	.354	.088
$3.0 \le t < 3.1$	0	22	.194	.083	4	44	.322	.091
$3.1 \le t < 3.2$	1	21	.185	.085	0	35	.322	.091
$3.2 \le t < 3.3$	0	18	.185	.085	0	30	.322	.091
$3.3 \le t < 3.4$	0	15	.185	.085	0	25	.322	.091
$3.4 \le t < 3.5$	0	9	.185	.085	0	18	.322	.091
$3.5 \le t < 3.6$	1	9	.164	.103	2	15	.279	.113
$3.6 \le t < 3.7$	0	4	.164	.103	0	7	.279	.113
$3.7 \le t$	0	1	.164	.103	0	1	.279	.113

survival function estimate $\hat{S}_i(t)$ and the standard error of the Kaplan–Meier estimate s.e.$\{\hat{S}_i(t)\}$ for treatments $i = 1, 2$. For example, to estimate $\hat{S}_i(t)$ for $.3 \le t < .4$ we apply (Eq. 9-26) and obtain:

$$\hat{S}_1(t) = [(257-15)/257]\cdot[(242-14)/242]\cdot[(228-16)/228]$$
$$= .825.$$

Calculated in a similar manner, from Table 9.7 for the midostaurin arm in the interval $2.0 \le t < 2.1$ the Kaplan–Meier estimated survival function $\hat{S}_2(t) = .475$. Then using n_{2j}, d_{2j} values

$$\sum_{j=1}^{k} \frac{d_{2j}}{n_{2j}(n_{2j}-d_{2j})} = .00431, \quad \text{(Eq. 9-32)}$$

where the (Eq. 9-32) sum is added over all values of d_{2j}, n_{2j} up to and including those in the $2.0 \le t < 2.1$ interval of Table 9.7. Therefore, using the Greenwood formula from (Eq. 9-26)–(Eq. 9-28) a 95% confidence interval on $S_2(t)$ in the interval $2.0 \le t < 2.1$ is given by:

$$\hat{S}_2(t) \pm z_{.025}\text{s.e.}\{\hat{S}_2(t)\} = .475 \pm 1.96 * .0312$$
$$= (.414,.536),$$

(Eq. 9-33)

where

$$\text{s.e.}\{\hat{S}_2(t)\} \approx [.475]\cdot[.00431]^{1/2} = .0312.$$

(Eq. 9-34)

For comparison purposes from (Eq. 9-29) and (Eq. 9-30) a 95% confidence interval on $S_2(t)$ in the interval $2.0 \le t < 2.1$ is given by:

$$\left[.475^{\exp\left[1.96\sqrt{.00745}\right]},\ .475^{\exp\left[-1.96\sqrt{.00745}\right]}\right] = (.414,.533),$$

(Eq. 9-35)

where

$$\text{var}\{\log[-\log \hat{S}_2(t)]\} = \frac{1}{\left[\log \hat{S}_2(t)\right]^2} \sum_{j=1}^{k} \frac{d_{2j}}{n_{2j}(n_{2j}-d_{2j})}$$
$$= \frac{.00413}{\left[\log(.475)\right]^2} = .00745.$$

(Eq. 9-36)

Note that the survival function estimate $\hat{S}_2(t) = .475$ is not near 0 or 1 and therefore the two confidence intervals from (Eq. 9-33) and (Eq. 9-35) are almost identical.

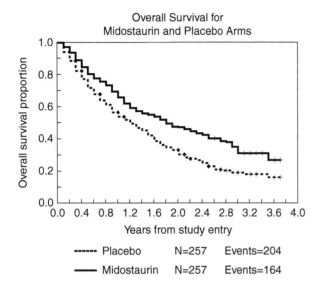

FIGURE 9.2 Kaplan–Meier estimated survival functions for the midostaurin and placebo arms using simulated data.

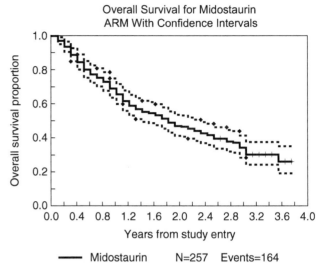

FIGURE 9.3 Kaplan–Meier estimated survival function plus confidence intervals for the midostaurin arm using simulated data.

Using the values of Table 9.7, Figure 9.2 provides the Kaplan–Meier estimated survival function for both treatments. Finally, Figure 9.3 provides the Kaplan–Meier estimated survival function for the midostaurin treatment arm with confidence bounds calculated using (Eq. 9-29).

REFERENCES

1. Simon R. Optimal two-stage designs for Phase II clinical trials. *Control Clin Trials.* 1988;10;1–10.
2. George SL, Desu MM. Planning the size and duration of a clinical trial studying the time to some clinical event. *J Chronic Dis.* 1974;27:15–24.
3. Rubenstein LV, Gail MH, Santner TJ. Planning the duration of a comparative clinical trial with loss to follow-up and a period of continued observation. *J Chronic Dis.* 1981;34:469–479.
4. Berger JO. *Statistical Decision Theory.* 2nd edn. New York, NY: Springer-Verlag; 1985.
5. Moser BK, *Linear Models: A Mean Model Approach.* San Diego, CA: Academic Press; 1996.
6. Collett D. *Modelling Survival Data in Medical Research.* Boca Raton, FL: Chapman and Hall; 1991.
7. Edelman MJ, Watson D, Wang X, et al. Eicosanoid modulation in advanced lung cancer: COX-2 expression is a positive predictive factor for Celecoxib + chemotherapy. *J Clin Oncol.* 2008;26(6):848–855.
8. Kindler H, Niedzwiecki D, Hollis D, Oraefo E. Summary report: a randomized Phase III trial of gemcitabine plus bevacizumab versus gemcitabine plus placebo in patients with advanced pancreatic cancer, CALGB July 2007 Summary Report; 2007.
9. Stone RM, Moser B, Sanford B, et al. High dose cytarabine plus gemtuzamab ozogamicin for patients with relapsed or refractory acute myeloid leukemia: cancer and leukemia group B study 19902. *Leukemia Research.* 2011;35(3):329–333. doi:10.1016/j.leukres.2010.07.017

Innovative Phase I Clinical Trials

Nolan A. Wages

INTRODUCTION

Historically, the primary objective of phase I clinical trials in oncology is to identify the maximum tolerated dose (MTD) of the agent being investigated from a discrete set of available doses. In a subsequent phase II trial, the agent is evaluated for efficacy at the recommended dose. In oncology trials of cytotoxic agents, identification of the MTD is often determined by considering dose-limiting toxicity (DLT) information only, with the assumption that the MTD is the highest dose that satisfies some safety requirement, and therefore provides the most promising outlook for efficacy. Numerous phase I designs (1) have been proposed for identifying the MTD from a set of I doses $\{d_1, \ldots, d_I\}$ in which toxicity is measured as a binary outcome, DLT (yes/no).

The current landscape of oncology drug development poses a challenge to widely accepted methods used in early-phase clinical trials. Dose-finding studies that aim to evaluate the safety of single agents are becoming less common, and advances in clinical research have complicated the paradigm of dose finding in oncology. In recent years, novel statistical methods have been developed in order to address more complex research questions in early-phase studies. However, broad implementation of novel methods has been limited, with traditional or modified 3 + 3 designs remaining in frequent use (2). A recent paper by Paoletti, Ezzalfani, and Le Tourneau (2) described the rigidity of the 3 + 3 design in meeting the challenges of studies involving combinations and/or biological agents, and called for wider use of more innovative methods to achieve the goals of contemporary research objectives. This call is present throughout the statistical and medical literature, with reviews, justification, and recommendations on the use of innovative designs (3–4). More complex problems, such as those involving targeted agents and immunotherapies, combination therapies, and stratification of patients by clinical or genetic characteristics, have created the need to adapt early-phase trial design

to the specific agents being investigated, and the corresponding endpoints. In this chapter, we describe the implementation of novel designs in several ongoing and recently completed early-phase studies for contemporary dose-finding problems.

COMBINATIONS OF AGENTS

Multiagent dose-finding trials present the significant challenge of finding an MTD combination, or combinations, of the agents being tested with the typically small sample sizes involved in phase I studies. In recent years, many methods have been proposed for locating the MTD combination of the multiple agents being investigated. Despite the emergence of new methodology, it is rare that innovative approaches are used in practice. A recent literature review revealed that the use of novel methods in practice is quite limited (5). A recent editorial in *Journal of Clinical Oncology* by Mandrekar (6) described the use of the method of Ivanova and Wang (7) in a phase I study of neratinib in combination with temsirolimus in patients with human epidermal growth factor receptor 2-dependent and other solid tumors (8), and called for more frequent use of novel designs. Wages et al. (9) added to the discussion of Riviere et al. (5) by describing the current implementation of novel methods in several ongoing early-phase combination studies, several of which are described in this chapter as illustrative examples.

In general, we consider multiagent trials to be testing I treatment combinations labeled d_i; $i = 1, \ldots, I$. Denote the probability of DLT at d_i with $R(d_i)$ and the target toxicity rate specified by physicians by θ. A key assumption to phase I methods for single-agent trials is the monotonicity of the dose–toxicity curve. In this case, the curve is said to follow a "simple order" because the ordering of DLT probabilities for any pair of doses is known and administration of greater doses of the agent can be expected to produce DLTs in increasing proportions of patients. In studies testing combinations, the probabilities of DLT often follow a "partial order" (10) in that there are pairs of combinations for which the ordering of the probabilities is not known. The monotonicity assumption lends itself to escalation along a single line of doses. Given the toxicity response (DLT; yes/no) for a particular patient, we either recommend the same dose for the next patient or move to one of two adjacent doses (i.e., either escalate one dose higher or de-escalate to one dose lower). In a multiagent trial, there will most likely be more than one possible treatment on which to enroll the next patient cohort in a decision of escalation, which implies a set, E, of "possible escalation combinations." As an illustration, consider the 3×3 matrix in Figure 10.1. Suppose the first cohort receives combination d_1 and no DLTs are observed. If d_1 is well tolerated, it is not clear which dose pair should be assigned to the next cohort of patients. The set of possible escalation combinations for d_1 would then consist of two combinations $E = \{d_2, d_3\}$. As demonstrated in Figure 10.1 (11), there are multiple directions in which the trial could move in deciding which combination the next entered cohort should receive. Because we make the assumption that each drug has been carefully investigated before being combined, we assume that the probability of DLT for each drug increases monotonically when the dose of the other drug is being held fixed (i.e., across rows and up columns of the matrix of drug combinations). It may be clear that dose d_2 is more toxic than d_1, but, in the off-diagonal direction, we may not know the ordering between d_2 and d_3 because we increased the dose of one agent and decreased the dose of the other agent. In terms of DLT probability, the conditions $R(d_1) < R(d_2)$ and $R(d_1) < R(d_3)$ may hold without it being possible to order $R(d_2)$ and $R(d_3)$ with respect to one another. It could be that $R(d_2) < R(d_3)$ or $R(d_3) < R(d_2)$.

A traditional approach to this problem is to preselect combinations with a known toxicity order, and apply a single-agent design by escalating and de-escalating along a chosen path. This could be done by, a priori, prespecifying a subset of combinations for which we know the toxicity ordering. For instance, in the 3×3 grid in Figure 10.1, a selected subset of combinations that satisfies the monotonicity assumption is given by

$$d_1 \to d_3 \to d_5 \to d_8 \to d_9.$$

This approach transforms the two-dimensional dose-finding space into a one-dimensional space, and it was the approach taken in much of the early work in combinations. Korn and Simon (12) present a graphical method, called the "tolerable dose diagram," based on single-agent toxicity profiles, for guiding the escalation strategy in combination. Kramar, Lebecq, and Candahl (13) also lay out an a priori ordering for the combinations, and estimate the MTD combo using a parametric model for the probability of a DLT as a function of the doses of the two agents in combination. The disadvantage of this approach is that it limits the number of combinations that can be considered and it can potentially miss promising dose combinations located outside of the path.

Rather than work with a single ordering, another approach to dealing with added complexity is to specify multiple possible orderings and appeal to established model selection techniques.

Taking into account known and unknown relationships between combinations using the assumption of monotonicity up columns and across rows of the matrix, this approach proceeds by laying out multiple possible simple orders of the dose–toxicity relationship. For instance, for the 3×3 grid in Figure 10.1, two *possible* orderings of the DLT probabilities, $R(d_i)$, are

$$R(d_1) < R(d_2) < R(d_3) < R(d_4) < R(d_5) < R(d_6) < R(d_7) < R(d_8) < R(d_9)$$

$$R(d_1) < R(d_3) < R(d_2) < R(d_6) < R(d_5) < R(d_4) < R(d_8) < R(d_7) < R(d_9).$$

One method making use of this approach is the partial order continual reassessment method (POCRM) (13), which we now describe.

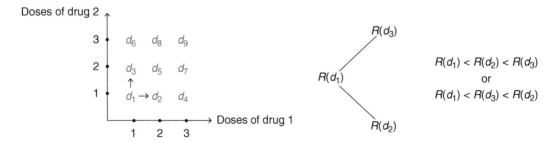

FIGURE 10.1 Illustration of a partial order between $R(d_1)$, $R(d_2)$, and $R(d_3)$, in a drug combination matrix. If d_1 is well tolerated, the set of possible escalation combinations is $E = \{d_2, d_3\}$. Two possible simple orders satisfy this partial order.

Source: Adapted from Wages NA, Ivanova A, Marchenko O. Practical designs for Phase I combination studies in oncology. *J Biopharm Stat.* 2016;26(1). Reprinted by permission of Taylor & Francis Ltd, http://www.tandfonline.com.

Partial Order Continual Reassessment Method (POCRM)

Trial Example 1 Using POCRM

A dose-escalation study was designed to determine the MTD/appropriate phase II dose combination of two small molecule inhibitors for refractory solid tumors and untreated metastatic disease. Agent 1 contained three doses (1.0, 1.5, 2.0 mg/day) and agent 2 contained three doses (1,000, 1,250, 1,500 mg/day), for a total of nine 3 × 3 drug combinations. This Food and Drug Administration/institutional review board (FDA/IRB) approved trial was designed using the two-stage POCRM (14). Each stage was to treat patients in single-patient cohorts, and the target toxicity rate for determining the MTD combination was $\theta = 30\%$.

Trial Example 2 Using POCRM

A phase I trial was designed to determine the MTD of a combination of long peptides plus toll-like receptor (TLR) agonists with or without a form of incomplete Freund's adjuvant (IFA) for the treatment of melanoma (NCT01585350). In this FDA/IRB-approved trial, TLR agonists had four dose levels (25, 100, 400, 1,600 EU) and IFA had three subgroups: 0—IFA is not administered with any vaccine, V1—IFA is administered with just the first vaccine, and V6—IFA is administered in all vaccines. This trial was also designed using the two-stage POCRM (14). There are a total of 12 combinations under consideration, and the target rate for determining the MTD combination was $\theta = 30\%$.

Specifying Possible Orderings

A prior specification for POCRM is to choose a subset of possible dose–toxicity orders. We rely on the guidance of Wages and Conaway (15) and choose approximately six to nine orderings based on ordering the combinations by rows, columns, and diagonals of the drug combination matrix. This provides an appropriate balance between choosing enough orderings so that we include adequate information to account for the uncertainty surrounding partially ordered dose–toxicity curves, without increasing the dimension of the problem so much so that we diminish performance. Since, in a large matrix, there could be many ways to arrange combinations along a diagonal, we restrict movements to only moving across rows, up columns, and up or down any diagonal. For instance, in the 3 × 3 grid in Figure 10.1, six orderings, indexed by m, arranged in this manner are given by:

1. Across rows ($m = 1$)
   $R(d_1) < R(d_2) < R(d_4) < R(d_3) < R(d_5) < R(d_7) < R(d_6) < R(d_8) < R(d_9)$.
2. Up columns ($m = 2$)
   $R(d_1) < R(d_3) < R(d_6) < R(d_2) < R(d_5) < R(d_8) < R(d_4) < R(d_7) < R(d_9)$.

3. Up diagonals ($m = 3$)
   $R(d_1) < R(d_2) < R(d_3) < R(d_4) < R(d_5) < R(d_6) < R(d_7) < R(d_8) < R(d_9)$.
4. Down diagonals ($m = 4$)
   $R(d_1) < R(d_3) < R(d_2) < R(d_6) < R(d_5) < R(d_4) < R(d_8) < R(d_7) < R(d_9)$.
5. Down–up diagonals ($m = 5$)
   $R(d_1) < R(d_2) < R(d_3) < R(d_6) < R(d_5) < R(d_4) < R(d_7) < R(d_8) < R(d_9)$.
6. Up–down diagonals ($m = 6$)
   $R(d_1) < R(d_3) < R(d_2) < R(d_4) < R(d_5) < R(d_6) < R(d_8) < R(d_7) < R(d_9)$.

POCRM Estimation Procedure

The continual reassessment method (CRM) for partial orders is based on utilizing a class of working models that correspond to the possible orderings. Specifically, suppose there are M possible orderings being considered, which are indexed by m. For a particular ordering, we model the true probability of toxicity, $R(d_i)$, corresponding to combination d_i via a single-parameter power model

$$R(d_i) \approx \Psi_m(d_i, a) = a_{mi}^{\exp(a)} \quad m = 1, \ldots, M; i = 1, \ldots, I$$

where a_{mi} represents the skeleton (16) of the model under ordering m. Other single-parameter working models common to the CRM class, such as a hyperbolic tangent function or a one-parameter logistic model, could be used, but there is little difference in the operating characteristics among the various model choices (17). For the skeleton values, we utilize the algorithm of Lee and Cheung (6) to generate reasonable skeleton values using the function **getprior** in **R** package **dfcrm**. We simply need to specify skeleton values at each combination that are adequately spaced (18), and adjust them to correspond to each of the possible orderings, in order for POCRM to have good performance in terms of identifying an MTD combo. The location of these skeleton values can be adjusted to correspond to each of the possible orderings using the **getwm** function in **R** package **pocrm** (19).

We let the plausibility of each ordering under consideration be described by a set of prior weights $\pi = \{\pi(1), \ldots, \pi(M)\}$, where $\pi(m) \geq 0$ and $\sum \pi(m) = 1; m = 1, \ldots, M$. Under ordering m, the log-likelihood for the parameter a after j patients is given by

$$L_{mj}(a) = \sum_{l=1}^{j} y_l \log\left(a_{mi}^{\exp(a)}\right) + \sum_{l=1}^{j} (1 - y_l) \log\left(1 - a_{mi}^{\exp(a)}\right).$$

Using the accumulated data from the first j eligible subjects accrued to the study, the maximum likelihood estimate (MLE), $\hat{a}_m$, of the parameter a can be computed for each of the m orderings, along with the value of the log-likelihood $L_{mj}(\hat{a}_m)$ at $\hat{a}_m$. Wages et al. (14) proposes an escalation method that first chooses the ordering that maximizes the updated model weight

$$\omega(m) = \frac{L_{mj}(\hat{a}_m)\pi(m)}{\sum_{m=1}^{M} L_{mj}(\hat{a}_m)\pi(m)}$$

before each patient inclusion. If we denote this ordering by m^*, the authors use the estimate $\hat{a}_{m^*}$ to estimate the toxicity probabilities for each combination under ordering m^* so that $\hat{R}(d_i) \approx \psi_{m^*}(d_i, \hat{a}_{m^*})$.

POCRM Dose-Finding Algorithm

Within the framework of sequential likelihood estimation, an initial escalation scheme is needed, since the likelihood fails to have a solution on the interior of the parameter space unless some heterogeneity (i.e., at least one DLT and one non-DLT) in the responses has been observed.

Stage 1. In Wages, Conaway, and O'Quigley (20), the POCRM is presented in a Bayesian framework, where the trial begins at the combination believed by the investigator to be the closest to the target. Wages, Conaway, and O'Quigley (14) described using an initial escalation stage in drug combination trials and discussed the need for a variant of the traditional escalation schemes due to the fact that, in partially ordered trials, the most appropriate dose to which the trial should escalate could consist of more than one treatment combination. A specification for two-stage POCRM is how rapidly to escalate in the early part of the trial, which is based on how many patients to include in each cohort of the initial escalation scheme. This could be done in groups of 1, 2, or 3 patients.

In the first stage, we make use of "zoning" the matrix of combinations according to the diagonals of the matrix in Figure 10.1. The trial begins in the zone $Z_1 = \{d_1\}$ and the first cohort of patients is enrolled on this lowest combination. At the first observation of a DLT in one of the patients, the first stage is closed and the second stage, based on the POCRM estimation procedure described previously, is opened. As long as no DLTs occur, cohorts of patients are examined at each dose within the currently occupied zone, before escalating to the next highest zone. If d_1 is tried and deemed safe, the trial would escalate to zone $Z_2 = \{d_2, d_3\}$. If more than one dose is contained within a particular zone, we can sample without replacement from the combinations available within the zone. Therefore, the next cohort is enrolled on a combination that is chosen randomly from d_2 and d_3. The trial is not allowed to advance to zone $Z_3 = \{d_4, d_5, d_6\}$ in the first stage until a cohort of patients has been observed at both combinations in Z_2. This procedure continues until a toxicity is observed or all available zones have been exhausted. Subsequent to a DLT being observed, the second stage of the trial begins.

Stage 2. Subsequent to a DLT being observed, the second stage of the trial begins.

1. Based on the accumulated data from j accrued subjects, the estimated toxicity probabilities $\hat{R}(d_i)$ are sequentially obtained for all combinations being tested, based on the estimation procedure described earlier.

2. The next entered patient is then allocated to the dose combination with estimated toxicity probability closest to the target rate so $|\hat{R}(d_i) - \theta|$ that is minimized.

3. There is no formal skipping restriction placed on model-based allocation in the POCRM method. That is, movement within the matrix is not restricted to a neighbor of the currently occupied combination in Stage 2. This is meant to allow for adequate exploration of the drug combination space. For instance, movement from d_4 to d_6 "skips" over d_5, yet it is unknown whether this move is actually an escalation or a de-escalation due to the partial order, so we allow such a move to encourage experimentation throughout the matrix and to avoid getting "stuck" in certain regions of the space.

4. The estimated MTD combination is defined as $\hat{v}$ such that

$$\hat{v} = \arg\min_i |\hat{R}(d_i) - \theta|$$

after a total sample size of n patients.

Single Trial Illustration

In this section, we illustrate the behavior of POCRM under a set of true DLT probabilities for Example 1. The method is illustrated using the true DLT probabilities in Table 10.1 with a target rate of $\theta = 30\%$, making d_2 and d_3 target combos. We utilized the set of six possible orderings described previously, and placed a uniform prior π on the orderings. The skeleton values were generated using the function **getprior(0.05,0.30,4,9)** in **R** package **dfcrm** (16). The location of these skeleton values was adjusted to correspond to each of the possible orderings using the **getwm** function in **R** package **pocrm** (19).

In the simulation of DLT outcomes in a trial, the tolerance of each patient can be considered a uniformly distributed random variable on the interval [0,1], which we term a patient's latent toxicity tolerance and denote

TABLE 10.1 A True DLT Probability Scenario for a Two-Agent Combination Trial

Doses of drug 2	Doses of agent 1		
	1	2	3
3	0.20	0.50	0.66
2	0.06	0.33	0.50
1	0.02	0.20	0.33

u_j for the jth entered patient (21). At the combination (d_i, as labeled in Figure 10.1) assigned to patient j, if the tolerance is less than or equal to its true DLT probability (i.e., $u_j \leq R(d_i)$), then patient j has a DLT; otherwise the patient has a non-DLT outcome. Of course, in a real trial, it is impossible to observe a patient's latent tolerance, but it is a useful tool in simulation and can be used to compare the operating characteristics of different designs within a single trial. In conducting this exercise to illustrate the POCRM, we generated the latent tolerance sequence in Table 10.2 for $n = 25$ patients using the function **runif(25)** in **R**. The method begins on the lowest combination so that patient $j = 1$ receives d_1. Because the tolerance $u_1 = 0.978$, he or she does not have a DLT, since $u_1 > 0.02$. Escalating in cohorts of size 1, the method then recommends that the second patient receive one of two combinations in the set $Z_2 = \{d_2, d_3\}$, and POCRM randomizes to d_3. The latent tolerance $u_2 = 0.5949$ is larger than $R(d_2) = 0.06$, resulting in a non-DLT outcome for the second subject. The first DLT occurs for each method at the fourth entered patient, based on a latent tolerance of $u_4 = 0.055$, which is less than the true DLT probability for the combination recommended to this patient. Notice at this point, POCRM would terminate Stage 1 of their designs due to heterogeneity in the DLT outcomes, and proceed with Stage 2.

There are some interesting features to each design as it sequentially allocates. With respect to movement around the drug combination space, it is of interest to note that POCRM allows movement at both ends of a diagonal of the matrix. In other words, after patient 6 receives d_3, the next combination recommended is d_4. This represents a two dose level increase in drug 1 and a one dose level decrease in drug 2, although it is unknown in practice whether this is actually an escalation or a de-escalation. After $n = 25$ patients, POCRM recommends d_5 as the MTD combo, which has an estimated DLT probability of $\hat{R}(d_5) = 0.303$. This is one of the true target dose combinations with a true DLT probability ($R(d_5) = 0.33$) closest to the target rate of $\theta = 30\%$. In the sections that follow, we highlight the implementation of POCRM in several ongoing and recently completed drug combination studies designed at the University of Virginia (UVA) Cancer Center (9).

TABLE 10.2 Simulated Sequential Trial Illustrating Each Approach Using Latent Toxicity Tolerance of 25 Patients

Patient j	u_j	d_i	$R(d_i)$	DLT (yes = 1; no = 0)
1	0.978	d_1	0.02	0
2	0.595	d_3	0.06	0
3	0.340	d_2	0.20	0
4	0.055	d_5	0.33	1
5	0.043	d_6	0.20	1
6	0.869	d_3	0.06	0
7	0.478	d_4	0.33	0
8	0.649	d_4	0.33	0
9	0.873	d_5	0.33	0
10	0.539	d_5	0.33	0
11	0.738	d_7	0.50	0
12	0.129	d_7	0.50	1
13	0.495	d_5	0.33	0
14	0.690	d_7	0.50	0
15	0.787	d_7	0.50	0
16	0.285	d_7	0.50	1
17	0.847	d_7	0.50	0
18	0.095	d_7	0.50	1
19	0.963	d_5	0.33	0
20	0.779	d_7	0.50	0
21	0.223	d_7	0.50	1
22	0.248	d_5	0.33	1
23	0.862	d_5	0.33	0
24	0.534	d_5	0.33	0
25	0.286	d_5	0.33	1
MTD estimate		d_5	$\hat{R}(d_5) = 0.333$	

EXTENSIONS TO OTHER COMPLEX DOSE-FINDING PROBLEMS

Combination Immunotherapies

Immunotherapy has emerged as an effective approach for many cancers, with particular promise for checkpoint blockade agents (e.g., antibodies blocking CTLA-4 and PD-1). Cancer vaccines have also been studied for decades, but with disappointing results in many trials. On the other hand, recent studies have shown clinical benefit and promise with vaccines for lymphoma, melanoma, and prostate cancer patients (22–24), with a cancer vaccine now FDA-approved for hormone-refractory prostate cancer. Vaccine-based immunotherapy offers potential low-toxicity alternatives or additions to chemotherapy, targeted molecular therapies, or other immunotherapies.

Immunotherapy is posing a challenge to the accepted methods of early-phase trial design (25). The FDA recently published a "Guidance for Industry: Clinical Considerations for Therapeutic Cancer Vaccines," which acknowledged the need for alternative dose-escalation methods in cancer vaccines (3). In contrast to chemotherapeutic agents, dose finding in immunotherapy often investigates treatments that demonstrate minimal toxicity overall, where higher doses may not induce greater immunologic effect. The biologic activity of the treatment may increase at low doses, and then begin to level off, or plateau, at higher doses (26–30). Rather than determining the MTD, the goal of dose finding with immunologic agents is to locate the optimal biological dose, which we define as the lowest safe dose, which demonstrates the greatest immunogenicity, based on some predefined measure of immune response. Protocol-specific immunological endpoints give the investigator a measure of biologic activity that serves as a driving factor in the trial design. Although the relationship between clinical outcome and immunologic activity is not clear at this point, it is generally assumed that the absence of biologic effect will accompany a lack of clinical efficacy. Before an immunologic agent can be taken into large-scale trials to test for clinical efficacy, early-phase trials are needed to establish that the therapy can produce an immunologic effect with the potential to translate to clinical benefit. Some published phase I/II methods (31,32) can reasonably be applied in a single-agent immunotherapy setting by replacing "efficacy" with "immune response" because most account for the potential plateau of biological effects at higher doses.

Studies involving combinations of agents are another area of trial design that challenges accepted methods in dose finding. Gao et al. (22) argue that the treatment benefits seen in patients who have received single-agent immunotherapies have reached a limitation and that trials combining multiple agents are necessary in order to advance cancer immunotherapy. Incorporation of adjuvants, such as TLR agonists, new or optimized peptide vaccines, and combining vaccines with immune modulators such as checkpoint blockade agents (e.g., blocking antibodies to CTLA-4 or PD-1/PD-L1) may aid in improving immune response, with the goal of improving clinical outcome (22,33). Innovative dose-escalation strategies are needed to establish the safety and immunogenicity of new immunologic combinations. Novel dose-finding designs for multiple immunologic agents could potentially have a significant impact on the growth of immunotherapy as a treatment for cancer. In subsequent sections, we describe the implementation of the method in an ongoing trial (Mel 63) investigating a helper peptide vaccine plus local and systemic adjuvant combinations for the treatment of melanoma (NCT02425306) designed at the UVA Cancer Center. The statistical modeling framework is outlined in Wages

and Conaway (34). This design extends the one outlined in Wages et al. (35) for Mel 60 (NCT02126579), a multisite, FDA/IRB-approved, phase I/II trial of a novel melanoma vaccination approach using long peptides plus TLR agonists. This design is also being used in a phase I/II trial to locate the optimal biological combination of two oral targeted inhibitors (NCT02419560). Recently published guidelines (36,37) for implementing novel early-phase methods were followed in executing the described design.

Mel 63 Trial

Mel 63 is an early-phase evaluation of the safety and immunogenicity of a vaccine composed of a mixture of 6 synthetic melanoma helper peptides (6MHP) (38) administered with one of two local adjuvant combinations, IFA or IFA + the TLR 3 agonist polyICLC, alone or with systematic low-dose cyclophosphamide (mCy), as shown in Table 10.3. Treatment combinations are grouped into "zones" based on the number of adjuvants. The trial was designed to find the range of optimal treatment combinations (OTC), defined as a combination with early and durable immunologic response and an acceptable level of toxicity. An adaptive design is being used to guide accrual decisions with toxicity assessments and the potential for a durable immune response characterizing the main decision measures. The decision endpoints are DLTs and durable immune response (dRsp) as measured by CD4+ T cell responses to 6MHP during the time period of vaccination administration.

In monitoring safety, adverse events are being assessed and acute toxicity graded using the National Cancer Institute (NCI) Common Terminology Criteria for Adverse Events (CTCAE) Version 4.03. A patient is classified as experiencing a DLT (yes/no) based on protocol-specific dose-limiting adverse events. A DLT is defined as any unexpected adverse event that is possibly, probably, or definitely related to treatment and meets the following criteria: (a) grade ≥ 3, (b) grade 1 ocular adverse events, and (c) grade 2 allergic/autoimmune reactions. An early dRsp is defined as at least a fivefold increase in immune response to the 6MHP peptide as measured by CD4+ T cells over two consecutive time periods during vaccination (days 0 to 85). As

TABLE 10.3 Treatment Arm/Combination/Zone Definitions for Mel 63 Trial

Zone	Arm/Combination	6MHP+
1	A	IFA
2	B	IFA + mCy
2	C	IFA + PolyICLC
3	D	IFA + PolyICLC + mCy

data accumulate, each patient is classified as experiencing a DLT (yes/no) and experiencing a dRsp (yes/no). Treatment-related grade 3 or higher adverse event data from our prior studies (39,40) (NCT01585350) are being used to gauge DLT rates. Using these data, the DLT tolerance level was chosen to be 25% (i.e., any optimal combination that we are satisfied has an estimated DLT probability ≤25% to be considered "acceptable" in terms of safety).

Allocation decisions presented depend on the definition (and measure) of an immune response as a yes/no (binary) endpoint. In particular, the endpoint must be defined prospectively and ideally as one that has biologic relevance and/or is associated with clinical response. Many immunologic endpoints depend on continuous variables, and, in this design strategy, it is important to define prospectively a criterion for defining a "positive" or "negative" result along a continuum of data values. In the present study, we have defined criteria based on prior reports (41). Another important consideration is that the result of the immune response measure must be available in a reasonable time frame if it is to be useful in guiding trial enrollment. Thus, it is important to select an immunologic endpoint that occurs early enough to be meaningful and to design processes for collecting samples and assaying them rapidly so that the data may guide patient enrollment in accordance with the study design.

Estimation. Model-based allocation is being based upon a CRM (42) that accounts for two binary endpoints (DLT, dRsp) in combinations of agents (34). Safety assessments are based on the assumption that, as the number of adjuvants increases, the probability of DLT is nondecreasing. It is reasonable to assume that regimens in higher zones do not have lower probabilities of DLT than regimens in lower zones. This assumption is based on data from previous melanoma studies in which these adjuvant preparations were combined with other peptide vaccines. It is unknown whether regimens have higher or lower DLT probabilities than other regimens within the same zone. It could be that B < C or C < B in terms of their respective DLT probabilities. We express this uncertainty through specification of multiple one-parameter power models in Table 10.4 that reflect different orderings of the DLT probabilities. We then rely on model selection techniques, as described in the POCRM estimation procedure, to choose the model most consistent with the data. Using the accumulated toxicity data, the CRM is fit for each DLT probability working model, and the parameter a is estimated for each model by maximum likelihood estimation. The working model with the largest likelihood is chosen and, using the selected model, DLT probability estimates are updated for each combination.

The working models for dRsp probabilities are formulated under two different assumptions: (a) the probabilities are increasing with increasing zone, or (b) the

TABLE 10.4 Working Models/Skeletons of DLT Probabilities

Zone	1	2	3
Working model	A	B	C	D
1	0.04^a	0.07^a	0.11^a	0.17^a
2	0.04^a	0.11^a	0.07^a	0.17^a

[a] Parameter of the working DLT probability model to be estimated from the data.

probabilities increase initially and then plateau after a certain zone, as displayed in Table 10.5. Like toxicity, these possible shapes for the dose–immune response curve are expressed through multiple skeletons of CRM models. We again rely on a class of one-parameter power models, governed by the parameter b, to formulate working models for the dRsp probabilities. Using the accumulated immune response data, the CRM is fit for each dRsp probability working model, and the parameter b is estimated for each model by maximum likelihood estimation. Again, the working model with the largest likelihood is chosen and, using the selected model, dRsp probability estimates are updated for each combination. Based on the probability estimates for both DLT and dRsp, we make allocation decisions.

TABLE 10.5 Working Models/Skeletons of dRsp Probabilities

Under the assumption of increasing dRsp probability across zones			
Zone	1	2	3
Working model	A	B	C	D
10.30^a	0.30^a	0.45^a	0.59^a	0.70^a
2	0.30^a	0.59^a	0.45^a	0.70^a
3	0.30^a	0.45^a	0.70^a	0.59^a
4	0.30^a	0.70^a	0.45^a	0.59^a
5	0.30^a	0.59^a	0.70^a	0.45^a
6	0.30^a	0.70^a	0.59^a	0.45^a
Under the assumption of plateau dRsp probability across zones			
7	0.45^a	0.59^a	0.70^a	0.70^a
8	0.59^a	0.70^a	0.70^a	0.70^a
9	0.70^a	0.70^a	0.70^a	0.70^a
10	0.45^a	0.70^a	0.59^a	0.70^a
11	0.45^a	0.70^a	0.70^a	0.59^a

[a] Parameter of the working dRsp probability model to be estimated from the data.

Accrual to arms occurred in two stages. The initial stage accrued eligible patients in cohorts of two on each arm, until a patient experienced a DLT. The second stage is allocating eligible patients in cohorts of one according to the estimation procedure described earlier.

Allocation in Completed Stage 1. The escalation plan for the first stage was based on the zones. With this design, patients could be accrued and assigned to other open arms within a zone but escalation would not occur outside the zone until the minimum follow-up period was observed for the first patient accrued to an arm. The minimum follow-up period for escalation between zones was 3 weeks after the initial vaccine. Initial allocation within a zone was based upon random allocation (1:1) between the possible arms. Escalation to a higher zone occurred only when all arms in the lower zone had been tried, and no DLT had been observed. Patient allocation to subsequent arms within the new zone followed the same accrual strategy. This allocation strategy was followed for accrual to increasing zones until a patient experienced a DLT or a stopping rule was triggered. The seventh patient accrued to the study experienced the first DLT on arm D, at which time the second stage using multidimensional CRM modeling began. The eighth patient had already been accrued to arm D in Stage 1 when the DLT occurred.

Allocation in Ongoing Stage 2. Stage 2 is allocating eligible patients based upon the multidimensional CRM modeling approach described earlier. Model-based estimation of DLT probabilities began for the accrual of the ninth patient to the study. After each new accrual in Stage 2, the estimated DLT probabilities are being updated and used to define a set of "acceptable" combinations in terms of safety. For arm combinations B to D, a one-sided 90% confidence interval is calculated using the estimated DLT probability for that arm, based on confidence interval estimation for CRM models (18). If the lower bound of this confidence interval exceeds the maximum toxicity tolerance of 25%, then this arm is deemed too toxic and excluded from the acceptable set of combinations. If arm A is excluded from the acceptable set then no arm is considered acceptable and the trial is stopped for safety. Therefore, for arm A the level of confidence is set at 95% instead of 90%. If the minimum follow-up period is not satisfied at the time a new patient is ready to be put on study, then the patient may be accrued to any arm, by random allocation, which has accrued at least one patient and is in the acceptable set.

Model-based estimation of dRsp probabilities started at the beginning of Stage 2, since a dRsp was observed in Stage 1 (patient 5). Once the set of acceptable combinations is determined, the recommended combination will be based upon how many patients have been entered into the study to that point. For the first third of the trial (i.e., 1/3 of the maximum sample size), the combination recommendation is based on randomization using a weighted allocation scheme. Randomization prevents the design from getting "stuck" at a suboptimal regimen based on limited data. The recommended combination for the next entered patient is chosen at random from the "acceptable" combinations with each acceptable combination weighted by its estimated dRsp probability. That is, acceptable combinations with higher estimated dRsp probabilities have a higher chance of being randomly chosen as the next recommended combination. For the latter third of the trial (i.e., final 2/3 of maximum sample size), the recommended combination for the next entered patient is defined as the "acceptable" combination with the highest estimated dRsp probability. After each patient, a new recommended combination is obtained, and the next entered patient is allocated to the recommended combination. The trial will stop once sufficient information about the optimal dose range has been obtained, according to the stopping rules outlined earlier. Currently, the trial has accrued 32 patients, with model-based allocation (Stage 2) having been utilized after the first eight patients.

Stopping the Trial. Accrual to the study will be halted and trigger a safety review by the study investigators and Data and Safety Monitoring Committee (DSMC) to determine if the study should be modified, or permanently closed to further accrual according to the following: (a) accrual would be halted for safety if the first two entered patients in zone 1 experience a DLT in Stage 1, (b) if at any point in Stage 2, the acceptable set is empty, the trial will stop for safety, (c) otherwise, accrual to the study will end if the recommendation is to assign the next patient to a combination that already has 30 patients treated at that combination.

Sample Size and Accrual. Target sample size for the optimal combination is based upon acquiring sufficient information to assess the objective of estimating dRsp rates, assuming at least one optimal combination has been found. Based upon results from the Mel 44 clinical trial (39), 30 eligible patients treated at the optimal combination will provide adequate data to assess dRsp. The target of 30 patients was chosen based on having sufficient information to determine if the optimal arm shows an increase in dRsp rate compared to the baseline rate observed in the 6MHP arms of Mel 44 of 18% (90% CI: 11–26). If at least 13/30 (43%; 90% CI: 28–60) patients on the optimal arm experience a dRsp the results will be considered promising since the lower limit of the confidence interval exceeds the upper limit from the Mel 44 estimated rate. Total study sample size is estimated from simulations that were conducted at the planning stage, and is determined by the stopping rules in the preceding section. We set the maximum total sample size to 70 eligible patients; however, the simulation results indicated that the maximum average trial size over all scenarios is 52 patients.

Patient Heterogeneity

Another complexity that may arise in early-phase dose-finding studies is encountering some patient heterogeneity, in which patients can be categorized into two or more prognostic groups. A straightforward example of the two-group structure is seen in the degree of previous treatment (heavily pretreated vs. no/lightly pretreated). Given the varying amounts of prior treatment, it is not unreasonable to assume that there could be a difference in the way the patients in each group tolerate and respond to a new treatment (or treatment regimen), and it may be important to incorporate this heterogeneity into the design of the trial. Most studies do not incorporate any group structure into the design. The resulting recommended dose is weighted in favor of the appropriate dose for the most frequently occurring group, and effectively moves away from personalized dosing for patients not in the dominant group. Within this scenario of heavily pretreated versus no/lightly pretreated example, it is reasonable to assume that a heavily pretreated patient may be more likely to experience a DLT than a no/lightly pretreated patient. Consequently, an objective of the trial may be to find an MTD within each group, and it would be beneficial for the trial design to reflect this goal. A simple solution would be to conduct parallel dose-finding studies, one for each group. This approach would not make use of any information common between the groups and, thus, may not be very efficient. There are many examples of these designs, including Ramanathan et al. (43), which stratifies patients into "none," "mild," "moderate," or "severe" liver dysfunction at baseline. A similar classification is used by LoRusso et al. (44). Dasari et al. (45) defined groups in terms of type of cancer, while Prados et al. (46) stratifies patients by prior therapies. Ura et al. (47) and Kim et al. (48) conduct phase I trials in groups defined by patient genetic characteristics. These examples use different dose-finding designs within groups; Ramanathan et al. (43) use the traditional 3 + 3 design, while Ura et al. (47) use the more efficient CRM (40), but they share the common feature that the MTD in each group is determined only from the data obtained within that patient group.

Given the typically small samples used in early-phase trials, a more efficient design that can borrow information in order to identify the most appropriate dose level for both groups is desirable. Several advanced design methods have been proposed in order to address the problem of patient heterogeneity in dose finding. O'Quigley, Shen, and Gamst (49) introduced a two-sample CRM, which allowed for the identification of the appropriate MTDs for two groups simultaneously. Legedza and Ibrahim (50) proposed a related method, augmenting the dose–toxicity model for a vector of patient characteristics and putting a prior on the coefficient in the dose–toxicity model. In O'Quigley et al. (49), no assumption was made regarding the order of tolerance toward the treatments between the two

groups. O'Quigley and Paoletti (51) proposed a two-parameter CRM for ordered groups that utilizes known differences between the groups. Yuan and Chappell (52) describe a generalization of up-and-down, isotonic and CRM designs for trials carried out in ordered groups. Ivanova and Wang (53) also incorporate isotonic estimates into designs for ordered groups that take into account both toxicity and efficacy endpoints. Morita (54) presented an application of the CRM that utilized information from Caucasian patients in order to design a phase I dose-finding study for Japanese patients. Most recently, Conaway and Wages (55) proposed a phase I design for ordered groups based on order restricted statistical inference (10).

In the usual single-group CRM, an underparameterized (one-parameter) working model is often utilized in modeling toxicity. In O'Quigley et al. (49) and O'Quigley and Paoletti (51), a two-parameter CRM model was introduced, with the additional parameter essentially measuring differences between the groups. The regression models described in O'Quigley et al. (49) and O'Quigley and Paoletti (51) allow for a large, possibly infinite, number of possible values for the second parameter. Recently, O'Quigley and Iasonos (56) outlined the potential for being more restrictive on the range of potential values for the "group" parameter and suggested using a very small, discrete set of values, which has been termed the "shift" model. The authors apply the shift model to the area of bridging, a problem closely linked to that of group heterogeneity. In this parameterization, suppose Group 1 is recommended dose level d_v, based on the minimization of the distance between its estimated DLT probability, $R(d_i)$, and some target DLT rate, θ (i.e., $v \equiv \arg \min |R(d_i) - \theta|$). Then, Group 2 will be recommended to receive either the same dose, or a dose that is "shifted" one, two, or more levels away from d_v. The investigators involved in the study can specify constraints on both the direction and magnitude of the difference between the two groups. The following section demonstrates a practical extension of the shift model as part of a phase I/II design for a trial of stereotactic body radiation therapy (SBRT) in patients with painful osseous metastatic disease classified into two prognostic groups. The safety objective in this current trial deviates from one of identifying the MTD in each group according to a target rate θ, to one of estimating an acceptable set of doses defining a set of acceptable doses with regard to safety. To this end, θ is redefined from a target DLT probability to a maximum acceptable toxicity tolerance that will guide the definition of safe doses. This set of acceptable doses is used to drive allocation toward doses that optimize a response endpoint.

An Ongoing Stereotactic Body Radiation Therapy Study

STAT-RT-1/2 (57) is an IRB-approved, phase I/II trial of rapid helical radiation therapy for patients with painful osseous metastatic disease that was designed, and is currently open to accrual, at the UVA Cancer Center. Patients are grouped into good and poor prognosis subjects, with poor prognosis patients having a shorter life expectancy. The poor prognosis patients are unlikely to require radiation retreatment for recurrent pain after treatment, and therefore may not require higher dose escalation for palliation, which is associated with more toxicity. At study entry, patients will be classified as having a good prognosis and stratified into Group 1 if they meet **all** of the following criteria: (a) limited metastatic disease in two or fewer organ systems especially bone-only disease; (b) have not completed second-line chemotherapy or are on hormonal therapy only; (c) indolent disease process with relatively stable disease on serial imaging over the past 3 to 6 months or reduced tumor burden due to systemic therapy; or (d) stable or improving performance status (PS) over the past 6 months with a current Eastern Cooperative Oncology Group (ECOG) PS of 0 to 2. Patients are classified as having a poor prognosis and stratified into Group 2 if they meet **any** of the following criteria: (a) diffuse metastatic disease in three or more organ systems; (b) completed second-line chemotherapy with persistent disseminated disease; (c) rapid progression of disease over the past 3 to 6 months or rapid decline in PS over the past 6 months with a current ECOG PS of 3 or 4. It was anticipated that 75% of the patient population will be from Group 1 and 25% from Group 2.

Design Considerations. STAT-RT-1/2 is evaluating $I = 4$ dose levels in each of the two prognostic groups, which are given in Table 10.6. The trial was designed to determine the optimal dose, defined as the dose with acceptable toxicity and that minimizes retreatment rate, in each group, among the available dose levels. A toxicity endpoint is defined as a binary random variable (i.e., DLT yes/no). Similarly, we define a "response" variable as a binary outcome (i.e., retreatment yes/no). Patients receive a radiation treatment via a novel real-time radiation oncology workflow for the delivery of high-dose single-fraction SBRT known as the Scan-Plan-QA-Treat STAT-RAD workflow. The overall goal of this workflow is to develop a more rapid, convenient,

and effective palliative SBRT approach for patients with osseous metastases that is less toxic and less expensive than current clinical treatment regimens. Therefore, this trial will attempt to establish whether conformal radiation dose escalation above 8 Gy can improve patient pain scores and reduce retreatment rates, since this is a major drawback of the standard of care 8 Gy single-fraction treatment. Based on pilot data from a previous clinical trial and data from other larger randomized clinical trials, the investigators believe that patients with osseous metastases treated with STAT-RAD-based single-fraction SBRT with dose escalation beyond 8 Gy will have a target lesion retreatment rate less than 20% with acceptable toxicity.

Adverse events are being assessed and acute toxicity graded using the NCI CTCAE Version 4. Late toxicity is being scored using the Radiation Therapy Oncology Group (RTOG) Late Radiation Toxicity Scoring System. A DLT is defined as any treatment-related grade ≥ 4 toxicity, within 90 days of treatment. For escalation decisions, subjects must be observed for a minimum of 30 days after the last radiation therapy treatment. However, any DLT observed through 90 days will be used in the modeling stage (see Stage 2 in the following) of this two-stage, model-based design. It is expected that patients in Group 1 will be more sensitive to the treatment and thus have a higher probability of DLT compared with those patients in Group 2. Therefore, the optimal dose for Group 1 should be lower than or at least as low as the optimal dose for Group 2. Due to the number of dose levels available in each group, the optimal dose in Group 1 will not be more than three levels below the optimal dose in Group 2 on the scale of prespecified doses. In other words, it is possible for the optimal dose to be 15 Gy in Group 2 and 8 Gy in Group 1. The overall strategy is, throughout the trial duration, to use a CRM-type "shift" model to continuously monitor safety data in order to adaptively update a set of acceptable (safe) doses in each group, with which to make allocation decisions based on retreatment rate.

Dose escalation will be conducted via a two-stage CRM that incorporates a "shift" model to account for the differences in toxicity among the two prognosis groups. Within each group more than one dose may satisfy the safety concerns, and therefore provide a range of optimal doses to assess secondary study objectives.

Trial conduct. In each group, the initial stage will accrue eligible patients in cohorts of two on each escalating dose level until a patient in either group experiences a DLT. The second stage will allocate eligible patients in cohorts of one based upon a CRM shift model illustrated in Table 10.7. In each group, the initial stage will accrue eligible patients in cohorts of two. The first two eligible patients in each group will be entered into dose level 1 in the patient's respective group. This initial stage differs slightly from the one previously described in the

TABLE 10.6 Four Dose Levels in Two Ordered Groups in the STAT-RT-1/2 Study

Prognosis Group	Doses in Gy			
	8	10	12.5	15
Group 2 dose levels	−1	(Start) 1	2	3
Group 1 dose levels	(Start) 1	2	3	4

TABLE 10.7 Working Models for Various Shifts in Dose Levels Between Two Prognosis Groups

	Prognosis Group	Doses in Gy			
		8	10	12.5	15
Model 1 (1-level shift)	Group 2 dose levels	0.01[a]	0.06[a]	0.13[a]	**0.20[a]**
	Group 1 dose levels	0.06[a]	0.13[a]	**0.20[θ₁]**	0.27[a]–
Model 2 (2-level shift)	Group 2 dose levels	0.01[a]	0.06[a]	0.13[a]	**0.20[a]**
	Group 1 dose levels	0.13[a]	0.20[a]	0.27[a]	0.34[a]
Model 3 (3-level shift)	Group 2 dose levels	0.01[a]	0.06[a]	0.13[a]	**0.20[a]**
	Group 1 dose levels	**0.20[a]**	0.27[a]	0.34[a]	0.41[a]

[a] Parameter of the working DLT probability model to be estimated from the data.

Mel studies because of the added complexity of conducting dose-escalation in groups.

- If 0/2 patients experience DLT, then the next cohort is treated at the next highest dose level within that group.
- If 1/2 patients experience DLT in either group, then Stage 2 of the study design begins.
- If 2/2 patients experience DLT:
  o In Group 1, study accrual to Group 1 is halted.
  o In Group 2, then the next cohort is treated at dose level 1 of Group 1.
- In the absence of DLTs, escalation will continue until dose level 3 is reached with the same allocation rules specified earlier. After two patients have been treated at each dose level within a group without DLT, the next cohort is treated at the dose with the lowest observed retreatment rate. Once a DLT has been observed in either group, Stage 2 modeling begins.

The second stage will allocate eligible patients based upon the CRM shift model. Specifically, eligible patients are accrued in cohorts of one and a CRM shift model fit from all the data accumulated is used to estimate DLT probabilities at each dose level for both groups. These DLT probabilities will be used to define a set of "acceptable" doses in each group, defined as any dose with estimated DLT probability less than or equal to 20%. This toxicity tolerance of 20% was chosen based on the expectedness of adverse events. Stage 2 modeling uses multiple working models that correspond to various "shifts" between the dose levels in the different groups. That is, the set of doses that is considered "acceptable" in one group may be shifted 1, 2, or 3 levels away from those considered acceptable in the other group. Table 10.7 illustrates the possible shift models used in modeling DLT probabilities, with Model 1 corresponding to a 1-level shift in acceptable doses between groups, Model 2 representing a 2-level shift between groups, and Model 3 representing a 3-level shift between groups. A set of working model values for the DLT probabilities under each model is also given in Table 10.7. This table also illustrates that the DLT probabilities under each possible shift model are estimated via the commonly used power model governed by the parameter a.

As the data accumulates, a is estimated for each model by maximum likelihood estimation. After each patient cohort inclusion, the model, m, that best fits the data (i.e., with the largest likelihood value) is chosen via model selection techniques, and used in the estimation of DLT probabilities. Within that model, updated estimates of the DLT probabilities at each available dose level are obtained *in each group*. These DLT probability estimates are then used to determine an acceptable set of safe doses in each group, which is defined by a dose with an estimated DLT probability ≤20%. Once the acceptable set is determined, the recommended dose for the next patient entered in each group is defined as the "acceptable" dose with the lowest observed retreatment rate. After each patient, a new recommended dose level is obtained for each group, regardless of the group to which the previous patient belonged. If the next entered patient is in Group 1, he or she is allocated to the recommended dose of Group 1. If the next entered patient is in Group 2, he or she is allocated to the recommended dose of Group 2.

Maximum sample size and stopping rules are based upon acquiring sufficient information to assess the secondary objective assuming at least one optimal dose has been identified. Sample size is estimated from the simulations in (57), but was determined by the stopping rules. The trial will stop once sufficient information about the optimal dose range has been obtained, according to the following:

1. The study will stop accruing patients in Group 1 and only treat eligible patients in Group 2 if two entered patients in Group 1 experience DLT on dose level 1.
2. The study will stop for safety if two entered patients in Group 2 experience DLT on dose level 1 of Group 1 in Stage 1.
3. The study will stop if the recommendation is to assign the next patient in Group 2 to a dose level that already has 17 patients in Group 2 treated at that dose level.

The maximum total sample size is set at 66 patients, based on a maximum of 5 at each dose level in Group 1 and a maximum of 17 at each dose level in Group 2. Although maximum accrual is 66, in the simulation results in Wages et al. (57), on average a total of between 39 and 42 patients were required to complete the study. The simulation results demonstrated the method's ability to effectively recommend optimal doses, defined by acceptable toxicity and low retreatment rates, in a high percentage of trials with manageable sample sizes within each group.

CONCLUSION

The development of novel methods in early-phase dose finding has been rapid in recent years, yet, the use of innovative designs remains infrequent. This can be attributed to several causes, not least of which includes (a) clinician skepticism, and (b) difficulty or assumed difficulty in obtaining approval of entities such as IRBs, pharmaceuticals, and the FDA. These complications are likely to be enhanced in the coming years as the recent paradigm of oncology drug development involves a shift to more complex dose-finding problems, such as combination or targeted therapies. In this chapter, we have outlined a novel early-phase adaptive design, implemented in ongoing or completed trials addressing contemporary research questions in early-phase studies. The methods presented serve as an alternative to the 3 + 3 design for early-phase trials, which are being called for by the FDA and by others (1–5). The methods we outline in this work can be viewed as an extension of the CRM, utilizing multiple skeletons for DLT and activity probabilities, increasing the ability of CRM designs to handle more complex dose-finding problems. We hope this increased flexibility will augment early-phase trial design in oncology.

REFERENCES

1. Iasonos A, O'Quigley J. Adaptive dose-finding studies: a review of model-guided phase I clinical trials. *J Clin Oncol.* 2014;32:2505–2511.
2. Paoletti X, Ezzalfani M, Le Tourneau C. Statistical controversies in clinical research: requiem for the 3 + 3 design for phase I trials. *Ann Oncol.* 2015;26:1808–1812.
3. Rahma OE, Gammoh E, Simon R et al. Is the "3+3" dose-escalation phase I clinical trial design suitable for therapeutic cancer vaccine development? A recommendation for alternative design. *Clin Cancer Res.* 2014;20:4758–4767.
4. Nie L, Rubin EH, Mehrotra N, et al. Rendering the 3+3 design to rest: more efficient approaches to oncology dose-finding trials in the era of targeted therapy. *Clin Cancer Res.* 2016;22:2623–2629.
5. Riviere M-K, Le Tourneau C, Paoletti X, et al. Designs of drug-combination phase I trials in oncology: a systematic review of the literature. *Ann Oncol.* 2015;26:669–674.
6. Mandrekar SJ. Dose-finding trial designs for combination therapies in oncology. *J Clin Oncol.* 2014;32:65–67.
7. Ivanova A, Wang K. A non-parametric approach to the design and analysis of two-dimensional dose-finding trials. *Stat Med.* 2004;23:1861–1870.
8. Gandhi L, Bahleda R, Tolaney SM, et al. Phase I study of neratinib in combination with temsirolimus in patients with human epidermal growth factor receptor 2-dependent and other solid tumors. *J Clin Oncol.* 2014;32:68–75.
9. Wages NA, Conaway MR, Slingluff CL, Jr, et al. Recent developments in the implementation of novel designs for early-phase combination studies. *Ann Oncol.* 2015;26:1036–1037.
10. Robertson T, Wright FT, Dykstra R. *Order Restricted Statistical Inference.* New York, NY: J. Wiley; 1988.
11. Wages NA, Ivanova A, Marchenko O. Practical designs for Phase I combination studies in oncology. *J Biopharm Stat.* 2016;26(1). Reprinted by permission of Taylor & Francis Ltd, http://www.tandfonline.com.
12. Korn EL, Simon R. Using the tolerable-dose diagram in the design of phase I combination chemotherapy trials. *J Clin Oncol.* 1993;11:794–801.
13. Kramar A, Lebecq A, Candalh E. Continual reassessment methods in phase I trials of the combination of two agents in oncology. *Stat Med.* 1999;18:1849–1864.
14. Wages NA, Conaway MR, O'Quigley J. Dose-finding design for multi-drug combinations. *Clin Trials.* 2011;8:380–389.
15. Wages NA, Conaway MR. Specifications of a continual reassessment method design for phase I trials of combined drugs. *Pharm Stat.* 2013;12:217–224.
16. Lee SM, Cheung YK. Model calibration in the continual reassessment method. *Clin Trial.* 2009;6:227–238.
17. Paoletti X, Kramar A. A comparison of model choices for the continual reassessment method in phase I clinical trials. *Stat Med.* 2009;28:3012–3028.
18. O'Quigley J, Zohar S. Retrospective robustness of the continual reassessment method. *J Biopharm Stat.* 2010;5:1013–1025.
19. Wages NA, Varhegyi N. pocrm: an R-package for phase I trials of combinations of agents. *Comput Methods Programs Biomed.* 2013;112:211–218.
20. Wages NA, Conaway MR, O'Quigley J. Continual reassessment method for partial ordering. *Biometrics.* 2011;67:1555–1563.
21. O'Quigley J, Paoletti X, Maccario J. Non-parametric optimal design in dose finding studies. *Biostatistics.* 2002;3:51–56.
22. Gao J, Bernatchez C, Sharma P, et al. Advances in the development of cancer immunotherapies. *Trend Immun.* 2012;34:90–98.
23. Marshall NA, Galvin KC, Corcoran AM, et al. Immunotherapy with PI3K inhibitor and Toll-like receptor agonist induces IFN-gamma+IL-17+ polyfunctional T cells that mediate rejection of murine tumors. *Cancer Res.* 2012;72:581–591.

24. Sikora AG, et al. IFN-alpha enhances peptide vaccine-induced CD8+ T cell numbers, effector function, and antitumor activity. *J Immunol.* 2009;182:7398–7407.
25. Petroni G. Design issues for early-stage clinical trials. In Disis M, ed. *Immunotherapy of Cancer.* Totowa, NJ: Humana Press; 2006, 479–485.
26. Simon R, Steinberg S, Hamilton M. Clinical trial designs for the early clinical development of therapeutic cancer vaccines. *J Clin Oncol.* 2001;19:1848–1854.
27. Korn E. Nontoxicity endpoints in phase I trial designs for targeted, non-cytotoxic agents. *J Natl Cancer Inst.* 2004;96:977–978.
28. Parulekar WR, Eisenhauer EA. Phase I trial design for solid tumors studies of targeted, non-cytotoxic agents: theory and practice. *J Natl Cancer Inst.* 2004;96:970–977.
29. Le Tourneau C, Lee JJ, Siu LL. Dose escalation methods in phase I cancer clinical trials. *J Natl Cancer Inst.* 2009;101: 708–720.
30. LoRusso P, Boerner S, Seymour L. An overview of the optimal planning, design, and conduct of phase I studies of new therapeutics. *Clin Cancer Res.* 2010;16:1710–1718.
31. Zang Y, Lee JJ, Yuan Y. Adaptive designs for identifying optimal biological dose for molecularly targeted agents. *Clin Trial.* 2014;11:319–327.
32. Wages NA, Tait C. Seamless phase I/II adaptive design for oncology trials of molecularly targeted agents. *J Biopharm Stat.* 2015;25:903–920.
33. Cannistra S. Challenges and pitfalls of combining targeted agents in phase I studies. *J Clin Oncol.* 2008;26:3665–3667.
34. Wages NA, Conaway MR. Phase I/II adaptive design for drug combination oncology trials. *Stat Med.* 2014;33:1990–2003.
35. Wages NA, Slingluff CL, Jr, Petroni GR. A phase I/II adaptive design to determine the optimal treatment regimen from a set of combination immunotherapies in high-risk melanoma. *Contemp Clin Trials.* 2015;41:172–179.
36. Iasonos A, Gönen M, Bosl GJ. Scientific review of phase I protocols with novel dose-escalation designs: how much information is needed? *J Clin Oncol.* 2015;33:2221–2225.
37. Petroni GR, Wages NA, Paux G, Dubois F. Implementation of adaptive methods in early-phase clinical trials. *Stat Med.* 2016;36(2):215–224.
38. Slingluff CL, Jr., Petroni GR, Olson W, et al. Helper T-cell responses and clinical activity of a melanoma vaccine with multiple peptides from MAGE and melanocytic differentiation antigens. *J Clin Oncol.* 2008;26:4973–4980.
39. Slingluff CL, Jr., Petroni GR, Chianese-Bullock KA, et al. A randomized multicenter trial of the effects of melanoma-associated helper peptides and cyclophosphamide on the immunogenicity of a multipeptide melanoma vaccine. *J Clin Oncol.* 2011;29:2924–2932.
40. Slingluff CL, Jr., Petroni GR, Olson W, et al. A randomized pilot trial testing the safety and immunologic effects of MAGE-A3 protein plus AS15 immunostimulant administered into muscle or into dermal/subcutaneous sites. *Cancer Immunol Immunother.* 2016;65:25–36.
41. Slingluff CL, Jr., Petroni GR, Chianese-Bullock KA, et al. Immunologic and clinical outcomes of a randomized phase II trial of two multipeptide vaccines for melanoma in the adjuvant setting. *Clin Cancer Res.* 2007;13:6386–6395.
42. O'Quigley J, Pepe M, Fisher L. Continual reassessment method: a practical design for phase I clinical trials in cancer. *Biometrics,* 1990;46:33–48.
43. Ramanathan R, Egorin M, Takimoto C, et al. Phase I and pharmacokinetic study of imatinib mesylate in patients with advanced malignancies and varying degrees of liver dysfunction: a study by the National Cancer Institute Organ Dysfunction Working Group. *J Clin Oncol.* 2008;26:563–569.
44. LoRusso P, Venkatakrishnan K, Ramanathan R, et al. Pharmacokinetics and safety of bortezomib in patients with advanced malignancies and varying degrees of liver dysfunction: phase I NCI organ dysfunction working group study NCI-6432. *Clin Cancer Res.* 2012;18:1–10.
45. Dasari A, Gore L, Messersmith W, et al. A phase I study of sorafenib and vorinostat in patients with advanced solid tumors with expanded cohorts in renal cell carcinoma and non-small cell lung cancer. *Invest New Drugs,* 2013;31:115–125.
46. Prados M, Chang S, Burton E, et al. Phase I study of OSI-774 alone or with temozolomide in patients with malignant glioma. *Proceed American Soc Clin Oncol.* 2003;22:abstract 394.
47. Ura T, Satoh T, Tsujinaka T, et al. Phase I study of irinotecan with individualized dosing based on UGT1A1 polymorphism in Japanese patients with gastrointestinal cancer. (UGT0601). *J Clin Oncol.* 2008;26(May 20 suppl; abstr 14502).
48. Kim T, Sym S, Lee S, et al. A UGT1A1 genotype-directed phase I study of irinotecan (CPT-11) combined with fixed dose of capecitabine in patients with metastatic colorectal cancer (mCRC). Journal of Clinical Oncology ASCO Annual Meeting Proceedings (Post-Meeting Edition) 2009; Vol 27, No 15S (May 20 Supplement): 2554.
49. O'Quigley J, Shen LZ, Gamst A. Two sample continual reassessment method. *J Biopharm Stat.* 1999;9:17–44.
50. Legezda A, Ibrahim J. Heterogeneity in phase I clinical trials: prior elicitation and computation using the continual reassessment method. *Stat Med.* 2001;20:867–882.
51. O'Quigley J, Paoletti X. Continual reassessment method for ordered groups. *Biometrics.* 2003;59:430–440.
52. Yuan Z, Chapell R. Isotonic designs for phase I cancer clinical trials with multiple risk groups. *Clinical Trials.* 2004;1:499–508.
53. Ivanova A, Wang K. Bivariate isotonic design for dose-finding with ordered groups. *Stat Med.* 2006;25:2018–2026.
54. Morita S. Application of the continual reassessment method to a phase I dose-finding trial in Japanese patients: East meets West. *Stat Med.* 2011;30:2090–2097.
55. Conaway MR, Wages NA. Designs for phase I trials in ordered groups. *Stat Med.* 2016;36(2):254–265.
56. O'Quigley J, Iasonos A. Bridging solutions in dose finding problems. *Stat Biopharm Res.* 2014;6:185–197.
57. Wages NA, Read PW, Petroni GR. A Phase I/II adaptive design for heterogeneous groups with application to a stereotactic body radiation therapy trial. *Pharm Stat.* 2015;14:302–310.

11

Pharmacokinetics in Clinical Oncology

Jill M. Kolesar

INTRODUCTION

Pharmacokinetics, also known as dose–concentration relationships, is the mathematical relationship describing the time course of absorption, distribution, metabolism, and excretion (ADME) of drugs and metabolites in the body (1). The biological, physiological, and physicochemical factors that influence the transfer processes of drugs in the body also influence the rate and extent of ADME of those drugs in the body.

Typically, pharmacokinetic parameters are determined by measuring plasma or other relevant distribution site drug concentrations.

Pharmacokinetics and pharmacokinetic modeling are important components of the clinical drug development process and are required as part of most new drug applications (NDAs). The initial guidance document describing the pharmacokinetic and bioavailability studies required in an NDA was published by the Food and Drug Administration (FDA) in 1987 (2). Since that time, the FDA has developed guidance documents that describe required pharmacokinetic studies and recommended study designs for special populations including hepatic dysfunction (3), renal impairment (4), pregnancy (5), and lactation (6) as well as drug interaction studies (7). In addition, guidance documents for use of population pharmacokinetics (8) and physiologically based pharmacokinetics (PBPK) (9) in clinical drug development are areas of recent interest.

BASIC PHARMACOKINETIC PRINCIPLES

Pharmacokinetic Vocabulary

The purpose of pharmacokinetics in clinical drug development is to assess relationships between plasma concentrations and clinical outcomes of interest, typically efficacy and adverse effects (10). The science of pharmacokinetics uses mathematical equations (regression) to model these effects and a working knowledge of pharmacokinetic parameters, constants, and variables is needed.

The basis for all pharmacokinetic analysis and modeling is a concentration versus time curve. See Figure 11.1. In this example, a patient received an oral medication at time 0 and blood samples were obtained at times 0, 0.5, 0.75, 1, 2, 4, 8, 12, 20, and 24 hours. Drug concentrations were analyzed and reported in nanogram (ng) of drug per milliliter (mL) of plasma. Many important pharmacokinetic parameters can be estimated by visual inspection of the plasma versus time–concentration curve. The maximum concentration of Cmax (see Table 11.1 and Figure 11.1) is the highest concentration we can observe, and is approximately 2,500 ng/mL. The time that the maximum concentration occurs is Tmax, and is at approximately 5 hours. Concentration and time are variables; time is the independent variable and concentration is the dependent or response variable. These variables are measured.

Observed concentration and time data are used to determine pharmacokinetic parameters, which may be primary or secondary. Primary pharmacokinetic parameters depend on the physiology of the body and the physiochemical properties of the drug and include clearance (Cl), volume of distribution (Vd), and bioavailability (F). Cl is the amount of drug eliminated per unit of time, Vd is a proportionality constant that relates the amount of drug in the body to the concentration of drug that was measured, while F is the proportion of drug that enters into the systemic circulation. Cl and Vd cannot be determined from the concentration versus time curve. It is likewise difficult to collect data to determine Cl and Vd. For example, to assess the Vd empirically, samples would need to be obtained from all possible body fluids and volumes of body fluids determined. Therefore, Cl and Vd are modeled from concentration versus time data.

Half-life (t1/2) and area under the curve (AUC) are secondary pharmacokinetic parameters because they can be calculated from primary parameters (if they are

TABLE 11.1 Pharmacokinetic Parameters

Parameter	Definition	Equation
Concentration maximum (Cmax)	The highest concentration of the drug	$C_{max} = \dfrac{FD}{V} e^{-\lambda_c t_{max}}$
Time of maximum concentration (Tmax)	The time the concentration is highest	$T_{max} = time\ point\ at\ C_{max}$
Half-life ($t_{1/2}$)	Time required for the drug concentration to decrease by 50%	$t_{\frac{1}{2}} = \dfrac{0.693.V}{CL}$
Area under the curve (AUC)	The concentration of drug, added up over a period of time	$AUC_{\infty} = AUC_{(0-t)} + \dfrac{C_n}{\lambda_z}$
Clearance (Cl)	The amount of drug eliminated per unit of time	$Cl = \dfrac{FD}{AUC_{\infty}}$
Volume (V)	The "tank" or the distribution of the drug	$V = \dfrac{FD}{AUC_{(0-t)}\lambda_z}$
Bioavailability (F)	For an oral drug, the amount of drug absorbed	Determined experimentally

*D, dose administered.

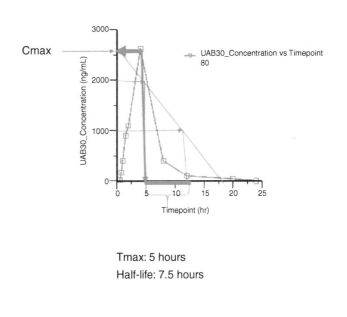

Time	Concentration (ng/mL)
0	0
0.5	198
0.75	569
1	869
2	1128
4	2630
8	470
12	55
20	10
24	0

Tmax: 5 hours

Half-life: 7.5 hours

a = 7.5 hr

b = 2750 ng/ml

= 1/2 a² √b²/a² -1/4 .

By hand AUC = 10,266 ng*hr/mL

Computer AUC = 11,677 ng*hr/mL

FIGURE 11.1 Assessing pharmacokinetic parameters from the concentration versus time curve.

known). They can also be determined from the concentration versus time curve (Figure 11.1). The half-life is the time required for the concentration to decrease by half. To go from 2,000 ng/mL to 1,000 ng/mL requires approximately 7.5 hours; therefore the half-life is 7.5 hours. The AUC can be calculated manually by using formulas for areas. In this example, the area of the triangle is 10,266 ng × hr/mL. While the tail of the curve is missed, this manual calculation approximates the software calculation of 11,677 ng × hr/mL.

Absorption

The starting point for any drug into the body is the administration. Common routes of administration include oral, intravenous (IV), intramuscular (IM), and subcutaneous (SC). The proportion of the drug that reaches the systemic circulation after administration is the pharmacokinetic parameter bioavailability (F). Historically, almost all anticancer agents were administered intravenously and the bioavailability of intravenously administered agents is defined as 1, or 100%, simplifying pharmacokinetic modeling for these agents. However, targeted agents are typically oral small molecules that are administered daily, making bioavailability an important consideration.

Drug absorption depends on the physiochemical properties of the drug and the physiological characteristics and habits of the patient, and two major considerations in drug development are food effects and drug interactions, which interfere with drug absorption.

Food Effect

Food can affect the pharmacokinetics of oral chemotherapy by changing both the rate and extent of absorption (2). Food can delay gastric emptying, change gastric pH, increase blood and bile flow, alter luminal metabolism, or physically interact with the drug. Food compositions most likely to change gastrointestinal physiology are those that are high in both fat and total calories; therefore high-fat and high-calorie meals are studied.

Physiochemical properties of drugs can also predict food effects. Drugs are categorized by permeability and solubility by the Biopharmaceutics Classification System (BCS). Drugs that have high permeability and high solubility are BCS class I, high permeability and low solubility are class II, low permeability and high solubility are class III, and low permeability and solubility are class IV. BCS class I drugs are least susceptible to food effects as their absorption is predicted to be independent of pH and site, although this is not always the case and food effect studies are generally required for all oral medications.

The overall goal of a food effect study is to determine if there is a difference in pharmacokinetic parameters under fed and fasting states. The most common study design is a single-dose, two-condition (fasted and fed) crossover design. Food effect studies outside of oncology are typically conducted in healthy volunteers; however,

due to safety concerns most oncology food effect studies are conducted in the oncology patient population. A high-fat, high-calorie meal is defined as 800 to 1,000 calories and 50% fat. Fasted condition is an overnight fast of 8 hours, followed by drug administration and subsequent 4 hours of additional fasting.

Food may increase, decrease, or not affect the extent of drug absorption, which is measured by Cmax and AUC ratio between the fed and fasted condition. Lack of clinically significant food effect on drug absorption is defined as the 90% confidence interval (CI) for the ratio between fed and fasted conditions falling between 80% and 125% for both AUC∞ and Cmax. If no food effect is determined from this experiment, the product labeling will indicate that the drug can be taken without regard to food. If a food effect is noted, administration on an empty stomach or with food will be advised.

Similar analysis is performed for Tmax, which if significantly prolonged, in the presence of no food effect, most likely indicates a delay in the rate absorption but not the extent. Tmax changes typically do not require administration of the drug under fasting conditions.

Drug Interactions Affecting Absorption

Concurrent medications that affect gastric pH or physically interact with the concurrent drug are the most common types of drug interactions affecting absorption.

pH-Dependent Absorption. Acid suppressive therapies are necessary treatments for individuals with duodenal or gastric ulcers and available over the counter for heartburn sufferers (11). Three marked types of acid reducing therapies are antacids, histamine H2 receptor antagonists (H2A), and proton pump inhibitors (PPIs). Antacids work by binding to and neutralizing stomach acid resulting in rapid onset and short duration of effect (approximately 2 hours). H2As reversibly compete with histamine at the H2 receptors to reduce gastric acid secretion, with effects lasting approximately 12 hours post dose. PPIs irreversibly bind to the proton pump that secretes gastric acid, resulting in 24 hours or more of gastric acid suppression. All therapies are able to increase gastric pH above 6.

Acid suppressive therapies can alter absorption of concurrently administered medications, especially those with pH-dependent solubility. If a drug is known to have reduced solubility above a pH of 6, drug interaction studies are typically required by the FDA and are of similar design as those described under food effects. The results of drug interaction studies also inform the product label; if the AUC or Cmax ratio falls outside of the 90% CI, a significant drug interaction between acid lowering therapies is determined. While this is generally considered a class effect of all acid suppressive therapies, from a practical standpoint, management of the drug interaction is different, given the different durations of acid suppression effects; antacid administration is staggered by 2 hours,

H2 antagonists by 12 hours, and PPIs are avoided. In addition, polyvalent cations found in antacids (Mg++, Ca++, etc.) can bind to some drugs forming insoluble chelates that limit drug absorption (12).

Distribution

The primary pharmacokinetic parameter that describes the distribution of a drug is the Vd. Conceptually, the Vd describes the location of the drug in the body. Total body water constitutes 55% to 65% of total body weight (see Table 11.2) and various other fluids make up the total body water. Drugs with a Vd of 3 L or less are considered confined to the plasma (see Table 11.2). If Vd is larger than 50 L, the drug is considered distributed to all tissues in the body, especially the fatty tissue. The larger the Vd, the more likely that the drug is found in the tissues of the body, typically the sites of action.

Mathematically, Vd is a proportionality factor that relates the amount of drug in the body to the amount of drug measured in the plasma. For example, let us assume 1,000 mg of drug is administered, and after 1 hour a plasma concentration is obtained of 10 mg/L and we know the Vd of this drug is 50 L. How much drug is left in the body after 1 hour = 10 mg/mL × 50 L = 500 mg, or about half the dose. We can use this information to estimate the half-life (1 hr) and infer the distribution of the drug goes beyond body water.

Metabolism

The majority of metabolism occurs in the liver and to a lesser extent in the gastrointestinal tract for orally absorbed drugs. Metabolism is divided into phase I and phase II types of reactions; phase I reactions are primarily carried out by cytochrome p450 enzymes and convert the parent drug to a more polar metabolite by adding functional groups. These metabolites may be inactive or active. A prodrug refers to the situation where the parent drug is inactive and the metabolite is active. Phase II reactions are performed by a variety of enzymes and result in the conjugation of the drug with an endogenous substance. These reactions are usually inactivation reactions that increase drug solubility and enhance excretion.

Drugs may be inducers, inhibitors, or substrates of drug metabolizing enzymes. Definitions are included in Table 11.3 (7). Observed changes arising from metabolic drug–drug interactions can be substantial—an order of magnitude or more decrease or increase in the blood and tissue concentrations of a drug or metabolite—and can include formation of toxic and/or active metabolites or increased exposure to a toxic parent compound. These large changes in exposure can alter the safety and efficacy profile of a drug and/or its active metabolites in important ways. This is most obvious and expected for a drug with a narrow therapeutic range (NTR), but is also possible for non-NTR drugs as well. In general, if a drug is a strong or moderate inducer, inhibitor, or a sensitive substrate, drug interaction studies will be required during clinical development.

In vitro studies can frequently serve as a screening mechanism to rule out the importance of a metabolic pathway and the drug–drug interactions that occur through this pathway so that subsequent in vivo testing is unnecessary. This opportunity should be based on appropriately validated experimental methods and rational selection of substrate/interacting drug concentrations.

In addition to in vitro metabolism and drug–drug interaction studies, appropriately designed pharmacokinetic studies, usually performed in the early phases of drug development, can provide important information about metabolic routes of elimination, their contribution to overall elimination, and metabolic drug–drug interactions. In cases where it is necessary to administer an interacting drug, it is crucial to have the adequate scientific background in order to adjust the dosage regimen, avoiding significant resultant toxicity.

It is important that metabolic drug–drug interaction studies explore whether an investigational agent is likely to significantly affect the metabolic elimination of drugs that are routinely taken concomitantly and, conversely, whether these drugs are likely to affect the metabolic elimination of the investigational drug. One example of this is the drug–drug interactions that occur in patients taking tamoxifen and selective serotonin reuptake inhibitors (SSRIs), which are often prescribed to alleviate tamoxifen-associated hot flashes. In a prospective clinical trial, coadministration of tamoxifen and the SSRI paroxetine, an inhibitor of CYP2D6, led to decreased plasma concentration of endoxifen, which is an active metabolite of tamoxifen. Another interesting point in this study was that women with differing CYP2D6 genotypes had significant metabolic differences. Endoxifen concentrations decreased by 64% (95% CI: 39–89) in women with a wild-type CYP2D6 genotype but by only 24% (95% CI: 23–71) in women with a variant CYP2D6 genotype ($p = .03$) (13).

TABLE 11.2 Composition of Total Body Water

Fluid	Volume (L)	Percentage of Body Weight
Extracellular water	13–16	18–22
Plasma	3	4
Blood	7	8
Interstitial fluids	10–13	4–18
Intracellular water	25–28	35–40
Transcellular water	0.7–2	1–3
Total body water	40–46	55–65

TABLE 11.3 Drug Interaction Definitions

Investigational drug	The drug(s) being evaluated in the clinical trial where CTEP holds the IND. In some cases these agents are commercially available, but for the purpose of this recommendation they will be considered investigational
Concurrent medications	Commercially available prescription and over-the-counter medications being taken by the study subject but not mandated by the study protocol
Drug metabolism enzymes	Primarily refer to CYP and UGT but others may be included if data is available
Narrow therapeutic index	Drugs for which there is little separation between therapeutic and toxic doses or the associated blood or plasma concentrations (i.e., exposures) and where a small change in plasma concentration may result in substantial clinical impact
Victim	The object of a drug–drug interaction, typically the substrate
Perpetrator	The precipitating cause of the drug interaction, typically the inducer or inhibitor
In vivo	Data available from clinical (human) pharmacokinetic studies
In vitro	Data available from animal models, cell lines, and isolated hepatocytes
Investigational drug brochure (IB)	A compilation of the clinical and nonclinical data on the investigational product(s) that are relevant to the study of the product(s) in human subjects
Inhibitors	
Strong inhibitor	Anticancer agent that causes a ≥5-fold increase in the plasma AUC values or more than 80% decrease in clearance
Moderate inhibitor	Anticancer agent that causes a ≥2-fold, but <5-fold increase in the plasma AUC values or 50%–79% decrease in clearance
Weak inhibitor	Causes a >1.25-fold but <2-fold increase in the plasma AUC values or 20%–49% decrease in clearance
Inducers	
Strong inducer	Anticancer agent that causes a ≥80% decrease in the plasma AUC
Moderate inducer	Anticancer agent that causes a 50%–79% decrease in plasma AUC
Weak inducer	Anticancer agent that causes a 20%–49% decrease in plasma AUC
Substrates	
Sensitive	Sensitive refers to drugs whose plasma AUC values have been shown to increase 5-fold when coadministered with a known inhibitor
Not sensitive	Not sensitive refers to drugs whose plasma AUC values have been shown to increase less than 5-fold when coadministered with a known inhibitor

AUC, area under the curve; CTEP, Cancer Therapy Evaluation Program; IB, Investigator's Brochure; IND, investigational new drug.

Not every drug–drug interaction is metabolism-based, but may arise from changes in pharmacokinetics caused by absorption, distribution, and excretion interactions. Drug–drug interactions related to transporters are of increasing interest and are important to consider in drug development.

Excretion

The primary pharmacokinetic parameter describing excretion is clearance (Cl), and is perhaps the most important of all pharmacokinetic parameters as it informs the dose and schedule of drug administration. Cl is assumed to be constant and is the process by which a drug is removed from the body, either as unchanged drug via renal elimination or by metabolism and subsequent elimination via the urine or feces. Clearance (Cl) is a proportionality factor that relates the concentration of drug measured in the body to the rate of elimination and is a function of renal or hepatic activity. Dosing and pharmacokinetics studies required to support dosing recommendations in hepatic or renal impairment are described in the Special Populations section.

PHASE I TRIALS

Pharmacokinetic evaluations are critical to phase 1 clinical trials and are used to characterize the dose–concentration relationships for new anticancer drugs (14). The primary purpose is to determine the dosing regimen that achieves target drug exposure in the relevant population. Phase I trials historically involved dose escalation with intensive pharmacokinetic sampling to determine the maximum tolerated dose (MTD), which would subsequently inform the recommended phase II dose (RP2D). Initial phase I studies require an intensive and extensive blood sampling schedule. Samples are obtained frequently, and over a period of five half-lives if possible. After samples are obtained, drug concentrations in plasma are determined by validated assay methodologies and data is typically analyzed by noncompartmental methods or nonlinear regression analysis.

The advantage of noncompartmental pharmacokinetic analysis is its model-independent pharmacokinetic parameters (15). See Table 11.1 for a description of pharmacokinetic parameters. The main assumption for noncompartmental analysis is pharmacokinetic linearity and the assumption that pharmacokinetic parameters do not vary with time or dose. Compartmental analysis requires the use of nonlinear regression and curve fitting and parameters, and is useful for estimating pharmacokinetic parameters as well as predicting plasma concentrations and simultaneous analysis of pharmacokinetics and pharmacodynamics data (16).

In addition to dose escalation studies, newer designs are being employed in early-phase studies (17). With the advent of targeted therapies and immunotherapies it is not always necessary to escalate the dose to the end of patient tolerability and some drugs may be dosed to reach a concentration associated with a therapeutic effect in preclinical studies (14). Drug interaction studies are often conducted in the phase I setting if it is the first time two anticancer agents are administered concurrently and drug interactions are anticipated based on preclinical studies (18).

PHASE II TRIALS

Biomarkers and Pharmacokinetic Relationships

Dose–concentration relationships may contribute to approval of different doses, dosing regimens, or dosage forms, or use of a drug in different populations, when effectiveness is already well established in other settings and the study demonstrates a pharmacodynamic relationship that is similar (9).

In some cases, measurement of systemic exposure levels (e.g., plasma drug concentrations) as part of dose–response studies can provide additional useful information (19). Systemic exposure data are especially useful when an assigned dose is poorly correlated with plasma concentrations, obscuring an existing concentration–response relationship. This can occur when there is a large degree of interindividual variability in pharmacokinetics or there is a nonlinear relationship between dose and plasma drug concentrations. Blood concentrations can also be helpful when (a) both parent drug and metabolites are active, (b) different exposure measures (e.g., Cmax, AUC) provide different relationships between exposure and efficacy or safety, (c) the number of fixed doses in the dose–response studies is limited, and (d) responses are highly variable and it is helpful to explore the underlying causes of variability of response.

Most required clinical pharmacology studies, including renal and hepatic impairment, food effect and drug interaction studies, are conducted in the phase II setting, after the RP2D is determined and preliminary activity of the new anticancer agents is established.

PHASE III TRIALS

The majority of clinical pharmacokinetic studies are conducted in the Phase I–II setting. However, sparse sampling approaches and population pharmacokinetic modeling can be useful in this setting as well.

Population Pharmacokinetics

Population pharmacokinetics is used to evaluate the sources and correlates of variability in drug concentrations among individuals who are the target patient population receiving clinically relevant doses of a drug of interest and is typically conducted as part of phase III clinical trials (20), although population pharmacokinetics modeling can be used in all phases of drug development. Patient-specific factors including ethnicity, renal and hepatic function, interacting medications, body weight, and gender can change dose–concentration relationships. Population pharmacokinetics may be able to identify the factors that cause changes in the dose–concentration relationship and if these changes have a clinical impact.

A key difference between the standard pharmacokinetic approach and population pharmacokinetics is interindividual variability. In the standard approach variability is a factor to be minimized via study design or strict inclusion criteria. The population pharmacokinetic approach embraces and attempts to explain interindividual variability, by collecting pharmacokinetic information in the target population likely to be treated with the drug, by identifying and measuring variability and correlating that variability with patient-specific factors.

Population pharmacokinetic data can often be used to modify dosing recommendations. One example of this in oncology is docetaxel, where Bruno and colleagues (21) demonstrated that individuals with mild to moderate liver function impairment (serum glutamic oxaloacetic transaminase [SGOT] and/or serum glutamic pyruvic transaminase [SGPT] >1.5 × upper limit of normal [ULN] concomitant with alkaline phosphatase >2.5 × ULN) had a decrease in docetaxel clearance by an average of 27% with an increased risk of toxicity. This information was used to provide recommendations for dose reduction of docetaxel for hepatic impairment.

PBPK Models

Physiologically based pharmacokinetic (PBPK) models have recently been accepted by the FDA (9) in support of INDs and NDAs. PBPK analysis builds on population pharmacokinetics and uses physiology, population parameters, and drug characteristics to describe pharmacokinetics and pharmacodynamics behaviors (19). PBPK modeling attempts to overcome one of the major issues in pharmacokinetics analysis, in that we only know drug concentrations in the plasma, by linking together submodels of target organs and tissues that may reproduce measurable physiological outcomes and target concentrations.

PBPK models can be used at all phases of drug development, and are useful for scaling across species to determine starting doses in humans based on animal data in the preclinical setting. PBPK modeling can also be used to predict many pharmacokinetic properties, including the propensity for drug interactions, impact of renal and hepatic failure and absorption, either decreasing or eliminating the need for human pharmacokinetics studies (22).

SPECIAL POPULATIONS

Renal impairment

Most drugs are cleared by elimination of unchanged drug by the kidney and/or by metabolism in the liver. For a drug eliminated primarily via renal excretory mechanisms, impaired renal function may alter its pharmacokinetics and PD to an extent that the dosage regimen needs to be changed from that used in patients with normal renal function (23). Although the most obvious type of change arising from renal impairment is a decrease in renal excretion, or possibly renal metabolism, of a drug or its metabolites, renal impairment has also been associated with other changes, such as changes in absorption, hepatic metabolism, plasma protein binding, and drug distribution (24). These changes may be particularly prominent in patients with severely impaired renal function and have been observed even when the renal route is not the primary route of elimination of a drug. Thus, for most drugs that are likely to be administered to patients with renal impairment, pharmacokinetic characterization should be assessed in patients with renal impairment to provide rational dosing recommendations.

Hepatic Impairment

The liver is involved in the clearance of many drugs through a variety of oxidative and conjugative metabolic pathways and/or through biliary excretion of unchanged drug or metabolites (20,25). Alterations of these excretory and metabolic activities by hepatic impairment can lead to drug accumulation or, less often, failure to form an active metabolite.

Hepatic disease can alter the absorption and disposition of drugs (pharmacokinetics) as well as their efficacy and safety (pharmacodynamics). Even though clinically useful measures of hepatic function to predict drug pharmacokinetics and pharmacodynamics are not generally available, clinical studies in patients with hepatic impairment, usually performed during drug development, can provide information that may help guide initial dosing in patients (3).

If hepatic metabolism and/or excretion accounts for a substantial portion (>20% of the absorbed drug) of the elimination of a drug or active metabolite in patients with impaired hepatic function or it accounts for a lesser amount (<20%), but the drug has a narrow therapeutic window, pharmacokinetic studies are recommended.

Pregnancy/lactation

As women delay childbearing, it is increasingly common to have cancer diagnosed during pregnancy. The diagnostic and therapeutic management of a pregnant patient with cancer is especially difficult because it involves two individuals, the mother and the fetus (21).

Few pharmacokinetic studies have been done in pregnant women receiving chemotherapy, and pregnant women are routinely excluded from clinical trials (5). When it is necessary to treat a pregnant woman, she receives similar weight-based doses as women who are not pregnant, adjusted with the continuing weight gain. The increased blood volume (by almost 50%), and increased renal clearance might decrease active drug concentrations compared with women who are not pregnant and who have the same weight. Increased drug clearance from the body can lead to a reduced drug exposure and effect. A faster hepatic mixed-function oxidase system might also lower drug concentrations, and changes in gastrointestinal function can affect drug absorption. The volume of distribution, peak drug concentration, and half-life of administration is also sometimes changed during pregnancy. Plasma albumin decreases, increasing the amount of unbound active drug; however, estrogen increases other plasma proteins, which might decrease active drug fractions. Additional considerations include the ability of the drug to pass the placenta.

Pediatrics

In the pediatric population, growth and development may alter the pharmacokinetics of a drug when compared to the adult population (26). Of note, the pharmacokinetics in adolescents >16 years of age and weight >50 kg is very similar to adults.

Developmental changes in the pediatric population that can affect absorption include effects on gastric acidity, rates of gastric and intestinal emptying, surface area of the absorption site, gastrointestinal enzyme systems for drugs that are actively transported across the gastrointestinal mucosa, gastrointestinal permeability, and biliary function. Distribution of a drug may be affected by changes in body composition as well as differences in protein binding.

Studies on drug metabolism of specific drugs in children are limited. In general, it is extrapolated that children will form the same metabolites as adults via pathways such as oxidation, reduction, hydrolysis, and conjugation, but rates of metabolite formation can be different. Similarly, drug excretion can vary according to the developmental stage, especially when a drug is predominantly excreted via renal mechanisms.

In addition, there are laws that regulate clinical studies and use of anticancer drugs in the pediatric oncology. The Pediatric Research Act of 2003 provides legislative authority for FDA to require companies to do pediatric testing for drugs and biologics.

Geriatrics

Usually, there are no significant differences in pharmacokinetics for cytotoxic agents based on age alone (27). A progressive decrease in physiologic reserve that affects each individual at a unique pace accompanies aging (28,29). Both cancer and its treatment can be considered physiologic stressors and the age-related decrease in physiologic reserve can affect tolerance to cancer treatment.

A number of age-related changes in drug ADME with aging can contribute to differences in treatment tolerance between older and younger patients. The absorption of drugs can be affected by decreased gastrointestinal motility, decreased splanchnic blood flow, decreased secretion of digestive enzymes, and mucosal atrophy (29). As a person ages, body composition changes, with an increase in body fat and a decrease in lean body mass and total body water. The increase in body fat leads to a rise in the volume of distribution for lipid soluble drugs and a diminution in the volume of distribution for hydrophilic drugs. In the cancer population, malnutrition and hypoalbuminemia can result in an increased unbound concentration of drugs that are albumin-bound (30).

Over a life span, renal mass decreases by approximately 25% to 30%, and renal blood flow decreases by 1% per year after age 50 (31). The decline in glomerular filtration rate (GFR) with age is estimated at 0.75 mL/min per year after age 40; however, approximately one third of patients have no change in creatinine clearance with age. This reduced renal function does not usually result in increased serum creatinine levels because of the simultaneous loss of muscle mass. Therefore, serum creatinine is not an adequate indicator of renal function in the older patient.

The decline in GFR with age translates into pharmacokinetic alterations of drugs or their active metabolites, which are excreted by the kidneys. Due to the physiologic decline in renal function with age, chemotherapy agents that are primarily renally excreted must be dosed with caution in older patients.

Despite increasingly widespread drug exposure with age, older patients did not have adverse outcomes with standard dose. Studies with docetaxel likewise did not find clinically relevant changes in pharmacokinetics in older adults (32).

Drugs that do not have different pharmacokinetics in older adults as compared to younger patients can have different toxicities. Myelosuppression in older adults is an important concern; also, with fluoropyrimidines, mucositis can be severe in older adults. These effects can be difficult to predict. The increased use of hematopoietic growth factors has led to a shift in the toxicity profile. The dose-limiting toxicity of many regimens has shifted to nonhematologic toxicity, particularly neuropathy and gastrointestinal toxicity, which remain significant problems for older patients (32)

In conclusion, there are few reasons to modify dosing based purely on age. If an elderly patient has an adequate performance status as well as renal and hepatic function, the dose that would be used in a younger patient should be used (33).

Obesity

As the number of obese individuals continues to increase in the United States, obesity-based changes in pharmacokinetic parameters are of increasing concern. Obese individuals typically have increased gastric emptying, which can impact oral absorption of medications (34). More importantly, the ratio of adipose tissue to lean body mass is significantly altered in obesity and can impact the Vd of lipid soluble medications. This is particularly important for anesthetics and altered dosing regimens are recommended for obese individuals. Clearance is controlled primarily by underlying physiology, and obese individuals have been shown to have enhanced clearance of cytotoxic chemotherapy, although this is thought to be balanced by body surface area (BSA) dosing. BSA dosing is commonly performed for cytotoxic agents in oncology and is based on the belief that larger patients have larger volumes of distribution, although the BSA is typically capped at 2 m^2.

There are currently no required pharmacokinetic studies addressing obesity in drug development, although this remains an area of research interest.

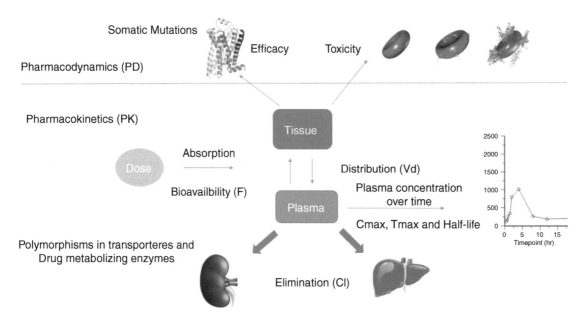

FIGURE 11.2 Overview of pharmacokinetics and pharmacodynamics.

CONCLUSIONS

The ultimate goal of pharmacokinetics and pharmacodynamics is to maximize the likelihood of response in the setting of minimal drug-related toxicity (Figure 11.2). Traditional practice has been based on administration of agents utilizing the MTD, and it is less clear whether this is the optimal dose, especially in the era of targeted agents.

REFERENCES

1. Wagner JG. Pharmacokinetics. *Annu Rev Pharmacol.* 1968;8:67–94.
2. Format and Content of the Human Pharmacokinetics and Bioavailability Section of an Application. www.fda.gov
3. Pharmacokinetics in Patients with Impaired Hepatic Function: Study Design, Data Analysis, and Impact on Dosing and Labeling. www.fda.gov
4. Pharmacokinetics in Patients with Impaired Renal Function: Study Design, Data Analysis, and Impact on Dosing and Labeling. www.fda.gov
5. Pharmacokinetics in Pregnancy: Study Design, Data Analysis, and Impact on Dosing and Labeling. www.fda.gov
6. Clinical Lactation Studies: Study Design, Data Analysis, and Recommendations for Labeling. www.fda.gov
7. Drug Interaction Studies: Study Design, Data Analysis, Implications for Dosing, and Labeling Recommendations. www.fda.gov
8. Population Pharmacokinetics. www.fda.gov
9. Physiologically Based Pharmacokinetic Analyses: Format and Content Guidance for Industry. www.fda.gov
10. Calvo E, Walko C, Dees EC, Valenzuela B. Pharmacogenomics, pharmacokinetics, and pharmacodynamics in the era of targeted therapies. *Am Soc Clin Oncol Educ Book.* 2016;35:e175–e184.
11. Zhang L, Wu F, Lee SC, et al. pH-dependent drug-drug interactions for weak base drugs: potential implications for new drug development. *Clin Pharmacol Ther.* 2014;96(2):266–277.
12. Ogawa R, Echizen H. Clinically significant drug interactions with antacids: an update. *Drugs.* 2011;71(14):1839–1864.
13. Stearns V, Johnson MD, Rae JM, et al. Active tamoxifen metabolite plasma concentrations after coadministration of tamoxifen and the selective serotonin reuptake inhibitor paroxetine. *J Natl Cancer Inst.* 2003;95(23):1758–1764.
14. Mathijssen RH, Sparreboom A, Verweij J. Determining the optimal dose in the development of anticancer agents. *Nat Rev Clin Oncol.* 2014;11(5):272–281.
15. Gillespie WR. Noncompartmental versus compartmental modelling in clinical pharmacokinetics. *Clin Pharmacokinet.* 1991;20(4):253–262.
16. Ranson MR, Scarffe JH. Population and Bayesian pharmacokinetics in oncology. *Clin Oncol (R Coll Radiol).* 1994;6(4):254–260.
17. Bhatt DL, Mehta C. Adaptive designs for clinical trials. *N Engl J Med.* 2016;375(1):65–74.
18. Riviere MK, Le Tourneau C, Paoletti X, et al. Designs of drug-combination phase I trials in oncology: a systematic review of the literature. *Ann Oncol.* 2015;26(4):669–674.
19. Upton RN, Foster DJ, Abuhelwa AY. An introduction to physiologically-based pharmacokinetic models. *Paediatr Anaesth.* 2016;26(11):1036–1046.
22. Ferl GZ, Theil FP, Wong H. Physiologically based pharmacokinetic models of small molecules and therapeutic antibodies: a mini-review on fundamental concepts and applications. *Biopharm Drug Dispos.* 2016;37(2):75–92.
23. Fabre J, Balant L. Renal failure, drug pharmacokinetics and drug action. *Clin Pharmacokinet.* 1976;1(2):99–120.
24. Rowland M, Benet LZ, Graham GG. Clearance concepts in pharmacokinetics. *J Pharmacokinet Biopharm.* 1973;1(2):123–136.
25. Levy RH, Bauer LA. Basic pharmacokinetics. *Ther Drug Monit.* 1986;8(1):47–58.
20. Cohen, A. Pharmacokinetic and pharmacodynamic data to be derived from early-phase drug development designing informative human pharmacology studies. *Clin Pharmacokinet.* 2008;47(6):373–381.
21. Pentheroudakis G. Cancer and pregnancy. *Ann Oncol.* 2008. 19(Suppl. 5):v38–v39.
26. General Clinical Pharmacology Considerations for Pediatric Studies for Drugs and Biological Products. www.fda.gov

27. Hurria A. Clinical trials in older adults with cancer: past and future. *Oncology (Williston Park)*. 2007;21(3):351–358;discussion 363–364, 367.
28. Green JM, Hacker ED. Chemotherapy in the geriatric population. *Clin J Oncol Nurs*. 2004;8(6):591–597.
29. Vincenzi B, Santini D, Spoto S, et al. The antineoplastic treatment in the elderly. *Clin Ter*. 2002;153(3):207–215.
30. Lichtman, SM. Pharmacokinetics and pharmacodynamics in the elderly. *Clin Adv Hematol Oncol*. 2007;5(3):181–182.
31. Karam Z, Tuazon J. Anatomic and physiologic changes of the aging kidney. *Clin Geriatr Med*. 2013;29(3):555–564.
32. Hurria A, Lichtman SM. Pharmacokinetics of chemotherapy in the older patient. *Cancer Control*. 2007;14:32–43.
33. Wasil T, Lichtman SM. Clinical pharmacology issues relevant to the dosing and toxicity of chemotherapy drugs in the elderly. *Oncologist*. 2005;10(8):602–612.
34. Hanley MJ, Abernethy DR, Greenblatt DJ. Effect of obesity on the pharmacokinetics of drugs in humans. *Clin Pharmacokinet*. 2010;49(2):71–87.

Dose Finding Using the Continual Reassessment Method

Mark R. Conaway

METHODS FOR A SINGLE CYTOTOXIC AGENT

In the standard statistical setup, the maximum tolerated dose (MTD) is to be chosen from a prespecified set of doses, $d_1 < d_2 < \ldots < d_k$, with the probability that a patient given dose level d_k experiences a dose-limiting toxicity (DLT) denoted by π_k. The majority of design methods are based on the assumption that the probability of a DLT increases with dose, $\pi_1 < \pi_2 < \ldots < \pi_k$. At any point in the trial, we will have observed a number of patients, n_k treated at dose level d_k, and of the patients treated, Y_k have experienced a DLT, $Y_k = 0, 1, \ldots, n_k$, and $k = 1, 2, \ldots, K$. The target level of toxicity is denoted by θ.

Methods in this situation are often broadly categorized as "rule-based," in which the dose chosen for the current patient is based on the observed number of toxicities in the most recently observed cohort of patients. Other designs are "model-based," in which an assumed parametric model is fit to all the accumulated data and used to guide dose allocation and the estimation of the MTD (1) at the end of the study. In practice, the distinction between rule-based and model-based is not completely clear, as there are methods that use rule-based allocation (2–5) but use a parametric model or isotonic regression at the end of the trial to estimate the MTD. Other methods (6,7) are model-based, but start with an initial rule-based stage before using the parametric model to guide the allocation of doses to patients and to estimate the MTD.

The continual reassessment method (CRM) (8) is the most widely recognized model-based method for dose-finding trials. The original CRM paper proposed a single-stage design; a later version (6) is a two-stage design using a rule-based algorithm in the first stage and maximum likelihood estimation in the second stage. An excellent overview of the theoretical properties and guidelines for the practical application of the method are given in (9) and (10). The CRM assumes a parametric model for the dose–toxicity curve, $F(x, b)$, but it does not require that the model be correct across all the doses under consideration. The model only needs to be sufficiently flexible so that, if x^* denotes the true MTD corresponding to a target value θ, there exists a parameter value b^* such that $F(x^*, b^*) = \theta$. The original CRM paper discussed one- and two-parameter models, but focused primarily on one-parameter models because the simpler models tended to have better properties in terms of identifying the correct MTD.

The most common implementation of the CRM uses the "empiric" model,

$$\pi_k = \psi_k^{exp(a)} \qquad \text{(Eq. 12-1)}$$

where $0 < \psi_1 < \psi_2 < \ldots < \psi_K < 1$ are prespecified constants, often referred to as the "skeleton" values and a is a scalar parameter. The parameterization $exp(a)$ ensures that the probability of toxicity is increasing in dose for all $-\infty < a < \infty$. The original CRM paper (8) provided guidance on eliciting a gamma prior for $exp(a)$ but noted that in many cases, the special case of an exponential prior with mean 1 gave satisfactory performance. The skeleton values can be based on the prior, as suggested in the original CRM paper, or by using the method of Lee and Cheung (11), where the skeleton values are calibrated in a way to give good performance for the CRM across a variety of true dose–response curves.

An alternative method for choosing a prior is to use a "pseudodata prior" (12,13) in which "toxicities" $(y_1^*, y_2^*, \ldots, y_K^*)$ and "patients treated" $(n_1^*, n_2^*, \ldots, n_K^*)$ are chosen prior to the study. The ratio $\dfrac{y_k^*}{n_k^*}$ reflects the prior belief about the toxicity probability at dose level k and n_k^* represents the strength of that belief. Once the prior and skeleton values are chosen, the first patient is assigned to the dose level with prior probability closest to the target θ. After that, the CRM allocates patients sequentially, with each patient assigned to the dose level with the model-based estimated probability of toxicity closest to the target. To be specific, suppose that $j-1$ patients have been observed on the trial, with $n_1, n_2, \ldots, n_k$ patients assigned to dose levels $1, 2, \ldots, K, \sum_{k=1}^{K} n_k = j - 1$ and with Y_k patients on dose level $k, k = 1, 2, \ldots, K$, having experienced a DLT. With the empiric model (Eq. 12-1) the likelihood, $L(a; n_k, Y_k)$ is

$$L(a; n_k, y_k) = \prod_{k=1}^{K} \psi_k^{y_k \exp(a)} (1 - \psi_k^{\exp(a)})^{n_k - y_k}. \quad \text{(Eq. 12-2)}$$

If we use a parametric form, g(a), for the prior distribution on a, the posterior density of a, $h(a)$, is proportional to

$$h(a) \propto \int L(a; n_k, y_k) g(a) da. \quad \text{(Eq. 12-3)}$$

If we use the pseudodata prior, the posterior $h(a)$, is proportional to

$$h(a) \propto \prod_{k=1}^{K} \psi_k^{(y_k + Y_k^*) \exp(a)} (1 - \psi_k^{\exp(a)})^{(n_k + n_k^*) - (y_k + y_k^*)}. \quad \text{(Eq. 12-4)}$$

The updated model-based toxicity probabilities are $\hat{\pi}_k = \psi_k^{\exp(\hat{a})}$, where $\hat{a}$ can be the posterior mean computed via numerical integration, an approximation to the posterior mean (8), the posterior mode, or the posterior median (14). The jth patient is assigned to the dose level k with the smallest value of $\Delta(\hat{\pi}_k, \theta)$, where $\Delta(u, v)$ is a prespecified measure of distance between u and v. The original paper uses a quadratic distance, $\Delta(u, v) = (u - v)^2$, but asymmetric distance functions, which give greater loss to deviations above the target than below, could also be used. The updating of a and the allocation of patients to the dose with updated toxicity probability closest to the target continues until a prespecified number of patients have been observed. At the end of the study, the MTD is taken to be the dose that the next patient would have received had the trial not ended.

A likelihood-based version of the CRM, conducted in two stages, is presented by (6). The first stage uses a rule-based design, and continues until there is heterogeneity in the responses from patients. Once heterogeneity is observed, the trial proceeds as in the original CRM, except that the estimate of the parameter a is based on maximizing the likelihood (Eqn. 12-2). Shen and O'Quigley use single-patient cohorts in the first stage: if a patient does not experience a DLT, the next patient is treated at the next highest dose level.

Cheung (9) defines the notion of "coherence" for a dose allocation method. For single-patient allocations, a method is coherent if it does not recommend escalation after a toxicity is observed and does not recommend a de-escalation if a DLT is not observed for the previous patient. Cheung shows that the one-stage Bayesian CRM is coherent, and that the two-stage CRM is coherent as long as it does not produce an incoherent transition at the seam between the rule-based and model-based stages. The operating characteristics of the CRM have been evaluated in numerous articles, and it has been shown to have excellent performance in terms of identifying the MTD (15–17).

Figure 12.1 gives an example of the two-stage CRM. There are five dose levels, with the trial data generated from true toxicity probabilities of (0.02, 0.04, 0.10, 0.20, 0.30). With a chosen target toxicity probability equal to 0.20, dose level 4 is the true MTD. The skeleton values are (0.05, 0.11, 0.20, 0.31, 0.42), chosen according to Cheung's recommendations with a prior MTD guess equal to 3 and a δ parameter equal to 0.25 times the target. The dark circles represent DLTs and open circles represent patients without a DLT. The identical diagram is found using the pseudodata prior of (13).

This trial illustrates many of the important features of the CRM. The MTD recommendation at the end of the trial is dose level 4, and many of the 30 patients are treated at the MTD.

There are a number of misperceptions concerning the CRM. One is that skeleton values are difficult to specify and that the performance of the method will suffer if the skeleton values are far from the true underlying toxicity probabilities. On the contrary, a change in the skeleton values from ψ_k to ψ_k^c, $c > 0$, does not affect the maximum of the likelihood (Eq. 12-2), meaning, for example, that using very different sets of skeleton values 0.1, 0.2, 0.3, 0.4, 0.5, 0.6, or $0.1^3, 0.2^3, \ldots 0.6^3$ can produce exactly the same results in the likelihood version and in the Bayesian version, as long as the prior is recalibrated for each change in the power (18).

This is not to say that the skeleton choice is irrelevant, but rather that skeleton spacing is more important than the actual skeleton values. For example, choosing a set of skeleton values that rise steeply, such as 0.01, 0.02, 0.05, 0.50, 0.90, 0.95 will tend to result in recommendations in the steep part of the skeleton. This skeleton will yield excellent properties when the true MTD is in the steep part of the skeleton and poor results otherwise. Skeletons like this can be avoided by using the method of Lee and Cheung (11), or simply spacing out skeleton values over the interval (0,1). Another option is to use the multiple skeleton approach of Yin and Yuan (19), who propose a Bayesian-model-averaging (BMA) version of the CRM. Rather than specifying a single skeleton, Yin and Yuan specify multiple skeletons, putting a prior on each set of values. Sequential allocations of patients to doses are made using the BMA estimates of the toxicity probabilities.

Another misperception is that the one-parameter power model is not sufficiently rich to allow accurate

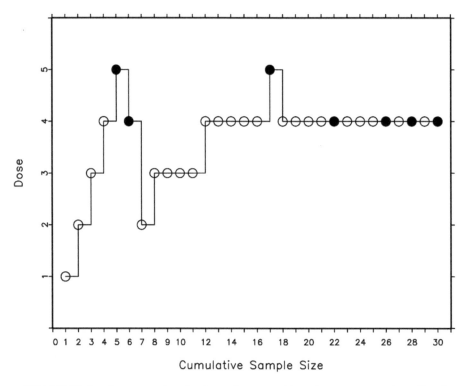

FIGURE 12.1 An example of a two-stage continual reassessment method

estimation of the MTD. The original CRM paper (8) compared one- and two-parameter versions of the method and found that the one-parameter version outperformed the two-parameter version, even when the data were generated from a two-parameter model. Chevret (20) found that the two-parameter model could give slight improvements in estimating the probability of toxicity at the chosen MTD, but only for specific scenarios and certain prior distributions. Paoletti and Kramar (17) generated 5,000 dose–toxicity curves and found that the one-parameter power model had superior properties to the two-parameter logistic model and other single-parameter models such as a logistic model with either a fixed slope or intercept.

A number of modifications have been proposed to address some of these perceived problems (21,22) including the recommendation to start at the lowest dose and to base allocations on cohorts of two or three patients rather than the single-patient cohorts originally proposed. These modifications are often used in practice (23–27).

TIME-TO-EVENT TOXICITY OUTCOMES

The original CRM paper (8) noted that the observation of a toxicity does not occur immediately and there may be patients to be enrolled in the study before all the observations have been completed on the prior patients. This paper suggested treating the new patients at the last allocated dose, or given the uncertainty in the dose allocations, treating patients one level above or one level below the most recent model-recommended dose.

Cheung and Chappell (28) proposed an extension known as the "time-to-event CRM" (TITE-CRM) that allowed for a weighted toxicity model, with weights proportional to the time that the patient has been observed. They consider a number of weight functions, but simulation results suggested that a simple linear weight function of the form $w(u) = u/T$, where T is a fixed length of follow-up observation time for each patient, is adequate. If a patient is observed to have a toxicity at time $u < T$, the follow-up time u is set to equal T.

In choosing the dose allocation for patient j, and using the empiric model (Eq. 12-1) for the CRM, the TITE-CRM likelihood is given by

$$L(a; y_1, \ldots y_{j-1}, x_1, \ldots x_{j-1} = \prod_{l=1}^{j-1} \left[\frac{t_l}{T} \psi_{x_l}^{exp(a)} \right]^{y_l} \quad \text{(Eq. 12-5)}$$
$$\left[1 - \frac{t_l}{T} \psi_{x_l}^{exp(a)} \right]^{1-y_l}$$

where $y_1, \ldots y_{j-1}$ are toxicity indicators and $x_1, \ldots x_{j-1}$ are the indices of the dose allocations for the first $j-1$ patients. Note that the likelihood (Eq. 12-5) is written in terms of the individual patient observations, whereas (Eq. 12-2) groups patients according to the dose received. If all the subjects were fully observed, $t_l = T$ for all $l = 1, \ldots, j-1$, the likelihood (Eq. 12-5) reduces to (Eq. 12-2). Cheung and Chappell investigate this generalization of both the one-stage Bayesian CRM (8) and the two-stage likelihood CRM (6).

Normolle and Lawrence (29) discuss the use of the TITE-CRM in radiation oncology studies, where the toxicities tend to occur late in the follow-up period. Polley (30) observes that in studies with rapid patient accrual and late toxicities, the TITE-CRM can allocate too many patients to overly toxic doses. The paper has a comparison of a modification of the TITE-CRM that was suggested in the original TITE-CRM paper, as well as a modification that incorporates wait times between patient accruals. A version of escalation with overdose control (EWOC) with time to event endpoints is described in Mauguen et al. (31) and Tighiouart et al. (32).

Extensions of the CRM

The CRM can be extended naturally to cover more complex dose-finding studies (33,34), including combinations of agents and heterogeneous groups of patients. Wages et al. (7,35) propose the CRM for partial orders (partial order continual reassessment method [POCRM]) that can estimate a single or multiple MTDs for a combination of agents. Wages et al. (36) extended the TITE-CRM to the studies involving combinations of agents.

In some dose-finding trials, there are several groups of patients, and the goal is to estimate an MTD within each group. For example, Ramanathan et al. (37) stratifies patients into none, mild, moderate, or severe liver dysfunction at baseline. A similar classification is used by LoRusso et al. (38). In each of these cases, the group structure was not used in the design, in that parallel phase I studies were conducted within each group and the design did not account for the expectation that the MTD would be lower in the more severely impaired patients at baseline.

O'Quigley et al. (39) proposed a generalization of the CRM (8) for two groups. Legezda and Ibrahim (12) proposed a related method, augmenting the dose–toxicity model for a vector of patient characteristics and putting a prior on the coefficient in the dose–toxicity model. The shift model (40,41) is a way of generalizing the CRM to two ordered groups. Yuan and Chappell (42) proposed a generalization of the CRM that is a hybrid of the single agent–single group CRM and isotonic regression methods described by Robertson et al. (43).

REFERENCES

1. Le Tourneau C, Lee J, Siu L. Dose escalation methods in Phase I clinical trials. *J Natl Cancer Inst.* 2009;101:708–720.
2. Ji Y, Li Y, Bekele B. Dose-finding in Phase I clinical trials based on toxicity probability intervals. *Clinical Trials.* 2007;4:235–244.
3. Storer B. Design and analysis of Phase I clinical trials. *Biometrics.* 1989;45(3):925–937.
4. Stylianou M, Flournoy N. Dose finding using the biased coin up-and-down design and isotonic regression. *Biometrics.* 2002;58:171–177.
5. Yuan J, Liu P, Li Y, Bekele B. A modified toxicity probability interval method for dose-finding trials. *Clinical Trials.* 2010;7:653–663.
6. Shen L, O'Quigley J. Continual reassessment method: a likelihood approach. *Biometrics.* 1996;52(2):673–684.
7. Wages N, Conaway M, O'Quigley J. Dose-finding design for multi-drug combinations. *Clinical Trials.* 2011;8:380–389.
8. O'Quigley J, Pepe M, Fisher L. Continual reassessment method: a practical design for Phase I clinical trials in cancer. *Biometrics.* 1990;46(1):33–48.
9. Cheung YK. *Dose Finding by the Continual Reassessment Method.* Boca Raton, FL: Chapman and Hall/CRC Biostatistics Series; 2011.
10. O'Quigley J, Iasonos A. Dose-finding designs based on the continual reassessment method. In: Crowley J, Hoering A, eds. *Handbook of Statistics in Clinical Oncology.* 3rd edn. Boca Raton, FL: Chapman and Hall/CRC Biostatistics Series; 2012:21–52.
11. Lee S, Cheung YK. Model calibration in the continual reassessment method. *Clinical Trials.* 2009;6:227–238.
12. Legezda A, Ibrahim J. Heterogeneity in Phase I clinical trials: prior elicitation and computation using the continual reassessment method. *Stat Med.* 2001;20:867–882.
13. Whitehead J, Thygesen H, Whitehead A. A Bayesian dose-finding procedure for Phase I clinical trials based only on the assumption of monotonicity. *Stat Med.* 2010;29:1808–1824.
14. Chu P-L, Lin Y, Shih WJ. Unifying CRM and EWOC designs for Phase I cancer clinical trials. *J Stat Plan Inference.* 2009;139:1146–1163.
15. Wages N, Conaway M, O'Quigley J. Performance of two-stage continual reassessment method relative to an optimal benchmark. *Clinical Trials.* 2013;10:862–875.
16. Ahn C. An evaluation of Phase I cancer clinical trial designs. *Stat Med.* 1998;17:1537–1549.
17. Paoletti X, Kramar A. A comparison of model choices for the continual reassessment method in Phase I cancer trials. *Stat Med.* 2009;28:3012–3028.
18. Iasonos A, O'Quigley J. Interplay of priors and skeletons in two-stage continual reassessment method. *Stat Med.* 2012;31(30):4321–4336.
19. Yin G, Yuan Y. Bayesian model averaging continual reassessment method in Phase I clinical trials. *J Am Stat Assoc.* 2009;104:954–968.
20. Chevret S. The continual reassessment method in cancer Phase I clinical trials: a simulation study. *Stat Med.* 1993;12:1093–1108.
21. Faries D. Practical modifications of the continual reassessment method for Phase I cancer clinical trials. *J Biopharm Stat.* 4:147–164, 1994.
22. Goodman S, Zahurak M, Piantadosi S. Some practical improvements in the continual reassessment method for Phase I studies. *Stat Med.* 1995;14:1149–1161.
23. Shah J, Jakubowiak A, O'Connor O, et al. Phase I study of the Novel Investigational NEDD8-Activating Enzyme Inhibitor Pevonedistat (MLN4924) in patients with relapsed/refractory multiple myeloma or lymphoma. *Clin Cancer Res.* 2016;22(1):34–43.
24. Sarantopoulos G, Shapiro GI, Cohen R, et al. Phase I Study of the Investigational NEDD8- Activating Enzyme Inhibitor Pevonedistat (TAK-924/MLN4924) in patients with advanced solid tumors. *Clin Cancer Res.* 2016;22(4):847–857.
25. Hohloch K, Zeynalova S, Chapuy B, et al. Modified BEAM with triple autologous stem cell transplantation for patients with relapsed aggressive non-Hodgkin lymphoma. *Ann Hematol.* 2016;95:1121–1128.

26. Gouy S, Ferronb G, Glehen O, et al. Results of a multicenter Phase I dose-finding trial of hyperthermic intraperitoneal cisplatin after neoadjuvant chemotherapy and complete cytoreductive surgery and followed by maintenance bevacizumab in initially unresectable ovarian cancer. *Gynecol Oncol*. 2016;142:237–242.

27. Pant S, Jones S, Kurkjian C, et al. A first-in-human Phase I study of the oral Notch inhibitor, LY900009, in patients with advanced cancer. *Eur J Cancer*. 2016;56:1–9.

28. Cheung YK, Chappell R. Sequential designs for Phase I clinical trials with late-onset toxicities. *Biometrics*. 2010;56:1177–1182.

29. Normolle D, Lawrence T. Designing dose-escalation trials with late-onset toxicities using the time-to-event continual reassessment method. *J Clin Oncol*. 2006;24:4426–4433.

30. Polley M-Y. Practical modifications to the time-to-event continual reassessment method for Phase I cancer trials with fast patient accrual and late-onset toxicities. *Stat Med*. 2011;30:2130–2143.

31. Mauguen A, Le Deleya M, Zohar S. Dose-finding approach for dose escalation with overdose control considering incomplete observations. *Stat Med*. 2011;30:1584–1594.

32. Tighiouart M, Liu Y, Rogatko A. Escalation with overdose control using time to toxicity for cancer Phase I clinical trials. *PLoS One*. 2014;9(3):e93070.

33. O'Quigley J, Conaway M. Extended model-based designs for more complex dose-finding studies. *Stat Med*. 2011;30:2062–2069.

34. O'Quigley J, Conaway M. Continual reassessment and related dose-finding designs. *Stat Sci*. 2010;25(2):202–216.

35. Wages, Conaway M, O'Quigley J. Continual reassessment method for partial ordering. *Biometrics*. 2011;67:1555–1563.

36. Wages N, Conaway M, O'Quigley J. Using the time-to-event continual reassessment method in the presence of partial orders. *Stat Med*. 2013;32:131–141.

37. Ramanathan R, Egorin M, Takimoto C, et al. Phase I and pharmacokinetic study of imatinib mesylate in patients with advanced malignancies and varying degrees of liver dysfunction: a study by the National Cancer Institute Organ Dysfunction Working Group. *J Clin Oncol*. 2008;26:563–569.

38. LoRusso P, Venkatakrishnan K, Ramanathan R, et al. Pharmacokinetics and safety of bortezomib in patients with advanced malignancies and varying degrees of liver dysfunction: Phase I NCI Organ Dysfunction Working Group Study NCI-6432. *Clin Cancer Res*. 2012;18(10):1–10.

39. O'Quigley J, Shen L, Gamst A. Two sample continual reassessment method. *J Biopharm Stat*. 1999;9:17–44.

40. O'Quigley J. Phase I and Phase I/II dose finding algorithms using continual reassessment method. In: Crowley J, Ankherst D, eds. *Handbook of Statistics in Clinical Oncology*. 2nd edn. Boca Raton, FL: Chapman and Hall/CRC Biostatistics Series; 2006.

41. O'Quigley J, Iasonos A. Bridging solutions in dose-finding problems. *J Biopharm Stat*. 2014;6(2):185–197.

42. Yuan Z, Chapell R. Isotonic designs for Phase I cancer clinical trials with multiple risk groups. *Clinical Trials*. 2004;1(6):499–508.

43. Robertson T, Wright FT, Dykstra R. *Order Restricted Statistical Inference*. New York, NY: J. Wiley; 1988.

Design of Phase II Trials

Hongkun Wang and Gina R. Petroni

The most common primary goal of a phase II trial is to assess the therapeutic efficacy of a new agent or treatment regimen, and decide if the biological activity of the new agent or regimen is sufficient to warrant further investigation. Historically most phase II trials used a one-sample design, in which all the patients accrued were treated with the new agent or treatment regimen. Based upon a current review of phase II trials published in the past 2 years in the *Journal of Clinical Oncology and Clinical Cancer Research*, approximately 45% of phase II trials include randomization, usually among two arms. Many methods of single-stage, multistage, and sequential designs and analyses have been proposed and are used in practice. In this chapter, we describe some of the most common designs and provide examples of the use of each approach in practice. We discuss designs with multiple arms and multiple endpoints and give some concluding remarks toward the end of the chapter.

In order to illustrate the different design choices, we apply all the methods we discuss to a common example based upon a phase II study by Rietschel et al. (1) of extended-dose temozolomide (TMZ) in patients with melanoma. Patients with stage IV or unresectable stage III melanoma were enrolled into the study and two cohorts of patients, M1c disease or not, were studied. Detailed information regarding patient entry criteria, dose and administration of TMZ, study design, and study results can be found in the original paper. The same study design and target rates were used within each cohort, and serve as the basis to illustrate many of the designs discussed. In some examples, cohort-specific data are identified to display sequential design strategies.

SINGLE-STAGE DESIGNS

Hypothesis Testing Framework

In a single-stage phase II trial, n patients are accrued and treated. Based on the anticipated number of responses, a statistical test is formulated to decide

whether the new therapy should be tested further for efficacy. It is common to define the response variable as a dichotomous outcome where patients are classified as having *responded* or *not responded* depending upon prespecified criteria. The population proportion of patients who respond to the new therapy is denoted by p. The population proportion of patients who respond to the standard therapy is denoted by p_0, which is assumed known. With this notation, the hypothesis test can be written as $H_0: p \leq p_0$ versus $H_a: p > p_0$. The null hypothesis, H_0, will be rejected if the number of observed responses is greater than a specified threshold; otherwise we fail to reject the null hypothesis. If X is the random variable that counts the number of responses in a sample of n patients, then the distribution of X follows a binomial (p) distribution with probability density function $P(X = k) = \binom{n}{k} p^k (1-p)^{n-k}$ where $\binom{n}{k} = \frac{n!}{k!(n-k)!}$. If we let r denote the number of observed responses, and assume p_a is the response rate in the alternative hypothesis that is "important not to miss" then the sample size n and critical value c should satisfy the following equations:

$$a = P(\text{reject } H_0 \mid p = p_0) = P(X \geq c \mid p_0)$$
$$= \sum_{k=c}^{n} \binom{n}{k} p_0^k (1-p_0)^{n-k} \tag{Eq. 13-1}$$

and

$$1 - \beta = P(\text{reject } H_0 \mid p_a) = P(X \geq c \mid p_a)$$
$$= \sum_{k=c}^{n} \binom{n}{k} p_a^k (1-p_a)^{n-k} \tag{Eq. 13-2},$$

where a and β are the maximum tolerable levels for the probability of type I (false positive) and type II (false negative) errors. The type I error a represents the probability that the study will incorrectly identify a new therapy as "sufficiently promising" when the new therapy is no more effective than the standard. The type II error β represents the probability that the study will incorrectly identify a truly promising therapy as "not sufficiently promising."

In the TMZ example, it was assumed that a null response rate of 10% would be considered "not sufficiently promising" while an alternative response rate similar to that of extended-dose TMZ with antiangiogenic agents of 30% would be considered "sufficiently promising." Type I and type II error rates were set at 0.10. Using the preceding formulas (Eq. 13-1) and (Eq. 13-2) with $p_0 = 0.1$ and $p_a = 0.3$, a sample of size 25 will yield $a = 0.098$ and $\beta = 0.090$ (power = 0.910) with a critical value $c = 5$ responses. Thus, at the end of the study we would reject the null hypothesis in favor of the alternative if five or more responses are observed among the 25 patients.

For large n and a moderate p, the test can be based on $\hat{p} = r / n$, which is asymptotically normally distributed. A test statistic for testing H_0 is given by

$$z = \frac{\hat{p} - p_0}{\sqrt{\dfrac{p_0(1 - p_0)}{n}}} = \frac{r - np_0}{\sqrt{np_0(1 - p_0)}} \qquad \text{(Eq. 13-3)}$$

which follows asymptotically a normal distribution. H_0 will be rejected if $z > z_{1-a}$, where z_{1-a} is the $(1 - a)$ percentile of the standard normal distribution. The p value is given by $P(Z \geq z \mid p_0) = 1 - \Phi(z)$, where Φ is the standard normal cumulative distribution function. The sample size n required to have a significance level a and power $1 - \beta$ can be calculated approximately from $n = \{z_{1-a} [p_0(1 - p_0)]^{\frac{1}{2}} + z_{1-\beta} [p_a(1-p_a)]^{\frac{1}{2}}\}^2 / (p - p_a)^2$, with z_{1-a} and $z_{1-\beta}$ the $(1 - a)$ and $(1 - \beta)$ percentiles of the standard normal distribution.

The sample size from the large-sample approximation can be quite different from the sample size calculated from binomial formulas (Eq. 13-1 and Eq. 13-2). Using the TMZ design parameters with a type I error rate of 0.1 and power of 0.9, the required sample size would be 30 using (Eq. 13-3).

Confidence Interval or Precision Framework

In a single-stage phase II trial, sample size can be chosen to satisfy a specified level of precision where a useful measure of precision is the confidence interval around the estimated parameter. Here the goal is estimation and not hypothesis testing. Consider the 95% confidence interval for p, the proportion of interest. At the end of the trial p is estimated by $\hat{p} \pm 1.96 \sqrt{\hat{p}(1 - \hat{p}) / n}$ where $\hat{p} = (\# \text{ responses} / n)$. For sample size estimation one must decide upon how narrow or *precise* a 95% confidence interval is desired at the final analysis (for example ±10%). Narrowness is defined by the

half-width of the 95% confidence interval, which is equal to $1.96 \sqrt{p(1 - p) / n}$. With an initial guess for p, the equation can be solved for n, or one can set $p = .5$ the maximal amount for $p(1 - p)$. This method uses the normal approximation to the binomial distribution. For extreme values of p (say, $p < .2$ or $p > .8$) estimation should be based upon exact binomial confidence limits.

In the TMZ example, we could assume that the response rate will be similar to that of extended-dose TMZ with antiangiogenic agents of 30%. Setting $p = .30$ then we would need $n = 36$ for a half-width of 15% or $n = 81$ for a half-width of 10%. For a one-sided 95% lower limit confidence interval with distance from the sample proportion to the lower limit of 15% and 10% would require $n = 26$ and $n = 57$, respectively.

MULTISTAGE DESIGNS

In a multistage setting, patients are accrued into the study in several stages. Testing is performed at each stage after a predefined target accrual has been completed. At each stage a decision of whether to terminate the trial early or to continue to the next stage is made. In the most commonly used multistage designs, accrual was to stop early only when the preliminary data supported inactivity of the new agent. A variety of early-stopping rules have been proposed.

Gehan's Two-Stage Designs

The two-stage design for phase II setting was first proposed by Gehan (2) in 1961. The goal was to identify the minimum number of patients to observe with a sequence of no responses before concluding that the new drug was not worthy of further study. It is important to note that Gehan proposed this design when the response rate for the new agent under investigation was expected to be low, for instance, no more than 20%.

In the first stage, n_1 patients are enrolled and X_1 responses are observed. If $X_1 = 0$, the trial is closed to accrual. If one or more patients respond ($X_1 > 0$), then accrual to the second stage begins. In the second stage, n_2 additional patients are accrued and X_2 responses are observed. The number of additional patients is chosen to estimate the response rate within a specified level of precision. With this design the true response rate, p, can be estimated by $\dfrac{X_1 + X_2}{n_1 + n_2}$, the total number of responders in both stages, divided by the number of patients accrued at each stage.

In Gehan's design, the first-stage sample size n_1 is chosen to give a small probability of early stopping (say, 5%) at a fixed target response rate p_a, considered to be the minimum response rate of interest, in a sequence of no responses. The first-stage sample size n_1 is found by solving $0.05 = P(\text{Stop early} \mid p_a) = P(X_1 = 0) = (1 - p_a)^{n_1}$. The second-stage sample size n_2 is chosen to give sufficient precision for estimating the response rate p after all patients are observed. The precision is based on choosing a desired value for the standard error, $\sqrt{\dfrac{p(1 - p)}{n_1 + n_2}}$.

For example, if one wants the precision of effectiveness to be no greater than s, then n_2 can be chosen to solve

$$s = \sqrt{\frac{\hat{p}_1(1 - \hat{p}_1)}{n_1 + n_2}}, \text{ where } \hat{p}_1 = X_1 / n_1. \quad \text{(Eq. 13-4)}$$

At the end of the trial, p is estimated by $\hat{p} = \dfrac{X_1 + X_2}{n_1 + n_2}$, with an approximate standard error given by $SE(\hat{p}) = \sqrt{\dfrac{\hat{p}_1(1 - \hat{p}_1)}{n_1 + n_2}}$. To be conservative, Gehan suggested using the upper 75% confidence limit for the true percentage of treatment success in the first sample in (Eq. 13-4).

In Gehan's design, the number of patients accrued in the second stage depends on the number of responses in the first stage and the desired standard error. In practice, Gehan's design is often used with 14 patients in the first stage and 11 patients in the second stage. This provides for estimation with approximately a 10% standard error. Higher precision provides better estimates but requires much larger sample sizes. Gehan's design is sufficient for the very specific context in which it was derived, for instance, low small expected response rate, but has practical and statistical disadvantages in other situations, and is not often used today.

In the TMZ design, the response rate of interest is defined as at least 0.3 ($p_a \geq 0.3$). Following Gehan's approach, in the first stage the $P(\text{Stop early} \mid p_a) \leq 0.1$ gives $n_1 = 7$; the probability of observing all seven consecutive failures is $(1 - 0.3)^7 = 0.082$. The chance of at least one success would be $1 - 0.082 = 0.918$ or 91.8%. Thus if 0/7 responses are observed, we would reject the new treatment and would be approximately 92% confident that the response rate with the new treatment is less than 30%. If at least one response is observed, then the trial would continue to accrue to the second stage. Assuming a standard error of 10% leads to a very broad 95% confidence interval and reducing it to 5% leads to very large second-stage sample sizes. The sample size for the second stage is approximately 16 or 83 patients for standard errors of 10% and 5%, respectively using (Eq. 13-4) with the upper 75% confidence limit of 0.34.

Fleming's *K*-Stage Designs

The design proposed by Gehan allowed for early termination only if preliminary data supported that the

new therapy was likely to be ineffective. Schultz et al. (3) defined a general multiple testing procedure as an alternative to the single-stage design. Fleming (4) continued the work of Schultz et al. and proposed the *K*-stage design to determine appropriate acceptance and rejection regions at each stage. In addition to allowing for early stopping if a treatment appears ineffective, Fleming's design allows for early stopping if the treatment appears overwhelmingly effective, while preserving (approximately) size and power characteristics of a single-stage design.

The study is done in K stages, with the kth stage sample size equal to n_k, $k = 1, \ldots, K$. The total sample size over all stages, $n = n_1 + n_2 + \ldots + n_k$, is guided by the fixed sample design using the exact binomial calculations (Eqs. 13-1 and 13-2) and the large-sample approximation. Fleming derived upper and lower boundaries that would allow investigators to make decisions based on the accumulated number of responses observed by the end of each stage. If the number of responses at the end of the kth stage exceeds the upper boundary for the kth stage, the study can be terminated with the conclusion that the treatment shows promise. If the accumulated number of responses is less than the lower boundary, the study can be terminated with the conclusion that the treatment is not effective. If neither boundary is crossed, the study continues by enrolling the next set of patients. The stage boundaries are chosen to preserve the type I and type II error rates of the fixed sample size design. Even though Fleming derived the boundaries based on normal approximations, he evaluated the properties via simulations for small sample cases and concluded that the approximations give close answers.

In Fleming's design, decisions in favor of or against the new agent occur only when initial results are extreme. In practice, investigators rarely choose to terminate a phase II trial early if the data supports that the treatment is effective. Instead, they want to continue to get supportive data and to plan the possible follow-up phase III trial, which will take time to develop.

Referring to the TMZ design parameters, a Fleming two-stage design with 25 total patients and 16 in the first stage would yield an exact a value of 0.095 and a β value of 0.097. In the first stage the trial would stop for futility if one or fewer responses are observed; or the trial would stop in favor of the new agent if at least five responses are observed; otherwise the trial would continue to a second stage. At the final analysis (i.e., the end of the second stage) if only three responses are observed among all the patients, we would fail to reject the null hypothesis and conclude that the new agent does not warrant further study. If four or more responses are observed we would reject the null hypothesis and conclude that the data supports that the new agent is worthy of further study. Note in this example that the final critical value to reject the null hypothesis is decreased by one compared to the single-stage decision rule.

Simon's Optimal Two-Stage Designs

Simon (5) proposed an optimal two-stage design, where optimality is defined in terms of minimizing the expected sample size when the true response probability is p_0. The trial is terminated early only for ineffective therapies. Simon argued that when the new agent has substantial activity, it is important for planning the larger comparative trial to estimate the proportion, extent, and durability of response for as many patients as possible in the phase II trial. The hypothesis to be tested is the same as in other phase II trials, $H_0: p \leq p_0$ versus $H_a: p > p_0$.

The Simon design consists of choosing stage sample sizes n_1 and n_2 along with decision rules c_1 and c_2, where c_1 and c_2 are critical values to guide decisions at each stage. At the first stage, patients are accrued and X_1 responses are observed. If too few responses are observed in the first stage $X_1 \leq c_1$, the trial is stopped and the treatment is declared "not sufficiently promising" to warrant further study in a comparative trial (fail to reject H_0). If the number of patients who respond exceeds the prespecified boundary $X_1 > c_1$, an additional n_2 patients will be accrued into the second stage of the study. Among the n_2 patients accrued in the second stage, X_2 responses are observed. If the total number of responders in both stages exceeds the prespecified boundary $X_1 + X_2 > c_2$, the null hypothesis is rejected and the treatment is deemed sufficiently promising. If there are too few observed responders $X_1 + X_2 \leq c_2$, then the null hypothesis is not rejected. The boundaries c_1 and c_2 are chosen to meet the following type I and type II error specifications:

$$(\text{size}) \ P[X_1 > c_1, X_1 + X_2 > c_2 \,|\, p_o] \leq a, \text{ and}$$
$$(\text{power}) \ P[X_1 > c_1, X_1 + X_2 > c_2 \,|\, p_a] \geq 1 - \beta.$$

There are many choices of (c_1, c_2) that meet the type I and type II error specifications. Among all sets of (c_1, c_2) that meet the requirements, Simon proposed to choose the boundaries that minimize the expected sample size under H_0. Intuitively, this is a sensible criterion in that, among all designs that meet the type I and type II error specifications, the *optimal* design is the one that on average treats the fewest number of patients with a therapy that is no better than the current standard therapy. Simon tabulated the optimal designs for various choices of design parameters $N = n_1 + n_2$, p_0, p_a, a, and β.

In addition, Simon tabulated designs for an alternate optimality criterion, which he called the "minimax design." This design has the smallest maximum sample size among all designs that satisfy the type I and type II error requirements. The stage sample size and the boundaries for the two optimality criteria can be very different. Simon pointed out that in cases when the difference in expected sample sizes is small and the patient

accrual rate is low, the minimax design may be more attractive than that with the minimum expected sample size under H_0.

The TMZ example was designed using the Simon minimax design. The study called for accrual of 16 patients in the first stage and 9 additional patients in the second stage for a maximum accrual of 25 patients. At the first stage, the trial would stop for futility if ≤1 response was observed, otherwise the trial would go on to the second stage. At the final analysis, if >4 responses were observed among all 25 patients, then they would reject the null hypothesis in favor of the alternative. In the TMZ study, the Simon's minimax design resulted in the same total sample size and final decision rule as the one determined from the single-stage design; that will not always be the case.

If Simon's optimal design had been chosen, then accrual to the first stage would have been set at 12 patients, and 23 additional patients would have been accrued to the second stage if the first-stage stopping criterion had not been met. With the optimal design the trial would stop at the first stage if ≤1 response is observed; otherwise it would continue to the second stage. At the final analysis, if >5 responses were observed among all 35 patients, then they would reject the null hypothesis in favor of the alternative. In this setting the stage and total sample sizes and critical values differed considerably among the two designs.

Modifications and Other Two-Stage Designs

Research in improving designs for two-stage phase II trials is ongoing. Examples include the following. Banerjee and Tsiatis (6) proposed an adaptive two-stage design, which allows the rejection rule and the sample size of the second stage to depend on the results of the first stage. Jin and Wei (7) modified Simon's optimal two-stage design and developed an alternative frequentist adaptive approach. Englert and Kieser (8) proposed optimal adaptive two-stage designs, in which the sample size in the second stage is also based on the number of responders from the first stage. Kieser and Englert (9) proposed specifying an interval of possible true response rate in a two-stage design. Shan et al. (10) proposed the branch-and-bound algorithm to search for the optimal adaptive design with the smallest expected sample size under the null hypothesis. Mander and Thompson (11) considered optimal designs that allow early stopping for efficacy. Mander et al. (12) also considered the admissible design that is optimal for a weighted sum of the expected sample size and maximum sample size. Under the Bayesian framework, Tan and Machin (13) proposed a Bayesian two-stage design in which the parameters are calibrated based on the posterior probability approach. Sambucini (14) extended Tan et al. and took into account the uncertainty of future data.

FULLY SEQUENTIAL DESIGNS

The multistage designs can be considered as group-sequential designs where patients are entered in cohorts. A decision of whether to terminate the trial early or to continue to the next stage is made after each cohort is accrued and the test statistic is calculated. In a fully sequential design, an analysis is performed after the outcome of each new patient is observed using a test statistic based on the accumulated data to that point. The test statistic is then compared with an upper and lower boundary. If the test statistic falls in the region between the boundaries, an additional patient is sampled and his or her response to the new treatment is observed. If, however, the test statistic falls above the upper (below the bottom) boundary, then accrual is stopped and the null (alternative) hypothesis is rejected. A fully sequential design requires continuous monitoring of the study results, patient by patient, and thus it is often difficult to implement.

Herson (15) proposed a fully sequential design for phase II trials. In this setting the null and alternative hypotheses were defined as $H_0: p \geq p_a$ versus $H_a: p < p_a$, where p_a is a "minimum acceptable response rate" chosen by the investigators. The technical details of Herson's method, which use Bayesian predictive distributions, are beyond the scope of this chapter, but the idea is intuitive. A fixed sample size trial would reject Herson's H_0 if at the end of the trial there were too few responders. At any point in the trial, given information on the number of patients treated so far and the number of observed responders, it is possible to predict the probability that the null hypothesis will be rejected after n patients have been observed. If this predicted probability is too low or too high, it is reasonable to stop the trial.

Thall and Simon (16) also proposed a fully sequential design using Bayesian methods. The design requires specification of the response rate for the standard therapy p_0, the experimental therapy p, the prior for p_0, the prior for p, a targeted improvement for new therapy δ_0, and bounds N_{min} and N_{max} on the allowable sample size. The priors for p_0 and p are chosen to be independent beta distributions. Thall et al. give recommendations as to choosing the parameters of the prior distributions. After the outcome from each patient is observed, Thall et al. calculate the posterior probability that the new therapy will be shown to be effective. The trial continues until the maximum sample size is reached, or the experimental therapy is shown with high probability to be effective. Thall et al. also calculate the posterior probability that the new therapy will meet the targeted improvement in response rate, and will terminate the trial early if this probability is too low.

One of the advantages of Thall et al.'s approach is that it allows for the uncertainty in response rate

with the standard therapy to be incorporated into the design. A disadvantage is that it requires monitoring the data continuously and needs numerous analyses. It can often arrive at "not convincing either way" decisions.

For the TMZ example responses were observed in the 12th, 15th, and 23rd patients in the first cohort and in the 2nd, 15th, and 21st patients in the second cohort. Using a targeted improvement of 0.20, and the priors recommended in Thall and Simon, the trial would be stopped in the first cohort at the maximum of 4 or the preselected minimum sample size N_{min}. In the second cohort, the trial would be stopped at the maximum of 9 or the preselected minimum sample size. In each case, the trial would be stopped because of a low posterior probability that the therapy would meet the targeted improvement in response rate.

Lee and Liu (17) proposed a predictive probability design for phase II cancer clinical trials based on a Bayesian predictive probability framework. The predictive probability is defined as the probability of observing a positive result by the end of the trial based on the cumulative information in the current stage. A higher (lower) predictive probability means that the new treatment is (is not) likely to be efficacious by the end of the study, given the current data. Given p_0, p, the prior distribution of response rate, and the cohort size for interim monitoring, they search for the maximum sample size N_{max}, threshold values θ_L, θ_T, θ_U (usually choose 1.0) for the predictive probability, to yield a design satisfying the type I and type II error rates constraints simultaneously. The smallest N_{max} that controls both the type I and type II error rates at the nominal level is the one to choose. Similar to the Thall et al. approach, the predictive probability design is computationally intensive.

Some recent developments in phase II designs under the Bayesian framework include the following. Wathen et al. (18) proposed a class of model-based flexible Bayesian single-arm phase II designs with two or more prognostic subgroups. The early-stopping rules are subgroup-specific, which allows the decision of trial termination to differ within each subgroup. In Johnson and Cook (19), formal Bayesian hypothesis tests were used to design single-arm phase II trials. A new class of prior densities was proposed, which provides exponential convergence of Bayes factors under both null and alternative models. Trials with both binary and time-to-event outcomes are considered and the proposed method was compared with Bayesian designs based on posterior credible intervals and Simon's two-stage design. Cai et al. (20) proposed a Bayesian trial design, which allows continuous monitoring in the presence of delayed response. The delayed responses were treated as missing data and imputed based on a piecewise exponential model, while the observed response was kept as binary.

OTHER PHASE II DESIGNS

Bivariate Designs

In some circumstances it is necessary to consider the use of multiple endpoints for determining sample size and stopping guidelines instead of a single endpoint. For example, in studies of high-dose chemotherapy it may be hypothesized that a more intensive therapy will induce more responders; however, more intensive therapy may also cause more unacceptable adverse events. An increase in the adverse event rate may be acceptable as long as the toxicities are not too severe or are reversible as long as the higher dose results in an increased response rate.

Similar in structure to Simon's two-stage designs, Bryant and Day (21) proposed methods that integrate toxicity monitoring into phase II designs. The trials are terminated at the initial stage if either the number of observed responses is inadequate or the number of observed toxicities is excessive. If there are both a sufficient number of responses and an acceptable toxicity rate in the second stage, then the new agent is considered to be worthy of further study. The design parameters are determined by minimizing the expected accrual for treatments with unacceptable rates of response or toxicity.

Conaway and Petroni (22) proposed similar designs. A new therapy may be acceptable if it can achieve a substantially greater response rate but with acceptable toxicity, or it has a slightly lower response rate but with substantially less toxicity. Conaway and Petroni (23) proposed two-stage designs to allow for early termination of the study if the new therapy is not sufficiently promising, and to allow for trade-offs between improvements in activity and increases in toxicity.

Thall et al. (24,25) took the Bayesian approach that allows for monitoring each endpoint on a patient-by-patient basis in the trial. They define for each endpoint in the trial a monitoring boundary based on prespecified targets for an improvement in efficacy and an unacceptable increase in the rate of adverse events. Thall and Cheng (26,27) proposed another approach for multi-endpoint designs by quantifying a two-dimensional treatment effect parameter for efficacy and safety.

Strategies that have been proposed within the past 10 years include Wu and Liu (28) who recommend specifying the odds ratio in monitoring simultaneously the response and toxicity rate of a therapeutic agent. The type I error rate can be inflated substantially if the specified value is considerably larger than the true odds ratio. To overcome the sensitivity of the error rates to the odds ratio, they proposed an adaptive procedure that allows the sample size to be reestimated based on the observed odds ratio.

Chen and Smith (29) propose an adaptive group-sequential design using a Bayesian decision theoretic approach when considering efficacy and toxicity as correlated bivariate binary endpoints. Interim evaluations are conducted group sequentially, but the number of interim looks and the size of each group are chosen adaptively based on current observations. A loss function is utilized, which consists of two components: the loss associated with accruing, treating, and monitoring patients, and the loss associated with making incorrect decisions.

Brutti et al. (30) proposed an extension of Tan and Machin (13) and incorporate safety considerations into the design. Ray and Rai (31) proposed a flexible bivariate single-arm clinical trial design that incorporates both response and toxicity. The design can monitor toxicity on a different schedule from the response. Bersimis et al. (32) considered reducing the sample size by proposing flexible designs that allow stopping the trial when high rates of favorable or unfavorable outcomes are observed early; thus a smaller number of patients could be used.

Phase II Design Using Time-to-Event Endpoints

All the designs discussed so far focused on a binary(s) endpoint, tumor response, as a measure of efficacy. However, in situations when tumor response is difficult or not possible to evaluate, or when the agents studied are not expected to reduce tumor response (i.e., cytostatic agents), response rate may not be an appropriate endpoint to evaluate the efficacy of the new agent. Endpoints that incorporate information of a time-to-event outcome such as disease free survival (DFS), progression-free survival (PFS), or overall survival (OS) may be reasonable choices in this situation.

The use of PFS estimates at a fixed time point, instead of the response rate as the primary endpoint, was proposed by Van Glabbeke et al. (33). Mick et al. (34) proposed a methodology for evaluating time to progression (TTP) as the primary endpoint in a single-stage design with each patient's previous response time serving as his or her own control. If it is reasonable to assume that the time-to-event outcome, say survival, follows a known distribution (such as the exponential) then under specified assumptions for accrual and minimum follow-up time, sample size can be estimated from a one-sample test for median survival rates (35). Owzar and Jung (36) recommended dichotomizing the time-to-event outcome at a clinically relevant landmark over the parametric and nonparametric methods for the design of phase II cancer studies. Wu and Xiong (37) proposed three nonparametric test statistics in designing single-arm group-sequential trials with a survival endpoint at a fixed time point. Whitehead (38) proposed extensions of one-stage and two-stage single-arm designs based on binary responses. The new method is based on a limited number of landmark time points, and the designs and analyses can use either normal approximations or exact calculations. Other proposed approaches include Zhao et al. (39) who proposed a Bayesian decision theoretic procedure for the two-stage design with a survival endpoint assuming that the survival times follow an exponential or Weibull distribution.

Randomized Designs

The outcomes from single-arm trials are greatly influenced by several factors including protocol-specific entry criteria, the definition of response, and patient selection bias. Randomized designs are considered when the aim of a phase II trial is to evaluate two or more regimens concurrently, adequate historical control data are not available, or to select which of the several new agents should be studied further. The standard single-arm paradigm may be inefficient in these settings.

The randomized selection design (40–43) allows multiple single-arm trials to be conducted at the same time with the same entry criteria. Typically patients are randomized to two or more experimental arms without a control arm. A test for activity using standard criteria for single-arm studies is conducted for each arm, and there is a selection rule for selecting the best arm(s) for further investigation. The advantages of this type of design include decreasing the patient selection bias, and the ability to ensure uniform evaluation criteria in each arm. The weakness is that the probability of selecting the better arm decreases if the difference between the arms decreases and if the number of arms increases (44).

In a randomized control design, patients are randomly assigned to an experimental or control arm and the results obtained from the two arms are compared. Comparison to a control arm is useful when there is little prior information of the expected response rate in a population, or when endpoints such as TTP and PFS, which are influenced by patient selection, are used. This design format is typical in the phase III setting, but has been proposed in the phase II setting as well (45–47). Compared with a standard single-arm phase II study, a potential weakness of this type of design often includes the need for a second larger study before moving on to a phase III study.

The randomized discontinuation design (48–50) was proposed to select a more homogeneous group of patients thus to provide smaller bias. All patients are initially treated with the experimental drug. Patients free of progression at some defined time point are randomized between continuing the experimental drug and receiving a placebo. The effectiveness of the design depends on the accuracy of identifying true treatment responders who are clearly benefiting on the basis of disease stabilization versus rapid progression. It may overestimate the treatment benefit and may require a larger sample size compared with other phase II designs. As pointed out by Freidlin and Simon (51), with careful planning, it can be useful in some settings in the early development of targeted agents where a reliable assay to select patients expressing the target is not available.

Jung (52) proposed a two-stage randomized design for evaluating the efficacy of an experimental therapy compared to a prospective control. Using exact binomial distributions, the proposed design allows for early termination of the study when the experimental arm does not show promising efficacy at the interim analysis. By defining the minimax and optimal designs to satisfy a prespecified restriction on type I and type II error probabilities, the designs are randomized phase II trial analogs of Simon's design for a single-arm trial. In Jung and Sargent (53), use of Fisher's exact test was proposed to be more powerful than the binomial test under certain circumstances.

Yin et al. (54) proposed a randomized design based on Bayesian adaptive randomization and predictive probability monitoring, and provided a detailed comparison with group-sequential methods in a two-arm trial.

Lei et al. (55) propose a Bayesian adaptive randomization procedure that accounts for both efficacy and toxicity outcomes. They model the efficacy as a time-to-event endpoint and toxicity as a binary endpoint, sharing common random effects to induce dependence between the bivariate outcomes. Early-stopping boundaries are constructed for toxicity and futility, and a superior treatment arm is recommended at the end of the trial.

Zhong et al. (56) propose a two-stage Bayesian design with sample size reestimation at the interim stage, which generalizes Whitehead et al. (57) method for exploratory studies on efficacy to a two-sample setting, and uses a fully Bayesian predictive approach to reduce an overly large initial sample size.

Song (58) illustrated the use of a patient enrichment adaptive design in a randomized phase II metastatic hepatocellular carcinoma trial. The design allows the evaluation of treatment benefits by the biomarker expression level and makes interim adjustment according to the prespecified rules.

The choice between using a single-arm or a randomized design is discussed in Gan et al. (59) and Lara et al. (60).

DISCUSSION

There are many design methods available for phase II clinical trials. It is important to note that the study objectives should define the choice of design to use and not the reverse. If the main objective is to assess clinical response rates, then one can choose from the classic design methods. However, for a more complicated study, it is recommended that a novel design method be used. This requires more interaction between the investigators and statisticians, and results in higher quality research.

In the genomic era, the use of genomic biomarkers to individualize cancer treatments has led to clinical trials designed to investigate the effects of targeted therapy on specific molecularly selected patients. Among the new and evolving trial designs are the "Basket" trials and "Umbrella" trials (61–64). Each cohort in the trial is considered as a phase II trial and within the master protocol, designs such as Simon's two-stage design or randomized designs discussed in this chapter are applied. Renfro et al. (65) describe and give examples of clinical trials where biomarker-based designs have been utilized.

The methods discussed here are only some of the methods available in the literature, but we hope it will serve as a good starting point when considering the design of phase II trials. Appropriate trial design remains an expanding field of research.

REFERENCES

1. Rietschel P, Wolchok JD, Krown S, et al. Phase II study of extended-dose Temozolomide in patients with melanoma. *J Clin Oncol*. 2008;26:2299–2304.
2. Gehan EA. The determination of number of patients in a follow-up trial of a new chemotherapeutic agent. *J Chronic Dis*. 1961;13:346–353.
3. Schultz JR, Nichol FR, Elfring GL, Weed SD. Multiple stage procedures for drug screening. *Biometrics*. 1973;29:293–300.
4. Fleming TR. One-sample multiple testing procedures for phase II clinical trials. *Biometrics*. 1982;38:143–151.
5. Simon R. Optimal two-stage designs for Phase II clinical trials. *Control Clin Trials*. 1989;10:1–10.
6. Banerjee A, Tsiatis AA. Adaptive two-stage designs in Phase II clinical trials. *Stat Med*. 2006;25:3382–3395.
7. Jin H, Wei Z. A new adaptive design based on Simon's two-stage optimal design for Phase II clinical trials. *Contemporary Clinical Trials*. 2012;33:1255-1260.
8. Englert S, Kieser M. Optimal adaptive two-stage designs for Phase II cancer clinical trials. *Biom J*. 2013;55:955–968.
9. Kieser M, Englert S. Performance of adaptive designs for single-armed Phase II oncology trials. *J Biopharm Stat*. 2015;25:602–615.
10. Shan G, Wilding GE, Hutson AD, Gerstenberger S. Optimal adaptive two-stage designs for early Phase II clinical trials. *Statist. Med*. 2016;35:1257–1266.
11. Mander AP, Thompson SG. Two-stage designs optimal under the alternative hypothesis for Phase II cancer clinical trials. *Contemp Clin Trials*. 2010;31:572–578.
12. Mander AP, Wason, JM, Sweeting MJ, Thompson SG. Admissible two-stage designs for Phase II cancer clinical trials that incorporate the expected sample size under the alternative hypothesis. *Pharm Stat*. 2012;11:91–96.
13. Tan SB, Machin D. Bayesian two-stage designs for Phase II clinical trials. *Stat Med*. 2002;21:1991–2012.
14. Sambucini V. A Bayesian predictive two-stage design for Phase II clinical trials. *Statist Med*. 2008; 27:1199–1224.
15. Herson J. Predictive probability early termination plans for Phase II clinical trials. *Biometrics*. 1979;35:775–783.
16. Thall PF, Simon R. Practical Bayesian guidelines for Phase IIB clinical trials. *Biometrics*. 1994;50:337–349.
17. Lee JJ, Liu DD. A predictive probability design for Phase II cancer clinical trials. *Clin Trials*. 2008;5:93–106.
18. Wathen JK, Thall PF, Cook JD, Estey EH. Accouting for patient heterogeneity in Phase II clinical trials. *Stat Med*. 2008;27:2802–2815.
19. Johnson VE, Cook JD. Bayesian design of single-arm Phase II clinical trials with continuous monitoring. *Clin Trials*. 2009;6:217–226.
20. Cai C, Liu S, Yuan Y. A Bayesian design for Phase II clinical trials with delayed responses based on multiple imputation. *Stat Med*. 2014;33:4017–4028.
21. Bryant J, Day R. Incorporating toxicity considerations into the design of two-stage Phase II clinical trials. *Biometrics*. 1995;51:1372–1383.
22. Conaway MR, Petroni GR. Bivariate sequential designs for Phase II trials. *Biometrics*. 1995;51:656–664.
23. Conaway MR, Petroni GR. Designs for Phase II trials allowing for trade-off between response and toxicity. *Biometrics*. 1996;52:1375–1386.
24. Thall PF, Simon RM, Estey EH. Bayesian sequential monitoring designs for single-arm clinical trials with multiple outcomes. *Stat Med*. 1995;14:357–379.
25. Thall PF, Simon RM, Estey EH. New statistical strategy for monitoring safety and efficacy in single-arm clinical trials. *J Clin Oncol*. 1996;14:296–303.
26. Thall PF, Cheng SC. Treatment comparisons based on two-dimensional safety and efficacy alternatives in oncology trials. *Biometrics*. 1999;55:746–753.
27. Thall PF, Cheng SC. Optimal two-stage designs for clinical trials based on safety and efficacy. *Stat Med*. 2001;20: 1023–1032.
28. Wu C, Liu A. An adaptive approach for biavariate Phase II clinical trial designs. *Contemp Clin Trials*. 2007;28:482–486.
29. Chen Y, Smith BJ. Adaptive group sequential design for Phase II clinical trials: a Bayesian decision theoretic approach. *Stat Med*. 2009;28:3347–3362.
30. Brutti P, Gubbiotti S, Sambucini V. An extension of the single threshold design for monitoring efficacy and safety in Phase II clinical trials. *Stat Med*. 2011;30:1648–1664.
31. Ray HE, Rai SN. Flexible bivariate Phase II clinical trial design incorporating toxicity and response on different schedules. *Stat Med*. 2013;32:470–485.
32. Bersimis S, Sachlas A, Papaioannou T. Flexible designs for Phase II comparative clinical trials involving two response variables. *Stat Med*. 2015;34:197–214.
33. Van Glabbeke M, Verweij J, Judson I, et al. Progression-free rate as the principal endpoint for Phase II trials in soft-tissue sarcomas. *Eur J Cancer*. 2002;38:543–549.
34. Mick R, Crowley JJ, Carroll RJ. Phase II clinical trial design for noncytotoxic anticancer agents for which time to disease progression is the primary endpoint. *Control Clin Trials*. 2000;21:343–359.
35. Lawless J. *Statistical models and methods for lifetime data*. New York, NY: Wiley & Sons; 1982.
36. Owzar K, Jung S. Designing Phase II studies in cancer with time-to-event endpoints. *Clin Trials*. 2008;5:209–221.
37. Wu J, Xiong X. Single-arm Phase II group sequential trial design with survival endpoint at a fixed time point. *Stat Biopharm Res*. 2014:6:289–301.
38. Whitehead J. One-stage and two-stage designs for Phase II clinical trials with survival endpoints. *Stat Med* 2014;33(22):3 830–3843.
39. Zhao L, Taylor JM, Schuetze SM. Bayesian decision theoretic two-stage design in Phase II clinical trials with survival endpoint. *Statist Med*. 2012;31:1804–1820.
40. Simon R, Wittes RE, Ellenberg SS. Randomized Phase II clinical trials. *Cancer Treat Rep*. 1985;69:1375–1381.
41. Simon RM, Stienberg SM, Hamilton M, et al. Clinical trial designs for the early clinical development of therapeutic cancer vaccines. *J Clin Oncol*. 2001;19:1848–1854.
42. Liu PY, Dahlberg S, Crowley J. Selection designs for pilot studies based on survival endpoints. *Biometrics*. 1993;49:391–398.
43. Scher HI, Heller G. Picking the winners in a sea of plenty. *Clin Cancer Res*. 2002;8:400–404.

44. Gray R, Manola J, Saxman S, et al. Phase II clinical trials: methods in translational research from the genitourinary committee at the eastern cooperative oncology group. *Clin Cancer Res.* 2006;12:1966–1969.

45. Herson J, Carter SK. Calibrated Phase II clinical trials in oncology. *Stat Med.* 1986;5:441–447.

46. Thall PF, Simon R. Incorporating historical control data in planning Phase II clinical trials. *Stat Med.* 1990;9:215–228.

47. Korn EL, Arbuck SG, Pluda JM, et al. Clinical trial designs for cytostatic agents: are new approaches needed? *J Clin Oncol.* 2001;19:265–272.

48. Stadler WM, Ratain MJ. Development of target-based antineoplastic agents. *Investigational New Drug.* 2000;18:7–16.

49. Rosner GL, Stadler W, Ratain MJ. Randomized discontinuation design: application to cytostatic antineoplastic agents. *J Clin Oncol.* 2002;20:4478–4484.

50. Ratain MJ, Eisen T, Stadler WM, et al. Phase II placebo-controlled randomized discontinuation trial of Sorafenib in patients with metastatic renal cell carcinoma. *J Clin Oncol.* 2006;24: 2505–2511.

51. Freidlin B, Simon R. Evaluation of randomized discontinuation design. *J Clin Oncol.* 2005;23:5094–5098.

52. Jung SH. Randomized Phase II trials with a prospective control. *Stat Med.* 2008:27:568–583.

53. Jung SH, Sargent D. Randomized Phase II cancer clinical trials. *J Biopharm Stat.* 2014:24:802–816.

54. Yin G, Chen N, Lee JJ. Phase II trial design with Bayesian adaptive randomization and predictive probability. *Appl Statist.* 2012:61:219–235.

55. Lei X, Yuan,Y, Yin G. Bayesian Phase II adaptive randomization by jointly modeling time-to-event efficacy and binary toxicity. *Lifetime Data Anal.* 2011;17:156–174.

56. Zhong W, Koopmeiners JS, Carlin BP. A two-stage Bayesian design with sample size reestimation and subgroup analysis for Phase II binary response trials. *Contemp Clin Trials.* 2013;36:587–596.

57. Whitehead J, Valdes-Marquez E, Johnson P, Graham G. Bayesian sample size for exploratory clinical trials incorporating historical data. *Stat Med.* 2008;27:2307–2327.

58. Song JX. A two-stage patient enrichment adaptive desing in Phase II oncology trials. *Contemp Clin Trials.* 2014;37:148–154.

59. Gan HK, Grothey A, Pond GR, et al. Randomized Phase II trials: inevitable or inadvisable? *J Clin Oncol.* 2010:28:2641–2647.

60. Lara PN, Redman MW. The hazards of randomized Phase II trials. *Annals of Oncology.* 2012:23:7–9.

61. Kim ES, Herbst RS, Wistuba II, et al. The BATTLE trial: personalizing therapy for lung cancer. *Cancer Discov.* 2011:1:44–53.

62. Menis J, Hasan B, Besse B. New clinical research strategies in thoracic oncology: clinical trial design, adaptive, basket and umbrella trials, new end-points and new evaluations of response. *Eur Respir Rev.* 2014:23:367–378.

63. Redig AJ, Janne PA. Basket trials and the evolution of clinical trial design in an era of genomic medicine. *J Clin Oncol.* 2015:33:975–977.

64. Simon R, Geyer S, Subramanian J, Roychowdhury S. The Bayesian basket design for genomic variant-driven Phase II trials. *Semin Oncol.* 2016;43:13–18.

65. Renfro LA, Mallick H, An M, et al. Clinical trial designs incorporating predictive biomarkers. *Cancer Treat Rev.* 2016;43:74–82.

Biomarkers in Confirmatory Clinical Trials

Thomas Gwise

PRECISION MEDICINE AND BIOMARKERS

Clinical trials using biomarker information play an important role in precision medicine. In 2008, before the current term precision medicine was adopted, the President's Council of Advisors on Science and Technology described personalized medicine as tailoring medicine to individuals. But they did not literally mean the goal was to create unique products for each member of the population. Rather, the goal of personalized medicine is to determine bounds for subpopulations, which once determined can be readily identified and treated effectively (1). The term precision medicine has gained favor over personalized medicine because it is thought to more closely represent the actual direction of the field. Precision medicine has been described as getting the right drug at the right dose to the right patient at the right time (2). While this latter description may already be a general expectation, the reality is that therapeutic drugs and biologics are typically developed on a large-scale basis. The vast majority of late-phase clinical trials supporting drug marketing are designed to evaluate therapeutic effects for populations, where populations are defined by trial inclusion criteria. Drugs shown to be effective on average in a population may, nonetheless, be ineffective for a considerable fraction of individuals within that population. Scientific advances, such as the mapping of the human genome, have allowed researchers new insight into the mechanisms of cancers. New understandings based on specific molecular processes, such as insight into the role certain genomic alterations play in some patients' lung cancers, have pointed to new treatments. When a treatment is designed by leveraging knowledge of one of the disease's underlying mechanisms, that same knowledge may also be useful to single out patients expected to benefit from the treatment. For example, rearrangements in the anaplastic lymphoma kinase (ALK) gene are thought to be important in non–small-cell lung cancer (NSCLC). The drug crizotinib was designed to inhibit several tyrosine kinases, including ALK. When ALK was found to be present in a subset of NSCLC patients, crizotinib was targeted to their treatment (3). In this example, ALK is a measurable dimension of patients that can be used to inform treatment decisions. Such a patient feature is an example of a kind of biomarker. This chapter considers aspects of late-phase trials designed to leverage biomarker information to support claims of efficacy in the specific context of marketing application.

BIOMARKERS

Predictive and Prognostic Biomarkers

A biomarker is an objectively measured characteristic of a person, which can be evaluated as an indicator of normal biological processes, pathogenic processes, or pharmacologic responses to therapeutic interventions (4). Biomarkers are divided into several categories, including diagnostic, monitoring, prognostic, predictive, and safety biomarkers. Our focus is primarily binary predictive biomarkers, but we briefly discuss prognostic biomarkers because they can also play an important role in clinical trials. Often, such as with human epidermal growth factor receptor 2 (HER2) discussed in the following, biomarkers are both predictive and prognostic. When considering biomarkers in clinical trials, the time of marker assessment relative to the study therapies is important. The clinical trial application of biomarkers discussed in this chapter, whether predictive or prognostic, require baseline evaluation. Posttreatment or midtrial biomarker values could be impacted by the study therapies thus confounding the trial results. A predictive biomarker is one that can be used to predict the effect of a therapy. An example of a predictive biomarker is the histological category of a patient's NSCLC when considering pemetrexed diosodium treatment. The product label (5) describes several clinical trials evaluating pemetrexed for treating NSCLC. Trial 14.1 is a comparison of pemetrexed combined with cisplatin to gemcitabine combined with cisplatin. A total of 1,725 patients with stage IIIb/IV

NSCLC were randomized equally to the two treatment arms. The hazard ratio (HR) comparing treatment arms with respect to overall survival (OS) was not significantly different from one when considering the overall population. A prospectively designed comparison of the treatment arms within the histologic subgroups squamous and nonsquamous NSCLC showed the biomarker to be predictive for pemetrexed treatment in this setting. The OS HR in the nonsquamous NSCLC treatment comparison (N = 1,252) was 0.84 with a 95% confidence interval of (0.74–0.96). The comparison in the squamous NSCLC group (N = 473) resulted in an HR of 1.23 with a 95% confidence interval of (1.00–1.51) for OS. There was also a statistically significant treatment by biomarker interaction (p = .001) (6). The differential treatment effect across the two subsets supports the claim that the biomarker is predictive in this setting. The trial described as 14.2 in the pemetrexed label (5) was a comparison of pemetrexed to placebo used to treat patients with stage IIIb/IV NSCLC who had not experienced disease progression after having received four cycles of platinum-based chemotherapy. A total of 663 patients were randomized in a 2:1 ratio to receive pemetrexed or placebo therapy, respectively. As in trial 14.1, the OS HR comparing the treatment arms was not significantly different from one. A prospectively planned analysis showed histological category to be predictive in the setting just described. The OS HR comparing treatment arms within the nonsquamous NSCLC group was 0.70 with a 95% confidence interval of (0.65–0.88). In the squamous NSCLC group, the OS HR was 1.07 with a 95% confidence interval of (0.77–1.50). There was also a statistically significant treatment by biomarker interaction (p = .011) (6). Again, the differential treatment effect across the two subsets supports the claim that the biomarker is predictive in this setting. A prognostic biomarker is one that can assist in assessing the natural history of a patient's condition independent of therapy effects. Breast cancer patients having a high expression of BRCA1 have worse prognosis than those not having high levels of the biomarker (7). Overexpression of HER2 is another prognostic marker for breast cancer patients. Patients overexpressing HER2 have a worse prognosis than those not overexpressing the biomarker (8). The biomarker HER2 is also used in a predictive fashion as a treatment selection biomarker for the drug trastuzumab (9). Trastuzumab is indicated for patients overexpressing HER2, as determined by a Food and Drug Administration (FDA) approved test (10). Prognostic biomarkers have been used to increase the efficiency of randomized controlled clinical trials (11). Consider for example, an event-driven randomized controlled trial. A differential effect between an effective treatment and a less effective control treatment will be more readily observable in a sample of patients having a relatively higher event risk than the entire population. Fisher et al. (12) showed that in a group of 13,388 women with relatively higher risk of breast cancer as determined

by a prognostic marker, tamoxifen reduced the risk of developing breast cancer from 42.5 to 24.8 per 1,000 with respect to a placebo. Because the standard error of the risk ratio increases as the event rates decrease, an even larger sample would have been necessary to observe the same risk ratio given lower event rates in the two treatment arms. The Kaplan–Meier plots (Figure 14.1) illustrate the differences between prognostic and predictive markers. The plot on the top is a display of simulated survival data for four sets of patients. The plots represent study subjects who received an experimental treatment (Drug) or placebo, stratified by their status with respect to a biomarker of interest (Marker). In this case, the biomarker is predictive because there is a clear difference in treatment effect across biomarker status, as well as superior survival in the drug subgroup compared to patients on placebo within the biomarker positive stratum.

The lower plot shows data simulated for a similar situation, but the biomarker in this case is prognostic and not predictive. The data show patients who are biomarker

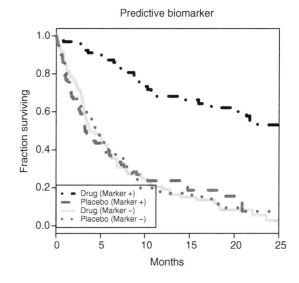

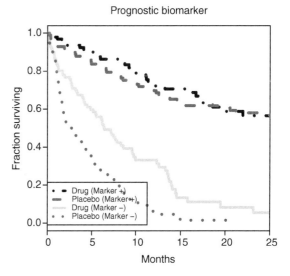

FIGURE 14.1 Prognostic and predictive biomarkers.

positive had better survival probabilities than those who were biomarker negative regardless of treatment. For this particular setting, biomarker negative patients who receive the treatment tend to have better survival outcomes than biomarker negative patients receiving placebo instead. The treatment appears to be effective in both biomarker positive and biomarker negative groups, but the effect is much more pronounced in the biomarker negative group. The effect in the biomarker positive group is small with the survival curves converging after approximately 16 months. The most notable feature of the plot is the biomarker positive patients tend to have better survival outcomes than the biomarker negative patients regardless of treatment. A prognostic biomarker like this one could potentially be useful in making treatment decisions. A patient who is biomarker positive in a setting similar to this might opt to avoid any risks associated with the drug treatment because the expected benefit is small relative to the survival probability in the biomarker positive group. To demonstrate that a biomarker is predictive with respect to some therapy, one should conclusively show that there is a difference in treatment effect across biomarker strata. One possible way to do this is to show there is a marker by treatment interaction using a model. For example, one could use logistic regression to model the logit of response rates as a function of the treatment, the biomarker, and a term for their interaction. On the logit scale, the interaction term being statistically significantly different from zero at a specified level would support the biomarker being predictive. In the pemetrexed example discussed earlier, a statistically significant interaction between the treatments and histological category was demonstrated in two trials evaluating treatments for patients with stage IIIb/IV NSCLC (6).

Simple Biomarker Clinical Trials

Evaluation of biomarker directed drugs for regulatory approval is a specialized experimental setting with unique design issues. Since 1998, when trastuzumab was first licensed for marketing, a wide range of targeted cancer therapies have been approved by the FDA. The labeled uses for more than 15 of these targeted therapies require biomarker information obtained using a test cleared or approved by FDA for that purpose (13). Targeted products whose labels require a companion diagnostic device to determine patient biomarker status include: vemurafenib for the treatment of patients with unresectable or metastatic melanoma with BRAF V600E mutation, crizotinib for the treatment of patients with metastatic NSCLC whose tumors are ALK positive, and venetoclax for the treatment of patients with chronic lymphocytic leukemia (CLL) with 17p deletion who have received at least one prior therapy. Before a drug can be marketed in the United States, it is necessary to demonstrate that the drug has a favorable benefit–risk relationship for its indicated use. When comparative studies were used,

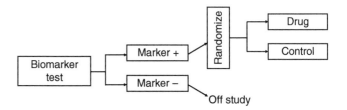

FIGURE 14.2 Enrichment design.

the data supporting most U.S. approvals of biomarker directed drugs were generated using enrichment designs, as described by Mandrekar and Sargent (14). This simple design, which can be viewed as a conventional randomized controlled trial using biomarker status as an inclusion criterion, is also known as a targeted design (15). Figure 14.2 is a schematic of an enrichment design. As patients are enrolled in the trial, they are tested for the presence of the biomarker of interest. Patients testing positive for the biomarker are randomized to either the targeted treatment or a control treatment. Patients who test negative for the biomarker are excluded from the study. The treated patients who remain on the study are followed according to the clinical protocol, and their outcomes are recorded for analysis.

While the enrichment design is a direct way to efficiently compare the targeted therapy to a control therapy, it cannot generate all information necessary to investigate the treatment by biomarker interaction, which is useful in demonstrating the biomarker is predictive or prognostic. More importantly, in the context of product approval, the enrichment design cannot generate data necessary to fully describe the diagnostic ability of the biomarker measuring device, termed its companion diagnostic device, with respect to its clinical application. Although predictiveness of the biomarker could be shown in other trials, the clinical trial evaluating a marker directed therapy may be the best opportunity to characterize the clinical classification performance of the companion diagnostic device. To estimate clinical predictive values and classification probabilities, it is necessary to have information about the impact of the targeted therapy on patients who test negative for the biomarker, as well as those who test positive and enter the trial. Certain information about in vitro diagnostic test performance must be stated in the device labels (16). A draft FDA guidance document (17) describes how information collected in a targeted therapeutic product's clinical trial partially determines how its companion diagnostic device may be described in the device label. For example, a companion diagnostic used in a targeted therapy clinical trial following an enrichment design could be described as a test for patient selection rather than a predictive test. The marker by treatment interaction design (18) shown in Figure 14.3 is a straightforward procedure that can generate data necessary to investigate the biomarker interaction and evaluate the companion diagnostic test performance.

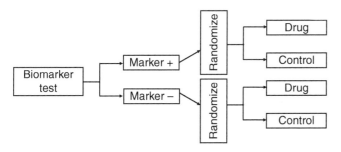

FIGURE 14.3 Marker by treatment interaction design.

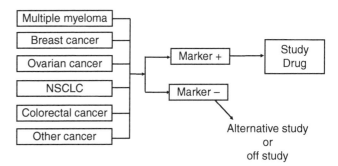

FIGURE 14.4 Simple basket trial.

Using the marker by treatment interaction design is similar to running a clinical trial stratified on biomarker status and can be viewed as running two clinical trials, one on biomarker positive patients and the other on biomarker negative patients (18). Notwithstanding the value of validating predictive biomarkers and estimating the diagnostic performance of companion diagnostic devices, ethics and limited resources often preclude using the treatment by interaction design. Simon and Maitournam show that the treatment by marker interaction design can require a sample size up to four times that required when using an enrichment design (19). Lack of equipoise is a major reason for excluding biomarker negative patients from studies of targeted therapies. The development and approval of trastuzumab is a case in point. Harries and Smith (20) trace the developmental history of trastuzumab, a monoclonal antibody drug indicated to treat patients with HER2 expressing breast cancer, from the early 1980s when HER2 was first isolated through the realization of the gene's implications for about 30% of breast cancer patients to the development of trastuzumab in the 1990s. In this and similar situations where drug developers believe they comprehend the targeted disease mechanism, it is understandable that they would expect their product to be effective only in the targeted group and opt to exclude others from the risks of clinical trials.

MORE COMPLEX DESIGNS

Basket Trials

Basket trials are designed to investigate therapies under the theory that diseases can be treated based on specific molecular characteristics independent of histological category. For example, a drug might be developed to treat patients having several different diseases believed to depend on a process associated with a biomarker. A simple version of a trial using tumor response as the endpoint could be described by Figure 14.4. Patients having certain diseases and testing positive for the biomarker would be assigned to the treatment and followed for evaluation. Patients testing negative for the biomarker would not be enrolled according to this specific simple

model. The design shown can be thought of as combining several single arm trials. More complex basket trials having common control arms and/or including strategies for the biomarker negative patients are possible.

An example of a phase 2 basket trial for one treatment that enrolled patients having NSCLC, multiple myeloma, cholangiocarcinoma, anaplastic thyroid cancer, and several other diseases is described by Hyman et al. (21). The Hyman study followed a design similar to that shown in Figure 14.4, under which design patients testing positive for the BRAF 600V mutation were treated with vemurafenib, except for some patients with colorectal cancer who were assigned to receive cetuximab in addition to vemurafenib. One goal of the study was to find signals for diseases in which vemurafenib therapy could be beneficial and thus worthy of follow-up in larger trials. The authors reported modest partial responses for several disease groups; one complete response in anaplastic thyroid cancer and one complete response in the Erdheim–Chester disease or Langerhans-cell histiocytosis cohort. The largest disease cohort was colorectal cancer with 37 patients between the vemurafenib and vemurafenib+cetuximab groups. A notable result of the study was the partial response rates in the colorectal cancer groups were not significantly different from zero, but the NSCLC group had a 42% partial response rate with 95% confidence interval of (20%–67%). The authors drew from this that BRAF 600V responses are heterogeneous across tumor types. See Hyman et al. (21) for details.

Umbrella Trials

Umbrella trials, in contrast to basket trials (22), aim to identify possible treatments for a molecularly heterogeneous disease. A simplified sketch of an umbrella is presented in Figure 14.5. Patients with a specific cancer enroll in the trial and are tested for a number of biomarkers. Depending on their status with respect to the various markers, they are randomized to a biomarker targeted treatment or a control arm. Depending on the setting, it is possible that the control could be a common control arm against which each of the treatment arms would be compared or individual control arms for each biomarker defined subset could be established. The latter is shown in Figure 14.5.

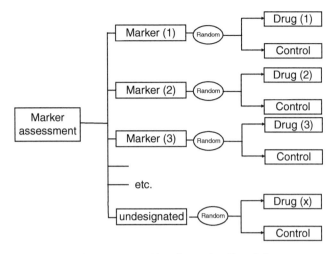

FIGURE 14.5 Simple umbrella trial.

LUNG-MAP, an innovative design resulting from the collaboration of a number of industry, academic, and government agencies, is an example of an umbrella trial. The study, as presented in Steuer et al. (23), is a phase-2–3 trial designed to compare four experimental therapeutic products with a control (docetaxel) for the treatment of patients with squamous cell carcinoma (SCC) of the lung who have progressed after having received first-line platinum-based chemotherapy. Three of the experimental treatment arms are for therapies targeted to specific biomarkers; the fourth experimental arm accepts patients not positive for any of the targeted biomarkers. Each experimental treatment is to be addressed as a separate substudy for which an interim progression-free survival (PFS) analysis will determine whether or not the treatment goes on to be evaluated in phase 3. Assuming a treatment continues through phase 3, both PFS and OS will be evaluated. We note that the LUNG-MAP protocol has been modified since the approval of nivolumab for NSCLC. An advantage of using umbrella designs is the sharing of resources to more efficiently evaluate multiple treatments simultaneously.

Adaptive Designs

A number of adaptive or flexible designs have been proposed for use in development of personalized medicine. The term adaptive design is general and applies to study designs that adapt depending on data accrued in the trial itself. Adaptive trial designs include the familiar sample size reestimation and group sequential designs (24), adaptive randomization (25), as well as Bayesian adaptive methods for these applications and others (26). The Biomarker-integrated Approaches of Targeted Therapy for Lung Cancer Elimination (BATTLE) trial (27) is an example of an umbrella trial that uses Bayesian response adaptive randomization with the goal of randomizing more patients to the better treatments. The biomarker-adaptive threshold design (28) was proposed for cases

in which investigators wish to evaluate a treatment in a population, but a biomarker for selecting patients is also plausible. In this design, a preliminary test of the therapy effect in a larger population is done with type I error probability (a_a) controlled at a level less than the allowable type I error probability (a). If the test in the unrestricted group is not significant, the subgroup defined to be those with biomarker positive status can then be tested at a level (a_b) chosen such that $a_a + a_a = a$. The authors also generalize the procedure to evaluate several cutoffs of a quantitative biomarker. It has been reported that the flexibility offered by this design can incur the cost of a larger sample size (29).

Simon and Simon (30) propose a set of procedures that sequentially restrict the enrollment criteria based on a function of patient covariates followed by a test designed to conserve type I error probability. The approach allows optimization of the target population considering several biomarkers. Because the procedure changes the study population gradually over the course of the trial, it may be difficult to describe the population sampled for the statistical test to be done at accrual completion.

BIOMARKER MEASUREMENT

The ability to correctly identify a targeted subgroup can impact the associated efficacy trial. We use the selection of HER2 positive patients for trastuzumab treatment to explore biomarker detection variability. Press et al. (31) estimated the diagnostic performance of several immunohistochemical (IHC) assays and fluorescence in situ hybridization (FISH) assays using 117 breast cancer specimens with known HER2 status. Forty-three of the specimens were known to be positive and 74 were negative. The authors reported significant differences between two of the ICH assays and one of the FISH assays. The estimated sensitivities, the conditional probabilities of a positive biomarker test results given the biomarker is present, ranged from 0.70 with 95% CI of (0.54–0.83) for one of the IHC assays to 0.95 with 95% CI of (0.84–0.99) for one of the FISH assays. Estimated specificities, the conditional probabilities of negative biomarker test results given the biomarker is absent, were 1.0 for all of the IHC assays with 95% CIs of (0.95–1.0). The lowest observed FISH assay specificity was 0.96 with 95% CI (0.89–0.99). In another example, Mass et al. (32), using a FISH assay, prospectively analyzed a set of archived breast cancer specimens that had all previously tested positive using IHC and reported that 22% of these tested negative with the FISH assay. This study was used to support FDA approval of the particular FISH assay. Similar comparison studies show variability in tests used to detect BRAF V600 mutations in melanoma and ALK rearrangements in lung cancer. One study showed two tests for the BRAF V600 mutation agreeing on 89% (105/118) of determinations (33). Neither BRAF test studied agreed perfectly with a third test, next-generation sequencing, considered to be a reference standard. In a 2015 comparison of ALK assays (34), using a set of 51 NSCLC specimens, of which approximately 13% were ALK positive by the next-generation sequencing reference standard, a FISH assay was found to have sensitivity and specificity of 42.9% and 97.7%. The IHC test in the study had sensitivity and specificity of 100% and 97.7% respectively. A companion diagnostic test's imperfect accuracy can negatively impact the statistical power of a biomarker directed clinical trial. Because clinical trials typically do not use probability sampling, their findings apply to the limited population represented by the sample, rather than a more general population. Trial interpretation therefore depends heavily on inclusion criteria. Biomarker tests essentially define one of the most important enrollment criteria in trials following enrichment designs. We consider now how the test variability, such as described earlier, can impact power. Under an enrichment design, for one to be enrolled in a trial evaluating a biomarker directed therapy, one must test positive for the biomarker. As we have seen, tests are not perfect and a positive test result has some probability of being incorrect. The probability of a patient who does not actually have positive biomarker status but receives a positive test result is the complement of the test's positive predictive value (PPV). From a slightly different perspective, the fraction of patients enrolled in the trial who are truly biomarker positive tends toward the PPV of the test as the number of patients enrolled gets large. To better understand the implications of test inaccuracies, we first review some facts about test performance metrics. PPV is the probability a person actually has biomarker positive status given he or she has received a positive test result for the biomarker. Negative predictive value (NPV) is the probability a person is truly biomarker negative given he or she has a negative biomarker test result. PPV is our focus in this example because we are interested in knowing the value of positive testing as an inclusion criterion. Classification probabilities, sensitivity (Se) and specificity (Sp), are preferred over predictive values as descriptors of diagnostic ability because the former are not dependent on biomarker prevalence whereas the latter do depend on prevalence. The importance of this will be apparent shortly. A diagnostic test's performance can be completely described by the test's sensitivity, specificity, and the prevalence of the marker in the population of interest. Alternatively, a test may be described using PPV, NPV, and the probability of a positive test (35). With test performance given as sensitivity and specificity, we can use the Bayes rule to calculate the predictive values in terms of prevalence and the classification probabilities, as is done in the following for PPV, the probability of a

patient being biomarker positive conditional on a positive test result:

$$P(BM^+ \mid T^+) = \frac{P(T^+ \mid BM^+)P(BM^+)}{P(T^+ \mid BM^+)P(BM^+) + P(T^+ \mid BM^-)P(BM^-)}$$

$$= \frac{\rho * Se}{\rho * Se + (1-\rho) * (1-Sp)},$$

where T^+, T^-, BM^+, and BM^- represent positive and negative test results and the actual presence or absence of the biomarker, respectively. Here r represents the prevalence of the biomarker. The plots in Figure 14.6 show

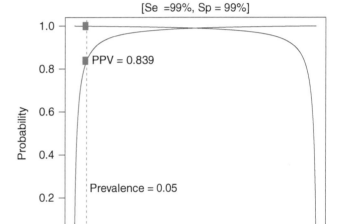

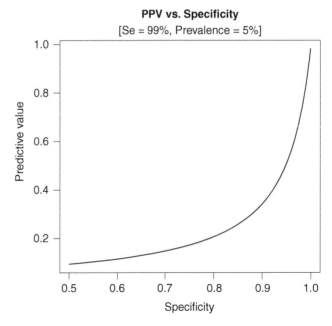

FIGURE 14.6 Predictive values depend on prevalence.

the relationship between test predictive values and biomarker prevalence, given fixed classification probabilities. The ALK gene rearrangement is an example of a low prevalence biomarker that is being used to direct an approved therapeutic drug. The prevalence of ALK in NSCLC patients has been reported to be between 4% and 5%. Notice that sensitivity and specificity in the plot are both 99% for the left-hand plot. Even with this high level of diagnostic performance, the test has PPV of 84% for a prevalence of 5%. The steep drop in PPV for low prevalence markers is intuitive. At such low prevalence there is a very low probability that a randomly chosen subject will be marker positive. So, even with high sensitivity and specificity, the probability of a false positive is 16%. The plot on the right shows the impact of specificity on PPV. We see that with prevalence of 5% and a highly sensitive test of 99%, as specificity decreases, PPV drops sharply. For example, with prevalence of 5% a test with sensitivity and specificity of 99% and 90% respectively will have PPV of 34.25%. To illustrate the impact imperfect biomarker tests can have on efficacy trials, we consider sample size estimation for a comparison of response rates using the normality approximation in a clinical trial following the enrichment design. The expression in (Eq. 14-1) shows the relationship between Δ, the difference between the two expected response rates $(P_t - P_c)$ assumed by the designers, and sample size, n. P_{Ave} is the average of the assumed proportions. The sample size calculations follow the example of Piantadosi (36) while also assuming equal patient allocation across treatment arms:

$$n = \frac{\left(Z_{1-\beta}\sqrt{P_t(1-P_t) + P_c(1-P_c)} + Z_a\sqrt{P_{Ave}(1-P_{Ave})}\right)^2}{\Delta^2}.$$

(Eq. 14-1)

As is customary, the normal distribution quantiles associated with power and type I error probability are Z_{1-b} and Z_a, respectively. We observe from (Eq. 14-1) that sample size is inversely proportional to the square of the effect we wish to detect. Although it may not be intuitively clear from the expression because the variance terms also depend on assumed response probabilities, a smaller Δ will cause an increase in sample size. Including patients in a biomarker-driven trial who are false positive can dilute an effect from a product only active in the biomarker positive patients. Viewed from the perspective of power, this means that not considering imperfections in test performance may underpower the trial. Consider the following example. Using (Eq. 14-1), we find that 93 patients per arm are required to detect a difference in response rates of 0.20 between an assumed response rate of 0.5 for the experimental treatment and 0.30 for the control with $a = 0.025$ and 80% power.

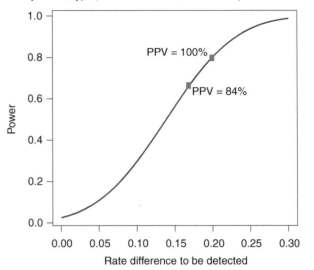

Rate difference to be detected
[N: 186, Type I Error Rate: 2.5%, Control response rate: 30%]

FIGURE 14.7 The impact of the biomarker test having PPV = 84% instead of PPV = 100% is a smaller treatment difference and therefore a loss of power from 80% to 67% in this setting if *n* is held constant.

We consider the hypothetical test described in Figure 14.6. Under the assumption that biomarker negative patients will have a response rate equal to that of the control, 30%, the effect of selecting patients with a test having PPV = 0.84 can be seen by taking a weighted average of biomarker positive and biomarker negative patients. The effective response rate for the experimental treatment therefore is (0.84 × 0.5 + 0.16 × 0.3) = 0.468.

The power to detect a difference between 0.47 and 0.30 holding all other assumptions constant is approximately 67% (Figure 14.7). We see that assigning patients based on the status of a biomarker with prevalence of 5% using a test with sensitivity and specificity each of 99%, and thus providing PPV of 84%, results in a study design underpowered by approximately 13% if the study were designed for 80% power and the naive PPV value of 100% were assumed.

CONCLUSION

This chapter has been a short overview of late-stage biomarker directed clinical trials of the type submitted to FDA as partial support for marketing applications. We noted that the most often used biomarker directed trial design is the simple enrichment design and that its efficiency also comes with the drawback of not providing adequate information for complete test device evaluation. A brief overview of several innovative and adaptive designs was presented. The references given at the end of the chapter provide more details on innovative trial designs. While biomarker-driven trials hold great promise and regulators look forward to using innovative designs (37), the last section of the chapter points out that measurement error should be considered in designing these trials. As the sizes of the subgroups defined by biomarkers grow smaller, the ability to properly measure them will grow in importance.

ACKNOWLEDGMENTS

I would like to acknowledge the helpful advice of Dr. Rajeshwari Sridhara, Dr. Estelle Russek-Cohen, and Dr. Meijuan Li of FDA.

REFERENCES

1. Report to the President; Priorities for Personlized Medicine, Presidents Council of Advisors on Science and Technology, Subcomittee on Personalized Medicine, September 2008.
2. Woodcock J. "Precision" drug development? *Clin Pharmacol The.* 2016;99:152–154.
3. Blackhall F, Cappuzzo F. Crizotinib: from discovery to accelerated development to front-line treatment. *Ann Oncol.* 2016;27:iii35–iii41.
4. FDA-NIH Biomarker Working Group. Terms and definitions. In: *BEST (Biomarkers, EndpointS, and Other Tools) Resource* [Internet]. http://www.ncbi.nlm.nih.gov/books/NBK338448/#glossary. Published 2016.
5. U.S. Food and Drug Administration. Pemetrexed. http://www.accessdata.fda.gov/drugsatfda_docs/label/2013/021462s045lbl.pdf. Published 2008.
6. U.S. Food and Drug Administration. FDA review of pemetrexed. http://www.accessdata.fda.gov/drugsatfda_docs/nda/2008/021462s015.pdf. Published 2008.
7. Mehta S, Shelling A, Muthukaruppan A, et al. Predictive and prognostic molecular markers for cancer medicine. *Ther Adv Med Oncol.* 2010;2:125–148.
8. Ross JS, Fletcher JA. The HER-2/neu oncogene in breast cancer: prognostic factor, predictive factor, and target for therapy. *Stem Cells.* 1998;16:413–428.
9. Mansfield EA. FDA perspective on companion diagnostics: an evolving paradigm. *Clin Cancer Res.* 2014;20:1453–1457.
10. U.S. Food and Drug Administration. Trastuzumab. http://www.accessdata.fda.gov/drugsatfda docs/label/2016/103792 s5330lbl.pdf. Published 2016.
11. U.S. Food and Drug Administration. Guidance for industry, enrichment strategies for clinical trials to support approval of human drugs and biological products: draft guidance. http://www.fda.gov/downloads/drugs/guidancecompliance regulatoryinformation/guidances/ucm332181.pdf. Published 2012.
12. Fisher B, Costantino JP, Wickerham DL, et al. Tamoxifen for the prevention of breast cancer: current status of the national surgical adjuvant breast and bowel project p-1 study. *J Natl Cancer Inst.* 2005;97(22):1652–1662.
13. U.S. Food and Drug Administration. List of cleared or approved companion diagnostic devices (in vitro and imaging tools). http://www.fda.gov/MedicalDevices/Products andMedicalProcedures/InVitroDiagnostics/ucm301431.htm. Published 2016.
14. Mandrekar SJ, Sargent DJ. Clinical trial designs for predictive biomarker validation: theoretical considerations and practical challenges. *J Clin Oncol.* 2009;27:4027–4034.
15. Fox E, Curt GA, Balis FM. Clinical trial design for target-based therapy. *Oncologist.* 2002;7(5):401–409.
16. Code of Federal Regulations. Food and drugs [Cite: 21cfr809.10(b)(12)]. Current as of April 1 2017. https://www.accessdata.fda.gov/scripts/cdrh/cfdocs/cfCFR/CFRSearch.cfm?fr=809.10
17. U.S. Department of Health and Human Services Food and Drug Administration. Principles for codevelopment of an in vitro companion diagnostic device with a therapeutic product: draft guidance for industry and food and drug administration staff. http://www.fda.gov/downloads/MedicalDevices/Device RegulationandGuidance/GuidanceDocuments/UCM510824.pdf. Published 2016.
18. Sargent DJ, Conley BA, Allegra C, Collette L. Clinical trial designs for predictive marker validation in cancer treatment trials. *J Clin Oncol.* 2005;23:2020–2027;2005.
19. Simon R, Maitournam A. Evaluating the efficiency of targeted designs for randomized clinical trials. *Clin Cancer Res.* 2004;10:6759–6763.
20. Harries M, Smith I. The development and clinical use of trastuzumab (herceptin). *Endocr Relat Cancer.* 2002;9:75–85.
21. Hyman DM, Puzanov I, Subbiah V, et al. Vemurafenib in multiple nonmelanoma cancers with braf v600 mutations. *N Engl J Med.* 2015;373:726–736.
22. Menis J, Hasan B, Besse B. New clinical research strategies in thoracic oncology: clinical trial design, adaptive, basket and umbrella trials, new end-points and new evaluations of response. *Eur Respir Rev.* 2014;23:367–378.
23. Steuer CE, Papadimitrakopoulou V, Herbst RS, et al. Innovative clinical trials: the lung-map study. *Clin Pharmacol Ther.* 2015;97:481–491.
24. Jennison C, Turnbull BW. *Group Sequential Methods With Applications to Clinical Trials.* Boca Raton, FL: Chapman & Hall/CRC; 2000.
25. Hu F, Rosenberger W. *The Theory of Response-Adaptive Randomization in Clinical Trials.* Hoboken, NJ: John Wiley and Sons, Inc.; 2006.
26. Berry SM, Carlin BP, Lee JJ, Müller P. *Bayesian Adaptive Methods for Clinical Trials..* Boca Raton, FL: CRC Press Taylor & Francis Group; 2010.
27. Kim ES, Herbst RS, Wistuba II, et al. The battle trial: personalizing therapy for lung cancer. *Cancer Discov.* 2011;1:44–53.
28. Jiang W, Freidlin B, Simon R. Biomarker-adaptive threshold design: a procedure for evaluating treatment with possible biomarker-defined subset effect. *J Natl Cancer Inst.* 2007;99:1036–1043.
29. Emerson SS, Fleming TR. Adaptive methods: telling "the rest of the story." *J Biopharm Stat.* 2010;20(6):1150–1165.
30. Simon N, Simon R. Adaptive enrichment designs for clinical trials. *Biostatistics.* 2013;14:613–625.
31. Press MF, Slamon DJ, Flom KJ, et al. Evaluation of HER-2/neu gene amplification and overexpression: Comparison of frequently used assay methods in a molecularly characterized cohort of breast cancer specimens. *J Clin Oncol.* 2002;20:3095–3105.
32. Mass RD, Press MF, Anderson S, et al. Evaluation of clinical outcomes according to HER2 detection by fluorescence in situ hybridization in women with metastatic breast cancer treated with trastuzumab. *Clin Breast Cancer.* 2005;6:240–246;2005.

33. Longshore J, Banawan S, Amidon H, et al. Comparison of molecular testing methods for detecting braf v600 mutations in melanoma specimens with challenging attributes. *J Molecular Biomarkers Diagnosis*. 2015;6:1–7.

34. Pekar-Zlotin M, Hirsch FR, Soussan-Gutman L, et al. Fluorescence in situ hybridization, immunohistochemistry, and next-generation sequencing for detection of eml4-alk rearrangement in lung cancer. *Oncologist*. 2015;20:316–322.

35. Pepe M. *The Statistical Evaluation of Medical Tests for Classification and Prediction*. New York, NY: Oxford University Press; 2003.

36. Piantadosi S. *Clinical Trials a Methodological Perspective*. 2nd edn. Hoboken, NJ: John Wiley and Sons, Inc.; 2005.

37. Bhatt DL, Mehta C. Adaptive designs for clinical trials. *New Eng J Med*. 2016;375(1):65–74.

Bayesian Designs in Clinical Trials

Gary L. Rosner, B. Nebiyou Bekele, and Yuan Ji

In this chapter, we discuss issues that arise when developing, reporting, and implementing clinical study designs that incorporate Bayesian models and calculations. We have had the opportunity to work with many such designs over our careers. We feel that incorporating Bayesian models in study designs offers many advantages over traditional frequentist designs, and we discuss these advantages in this chapter. At the same time, Bayesian models require considerable thought and close collaboration between statisticians and clinical investigators. Also, there may still be some reluctance on the part of some clinical investigators to accept a study design that is built on Bayesian considerations. We provide some arguments and real examples that may help clinical researchers in oncology overcome such reluctance. Although our examples come from the field of oncology, the lessons and underlying ideas have broad applications.

WHY BAYESIAN DESIGNS?

Types of Bayesian Designs

First, we need to define "Bayesian statistics." Bayesian statistical inference derives its name from Bayes' rule, a basic theorem in mathematical probability. Bayes' rule shows how one can calculate the probability of an outcome, conditional on an event, based on the probability of the event, conditional on the outcome. For example, a diagnostic test for some disease often is characterized by its sensitivity and specificity. The sensitivity is the probability the test is positive, given that the person has the disease in question. Specificity is the probability the test is negative for the disease, given that the person does not have the disease. If you or I undergo the diagnostic test, however, we are interested in the probability that we have the disease, given a positive test result, that is, the positive predictive value of the diagnostic test. Bayes' rule tells us how to reverse the conditioning to determine the positive predictive value from the test's sensitivity and specificity.

In Bayesian statistics, we use information about variation in the data and a characterization of the uncertainty about parameters in a mathematical model of the variation in the data to increase our knowledge about the underlying mechanisms that give rise to the data. Each of these elements of Bayesian statistics has a mathematical formulation. The information about the variation or distribution of observations in the data is characterized by a probability distribution often called the sampling distribution or the likelihood. For example, if we study a new drug for treating cancer patients, we may think that each patient in our study has an unknown chance of responding to the drug. We carry out the study to learn what this chance or probability of response is with the drug, often called the drug's response rate. We estimate this chance of a clinical response by the proportion of patients who respond in our study. This chance is a parameter in the model that we may use to describe the heterogeneity of responses across the patients in our study. Before we analyze the study's data, we may have some idea of likely values this chance may take. Some values may be more likely than others. We can characterize this distribution of likely values with another probability distribution. We call this distribution the prior distribution for the probability a patient will achieve a clinical response if the patient takes the new drug. The goal of the study is to learn about this probability and, hopefully, make our estimate more precise than one based solely on information coming from outside of the study. The (hopefully more precise) characterization of our uncertainty about the drug's response rate is called the posterior distribution. Bayesian statistical inference applies Bayes' rule to the sampling distribution and the prior distribution to determine the posterior distribution for the probability a patient will achieve a clinical response with the new drug.

What do we mean by a Bayesian design? In the first sentence, we specifically avoided writing the term "Bayesian design," choosing instead the phrase "clinical study designs that incorporate Bayesian models and calculations." The latter phrase allows us to include many designs that are not fully Bayesian, meaning that the designs are not based solely on Bayesian considerations, such as minimizing an expected risk. Instead, many of these "calibrated Bayes"(1) designs incorporate a Bayesian model, possibly considering prior information, in the stopping rules of the study, but the choice of design depends on its having good properties according to common frequentist considerations (e.g., control of the type I error rate, appropriate power, etc.). These calibrated Bayes designs are called Bayesian designs in many applied settings.

An example of this calibration is the following. The statistician and clinical investigators decide on the general form of a criterion for decisions at interim analyses, such as basing stopping decisions on the posterior probability that the treatment's success probability exceeds a threshold value (or falls below a different cutoff). Next, the statistician carries out a large number of simulations under various scenarios. The statistician reviews the simulation results with the clinical investigators, allowing them to decide on the criteria that yield the best (to their minds) operating characteristics. The operating characteristics of the proposed design include the relative frequency of deciding that the new treatment is beneficial under different hypothetical treatment effects, including no benefit; the average number of patients enrolled in the study for each scenario; and other aspects that relate to the design's performance. This review-and-revise process may include changing the benchmark values against which one compares the posterior treatment-related success probability or the degree of certainty (e.g., 80% or 90%) that one will require before deciding to stop the study.

There also exist more formal Bayesian designs for clinical trials. Berry argues for the application of decision theory in clinical trial design (2,3). Even if one takes a fully Bayesian view, one will still find that reviewing these simulations during the design stage serves to make the transition from frequentist designs to Bayesian ones easier for investigators. Simulations under various scenarios also help reveal the sensitivity of the study's decisions and inference to prior assumptions. We discuss these ideas later in this chapter through our examples.

Advantages of Bayesian Designs

Why is one interested in Bayesian designs for clinical trials? One can view a clinical trial as an experiment that will lead to a decision (use the new treatment or do not use the new treatment) or prediction (the new treatment regimen will provide a benefit of so much over the standard treatment). Bayesian methods are ideal for decision making (i.e., minimizing risk or maximizing utility) and for prediction.

Additionally, Bayesian methods are ideal for combining disparate sources of information. With Bayesian statistical models, one can construct a coherent probability model to combine the information from the current study with historical data and with any information available from ongoing studies. Perhaps the current interest in Bayesian designs derives impetus from the fact that the Bayesian inference obeys the likelihood principle, a basic concept of statistical inference. The likelihood principle requires that data that lead to the same likelihood (viz., the functional form of the sampling distribution for the observations) for the parameter of interest should lead to the same inference (4). The likelihood principle highlights a difference between Bayesian inference and frequentist inference when we consider interim analyses of an ongoing study. Many clinical studies include interim analyses to allow stopping the study early if the treatment shows exceptional efficacy or if it appears unlikely that the study will show a treatment benefit. When reviewing a study's protocol, we often suggest interim analyses if not already included. Often, studies incorporate frequentist stopping rules, such as group-sequential designs (5). These rules preserve the overall type I error probability, which is the probability of incorrectly rejecting the null hypothesis. Such modifications to the designs account for the fact that carrying out multiple statistical hypothesis tests increases the probability of a type I error. As a result of such adjustments, a treatment effect that might have been statistically significant without any prior interim analyses may not be significant after accounting for the number of prior analyses. A consequence of the likelihood principle is that the number of interim analyses should not affect inference, since the likelihood is the same whether the current analysis had been the first or the most recent of several earlier analyses. All that matters to the Bayesian (and anyone else whose school of inference is consistent with the likelihood principle) are the data at hand and not what happened before, unless earlier analyses somehow alter the likelihood.

Another reason more and more clinical trials are incorporating Bayesian ideas is the desire in many situations to include adaptive randomization. Such clinical trials change the randomization probabilities in light of the accruing data. The study may start randomizing patients to the different treatments with equal probability. Then, perhaps after enrolling some minimum number of patients, the randomization probabilities adapt to favor the better performing treatments. Bayesian methodology may enter the study by way of using posterior probability calculations to influence the randomization probabilities (6). The use of adaptive randomization is based on an ethical argument that attempts to balance two competing goals: (a) reduce the number of patients who receive inferior treatment; and (b) still accrue convincing evidence within the clinical trial. There have been interesting debates on the ethics of randomization and adaptive randomization (7–12), but we do not discuss this aspect of clinical trial design here. We discuss an example of Bayesian adaptive randomization later in this chapter.

Another area of current interest is precision medicine. Because of unprecedented recent breakthroughs in cancer genomics and immuno-oncology, the traditional histology-stage-based approach for classifying cancers and one-size-fits-all approach for treating tumors are being rapidly challenged by genomics-based cancer subtyping and availability of drugs that target specific molecular pathways in tumors. In precision oncology, a targeted therapy is no longer deemed effective for an entire histology, such as lung cancer. Instead, a subgroup of lung cancer patients bearing specific tumor DNA mutations will receive therapy targeting these genomic aberrations. Development of precision medicine approaches calls for clinical trials that enrich study populations for known or even unknown subgroups (13). Moreover, a genomic-aberration-based drug for lung cancer might be effective for other cancers with the same genomic aberration. The so-called umbrella trials evaluate a drug for multiple cancer subtypes sharing the same genomic aberration. An alternative approach, called a platform trial, leverages genomics-based cancer subtyping by matching a set of targeted drugs to a corresponding set of genomic aberrations and simultaneously testing these drugs within one cancer type. This design allows more drugs to be used for the same histology-based cancer. An example of a platform trial is the I-SPY 2 trial (14) that has found active drugs in molecularly defined subpopulations of women with breast cancer (15–17). Last, when multiple genomic aberrations, multiple drugs, and multiple cancer types are considered simultaneously, a platform umbrella clinical trial is needed. Bayesian designs can be used for all of these new clinical trial designs, because of their ability to borrow information across drugs and patient populations (16,18). Rapid development of subgroup-based statistical designs is under way, including many Bayesian designs (19–21).

REQUIREMENTS FOR A SUCCESSFUL BAYESIAN DESIGN

As with all clinical studies, considerable work has to go into the preparation of the study design. The statistician and the clinical investigators need to discuss the study's aims and objectives. Care must go into selecting endpoints for the primary and secondary aims of the study. Much of these considerations are discussed elsewhere in this volume, so we will focus more on the aspects that relate to the Bayesian part of the design. In particular, we will talk about the prior distribution and stopping rules. Additionally, if one takes a decision-theoretic approach, one will have to consider the utility function that accounts for the study's aims. If one wishes to calibrate the design, then one will have to

review with the other investigators the implication of various decision-rule parameters on the design's operating characteristics.

Software for Real-Time Updating

Real-time updating is an important aspect of many Bayesian study designs. These designs incorporate early stopping rules, allowing the investigator to stop early for lack of efficacy, for superiority over a comparator, or because of excessive toxicity. For example, in a single-arm phase II study that will compare the progression-free survival (PFS) associated with a new treatment to historical information relating to one or several standard treatments, an investigator may desire to stop the study early if there is evidence that the new treatment results in worse outcomes than the historical standard. A Bayesian approach to this problem might assume that PFS follows an exponential probability distribution that has rate parameter r. This parameter indicates the expected number of events per follow-up time unit at risk. If one assumes a gamma prior distribution for r, then the parameter's updated probability distribution is also a gamma distribution but with parameters that incorporate the new information. A common stopping rule under this setup is to stop the trial if at any point $\Pr(r > r^* | \text{Data}) > C$, where r^* usually represents some historical event rate. In words, this rule calls for stopping the study if the data suggest that the rate (r) exceeds the historical benchmark rate (r^*) with probability C or more. One may compute this probability each time a new patient (or group of patients) enters the study or when a patient already enrolled experiences disease progression.

Typically, calculation of this probability requires numerical integration. One may have to develop statistical software to carry out these calculations. These computer programs would allow one to monitor the accruing data relative to the stopping rules to assess if the boundaries have been crossed. This computation would also have to be part of the computer programs that one uses to estimate the operating characteristics, since one has to run the study *in silico* to estimate the design's operating characteristics. By "software," we include programs written in either R (22) or SAS and used by the collaborating statistician, a stand-alone desktop computer program written for use by other statisticians, or even a web-based application for use by nonstatistical research staff. The kind of application one develops is a function of who the end user will be and how often future studies may use the same sort of design. When carrying out a single-institution study, it may be sufficient for the collaborating statistician to develop a function that runs within a general purpose statistical or mathematical package. Such a study may experience slow accrual and require infrequent posterior updating, perhaps only every 4 to 6 weeks. In contrast, a rapidly accruing multicenter, multiarm trial may require real-time updating via a web-based application or a telephone voice-response system. Part of the work involved in implementing Bayesian methods is to determine the exact software needs of the particular study's design. In what follows, we describe some common types of clinical studies that require real-time updating.

Types of Studies

Phase I Oncology Dose-Finding Study. Many drugs used in oncology are associated with severe toxicities and have a narrow therapeutic window, meaning that there is only a small range of doses that may be efficacious without being overly toxic. Therefore, the initial step in assessing these compounds in humans usually focuses on finding a dose that has an acceptable level of toxicity. Because one of the most important constraints on the conduct of these initial trials is the desire to limit the number of patients who experience severe toxicity, these studies are conducted with dose escalation proceeding carefully and sequentially. The study enrolls small cohorts of patients (often three to six) and does not assign a higher dose until each patient in a given cohort has been through at least one cycle of treatment and their outcomes assessed. The toxicity outcomes observed from these (and earlier) patients may enter into an algorithm that the investigators use to select the dose for the next cohort. The purpose of this sequential approach is to decrease the chance that large numbers of patients receive doses that are too toxic.

The assumption underlying this approach, in oncology at least, is that toxicity and response are correlated *through dose.* That is, higher doses lead to an increase in the toxicity risk and an increase in the probability that the treatment will harm the tumor. This assumption was historically reasonable in oncology, where one defined activity in terms of killing cancer cells. Thus, phase I oncology studies have traditionally attempted to determine the highest dose that has an acceptable toxicity level, the maximally tolerated dose (MTD), since by assumption this dose will also lead to greater efficacy than lower doses. It is worth noting that this assumption may not be appropriate when considering newer targeted agents, particularly immunologic drugs.

Bayesian phase I designs treat a patient's risk of toxicity at a given dose as a quantity about which the investigator has some degree of uncertainty. One quantifies this uncertainty via a probability distribution. Decisions to escalate the dose, continue with the current dose, or de-escalate from the current dose incorporate all data available at the time the investigators need to make the decision. Given what one has learned to date, one may choose to treat the next patient with the dose for which the expected risk of toxicity is closest to a predefined target toxicity risk. In such a setting, Bayesian methods offer clear advantages. The Bayesian framework provides a means by which one can learn about toxicity risks at the different doses and naturally make decisions based on the data observed, applying the calculations in a sequential manner. The increase in knowledge is reflected by a decrease in uncertainty about which dose to recommend as one moves from prior to posterior. Several Bayesian proposals for designing dose-finding studies in oncology have appeared in the literature, including the continual reassessment method (CRM) (23), extension of the CRM for late-occurring toxicities (24), Bayesian logistic regression (25), and modified toxicity probability intervals (mTPI) (26,27), to name a few. Many of these proposals include considerations to control the possibility of overdosing patients (28). For a comprehensive review of phase I dose-finding designs, including Bayesian and non-Bayesian designs, we refer to the work of Sverdlov et al. (29).

We describe two representative Bayesian designs that highlight different aspects of Bayesian philosophy. The CRM design takes advantage of the power of Bayesian models that allow aggregating information at different dose levels to be shared in making statistical inference and dose-finding decisions. It uses a parametric function to describe the relationship of dose levels and toxicity probabilities at the dose levels. Typically, the higher the dose level, the higher the risk of toxicity. The parametric function uses one or two parameters to describe the dose–toxicity relationship. The CRM then relies on the posterior distributions of the parameters based on the observed trial data to update dose-specific estimates of risk. As more patients are enrolled and their toxicity responses observed, the posterior distributions are estimated and updated. Toxicity data across all the dose levels are aggregated for the estimation of the posterior, helping Bayesian inference to achieve better accuracy.

The mTPI design takes a different approach. It takes advantage of the Bayesian decision framework and casts the dose-finding inference as a problem of making multiple optimal decisions. The mTPI design first breaks the whole interval of possible toxicity risks (i.e., a number between 0 and 1) into three subintervals: $(0, a)$, (a, b), and $(b, 1)$. The target MTD is believed to have risk of toxicity in the middle interval (a, b). For example, if the study targets a dose as the highest dose with a risk of toxicity equal to 0.3, then the three subintervals might be $(0.0, 0.25)$, $(0.25, 0.35)$, and $(0.35, 1.0)$. When patients are treated at a given dose, mTPI infers whether the dose's risk falls in the left interval $(0, a)$, the middle interval (a, b), or the right interval $(b, 1)$, based on a Bayesian decision framework that maximizes a posterior expected loss. The loss function assigns a penalty when a wrong decision is made. For example, if a dose's risk falls in $(0, a)$, suggesting that the dose is below the MTD, a decision to decrease the dose level will be penalized while a decision to increase the dose level will not. After determining the optimal decision that minimizes the posterior expected loss, mTPI chooses one of three decisions: (a) escalate, (b) stay at the current dose, or (c) de-escalate, to enable an up-and-down dose-finding algorithm. Such decisions are sequentially applied when new patient data are available.

Both designs have been shown to perform well in the literature (23,26). The CRM design has been implemented in R packages, such as the dfCRM package (https://cran.r-project.org/web/packages/dfcrm/index.html) (30). The mTPI design is available online at (31).

Phase II Adaptive Randomization Trials. Bayesian adaptive randomization designs modify the randomization probabilities for patients entering the trial based on either posterior or predictive probabilities that incorporate observed outcomes for patients already treated. The effect is that the randomization probabilities may tend to favor one treatment over another if the evidence in the trial suggests that patients are having better outcomes if treated with one treatment relative to the other. In essence, data from patients previously enrolled and evaluated in a study inform future treatment assignments, so that patients currently enrolling onto the trial will have a higher probability of being randomized to the more (or most) efficacious treatment(s). In many of these designs, patients are initially randomized fairly (i.e., with equal probability) to the various (at least two) treatment arms. Since many trials with adaptive randomization usually have a period in which patients are equally randomized prior to the implementation of adaptive randomization, it is important that the statistician monitor the actual randomization versus expected randomization. If the randomization probabilities change earlier than expected or in a manner that seems inconsistent with the data, there may be a problem with the design or the software. Extensive simulations under many scenarios during the design stage will help avoid such problems.

Other Bayesian Trial Designs. Other interesting and useful examples of successful Bayesian applications in the design of clinical trials include single-treatment phase II studies that consider efficacy and toxicity, with stopping rules based on both endpoints (32–35). Another interesting innovation is the so-called seamless phase II–III design (36,37). With this design, randomization begins within the context of a small phase II study that collects survival information but has an intermediate endpoint as the primary outcome. Based on early results with respect to the intermediate endpoint, the study may expand to a large randomized phase III study with survival as the primary outcome. Berry et al. discuss a design that simultaneously sought the best dose of a drug in an adaptive way and maintained a randomized comparison with placebo (38).

As mentioned earlier, the Bayesian inferential machinery fits well with decision theory. Once one has determined an appropriate utility function, one can set up the design to optimize the expected or average utility. Furthermore, one can carry out sequential decision making by looking ahead one or a few steps or in a fully sequential design. The computation can get very complex, especially for fully sequential designs, since they often require algorithms based on backward induction (39). In all cases, one maximizes the utility, taking into account posterior uncertainty. There also exist more formal Bayesian designs for clinical trials. Berry argues for the application of decision theory in clinical trial design (2,3). Kadane (40) describes an interesting case study of a clinical trial, describing the background and development of the study. The literature includes other examples of formal Bayesian designs (41–44). Rossell et al. (45) and Ding et al. (46) present decision-theoretic designs for phase II studies that screen out active therapies from among a sequence of new treatments.

Realistic Priors

Historical Priors

Often, the current study may include one or more agents that were included in earlier studies. These data usually inform the study's design, either informally (as in determining the null and alternative hypotheses in frequentist designs) or formally via a prior distribution. If one assumes that the current study's patients will be exchangeable with the historical patients (i.e., patients in both groups give rise to the same sampling distribution, regardless of how one orders their data), the historical information will be extremely informative with respect to inference during the current study. Such a situation may arise if the historical information comes from studies that enrolled many more patients than planned for the current study. (In many situations, it may well be appropriate to consider whether there really is a need for the current study, given the strength of historical evidence. That is a topic for another discussion, however.) Since the current study will go forward, one has to find a way to discount the historical information or choose to assume that the patients in the current study are not fully similar to those enrolled in the earlier studies.

Consider a clinical study in which the primary outcome is binary, such as treatment success or failure, however defined. The parameter of interest in the statistical model of the study's data is the probability that a patient has a successful treatment outcome with the therapy. In this situation, we might characterize the probability of a treatment success in the historical data by means of a probability distribution that takes values between 0 and 1, such as the beta distribution. For example, if an early study enrolled 50 patients and 30 patients experienced a treatment success, we might characterize the uncertainty about the treatment's underlying success probability by a beta distribution with parameters equal to 30 and 20. One might think of this prior as the posterior distribution arising from an experiment that gave rise to these data and a distribution representing no prior data. (Alternatively, one could consider an initial uniform(0,1) prior or Jeffreys' beta(0.5, 0.5) prior and determine a posterior beta distribution with slightly different parameters.)

One may feel, however, that the beta(30,20) prior is too informative for this study. For example, this distribution has 95% of the central mass between 0.46 and 0.73. If one wants to entertain the possibility of smaller success probabilities than 0.4, then one may want to discount this prior data in some way. A natural way to keep the prior mean 0.6 but increase the uncertainty is to decrease the "prior sample size." For the beta distribution, the sum of the two parameters can be thought of as comparable to a prior sample size. The smaller the parameters are, the larger the variance becomes, which is similar to the change in precision with sample size. The historical data consist of 50 patients in our example, and the beta distribution's two parameters (30 and 20) sum to 50. Instead of using a prior with precision corresponding to a sample of 50 patients, one might choose to reduce the prior information to the equivalent of a prior sample size of 5 by using a beta(3, 2) distribution. Now the central 95% of the mass lies between 0.19 and 0.93.

A related approach for discounting the historical information is with a power prior (47,48). The power prior extends the notion of discounting to a general class of distributions and allows for inference with respect to the degree of discounting. Briefly, one considers a parameter in the probability model that will characterize the level of discounting for the historical information. The basic idea of the power prior is that the more similar the prior and current data are, the less discounting that takes place and vice versa. Let $L(\theta|D)$ represent the sampling distribution or likelihood function that will characterize the data at the end of the current study (i.e., after collecting the data represented by D). Using the same likelihood function with the historical data D_H, the power prior for the current study is $p(\theta|D_H,\delta) \propto L(\theta|D_H)^\delta p(\theta|c)$. The parameter δ will discount or downweight the information content of the historical data when one will apply this prior to carry out posterior inference in the analysis of the current study. Another approach with advantages over the power prior is the so-called commensurate prior (49).

Another way people have discounted prior information is less direct: they have modified parameters in the stopping rules to make it more difficult to stop early. In other words, one uses the historical information to generate an informative prior but makes the cutoff for early stopping more stringent than perhaps one would normally consider reasonable. For example, if one proposes a stopping rule criterion based on the posterior probability that some parameter or function of model parameters exceeds a threshold, one may require a very high probability (e.g., 99%) of this event before considering

early stopping. Making the stopping rule more stringent basically provides a way to keep the prior from dominating the posterior distribution and allows the current study to continue accumulating data.

The process of determining the boundary criteria often proceeds iteratively. One determines the criteria for early stopping by carrying out simulations under various scenarios and then deciding which stopping rules lead to satisfactory operating characteristics. While such devices tend to make the designs acceptable to frequentists, because of the calibrated operating characteristics, they also may tend to undermine the benefit of the underlying Bayesian model. The historical information may become almost neglected or, at most, these data enter into the design as a formality without giving full consideration of their importance to the overall inferential question under investigation.

Elicitation of Experts

Elicitation of priors from experts would seem a reasonable approach, especially in the absence of directly relevant historical data. Carlin et al. (50) describe their experience eliciting prior information for a clinical trial. Problems may occur, however. The experts' opinions may have led to a prior distribution that subsequently appears to be at odds with the data. An informative example is discussed by Carlin et al. in the context of a randomized clinical trial evaluating the benefit of prophylaxis against possible infection with toxoplasmic encephalitis (TE) (51). In this study, the five experts whose opinions went into the prior distribution turned out to have been overly optimistic. Each expert anticipated a treatment benefit. Although there was widespread disagreement among these five individuals, none considered the possibility that the treatment might not be better than placebo, let alone worse.

The key points resulting from these investigators' experience with this study are instructive. In particular, the experts may provide point estimates of the treatment's efficacy, but there is underlying uncertainty in each expert's opinion. Perhaps a mixture of these separate prior distributions will be more robust to the analysis than combining the experts' point estimates into a single prior distribution. Another point brought out in this study was that different experts might find it easier to specify priors for the effect of the treatment on different endpoints. For example, one expert was not able to provide a prior estimate of the effect of the treatment on the risk of death or TE, whereas the other four could and did.

In our experience, it is important that those experts also see the consequences of their a priori estimates. Graphical displays of uncertainty distributions or of possible observations, given prior specification of underlying parameters, allow the experts to gain insight into the implications of their stated beliefs (35,52). Quite often, this feedback reveals inconsistencies and leads to revisions by the experts.

Thus, one has to be careful about incorporating expert opinion into a prior distribution for a clinical trial's design.

Operating Characteristics

One of the biggest challenges to utilizing Bayesian methods when designing studies is having software available to assess the operating characteristics of a design. For any Bayesian design used in practice, the collaborating statistician must provide operating characteristics that summarize the average behavior of the proposed method under a wide variety of situations or scenarios. Because these designs typically involve complex models and decision rules, one usually has to carry out simulations to evaluate the operating characteristics of a study's design. The scenarios typically cover a wide variety of possibilities, ranging from very pessimistic, such as the case in which no treatment provides any benefit, to optimistic cases, in which several of the treatments are highly effective. Some of the characteristics that one typically summarizes are the number of patients assigned to each treatment, the probability of selecting each dose as most efficacious, the probability of stopping a trial if all treatments are too toxic, the average number of patients enrolled, and so on.

Purpose of Checking Operating Characteristics (Calibration)

Controversy Surrounding Evaluation of Frequentist Properties. If one has chosen to demonstrate the frequentist characteristics of the Bayesian design, then one will have to simulate the design under different scenarios. It may seem odd to want to evaluate frequentist characteristics, such as the proportion of false declarations of treatment efficacy of a proposed Bayesian design, but there are some reasons for this. First, one may want to convince a non-Bayesian audience that the proposed design offers benefits over standard frequentist designs without incurring a loss in terms of the frequentist characteristics. For example, some sequential designs base their stopping rules on posterior probability calculations, such as the magnitude of the probability that the treatment difference is larger than a prespecified threshold delta, given the current study data. If this probability exceeds a cutoff value, then one might consider stopping. One can certainly view these posterior probabilities as test statistics, even though they differ from more common test statistics like the chi-square test. If one considers the posterior probabilities in decision rules as test statistics, then one can evaluate their operating characteristics. Another reason one might want to estimate the operating characteristics of the proposed design is to evaluate how robust the design is under different scenarios. If one feels that the prior distribution is based on rather limited historical information, for example, then one might want to ensure that the prior does not overly

dominate inference in situations that may appear to be consistent with the earlier study.

Potential Pitfalls

Potential pitfalls include not stopping when one should, stopping a study and later regretting it, and the often perceived possibility that the study's Bayesian analysis will not receive widespread acceptance. The surest way to avoid these problems is to carry out simulations under many, many different scenarios.

EXAMPLES OF BAYESIAN DESIGNS

What Worked and Why

We have seen dozens of successful Bayesian clinical trials. One characteristic that has contributed to successful implementation is a schedule of regular meetings between the statisticians and the clinical research staff during the trial's design stage. The meetings serve to educate each group to the other's needs and perspectives. After initiation of patient enrollment, meetings between the research staff and the statistician continue for the purpose of interim review of the trial's progress. Also, the statistician should provide appropriate data-management oversight to ensure that the database accurately reflects the trial data.

Clear communication between the clinical investigators and statisticians with respect to what a design can and cannot do is essential. It is also vitally important for the statistician to test the computer code and its interface to ensure that everything is working properly. Is the program computing the posterior probabilities correctly? Do the results and recommendations under different hypothetical situations make sense, mathematically and clinically? Is the user interface (for example, a stand-alone graphical user interface or a web-based application) intuitive and easily navigated by the individuals who will be using it? Does the interface perform appropriately? These are important questions to address while preparing the protocol. One should carry out these evaluations well before the study enrolls the first patient if one wants to realize the full potential of the Bayesian design. When clinical studies with Bayesian designs work well, the benefits of these designs are very much appreciated by the collaborating investigators. Four examples of clinical studies that incorporated Bayesian considerations in their designs follow.

Correlated Ordinal Toxicity Monitoring in Phase I

In this example, investigators used a Bayesian design within a new statistical framework for dose finding based on a set of qualitatively different ordinal-valued toxicities (53). The objective of this trial was to assess the toxicity profile associated with the anticancer drug gemcitabine when combined with external beam radiation to treat patients with soft-tissue sarcoma. The study's design allowed for possible evaluation of a total of 10 gemcitabine doses, combined with a fixed dose of radiation. Traditionally, phase I studies in oncology consider a binary endpoint as the primary outcome. This binary endpoint is an indicator of whether or not each patient experienced a dose-limiting toxicity, as defined in the protocol. This single endpoint reduces all toxicity information across grade or severity of the toxicity and across organ systems into a single yes-or-no outcome. Berry and Berry (54) consider toxicities categorized by organ systems and propose a hierarchical model to borrow strength across types of toxicities within organ systems in the context of drug safety monitoring. In most phase I oncology settings, however, the patient is at risk of several qualitatively different toxicities, each occurring at several possible levels of severity. The different toxicities often are not of equal clinical importance, however.

The design of this soft-tissue sarcoma phase I study represented a radical departure from conventional phase I study design in oncology. It was based on an underlying probability model that characterized the relationship between dose and the severity of each type of toxicity. The model included a set of correlated normally distributed latent variables to induce associations among the risks associated with the different toxicities. Additionally, there were weights or numerical scores to characterize the importance of each level of each type of toxicity. The statistician met with the physicians prior to initiation of the trial to elicit from them these scores. An algorithm combined the scores associated with each type and level of toxicity with the probability of observing each particular type and level of toxicity. This algorithm produced a weighted average toxicity score i. This weighted average toxicity score informed decisions about doses for successive cohorts of patients in this phase I study.

Concerns expressed by the oncologists motivated the development of this design. The clinicians wanted a dose-finding method that would account for the fact that, clinically, the toxicities that they had identified are not equally important. Additionally, the different toxicities do not occur independently. The investigators also requested that the dose-finding method utilize the information contained in the grade or severity of an observed toxicity. That is, if patients experience a low-grade toxicity at a given dose, while not dose limiting, this event suggests that higher doses may be more likely to lead to a higher grade of that toxicity. The Bayesian framework of this study's design was capable of addressing all of the investigators' concerns regarding the characterization of toxicity while also incorporating key design aspects required for institutional approval of the protocol, such as early trial termination for excessive toxicity at the lowest dose. At the end of the study, the model recommended a dose to take forward into phase II, and the investigators were in complete agreement with this choice as the appropriate dose (55).

Joint Modeling Toxicity and Biomarker Expression in a Phase I/II Dose-Finding Trial

In this example, the investigators used a Bayesian framework to model jointly a binary toxicity outcome and a continuous biomarker expression outcome in a phase I/II dose-finding study of an intravesical gene therapy for treating superficial bladder cancer (56). Since the toxicity and efficacy profiles of the gene therapy were unknown, the investigators proposed a phase I/II dose-finding study with four possible doses.

This trial's motivation was partially attributable to the increasing use of biomarkers as indicators of risk or as surrogate outcomes for activity and efficacy. In many contexts, the biomarker is observable immediately after treatment, allowing the investigators to learn about the therapeutic potential of the compound without having to wait months or even years as survival data mature. Unlike conventional phase I studies, this study's objective was to determine the "best" dose based on both biomarker expression and toxicity. This dual outcome required a joint model for the two endpoints. For ethical reasons, the study escalated doses between patients sequentially. An algorithm based on the joint model chose the dose for each successive patient using both toxicity and activity data from patients previously treated in the trial. The modeling framework incorporated a correlation between the binary toxicity endpoint and the continuous activity outcome via a latent Gaussian random variable. The dose-escalation/de-escalation decision rules were based on the posterior distributions of model parameters relating to toxicity and to activity. The study's stopping rule called for it to stop if the estimated risk of toxicity appeared excessive or if there was clear evidence that the treatment was not modulating the biologic marker.

The Bayesian framework used in this study allowed for flexible modeling of some rather complicated outcomes. In addition, this framework provided a coherent mechanism for incorporating prior information into the modeling process. The study ended, in fact, when it became evident that the drug was not modulating the biologic marker.

Adaptive Randomization

Investigators wished to evaluate the effectiveness of combinations of three drugs (an immunosuppressive agent, a purine analog antimetabolite, and an antifolate) to prevent graft-versus-host disease (GVHD) after transplantation. The study design included adaptive randomization and was to enroll a maximum of 150 patients. A success was defined in this study as "alive with successful engraftment, without relapse, and without a GVHD 100 days after the transplant." The design called for comparing each treatment to the control arm (i.e., the combination treatment with the immunosuppressive agent and antifolate) in terms of the probability of success in the following manner. As information accrues about the treatments, the randomization probabilities will change from equal randomization to randomization biased in favor of better performing treatment arms. The altered randomization probabilities will be functions of the posterior probabilities that each treatment-specific success probability exceeds that of the control arm.

In addition, the study's design allowed for early stopping based on predictive probabilities. Specifically, the design would suggest dropping a treatment arm if the predictive probability that its success probability will be greater than p_0 was less than 0.05, given the data at hand and predictions for data yet to accrue. The design was successful in that it limited the number of patients who received the inferior treatments to 18.2% of all of the 110 patients randomized to one of the four experimental arms. By contrast, a design that randomized patients equally to the treatments and did not allow for early stopping would have exposed 50% of patients to these ineffective therapies.

A Subgroup-Based Bayesian Adaptive Trial

We consider a novel clinical trial in gastroesophageal adenocarcinoma (GEC). GEC is the fourth most common malignancy and the second most common cause of death worldwide. It is a molecularly heterogeneous disease, and tumor heterogeneity (TH) between patients may be an important consideration for treatment selection (57). Failure to account for TH has likely contributed to negative results in a number of recent clinical trials testing novel molecularly targeted therapies with designs that used a one-size-fits-all approach. We proposed an adaptive design based on inference for TH for the PANGEA trial (funded by National Institutes of Health, NCT02213289). Currently, PANGEA is based on a design that addresses TH by assigning treatments according to predefined predictive molecular "oncogenic driver" categories, namely, genes *HER2*, *MET*, *FGFR2*, *EGFR/HER3*, and *KRAS/PI3K*. The protocol includes comprehensive molecular profiling at enrollment of patients' tumor tissue at a metastatic disease site (liver, lung, or peritoneum). The study assigns each patient to one of five specific treatments based on the metastatic tumor molecular profile. We proposed enhancing the design of the PANGEA trial, aiming for an improved patient allocation strategy after first-line targeted therapy.

The existing PANGEA protocol uses fixed rules to allocate targeted molecular therapies to patients based on their baseline genomic and proteomic profiles. In the next iteration of the trial's design, we will replace the existing fixed rules with the Subgroup ClUster-based Bayesian Adaptive (SCUBA) design (19) to guide second-line treatment assignments in cases of disease progression after first-line therapy. The SCUBA design forms random partitions of the range of biomarker values, along with Bayesian modeling, to learn about which biomarker–treatment pairs show promise. Treatment assignments will be based on the protein expression of several biomarkers, and assignments will adapt to treat patients with what appear to be their optimal treatments as predicted by the SCUBA design. Simulations under various scenarios will allow assessments of how well the design will work.

In practice, implementation of a trial that uses SCUBA requires an online tool that allows nurses and physicians to input the baseline covariate values. This tool then provides a treatment assignment based on a posterior inference that uses all previous trial data and the patient's covariate values. Availability of such software will be the key to the success of such adaptive trials.

What Did Not Work and Why

When designing clinical studies, the collaborating statistician should be aware of potential pitfalls associated with the design or designs of choice. This is true of Bayesian designs, which may have some unique issues to consider. The most common difficulties include problems with the computer code, such as bugs that lead to incorrect posterior probability calculations; human error in data entry and management; and reconciling differences in how statisticians (or statistical models) define adequate evidence of treatment effects and how physicians define these effects. In what follows, we give examples of three of these potential problems and discuss steps one can take to avoid them.

Over time, Bayesian designs have found more application and become more complicated. While most of the designs developed in the early 1990s focused on binary endpoints, current implementations include models for time-to-event endpoints that include parameter effects for treatment, patient-specific covariate (e.g., patient's risk of death) and covariate-by-treatment interaction (e.g., Zhou et al. [(58)]). For very simple designs based on a binary endpoint, the data-management requirements for posterior updating were relatively straightforward. These types of models only require keeping track of the number of patients in the trial and the total number of patients who have experienced the event of interest. In contrast, as the models become increasingly complex, studies require more data (and more data management) for calculation of posterior probabilities. As a consequence, an increase in data management can lead to data entry errors.

For example, Maki et al. (59) describe a two-arm open-label phase II clinical study in sarcoma with tumor response as the primary endpoint. The study employed a Bayesian adaptive randomization procedure that accounted for treatment-by-sarcoma-subgroup interactions. Specifically, the adaptive randomization scheme incorporated information on the type of sarcoma. After randomizing the first 30 patients equally to the two treatment regimens, the design called for adapting the randomization probabilities for subsequent patients to favor the better performing treatment, according to the accrued data. The investigators subsequently found that the initial recorded sarcoma subtypes for some patients were incorrect. The consequence of this incorrect labeling was that, for one sarcoma subtype, the probability of randomization to the top performing arm was less than it should have been, relative to the other treatment arms. While all patients continued to have a higher probability of randomization to the better performing treatment arm, it is conceivable that if such an error were not discovered early, patients could have been randomized to inferior treatments. Therefore, it is extremely important that the statistician be involved with data-management oversight to ensure that such errors do not occur.

One of the key considerations in designing Bayesian clinical trials involves navigating the relationship between the proposed Bayesian model and the realities of medical research. A model may indicate that one treatment confers benefit over another (calculated via posterior probabilities), but if the study investigators are claiming this benefit on a very small number of patients, they are going to have a hard time convincing a medical audience that the results are "robust" (robust in an English and not statistical sense). For example, Giles et al. (60) reported a phase II trial that randomized patients to receive one of three treatment regimens: idarubicin and Ara-C (IA); troxacitabine and Ara-C (TA); and troxacitabine and idarubicin (TI). The study's Bayesian design adaptively randomized patients to the treatments. Initially, there was an equal chance for randomization to IA, TA, or TI, but treatment arms with a higher success rate progressively received a greater proportion of patients. The adaptive randomization led to a total of 18 patients randomized to the IA arm; 11 patients randomized to the TA arm; and just 5 patients randomized to the TI arm. The small sample size associated with the TI arm left this trial open to concerns that the results were not conclusive.

This story is reminiscent of the controversy surrounding the early randomized trials of extracorporeal membrane oxygenation (ECMO) for neonates in respiratory failure. Two early ECMO trials (61,62) included adaptive randomization algorithms that led to very few babies receiving the non-ECMO treatment. In the end, a vocal part of the medical community seemed to think that these trials included too few patients treated conventionally (i.e., without ECMO) to justify making ECMO the standard treatment for neonates in respiratory distress (see Ware and related discussion for more information about the ECMO trials [(63)]). Eventually, a randomized clinical trial without adaptive randomization in the United Kingdom demonstrated the benefit of ECMO (64). The lesson to learn is that one should ensure that the trial will include a minimum number of patients in all treatments (subject to safety assurances) before it begins to adapt the randomization in light of the accruing evidence.

A common criticism voiced by some investigators reflects a perceived disconnect between recommendations based on Bayesian models and the investigator's intuition. This disconnect is exemplified in the context of phase I studies in oncology. Although we described and illustrated Bayesian phase I oncology trials earlier in this chapter, most phase I clinical trials in oncology use non-Bayesian algorithms for dose finding, such as the 3 + 3 design (65). Their popularity is driven by the fact that clinicians can easily understand these trial designs and the decision rules employed make intuitive sense. Yet, much is left unspecified in the implementation of these methods. For example, algorithmic designs *implicitly* target toxicity rates of around 17% (1 in 6) as being acceptable. In contrast, while Bayesian phase I designs seem (to some clinicians) to be black boxes, these models make explicit the outcomes being targeted. Specifically, all Bayesian designs *explicitly* specify a target probability of toxicity (usually between 25% and 33%). We believe that one of the main reasons for this disconnect is lack of communication between the statistician and the clinical investigator. Partly, this lack of communication may result from difficulty explaining these methods to nonstatisticians (66). One way to overcome these difficulties is by making the underlying assumptions of the Bayesian model explicit to the investigator. One can illustrate these assumptions by providing the investigator with sample trajectories of virtual trials simulated under different scenarios, in addition to providing the operating characteristics of the trial's average behavior (as discussed earlier in this chapter). While potentially time-consuming, this type of upfront examination and assessment before the study begins will help the clinician understand both the merits and limitations of the design and the underlying model contained in the protocol.

SUMMARY OF RECOMMENDATIONS

In this chapter, we have illustrated the use of Bayesian methods in the design of clinical studies. Although we work with investigators interested in treating cancer, the examples illustrate ideas that are applicable in all disease areas. The main advantages of incorporating Bayesian ideas in the design of clinical trials are the inherent flexibility of Bayesian inference; the ease with which one can incorporate information from outside of the study, including measured outcomes of mixed types (e.g., continuous and discrete); the natural notion of evolving knowledge evinced by the transformation from prior uncertainty to posterior uncertainty based on observations; and the way the Bayesian methodology allows one to make decisions and maximize utility, taking into account all uncertainty captured in the basic probability model. Although our examples concerned novel designs and new methodology, Bayesian ideas are applicable when designing any clinical study.

REFERENCES

1. Little RJ. Calibrated Bayes: a Bayes/frequentist roadmap. *Am Stat.* 2006;60(3):213–223.
2. Berry DA. A case for Bayesianism in clinical trials. *Stat Med.* 1993;12(15–16):1377–1393; discussion 1395–1404.
3. Berry DA. Decision analysis and Bayesian methods in clinical trials. In: Thall PF, ed. *Recent Advances in Clinical Trial Design and Analysis.* Boston, MA: Kluwer Academic Publishers; 1995:125–154.
4. Berger JO, Wolpert RL. *The Likelihood Principle.* Vol 6. Hayward, CA: Institute of Mathematical Statistics; 1984.
5. Jennison C, Turnbull BW. *Group Sequential Methods with Applications to Clinical Trials.* Boca Raton: Chapman & Hall/CRC; 1999.
6. Thall PF, Wathen JK. Practical Bayesian adaptive randomisation in clinical trials. *Eur J Cancer.* 2007;43(5):859–866.
7. Anscombe FJ. Sequential medical trials (Com: pp. 384–387). *J Am Stat Assoc.* 1963;58,365–383.
8. Armitage P. Sequential medical trials: some comments on F. J. Anscombe's paper. *J Am Stat Assoc.* 1963;58(302):384–387.
9. Armitage P. The search for optimality in clinical-trials. *Inter Stat Rev.* 1985;53(1):15–24.
10. Bather JA. On the allocation of treatments in sequential medical trials. *Inter Stat Rev.* 1985;53(1):1–13.
11. Royall RM. Ethics and statistics in randomized clinical trials. *Stat Sci.* 1991;6(1):52–62.
12. Hey SP, Kimmelman J. Are outcome-adaptive allocation trials ethical? *Clin Trial.* 2015;12(2):102–106.
13. Simon R. Genomic alteration-driven clinical trial designs in oncology. *Ann Inter Med.* 2016;165(4):270–278.
14. Barker AD, Sigman CC, Kelloff GJ, et al. I-SPY 2: an adaptive breast cancer trial design in the setting of neoadjuvant chemotherapy. *Clin Pharm Therap.* 2009;86(1):97–100.
15. Carey LA, Winer EP. I-SPY 2: toward more rapid progress in breast cancer treatment. *New Engl J Med.* 2016;375(1):83–84.
16. Park JW, Liu MC, Yee D, et al. Adaptive randomization of neratinib in early breast cancer. *New Engl J Med.* 2016;375(1):11–22.
17. Rugo HS, Olopade OI, DeMichele A, et al. Adaptive randomization of veliparib–carboplatin treatment in breast cancer. *New Engl J Med.* 2016;375(1):23–34.
18. Berry DA. The brave new world of clinical cancer research: adaptive biomarker-driven trials integrating clinical practice with clinical research. *Mol Oncol.* 2015;9(5):951–959.
19. Guo W, Ji Y, Catenacci DV. A subgroup cluster-based Bayesian adaptive design for precision medicine. *Biometrics.* 2016.
20. Schnell PM, Tang Q, Offen WW, et al. A Bayesian credible subgroups approach to identifying patient subgroups with positive treatment effects. *Biometrics.* 2016.
21. Xu Y, Trippa L, Müller P, et al. Subgroup-Based Adaptive (SUBA) designs for multi-arm biomarker trials. *Stat Biosci.* 2016;8(1):159–180.
22. R Development Core Team. *R: A Language and Environment for Statistical Computing* [computer program]. Vienna, Austria: R Foundation for Statistical Computing; 2014. http://www.R-project.org

23. O'Quigley J, Pepe M, Fisher L. Continual reassessment method: a practical design for phase I clinical trials in cancer. *Biometrics.* 1990;46:33–48.
24. Cheung YK, Chappell R. Sequential designs for phase I clinical trials with late-onset toxicities. *Biometrics.* 2000;56(4):1177–1182.
25. Neuenschwander B, Branson M, Gsponer T. Critical aspects of the Bayesian approach to phase I cancer trials. *Stat Med.* 2008;27(13):2420–2439.
26. Ji Y, Liu P, Li Y, et al. A modified toxicity probability interval method for dose-finding trials. *Clin Trials.* 2010;7(6):653–663.
27. Ji Y, Wang SJ. Modified toxicity probability interval design: a safer and more reliable method than the 3 + 3 design for practical phase I trials. *J Clin Oncol.* 2013;31(14):1785–1791.
28. Babb J, Rogatko A, Zacks S. Cancer phase I clinical trials: efficient dose escalation with overdose control. *Stat Med.* 1998;17(10):1103–1120.
29. Sverdlov O, Wong WK, Ryeznik Y. Adaptive clinical trial designs for phase I cancer studies. 2014:2–44.
30. Cheung YK. *Dose-finding by the continual reassessment method* [computer program]. 2013.
31. U-Design. http://udesign.laiyaconsulting.com (accessed January 8, 2018).
32. Thall PF, Sung HG. Some extensions and applications of a Bayesian strategy for monitoring multiple outcomes in clinical trials. *Stat Med.* 1998;17(14):1563–1580.
33. Thall PF, Simon RM, Estey EH. New statistical strategy for monitoring safety and efficacy in single-arm clinical trials. *J Clin Oncol.* 1996;14(1):296–303.
34. Thall PF, Simon RM, Estey EH. Bayesian sequential monitoring designs for single-arm clinical trials with multiple outcomes. *Stat Med.* 1995;14(4):357–379.
35. Thall PF, Cook JD. Dose-finding based on efficacy-toxicity trade-offs. *Biometrics.* 2004;60(3):684–693.
36. Inoue LYT, Thall PF, Berry DA. Seamlessly expanding a randomized phase II trial to phase III. *Biometrics.* 2002;58(4):823–831.
37. Thall PF. A review of phase 2-3 clinical trial designs. *Lifetime Data Anal.* 2008;14(1):37–53.
38. Berry DA, Müller P, Grieve AP, et al. Adaptive Bayesian designs for dose-ranging drug trials. In: Gatsonis C, Carlin B, Carriquiry A, eds. *Case Studies in Bayesian Statistics V.* New York, NY: Springer-Verlag; 2001:99–181.
39. DeGroot MH. *Optimal Statistical Decisions.* New York, NY: McGraw-Hill, Inc.; 1970.
40. Kadane JB, ed. *Bayesian Methods and Ethics in a Clinical Trial Design.* New York, NY: John Wiley & Sons; 1996.
41. Berry DA, Wolff MC, Sack D. Decision making during a phase III randomized controlled trial. *Control Clin Trials.* 1994;15(5):360–378.
42. Carlin BP, Kadane JB, Gelfand AE. Approaches for optimal sequential decision analysis in clinical trials. *Biometrics.* 1998;54(3):964–975.
43. Stallard N, Thall PF. Decision-theoretic designs for pre-phase II screening trials in oncology. *Biometrics.* 2001;57(4):1089–1095.
44. Stallard N, Thall PF, Whitehead J. Decision theoretic designs for phase II clinical trials with multiple outcomes. *Biometrics.* 1999;55(3):971–977.
45. Rossell D, Müller P, Rosner GL. Screening designs for drug development. *Biostatistics.* 2007;8(3):595–608.
46. Ding M, Rosner GL, Müller P. Bayesian optimal design for phase II screening trials. *Biometrics.* 2008;64(3):886–894.
47. Chen M-H, Ibrahim JG. The relationship between the power prior and hierarchical models. *Bayesian Anal.* 2006;1(3):551–574.
48. Ibrahim JG, Chen MH. Power prior distributions for regression models. *Stat Sci.* 2000;15(1):46–60.
49. Hobbs BP, Carlin BP, Mandrekar SJ, et al. Hierarchical commensurate and power prior models for adaptive incorporation of historical information in clinical trials. *Biometrics.* 2011;67(3):1047–1056.

50. Carlin BP, Chaloner K, Church T, et al. Bayesian approaches for monitoring clinical trials with an application to toxoplasmic encephalitis prophylaxis. *Statistician*. 1993;42(4):355–367.

51. Carlin BP, Chaloner KM, Louis TA, et al. Elicitation, monitoring, and analysis for an AIDS clinical trial (with discussion) In: Gatsonis C, Hodges JS, Kass RE, Singpurwalla ND, eds. *Case Studies in Bayesian Statistics, Vol. II*. New York, NY: Springer-Verlag; 1995:48–89.

52. Chaloner K, Church T, Louis TA, et al. Graphical elicitation of a prior distribution for a clinical trial. *Statistician*. 1993;42(4):341–353.

53. Bekele BN, Thall PF. Dose-finding based on multiple toxicities in a soft tissue sarcoma trial. *J Am Stat Assoc*. 2004;99(465):26–35.

54. Berry SM, Berry DA. Accounting for multiplicities in assessing drug safety: a three-level hierarchical mixture model. *Biometrics*. 2004;60(2):418–426.

55. Tseng WW, Zhou S, To CA, et al. Phase 1 adaptive dose-finding study of neoadjuvant gemcitabine combined with radiation therapy for patients with high-risk extremity and trunk soft tissue sarcoma. *Cancer*. 2015;121(20):3659–3667.

56. Bekele BN, Shen Y. A Bayesian approach to jointly modeling toxicity and biomarker expression in a phase I/II dose-finding trial. *Biometrics*. 2005;61(2):343–354.

57. Catenacci DV. Next-generation clinical trials: novel strategies to address the challenge of tumor molecular heterogeneity. *Mol Oncol*. 2015;9(5):967–996.

58. Zhou X, Liu S, Kim ES, et al. Bayesian adaptive design for targeted therapy development in lung cancer--a step toward personalized medicine. *Clin Trials*. 2008;5(3):181–193.

59. Maki RG, Wathen JK, Patel SR, et al. Randomized phase II study of gemcitabine and docetaxel compared with gemcitabine alone in patients with metastatic soft tissue sarcomas: results of sarcoma alliance for research through collaboration study 002 [corrected]. *J Clin Oncol*. 2007;25(19): 2755–2763.

60. Giles FJ, Kantarjian HM, Cortes JE, et al. Adaptive randomized study of idarubicin and cytarabine versus troxacitabine and cytarabine versus troxacitabine and idarubicin in untreated patients 50 years or older with adverse karyotype acute myeloid leukemia. *J Clin Oncol*. 2003;21(9): 1722–1727.

61. Bartlett RH, Roloff DW, Cornell RG, et al. Extracorporeal circulation in neonatal respiratory failure: a prospective randomized study. *Pediatrics*. 1985;76(4):479–487.

62. O'Rourke PP, Crone RK, Vacanti JP, et al. Extracorporeal membrane oxygenation and conventional medical therapy in neonates with persistent pulmonary hypertension of the newborn: a prospective randomized study. *Pediatrics*. 1989;84(6):957–963.

63. Ware JH. Investigating therapies of potentially great benefit: ECMO (with discussion). *Stat Sci*. 1989;4(4):298–340.

64. UK Collaborative ECMO Trial Group. UK collaborative randomised trial of neonatal extracorporeal membrane oxygenation. *Lancet*. 1996;348(9020):75–82.

65. Korn EL, Midthune D, Chen TT, et al. A comparison of two phase I trial designs. *Stat Med*. 1994;13:1799–1806.

66. Rosenberger WF, Haines LM. Competing designs for phase I clinical trials: a review. *Stat Med*. 2002;21(18):2757–2770.

Selection Designs

Suzanne E. Dahlberg

INTRODUCTION

Phase II clinical trials are generally used to demonstrate efficacy of a new therapeutic regimen with the goal that a sufficient magnitude of benefit be demonstrated to warrant further testing of that regimen definitively in a randomized phase III clinical trial. A variety of treatments may be available for testing, but prioritizing promising agents and resources is often necessary, for example, due to restricted financial resources or due to the rarity of a disease.

Selection designs represent an appropriate way to simultaneously evaluate and screen multiple novel single-agent therapies or combinations of therapies, particularly if formal comparison of each of those regimens against the standard of care is impractical. Standard-of-care control arms are generally not included as part of selection designs, which are generally implemented in the phase II setting with the understanding that one regimen will be selected for further testing against a standard control in a phase III clinical trial.

This chapter discusses issues pertaining to the design and conduct of phase II selection trials. The examples discussed throughout this chapter illustrate published studies in which these designs were used in oncology.

STATISTICAL CONSIDERATIONS

With a selection design, patients are randomized to one of several available novel therapies or combinations, but the key aspect of these designs is that a reference standard control arm is not implemented in the design, and that the observed best treatment will be selected regardless of the margin of benefit demonstrated relative to the other agents studied in the trial (Figure 16.1). This type of design might be appropriate for selection from a suite of available single-agent therapies or from a compendium of novel combinations sharing a common standard-of-care backbone. In the situation where the adverse event profile of a particular agent was not

known to vary substantially across dose or schedule, the selection design could also be used to evaluate and select dose or schedule. The statistical principles for these designs are rather simple, and can be performed with conventional nonrandomized trial designs within each arm; however, the appropriate application and interpretation can be challenging. Direct statistical comparisons via hypothesis testing between arms are neither planned within the study design nor performed because these studies are generally underpowered for comparisons of endpoints across arms. As such, the reporting of p values for such comparisons is also not standardly done or viewed as acceptable since the type I error rate of selection designs is 50% (1).

Efficiency in trial conduct is achieved by selection designs when compared to the alternative strategy of conducting several independent phase II trials. Logistically, the single-protocol infrastructure is easier for principal investigators and sites to maintain, particularly after considering the consent processes associated with a single trial as well as the burden of protocol amendments for minor modifications and clarifications over time. From a research perspective, randomization also provides some assurance that observed differences in efficacy or toxicity are not attributable to patient

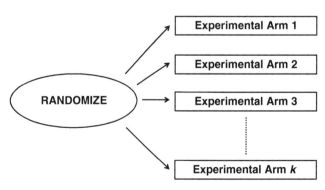

FIGURE 16.1 General schema for a selection design in which patients are randomized to one of *k* experimental arms.

selection bias, interobserver variability in tumor measurement, protocol compliance, institutional reporting procedures, and differences in sample size. Sample sizes also tend to be lower than they would otherwise be when direct comparison between a control and experimental therapy is of interest.

Binary Endpoints

The concept of selection design was first introduced in oncology for ranking and selection of therapies under the premise that sample sizes are chosen with a high probability of selecting the best treatment arm when it is superior by a fixed margin (2). The observed ranking is therefore not conclusive, which implies that promising agents could be discarded and never tested in a phase III trial. The use of randomization, while beneficial for balancing patient demographics and disease characteristics across arms, can give a false sense of security when selecting the "best" regimen. In situations where a reliable standard therapy or an adequate historical control does not exist for a particular disease, there is also concern for falsely identifying the treatment of choice for further study. As such, these designs underscore the need to minimize the probability that an inferior regimen will be carried forward to a phase III trial (3). In practice, this can be challenging because of the relatively small sample sizes of these trials, and because the type I error rate is not well controlled in this setting.

This design assumes that if the true but unknown measure of the primary endpoint of interest exceeds that of any other arm by some fixed margin, Δ, then it will be chosen as the best regimen with high probability, preferably .90 or higher. The selection criteria requires that the treatment with the greatest or best value in the primary endpoint be chosen for further study regardless of how small or insignificant its advantage over other regimens appears to be. This explains why these types of designs are also often referred to as "pick-the-winner" designs.

A common endpoint for selection designs in oncology is response rate. However, they provide less information and precision than time-to-event endpoints, which report both the binary indicator of an event and the time of that event. The criteria used to measure response should be the standard criteria established for that disease: for example, Response Evaluation Criteria in Solid Tumors (RECIST), Response Assessment in Neuro-Oncology (RANO) Criteria, or Cheson Criteria for Lymphoma (4–6).

The most common approach to randomized selection designs involves the statistical methods of ranking and selection such that patients are randomized to multiple single-stage arms and the winner is identified as the arm with the highest estimated response rate. Simon et al. presents sample size requirements for selection designs with response as a primary endpoint and when one treatment is inferior to another treatment by a margin

of 15% (2). For example, in a selection design involving randomization to three different experimental therapies, the probability of correctly selecting the best treatment is 0.90 when 37 patients are enrolled to each arm, and when the lowest response rate among those arms is 10%.

A variation in this approach was derived by Thall et al. who consider trials in which patients are randomized to some number of experimental arms or a control arm; however, patients are assigned to the experimental arms only in a first stage of accrual from which a winner is selected for a second stage only if its observed efficacy is superior to that for the historical control by 10% (7). If the winning arm's efficacy does not meet this threshold then the trial is stopped early; otherwise, a second stage of accrual is opened so that patients can be randomized between the winning experimental arm and the control arm.

Alternatively, Steinberg and Venzon proposed a two-stage two-arm design in which patients are randomized between two arms in an initial stage of accrual, and if the difference in the number of responders between the two arms is larger than some fixed margin, which is selected so that the two arms have a difference in response rate of 0.15, then the trial stops early with a clear winner (8). Otherwise, accrual proceeds to a second stage and patients continue to be assigned between the two arms and a winner is chosen based on the total number of responses observed across the two stages.

At times it might be desirable to factor other considerations into the selection of the winner. Sargent and Goldberg proposed a framework for when it is more critical that an inferior regimen not be selected when a superior therapy exists (9). Their design offers the flexibility to select a therapy based on a prespecified decision rule that states that if the observed difference in response rates exceeds a prespecified margin, then the treatment with the highest observed response rate is chosen. If the difference is lower than the prespecified margin, then other factors such as toxicity, cost, or quality of life may be factored into the choice of a winner.

Time-to-Event Outcomes

An alternative endpoint for selection designs is a time-to-event outcome such as progression-free survival (PFS) or overall survival. For such endpoints, Cox proportional hazards models can be fitted to the data as: $h(t, z) = h0(t)\exp(\beta' z)$, where z is the (K – 1) vector of treatment group indicators and β is the vector of log hazard ratios (10). In this manner, the best treatment is selected based on the event time endpoint, though it is worth noting that the survival probability of the regimen chosen as "best" may not be uniformly better than that of other regimens across time. Advantages of this design over those with binomial endpoints include the opportunity to garner enough information on the time-to-event outcomes to inform future trial designs since response endpoints are not commonly used as primary endpoints in the phase III setting. Rubenstein also showed that the required sample size for such trials are generally reduced by a factor of 4 when compared to randomized controlled studies (11–12).

Alternative Approaches

In practice, sample size calculations for selection designs are more commonly structured so that each individual experimental arm is conducted as though it were its own one-armed two-stage study; such designs are appropriate when reliable historical control data are available (12). When a historical control arm is not well established, it may be difficult to define a clinically meaningful level of efficacy that is worthy of further study. Regardless, this approach allows for early termination of an arm due to lack of efficacy, while allowing for comparison of the response rate or the other binary endpoint of each arm to the stated historical control with prespecified power and type I error rate (13).

EXAMPLES OF STUDY DESIGNS

Overall Survival Endpoint in Lung Cancer

One study that implemented a selection design is the Southwestern Oncology Group study, S0342, which compared concurrent chemotherapy and cetuximab to chemotherapy followed by cetuximab in advanced-stage non–small-cell lung cancer (14). At the time, standard first-line therapy for patients with advanced non–small-cell lung cancer was platinum-based doublet, which could be combined with bevacizumab for a subset of patients with nonsquamous histology, thereby providing proof of concept that addition of a third agent to platinum chemotherapy doublet has a role in improving outcomes for this patient population. That being said, many other trials combining novel agents with chemotherapy have failed, raising the question of whether or not mechanistic differences require that some novel agents be administered sequentially, rather than concurrently with chemotherapy. Prior to the conduct of this trial, two small single-arm trials that combined cetuximab with paclitaxel and carboplatin or gemcitabine and carboplatin demonstrated that the triplet combination was safe and promising for further study. Another randomized study had demonstrated activity of cetuximab administered concurrently with cisplatin and vinorelbine. The S0342 study was designed with a selection design to evaluate the sequential and concurrent administration of cetuximab in a single trial, with the goal of ultimately pursuing a phase III study of the superior regimen.

The primary endpoint of this trial was overall survival, and the regimen with the superior observed median overall survival was to be selected if it had met a minimum median overall survival of 10 months. Using

the design by Liu described previously, the planned sample size was 90 eligible patients per arm. The study design planned for an accrual period of 9 months with 10 additional months of follow-up. These calculations assumed a historical control of 10 months for the median event time, and the probability of correctly choosing the superior arm if the true but unknown overall survival hazard ratio was 1.3 in favor of the superior novel arm was 91%. A total of 224 eligible patients were ultimately randomized on this trial. At the median follow-up time of 32 months, the median overall survival for cetuximab administered concurrently with paclitaxel and carboplatin was 10.9 months (95% CI: 9.2–13.0); the median overall survival associated with sequential administration of cetuximab after paclitaxel and carboplatin was 10.7 months (95% CI: 8.5–12.8). The median PFS associated with concurrent administration of cetuximab was 4.3 months (95% CI: 3.7–4.7), and was slightly higher at 4.4 months (95% CI: 4.0–5.3) for patients on the sequential arm. We also note that overall grade 3 or 4 toxicities were significantly higher among patients receiving the concurrent regimen (82%) compared with patients treated with the sequential regimen (63%; $p = .002$). Despite that, and noting that both arms of the study met the predefined threshold of 10 months median overall survival, the regimen selected for further study in the phase III trial was that associated with the higher median overall survival: concurrent cetuximab.

Toxicity Endpoint in Patients With Different Cancer Types

A second example of the implementation of selection design is the randomized phase II trial comparing the activity of two different escalating strategies for pregabalin and oxycodone for the treatment of neuropathic pain in cancer patients, which was conducted by Garassino et al. (15). Neuropathic pain is commonly experienced by cancer patients and is thought to be caused by a tumor compressing nerve or occurs as a side effect of chemo- or radiation therapy. Because monotherapy generally does not control neuropathic pain very well, new therapies are needed. Pregabalin had demonstrated efficacy for relief of neuropathic pain and was thought to have synergy with oxycodone without exacerbating adverse events; the strategy for increasing the dose of opioids had not been established at the time this study was conducted. Therefore, this study aimed to establish the role of two different dose escalation strategies with the combination of pregabalin and oxycodone for neuropathic pain. Patients were randomly assigned to receive oxycodone controlled release, 20 mg/day, plus increasing doses of pregabalin, starting at 50 mg/day (arm A), or pregabalin, 50 mg/day, plus increasing doses of oxycodone, starting at 20 mg/day (arm B). Using the method of Simon et al., the minimum expected response rate was estimated to be 45%, and 74 patients were required to maintain a 90% probability of correctly selecting the best schedule when the true but unknown response difference was at least 15%.

The primary endpoint was analgesia, defined as at least a 1/3 reduction in pain intensity. This was achieved in 76.5% of patients on arm A, and 63.9% of patients on arm B; this result was also upheld in multivariable modeling adjusting for other known prognostic factors. The median time to analgesia was 10 days (95% CI: 5–14) in arm A and 11 days (95% CI: 5–18) in arm B. Both regimens were considered to be tolerable, albeit with slightly fewer side effects associated with arm A: constipation, nausea, drowsiness, confusion, and itching. As such, the authors concluded that arm A, oxycodone controlled release plus increasing doses of pregabalin was preferable for pain control.

Response Endpoint in Melanoma

Another trial that utilized a selection design was published by Dudley et al. who reported the results of a trial evaluating CD8+-enriched versus unselected tumor-infiltrating lymphocytes (TILs) for adoptive cell therapy (ACT) for patients with melanoma. At the time this trial was conducted, TILs were known to mediate durable regression of metastatic melanoma when administrated with interleukin-2 therapy to autologous patients following a lymphodepleting preparative regimen (16). Additional studies demonstrated the value of ACT as a salvage therapy for patients with melanoma but also established that a simpler, more reliable TIL production method was needed. This study leveraged new production methods for individualized TIL therapies to initiate a selection design with ACT. To determine whether CD8+-enriched TILs or unselected young TILs containing CD4+ cells represented a better product for ACT, the study planned to randomize 70 patients with measurable metastatic melanoma who had TILs available to these two regimens to maintain a 91% probability of correctly selecting the superior arm if the true probability of a clinical response was 25% in the arm with lower true probability of response and 40% in the arm with greater probability of response. The randomization was stratified by stage (M1a, M1b, or M1c). Patient response was assessed via the RECIST 1.0 criteria and radiographic studies were conducted at 4 to 6 weeks following TIL administration and at regular intervals thereafter.

The study reported that 35% of patients randomized to therapy with unselected young TILs and 20% of patients randomized to therapy with CD8+-enriched TILs responded to treatment; overall survival and side effects were not notably different between the two arms. The study therefore concluded overall that future studies should focus on therapy with unselected young TILs since the evidence indicated that CD8+-enriched TILs were not more effective with respect to RECIST response and were more laborious to prepare.

Response Endpoint With Two-Stage Design in Esophageal Cancer

The randomized phase II study of two regimens of sequentially administered mitomycin C (MMC) and irinotecan in patients with unresectable esophageal and gastroesophageal adenocarcinoma is another trial that implemented selection design (17). Irinotecan has been shown to have antitumor activity in many cancers, and the investigators had shown that MMC upregulates topoisomerase I, a cellular target of irinotecan. Therefore, it was of interest to conduct a clinical trial in which patients were randomized to two doses (modulatory and nonmodulatory) of MMC in combination with irinotecan using a two-stage pick-the-winner approach.

The primary objective of the trial was to select the best regimen based on objective response. The randomization was stratified by locally advanced or metastatic disease with a fixed block design, and each arm was conducted with a minimax two-stage design. Either regimen was considered ineffective if the true but unknown response rate was less than 30%, the historical control rate for irinotecan in stomach cancer. This design had 90% power to detect the target response rate of 50% or greater in each arm while controlling the one-sided type I error rate at 10%. If 7 or fewer patients demonstrated response among the first 28 patients in stage I, the regimen was terminated early and deemed ineffective. If 8 or more patients showed responses in the first 28 patients, 11 additional patients were treated for a total enrollment of 39 patients overall. A regimen would be considered worthy of further study if 16 or more responses were observed among those 39 patients.

A total of 76 patients were randomized to either 6 mg/m^2 MMC on day 1 and 125 mg/m^2 irinotecan on days 2 and 9 (arm A) or 3 mg/m^2 MMC on days 1 and 8 and 125 mg/m^2 irinotecan on days 2 and 9 (arm B). The Data Safety Monitoring Board recommended stopping enrollment to arm B when it realized that the prespecified criteria for response would not be met. Overall, 42 patients received treatment on arm A and 35 on arm B. The observed response rate was 52% on arm A, and 33% on arm B, and major differences in moderate to severe adverse events were not reported. Because arm B stopped early and because arm A met the criteria for success with a total of 21 responses among 40 patients, it was determined that MMC (6 mg/m^2) every 28 days for up to six cycles was the recommended modulatory dose for irinotecan.

Evaluating Different Schedules of Monotherapy in Ovarian Cancer

Baumann et al. conducted a phase II study of sunitinib in platinum-resistant ovarian cancer using response as the primary endpoint (18). The unique feature of this trial was that it evaluated two different schedules of sunitinib monotherapy: 50 mg sunitinib daily orally for 28 days followed by 14 days off drug; and 37.5 mg sunitinib administered daily continuously. A total of 36 patients were required for each arm of the trial in order to achieve a 90% probability of identifying the superior schedule, when the difference between the two was at least 11%. The observed response rate on the noncontinuous arm was 16.7%; on the continuous arm the response rate was 5.4%. With this design, the "best" regimen was chosen as the winner in noncontinuous dosing of sunitinib even though the result was relatively modest when compared to what the research community has come to expect as successful when evaluating response to single-agent targeted therapies. Because the prognosis of this disease is particularly poor, historical controls had not set expectations very high; but the small sample limits the level of precision of the observed response rates overall.

ACKNOWLEDGMENTS

This work was based on experience gained through the ECOG-ACRIN Cancer Research Group (Robert L. Comis, MD and Mitchell D. Schnall, MD, PhD, Group Co-Chairs), which is supported by the National Cancer Institute of the National Institutes of Health under the following award numbers: CA180820, CA21115, CA180794, CA23318, and CA66636.

REFERENCES

1. Korn EL, Freidlin B, Abrams JS, Halabi S. Design issues in randomized phase II/III trials. *J Clin Oncol*. 2012;30(6):667–671.
2. Simon R, Wittes RE, Ellenberg SS. Randomized phase II clinical trials. *Can Treat Report*. 1985;69:1375–1381.
3. Sargent DJ, Goldberg RM. A flexible design for multiple armed screening trials. *Stat Med*. 2001;20:1051–1060.
4. Eisenhauer EA, Therasse P, Bogaerts J, et al. New response evaluation criteria in solid tumours: revised RECIST guideline (version 1.1). *Eur J Cancer*. 2009;45:228–247.
5. Cheson BD, Pfistner B, Juweid ME, et al. Revised response criteria for malignant lymphoma. *J Clin Oncol*. 2007;25(5):579–586.
6. Wen PY, Macdonald DR, Reardon DA, et al. Updated response assessment criteria for high-grade gliomas: response assessment in neuro-oncology working Group. *J Clin Oncol*. 2010;28(11):1963–1972.
7. Thall PF, Simon R, Ellenberg SS. A two-stage design for choosing among several experimental treatments and a control in clinical trials. *Biometrics*. 1989;45(2):537–547.
8. Steinberg SM, Venzon DJ. Early selection in a randomized phase II clinical trial. *Stat Med*. 2002;21(12):1711–1726.
9. Sargent DJ, Goldberg RM. A flexible design for multiple armed screening trials. *Stat Med*. 2001;20(7):1051–1060.
10. Liu PY, Dahlberg S, Crowley J. Selection designs for pilot studies based on survival. *Biometrics*. 1993;49:391–398.
11. Rubinstein L, Crowley J, Ivy P, et al. Randomized phase II designs. *Clin Cancer Res*. 2009;15(6):1883–1890.
12. Rubinstein LV, Gail MH, Santner TJ. Planning the duration of a clinical trial with loss to follow-up and a period of continued observation. *J Chron Dis*. 1981;34:469–479.
13. Rubinstein LV, Korn EL, Freidlin B, et al. Design issues of randomized phase II trials and a proposal for phase II screening trials. *J Clin Oncol*. 2005;23(28):7199–7206.
14. Herbst RS, Kelly K, Chansky K, et al. Phase II selection design trial of concurrent chemotherapy and cetuximab versus chemotherapy followed by cetuximab in advanced-stage non-small-cell lung cancer: Southwest Oncology Group study S0342. *J Clin Oncol*. 2010;28(31):4747–4754.
15. Garassino MC, Piva S, La Verde N, et al. Randomised phase II trial (NCT00637975) evaluating activity and toxicity of two different escalating strategies for pregabalin and oxycodone combination therapy for neuropathic pain in cancer patients. *PLoS One*. 2013;8(4):e59981.
16. Dudley ME, Gross CA, Somerville RP, et al. Randomized selection design trial evaluating CD8+-enriched versus unselected tumor-infiltrating lymphocytes for adoptive cell therapy for patients with melanoma. *J Clin Oncol*. 2013;31(17):2152–2159.
17. Lustberg MB, Bekaii-Saab T, Young D, et al. Phase II randomized study of two regimens of sequentially administered mitomycin C and irinotecan in patients with unresectable esophageal and gastroesophageal adenocarcinoma. *J Thorac Oncol*. 2010;5:713–718.
18. Baumann KH, du Bois A, Meier W, et al. A phase II trial (AGO 2.11) in platinum-resistant ovarian cancer: a randomized multicenter trial with sunitinib (SU11248) to evaluate dosage, schedule, tolerability, toxicity and effectiveness of a multitargeted receptor tyrosine kinase inhibitor monotherapy. *Ann Oncol*. 2012;23(9):2265–2271.

17

Phase III Oncology Clinical Trials

Antje Hoering and John Crowley

INTRODUCTION

The goal of phase III clinical trials is to compare the efficacy of an agent or an entire treatment strategy with the standard of care. In traditional clinical trial development, a phase III trial is performed after an appropriate dose was determined in the phase I setting and preliminary efficacy was confirmed in the phase II setting in a smaller and possibly slightly different cohort of patients. Several considerations go into designing a well-thought-out phase III clinical trial. These considerations include the choice of primary and secondary endpoints, the patient population under study, randomization strategies including stratification, appropriate sample size, study duration, the number of comparisons to be made, and the inclusion of potential prognostic or predictive biomarkers.

GENERAL DESIGN CONSIDERATIONS

Endpoints

Endpoint considerations, especially the selection of the primary endpoint, are very important. The gold standard for a primary endpoint to prove definitive efficacy remains overall survival (OS). However, sometimes it is not possible to use OS as the primary endpoint. In disease settings where the survival of patients is long, such as in early-stage breast cancer, it may not be feasible to wait for the outcome of a trial based on OS, and disease-free survival (DFS) is often used instead. In disease settings where many treatment options are available after progression of disease, patients may receive several different lines of therapy after progressing on the phase III trial of interest, and it will be difficult if not impossible to decipher which treatment was responsible for a longer survival. In some of these settings progression-free survival (PFS) may be an appropriate primary endpoint. However, one needs to be careful when determining disease assessment schedules, particularly for PFS. When

the time window between assessments is too large, we do not know with accuracy when a patient progressed, and when disease assessment times vary between treatment arms, artificial bias can result. See the series of papers on the pros and cons of PFS as an endpoint in Bates (1). Response or response maintained after a specific time point are common primary endpoints in phase II trials, but are rarely utilized as the primary endpoint in the phase III setting. For a more detailed discussion of endpoints, see Chapter 8.

Patient Population

Careful consideration needs to be given to the population of patients to which the results of a trial are to be generalized. Such considerations are embedded in the eligibility section of the protocol, which defines the types of patients who may enroll in the trial. Eligible patients should be those for whom the treatments are likely to benefit, and for whom the treatments are judged not to be too toxic. Thus considerations of tumor stage, histology, and lately genetics come into play, as well as descriptions of adequate organ function to minimize side effects. As is often the case there is tension between having broad and inclusive eligibility criteria, which increases generalizability but also may increase variability, and stricter criteria, which reduce variability but restrict generalizability. Care should be taken not to have exclusions based merely on what has been done in other trials in the past.

Randomization

The most common phase III trial is a randomized trial randomizing patients to an experimental and a control arm. The control arm is the currently acceptable standard of care and the experimental arm includes the new agent of interest. Frequently patients are randomized to the standard of care plus or minus the new experimental agent. Randomization is important to ensure that the patient populations in the two treatment arms are as comparable as possible. Randomization yields comparable patient populations in treatment arms for large trials; for more moderate size studies there can still be imbalances and it is helpful to stratify patients by known important prognostic factors. A detailed description of randomization strategies is given in Chapter 21.

Sample Size and Study Duration

When powering a study with time-to-event endpoints, such as OS, DFS, or PFS, it is important to keep in mind that the overall power is driven by the number of observed events (deaths or recurrences or progressions) at the time of final analysis. In turn, the number of events is a function of the overall sample size and sample size ratio between arms, the accrual rate, and the follow-up time. We return to this issue in more detail in the section Analysis of Time-to-Event Data.

There are several complicating factors that can dilute the overall treatment effect and should be avoided if at all possible. One of those factors is loss to follow-up before the final assessment. In such a case the patient is censored at the last time the patient was known to be alive (for OS) or known to be disease- or progression-free (for DFS or PFS). Other complicating factors include dropouts, that is, patients stopping treatment therapy early, as well as drop-ins, that is, patients taking therapy that is not part of the treatment protocol.

ANALYSIS OF TIME-TO-EVENT DATA

Notation and Background

A minimum of notation will help set the stage for the rest of this section. Let the time to event be denoted by a random variable X, with cumulative distribution function $F(t)$, density $f(t)$, and survival function $S(t) = 1 - F(t) = P(X > t)$. The event could be death, for the analysis of OS, or time to the minimum of progression or death, for the analysis of PFS, and so on but for simplicity we adopt the language of survival analysis; the statistical formulation is the same regardless. The hazard function, or instantaneous rate of death, is given by $\lambda(t) = f(t)/S(t)$. Furthermore, define the cumulative hazard by $\Lambda(t) = \int_0^t \lambda(s)ds$. Mathematically, $S(t) = \exp(-\Lambda(t))$. The simplest model for the survival functions is the exponential distribution, for which the hazard is constant, $\lambda(t) = \lambda$, and thus $S(t) = \exp(-\lambda t)$. This is an important central case, but the bulk of the analysis of time-to-event data is done without relying on such parametric assumptions.

Observations on the event time X will in general be incomplete due to practical constraints on the amount of possible follow-up time, resulting in an incompleteness called right censoring. We focus for ease of exposition on the random censorship model, in which subjects have a maximum observation time governed by a random variable C with cumulative distribution function $G(t)$. The observable random variable is $T = \min(X, C)$, as well as an indicator Δ, which is 1 when $X \leq C$ (true survival time observed) and 0 otherwise (censoring time observed).

Consider first the data from a single sample, consisting of N patients, n of whom are observed to die. The observed data consist of doublets (t_i, δ_i), $i = 1, \ldots, N$, where t_i are the observed event times (assumed measured continuously, and thus no tied observations) ordered from smallest to largest, whether censored or not, and δ_i is 0 for censored observations and 1 for true death times. The product limit estimator $\hat{S}(t_i)$ of the population quantity $S(t)$ at a given event time t_i is given by $\hat{S}(t_i) = \prod_{j=1}^{i}(1 - \delta_j/n_j)$, where n_j represents the number still alive and on study just before time t_j. This is also called the Kaplan–Meier estimator (2) but it has a history that goes back to Greenwood (3). Statistical properties of this estimator were derived rigorously by Breslow and Crowley (4), including the verification of asymptotic normality, with an estimator of the variance of $\hat{S}(t_i)$ given by Greenwood's formula as $\left[\hat{S}(t_i)\right]^2 * \sum_{j=1}^{i} \delta_j/n_j(n_j - \delta_j)$. Note that the product limit estimator steps down only at the true death times, corresponding to $\delta = 1$, and that the variance estimator increases with increasing event times.

Now consider the case of two samples, as would arise from a randomized trial of two different treatment regimens. The log-rank test (5,6) for comparing the survival curves $S_1(t)$ and $S_2(t)$ of two groups with samples sizes N_1 and N_2 and numbers of true deaths n_1 and n_2 is one of the most commonly used procedures in survival analysis. Let the ordered event times from the combined sample of $N = N_1 + N_2$ patients be given by $t_1 < \cdots t_N$. At time t_j, with numbers still at risk in the two samples n_{1j} and n_{2j} and numbers of deaths δ_{1j} and δ_{2j}, consider the

$$2 \times 2 \text{ table} \begin{pmatrix} \delta_{1j} & n_{1j} - \delta_{1j} \\ \delta_{2j} & n_{2j} - \delta_{2j} \end{pmatrix}.$$

Denote the total number at risk and dying at t_j as n_j and δ_j. Define the expected number of deaths in sample i from standard contingency table arguments to be $E_{ij} = n_{ij}\delta_j/n_j$. Further define the variance term $V_j = n_{1j}R_{2j}\delta_j\left(n_j - \delta_j\right)/n_j^2\left(n_j - 1\right)$. Then the numerator of the log-rank test for comparing groups 1 and 2 is given by $L_{12} = D_{1j} - E_{1j}$ and the log-rank test is $\left\{\sum_{j=1}^{N}\delta_j L_{12}\right\}^2 \bigg/ \sum_{j=1}^{N}\delta_j V_j$. Crowley (7) proved that the log-rank test has an asymptotic X^2 distribution with one degree of freedom; see also Aalen (8), Anderson et al. (9), and Gill (10). Note that there are contributions to the sums defining the log-rank test only for those event times that are uncensored ($\delta_j = 1$).

Sample Size and Power Calculations

The most common paradigm for the calculation of sample size and power in phase III trials in oncology is that of hypothesis testing, and the assessment, in hypothetical replications of the experiment, of the probabilities of a false-positive (type I error, a) or a false-negative (type II error, β) result. Thus we define a null hypothesis H_0 as an expression of the status quo that we wish to disprove, for example, that the new treatment is no better than the standard, versus an alternative hypothesis H_A that the new treatment differs from the standard. Then the type I error rate, or a, is the probability of rejecting H_0, in favor of H_A, when in fact H_0 is true. The type II error rate, or β, is the probability of *not* rejecting H_0, in favor of H_A, when in fact H_A is true. The *power* of a test of hypothesis is defined to be the probability of rejecting H_0 when H_A is true, or $1-\beta$.

With survival (or PFS, or DFS, etc.) as the primary outcome, the hypothesis test can be expressed symbolically as $H_0: S_1(t) = S_2(t)$ versus $H_A: S_1(t) \neq S_2(t)$. Expressing the alternative hypothesis in this way, via an inequality, is called a two-sided hypothesis test, and implies a difference in either direction (new treatment is better or worse than the standard) is of interest. Clearly the interest in most (all?) phase III trials is in a difference only in favor of the new treatment, a one-sided test, $H_0: S_1(t) = S_2(t)$ versus $H_A: S_1(t) \leq S_2(t)$, where we take $S_1(t)$ to be the survival in the standard arm, and $S_2(t)$ to be the survival with the new treatment. There is a very strong convention, with journals as well as with the Food and Drug Administration, that hypotheses are to be considered two-sided. However, a one-sided test with type I error $a/2$ leads to the same statistical properties as a two-sided test with type I error a; in what follows we will assume one-sided testing, noting that by convention the false-positive rate in the direction of interest needs to be doubled for most scientific communication.

The calculation of the false-negative probability, or type II error rate, β, or equivalently the power, requires several more assumptions, the first being a specification of *how much* better the new treatment is than the standard. This is most often specified in terms of the hazard function $\lambda(t)$ and in particular the ratio of hazard functions in the two groups, further assumed to be a constant. Thus we can specify $H_0: \lambda_1(t) = \lambda_2(t)$ and $H_A: \lambda_1(t) = \Delta\lambda_2(t)$, where the interest lies in the direction $\Delta < 1$, meaning a lower rate of dying, or better survival. Note that if survival is exponential, $S_i(t) = \exp(-\lambda_i t)$, then the ratio of hazards is constant, being λ_1/λ_2, but the assumption of a constant hazard ratio is more general than the exponential model. For example, the two-parameter Weibull distribution for survival is given by $S(t) = \exp(-\lambda t^\rho)$ if survival in the two groups follow a Weibull distribution with the same shape parameter ρ (not necessarily equal to 1) then the ratio of hazards is constant. Note also that for the exponential model there is a convenient interpretation of the hazard ratio in terms of

the inverse of the ratio of median survival in the two groups. The median m is the time at which $S(t) = \frac{1}{2}$; thus for the exponential distribution this is in $2/\lambda$, so that if $\lambda_1/\lambda_2 = \Delta$, $m_1/m_2 = 1/\Delta$.

Further input required for the calculation of power for a given sample size, or sample size for a given power, includes the expected rate of accrual and the length of follow-up after the last patient is accrued. There is a publicly available website for these calculations, maintained jointly by Cancer Research And Biostatistics (CRAB) and the National Cancer Institute (NCI) funded cooperative group Southwest Oncology Group (SWOG). The site can be entered through the CRAB website (crab.org), then finding the Biostatistical Tools tab at the bottom of the page, and then selecting Two Arm Survival. A direct link is at https://stattools.crab.org/Calculators/twoArmSurvivalColored.htm. The calculations are done according to the formulas given in Bernstein and Lagakos (11) and assume a uniform accrual rate over the accrual period and an exponential model for the survival distribution. However the results hold to a good approximation under the more general assumption of a constant hazard ratio, and use of the log-rank test (Schoenfeld, [12]). If the constant hazard ratio assumption is felt not to be a good approximation for a given clinical situation, other methods need to be employed (see e.g., Lakatos and Lan, [13]).

The initial page from the Two Arm Survival tool is given in Figure 17.1. It can be found on the CRAB and SWOG web pages. Yellow highlights the user input data and blue highlights the program output data. Please note that input and output change depending on what type of calculation is desired (sample size or power) and what type of input is used for the control group per stratum (hazard rates or survival proportion at a specific time point). Notice that defaults are set for the number of strata (2) and the proportion in the standard group $N_1/(N_1 + N_2) = .5$; we return to these options later. Note also that the hazard ratio given in the tool is $1/\Delta$, which has the interpretation within the exponential distribution of the ratio of medians, experimental to standard. Figures 17.2 and 17.3 show some example sample size calculations. Specifically, Figure 17.2A shows a randomized phase III design with standard error rates (one-sided significance level $a = .025$, which corresponds to a two-sided $a = .05$, and a power $= .90$), an accrual period of 2 years, and a follow-up period of 1 year. The median survival in the control group is estimated to be 1 year and the hazard ratio to be tested is 1.33, which corresponds to a 33% improvement in median OS from 1 year in the control group to 1.33 years in the experimental group. Entering all this information yields a total sample size of 764. Figure 17.2B explores the effect of increasing a to a one-sided $a = .05$. Leaving everything else the same, the total sample size reduces to 624. Similarly, if the power is reduced while keeping the significance level unchanged, the total sample size is reduced (not shown in

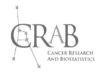 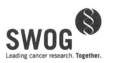

STATISTICAL TOOLS   🖊 DESIGN ˅   🔍 ANALYSIS ˅   ▁▍ PROBABILITIES ˅   𝒮 ABOUT US ˅

Two Arm Survival

Two Arm Survival is a program to calculate either estimates accrual or power for differences in survival times between two groups. The program allows for unequal sample size allocation between the two groups. The survival time estimates also allow for multiple strata or risk groups.

User Input	Program Output

Select Parameters

Type calculation	Type input	Sided
○ Sample Size	○ Hazard Rates	◉ 1 Sided
◉ Power	◉ Survival Proportion	○ 2 Sided

Number strata	Proportion in standard group	Alpha
1	.5	.05

Years of accrual	Years of follow-up	Accrual rate	Hazard ratio	Total accrual	Power

Calculate

Stratum	Proportion	Hazard rate, std.	Hazard rate, exp.	Proportion surviving	Survival time
1	1.0				

FIGURE 17.1 Two Arm Survival tool from the CRAB (www.crab.org) and SWOG web pages.
CRAB, Cancer Research And Biostatistics; SWOG, Southwest Oncology Group.
Source: Cancer Research and Biostatistics, CRAB and SWOG.

the figure). Figure 17.2C investigates a more aggressive hazard ratio of 1.5, which corresponds to an increase in median OS from 1 year in the control arm to 1.5 years in the experimental arm. The total sample size required in this example reduces to 392. Similarly, if the hazard ratio is reduced to 1.25 (Figure 17.2D), which corresponds to an increase in median OS from 1 year to 1.25 years in the experimental arm, the total sample size is increased to 1,225. Figure 17.3A explores the effect of a 2:1 randomization, which can be achieved in our tool by changing the proportion in the standard group from 0.5 to 0.33. Doing so increases the sample size slightly from 764 to 800. Another issue with uneven randomization is the fact that equipoise is violated. In general, such a randomization should be avoided, especially in the phase III setting. Figure 17.3B explores the effect of having more than one stratum. In this example we assume two strata: one with a median survival time of 1.5 years and the other with a median survival time of 0.5 years so that the overall median survival time is again 1 year. This assumes the use of a stratified log-rank test and results in a slight increase of the total sample size from 764 to 800. Finally, Figures 17.3C and 17.3D explore the effect of a longer median survival time as is the case in less aggressive cancers. We chose a median survival of 5 years. Leaving everything

else unchanged (Figure 17.3C) compared to our original example in Figure 17.2A, this yields a sample size of more than twice the original sample size (1,761 vs. 764). We then explored the effect of also increasing the follow-up time from 1 year to 5 years. This reduces the sample size to 922. These last two examples demonstrate the fact that power and sample size in the setting of survival endpoints is governed by the number of overall events observed.

General Analysis Considerations

The Intent-to-Treat Principle

An important concept in the analysis of phase III trials is the intent-to-treat (ITT) principle, which states that one should analyze all patients on the treatment group to which they were randomly assigned, even if they actually received a different treatment. This is widely accepted as the appropriate strategy for analyzing the primary and secondary outcome measures, because any exclusions or reassignment based on factors after randomization, such as treatment deviations, can reintroduce bias that randomization is meant to eliminate. Further in support of this principle is the notion that clinical trials address practical questions, and treatment deviations occur in practice.

Two Arm Survival

Two Arm Survival is a program to calculate either estimates accrual or power for differences in survival times between two groups. The program allows for unequal sample size allocation between the two groups. The survival time estimates also allow for multiple strata or risk groups.

User Input	Program Output

Select Parameters

Type calculation	Type input	Sided
○ Sample Size	○ Hazard Rates	⦿ 1 Sided
⦿ Power	⦿ Survival Proportion	○ 2 Sided

Number strata	Proportion in standard group	Alpha
1	.5	.025

Years of accrual	Years of follow-up	Accrual rate	Hazard ratio	Total accrual	Power
2	1	382	1.33	764	0.9001

[Calculate]

Stratum	Proportion	Hazard rate, std.	Hazard rate, exp.	Proportion surviving	Survival time
1	1	0.693	0.521	0.5	1
2					

(A)

Two Arm Survival

Two Arm Survival is a program to calculate either estimates accrual or power for differences in survival times between two groups. The program allows for unequal sample size allocation between the two groups. The survival time estimates also allow for multiple strata or risk groups.

User Input	Program Output

Select Parameters

Type calculation	Type input	Sided
○ Sample Size	○ Hazard Rates	⦿ 1 Sided
⦿ Power	⦿ Survival Proportion	○ 2 Sided

Number strata	Proportion in standard group	Alpha
1	.5	.05

Years of accrual	Years of follow-up	Accrual rate	Hazard ratio	Total accrual	Power
2	1	312	1.33	624	0.9006

[Calculate]

Stratum	Proportion	Hazard rate, std.	Hazard rate, exp.	Proportion surviving	Survival time
1	1	0.693	0.521	0.5	1
2					

(B)

FIGURE 17.2 Example sample size calculations. (*continued*)

Source: Cancer Research and Biostatistics, CRAB and SWOG.

Two Arm Survival

Two Arm Survival is a program to calculate either estimates accrual or power for differences in survival times between two groups. The program allows for unequal sample size allocation between the two groups. The survival time estimates also allow for multiple strata or risk groups.

User Input	Program Output

Select Parameters

Type calculation	Type input	Sided
● Sample Size ○ Power	○ Hazard Rates ● Survival Proportion	● 1 Sided ○ 2 Sided

Number strata	Proportion in standard group	Alpha
1	.5	.025

Years of accrual	Years of follow-up	Accrual rate	Hazard ratio	Total accrual	Power
2	1	196.22	1.5	392	0.9

Calculate

Stratum	Proportion	Hazard rate, std.	Hazard rate, exp.	Proportion surviving	Survival time
1	1	0.693	0.462	0.5	1
2					

(C)

Two Arm Survival

Two Arm Survival is a program to calculate either estimates accrual or power for differences in survival times between two groups. The program allows for unequal sample size allocation between the two groups. The survival time estimates also allow for multiple strata or risk groups.

User Input	Program Output

Select Parameters

Type calculation	Type input	Sided
● Sample Size ○ Power	○ Hazard Rates ● Survival Proportion	● 1 Sided ○ 2 Sided

Number strata	Proportion in standard group	Alpha
1	.5	.025

Years of accrual	Years of follow-up	Accrual rate	Hazard ratio	Total accrual	Power
2	1	612.68	1.25	1225	0.9

Calculate

Stratum	Proportion	Hazard rate, std.	Hazard rate, exp.	Proportion surviving	Survival time
1	1	0.693	0.555	0.5	1
2					

(D)

FIGURE 17.2 *(continued)*

Two Arm Survival

Two Arm Survival is a program to calculate either estimates accrual or power for differences in survival times between two groups. The program allows for unequal sample size allocation between the two groups. The survival time estimates also allow for multiple strata or risk groups.

User Input	Program Output

Select Parameters

Type calculation	Type input	Sided
○ Sample Size	○ Hazard Rates	● 1 Sided
● Power	● Survival Proportion	○ 2 Sided

Number strata	Proportion in standard group	Alpha
1	.33	.025

Years of accrual	Years of follow-up	Accrual rate	Hazard ratio	Total accrual	Power
2	1	400	1.33	800	0.8847

Calculate

Stratum	Proportion	Hazard rate, std.	Hazard rate, exp.	Proportion surviving	Survival time
1	1	0.693	0.521	0.5	1
2					

(A)

Two Arm Survival

Two Arm Survival is a program to calculate either estimates accrual or power for differences in survival times between two groups. The program allows for unequal sample size allocation between the two groups. The survival time estimates also allow for multiple strata or risk groups.

User Input	Program Output

Select Parameters

Type calculation	Type input	Sided
○ Sample Size	○ Hazard Rates	● 1 Sided
● Power	● Survival Proportion	○ 2 Sided

Number strata	Proportion in standard group	Alpha
2	.5	.025

Years of accrual	Years of follow-up	Accrual rate	Hazard ratio	Total accrual	Power
2	1	400	1.33	800	0.9244

Calculate

Stratum	Proportion	Hazard rate, std.	Hazard rate, exp.	Proportion surviving	Survival time
1	0.5	0.462	0.347	0.5	1.5
2	0.5	1.386	1.042	0.5	0.5

(B)

FIGURE 17.3 More example sample size calculations. (*continued*)

Source: Cancer Research and Biostatistics, CRAB and SWOG.

Two Arm Survival

Two Arm Survival is a program to calculate either estimates accrual or power for differences in survival times between two groups. The program allows for unequal sample size allocation between the two groups. The survival time estimates also allow for multiple strata or risk groups.

User Input	Program Output

Select Parameters

Type calculation ◉ Sample Size ○ Power	Type input ○ Hazard Rates ◉ Survival Proportion	Sided ◉ 1 Sided ○ 2 Sided

Number strata 1	Proportion in standard group .5	Alpha .025

Years of accrual 4	Years of follow-up 1	Accrual rate 440.31	Hazard ratio 1.33	Total accrual 1761	Power 0.9

Calculate

Stratum	Proportion	Hazard rate, std.	Hazard rate, exp.	Proportion surviving	Survival time
1	1	0.139	0.104	0.5	5
2					

(C)

Two Arm Survival

Two Arm Survival is a program to calculate either estimates accrual or power for differences in survival times between two groups. The program allows for unequal sample size allocation between the two groups. The survival time estimates also allow for multiple strata or risk groups.

User Input	Program Output

Select Parameters

Type calculation ◉ Sample Size ○ Power	Type input ○ Hazard Rates ◉ Survival Proportion	Sided ◉ 1 Sided ○ 2 Sided

Number strata 1	Proportion in standard group .5	Alpha .025

Years of accrual 4	Years of follow-up 5	Accrual rate 230.5	Hazard ratio 1.33	Total accrual 922	Power 0.9

Calculate

Stratum	Proportion	Hazard rate, std.	Hazard rate, exp.	Proportion surviving	Survival time
1	1	0.139	0.104	0.5	5
2					

(D)

FIGURE 17.3 (*continued*)

A modified ITT principle, often employed in the trials conducted in the U.S. cooperative group system, is to analyze all *eligible* randomized patients on the arm to which they are randomized. The logic is that the eligibility criteria describe the patient population to which the results of the trial may be generalized, and that eligibility is in principle known at the time of randomization, so that their exclusion has less risk of introducing bias. The Food and Drug Administration, however, is quite clear that this modification to the ITT principle is not acceptable for trials used for registration.

In addition to the all randomized population as embodied in the ITT principle, other patient populations often included for analysis include the safety population, defined as all patients starting therapy and often used in toxicity analysis; and the as-treated population, used as a sensitivity analysis of the conclusions reached by ITT.

Subset Analyses

It is very tempting to perform subset analyses for both positive as well as negative trials. In trials with no statistically significant overall difference between treatment arms there is the hope that the new therapy may be beneficial for a certain subset of patients, such as older patients, younger patients, males, females, or patients who test positive for a specific biomarker. On the other hand, in a positive trial one is tempted to find subsets of patients in which the new treatment is particularly effective and the hazard ratio between arms particularly striking. There are two basic problems with such unplanned subset analyses. Most trials are designed such that the overall sample size yields a statistical test with a power just large enough to test the overall difference between arms; any subset analysis that by definition has a smaller sample size does not have adequate power (unless designed appropriately ahead of time) and thus yields high false-negative rates. On the other hand, often many subsets are tested with no appropriate adjustments for multiple comparisons, so that one is likely to find a significant difference for a subset if enough such subsets are tested, meaning that collectively there is a high false-positive rate. This is the worst of both worlds.

Subset analyses that were not predefined with specific hypotheses in mind and properly powered with adequate sample sizes in each subset should always be viewed as exploratory and need to be confirmed in a future trial that is powered to test treatment difference in the specific subset. A similar issue with multiple comparisons can be found in multiarm trials if no proper adjustments for multiple comparisons are being implemented, as we explain in the next section.

MULTIARM TRIALS

Several Experimental Treatments Versus Control

Sometimes trials are designed to test multiple experimental treatments versus a single control therapy. The overall goal is to determine whether one of the promising new experimental treatments is superior to the current standard of care (control therapy).

The main issues with multiarm trials are related to power and significance due to testing multiple hypotheses. If each hypothesis is tested at a significance level a, the probability of an overall false-positive significance level is much greater than a. One way to reduce the probability of false positives is to do a global test first, followed by individual subset tests only if the global test is positive. Another possibility is to adjust a for multiple

comparisons, for example using the Bonferroni adjustment, where each of the n hypotheses is tested at a level a/n to ensure an overall experimentwise significance level of a. For example, with K treatments the number of possible pairwise comparisons is $n = \binom{K}{2}$; if only the comparisons of each experimental treatment with the control are of interest, then $n = K - 1$.

The power for pairwise comparisons in multiarm trials can be calculated the same way as for two-arm trials, with a adjusted as in the preceding, but the differences to be tested between the different pairs may not be the same. Thus the number of patients required per arm is higher in multiarm than in two-arm trials.

Factorial designs

A special form of multiarm trials is factorial designs in which new therapies are tested alone and in combination with the other therapies. The simplest factorial design is the 2 × 2 factorial design with two factors (treatments) A and B. In such a trial, subjects are being randomized to observation O, treatment A, treatment B, and treatment AB. The appeal of such a design is that arms can be collapsed to compare A versus no A (or B versus no B), if there are no treatment interactions, meaning that A is not influenced by B and vice versa when given in combination. Unfortunately, that is rarely the case in practice and treatments; when given in combination, this does not typically have a simple additive effect. Unfortunately, testing for significant interactions suffers from small power and even if a significant interaction is being detected it is not clear how to best analyze such a study. Several analytic strategies are possible, including ignoring the possibility of interactions and testing only main effects; first doing a global test as previously before proceeding to further testing; and testing first for interactions and then proceeding according to whether that test is significant or not. These strategies are compared in the text by Green et al. (14), who conclude by recommending against factorial designs unless treatment interactions can be excluded. If there is a true interaction, more than twice the sample size is being required in order to achieve appropriate power, in fact up to four times that of a two-arm trial (15). Finally, a gatekeeping strategy is explored by Korn and Friedlin (16).

TRIAL MONITORING

The ongoing results of phase III trials in oncology are almost always available only to a few key individuals, often a completely independent data and safety monitoring committee. This is to guard against premature and perhaps erroneous judgments being made during the conduct of the trial. This is not a completely academic concern; see for example Green and Crowley (17) and Crowley et al. (18) for some history. Formal guidelines are provided in advance about how such interim analyses should be done. As with subset analysis, and multiarm trials, repeated formal interim analyses raises concerns of multiple comparisons. Use of very conservative testing procedures (very small type I error) for the interim analyses, perhaps with a Bonferroni correction for the final analysis, is one simple way to minimize these concerns (19). See Chapter 30 for a detailed discussion of interim analysis procedures that preserve overall type I error.

DESIGNS INCORPORATING BIOMARKERS (SEE ALSO CHAPTER 14)

Better understanding of underlying biology and molecular pathways in combination with new therapeutic agents that target a specific mechanism of action has made precision medicine in oncology a reality. Initially, the clinical development of targeted agents was similar to that of cytotoxic agents. In the phase II setting such an agent was typically being tested in patients who tested positive for a specific biomarker and in the phase III setting traditional trial designs were typically based on a randomize-all (all-comers) or a targeted or enrichment design (20).

MASTER PROTOCOLS

With the increasing number of biomarkers based on genetic and molecular profiling, master protocols have become popular. Patients are tested for several biomarkers, often using a multiplex diagnostic assay, to determine which therapeutic approach may be best for a specific patient. Substudies are available for patients with a particular molecular profile, all within the same master protocol. Such a protocol allows maximal flexibility, as individual substudies or arms can be stopped early, extended based on emerging results, or new ones added as new actionable targets become available. The premise is that such a trial increases trial participation and decreases the timeline for drug–biomarker testing and ultimately for drug development.

Master protocols for patients with the same type of cancer are referred to as umbrella studies. Umbrella protocols have been implemented in cancers with high prevalence, such as Lung-MAP in squamous cell lung cancer (www.lung-map.org/about-lung-map), Biomarker-integrated Approaches of Targeted Therapy for Lung Cancer Elimination (BATTLE) in non–small-cell lung cancer (NSCLC) (21), and I-Spy 2 in breast cancer (22), to name just a few. The SWOG Statistics and Data Management Center, colocated at the Fred Hutch Cancer Research Center and CRAB has implemented Lung-MAP. This is a complex and complicated

undertaking with many logistical challenges. Lung-MAP opened to accrual in June 2014 and there have been many changes since then, many of those due to external circumstances.

The complexities inherent with such a trial design include selection of a platform for biomarker testing; logistics of how to automate the capture of the biomarker results into the database and automate treatment assignment based on the results; selection of drugs and biomarkers for the first set of studies and associated negotiations of design, budgets, and contracts with several pharmaceutical companies. In addition, since precision medicine is such a fast-moving field, there will be unexpected changes. In the Lung-MAP trial, the standard of care changed within a few months into the study, making some of the control arms obsolete. In addition, one of the participating drug companies terminated all sponsored trials for one of their agents used in a substudy. This resulted in closing some of the substudies early and drastically redesigning the different substudies. Changes like this are a reality in this fast-moving field and we have to be prepared to rapidly change and adapt to new challenges.

REFERENCES

1. Bates S. PFS: The endpoint we love and love to hate. In Crowley J, ed. (Guest Editor). *Clinical Cancer Research Focus Issue*. 2013;19(10):2606–2656.
2. Kaplan EL, Meier P. Nonparametric estimation from incomplete observations. *J Am Stat Assoc*. 1958;53:457–481.
3. Greenwood M. *The natural duration of cancer. Reports on Public Health and Medical Subjects*. London, UK: His Majesty's Stationery Office. 1926;33:1–26.
4. Breslow N, Crowley J. A large sample study of the life table and product limit estimates under random censorship. *Ann Stat*. 1974;2:437–453.
5. Mantel N. Evaluation of survival data and two new rank order statistics arising in its evaluation. *Cancer Chemother Reports*. 1966;50:163–170.
6. Peto R, Peto J. Asymptotically efficient rank invariant test procedures. *J Royal Stat Society, Series A*. 1972;135:185–198.
7. Crowley J. *Non-parametric analysis of censored survival data, with distribution theory for the k-sample generalized savage statistic*. Ph. D. Thesis, University of Washington, 1973.
8. Aalen O. Nonparametric inference in connection with multiple decrement models. *Scand J Stat*. 1976;3:15–27.
9. Anderson PK, Borgan O, Gill R, Keiding N. Linear nonparametric tests for comparison of counting processes, with application to censored survival data. *Inter Stat Rev*. 1982;50:219–244.
10. Gill R. *Censoring and Stochastic Integrals. Mathematics Centre Tracts 124*. Amsterdam: Mathematisch Centrum. 1980.
11. Bernstein D, Lagakos SW. Sample size and power determination for stratified clinical trials. *J Stat Comput Simul*. 1978;8:65–73.
12. Schoenfeld DA. Sample-size formula for the proportional-hazards regression model. *Biometrics*. 1983;39(2):499–503.
13. Lakatos E Lan KK. A comparison of sample size methods for the log-rank statistic. *Stat Med*. 1992;11(2):179–191.
14. Green S, Benedetti J, Smith A, Crowley J. *Clinical Trials in Oncology*. 3rd edn. London, UK: CRC Press/Chapman and Hall; 2012.

15. Peterson B, George SL. Sample size requirements and length of study for testing interaction in a 2 x k factorial design when time to failure is the outcome. *Control Clin Trial.* 1993;14:511–522.

16. Korn EL, Friedlin B. Non-factorial analysis of two-by-two factorial trial designs. *Clinical Trials.* 2016;13(6):1–9.

17. Green S, Crowley J. Data monitoring committees for Southwest Oncology Group trials. *Stat Med.* 1993;11:451–455.

18. Crowley J, Green S, Liu P-Y, Wolf M. Data monitoring committees and early stopping guidelines. *Stat Med.* 1994;13: 1391–1399.

19. Haybittle JL. Repeated assessments of results in clinical trials of cancer treatment. *Br J Radiol.* 1971;44:793–797.

20. Hoering A, LeBlanc M, Crowley J. Randomized phase III clinical trial designs for targeted agents. *Clin Cancer Res.* 2008;14:4358–4367.

21. Kim ES, Herbst RS, Wistuba II, et al. The BATTLE trial: personalized therapy for lung cancer. *Cancer Discov.* 2011;1:44–53.

22. Barker AD, Sigman CC, Kelloff GJ, et al. I-SPY 2: an adaptive breast cancer trial in the setting of neo adjuvant chemotherapy. *Clin Pharmacol Ther.* 2009;86:97–100.

Design of Noninferiority Trials in Oncology

Lei Nie and Zhiwei Zhang

INTRODUCTION

Before a drug can be marketed in the United States, according to regulation, it must be shown to be safe and effective for its labeled uses. Substantial evidence that a drug is safe and effective should be derived from adequate and well-controlled clinical trials. Obtaining a quantitative estimate of the effect an experimental treatment has on patients is an expected result of a controlled trial. This chapter discusses active control noninferiority trials. These trials are designed:

- To show that a drug is effective, meaning that the difference between the drug and the control on patients is small and its effect is superior to that of a placebo
- To estimate the drug's effect without including a control group receiving a placebo

It is well established that simply treating a patient, even with a benign substance, can provide a positive outcome with respect to some diseases. This phenomenon is known as the placebo effect. This effect indicates the underlying need to have a control group in a clinical trial. Without a control group against which to compare experimental treatment outcomes, it is impossible to determine whether outcomes seen after administering the treatment are due to the treatment or the placebo effect. In cancer clinical trials, it is not uncommon to compare several standard treatments used concurrently plus a placebo with the same standard treatments plus an experimental drug. In such cases, the term *placebo arm* is commonly applied to the control arm.

Noninferiority designs can provide indirect comparison of the experimental treatment to the placebo. There are situations in which a placebo-controlled trial would be unethical or impractical. For example, for a given disease, several treatments, each having considerable side effects, may be available. The developer of a drug offering a new treatment for this disease, one that cannot be combined with the existing treatments, faces a challenge in showing the product is more effective than placebo; it is unethical to assign patients to a placebo arm when effective treatments are available. In such a case, a trial showing that the new treatment is more effective than one of the existing treatments could be a viable option for demonstrating effectiveness of the new treatment. Although viable, this option could be considered excessively resource demanding if (1) the new treatment has a better safety profile than the existing treatment and (2) the community, including physicians and patients, could consider an equivalent effect or even a lesser effect desirable if the side effects of the existing product could be avoided. This is the prototypical noninferiority situation. One wishes to show that an experimental product is comparable in effectiveness to a currently marketed product while ensuring that it is more effective than a placebo, without including a placebo control group in the trial.

A general approach to noninferiority is to show that the effectiveness of an experimental product is not excessively inferior to an active control product and more effective than a placebo. Comparisons are commonly done through the use of ratios and differences. For simplicity, we consider comparisons using differences. Let T be some measure of effectiveness for an experimental treatment and C be the same measure for an active control. These could be survival time or response rate, for example. Define the difference $\Delta = T - C$. We wish to show that the difference Δ is greater than some predetermined value we will call δ, the noninferiority margin. A successful noninferiority inference can be achieved by showing the lower bound of the 100% a confidence interval of the difference $T - C$ is greater than δ, corresponding to a hypothesis test at the one-sided $a/2$ level.

Examples of Confidence Intervals for $T - C = \Delta$

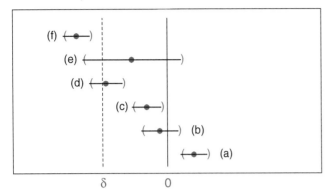

FIGURE 18.1 Possible outcomes of a noninferiority trial using the difference as the comparison metric.

Figure 18.1 illustrates several situations that can occur in noninferiority testing. Note that all point estimates except for (a) are negative. The interval (a) is completely greater than 0, indicating that T is superior to C at the selected α level. Interval (f) is entirely less than δ and clearly cannot support noninferiority. The lower bounds of (b) and (c) are greater than δ and would support noninferiority, although the point estimates are negative. The lower bounds of intervals (d) and (e) are less than δ. These intervals do not support noninferiority.

This chapter mainly focuses on aspects of noninferiority studies as they are applied to the setting of therapeutic drug and biologic products for cancer. Specifically, the issues include time-to-event endpoints and censoring, multiplicity adjustments, treatment effect estimation complicated by censoring and incomplete follow-up, and noninferiority margin determination when limited historical information is available.

ENDPOINTS AND METRICS

Clinical trial endpoints are clinical outcomes or laboratory measurements that provide information about patient treatment results. Endpoints allow investigators to evaluate whether a drug provides a clinical benefit, such as prolongation of survival or improvement in symptoms. Under regulations for regular drug approval, a common endpoint, and one regarded as the most reliable measure of treatment effect in oncology clinical trials, is survival. Generally endpoints used to support regular approval should be measures of how a patient feels, functions, or survives. More specialized regulatory pathways allow other endpoints to be used. For example, a drug may be approved under the accelerated approval regulation for a serious and life-threatening disease if it can be shown to be more effective than currently available therapies or provide therapy where none exists. In this setting, the Food and Drug Administration (FDA) may grant approval based on an effect demonstrated using a surrogate endpoint that is reasonably likely to predict clinical benefit (1).

Overall survival (OS) is one of the most commonly used endpoints in oncology noninferiority trials. OS is considered to be the most reliable endpoint because it is precise and easily measured. However, use of OS as an endpoint is not without problems. Situations in which patients are expected to have long survival times make OS less feasible as an endpoint because of confounding because of patients' changing therapies during the trial. Motivation to change therapies could be the result of any number of things, including another treatment becoming available or the patients' disease progression.

Objective response rate (ORR) has been a commonly used surrogate endpoint in oncology. However, it is more challenging to justify ORR as the primary endpoint for a noninferiority trial to demonstrate a meaningful advantage over available therapy than a primary endpoint for a superiority trial. Using noninferiority in a situation requiring an improvement in therapy may be theoretically possible, if dimensions of patients' experience beside ORR have improved. For example, if noninferiority of an experimental treatment with respect to ORR were demonstrated, but the duration of the responses for the experimental treatment surpassed those attributed to the control, one might judge the experimental therapy to be a net improvement. Of course, such a determination would depend on numerous factors, including the disease setting, available therapies, and their side effects.

Progression-free survival (PFS), defined as the time from randomization until death or disease progression, where disease progression is defined by the study protocol, has been used as an endpoint to support accelerated approval in some oncology settings or regular approval in some others. One main benefit of using PFS as a primary endpoint compared to OS is the reduction in time necessary to complete a clinical trial. While progression usually precedes death, it has been difficult to validate PFS as a surrogate for OS. Progression time is usually not confounded by subsequent cancer therapies or by discontinuation of treatment that occurs after disease progression, unlike OS. Whether an improvement in PFS in a superiority trial represents a direct clinical benefit of a surrogate for clinical benefit depends on the disease area, the magnitude of the effect, and the risk-benefit relationship of the experimental treatment compared to available therapies. For example, if a clinical trial demonstrates that an experimental treatment has a substantially larger median PFS than the control therapy, concerns about surrogacy may be mitigated somewhat, depending on the disease setting. On the other hand, the clinical benefit of an experimental therapy may be in question if when it compared to standard therapy through PFS, the hazard ratio is not statistically significantly less than one. Because surrogacy is difficult to establish for PFS, noninferiority is difficult to interpret with respect to clinical benefit. Other concerns include the dependence of PFS on frequency of progression assessment, method of progression measurement, and differences in censoring patterns between the noninferiority trial and the historical trials on which the non-inferiority margin is based. Any one of these concerns can lead investigators to question the ability of the trial to detect a difference between treatments, assuming one exists. This property of clinical trials has been called assay sensitivity. For a noninferiority trial, assay sensitivity is the ability of the trial to detect a difference of a specified magnitude between the treatments that would imply the experimental therapy is not effective.

Inherent to survival analysis are the issues of censoring and inadequate follow-up time. While informative censoring can cause bias and have an impact on one's ability to determine superiority using survival analysis, noninformative censoring in a superiority trial tends to cause treatment effect estimates to be similar. This latter point means even noninformative censoring, in large amounts, can be problematic from the investigator's point of view because trials with large amounts of censoring provide little information. Noninformative censoring will not lead to a bias in favor to the experimental treatment in a superiority trial. That is not true for noninferiority studies. If the sample size is large enough to drive down the variance of the hazard ratio estimate, increasing amounts of noninformative censoring will tend to drive the hazard ratio toward one and possibly imply noninferiority. This phenomenon is not restricted to noninformative censoring. Any trial conduct that tends to cause treatment effect estimates to appear similar, such as patients' switching treatments or missing data, may lead to inappropriately rejecting the null hypothesis in favor of noninferiority.

The hazard ratio is typically used as a comparison metric in clinical trials using time to event endpoints. The Cox proportional hazards model is the most common approach used to estimate the hazard ratio. A reasonable definition of a noninferiority margin may rely on the proportional hazards assumption. If any of the historical clinical trials supporting noninferiority margin determination violate the proportional hazards assumption, the resulting margin may be questioned. Note that the typical log rank test used in superiority trials is a nonparametric test that does not rely on the proportional hazards assumption. A noninferiority log-rank test was introduced as an alternative to testing based on the hazard ratio (2,3).

Several metrics are available to compare treatment effects when considering binary endpoints, such as objective response rate. The three commonly used metrics are the absolute risk difference (RD), relative risk (RR), and odds ratio (OR). The choice of metric depends on the clinical trial setting and assumed event rate. Because the metrics behave differently under different conditions, the choice of metric can have an impact on the quantification of the control effect on which the noninferiority

margin depends and thus can affect the sample size of the trial. For example, when the event rate is very low, the variance of RR, which is approximately inversely proportional to the number of events, is small only when a sufficient number of events occurs. The large variance causes the estimated sample size to also be large. The choice of metric should be based on scientific rationale. Similar discussion could extend to the comparison among hazard ratio, restricted mean, and survival rate at a certain time point since randomization.

NONINFERIORITY MARGIN

The noninferiority margin is set to achieve two main goals:

Goal 1: to demonstrate that the experimental treatment is more effective than placebo

Goal 2: to demonstrate that the experimental treatment is not unacceptable in comparison to the active control.

It is difficult to overstate the role the noninferiority margin plays in the design of noninferiority trials and the interpretation of their results. On one hand, an inappropriately large margin could result in falsely concluding an ineffective drug is effective. On the other hand, an overly conservative margin can unnecessarily inflate the sample size of a noninferiority trial. Although the noninferiority margin is often determined through data-driven techniques, it should be justified both on clinical and statistical grounds.

In the first goal (Goal 1), one could demonstrate that the experimental treatment effect T is superior to the placebo effect P by rejecting the null hypothesis H_0: $\mu_T - \mu_P \leq 0$, where μ_T and μ_P are the mean responses under the experimental treatment and placebo, respectively. As mentioned earlier, several comparison metrics can be used in noninferiority testing. Here, for simplicity of illustration, we consider the difference in means. We will consider the fixed margin approach to noninferiority. In this approach, a margin δ is predefined based on the effect size of the active control, which is estimated considering historical trials in which the active control product was previously compared to a placebo. Under the fixed margin approach, we implicitly reject the null hypothesis H_0: $\mu_T - \mu_P \leq 0$ when the hypothesis K_0: $\mu_T - \mu_C \leq \delta$ is rejected (where μ_C is the mean response under the control of the noninferiority trial).

To achieve Goals 1 and 2, a margin that is no more than δ should be used, generally based, in part, on clinical judgment. The decision relies on how much of the treatment effect must be shown to be preserved, considering the seriousness of disease, the treatment options patients may have, the benefit of the active comparator, and the expected safety profiles of the treatment and control. Note that a smaller hazard for time-to-event endpoints corresponds to a better outcome. In this example, hazards can be considered by defining μ_T, μ_C, and μ_P to be the negative logs of the respective hazards.

Derivation of the noninferiority margin is critical to achieving the goals of noninferiority studies. The margin δ must be chosen so that rejection of K_0: $\mu_T - \mu_C \le \delta$ implies rejection of H_0: $\mu_T - \mu_P \le 0$. For example, δ may be chosen as $\hat{\mu}_{CP} - z_a \sigma_{CP}$, the lower bound of the $100(1 - 2a)\%$ confidence interval of the treatment effect of the active control versus placebo. Here $\hat{\mu}_{CP} = \hat{\mu}_C - \hat{\mu}_P$, σ_{CP} is the standard error, and z_a is the $100(1 - a)\%$ quantile of a standard normal distribution. Determining a noninferiority margin following this procedure relies on an assumption of constancy—the assumption that the treatment effect estimated from historical controlled trials would be the same treatment effect estimated if it were possible to run identical clinical trials under the current standard of care. A popular way of determining the noninferiority margin is to estimate the treatment effect using historical information available for the control therapy. Once that effect is estimated, the margin is set to ensure the difference between the experimental treatment and the control treatment; if this is greater than δ, it rules out the possibility of the experimental product's being less effective than placebo by some preselected amount. This has been referred to as discounting the initial calculation of the control product's effect to provide some assurance that the noninferiority test will be valid in the event constancy does not hold. We note that using the point estimate of the treatment effect $\hat{\mu}_{CP}$ as a basis of deriving the noninferiority margin would not incorporate the variability of the treatment effect estimator and doing so is not recommended because of the effect it would have on the margin derivation.

In addition to ensuring that rejecting the null hypothesis in favor of noninferiority will be valid in the event constancy does not hold, discounting the estimated control effect when determining the margin is done to achieve the second goal (Goal 2). Clinical opinion may dictate that regardless of the magnitude of the control effect, declaring a treatment to be noninferior to the control would only be reasonable if the difference between the experimental treatment and the control treatment were fixed at a clinically defined margin. One way to address this goal in a fixed margin approach is to choose δ to be a fraction of the control effect size. For example, letting $\delta = 50\%$ of $(\hat{\mu}_{CP} - z_a \sigma_{CP})$ corresponds to a tighter noninferiority margin that aims to preserve $50\% = 1 - 50\%$ of the control effect size relative to placebo. Discounting the estimated control effect has also been used to set a clinical margin to achieve Goal 2, to ensure that the treatment is not too much worse than the active control.

In some special cases, there is no need to derive the noninferiority margin based on historical data of the effect size that the active controlled demonstrated over placebo. For example, if the treatment effect of the

placebo in response rate is known as 0%, then rejection of K_0: $p_T - p_C \le 0$ will meet Goal 1 to demonstrate that the new treatment is better than placebo and Goal 2 that the new treatment preserves 75% of the control treatment effect over placebo.

Many authors have expressed concern over noninferiority trials in oncology, citing the determination of and use of a large margin as a major issue. For example, "the margin of non-inferiority is often not clearly justified and there is large variability in this metric" (4) and in clinical trials "often use large non-inferiority margin and frequently present serious methodological problems" (5). Below we provide some challenges that could explain the reasons behind the difficulty in selecting a reasonable margin.

Challenge 1: Determining Margin Based on Limited Historical Data

There is little historical information available from which the control effect can be estimated and thus a noninferiority margin can be derived. There have been oncology treatments approved based on one randomized controlled trial. Also, in some cases, oncology treatments are approved using single-arm trials. Basing margin determination on the control treatment's effect size is difficult in these situations because of the lack of information. The consequence of using sparse data to estimate μ_{CP} could be a poor estimation with large variability σ^2_{CP}, leading to a very small margin and thus a very large noninferiority study.

Challenge 2: Defining Margin for Time to Event Endpoint

It is typically challenging to determine noninferiority margins for time-to-event endpoints, which could be the primary endpoint in oncology. The metric is usually the hazard ratio. Data obtained from historical trials, which are essential to quantify the effect size of the control, may not be reliable enough for time-dependent endpoints, including overall survival and PFS. Differences between historical trials and noninferiority trials include differences in patient populations, improved supportive care, different censoring patterns, and different study follow-up. For time-to-event endpoints based on tumor assessments, the difference further includes improved imaging techniques over the time, frequency of assessment, criteria for progression, and method of measurements. When the proportional hazard model assumption is not true or the hazard is not constant over time, the definition of the margin could be problematic. For example, if the historical trial of a 2-year study (e.g., approved based on interim analysis) showed a hazard ratio of 0.7 of control over placebo, the margin defined based on the short follow-up may not apply to a noninferiority trial requiring a much longer follow-up (e.g., 5 years), because the effect size measured during the 2-year period may not be the same as the effect size that would have been observed had the historical trial follow-up been 5 years.

It is even more challenging to determine noninferiority margins when the effect size of the control over placebo is relatively small. Consider the example of capecitabine for metastatic breast cancer. The historical data showed a hazard ratio of 0.7 with a 95% confidence interval (CI) of (0.5, 0.8) for capecitabine + docetaxel versus docetaxel after failure of a prior anthracycline-containing regimen for time to progression, with the absolute gain of 1.9 months in median PFS (6). It remains unclear if a noninferiority margin defined using hazard ratio would be reliable and not a result of censoring and assessment window differences between trials.

Challenge 3: Addressing the Constancy Assumption

Noninferiority trials also rely on the constancy assumption, which states that the effect size in the current noninferiority trial is equal to the effect size in the historical trials. Many factors may affect constancy assumption, including changes of standard care and general health care over the time, population difference in key predictive factors, study conduct including duration, follow-up, missing data patterns, and differences in assessment of primary endpoints. In the literature, two approaches, discounting Ng (7,8), Rothmann (9) and the covariate adjustment approach (10–12), were proposed to deal with potential violations of the constancy assumption. To implement discounting in a fixed margin approach, δ may be chosen as a fraction (e.g., 50%) of $(\hat{\mu}_{CP} - z_a \sigma_{CP})$, which corresponds to a tighter noninferiority margin with 50% as the discounting factor. Another approach to deal with potential constancy assumption violation due to population difference is covariate adjustment.

To prevent constancy assumption violations, we intend to make sure the design of the active control trial is as close to the design of the historical trial as possible. However, a rigorous requirement of the same design and study conduct are rarely fulfilled in practice and may be unnecessary as well. When there is known heterogeneity of the active control treatment effect related to patient characteristics, and that heterogeneity can be quantified, we may adjust the estimate of the size of the active control effect in the noninferiority study (13). The covariate-adjustment approach aims to achieve two goals: (a) to quantify the impact of population difference between the historical trial and the active control trial to the degree of constancy assumption violation and (b) to redefine the active control treatment effect with respect to the active control trial population if the quantification suggests an unacceptable violation. Readers are referred to several references for further details (10–12).

PRACTICAL CONSIDERATIONS

In a superiority trial, intent-to-treat (ITT) analysis (or modified ITT, which excludes patients who were not dosed in double-blind trials) is intended to protect against bias in favor of the treatment. When use appropriately, it maintains randomization and permits a conservative estimate of treatment effect while usually guiding investigators to minimize unnecessary violations of protocol and also to minimize missing data. However, it has been argued that addressing problems such as nonadherence, misclassification of primary endpoints, missing data, or many dropouts who must be assessed as part of the treated group can bias noninferiority trial estimates toward no treatment difference. On the other hand, the per-protocol analysis does not necessarily maintain the randomization. Generally, ITT analysis is performed as the primary analysis, and per-protocol analysis is conducted as sensitivity analysis in noninferiority studies. Differences in results using the two analyses will need close examination.

When a noninferiority test is significant, a subsequent superiority test can be performed. This is because in the closed test procedure, the type I error rate is controlled as in the hierarchical testing procedure (often used to test primary and subsequent secondary endpoints) (14). However, one needs to be careful when the intention is to test superiority and some secondary endpoints after the noninferiority test is significant. For example, if a test of noninferiority in the primary endpoint is significant at level a, the test of superiority in the primary endpoint can be tested at level a. Following the closed test procedure (14), the familywise type I error rate is controlled at level a. However, if the test of superiority fails, continuing to test any secondary endpoints may inflate the familywise type I error rate. Thus, the specific order of the testing needs to be specified or, alternatively, a could be split between superiority and secondary endpoints following successful noninferiority testing of the primary endpoint. Note that only successful testing leads to further testing down the list of the hieratical order. Thus, testing noninferiority cannot be followed after failing superiority testing. A situation that appears similar is the wish to change the trial test from superiority to noninferiority before unblinding the data but without having designed the trial for noninferiority testing. This is an example of poor planning. See also (15).

The use of P values is often avoided in noninferiority trials because P values depend on the specific noninferiority margin and thus they are difficult to practically interpret. Comparing the CI of the treatment difference to the preset margin is a more transparent way to view the trial results. The treatment difference is the result of the trial, and it may be interpreted independently of the noninferiority margin as well as in the context of the margin. The P values of a noninferiority test takes the margin, which is not based on the noninferiority trial data, into account.

REMARKS

An active controlled noninferiority trial is an important alternative. With successful development in many cancer indications, we expect more noninferiority trials to develop new treatments that are anticipated to have similar efficacy as the active control but may have other advantages in safety, in convenience and associated improved adherence, or in fighting against drug resistance or drug shortage. Due to the "expedited" development of oncology drugs, often using surrogate endpoints, development of new treatment in oncology through noninferiority trials faces more challenges than some other disease areas. On the other hand, although all of these challenges test our limit in wisdom, none of the barriers should be unsurmountable.

ACKNOWLEDGMENT

The authors would like to thank Dr. Thomas E. Gwise and Dr. Rajeshwari Sridhara for their valuable comments and suggestions, which greatly and substantially improved the quality of this chapter.

REFERENCES

1. FDA. Guidance for Industry Clinical Trail Endpoints for the Approval of Cancer Drugs and Biologics; 2007.
2. Chow SC, Shao J, Wang H. *Sample Size Calculation in Clinical Research*. New York, NY: Marcel Dekker; 2003.
3. Jung SH, Kang SJ, McCall LM, Blumenstein B. Sample sizes computation for two-sample noninferiority log-rank test. *J Biopharm Stat*. 2005;15:969–979.
4. Mauricio B, Vinay P, Tito F. Non-inferiority trials: why oncologists must remain wary. *Lancet*. 2015;16(4):364–366.
5. Riechelmann RP, Alex A, Cruz L, et al. Non-inferiority cancer clinical trials: scope and purposes underlying their design. *Ann Oncol*. 2013;24:1942–1947.
6. Buzdar AU, Xu B, Digumarti R, et al. Randomized phase II non-inferiority study (NO16853) of two different doses of capecitabine in combination with docetaxel for locally advanced/metastatic breast cancer. *Ann Oncol*. 2012;23:589–597.
7. Ng T-H. Choice of delta in equivalence testing. *Drug Informat J*. 2001;35:1517–1527.
8. Ng TL. Equivalency and non-inferiority testing in clinical trials: issues and challenges. 2015.
9. Rothmann MD, Wiens BL, Chan ISF. *Design and Analysis of Non-Inferiority Trials*. Chapman Hall/CRC; 2010.
10. Zhang, Z. Estimating the current treatment effect with historical control data. *JP J Biostat*. 2007;1:217–247.
11. Nie L, Soon G. A covariate-adjustment regression model approach to non-inferiority margin definition. *Stat Med*. 2010;29:1107–1113.
12. Nie L, Zhang Z, Rubin D, Chu J. Likelihood reweighting methods to reduce potential bias in non-inferiority trials which rely on historical data to make inference. *Ann Appl Stat*. 2013;7(3):1796–1813.
13. FDA. Guidance for Industry: Non-Inferiority Clinical Trials to establish effectiveness; 2016.
14. Marcus R, Peritz E, Gabriel KR. On closed testing procedures with special reference to ordered analysis of variance. *Biometrika*. 1976;63:655–660.
15. Committee for Proprietary Medicinal Products (CPMP). *Points to Consider on Switching Between Superiority and Non-Inferiority*; 2000.

Design of Quality of Life Studies

Amylou C. Dueck and Katie L. Kunze

INTRODUCTION

Quality of life (QOL) has long been identified as an important endpoint in oncology clinical trials (1) with some identifying it as second in importance only to survival. The term "quality of life" is used here and historically as an umbrella term to include a variety of outcomes captured via patient self-report but is technically defined in health research as "a reflection of the way that people perceive and react to their health status and to other, non-medical aspects of their lives"(2). Health-related QOL (HRQOL) refers to the subset of QOL outcomes related to health aspects and reflecting the impact of disease and treatment on disability and daily functioning (2). QOL as an umbrella term in recent years has been replaced in some contexts by the term "patient-reported outcome" (PRO), which is defined as any report directly from the patient about his or her health status or condition without interpretation by a clinician or anyone else. PROs may be collected via self-report or interview but must contain the responses of only the patient with no interpretation or revision by the interviewer. The Food and Drug Administration (FDA) categorizes PROs as one of four clinical outcome assessments (COAs) (3), with the other three COAs being clinician-reported outcomes (ClinROs; e.g., clinician-reported Eastern Cooperative Oncology Group [ECOG] performance status), observer-reported outcomes (ObsROs; e.g., a parent's report of a child's vomiting episodes), and performance outcomes (PerfOs; e.g., 6-minute walk test). All COAs measure treatment benefits or harms either directly or indirectly from patients.

QOL endpoints in oncology clinical trials in the past have been hampered by issues such as lack of available measurement tools, no guidance for integrating QOL into oncology clinical trial protocols, high rates of informative missing data, difficulty in interpreting results relative to clinical meaningfulness, and variability in statistical analysis and reporting approaches. Essentially all of these issues have been resolved in recent years with many resources available to investigators interested in assessing QOL in their trials. For example, the FDA (4) and European Medicines Agency (EMA) (5) communications have become the gold standard for QOL endpoints in clinical trials intended to support a label claim in the United States and Europe, respectively. Though narrowly focused on the regulatory setting, the considerations detailed within these documents are also applicable to QOL in clinical trials not intended for registration. If the intent of your study is to support a label claim based on a QOL endpoint, regulatory officials should be consulted as early in the drug development process for context-specific QOL recommendations. The goal of this chapter is to provide an overview with key references for further reading of design, statistical analysis, interpretation, and reporting considerations for QOL in oncology clinical trials.

ANATOMY AND DEVELOPMENT OF A QOL QUESTIONNAIRE

A QOL questionnaire or instrument can measure effects of medical interventions on one or more concepts. A typical QOL instrument includes specific elements, which are defined here using the example of the Myeloproliferative Neoplasm Symptom Assessment Form (MPN-SAF) (6), which was developed to assess symptoms and QOL of patients with essential thrombocythemia, polycythemia, and myelofibrosis shown in Figure 19.1. Common elements include (a) items or questions (MPN-SAF items share a common stem but each item covers a specific symptom or concept); (b) measurement scales (i.e., response options), which may appear in a variety of formats such as a verbal rating scale (a scale consisting of ordered descriptive categories; e.g., "none," "mild," "moderate," "severe," and "very severe"), visual analog scale (a line, ruler, or bar, which allows a patient to identify a numeric rating on a continuum), or numeric rating scale (as in the MPN-SAF with integers over a range often anchored on

Myeloproliferative Neoplasm Symptom Assessment Form (MPN-SAF) ©

Circle the one number that describes how, during the past Week how much difficulty you have had with each of the following symptoms	
Filling up quickly when you eat (Early satiety)	(Absent) 0 1 2 3 4 5 6 7 8 9 10 (Worst Imaginable)
Abdominal pain	(Absent) 0 1 2 3 4 5 6 7 8 9 10 (Worst Imaginable)
Abdominal discomfort	(Absent) 0 1 2 3 4 5 6 7 8 9 10 (Worst Imaginable)
Inactivity	(Absent) 0 1 2 3 4 5 6 7 8 9 10 (Worst Imaginable)
Problems with headaches	(Absent) 0 1 2 3 4 5 6 7 8 9 10 (Worst Imaginable)
Problems with concentration - Compared to prior to my MPD	(Absent) 0 1 2 3 4 5 6 7 8 9 10 (Worst Imaginable)
Dizziness/ Vertigo/ Lightheadedness	(Absent) 0 1 2 3 4 5 6 7 8 9 10 (Worst Imaginable)
Numbness/ Tingling (in my hands and feet)	(Absent) 0 1 2 3 4 5 6 7 8 9 10 (Worst Imaginable)
Difficulty sleeping	(Absent) 0 1 2 3 4 5 6 7 8 9 10 (Worst Imaginable)
Depression or sad mood	(Absent) 0 1 2 3 4 5 6 7 8 9 10 (Worst Imaginable)
Problems with sexual desire or Function	(Absent) 0 1 2 3 4 5 6 7 8 9 10 (Worst Imaginable)
Cough	(Absent) 0 1 2 3 4 5 6 7 8 9 10 (Worst Imaginable)
Night sweats	(Absent) 0 1 2 3 4 5 6 7 8 9 10 (Worst Imaginable)
Itching (pruritus)	(Absent) 0 1 2 3 4 5 6 7 8 9 10 (Worst Imaginable)
Bone pain (diffuse not joint pain or arthritis)	(Absent) 0 1 2 3 4 5 6 7 8 9 10 (Worst Imaginable)
Fever (>100 F)	(Absent) 0 1 2 3 4 5 6 7 8 9 10 (Daily)
Unintentional weight loss last 6 months	(Absent) 0 1 2 3 4 5 6 7 8 9 10 (Worst Imaginable)
What is your overall quality of life?	(As good as it can be) 0 1 2 3 4 5 6 7 8 9 10 (As bad as it can be)

© Mayo Clinic

FIGURE 19.1 The Myeloproliferative Neoplasm Symptom Assessment Form (MPN-SAF).

Source: From Scherber R, Dueck AC, Johansson P, et al. The Myeloproliferative Neoplasm Symptom Assessment Form (MPN-SAF): international prospective validation and reliability trial in 402 patients. *Blood.* 2011;118(2):401–408. Used with permission of Mayo Foundation for Medical Education and Research. All rights reserved.

either end by descriptive text; e.g., integers from 0 to 10 anchored by "absent" and "worst imaginable"); (c) a specified recall period (e.g., "during the past week"); and (d) copyright information.

A QOL instrument typically undergoes a rigorous multistep development process to ensure that the instrument has adequate measurement (or psychometric) properties and other characteristics in a given patient population. Minimum standards for development of QOL instruments have been established (7). Standard measurement properties or characteristics that are typically explored during development include validity (the instrument measures the construct[s] it intends to measure), reliability (the instrument's score or scores have no measurement error), responsiveness (the instrument's score or scores change over time when the construct(s) being measured changes over time), and interpretability (the instrument's score or scores have qualitative meaning) (8). Measurement properties and characteristics are generally considered to be setting specific (i.e., established only in the patient population or disease and/or treatment setting in which the instrument was tested during its development).

During the development process, a scoring algorithm is commonly developed for the QOL instrument. The scoring algorithm may result in a single overall score across all items and/or one or more subscale scores each computed from a subset of one or more related items. The way in which items within a QOL instrument are combined to measure constructs is often depicted in a conceptual framework.

After the development process, a validated QOL instrument may undergo language translation and cross-cultural adaptations and/or adaptations for administration via a different modality (e.g., a pen-and-paper questionnaire may be adapted for administration on a tablet or smartphone). Recommended procedures for language/cultural (9,10) and mode adaptations (11) have been developed.

DESIGN CONSIDERATIONS

In order to integrate QOL endpoints into an oncology clinical trial, the study team must establish the "who," "what," "where," "when," "why," and "how" of the trial. These six elements are interrelated with decisions made in one impacting one or more of the others as described in the following. Beginning with the first of these elements, the target patient population (i.e., the "who") must be identified including the specific disease setting and treatments being researched. Other patient characteristics (e.g., languages spoken, age range, stamina, ability to complete questionnaires on their own, and access to technology) or protocol characteristics (e.g., timing of clinic visits or disease evaluations) may also be important for downstream design decisions. The patient population, disease setting, and treatment will in part inform such design features as selection of a QOL instrument, the location of the administration, the mode by which questionnaires are administered, and timing of the assessments. If necessary, eligibility criteria should be considered. If the goal of the clinical trial is to show symptom improvement, then eligibility criteria should specify the minimum level of the symptom required at

the time of registration to ensure a symptomatic patient population (e.g., see Dworkin et al. [12] for a recommendation to require patients to report a baseline pain level of at least 4 or 5 on a scale from 0 [no pain] to 10 [worst pain imaginable] in pain trials). If the QOL instrument is only available in English, then the study team could consider requiring English literacy if QOL is the primary or key secondary outcome of the trial. If the selected mode of administration is telephone- or web-based, then at-home access to a telephone and/or Internet-connected computer could be specified in the eligibility criteria.

Next, the study team must identify "what" should be measured (i.e., the intended constructs or concepts to be measured) and "how" these constructs or concepts will be measured (i.e., which QOL instrument[s] will be used and by which mode they will be administered). Intended constructs or concepts to be measured are related to the objectives/hypotheses and may be based on the constructs or concepts that are likely to change or differ between treatment arms in the given clinical trial. Constructs can be identified through, for example, review of the literature on preceding early-phase clinical trial or clinical trials of the same or similar treatments tested in a related patient population, patient focus groups, clinician input, or, if available, published standards for the given disease context (e.g., see Donovan et al. [13]).

The selected QOL instrument(s) should have a conceptual framework that supports the intended research objectives and have suitable measurement properties and supporting development work that is appropriate for the current clinical trial's patient population. Other considerations in selecting a QOL instrument(s) could be availability of desired language translations and mode adaptations (i.e., be adapted for the intended mode of administration), age appropriateness, cost, consistency with comparator trials, and overall patient burden. If a QOL instrument that measures all constructs or concepts of interest is not available, multiple instruments can be selected but care should be taken to ensure the total length of the combined assessments does not put undue burden on the patients. While ad hoc selection or deletion of items from a questionnaire is not recommended, a reasonable strategy to limit burden is to use only the validated subscales from a questionnaire that measure the constructs or concepts of interest. However, creating an ad hoc summary measure across instruments or across subscales is not recommended unless adequate psychometric testing of the combined score has been undertaken. Before finalization of the QOL battery, every item should be reviewed to ensure appropriateness for the patient population. Avoid instruments that will suffer from floor/ceiling effects in your patient population (e.g., asking about ability to complete very low-intensity activities in a relatively young and healthy population will result in most or all scores being at one extreme end of the range) or which include nonapplicable items or subscales (e.g., asking about injection site reactions when patients are only taking oral medications). Another useful exercise is to ask colleagues and patient advocates to review the planned QOL battery and ask for feedback about whether the length is appropriate, whether anything is unclear or not relevant, or if there are any key constructs or concepts that are missing.

In terms of patient burden, administering 25 or fewer questions is ideal and 100 or more questions would be unacceptable in most clinical trial participants. A general upper limit for acceptability is 50 questions in most patient populations. Based on the 75th percentile of item completion times in a study reported by Bennett et al. (14) patients can complete relatively simple questions in about 12 to 18 seconds per item depending on the mode of administration. This suggests that most patients can complete a 50-item questionnaire in approximately 10 to 15 minutes. Patient burden can be minimized by including only relevant subscales, using single-item or short-form versions of questionnaires when available, and administering questionnaires at relevant time points only. This includes the approach of not administering all questions at every time point (e.g., measuring the primary QOL outcome weekly over an 8-week trial with secondary/exploratory QOL outcomes assessed at baseline and after 8 weeks only).

If an appropriate QOL instrument (or combination of instruments) has not previously been developed to measure the constructs or concepts of interest in the chosen patient population and disease/treatment(s) setting then researchers may be tempted to develop a new QOL instrument. The choice to develop a new QOL instrument should be approached cautiously as development of a new instrument when done properly (see the Anatomy and Development of a QOL Questionnaire section) can be both time and resource intensive. An alternative strategy could be to use an instrument that has been validated in a related population or modify an existing validated instrument. In this situation, a study team might consider integrating the instrument in a phase II trial prior to the phase III trial to test the instrument. Alternatively, the study team can consider collecting additional data in the current (phase III) clinical trial to allow for confirming measurement properties concurrently with carrying out the planned statistical analysis related to the QOL objectives (see the Other QOL Statistical Analyses section).

Common modes of questionnaire administration include paper-and-pencil, electronic (web-based on Internet-enabled devices, app-based on personal or provided tablets or smartphones, or dedicated handheld devices), automated telephone, and in-person or telephone-based interview administrations. Considerations in selecting a mode of administration are discussed by Eremenco et al. (11). Electronic modes are generally preferred due to flexibility in scheduling (no restriction for assessments to be tied to clinic visits), automatic reminders to patients, automatic alerts to study and clinical staff, ability to monitor real-time compliance, elimination of data entry costs, and time-stamped entries. However, electronic modes can be expensive to implement with the potential added costs associated with distributing, tracking, and collecting devices if provided to sites and/or patients. Also, the study team should consider how technical issues will be identified and handled (e.g., whether a backup paper-and-pencil option or telephone-based interview option will be established). Location of reporting is an important factor in selecting the mode of administration. If the administration time points occur at clinic visits, paper-and-pencil administration may be an appropriate option. For frequent at-home reporting, an electronic mode of administration is almost a necessity. Two recent meta-analyses suggest that limited bias existed among various modes of administration (15,16).

The study team must also decide "why" the selected constructs or concepts should be measured (i.e., the objectives and hypotheses, if applicable, related to the QOL endpoint[s]). QOL assessment may be undertaken for a variety of reasons in a clinical trial. QOL may be measured as an outcome of treatment and as such, specified as the primary, secondary, or exploratory endpoint of the clinical trial. QOL assessment may be a component of safety monitoring (e.g., through patient self-reporting of symptomatic adverse events). QOL assessment may also be incorporated as an eligibility screener (e.g., to ensure enrollment of a symptomatic population). Finally, the intention of QOL assessment may be to measure mediators or moderators of treatment on another clinical outcome. The relationship among constructs, concepts, and objectives/hypotheses are often depicted in a conceptual model (17). Defining the objectives/hypotheses will likely inform selection of a QOL instrument as well as planned statistical analyses.

The study team must finally decide "where" and "when" the QOL instruments will be administered. Timing of assessments may depend on what is being measured and when the within-arm changes or between-arm differences are expected to be observed, but typically include prior to treatment (i.e., baseline) and at the end of treatment and may include additional administrations at one or more times during treatment and one or more times after the end of treatment (i.e., during longer term follow-up). Time points are commonly consistent with collection time points of other clinical data. A pretreatment baseline assessment is recommended. Further, assessment time points should be the same for all arms in a randomized study. Timing may also be influenced by the length of recall period of the QOL instrument and consideration of patient and administrative burden. Researchers may decide to request responses to QOL instrument(s) while the patient is at home or in clinic (or both). As previously discussed in considerations for mode selection, location of reporting is a key consideration in selecting the mode of administration. QOL instruments when administered at clinic visits should be administered to the patient prior to discussions of test results or health status to avoid bias. See Fairclough (18) for further reading about selection of appropriate QOL instrument administration time points.

Other Design Considerations

When integrating QOL instruments in oncology clinical trials, additional considerations may be necessary regarding blinding and randomization. Like most endpoints in oncology clinical trials, QOL endpoints in open-label and nonrandomized trials may be subject to various biases or issues in interpretation. When QOL is the primary or key secondary endpoint in a randomized trial, the baseline score should be used in stratification to ensure balance.

In addition to the collection of item scores on QOL questionnaires, the study team should consider at the design stage additional data that are needed for analysis. Such data may include reasons for missing data, auxiliary data to be used in imputation models to handle missing data, features of the administration (e.g., language, mode), and data needed for concurrent validation analyses (see the Other QOL Statistical Analyses section).

Integrating QOL Into the Protocol

Calvert et al. (19) systematically reviewed PRO-specific guidances for integrating PROs (including QOL) into research protocols and found 162 recommendations. Common recommendations included: (a) providing a rationale for measuring QOL/PRO; (b) stating QOL/PRO hypothesis and objectives; (c) specifying the timing of administering the QOL/PRO instrument(s); (d) stating the intended analyses (including missing data handling), sample size, and power; (e) specifying the questionnaire with the mode of administration; and (f) providing guidance on data collection and identifying site staff responsible for data collection elements. Development of international consensus standards for integrating QOL into protocols is ongoing. This effort has an eventual goal of releasing a PRO-specific extension called SPIRIT-PRO to existing protocol standards called Standard Protocol Items: Recommendations for Interventional Trials (SPIRIT; www.spirit-statement.org).

In order to prospectively minimize missing data, another protocol recommendation is to include QOL in the main study protocol with as much prominence as any other clinical endpoint. In particular, the QOL assessments should be integrated into the main study calendar of clinical tests and assessments. This emphasizes the importance of data collection for the QOL portion of the study to all study staff. The impact of missing data cannot be completely mitigated during analysis, so the best method for preventing the bias that missingness

may introduce is to design the QOL aspects of a trial in a way that will support collecting the most complete data possible. Other strategies include identifying staff members at each site who will be responsible for QOL aspects of the study and providing standardized training about QOL administration at each site. Site staff can be trained to check for skipped items and blank pages in paper-based questionnaires and to use backup methods (if available) to capture data for missed administrations. Using professional-looking paper booklets or electronic screens, convenient timing, applicable and understandable questions, and reasonably short questionnaires can also encourage patient completion. Real-time monitoring of completion rates can identify site-specific issues that can be addressed to improve completion rates for the remainder of the trial. Additional design considerations and strategies for minimizing missing data are detailed by Sloan et al. (20), Little et al. (21,22), Mercieca-Bebber et al. (23), and Mallinckrodt (24).

STATISTICAL ANALYSIS STRATEGIES

Statistical analysis strategies for QOL data are similar to those for any other clinical endpoint. The general recommendation is to craft an analysis plan around clearly specified hypotheses and endpoints while incorporating the design features of the clinical trial. However, in the case of QOL data, special care must be taken with regard to multiplicity and missing data, as described in subsequent sections. Like other endpoints in clinical trials, the recommended approach to statistical analysis of QOL data is the intent-to-treat (ITT) approach in which all enrolled patients are included in the analysis according to the randomized treatment assignment. In practice, because of lack of consent or noncompliance, a modified ITT approach is commonly employed in QOL analysis in which only patients with at least some minimum amount of QOL data are included in analysis according to the randomized treatment assignment (see the Missing Data section for more information regarding the assessment of selection bias related to exclusion of patients due to missing QOL data). Per-protocol analyses, which include only patients who receive treatment as specified in the protocol, may be warranted in some situations but should be considered as descriptive in nature only with statistical comparisons carried out with extreme caution due to the potential for selection bias.

Defining the Endpoint

Before developing the statistical analysis plan but after the QOL instrument, specific score of interest (which measures the construct or concept of interest), and time points are identified, the endpoint should be clearly defined from among several options (Figure 19.2). In a trial of adjuvant chemotherapy administered for 1 year

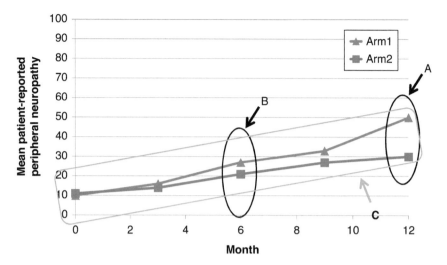

FIGURE 19.2 Selection of possible endpoints in a 12-month chemotherapy trial with peripheral neuropathy assessed using a validated patient questionnaire at baseline (prechemotherapy) and after 3, 6, 9, and 12 months of chemotherapy. Possible endpoints include: (A) peripheral neuropathy at the end of treatment assessment (12-month time point); (B) intermediate peripheral neuropathy at the 6-month time point; and (C) longitudinal peripheral neuropathy across all time points.

with patient-reported peripheral neuropathy assessed at baseline and after 3, 6, 9, and 12 months of treatment, numerous endpoints can be constructed. For example, the endpoint can be constructed as the peripheral neuropathy score at a fixed time point (e.g., after 12 months of treatment). Alternatively, a summary measure could be constructed as the average peripheral neuropathy score across the 3-, 6-, 9-, and 12-month time points or the endpoint could be defined as the collection of longitudinal assessments over time. In trials testing treatments given for a limited duration as in the previous adjuvant chemotherapy example or for a primary symptom management trial such as a 4-week hot flash study, the appropriate endpoint typically reflects the final outcome of the trial (e.g., the final time point at which QOL was assessed). Assessments during treatment may still be needed to capture intermediate outcomes or to describe side effects. In extended-duration trials where cancer treatments are administered indefinitely until the patient's cancer progresses, the appropriate endpoint may be a fixed time point that is both early enough in the trial so that most patients are still expected to be receiving treatment and late enough so that the treatment's impact is detectable. Summary measures across time points or longitudinal measurements over time may also be acceptable alternatives. The selected endpoint should reflect the objective of the clinical trial and should be clearly specified in the protocol. The nature and distribution of the endpoint is the basis for selecting the appropriate statistical analysis strategy from among options presented in the following sections.

Cross-Sectional Analysis

The types of cross-sectional analyses may include parametric (e.g., two-sample *t*-test or analysis of variance) or nonparametric (e.g., Wilcoxon rank-sum test or Kruskal–Wallis test) analysis, which compares ordinal or continuous QOL scores between two or more arms of the clinical trial at a fixed time point. Parametric approaches are appropriate for even ordinal QOL scores with limited response options and with large floor/ceiling effects for sample sizes as small as five observations per group based on the Central Limit Theorem (25,26) and may be preferred to ordinal approaches (27).

Analysis of covariance can be used to compare PRO scores at a fixed time point between arms while including the baseline QOL score as a covariate. This is generally regarded as the recommended approach due to providing the most power among all basic approaches for the comparisons of an ordinal or continuous QOL score between arms at a fixed time point (28). Multivariable linear regression can also be considered for analysis to account for other baseline patient characteristics in addition to baseline QOL score. Binary QOL endpoints can be compared between arms at a fixed time point using a chi-square or similar test, or using logistic regression to include baseline patient characteristics as covariates.

Summary Measures and Statistics

Summary measures and summary statistics are values that aggregate data across different time points within individual patients or across patients within the same arm, respectively, and can be calculated to examine differences between arms or time points. Summary measures are also sometimes called "composite endpoints." The area under the curve (AUC) is one such summary statistic that is computed for each patient by connecting observed scores at multiple time points, computing the areas of each resulting trapezoid, and summing the areas across time points. The AUC values (one per patient) can be compared between arms using the cross-sectional methods described in the previous section.

Another method is responder analysis, which classifies a patient as a responder if his or her change in QOL score is greater than a prespecified threshold value, where the threshold is often established using the methods described in the Interpretation section. The binary outcome of QOL response is a similar approach to how solid tumor measurements are handled through Response Evaluation Criteria in Solid Tumors (RECIST). The dichotomized endpoint can be compared across arms using chi-square or another similar test and supplemental analysis should include comparisons of the cumulative distribution functions (CDF) or cumulative response curves (29). Visual comparison of the CDFs allows for investigation of robustness of results across all possible change thresholds. Transforming longitudinal PRO data into time-to-event endpoints is another option, which allows for estimation and comparison of time from baseline to a clinically meaningful event such as worsening or improvement of symptoms. The subsequent time-to-event data can be analyzed using standard statistical approaches including Kaplan–Meier plots with log-rank tests or Cox regression. If including progression and/or death as events in a time-to-symptom-worsening endpoint (e.g., see Benzo et al. [30] or Bukowski et al. [31]), the types of events that are contributing to an observed difference between arms should be examined.

Use of summary measures and statistics can be useful tools when applied thoughtfully because they can aid in interpretation; be an approach to multiplicity by combining data across instruments, subscales, and/or time points into a single score and hypothesis test; and be an approach for handling missing data because a patient can often be evaluable even if a patient misses a QOL questionnaire at a limited number of assessment time points. Care when using summary measures or statistics should always be taken to ensure that high-level summarization does not mask important differences in individual constructs and/or time points and to consider any bias introduced by missing data on these endpoints. For example, Bell et al. (32) showed how missing data due to dropout can impact an AUC summary measure computed per patient, as previously described, versus an AUC summary statistic estimated per arm using a linear combination of estimated means from a general linear mixed model (see the next section).

Longitudinal Analysis

Regression-based longitudinal analyses are also a common, and by some considered to be the preferred method for analyzing longitudinal QOL data over the fixed time point analyses described in the previous section (33). These analyses can incorporate contrasts to estimate and test within-arm changes or between-arm differences (see Vogel [34] for a handy trick for coding

contrasts within SAS). The two broad types of longitudinal models within the general linear mixed model framework with maximum likelihood estimation include event-driven and time-driven models. In event-driven models, timing of the QOL assessment is considered as an ordered discrete or categorical predictor variable, such as in repeated measures models. In time-driven models, timing of the assessment is considered as a continuous predictor variable, such as in random coefficient or mixed effects growth curve models. If sample size permits, use of an unstructured covariance matrix is the most flexible option in event-driven and time-driven longitudinal models because this approach does not assume any pattern among errors. If sample size necessitates a reduction in the number of parameters being estimated, an alternative covariance structure can be selected from among plausible structures (e.g., first-order autoregressive structure when time points are equally spaced in an event-driven model) based on optimization of model fit criteria such as Akaike information criterion (AIC; see Littell et al. [35] for an example). Finally, general estimating equations (GEEs), which are an extension of generalized linear models, are another approach to modeling longitudinal continuous, binary, or count-based QOL data (36). Longitudinal models can range from rather simple to highly complex in form and can incorporate a variety of design elements such as stratification and clustering. Many common statistical programs such as SAS, SPSS, Stata, R, and Mplus can carry out longitudinal modeling. See Cappelleri et al. (37) for examples of longitudinal models with corresponding SAS code.

Other QOL Statistical Analyses

In clinical trials where measurement properties of the QOL instrument may not be fully understood in the given patient population and trial setting, confirmation of the measurement properties of the QOL instrument may be undertaken concurrently with the primary between-arm comparisons of QOL outcomes or other QOL objectives in the clinical trial. These types of analyses are often called concurrent validation analyses. For example, Mesa et al. (38) reported on the measurement properties of the Myelofibrosis Symptom Assessment Form (MFSAF) v2.0, which was adapted from the original MPN-SAF within the COMFORT-I trial, in which the MFSAF v2.0 was also a key secondary endpoint compared between arms (39). These analyses often require supplemental data collection (e.g., patient global impression of change or patient global impression of severity scales).

Another type of analysis involving QOL data is the computation and comparison of quality-adjusted life years (QALYs). QALY is a value that weights the quantity of survival by the quality of survival where quality is commonly measured using the EuroQoL's EQ-5D or other health utility questionnaire. Health utility values typically range from 0 (death) to 1 (perfect health), though some instruments such as the EQ-5D produce values between 0 and –1 representing health states that are worse than death. A basic patient-level QALY can be computed as the weighted sum of times spent at each utility level (i.e., the AUC of the utility measure) (18), though in many settings, modifications to this basic approach may be warranted, for example, to incorporate discounting of later benefits or to handle change in utility measures between assessments (40). QALYs in the absence of censored survival times can be compared between arms using standard two-group approaches (e.g., two-sample t-test, Wilcoxon rank-sum test, or analysis of covariance). If survival times are censored, then QALYs can be computed for each patient over the same fixed time period prior to any censoring and compared between arms using standard two-group approaches. An alternative approach incorporating all follow-up is a model-based approach in which the arm-level QALY can be computed using survival estimates from the Kaplan–Meier curve and mean utility scores from a repeated measures model. The arm-level QALYs can then be compared between arms using a bootstrap or similar approach (41).

Another analysis related to QALYs is called the quality-adjusted time without symptoms or toxicity (Q-TWiST) method, which partitions survival time by three health states: time with symptoms or toxicity (i.e., time during initiating treatment), time without symptoms or toxicity (i.e., time in between toxic time and relapse), and time with relapse (i.e., time between relapse and death) (42,43). Many other QOL analyses exist such as correlative and supplemental analyses to investigate the relationships among QOL constructs using Pearson or Spearman correlations or between QOL constructs/concepts and clinical outcomes using various regression-based approaches. Finally, mediation models may be used to investigate the mediating effects of QOL constructs/concepts on other outcomes; (37) or joint models of QOL and survival data to investigate the dependencies and relationship between both (44).

Multiplicity

Multiplicity describes a scenario in which multiple hypothesis tests are conducted resulting in inflation of the type I error rate. Multiplicity is a concern in QOL data due to common practices of using multiple questionnaires within the same study, using instruments that generate multiple subscale scores, and the measurement of QOL at multiple time points. In some clinical trials, strict control (e.g., control across all clinical endpoints measuring treatment benefit of which some are QOL endpoints) of the type I error rate may be desired, as in trials intended to support label claims. Outside of the label claim setting, multiplicity is commonly considered for the set of QOL endpoints separately from other clinical endpoints. Like with other clinical endpoints,

relaxation of type I error in early-stage clinical trials may be appropriate for QOL endpoints as confirmation of results is expected in subsequent trials. If a method for handling multiplicity is needed, methods have been developed for use with analysis of QOL data including common practices such as specifying a hierarchy of endpoints (primary, secondary, and exploratory QOL endpoints) or using an alpha-adjustment method such as Bonferroni, resampling methods, or multivariate tests. Summary scores and measures are another alternative for reducing the number of hypothesis tests (see the Summary Measures and Statistics section).

Missing Data

Like with any clinical endpoint, missing QOL data can be pervasive and lead to bias in results within a clinical trial. Missing data may also reduce power for statistical tests of interest. Patients may miss items within a questionnaire, or may miss an entire questionnaire at one or more time points during a clinical trial. Reasons for missed items and missed questionnaires can be quite variable including but not limited to patient or staff error/oversight; patient felt uncomfortable answering the question(s), felt that the question(s) was not applicable, or did not understand the question(s); missed clinic appointments; hospitalizations; patient feeling too ill to complete some or all of the questionnaire; or patient dropped out due to recovery, relapse/progression, or death. Reasons for missed questionnaires should be recorded to aid in understanding the potential biases that may be introduced by the missing data. Reasons for missed questionnaires when patients are filling out questionnaires at home (typically by electronic means) may be more challenging to capture than when patients are completing questionnaires at clinical visits.

The singly best approach to missing data is to minimize missing data prospectively through careful design, protocol implementation, staff training, and real-time monitoring (see Integrating QOL into the Protocol section). Despite the very best efforts to avoid missing data, missing data may still persist and subsequently require management in the analysis phase. For missing items, a limited number of missed items (typically less than half of the total number of items used to compute the score) are commonly accommodated within the published scoring algorithms of many QOL instruments using mean imputation. If the scoring algorithm is unclear regarding handling of missed items for the selected QOL instrument, the previously described mean imputation approach may be appropriate depending on the instrument. For some instruments, like the Patient-Reported Outcomes version of the Common Terminology for Adverse Events (PRO-CTCAE) (45,46), alternative imputation strategies may include logical imputation. The PRO-CTCAE asks up to three questions about the frequency, severity, and interference with usual or daily activities of a given symptom. If the patient responds as not having the symptom of interest in the first question and omits responses to the follow-up questions about the same symptom, a reasonable approach is to impute a value of 0 (for severity and interference) for the missing items. Fayers et al. (47) describe other approaches and provide a framework for handling missing data at the item level.

If missingness occurs at the instrument or subscale level, then the mechanism for missingness influences which method(s) is appropriate to handle the missingness. Different approaches may be appropriate depending on whether the instrument- or subscale-level missing data are missing completely at random (MCAR), missing at random (MAR), or missing not at random (MNAR). Prior to any testing of hypotheses, the amount and patterns of missing data and the reasons for missingness should be tabulated. Baseline covariates can also be compared using standard statistical methods (e.g., two-sample t-tests and chi-square tests) between patients with and without missing data for a given analysis to assess for bias. Other analyses may include modeling of the likelihood of missing data using logistic regression or time to dropout using time-to-event analyses.

The recommended approach to handle missing data is to incorporate all patient data that is available and use a method that assumes MAR (such as the previously described general linear mixed modeling as well as multiple imputation) in primary analysis, followed by various sensitivity analyses that assume other missing data mechanisms. Results across sensitivity analyses should be descriptively compared to assess the robustness of trial results across varying missing data assumptions. Methods that assume MCAR, such as methods requiring each patient to have complete data, and approaches that exclude a large number of patients should be avoided. While MAR methods may result in some bias when data are not missing at random, MAR methods are often robust when estimating differences between arms if observed covariates or earlier scores reflect the likelihood of subsequent missingness (48).

While missing data in QOL studies are often MNAR, imputation incorporating auxiliary data (e.g., physician, caregiver, or proxy data), pattern mixture modeling, and joint modeling convert the MNAR problem into a lesser MAR problem. Finally, an alternative flexible approach involves searching for the tipping point at which study conclusions are reversed (49). For further reading regarding approaches to missing QOL data, see Bell and Fairclough (50) or Fairclough (18).

INTERPRETATION

Some of the previously described analyses require a priori specification of a clinically significant or clinically meaningful change. For other analyses, while carrying out the statistical tests does not explicitly require specification of a threshold for clinical significance, proper interpretation of the results (e.g., mean differences between arms) requires understanding of its clinical significance or meaningfulness in addition to the statistical significance. Methods for interpreting the QOL changes over time or differences between arms fall into two broad categories: anchor-based and distribution-based methods (51). Anchor-based methods determine clinical significance by comparing QOL scores to other clinically relevant measures (called anchors). This can either be, for example, a comparison of cross-sectional QOL scores or a comparison of within-patient change scores between two clinically distinct groups. The grouping of patients can be based on clinical features or events or based on patients' own reported global impressions of severity or global impressions of change. Distribution-based methods rely on measures of variability of QOL scores. One common approach deems a half standard deviation as universally (though not minimally) clinically meaningful (52). Smaller effects such as 0.3 standard deviations may also be clinically meaningful.

Wyrwich et al. (53) provide an overview of anchor-based and distribution-based methods for establishing a threshold for within-patient clinically significant change. Such a threshold is typically specified in the protocol prior to initiation of analysis and is not determined concurrently using clinical trial data. For between-arm comparisons, clinical significance can be incorporated into a protocol a priori using published estimates, which can be used to interpret the observed mean differences at the time of analysis. If such estimates are not available for the selected QOL instrument, another approach at the time of analysis is to report the magnitude of each effect using a standardized effect size. Cohen (54) provides several cutoffs for interpreting standardized effect sizes, including the often used effect size demarcation of 0.2, 0.5, and 0.8 as representing small, medium, and large effects for within-arm (between two time points) and between-arm (between two arms) mean comparisons where within-arm standardized effect sizes are computed as in Equation 3 in Dunlap et al. (55) and between-arm standardized effect sizes are computed as the difference in means between two arms divided by the pooled standard deviation.

REPORTING OF RESULTS

The CONSORT statement is a minimum set of standards for reporting randomized clinical trials. In 2013, the CONSORT-PRO extension expanded upon CONSORT to include key concepts related to the reporting of QOL endpoints (56). The five additional checklist items specific to QOL include that (a) QOL be identified as a primary or secondary outcome in the abstract; (b) QOL hypotheses be stated; (c) validity and reliability of the QOL instrument be provided or cited;

(d) statistical approach for dealing with missing data be explicitly stated; and (e) QOL-specific limitations and generalizability be discussed. The modified CONSORT diagram published by Calvert et al. (56) includes reporting the reasons why QOL assessments were not completed and the samples size for QOL analyses.

CONCLUDING REMARKS

Many of the issues that have plagued the incorporation of QOL in oncology clinical trials in the past have been overcome in recent years by advancements in how we measure, incorporate, and analyze QOL. Further, growing importance and acceptance of QOL endpoints in oncology clinical trials is highlighted by the FDA approval of the cancer therapeutic rux-olitinib in 2005 in which patient-reported symptoms were a key secondary endpoint. Many resources exist to assist investigators now in incorporating QOL into oncology clinical trials, including several publications (18,37,57) and a recent webinar codeveloped by the U.S. National Cancer Institute and the International Society for Quality of Life Research (https://ncorp. cancer.gov/resources/materials.html#best). For the future, newly developed QOL instruments such as the PRO-CTCAE and Patient-Reported Outcomes Measurement Information System (PROMIS) along with ongoing efforts to develop standardized QOL instruments or identify constructs to be measured for individual cancer populations will further facilitate incorporation of the patient voice through QOL measurement into oncology trials. Finally, the ongoing SPIRIT-PRO and Setting International Standards in Analyzing Patient-Reported Outcomes and Quality of Life Endpoints Data for Cancer Clinical Trials (SISAQOL) (58) will also advance the field by defining standardized approaches for the incorporation of QOL into protocols and for the statistical analysis of QOL data, respectively.

REFERENCES

1. Outcomes of cancer treatment for technology assessment and cancer treatment guidelines. American Society of Clinical Oncology. *J Clin Oncol.* 1996;14(2):671–679.
2. Mayo NE. *Dictionary of Quality of Life and Health Outcomes Measurement.* 1st ed. International Society for Quality of Life Research; 2015.
3. U.S. Food and Drug Administration, U.S. National Cancer Institutes of Health. *BEST (Biomarkers, EndpointS, and other Tools).* Silver Spring, MD; 2016.
4. U.S. Food and Drug Administration. *Guidance for industry: patient-reported outcome measures: use in medical product development to support labelling claims [interent].* Silver Spring, MD; 2009.
5. Agency EM. *Reflection paper on the regulatory guidance for the use of health-related quality of life (HRQL) measures in the evaluation of medicinal products.* London, UK; 2005.
6. Scherber R, Dueck AC, Johansson P, et al. The Myeloproliferative Neoplasm Symptom Assessment Form (MPN-SAF): international prospective validation and reliability trial in 402 patients. *Blood.* 2011;118(2):401–408.
7. Reeve BB, Wyrwich KW, Wu AW, et al. ISOQOL recommends minimum standards for patient-reported outcome measures used in patient-centered outcomes and comparative effectiveness research. *Qual Life Res.* 2013;22(8):1889–1905.
8. Mokkink LB, Terwee CB, Patrick DL, et al. The COSMIN study reached international consensus on taxonomy, terminology, and definitions of measurement properties for health-related patient-reported outcomes. *J Clin Epidemiol.* 2010;63(7):737–745.
9. Wild D, Grove A, Martin M, et al. Principles of Good Practice for the Translation and Cultural Adaptation Process for Patient-Reported Outcomes (PRO) measures: report of the ISPOR Task Force for Translation and Cultural Adaptation. *Value Health.* 2005;8(2):94–104.
10. Wild D, Eremenco S, Mear I, et al. Multinational trials-recommendations on the translations required, approaches to using the same language in different countries, and the approaches to support pooling the data: the ISPOR Patient-Reported Outcomes Translation and Linguistic Validation Good Research Practices Task Force report. *Value Health.* 2009;12(4):430–440.
11. Eremenco S, Coons SJ, Paty J, et al. PRO data collection in clinical trials using mixed modes: report of the ISPOR PRO mixed modes good research practices task force. *Value Health.* 2014;17(5):501–516.
12. Dworkin RH, Turk DC, Peirce-Sandner S, et al. Research design considerations for confirmatory chronic pain clinical trials: IMMPACT recommendations. *Pain.* 2010;149(2):177–193.
13. Donovan KA, Donovan HS, Cella D, et al. Recommended patient-reported core set of symptoms and quality-of-life domains to measure in ovarian cancer treatment trials. *J Natl Cancer Inst.* 2014;106(7).
14. Bennett AV, Dueck AC, Mitchell SA, et al. Mode equivalence and acceptability of tablet computer-, interactive voice response system-, and paper-based administration of the U.S. National Cancer Institute's Patient-Reported Outcomes version of the Common Terminology Criteria for Adverse Events (PRO-CTCAE). *Health Qual Life Outcomes.* 2016;14:24.
15. Gwaltney CJ, Shields AL, Shiffman S. Equivalence of electronic and paper-and-pencil administration of patient-reported outcome measures: a meta-analytic review. *Value Health.* 2008;11(2):322–333.
16. Rutherford C, Costa D, Mercieca-Bebber R, et al. Mode of administration does not cause bias in patient-reported outcome results: a meta-analysis. *Qual Life Res.* 2016;25(3):559–574.
17. Rothman ML, Beltran P, Cappelleri JC, et al. Patient-reported outcomes: conceptual issues. *Value Health.* 2007;10(Suppl 2):S66–S75.
18. Fairclough DL. *Design and Analysis of Quality of Life Studies in Clinical Trials.* 2nd ed. Boca Raton, FL: Chapman & Hall/CRC; 2010.
19. Calvert M, Kyte D, Duffy H, et al. Patient-reported outcome (PRO) assessment in clinical trials: a systematic review of guidance for trial protocol writers. *PloS One.* 2014;9(10):e110216.
20. Sloan JA, Dueck AC, Erickson PA, et al. Analysis and interpretation of results based on patient-reported outcomes. *Value Health.* 2007;10(Suppl 2):S106–S115.
21. Little RJ, Cohen ML, Dickersin K, et al. The design and conduct of clinical trials to limit missing data. *Stat Med.* 2012;31(28):3433–3443.
22. Little RJ, D'Agostino R, Cohen ML, et al. The prevention and treatment of missing data in clinical trials. *New Engl J Med.* 2012;367(14):1355–1360.
23. Mercieca-Bebber R., Palmer MJ, Brundage M, et al. Design, implementation and reporting strategies to reduce the instance and impact of missing patient-reported outcome (PRO) data: a systematic review. *BMJ open.* 2016;6(6):e010938.

24. Mallinckrodt CH. *Preventing and Treating Missing Data in Longitudinal Clinical Trials.* New York, NY: Cambridge University Press; 2013.

25. Norman G. Likert scales, levels of measurement and the "laws" of statistics. *Adv Health Sci Educ Theory Pract.* 2010;15(5):625–632.

26. Murray J. Likert data: what to use, parametric or non-parametric? *Inter J Bus Soc Sci.* 2013;4(11):258–264.

27. Sullivan LM, D'Agostino RB Sr. Robustness and power of analysis of covariance applied to ordinal scaled data as arising in randomized controlled trials. *Stat Med.* 2003;22(8):1317–1334.

28. Vickers AJ. The use of percentage change from baseline as an outcome in a controlled trial is statistically inefficient: a simulation study. *BMC Med Res Methodol.* 2001;1:6.

29. Cappelleri JC, Zou KH, Bushmakin AG, et al. Cumulative response curves to enhance interpretation of treatment differences on the self-esteem and relationship questionnaire for men with erectile dysfunction. *BJU Int.* 2013;111(3 Pt B):E115–E120.

30. Benzo R, Farrell MH, Chang CC, et al. Integrating health status and survival data: the palliative effect of lung volume reduction surgery. *Am J Respir Crit Care Med.* 2009;180(3):239–246.

31. Bukowski R, Cella D, Gondek K, et al. Effects of sorafenib on symptoms and quality of life: results from a large randomized placebo-controlled study in renal cancer. *Am J Clin Oncol.* 2007;30(3):220–227.

32. Bell ML, King MT, Fairclough DL. Bias in area under the curve for longitudinal clinical trials with missing patient reported outcome data: summary measures versus summary statistics. *SAGE Open.* 2014;4.

33. Mallinckrodt CH, Lane PW, Schnell D, et al. Recommendations for the primary analysis of continuous endpoints in longitudinal clinical trials. *Drug Inform J.* 2008;42:303–319.

34. Vogel RL. An easy and convenient method for constructing contrasts. *Proceed Southeast SAS Users Group.* 2009;1(5):Paper SD-013.

35. Littell RC, Pendergast J, Natarajan R. Modelling covariance structure in the analysis of repeated measures data. *Stat Med.* 2000;19(13):1793–1819.

36. Fitzmaurice GM, Laird NM, Ware JH. *Applied Longitudinal Analysis.* 2nd ed. Hoboken, NJ: John Wiley & Sons; 2011.

37. Cappelleri JC, Zou KH, Bushmakin AG, et al. *Patient-Reported Outcomes: Measurement, Implementation, and Interpretation.* Boca Raton, FL: Chapman & Hall/CRC; 2013.

38. Mesa RA, Gotlib J, Gupta V, et al. Effect of ruxolitinib therapy on myelofibrosis-related symptoms and other patient-reported outcomes in COMFORT-I: a randomized, double-blind, placebo-controlled trial. *J Clin Oncol.* 2013;31(10):1285–1292.

39. Verstovsek S, Mesa RA, Gotlib J, et al. A double-blind, placebo-controlled trial of ruxolitinib for myelofibrosis. *New Engl J Med.* 2012;366(9):799–807.

40. Billingham LJ, Abrams KR, Jones DR. Methods for the analysis of quality-of-life and survival data in health technology assessments. *Health Technol Assess.* 1999;3(10):1–152.

41. Khan I. *Design & Analysis of Clinical Trials for Economic Evaluation & Reimbursement: An Applied Approach Using SAS & STATA.* Boca Raton, FL: Chapman & Hall/CRC Biostatistics Series; 2016.

42. Gelber RD, Goldhirsch A. A new endpoint for the assessment of adjuvant therapy in postmenopausal women with operable breast cancer. *J Clin Oncol.* 1986;4(12):1772–1779.

43. Glasziou PP, Cole BF, Gelber RD, et al. Quality adjusted survival analysis with repeated quality of life measures. *Stat Med.* 1998;17(11):1215–1229.

44. Ibrahim JG, Chu H, Chen LM. Basic concepts and methods for joint models of longitudinal and survival data. *J Clin Oncol.* 2010;28(16):2796–2801.

45. Basch E, Reeve BB, Mitchell SA, et al. Development of the National Cancer Institute's patient-reported outcomes version of the common terminology criteria for adverse events (PRO-CTCAE). *J Natl Cancer Inst.* 2014;106(9).

46. Dueck AC, Mendoza TR, Mitchell SA, et al. Validity and Reliability of the US National Cancer Institute's Patient-Reported Outcomes Version of the Common Terminology Criteria for Adverse Events (PRO-CTCAE). *JAMA Oncol.* 2015;1(8):1051–1059.

47. Fayers PM, Curran D, Machin D. Incomplete quality of life data in randomized trials: missing items. *Stat Med.* 1998;17(5–7):679–696.

48. Donaldson GW, Moinpour CM. Learning to live with missing quality-of-life data in advanced-stage disease trials. *J Clin Oncol.* 2005;23(30):7380–7384.

49. Ratitch B, O'Kelly M, Tosiello R. Missing data in clinical trials: from clinical assumptions to statistical analysis using pattern mixture models. *Pharmaceut Stat.* 2013;12(6):337–347.

50. Bell ML, Fairclough DL. Practical and statistical issues in missing data for longitudinal patient-reported outcomes. *Stat Method Med Research.* 2014;23(5):440–459.

51. Guyatt GH, Osoba D, Wu AW, et al. Methods to explain the clinical significance of health status measures. *Mayo Clinic Proceed.* 2002;77(4):371–383.

52. Norman GR, Sloan JA, Wyrwich KW. The truly remarkable universality of half a standard deviation: confirmation through another look. *Exp Rev Pharmacoecon Outcomes Res.* 2004;4(5):581–585.

53. Wyrwich KW, Norquist JM, Lenderking WR, et al. Methods for interpreting change over time in patient-reported outcome measures. *Qual Life Res.* 2013;22(3):475–483.

54. Cohen J. *Statistical Power Analysis for the Behavioral Sciences.* Hillsdale, NJ: Lawrence Erlbaum Associates; 1988.

55. Dunlap WP, Cortina JM, Vaslow JB, Burke MJ. Meta-analysis of experiments with matched groups or repeated measures designs. *Psycholog Methods.* 1996;1(2):170–177.

56. Calvert M, Blazeby J, Altman DG, et al. Reporting of patient-reported outcomes in randomized trials: the CONSORT PRO extension. *JAMA.* 2013;309(8):814–822.

57. Sloan JA. Challenges in QOL assessment. Overview and introduction. *Curr Prob Cancer.* 2005;29(6):274–277.

58. Bottomley A, Pe M, Sloan J, et al. Analysing data from patient-reported outcome and quality of life endpoints for cancer clinical trials: a start in setting international standards. *Lancet Oncol.* 2016;17(11):e510–e514.

20

Adaptive Designs

Tze L. Lai, Ying Lu, and Ka Wai Tsang

In his 2010 budget request, the Director of the National Cancer Institute earmarked "reengineering" cancer clinical trials as a research initiative. The reason why reengineering is needed is that although remarkable progress in biomedical sciences has raised new hope for cancer treatment, the hope has not materialized because of the relatively small number of new anticancer agents that were demonstrated to be efficacious in phase III clinical trials. Critical barriers to clinical and translational progress in cancer therapeutics arise from the inadequacy of traditional clinical trial designs—from initial dose determination to confirmatory trials for regulatory approval. This chapter describes adaptive clinical trial designs to address these critical barriers and provide methodologic advances toward the envisioned reengineering in all phases of therapeutic development. The year 2010 also marked the appearance of the much awaited Food and Drug Administration Draft Guidance for Industry on Adaptive Design. Two years later, the President's Council of Advisors on Science and Technology (PCAST) issued a report on "Propelling Innovations in Drug Discovery, Development, and Evaluation" and argued for using "innovative new approaches for trial design that can provide more information more quickly" as "it is increasingly possible to obtain clear answers with many fewer patients and with less time" by focusing studies on "specific subsets of patients most likely to benefit, identified based on validated biomarkers." At the planning stage, there is usually inadequate information about the heterogeneity of subjects in their response to the cancer treatment being tested, but the information becomes increasingly available during the course of the trial. The basic idea of an adaptive design is to adapt at prespecified times the trial to the increasing information set, thereby improving its efficiency. In this chapter we describe important developments, many of which are still ongoing, in adaptive clinical trial designs for cancer treatments.

ADAPTATION IN PHASE I DESIGNS

In typical phase I studies in the development of relatively benign drugs, the drug is initiated at low doses and subsequently escalated to show safety at a level where some positive response occurs, and healthy volunteers are used as study subjects. This paradigm does not work for chemotherapies in cancer, for which a non-negligible probability of severe toxic reaction can be accepted to give the patient some chance of a favorable response to the treatment. Therefore, patients are used as study subjects, and it is widely accepted that some degree of toxicity must be tolerated to experience any substantial therapeutic effects. In particular, for cytoxic treatments, an acceptable proportion p of patients experiencing dose-limiting toxicities (DLTs) is generally agreed on before the trial, which depends on the type and severity of the DLT; the dose resulting in this proportion is thus referred to as the maximum tolerated dose (MTD). Commonly used designs in phase I cancer trials are up-and-down designs that implicitly place their focus on the safety of the patients in the trial, beginning from a conservatively low starting dose and escalating cautiously. Basically, they are sequential first-order Markov schemes choosing from a discrete dose set in which the next dose is equal or adjacent to the current dose. The widely used 3 + 3 design can be viewed as a cohort-by-cohort up-and-down scheme, but it has been recognized as unsatisfactory on both ethical and efficiency grounds because it results in mostly subtherapeutic doses and provides inadequate information to estimate the MTD for a subsequent phase II trial. To address this difficulty, Eisenhauer et al. (1) pointed out the need for (1) methods to determine more informative starting doses, (2) pharmacokinetic-guided dose-finding methods, and (3) model-based methods for dose escalation/deescalation. Chapters 10 to 12 have given overviews of these methods that have been steadily replacing the 3 + 3 designs. Here we describe some recent developments in adaptive phase I designs. Because the sample size is typically small, model-based designs are basically Bayesian sequential designs, an overview of which is already given in Chapter 15. We therefore focus in the rest of this section on (1) adaptive enhancement of these Bayesian designs, (2) their extensions to combination therapies, and (3) their modifications for cytostatic agents.

Global Risk-Benefit Function and Adaptive Designs Via Approximate Dynamic Programming

A commonly used model-based approach to phase I cancer clinical trial design assumes the usual logistic regression model $F_\theta(x) = 1/(1 + e^{-(a + \beta x)})$ for the probability $F_\theta(x)$ of DLT at dose level x, in which $\beta > 0$ and $\theta = (a, \beta)$ is unknown and to be estimated from the observed pairs (x_i, y_i), where $y_i = 1$ if the ith subject, treated at dose x_i, experiences DLT and $y_i = 0$ otherwise. The most frequent approach to inference on θ uses the likelihood function and estimates θ by maximum likelihood, whereas the Bayesian approach assumes a prior distribution of θ and uses the posterior distribution for inference on θ. One could denote the MTD by $\eta = F_\theta^{-1}(p)$ and the posterior distribution of θ based on $(x_1, y_1), \ldots, (x_k, y_k)$ by Π_k and let Π_0 denote the prior distribution. The Bayes estimate of η with respect to squared error loss is the posterior mean $E_{\Pi_k}(\eta)$, which is used in the continual assessment method proposed by O'Quigley, Pepe, and Fisher (2) to set the dose for the next patient; i.e., $x_{k+1} = E_{\Pi_k}(\eta)$. Instead of the posterior mean, the escalation with overdose control (EWOC) scheme proposed by Babb, Rogatko, and Zacks (3) sets x_{k+1} equal to the ω-quantile of the posterior distribution, where $0 < \omega < 1/2$ is chosen to be slightly less than p and is called the "feasibility bound." Instead of squared error loss, EWOC with feasibility bound ω uses the functional $x = x(\Pi)$ that minimizes the asymmetric loss function $E_\Pi[l(\eta, x)]$, where

$$\ell(\eta, x) = \begin{cases} \omega(\eta - x), & \text{if } x \le \eta \\ (1-\omega)(x - \eta), & \text{if } x \ge \eta. \end{cases} \quad \text{(Eq. 20-1)}$$

Note that the dose for the nth patient in CRM or EWOC depends only on the posterior distribution Π_{n-1}; that is, x_n is a functional $f(\Pi_{n-1})$ of Π_{n-1}. This functional defines $\{\Pi_k: k \ge 0\}$ as a Markov chain whose states are distributions on the parameter space Θ and whose state transitions are given by the Bayesian updating scheme: Given current state Π (which is a prior distribution of θ), let $x = f(\Pi)$ and generate first θ from Π and then y ~ Bern($F_\theta(x)$). The new state is the posterior distribution of θ given (x, y).

If the objective of a phase I cancer trial is just to estimate the MTD, then one should consider Bayesian sequential designs that are optimal, in some sense, for this estimation problem. See Whitehead and Brunier (4) and Haines, Perevozskaya, and Rosenberger (5), who

used the theory of optimal design of experiments to construct Bayesian c- and D-optimal designs and further impose a relaxed Bayesian feasibility constraint on the design to avoid highly toxic doses. We have pointed out that CRM or EWOC treats the next patient at the dose x that minimizes $E_\Pi[l(\theta, x)]$ for $l(\eta, x)$ given by $(\eta - x)^2$ or by (Eq. 20-1), where Π is the current posterior distribution. This is tantamount to dosing the next patient at the best guess of η, where "best" means "closest" according to some measure of distance from η. On the other hand, a Bayesian c- and D-optimal design aims at generating doses that provide most information for estimating the dose-toxicity curve to benefit future patients. To resolve this dilemma between treatment of patients in the trial and efficient experimental design for posttrial parameter estimation, Bartroff and Lai (6) considered the finite-horizon optimization problem of choosing the dose levels $x_1, x_2, \ldots, x_n$ sequentially to minimize the global cost function

$$E_{\Pi_0}\left[\sum_{i=1}^n h(\eta, x_i) + g(\hat{\eta}_n, \eta) \right], \quad \text{(Eq. 20-2)}$$

in which Π_0 denotes the prior distribution of θ, $h(\eta, x_i)$ represents the loss for the ith patient in the trial, $\hat{\eta}_n$ is the terminal estimate of the MTD (of benefit to future patients), and g represents a terminal loss function. They show how approximate dynamic programming can be used to compute the optimizing doses x_i that depend on $n - i$, where the horizon n is the sample size of the trial. Therefore, these are not of the form $x_i = f(\Pi_{i-1})$ considered previously.

In terms of "individual" and "collective" ethics, note that (Eq. 20-2) measures the individual effect of the dose x_k on the kth patient through $h(\eta, x_k)$, and its collective effect on future patients through $\sum_{i>k} h(\eta, x_i) + g(\hat{\eta}_n, \eta)$. By using a discounted infinite-horizon version of (Eq. 20-2), Bartroff and Lai (7) provided solutions of the form $x_i = f(\Pi_{i-1})$ for some functional f that only depends on Π_{i-1}. Specifically, take a discount factor $0 < \delta < 1$ and replace (Eq. 20-2) by $E_{\Pi_0}\left[\sum_{i=1}^\infty h(\eta, x_i) \delta^{i-1} \right]$ as the definition of global risk. The main complexity of the infinite-horizon problem is that the dose x for the next patient involves also consideration for future patients who will receive optimal doses themselves; these future doses depend on the future posterior distribution. Bartroff and Lai (8) reduced the complexity by considering two (instead of infinitely many) future patients, and use MATLAB to implement the procedure that chooses the next dose x to minimize $E_\Pi l(\eta, x, \Pi)$ when the current posterior distribution of θ is Π, where

$$l(h, x; \Pi) = h(\eta, x) + \lambda E_\Pi\{E_\Pi[h(\eta', x') \mid x_1 = x, y_1]\}. \quad \text{(Eq. 20-3)}$$

In (Eq. 20-3), $\eta' = F_{\theta'}^{-1}(p)$ with $\theta' \sim \Pi'$, and Π' and x' defined as follows. The first summand in (Eq. 20-3) measures the (toxicity) effect of the dose x on the patient receiving it. The second summand considers the patient who follows and receives a myopic dose x', which minimizes the patient's posterior loss; the myopic dose is optimal because there are no more patients involved in (Eq. 20-3). The effect of x on this second patient is through the posterior distribution Π' that updates Π after observing (x_1, y_1), with $x_1 = x$. Because y_1 is not yet observed, the expectation outside the curly brackets is taken over $y_1 \sim \text{Bern}(F_q(x))$, with $\theta \sim \Pi$.

A closely related approach is used in the "Bayesian decision-theoretic design" of Fan, Lu, and Wang (9). They assume a "working" Bayesian model with beta priors $\text{Beta}(a_i, b_i)$ for the toxicity rates p_i at increasing doses x_i belonging to a prescribed discrete set. Monotonicity in the means $\mu_i = a_i/(a_i + b_i)$ is achieved by fixing $c = a_i + b_i$ and choosing $a_i = r_i c$ with increasing r_i such that the MTD x_{i*} corresponds to $r_{i*} = p$. From this conjugate family of Beta prior distributions, they also apply a "working" adjustment of the data via the Pool Adjacent Violators Algorithm in isotonic regression to ensure that the adjusted sample toxicity rates also satisfy the monotonicity constraint. Analogous to the global cost function, they use a utility function that reflects an individual's payoff by participating in the trial and the gain for future patients in terms of the accuracy of the MTD estimate. They initialize by assigning a cohort to the lowest dose and then escalate the dose, one increment at a time, until the first toxicity occurs. Then they use a two-step look-ahead rule similar to (Eq. 20-3) but for the finite-horizon setting (with no more than n patients). They also allow for early termination "whenever the evidence for the current conclusion is considered sufficient," similar to a stopping criterion for CRM proposed by Heyd and Carlin (10).

Extension to Combination Therapies

Lee, Fan and Lu (11) have considered extending the approach in the preceding paragraph to a combination therapy involving two cytotoxic anticancer agents. They still use Beta prior distribution $\text{Beta}(a_j, b_j)$ for agent $j = 1$, 2 and a partial order $\prec$ of the dose-agent combinations such that $p_{ij} < p_{hk}$ whenever $(i,j) \prec (h,k)$. They also describe how the prior parameters can be elicited from clinicians and adjusted to satisfy the partial ordering as follows. The clinician provides his or her best estimate of $\mu_{ij} = a_{ij}/(a_{ij} + b_{ij})$ at each dose-agent combination and is asked to adjust the estimate so that the order restriction $\mu_{ij} \leq \mu_{hk}$ for $(i,j) \prec (h,k)$ is satisfied. A statistical default option that assumes independent toxicities of the agents is also provided. Extrapolating a subject's response at a single dose-agent combination to worse (respectively, better) combinations by the partial ordering if the subject experiences (respectively, does not have) a DLT, one obtains the following updates of the parameters

of the posterior Beta distribution. Suppose a cohort of n_{ij} patients were tested at (i, j), in whom t experienced DLTs. Then $a_{ij}^{new} = a_{ij}^{old} + t$ and $b_{ij}^{new} = b_{ij}^{old} + n_{ij} - t$, and

$$(a_{b,k}^{new}, b_{b,k}^{new}) = \begin{cases} (a_{bk}^{old} + t, b_{bk}^{old}), & \text{for } (h,k) \succ (i,j) \\ (a_{bk}^{old}, b_{bk}^{old} + n_{ij} - t), & \text{for } (h,k) \prec (i,j) \\ (a_{bk}^{old}, b_{bk}^{old}), & \text{for all other } (h,k). \end{cases}$$

(Eq. 20-4)

These posterior means satisfy the order restrictions. Because of the complexity of the problem, Lee, Fan, and Lu (11) only consider myopic rules and only provide a partial extension of the single-agent case. Other adaptive phase I designs for combination therapies have been proposed by Mandrekar, Cui, and Sargent (12), Yin and Yuan (13), Yuan and Yin (14), Braun and Wang (15) and Wages, Conaway, and O'Quigley (16).

Modifications for Cytostatic Therapies

A cytostatic therapy works by stopping the cancer cells from multiplying. The usual clinical trial design for a cytotoxic agent aims at a MTD for the agent to shrink the tumor. In contrast, cytostatic agents may slow or stop the growth of tumors without shrinking existing tumors. Therefore, the standard cytotoxic trial designs are unsuitable for cytostatic agents. New challenges have been pointed out by Freidlin and Simon (17):

In the early stages of development, reliable assays to identify the sensitive patients that express the target are often not available. This complicates evaluation of targeted agents as a result of the dilution of the treatment effect by the presence of the patients who do not benefit from the agent. Furthermore, some of these agents are thought to be cytostatic and are only expected to inhibit tumor growth without shrinking existing tumors. Traditionally, clinical development of cytotoxic agents involved a single arm phase II evaluation of the response rate. In most cases, this approach is no longer adequate for the development of cytostatic agents.

Millar and Lynch (18) and Korn et al. (19) have pointed out the urgency of developing new designs to avoid rejecting a clinically useful cytostatic agent because it is tested using standard cytotoxic trial designs. Rosner, Stadler, and Ratain (20) propose a randomized discontinuation design that initially treats all patients with the agent and then randomizes in a double-blind fashion to continuing therapy or placebo only for those patients whose disease is stable. They claim that by doing this, investigators can determine whether the slow tumor growth is due to the drug or to patients with naturally slow-growing tumors. In their evaluation of the randomized discontinuation design, Freidlin and Simon (17) agree that the design "can be useful in some settings in the early development of targeted agents where a reliable assay to select patients expressing the target is not available." Stone, Wheeler, and Barge (21), however, advocated randomized controlled (rather than single-arm) trials, and furthermore, they suggest that the endpoint for testing the activity of cytostatic agents should be progression-free survival instead of tumor response in cytotoxic trial designs. Xu et al. (22) have recently proposed a two-stage Bayesian adaptive design for cytostatic agents via model adaptation. Stage I uses the standard Bayesian approach to search for the MTD, and stage 2 uses a Bayesian outcome-adaptive randomization scheme to search for the optimal biological dose under the constraint that it does not exceed the MTD, randomizing according to the posterior probabilities of the effectiveness of the candidate doses.

ADAPTATION IN PHASE II DESIGNS

The MTD determined from a phase I study is used in a subsequent phase II study, in which a cohort of patients is treated, and the outcomes are related to the prespecified target or bar. If the results meet or exceed the target, the treatment is declared worthy of further study; otherwise, further development is stopped. The most widely used designs for these single-arm phase II trials are Simon's (23) two-stage design, which allows stopping of the trial at the first stage if the treatment has not shown beneficial effect that is measured by the response probability. Simon's design requires specification of the proportion p_0 for the null hypothesis $H_0: p = p_0$ and of $p_1 > p_0$. The design has been generalized by Jung et al. (24,25) and Lu et al (26) to allow for partial responses. Whether the new treatment is declared promising in a phase II trial depends strongly on the prescribed p_0 and p_1. Vickers, Ballen, and Scher (27) concluded that uncertainty in the choice of p_0 and p_1 can increase the likelihood that a treatment with no viable positive treatment effect proceeds to phase III, or a treatment with positive treatment effect is abandoned at phase II. Still within the single arm framework, Bartroff and Lai (6) proposed an adaptive design that uses generalized likelihood ratio (GLR) statistics for testing $H_0: p \leq p_0$, without specification of the alternative p_1 (which the GLR statistic uses the observations collected during the trial to estimate).

Bartroff and Lai's adaptive design is a three-stage design, which (1) allows early stopping for either efficacy or futility, (2) uses the data from the first stage to estimate the second-stage sample size (hence adaptive midcourse sample size reestimation), and (3) adds a third stage that terminates at the maximum sample size prescribed in the protocol. The maximum sample size uses an idea introduced by Lai and Shih (28) in

their development of the theory of group sequential tests. To test the one-sided hypothesis $H_0: \theta \leq \theta_0$ in an exponential family, suppose the significance level is α and no more than M observations $X1, X2, \ldots$ are to be taken. The fixed sample size test that rejects H_0 if $\sum_{i=1}^{M} X_i \geq c_a$ has maximal power at any alternative $\theta > \theta_0$. Although funding and administrative considerations often play an important role in the choice of M, justification of this choice in clinical trial protocols is typically based on some prescribed power $1 - \beta$ at an alternative $\theta(M)$ "implied" by M. The implied alternative is defined by that M and can be derived from the prescribed power $1 - \beta$ at $\theta(M)$. Banerjee and Tsiatis (29) have proposed a two-stage adaptive phase II design using Bayesian decision theory that uses simulated annealing to implement, and Englert and Kieser (30) and Shan et al. (31) have used conditional power and alternative search algorithms to develop alternative two-stage adaptive designs. In comparison, Bartroff and Lai's (6) design is much simpler and more efficient according to their theory of adaptive designs, which shows two-stage designs using sample size reestimation can have low power while the three-stage designs are nearly optimal.

To avoid the problem of choosing an artificially small p_0, whether intentionally by a practitioner wanting to give the treatment the "best chance" of showing a positive effect if one exists, or unintentionally because of inaccurate information about the control, Thall et al. (32) have extended Simon's two-stage design to randomized two-arm phase II trials. Bartroff and Lai (6) showed that the adaptive three-stage design can also be readily extended to randomized phase II cancer trials for testing $H_0: p \leq q$, where q is the response rate of the control that is also to be estimated besides p from the trial data.

SEAMLESS PHASE I/II-DESIGNS

Gooley et al (33) proposed to use efficacy and toxicity data and study three ad hoc designs. Thall and Russell (34) proposed a design combining binary toxicity data and trinomial (no, moderate, severe) response data into a single variable that can be modeled by proportional odds regression with a prior distribution on its parameters. Subsequent proposals to combine efficacy and toxicity outcomes included Ivanova (35), Braun (36), Thall and Cook (37), and Thall, Nguyen, and Estey (38). These designs are basically of the phase I dose-finding type but also include efficacy considerations to determine the dose for phase II efficacy testing.

While the traditional phase I/II designs are of the form that finding estimate $\hat{\eta}_0$ of MTD η in phase I and then test the null hypothesis $K_0: p(\hat{\eta}_0) \leq p_0$ in phase II, Bartroff, Lai, and Narasimhan (39) propose an integrated approach in designing early-phase dose-finding trials. In their design, a joint efficacy-toxicity model is chosen to model toxicity y_i and efficacy z_i, which can be dependent, and a phase I design is chosen to estimate MTD. In phase II, a group-sequential, test of H_0: $P(\text{efficacy}|x = \eta) \le p_0$ rather than $K_0: p(\hat{\eta}_0) \le p_0$ is used. The MTD estimate $\hat{\eta}$ is updated at each stage and always dose patients at the current estimated MTD "eta hat". If H_0 is rejected, $\hat{\eta}$ is updated with all phase I/II data as the recommended dose. In many dose-finding trials, however, there are only finitely many dose levels $\lambda_1 < \lambda_2 < \dots < \lambda_d$. Let the toxicity and efficacy probabilities be

$$\phi = P(y = 1 \mid x = \lambda_i), \pi_i = P(z = 1 \mid x = \lambda_i), i = 1, \dots d.$$
(Eq. 20-5)

The MTD is set to be $\eta = \lambda_{i^*}$, where $i^* = \max\{i: \phi_i \le q\}$ if $\phi_i \ge q$ for some i or $i^* = 1$ if otherwise. Therefore, the phase II hypotheses can be expressed as $H_0: \pi_{i^*} \le p_0$ versus $H_1: \pi_{i^*} \ge p_1$. Bartroff, Lai, and Narasimhan (39) have extended the seamless phase I/II design to this setting. They also consider the more general case where the toxicity and efficacy observations may not be independent by introducing d additional parameters in the form of the global cross ratios

$$\rho_i = \frac{\Pi_i(0,0)\Pi_i(1,1)}{\Pi_i(1,0)\Pi_i(0,1)}, i = 1 \dots, d,$$
(Eq. 20-6)

where $\Pi_i(y, z) = P(y_t = y, z_y = z \mid x_t = \lambda_i)$. The log-likelihood at the kth interim analysis in phase II for this general case can be computed as a function $l_k(\pi, \varphi, \rho)$. For $j = 0,1$, the GLR statistic associated with H_j is $\ell_{k,j} = \ell_k(\pi, \phi, \rho) - \ell_k(\tilde{\pi}_k^j, \tilde{\phi}_k^j, \tilde{\rho}_k^j)$, where $\hat{\pi}, \hat{\phi}, \hat{\rho}$ are the MLEs subject to the order restrictions $\pi_1 \le \dots \le \pi_d$ and $\phi_1 \le \dots \le \phi_d$, and $\tilde{\pi}_k^j, \tilde{\phi}_k^j, \tilde{\rho}_k^j$ are the MLEs subject to these order restrictions plus the constraints $\pi_{i_k^*}^j \le p_0$ for $j = 0$ and $\pi_{i_k^*}^j \ge p_1$ for $j = 1$.

Phase I/II Designs for Combination Therapies

The first section of the chapter, Adaptation in Phase I Designs discussed adaptive designs for phase I trials to determine the doses of combination therapies for use in phase II trials. Harrington et al. (40) pointed out that the need to design "smarter, faster clinical trials, appropriate for the era of molecularly targeted therapies" is particularly pressing for early-phase trials of combination therapies, especially those involving targeted therapies, and the authors advocate for the development and use of adaptive designs to meet this need. Standard rule-based dose-finding designs such as up-and-down rules that only consider the last cohort to guide escalation or deescalation to the nearest neighbor typically lead to high subtheapeutical doses for combination therapies that are considerably more complex than single agents. The investigators argue that a promising future lies in model-based designs that

can combine trial data (which include measurements of toxicity, efficacy, pharmacokinetics, and pharmacodynamics) with prior knowledge from the literature and previous related studies. In particular, these are adaptive model-based designs that allow investigators to use accumulated information during the course of the trial to learn the toxicity contour (formed by dose combinations that all have a prescribed target probability of DLT) and choose the most efficacious dose on the contour. Harrington et al. reviewed some adaptive designs in this direction already developed and used, including Houede et al. (41) and Whitehead, Thygesen, and Whitehead (42), which are phase I/II trials, and the adaptive phase I designs of Dragalin, Federov, and Wu (43) for selecting drug combinations based on efficacy-toxicity response. In fact, the approach used by Bartroff, Lai, and Narasimhan (39) in the preceding paragraph can be extended to modify this kind of adaptive phase I designs for combination therapies to develop seamless phase I/II designs to test for efficacy in phase II.

ADAPTIVE PHASE III (SURVIVAL-ENDPOINT) TRIALS

Overall survival (and occasionally progression-free survival) has been a definitive endpoint for a phase III cancer trial, which usually has a Data and Safety Monitoring Committee that conducts interim analysis. As pointed out by Lan and DeMets (44), survival trials have two timescales—calendar time t and information time $V(t)$, which is the null variance of the test statistic at t. The information time $V(t)$ is the intrinsic timescale for interim data but is typically unknown before time t unless restrictive assumptions are made a priori. Let $n = n' + n''$ be the total sample size, with n' patients randomized to treatment X and n'' to treatment Y; let $T_i \ge 0$ denote the entry time and $X_i > 0$ the survival time after entry of the ith subject in treatment group X; and $T_{j'}$ and Y_j denote the entry time and survival time after entry of the jth subject in treatment group Y. The subjects are followed until they fail or withdraw from the study or until the study is terminated. Let $\xi'_{i'}$ (or $\xi''_{j'}$) denote the time to withdrawal, possibly infinite, of the ith (or jth) subject in the treatment group X (or Y). Thus, the data at calendar time t consist of $(X_i(t), \delta'_{i'}(t))$, $i = 1, \dots, n'$, and $(Y_j(t), \delta''_{j'}(t))$, $j = 1, \dots, n''$, where $X_i(t) = \min(X_i, \xi'_{j'}(t - T'_{j'})^+)$, $\delta'_{i'}(t) = I(X_i(t) = X_i)$, and $Y_j(t)$ and $\delta''_{j'}(t)$ are defined similarly in terms of Y_j, $\xi''_{j''}$ and $T''_{j''}$. Let $H_{n,t}$ be the left-continuous version of the Kaplan-Meier estimator of the distribution function of the combined sample, defined by

$$1 - H_{n,t}(s) = \prod_{u < s}\left\{1 - \frac{\Delta N_{n,t}'(u) + \Delta N_{n,t}''(u)}{m_{n,t}'(u) + m_{n,t}''(u)}\right\}$$
(Eq. 20-7)

where $N'_{n,t}(s) = \sum_{i=1}^{n'} I\left(X_i \leq \xi'_i \wedge (t - T'_i)^+ \wedge s\right)$, $N''_{n,t}(s) = \sum_{j=1}^{n''} I(Y_j \leq \xi''_j \wedge (t - T''_j)^+ \wedge s)$, $\Delta N(s) = N(s) - N(s-)$, $m'_{n,t}(s) = \sum_{i=1}^{n'} I\left(X_i(t) \geq s\right)$, $m''_{n,t}(s) = \sum_{j=1}^{n''} I\left(Y_j(t) \geq s\right)$, and we use the convention 0/0 = 0. The time-sequential versions of commonly used censored rank statistics to test the null hypothesis of equal survival distributions for the new and control treatments have the general form

$$S_n(t) = \sum_{i=1}^{n'} \delta_{i'}(t)\psi\left(H_{n,t}\left(X_i(t)\right)\right)\left\{1 - \frac{m_{n,t}'(X_i(t))}{m_{n,t}'(X_i(t)) + m_{n,t}''(X_i(t))}\right\}$$
$$- \sum_{j=1}^{n''} \delta_{j''}(t)\psi\left(H_{n,t}\left(Y_j(t)\right)\right)\frac{m_{n,t}''(Y_j(t))}{m_{n,t}'(Y_j(t)) + m_{n,t}''(Y_j(t))}.$$

(Eq. 20-8)

In (5), ψ is a nonrandom function on [0,1]. Gu and Lai (45) have shown that $\left\{S_n(t)/\sqrt{n}, t \geq 0\right\}$ converges weakly to a Gaussian process with independent increments and variance function $V(t)$ under the null hypothesis and contiguous alternatives and have also provided consistent estimators $V_n(t)$ of $V(t)$. In particular, for the logrank statistic that corresponds to $\psi \equiv 1$, the commonly used estimate is $V_n(t)$ = (total number of deaths up to time t)/4. The case $\psi(u) = u^\rho$ corresponds to the G^ρ statistics proposed by Harrington and Fleming (46), with $\rho = 0$ corresponding to the logrank statistic and $\rho = 1$ corresponding to the Peto-Prentice generalization of Wilcoxon's statistic (47,48). Group sequential tests typically use the normalized statistics $W_i = S_n(t_i)/\sqrt{V_n(t_i)}$, where $t_1, \ldots, t_k$ are the calendar times of the interim analyses. Because $V_n(t_k)$ is not available until time t_k, it is difficult to apply the widely used "error spending" approach introduced by Lan and DeMets (49) to specify the stopping boundaries of group sequential tests. Gu and Lai (50) propose to use the modified Haybittle-Peto (modHP) boundaries that depend on a user-specified value of b for $b_1 = \ldots b_{k-1} = b$ so that $b_k = c$ can be determined by

$$P\left\{\left|W(V_n(t_j))\right| \geq bV_n^{1/2}(t_j) \text{ for some } j < k\right.$$
$$\text{or } |W\left(V_n(t_k)\right)| \geq cV_n^{1/2}(t_k)|V_n(t_1), \ldots, V_n(t_k)\right\} = a;$$

(Eq. 20-9)

see Haybittle (51) and Peto et al. (52) who use $b = 3$ and conventional critical values of c for the final analysis at t_k and therefore may fail to maintain the prescribed type I error probability. Lai and Shih (24) use (6) to guarantee the type I error probability constraint and have developed a theory of group sequential tests showing that the modHP test has nearly optimal power and expected sample size under the constraints α for type I error and n for maximum sample size.

The logrank statistic, together with the closely related hazard ratio and the proportional hazards model, has become the most widely used test statistic and endpoint for survival trials. Its popularity is partly due to the conceptual simplicity of the hazard ratio as a summary measure to compare two survival distributions, whose Kaplan-Meier estimates are typically also plotted in the report of a survival trial. Although the time-sequential logrank statistic $S_n(t)$ is indeed asymptotically efficient under the proportional hazards model, it can have a flattening (or eventually decreasing) drift $\sqrt{n}\mu(t)$ under local alternatives, as shown by Gu and Lai (50). In this case, functionals of the Kaplan-Meier curve that capture the key features of the curve are more appropriate, and He, Lai, and Su (53) have recently introduced an adaptive design that uses these functionals in conjunction with the logrank statistic for the terminal analysis at the prescheduled end $t^*(=t_k)$ of a time-sequential survival trial. At the planning stage and at interim analyses, the adaptive design follows the popular practice of carrying out repeated log-rank tests, and uses the modified Haybittle–Peto (modHP) boundary for early stopping, as in Gu and Lai (50) and Lai and Shih (28). Even when interim data show clear departures from the proportional hazards model, early efficacy stopping of the time-sequential log-rank test can actually have both increase in power and reduction in sample size if the mean $\mu(t)$ of $S_n(t)/\sqrt{n}$ decreases with increasing $V(t)$, as shown in Gu and Lai (50). What can really hurt by using the inefficient logrank statistic in such cases is when early stopping has not occurred during interim analyses, and one can end up with substantial loss of power with the log-rank test at the prescheduled end t^* of the trial.

Instead of Kaplan-Meier curves, He, Lai, and Su (53) consider the Studentized cumulative hazard differences at selected survival times $s_1, \ldots s_L$ (eg, 1-year, 2-year, 5-year survival). Let $\hat{\Lambda}_X(s) = \Sigma_{u \leq s}\left(\Delta N'_{n,t^*}(u)/m'_{n,t^*}(u)\right)$, $\hat{\Lambda}_Y(s) = \Sigma_{u \leq s}\left(\Delta N''_{n,t^*}(u)/m''_{n,t^*}(u)\right)$ be the Nelson-Aalen estimators of the cumulative hazard functions of the two groups at the prescheduled termination time t^* of the trial. Let $\hat{V}_X(s) = \Sigma_{u \leq s}\Delta N'_{n,t^*}(u)/(m'_{n,t^*}(u))^2$ be the estimate of Var $(\hat{\Lambda}_X(s))$ and define $V_Y(s)$ similarly. Define the Studentized cumulative hazard difference at s_l ($l = 1, \ldots L$) by

$$\Delta_l = \left(\hat{\Lambda}_X(s_l) - \hat{\Lambda}_Y(s_l)\right)/\left(\hat{V}_X(s_l) - \hat{V}_Y(s_l)\right)^{1/2}.$$

(Eq. 20-10)

The test statistics $\Delta_1, \ldots, \Delta_L$ defined by (7) or its survival variant are used to supplement the Studentized logrank statistic $S_n(t^*)/\hat{\sigma}_n(t^*)$, where $\hat{\sigma}_n^2(t)$ = (total number of deaths up to time $t/4$). Thus, the time-sequential test statistics W_i now take the form

$$W_i = \begin{cases} S_n(t_i)/\hat{\sigma}_n(t_i) & \text{for } i \leq i < k, \\ \max(S_n(t^*)/\hat{\sigma}_n(t^*), \Delta_1, \ldots, \Delta_L) & \text{for } i = k \end{cases}$$

(Eq. 20-11)

With W_i defined by (8), the determination of c in (6) becomes considerably more difficult after introducing the additional test statistics $\Delta_1, \ldots, \Delta_L$ because $(\Delta_1, \ldots, \Delta_L, S_n(t_i) / \hat{\sigma}_n(t_i), 1 \leq i \leq k)$ does not have an independent increments correlation structure. Instead of multivariate integration after applying the joint limiting normal distribution of the random vector under $F = G$ to evaluate the probability in (6), He, Lai, and Su (53) compute the probability by Monte Carlo simulations, using the procedure of Lai and Li (54, p. 644). However, the threshold c in the modHP test does not need to be computed explicitly because checking whether the observed values W_k^{obs} of W_k exceeds c if the trial has not stopped prior to t_k is equivalent to checking whether $\hat{P}\{(t_{i^*}, W_{i^*}^*) > (t_k, W_k^{obs})\} \leq a$, where the ordering $>$ is that introduced in Lai and Li (54), i^* represents the time index of the interim analysis at which the modHP test based on the random variables W_i^* (generated from $\hat{P}$) stops, and $\hat{P}$ is the probability measure corresponding to the estimated common survival distribution of the two groups.

Another issue with early stopping for futility, which involves $V_n(t^*)$ rather than the sample size n, in these group sequential trials is the lack of information about $V_n(t^*)$ (which is total number of deaths at time t^* in the case of the log-rank test) at interim analyses prior to t^*. To address this difficulty, He, Lai, and Liao (55) have developed a theory for futility stopping that uses a Bayesian approach to estimate $V_n(t^*)$ during the course of the trial.

SEAMLESS PHASE II/III DESIGNS

Seamless phase II/III trial designs with bivariate endpoints consisting of tumor response and survival time have been introduced by Inoue, Berry, and Thall (56) and Huang et al (57) using the Bayesian approach to relate survival to response. Let z_i denote the treatment indicator (0 = control, 1 = experimental), τ_i denote survival time, and y_i denote the binary response for patient i. Their Bayesian approach assumes that the responses y_i are independent Bernoulli variables and that the survival time τ_i given y_i follows an exponential distribution, denoted $\text{Exp}(\lambda)$ in which $1/\lambda$ is the mean:

$$y_i \mid z_i = z \overset{i.i.d.}{\sim} \text{Bern}(\pi_z), \tau_i \mid \{y_i = y, z_i = z\} \overset{i.i.d.}{\sim} \text{Exp}(\lambda_{z,y}).$$

It then follows that the conditional distribution of τ_i given z_i is a mixture of exponentials:

$$\tau_i \mid z_i = z \overset{i.i.d.}{\sim} \pi_z \text{Exp}(\lambda_{z,1}) + (1 - \pi_z)\text{Exp}(\lambda_{z,0}).$$

(Eq. 20-12)

Instead of the parametric assumption of $\exp(\lambda_{z,y})$ for the conditional distribution of τ_i, semiparametric methods such as Cox regression, however, are often preferred for reproducibility considerations and because of the relatively large sample sizes in phase III studies. This

led Lai, Lavori, and Shih (58) to develop an alternative seamless phase II/III design that uses a semiparametric model to relate survival to response and is directly targeted toward frequentist testing with GLR or partial likelihood statistics. Their basic idea is to replace the stringent parametric model involving exponential distributions by a semiparametric counterpart that generalizes the Inoue-Thall-Berry model.

Let y denote the response and z denote the treatment indicator, taking the value 0 or 1. Consider the proportional hazards model $\lambda(t|y, z) = \lambda_0(t) \exp(ay + \beta z + \gamma yz)$. The Inoue-Thall-Berry exponential model is a special case, with $\lambda_0(\cdot)$ being the constant hazard rate of an exponential distribution. Let $\pi_0 = pr(y = 1|\text{control})$ and $\pi_1 = pr(y = 1|\text{treatment})$. Let $a = e^\alpha$, $b = e^\beta$ and $c = e^\gamma$, and let S be the survival function and f be the density function associated with the hazard function λ_0 so that $\lambda_0 = f/S$. In this augmented proportional hazards model, the survival distribution of τ is

$$P(\tau > t) = \begin{cases} (1 - \pi_0)S(t) + \pi_0(S(t))^a \\ \qquad \text{for the control group } (z = 0), \\ (1 - \pi_1)(S(t))^b + \pi_1(S(t))^{abc} \\ \qquad \text{for the treatment group } (z = 1). \end{cases}$$

Because of this mixture form of the survival distribution, the hazard ratio of the treatment to control group varies with t. Let $\pi = (\pi_0, \pi_1)$, $\xi = (a, b, c)$. Lai, Lavori, and Shih (58) formulate the null hypothesis as $H_0: \pi_0 \geq \pi_1$, or $\pi_0 < \pi_1$ and $d(\pi, \xi) < 0$, and use time sequential GLR and partial likelihood ratio statistics to test H_0, where $d(\pi, \xi)$ is the limiting hazard ratio (which does not depend on t) as $a \to 1$ and $c \to 1$.

Seamless Phase II/III Designs for Cytostatic Therapies

Yin, Zhang, and Xu (59) have pointed out the advantages of seamless phase I/II designs over designing two separate single-arm early-phase cancer trials. They state, however, that for cytostatic agents, phase I trials are single-arm, whereas "phase II trials are often randomized with multiple treatment arms," making it difficult to combine the two phases. On the other hand, because the phase II trial is already a randomized trial with a control arm and treatment arm(s) corresponding to the selected dose(s) of the phase I trial, it already has the patient pool to be incorporated into a seamless phase II/III trial via an adaptive design. How this differs from the Lai-Lavori-Shih design described previously for cytotoxic drugs lies mainly in the lack of a phase I/II trial to first determine a safe and efficacious dose. Because cytostatic agents can slow or stop the growth of tumors without shrinking the existing ones, we also do not have tumor response as the phase II endpoint that Lai, Lavori, and Shih have related to the survival endpoint. Hence Yin, Zhang, and Xu (59) propose to carry out dose-finding in simple-arm phase I trials for cytotoxic therapies by first escalating to the MTD "by solely monitoring toxicity" and then deescalating to find the "optimum biological dose" based on the probability of surviving at least a prespecified unit of time. In the next section, we discuss an alternative seamless phase II/III to this design by including multiple doses in phase II and using an adaptive design that allows midcourse dose selection.

DISCUSSION AND ONGOING WORK

The adaptive phase II/III design referred to in the preceding sentence involves adaptive dose selection among multiple doses, which we are currently developing. It is closely related to the adaptive designs that allow midcourse choice of patient subgroup in the comparative study of a new treatment with a control recently introduced by Lai, Lavori, and Liao (60). It is widely recognized that the comparative efficacy of treatments can depend on certain characteristics of the patients that are difficult to prespecify at the design stage. In a randomized trial, ignoring the characteristics that account for patient heterogeneity in response may yield a false-negative result. On the other hand, narrowly defining the patient characteristics for inclusion and exclusion limits the proven usefulness of the treatment to a small patient subpopulation. A trial may also encounter difficulties in patient accrual when relatively few patients satisfy the stringent inclusion/exclusion criteria. Adaptive (data-dependent) choice of the patient subgroup to compare the new and control treatments is a natural compromise between ignoring patient heterogeneity and using stringent inclusion/exclusion criteria in the trial design and analysis. Methods have been developed by Lai, Lavori, and Liao (60) for adaptively choosing the patient subgroup and testing the efficacy of the new treatment on the chosen subgroup, with prescribed type I error probability for the data-dependent choice. Besides the ability to stop early for futility or for efficacy when the data warrant, incorporating interim analysis in a group sequential design also allows subgroup selection at interim analyses and thereby takes advantage of the opportunity to shift future recruitment (and subsequent testing) to the selected subpopulation as in an enrichment design.

To illustrate the basic ideas, suppose that there are two interim analyses before a terminal analysis in a group sequential trial with a maximum sample size n and that the responses are normally distributed, with mean μ_i for the new treatment and μ_{0i} for the control treatment if the patient falls in a predefined subgroup Π_i for $i = 1, \ldots, J$, and with common known variance σ^2, in which Π_J denotes the entire patient population. For $l = 1, 2, 3$, let

$$Z_i^l = \{n_i^l n_{0i}^l / (n_i^l + n_{0i}^l)\}^{1/2} \left(\hat{\mu}_i^l - \hat{\mu}_{0i}^l \right) / \sigma$$

denote the t-statistic for testing H_i: $\mu_i \leq \mu_{0i}$ at the lth interim analysis, where $\hat{\mu}_i^l(\hat{\mu}_{0i}^l)$ is the mean response

of patients in Π_i from the treatment (control) arm and $n_i^l(n_{0i}^l)$ is the corresponding sample size. At the lth interim analysis, the Lai-Lavori-Liao test rejects H_J if $Z_J^l \geq b$ or accepts H_J and proceeds to the subgroup selection if $\tilde{Z}_J^l \leq \tilde{b}$, where

$$\tilde{Z}_i^l = \{n_i^l n_{0i}^l / (n_i^l + n_{0i}^l)\}^{1/2} (\mu_i^l - \mu_{0i}^l - \delta) / \sigma,$$

is the t-statistic for testing the alternative hypothesis K_i: $\mu_i \geq \mu_{0i} + \delta$. In case $\tilde{Z}_J^l > \tilde{b}$ but $Z_J^l < b$, one should continue to the next stage and repeat the procedure. Once H_J is accepted at stage l and a subgroup $\hat{I}$ with the largest values of Z_i^l for $i \neq J$ is chosen, the future enrollment of the trial will include patients of this subgroup only, while the maximum total sample size n remains the same. Moreover, at the next stage, it is necessary to repeat the procedure with J replaced by $\hat{I}$. If no acceptance or rejection occurs before the final stage, H_J is rejected if $Z_J^3 \geq c$ and is accepted otherwise. By making use of the closed testing principle in multiple testing, Lai, Lavori, and Liao (60) have shown that the test indeed has type I error probability no larger than a prescribed bound α.

Lai, Liao, and Kim (61) have introduced another adaptive design for the development and testing of biomarker-guided treatment strategies that attempt to select the best of k treatments for each biomarker-classified subgroup of cancer patients in phase II studies. The clinical trial has several objectives, which include (a) treating accrued patients with the best (yet unknown) available treatment, (b) developing a biomarker-guided treatment strategy for future patients, and (c) demonstrating that the strategy developed indeed has significantly better treatment effect than some predetermined threshold. The group sequential design uses an outcome-adaptive randomization rule, which updates the randomization probabilities at interim analyses and uses GLR statistics and modHP rules to include early elimination of significantly inferior treatments from a biomarker class. It is shown to provide substantial improvements, besides being much easier to implement, over the Bayesian outcome-adaptive randomization design used in the Biomarker-integrated Approaches of Targeted Therapy for Lung Cancer Elimination (BATTLE) trial of personalized therapies for non–small cell lung cancer (62). An April 2010 editorial in *Nature Reviews in Medicine* pointed out that the BATTLE design, which "allows researchers to avoid being locked into a single, static protocol of the trial" that requires large sample sizes for multiple comparisons of several treatments across different biomarker classes, can "yield breakthroughs, but must be handled with care" to ensure that "the risk of reaching a false positive conclusion" is not inflated (63). Besides BATTLE, another design mentioned in the editorial is that of the Investigation of Serial Studies to Predict Your Therapeutic Response with Imaging and Molecular Analysis (I-SPY2) trial (64). We are currently extending the methodology developed by Lai, Liao, and Kim (61) to survival outcomes, particularly for cytostatic therapies, for which GLR statistics are replaced by partial likelihood or Studentized score statistics.

REFERENCES

1. Eisenhauer EA, O'Dwyer PJ, Christian M, Humphrey JS. Phase I clinical trial design in cancer drug development. *J Clin Oncol.*2000;18:684–692.
2. O'Quigley J, Pepe M, Fisher L. Continual reassessment method: a practical design for phase 1 clinical trials in cancer. *Biometrics.* 1990;46:33–48.
3. Babb J, Rogatko A, Zacks, S. Cancer phase I clinical trials: efficient dose escalation with overdose control. *Stat Med.* 1998;17:1103–1120.
4. Whitehead J, Brunier H. Bayesian Decision procedures for dose determining experiments. *Stat Med.* 1995;14:885–893.
5. Haines LM, Perevozskaya I, Rosenberger WF. Bayesian optimal designs for phase I clinical trials. *Biometrics.* 2003;59:591–600.
6. Bartroff J, Lai, TL. Generalized likelihood ratio statistics and uncertainty adjustments in efficient adaptive design of clinical trials. *Sequential Anal.* 2008;27:254–276.
7. Bartroff J, Lai TL. Incorporating individual and collective ethics into Phase I cancer trial designs. *Biometrics.* 2011;67:596–603.
8. Bartroff J, Lai TL. Approximate dynamic programming and its applications to the design of Phase I cancer trials. *Statist Sci.* 2010;25:245–257.
9. Fan SK, Lu Y, Wang YG. A simple Bayesian decision-theoretic design for dose-finding trials. *Stat Med.* 2012;31:3719–3730.
10. Heyd JM, Carlin BP. Adaptive design improvements in the continual reassessment method for phase I studies. *Stat Med.* 1999;18:1307–1321.
11. Lee BL, Fan S, Lu Y. A curve-free Bayesian decision-theoretic design for two-agent Phase I trials. *J Biopharm Stat.* 2016;16:1–10.
12. Mandrekar SJ, Cui Y, Sargent DJ. An adaptive phase I design for identifying a biologically optimal dose for dual agent drug combinations. *Stat Med.* 2007;26:2317–2330.
13. Yin G, Yuan Y. Bayesian dose finding in oncology for drug combinations by copula regression. *J Roy Statist Soc Ser C.* 2009;58:211–224.
14. Yuan Y, Yin G. Bayesian phase I/II adaptively randomized oncology trials with combined drugs. *Ann Appl Stat.* 2011;5:924–942.
15. Braun TM, Wang S. A hierarchical Bayesian design for phase I trials of novel combinations of cancer therapeutic agents. *Biometrics.* 2010;66:805–812.
16. Wages NA, Conaway MR, O'Quigley J. Dose-finding design for multi-drug combinations. *Clin Trial.* 2011;8:380–389.
17. Freidlin B, Simon R. Evaluation of randomized discontinuation design. *J Clin Oncol* 2005;23:5094–5098.
18. Millar AW, Lynch KP. Rethinking clinical trials for cytostatic drugs. *Nat Rev Cancer.* 2003;3:540–545.
19. Korn EL, Arbuck SG, Pluda JM, et al. Clinical trial designs for cytostatic agents: are new approaches needed? *J Clin Oncol.* 2001;19:265–272.
20. Rosner GL, Stadler W, Ratain MJ. Randomized discontinuation design: application to cytostatic antineoplastic agents. *J Clin Oncol.* 2002;20:4478–4484.
21. Stone A, Wheeler C, Barge A. Improving the design of phase II trials of cytostatic anticancer agents. *Contemp Clini Trial.* 2007;28:138–145.
22. Xu J, Yin G, Ohlssen D, Bretz F. Bayesian two-stage dose finding for cytostatic agents via model adaptation. *J Roy Stat Soc Ser C (Applied Atat.).* 2016;65:465–482.
23. Simon R. Optimal 2-stage designs for phase II clinical trials. *Contemp Clin Trial.* 1989;10:1–10.
24. Jung SH, Carey M, Kim KM. Graphical search for two-stage designs for phase II clinical trials. *Control Clin Trial.* 2001;22:367–372.
25. Jung SH, Lee T, Kim KM, George SL. Admissible two-stage designs for phase II cancer clinical trials. *Stat Med.* 2004;23:561–565.
26. Lu Y, Jim H, Lamborn KR. A design of phase II cancer trials using total and complete response endpoints. *Stat Med.* 2005;24:3155–3170.
27. Vickers AJ, Ballen V, Scher HI. Setting the bar in phase II trials: the use of historical data for determining "go/no go" decision for definitive phase III testing. *Clin Cancer Res.* 2007;13:972–976.
28. Lai TL, Shih MC. Power, sample size and adaptation considerations in the design of group sequential trials. *Biometrika.* 2004;91:509–528.
29. Banerjee A, Tsiatis AA. Adaptive two-stage designs in phase II clinical trials. *Stat Med.* 2006;25:3382–3395.
30. Englert S, Kieser M. Improving the flexibility and efficiency of phase II designs for oncology trials. *Biometrics.* 2012;68:886–892.
31. Shan G, Wilding GE, Hutson AD, Gerstenberger S. Optimal adaptive two-stage designs for early phase II clinical trials. *Stat Med.* 2016;35:1257–1266.
32. Thall PF, Simon R, Ellenberg SS, Shrager, R. Optimal two-stage designs for clinical trials with binary response. *Stat Med.* 1988;7:571–579.
33. Gooley TA, Martin PJ, Fisher LD, Pettinger M. Simulation as a design tool for phase I/II clinical trials: an example from bone marrow transplantation. *Controlled Clin Trial.* 1994;15:450–462.
34. Thall PF, Russell KT. A strategy for dose finding and safety monitoring based on efficacy and adverse outcomes in phase I/II clinical trials. *Biometrics.* 1998;54:251–264.
35. Ivanova A. A new dose-finding design for bivariate outcomes. *Biometrics.* 2003;59:1001–1007.
36. Braun TM. The bivariate continual reassessment method extending the CRM to phase I trials of two competing outcomes. *Control Clin Trial.* 2002;23:240–256.
37. Thall PF, Cook JD. Dose-finding based on efficacy-toxicity trade-offs. *Biometrics.* 2004;60:684–693.
38. Thall PF, Nguyen HQ, Estey EH. Patient-specific dose-finding based on bivariate outcomes and covariates. *Biometrics.* 2008;64:1126–1136.
39. Bartroff J, Lai TL, Narasimhan B. A new approach to designing phase I–II cancer trials for cytotoxic chemotherapies. *Stat Med.* 2014;33:2718–2735.
40. Harrington JA, Wheeler GM, Sweeting MJ, et al. Adaptive designs for dual-agent phase I dose-escalation studies. *Nat Rev Clin Oncol.* 2013;10:277–288.
41. Houede N, Thall PF, Nguyen H, et al. Utility-based optimization of combination therapy using ordinal toxicity and efficacy in phase I/II trials. *Biometrics.* 2010;66:532–540.
42. Whitehead J, Thygesen H, Whitehead A. Bayesian procedures for phase I/II clinical trials investigating the safety and efficacy of drug combinations. *Stat Med.* 2011;30:1952–1970.
43. Dragalin V, Fedorov V, Wu Y. Adaptive designs for selecting drug combinations based on efficacy-toxicity response. *J Stat Plan Infer.* 2008;2:352–373.
44. Lan KKG, DeMets DL. Group sequential procedures: Calendar versus information time. *Stat Med.* 1989;8:1191–1198.
45. Gu MG, Lai TL. Weak convergence of time-sequential censored rank statistics with applications to sequential testing in clinical trials. *Ann Statist.* 1991;19:1403–1433.
46. Harrington DP, Fleming TR. A class of rank test procedures for censored survival data. *Biometrika.* 1982;69:553–566.
47. Peto R, Peto J. Asymptotically efficient rank invariant test procedures. *J Roy Statist Soc Ser A.* 1972;135:185–207.
48. Prentice RL. Linear rank tests with right censored data. *Biometrika.* 1978;65:167–179.

49. Lan KKG, DeMets DL. Discrete sequential boundaries for clinical trials. *Biometrika*. 1983;70:659–663.
50. Gu MG, Lai TL. Repeated significance testing with censored rank statistics in interim analysis of clinical trials. *Stat Sinica*. 1998;8:411–423.
51. Haybittle J. Repeated assessment of results in clinical trials of cancer treatment. *Brit J Radiol*. 1971;44:793–797.
52. Peto R, Pike M, Armitage P, et al. Design and analysis of randomized clinical trials requiring prolonged observation of each patient 1. Introduction and design. *Br J Cancer*. 1976;34:585–612.
53. He P, Lai TL, Su Z. Design of clinical trials with failure-time endpoints and interim analyses: An update after fifteen years. *Contemp Clin Trials*. 2015;10th Anniversary Special Issue(45 Part A):103–112.
54. Lai TL, Li W. Confidence intervals in group sequential trials with random group sizes and applications to survival analysis. *Biometrika*. 2006;93:641–654.
55. He P, Lai TL, Liao OY. Futility stopping in clinical trials. *Stat Its Inter*. 2012;5:415–424.
56. Inoue LYT, Berry DA, Thall PF. Seamlessly expanding a randomized Phase II trial to Phase III. *Biometrics*. 2002;58:823–831.
57. Huang X, Ning J, Li Y, et al. Using short-term response information to facilitate adaptive randomization for survival clinical trials. *Stat Med*. 2009;28:1680–1689.
58. Lai TL, Lavori PW, Shih MC. Sequential design of phase II–III cancer trials. *Stat Med*. 2012;31:1944–1960.
59. Yin G, Zhang S, Xu J. Two-stage dose finding for cytostatic agents in phase I oncology trials. *Stat Med*. 2013;32:644–660.
60. Lai TL, Lavori PW, Liao OYW. Adaptive choice of patient subgroup for comparing two treatments. *Contemp Clin Trial*. 2014;39:191–200.
61. Lai TL, Liao OYW, Kim DW. Group sequential designs for developing and testing biomarker-guided personalized therapies in comparative effectiveness research. *Contemp Clin Trial*. 2013;36:651–663.
62. Kim ES, Herbst RS, Wistuba II, et al. The BATTLE trial: Personalizing therapy for lung cancer. *Cancer Discov*. 2011;1:44–53.
63. Ledford H. Clinical drug tests adapted for speed. *Nature*. 2010;464(7293):1258. doi:10.1038/4641258a
64. Barker AD, Sigman CC, Kelloff GJ, et al. I-SPY 2: an adaptive breast cancer trial design in the setting of neoadjuvant chemotherapy. *Clin Pharmacol Theor*. 2009;86:97–100.

Conducting Oncology Clinical Trials

21

Randomization

Susan Groshen

INTRODUCTION

In the perfect and ideal clinical trial that is designed to compare the effects of two or more interventions, all study participants would be alike and would be the same as all other patients in the target population to which the conclusions will be applied. In this perfect and ideal trial, each intervention or treatment would be delivered to the assigned patients in exactly the same way, the effect would be the same on each patient, and this effect would be measured correctly and exactly. Thus the only difference from patient to patient would be the real effect of the intervention. In contrast in a typical oncology trial, patients are heterogeneous, treatment cannot be delivered in a completely reproducible fashion, and the effect of the treatment is not the same from patient to patient. Furthermore not all factors affecting the outcome can be adequately controlled and the measurement of effect is often difficult. To deal with the realities of clinical research, as in all scientific research, the design of an experiment involves control, randomization, and replication (1). The objective is to have patients in the treatment groups to be similar on average in all important aspects, except for the treatment assigned; and in this way, observed differences can be attributed to treatment.

The first step in designing a clinical trial is to identify sources of patient heterogeneity, treatment variability, and outcome assessment measurement error. To the extent possible, all known sources' heterogeneity and variability should be controlled or limited. For those sources of heterogeneity that are either not known or that cannot be directly controlled, randomization is used to reduce and limit the impact of nonrandom differences between patients in the treatment arms. Replication is the mechanism by which the impact of random error or noise is controlled; sample sizes are calculated to ensure that there is a high probability of detecting a specified signal-to-noise ratio. Issues of control and replication are discussed in other chapters of this book; the purpose of this chapter is to discuss the application of randomization and to describe some common and effective randomization procedures.

In this chapter, the terms "treatment" and "intervention" are used interchangeably, as are "patient" and "study participant." In addition, we use the phrase "assign each patient to a treatment arm" and "assign a treatment to each study participant" to mean the same thing.

Bias

Bias is the term used to describe systematic error, in contrast to random error. In the context of clinical trials, serious bias arises when systematic, nonrandom, differences in patient characteristics are confused with treatment effect. An illustration of bias, that is, systematic error, can be found in a registry of patients with muscle invasive transitional cell bladder cancer who have undergone radical cystectomy (2). In this series, many patients with involved lymph nodes were treated off protocol with adjuvant chemotherapy. When the survival of patients who received chemotherapy was compared to the survival of patients who did not receive chemotherapy (all with involved lymph nodes), the patients who received adjuvant chemotherapy had inferior survival. This was not because chemotherapy had a detrimental effect on survival, but rather because patients with other unfavorable features (not all easily specified) were more likely to receive adjuvant chemotherapy. Because patients were not randomly assigned to receive chemotherapy, the assignment to chemotherapy depended on factors that are not all readily apparent. The resulting comparison of survival between the chemotherapy and nonchemotherapy groups was biased because the differences observed were not due to the chemotherapy, but rather to patient or disease characteristics.

There are other potential sources of bias, such as those that occur during the assessment of response to treatment, that cannot be reduced or eliminated by randomization. Many trials are single blind (when the patient does not know which treatment he or she is receiving) or double blind (when the patient and the individual evaluating the response, often the physician, do not know the treatment assignment) in order to reduce potential bias in outcome measurement. Thus even with randomization, there is still a need to exercise as much control as possible in the design of the trial in order to reduce bias. This systematic error, this bias, cannot be overcome or corrected by increasing the sample size. If the cause of the bias can be identified, then possibly the error can be corrected with careful analysis. But this is often not possible, and often the study investigators may not be aware of the bias. And this, finally, is the problem with bias: it is usually undetected. One can never say that there is no bias in a trial; one can only say that every precaution was taken to reduce the possibility of bias.

Goals of Randomization

For all the considerations discussed previously, trials using randomization to assign treatment to study participants are regarded as the most credible type of investigation for generating experimental data to compare the benefit and safety of therapies for the treatment of cancer. Randomization, properly implemented achieves two goals. The first goal is to assign a treatment to each study participant. The second, equally important goal of randomization is to reduce the chance of bias (as summarized in Table 21.1). This is done by ensuring that each patient is as likely to be assigned a particular treatment as any other patient. That is, a patient with feature X is just as likely as a patient with feature Y, to be assigned to a specific treatment. With randomization correctly executed, there is no systematic preference to assigning one treatment over the other, based either on patient characteristics or physician preference or (often) subconscious opinion.

Randomization does not guarantee that at every stage, the treatment arms will be exactly equally balanced in terms of known and unknown patient characteristics that could impact the patient response to treatment; the randomization process will decrease the

chances that this deleterious imbalance occurs with small numbers of patients, and has a high chance of achieving balance with large numbers of patients. Thus randomization has the feature that in the long run, the patients in one treatment group will be similar (on average) to patients in another treatment group. It is this long-run balance that will permit the conclusion that observed differences between treatment groups are due to treatment.

Finally, randomization can confer robustness to the statistical analysis. That is, the set of all possible randomization outcomes provides a context by which to evaluate the observed treatment differences; often this will suggest that standard (parametric) tests can be used to calculate p values to summarize the strength of the evidence refuting the null hypothesis.

From a practical perspective, the randomization scheme should be easy to use, it should be unpredictable, and it should be truly random; wherever possible it should assign individual patients and not groups of patients. For example, a scheme that assigns patients registered on Mondays to one treatment and those registered on Wednesdays to another treatment will invite bias. Patients making appointments for Monday may differ from those making appointments for Wednesday (e.g., traveling from out of town and/or attempting to minimize work days missed); this is sometimes called *experimental bias*. In addition, this form of assignment allows physician preference to intervene; this is sometimes called *selection bias*. Other forms of systematic assignment of patients to one treatment or another are also vulnerable to (often subconscious) selection bias of patients. Hence a treatment assignment scheme that assigns patients with a medical record number ending in an even digit to one treatment and assigns all other patients to a second treatment, invites patient selection bias if the scheme becomes known.

In 1930, the Department of Health for Scotland undertook a nutritional experiment in the schools of Lanarkshire (3). Ten thousand children received free milk for 4 months and 10,000 children were observed as controls. Assignment was done by ballot or alphabetically, although "adjustment" by the head teacher at each school was allowed if it appeared that "an undue proportion of well fed or ill nourished children" was assigned to one group. At the end of the experiment, it was observed that the "control" group weighed more than the "milk" group. Analysis of baseline heights and weights demonstrated that children assigned to the "milk" group had, on average, weighed less both at the start of the experiment and at the end, although they had gained more weight during the 4 months of the study. This example demonstrates the bias in personal selection of subjects for treatment or control; randomization is needed to ensure that assignment is free of bias and to maximize the likelihood that the comparison groups are similar on average.

TABLE 21.1 Goals of Randomization

1. Assign treatment to study participants
2. Ensure that each study participant is as likely to receive each of the trial treatments as any other participant
3. Ensure that in the long run, on average, the treatment groups are similar in terms of the participants' characteristics
4. Justify statistical analysis of results

Deciding Whether to Randomize

Two issues must be considered in deciding whether a planned trial should include randomization. One consideration is scientific: Can the potential problem of bias be managed without randomization? The other consideration is ethical: Will it be ethical to randomly assign one of several treatments to a study participant, rather than use medical opinion?

There are disadvantages and logistic difficulties to using randomization to assign treatment. These are not usually insurmountable, but they can complicate the conduct of the trial. Explaining the choice of treatments and the randomization process to patients is difficult to do well; many patients, as well as their physicians, would rather that the treating physician select the treatment option thought/believed to be best for the patient. As a result, some patients will not enroll in a trial that involves randomization, resulting in slower accrual and longer lasting studies. To mitigate the reluctance of patients to enroll in a trial with a not-yet-determined treatment, Zelen introduced the randomized consent design (4). In this design, the treatment assignment is obtained (by randomization) prior to the consent process and the patient is presented with the study knowing the treatment assignment. The goal of this design was to increase participation; however, if a sizable portion of patients decline participation after randomization, then interpretation of the results will be more complicated and possibly compromised (see the discussion on intention to treat [ITT] in the following). As a result, this approach has not been used often. Acceptance of randomization remains an obstacle for many patients and physicians.

Randomized trials are recognized as the most scientifically sound mechanism for establishing which of two or more treatments is superior. This is especially true in oncology clinical research, where phase III trials aim to establish standard-of-care options and therefore require a control group or comparator in order to compare the "new" therapeutic regimen to a standard-of-care option, that is, the control. In this setting, historical controls or concurrent nonrandomized controls are almost always unacceptable due to vulnerability to substantial bias. Because for most cancers, therapies now exist that offer palliation if not cure, differences needed to establish superiority or equivalence will be incremental and not large; treatment effect differences may not be substantially larger than differences resulting from changes in referral patterns or changes in ancillary care procedures. In addition, supportive care and diagnostic procedures have evolved substantially over the past decades and continue to do so. Hence the use of historical series is, at best, problematic and often invalid; concurrent, nonrandomized controls are usually subject to even more bias than historical controls. The onus will be on the study investigators to convincingly demonstrate to the skeptical reviewer that differences observed between the new treatment and the historical control group (or nonrandomized concurrent control group) are not due to bias. This will be, at best, difficult. Thus definitive trials that aim to change the standard or care, or convincingly compare two or more standard treatment options, should incorporate concurrent controls and randomization.

While the scientific justification for randomly assigning treatment to patients is rarely disputed, the ethical justification is not straightforward. The term *clinical equipoise* provides the ethical justification for clinical trials with randomization. Clinical equipoise is satisfied when there is "genuine uncertainty in the expert medical community...about the preferred treatment" (5). This occurs when there are no clear and definitive data supporting or refuting the hypothesis of benefit or superiority and individual clinicians and clinical investigators are either unsure or have conflicting opinions regarding the new treatment. It is not the purpose of this chapter to review all the ethical arguments for and against using randomization. However, these issues must be carefully discussed before initiating a randomized trial, by evaluating the potential harm to study participants and weighing the risks and benefits of undertaking the study, to study participants and to society. Much has been written on this subject (6–8).

PRACTICAL CONSIDERATIONS

There are many practical and logistic issues that must be resolved in order to correctly and effectively incorporate randomization into a clinical trial. To begin with, randomization should not be done by involved investigators; a separate office (possibly with telephone randomization) should be used. A document should be created and saved for each randomization, indicating the time and date of the randomization, the individual initiating the randomization, the pertinent patient information, and the randomization outcome.

Timing of Randomization

Randomization should not take place until after the patient is confirmed to be eligible and has signed the informed consent. In addition, randomization should be delayed until the latest practical moment before the intervention is to begin (see Durrleman and Simon for a discussion of this issue) (9). In general, it is reasonable for the intervention to begin within 1 or 2 weeks of randomization. This narrow window reduces the likelihood of intervening events to cause the patient to discontinue trial participation or fail to adhere to the treatment schedule as required. Noncompliance and dropouts can introduce bias and may complicate the final interpretation of the results.

In 1991, the Children's Cancer Group began a trial for the treatment of children with high-risk neuroblastoma (10). All patients were treated with the same initial regimen of chemotherapy. Those without disease progression at the completion of the initial therapy were then randomly assigned to receive either three cycles of intensive chemotherapy, or to receive myeloablative therapy with autologous bone marrow rescue. Patients who completed the second phase of cytotoxic therapy without disease progression were then randomized to no further treatment or 6 months of 13-*cis*-retinoic acid. In this study, both randomizations were delayed until patients were ready to begin the next phase of treatment. Had randomization taken place prior to the start of the initial chemotherapy with all 539 eligible patients randomized, then only 379 of the 539 patients would have begun the three cycles of intensive chemotherapy or myeloablative therapy, with 160 patients not receiving the randomly assigned treatment. Only 258 of the initial 539, who were still free of progression after all cytotoxic therapy, would have been able to comply with the second randomization. By delaying the randomization until patients were ready to begin the treatment, the investigators clearly defined the appropriate comparison groups and eliminated, upfront, those patients who would not contribute meaningful data to the planned comparisons.

Intention-to-Treat Analysis

In a randomized trial, an ITT analysis is one in which all eligible patients who are randomized are included in the analysis of the results and are classified according to the treatment assigned, regardless of whether this was the treatment actually received. The ITT analysis should be the primary analysis in a randomized trial designed to show the superiority of one regimen. The Children's Cancer Group, by delaying the randomization, was able to focus the ITT analysis on those patients who were still able to benefit from the second phase or third phase of therapy.

When some of the randomized patients fail to receive the assigned treatment, there is no "correct" way to include or exclude these patients in the analysis. Nor is there a way to correctly adjust the statistical analysis. This is because the outcome of these patients, had they received the assigned treatment, is unknown; furthermore it is often the case that these patients are different from those who received the assigned treatment, but it is not usually known how they differ. In the presence of noncompliance, any analysis will lead to a biased estimate of the true treatment difference. The ITT analysis is advocated in the case of trials designed to establish a difference (that one treatment arm is superior) because the bias, to the degree that it exists, will lead to an underestimate of the magnitude of the treatment difference. With other approaches, such as the "as-treated"

analysis or inclusion of only the compliant patients, the impact of the bias is not known: the resulting observed treatment difference could be either too large or too small, so the direction is not known. The ITT analysis is known to be a conservative strategy, and if the ITT results indicate a clear difference (i.e., statistically significant at the planned level), then the results can be considered conclusive. If the ITT analysis does not result in a clear (statistically significant) difference, but the "as-treated" or another analysis does, then interpretation of the results will be inconclusive.

Balanced Versus Unbalanced Randomization

Generally, it is most efficient to assign the same number of patients to each of the treatment groups under comparison in the clinical trial. That is, for the same total number of patients, the power will be greatest when the treatment arms have equal numbers. On some occasions however, it may be appropriate to assign more patients to one treatment arm. In some trials, more patients will be required for secondary objectives; additional studies may be performed on patients assigned to one of the treatments. In randomized pilot studies, there may be a need to obtain more data on the new or experimental arm, while sufficient experience exists for the arm that represents the standard of care. On occasion, one treatment may be substantially more expensive than the other. Sometimes, there might be more variability associated with one arm compared to the other, and in this case it would be more efficient to randomize more patients to the treatment with greater variability. In a related situation, Sposto and Krailo discuss unequal allocation when the primary outcome is time to an event and fewer events are expected in one arm (11). It is not appropriate, however, to design a study with fixed unequal allocation that will assign fewer patients to an arm that is thought to be inferior; this would suggest that clinical equipoise is not satisfied.

METHODS OF RANDOMIZATION

There are many ways to randomly assign treatments to patients (12,13). Kalish and Begg provide a comprehensive review of different schemes that are available for randomization in a clinical trial (14). In this section, several methods are described; simple randomization and the permuted block design are by far the more commonly used methods, but the others can be very useful in selected situations and are presented briefly to indicate the range of randomization options. For illustration purposes, it is assumed that there are two treatments (A and B) and that a balanced allocation is used (i.e., 50% of patients are assigned treatment A and 50% are assigned treatment B). However, each of the methods presented can easily be adapted to three or more treatment arms and to unequal allocation. Computer programs exist and are easy to create, in order to generate the random treatment assignments. For many of the randomization designs, a list can be prepared in advance, although this is not feasible for adaptive or minimization randomization schemes.

Simple Randomization (Completely Randomized Design)

Simple randomization is equivalent to flipping a coin or rolling a die every time a patient is randomized. If the coin is fair, that is, the probability of getting a head is equal to getting a tail, Pr{head} = Pr{tail} = 1/2, then the randomization is balanced. With this form of randomization, the outcome, heads or tails, does not depend on the number of previously randomized patients or their characteristics. That is, if the last five flips all resulted in heads, the probability that the next flip is a head is still 1/2. Although computers can quickly create a list of treatment assignments using simple randomization, a table of random digits is used here to illustrate the process.

Table 21.2 contains 300 random digits; that is, each of the 10 digits (0–9) appears in about 10% of the entries in the table, in no order. If even digits (0, 2, 4, 6, 8) are used to correspond to treatment A and odd digits (1, 3, 5, 7, 9) correspond to treatment B, then Table 21.2 can be used to assign treatment to 15 patients. First it is necessary to identify a starting point in Table 21.2, and then read a sequence of 15 digits originating at the starting point. Selection of the starting point should also be done randomly. If the starting point is column 8, row A, and 15 digits down column 8 are read, then the assignment of treatment to 15 patients will be:

Pt. Seq.	1	2	3	4	5	6	7	8	9	10	11	12	13	14	15
Random Digit	8	5	5	6	4	2	2	7	5	2	6	9	6	5	9
Treatment	A	B	B	A	A	A	A	B	B	A	A	B	A	B	B

TABLE 21.2 300 Random Digits

	1	2	3	4	5	6	7	8	9	10	11	12	13	14	15	16	17	18	19	20
A	5	6	1	0	6	2	1	8	7	9	4	2	4	5	2	8	2	1	0	4
B	0	8	7	4	5	6	2	5	3	9	2	4	6	5	8	7	5	7	3	4
C	1	3	3	8	1	9	2	5	8	4	9	5	1	3	6	7	1	7	4	1
D	6	1	2	8	7	8	1	6	8	4	5	8	0	6	9	3	5	4	1	6
E	7	9	5	0	1	8	2	4	7	5	4	7	7	2	9	8	2	1	9	0
F	4	8	8	3	5	0	2	2	3	4	9	8	8	8	0	4	1	7	9	9
G	5	6	0	7	4	4	5	2	3	1	8	3	5	0	9	5	2	2	9	4
H	9	1	3	0	2	7	1	7	3	9	4	9	3	8	4	7	7	0	3	7
I	0	9	8	9	0	9	2	5	0	0	5	7	7	6	1	7	6	9	4	1
J	3	9	5	8	4	2	3	2	2	1	7	4	4	9	9	0	4	3	4	8
K	6	8	3	5	7	6	7	6	2	1	5	9	9	4	5	0	7	7	9	0
L	2	8	6	8	6	6	1	9	6	9	2	6	5	7	5	9	8	1	9	7
M	6	6	5	8	8	5	1	6	0	2	6	1	0	4	8	1	0	1	6	3
N	7	6	3	5	2	0	7	5	7	8	3	4	1	7	5	1	6	0	3	9
O	7	8	7	0	1	2	3	9	4	0	7	4	8	6	9	4	1	3	7	3

In this case, treatment A was assigned to 8 patients and treatment B was assigned to 7 patients. The features of simple randomization can be summarized as:

Features of Simple Randomization	• Completely unpredictable (eliminates selection bias)
	• Eliminates experimental bias
	• In the short run, can lead to serious imbalance
	• Rarely exactly balanced, but balance is good in the long run
	• Procedure is flexible and easy
	• Resulting statistical analysis is easy

Replacement Randomization

It is possible that the randomization scheme described previously will produce substantial imbalance in the early part of the trial. A simple fix to avoid this problem is to specify a requirement in advance. For example, a possible requirement might be: in the first 40 patients, the difference in the numbers of patients assigned to receive A versus assigned to receive B should not exceed 8. The randomization list is prepared in advance; if the list does not fulfill the requirement, the entire list is rejected and another randomization list is prepared. As long as the entire randomization list is replaced and as long as this is done before the first patient is enrolled, this is one reasonable way to overcome the potential short-run imbalance of the simple randomization scheme.

Biased Coin Randomization

The biased coin randomization (15) begins with simple randomization: for each new patient, the probability of being assigned treatment A is 1/2. If the difference in the number of patients assigned to A minus the number of patients assigned to B differs by some prespecified number, D (or –D), then the probability of assignment to A is changed. If D more patients have been assigned to A, then the probability of assigning A to the next patient is changed to "p" where $p < 1/2$. If D more patients have been assigned to treatment B, then the probability of assigning A to the next patient is changed to "$1 - p$" where $1 - p > 1/2$. In general, $p = 1/3$ is reasonable;

smaller values will result in assignments that are too predictable. The choice of D should depend on the total number of patients planned and the timing of interim analyses. The features of the biased coin randomization can be summarized as:

Features of Biased Coin Randomization	• Largely unpredictable (eliminates selection bias)
	• Eliminates experimental bias
	• Better balance in the short run
	• Rarely exactly balanced, but close to exactly balanced; balance is good in the long run
	• Flexible but a little more complicated to set up
	• Resulting statistical analysis can be somewhat more complicated

Permuted Block Design

The permuted block design is one of the most commonly used methods for randomly assigning treatment to patients. The advantage of this method is that it forces exact balance at very regular intervals during the accrual phase of the trial, and not just at the end.

To construct a randomization list using the permuted block design, the first step is to select the "block size," which will be a multiple of K (2K, 3K, 4K, etc.) where K is the number of treatments in the trial. To illustrate this scheme for K = 2, block sizes of 6 = 3 × 2 will be used. In a block of 6 units (or patients), there are 20 different orders that the two treatments can be assigned with each treatment assigned to three patients (e.g., AAABBB or ABBAAB or ABABBA, etc.).

There are two ways to construct the randomization list. The first way is to randomly select blocks from a list of all 20 possible blocks; this is probably the fastest method. The second way is to randomly assign treatment to patients in groups of 6. This second method is demonstrated in the following for 30 patients, which will require 5 blocks with 6 patients per block. Taking random digits from Table 21.2, using row F for Block #1, row G for Block #2, through row J for Block #5, 6 digits will be read across each row, beginning in column 11. As before, even digits will correspond to treatment A and odd digits to treatment B.

	Block 1						Block 2						Block 3					
Pt. Seq.	1	2	3	4	5	6	7	8	9	10	11	12	13	14	15	16	17	18
Random #	9	8	8	8	0	4	8	3	5	0	9	5	4	9	3	8	4	7
Treatment	B	A	A	A	B	B	A	B	B	A	B	A	A	B	B	A	A	B

(continued)

(*continued*)

Pt. Seq.	Block 4						Block 5						Note: The numbers in the shaded cells with the strikethrough lines indicate that those treatment assignments were required to ensure that three patients were assigned to A and to B.
	19	20	21	22	23	24	25	26	27	28	29	30	
Random #	5	7	7	~~6~~	~~4~~	~~7~~	7	4	4	9	9	~~0~~	
Treatment	B	B	B	A	A	A	B	A	A	B	B	A	

At the end of each block, both treatment arms have exactly the same number of patients assigned. This short-run balance, as well as the ease of implementation, is a very favorable characteristic of this method of randomization. However, this randomization scheme is not as unpredictable as simple randomization, replacement randomization, or the biased coin method, since if the block size is known, one could anticipate the assignment of the last patient in the block. For this reason, a variation on this randomization scheme is frequently adopted in which the block sizes are also varied. For example, with K = 2 treatments, the block size of 4, 6, or 8 could be randomly chosen. The features of the permuted block design randomization can be summarized as:

Features of the Permuted Block Design	• Largely unpredictable, except at the end of each block (can vary block size to decrease predictability)
	• Eliminates experimental bias
	• Very good balance in the short run
	• Closely balanced at the end (exactly balanced if the total number of patients is a multiple of the block size)
	• Flexible but a little more complicated to set up
	• Resulting statistical analysis is easy

Outcome-Adaptive Randomization for Treatment Assignment

In this class of treatment assignment schemes, the probability that the next patient is assigned to treatment A or B will depend on the outcomes of the previously randomized and treated patients. It is for this reason that the methods are called adaptive, since the probability of assigning treatment A will be adapted to the data observed to date. Zelen first described the adaptive "play-the-winner" strategy in 1969 (16) for clinical trials; the statistical properties of these designs are reviewed by Simon (17).

These randomization schemes are controversial with proponents citing that in the long run, patients are more likely to be assigned to the regimen with the better outcome. Concerns regarding these designs involve practical and ethical issues (18–20). From a practical perspective, these designs can lead to early imbalance in treatment assignment, which may compromise the ability to perform an adequate comparison; that is, they are not efficient in terms of estimating the difference between treatments. In addition, for many of these designs, the treatment assignments can become nearly completely predictable quickly, exposing the trial to selection bias.

Those that cite ethical concerns state that if clinical equipoise is not maintained, then it is not appropriate to assign even a few patients to the inferior treatment; that is, one should be prepared to use balanced randomization or not randomize at all. Trials of neonatal extracorporeal membrane oxygenation (ECMO) used adaptive randomization and provide a fascinating discussion of the issues involved with randomization in general and adaptive randomization, in particular (6). On a practical note, adaptive designs may not be feasible in many oncology trials that involve time-to-event outcomes such as survival or time to recurrence that is not expected for several years. In general, these designs are not used in oncology clinical trials (17).

Cluster Randomization

The concept of cluster randomization has been formally discussed in statistical circles for over 40 years (21), and is now an important tool in the design of intervention studies in health services research (22). Cluster randomization assigns the intervention to groups (clusters) of patients, rather than to individual patients. Randomization can be done on a per-doctor (each doctor with multiple patients) basis, on a per-classroom basis, on a per-clinic basis, or even on a per-community basis. In using cluster randomization, it is necessary to distinguish between the "unit of interest" (UI: the unit to which inference will be applied) and the "unit of analysis" (UA: the unit on which the outcomes are measured). For example, to evaluate an intervention to modify practice among pediatricians, the UA may be the patient (Did he or she receive X?) but the UI may be the pediatrician (To what proportion of patients did the MD prescribe X?).

If the UI is the doctor or clinic or community, then it is reasonable that the UI should be the unit of randomization; if the UA is the individual the sample size and analysis plans may become complicated by the number of patients in each cluster and this is an area of statistical research (23). In contrast, if the UI is the individual patient, then if not done carefully, a cluster randomized design could result in substantial loss of efficiency; the primary reasons for adopting cluster randomization when the UA is the patient, should be (a) to ensure logistic feasibility, and (b) avoid contamination. Contamination arises when features of one intervention are adopted (at least in part) by participants assigned to the other intervention. For example, it may be logistically difficult to evaluate a modification to nursing practice in a hospital ward when two or more patients share a room or one nurse is responsible for multiple rooms, or when the intervention cannot be masked and patients have the opportunity to compare notes. Cluster randomization (by classroom) might have avoided the bias that arose in the Lanarkshire milk experiment (3). While cluster randomization can substantially reduce the risk of contamination, it introduces other challenges (24,25). There is an increased risk of selection bias if the randomization is completed and the intervention is assigned to the cluster, before patients are enrolled on the study. There are ethical issues in terms of ensuring that the study participant understands the trial and the potential interventions. The analysis of the results may not be as straightforward. While an important and sometimes necessary option, cluster randomization should not be adopted without a careful evaluation of the advantages and disadvantages of this strategy, as well as ways to improve efficiency (26).

STRATIFICATION AND RANDOMIZATION

In most clinical trials, there are patient and tumor characteristics that are known to influence the response to treatment. Randomization can be expected, in the long run, to yield treatment arms that are balanced in terms of these characteristics. Furthermore, statistical methods exist to adjust for these factors at the time of the final analysis. However, this may not be sufficient: interim analyses are planned, studies are terminated early, and sometimes "in the long run" implies a very large trial. Hence it is often desirable to control the randomization process to increase balance across the treatment arms in terms of these patient characteristics. This is done by stratification. While often successfully used, stratification can lead to loss of power and efficiency if not done properly. The patient and tumor characteristics used for stratification should be available at the time of randomization and based on objective data free of interpretation. Care should be taken not to "overstratify" and create too many subsets of patients with very small numbers. The statistical analyses should incorporate the stratification that was used at the time of randomization. Byron Brown summarized the rationale for stratification (27) with

> . . . .there is much to be gained in persuasiveness or credibility by presentation of data that show the numbers of patients assigned to the several treatments to be closely balanced with regard to the variables commonly felt to be related to the course of the disease and the response to treatment. No amount of post-stratification and covariance analysis, particularly if the techniques used are complex in nature, will be as convincing as the demonstration that the groups were *balanced in the beginning*. . . ..

Simple Stratification

Simple stratification works well when there are one or two patient or disease characteristics and these can each be grouped into two to four categories. The stratification variables will be cross-classified to create strata. For example, if there are two stratification variables, one with two classes (e.g., good performance status vs. poor performance status) and one with three classes (e.g., no prior chemotherapy, prior chemotherapy but no taxanes, prior treatment with a taxane), then there will be a total of $6 = 2 \times 3$ strata. Within each stratum, a separate randomization list (on paper or in the computer) will be created to assign treatment to the patients in that stratum. Operationally, each patient is first classified into one stratum and then randomized within that stratum. In the neuroblastoma example, at the first randomization, patients were stratified according to whether they had metastatic disease or not; at the second randomization, patients were stratified according to the treatment they had been assigned at the first randomization (10). A permuted block design was used for random treatment assignment within each stratum.

The replacement, biased coin, and permuted block randomization schemes can all be easily adapted to this type of stratification. Balance, or near balance should be achieved within each stratum. While there are no set rules for the maximum number of strata permitted, practical considerations would suggest that there should be on average, at least 10 patients per stratum, and at least 20 is better.

Adaptive Randomization to Minimize Imbalance: Minimization Randomization

Stratified randomization, as described previously, is attractive for its simplicity and general effectiveness within each stratum. However, this approach can lead to troublesome imbalance across strata during the early stages of a trial. Consider the hypothetical example in Figure 21.1 where there are three strata, two treatments, and within each stratum, a permuted block design with block size 4 is used. In Figure 21.1, after the first 10 patients, with 6, 3, and 1 patients in stratum 1, 2, and 3 respectively, 3 patients have been assigned A and 7 have been assigned B. Within each stratum, there is only slight imbalance, but the cumulative effect is more pronounced. This example highlights the potential problem with simple stratification when there are many strata, especially early in the trial.

Stratum 1	Stratum 2	Stratum 3
B	A	B
A	B	B*
B	B	A
A	A*	A
B	A	B
B	B	A
A*	A	B
A	B	A

*Treatment assignments for future patients. Only 6, 3, and 1 patient randomized in strata 1, 2, 3 respectively

FIGURE 21.1 Example of cumulative imbalance across strata with simple stratification.

In 1974, Taves published a method to minimize imbalance over the entire study, and within each of the subgroups dictated by the individual patient characteristics (i.e., each stratification variable) separately, but not within the strata formed by cross-classifying all the stratification variables (28). His method was deterministic and did not incorporate randomization. Pocock and Simon independently and subsequently published an extension of the Taves method, which included randomization (29). Their method is illustrated with the following simplified example. Suppose that 50 patients have already been enrolled and randomized in a trial with 2 treatments and 3 stratification variables giving rise to 12 strata, as displayed in Figure 21.2A. The minimization method considers the stratification variables separately, as displayed in Figure 21.2B.

Figure 21.2C shows the impact on the treatment assignment balance when the next patient, a male with low performance status and no prior therapy is assigned to either A or B. In Figure 21.2C, the imbalance for each level of each stratification variable is calculated (bottom line). A summary of the imbalance is then calculated either by squaring the differences and adding them or by taking the absolute values and adding them. Squaring

Gender:	Males						Females					
Prior therapy:	No			Yes			No			Yes		
Performance status*	H	M	L	H	M	L	H	M	L	H	M	L
Assigned to A:	2	2	4	1	1	0	2	4	5	0	2	2
Assigned to B:	2	4	5	1	2	0	1	2	7	0	1	0

*H = high (KPS = 100), M = middle (KPS = 90–80), L = low (KPS = 70–60

(A)

	Gender:		Prior therapy		Performance status		
	Male	Female	No	Yes	High	Mid	Low
A	10	15	19	6	5	9	11
B	14	11	21	4	4	9	12

(B)

	Gender: Male		Prior therapy: No		Performance status: Low	
New Patient Assigned to:	A	B	A	B	A	B
New # in A:	11	10	20	19	12	11
New # in B:	14	15	21	22	12	13
Difference: A-B	−3	−5	−1	−3	−0	−2

(C)

FIGURE 21.2 (A) Status of trial with 3 stratification variables after 50 patients—number of patients assigned to treatments A and B within each of the 12 Strata. (B) Balance of treatment assignments within each of the stratification variables—number of patients assigned to A or B. (C) Impact of assigning the next patient (Male, No Prior Therapy, and Low Performance Status) to A or B.

KPS, Karnofsky performance status.
*H, high (KPS = 100); M, middle (KPS = 90–80); L, low (KPS = 70–60).

the differences will put greater weight on large differences; taking the absolute value tends to weight all the differences more equally. Using the squared differences, if the next patient is assigned to A, the summary of imbalance becomes $(-3)^2 + (-1)^2 + (0)^2 = 10$; if this next patient is instead assigned to B, the summary of imbalance becomes $(-5)^2 + (-3)^2 + (-2)^2 = 38$. Assigning this patient to receive treatment A will minimize the imbalance at this point. The Taves procedure would assign the treatment A; the Pocock–Simon approach would randomly assign treatment with probability $p^* > 1/2$, for treatment A. Variations exist: stratification variables can be weighted and a term can be added that accounts for the overall balance across all strata. With available computer programs, both the simple stratification and the minimization randomization are easy to implement. Simple stratification achieves balance within each of the strata, while minimization is more likely to achieve balance across the stratification variables and overall.

SUMMARY

Randomized clinical trials remain the most robust and credible method for generating data to formally compare treatments for patients with cancer. In planning the technical aspects of the randomization during the design of the clinical trial, the stratification variables and the randomization scheme must be selected. Choice of the number of stratification variables represents a trade-off between controlling as much as possible and striving for simplicity to the extent that it is possible. Criteria for using a stratification variable in the design should include the strength of the association between the variable and the outcome measures, its known ability to affect the response to treatment, and the reliability with which it can be measured prior to the start of treatment. If there are only one or two stratification variables and the final study size will be large, then simple stratification will be sufficient. In this case, randomization using the permuted block design is both easy and effective. If there are many stratification variables or if there will be early interim analysis or the study is relatively small, then minimization randomization will be more effective for achieving short-term balance across the stratification variables.

All three elements of trial design are essential: control, randomization, and replication. Properly designing and executing the randomization is critical for the success of the trial.

REFERENCES

1. Fisher RA. *The Design of Experiments*. Edinburgh: Oliver and Boyd; 1935.

2. Stein JP, Stein JP, Lieskovsky G, et al. Radical cystectomy in the treatment of invasive bladder cancer: long-term results in 1,054 patients. *J Clin Oncol*. 2001;19:666–675.

3. Student. The Lanarkshire milk experiment. *Biometrika*. 1931;23:398–406.

4. Zelen M. Randomized consent designs for clinical trials: an update. *Statist Med*. 1990;9:645–656.

5. Freedman B. Equipoise and the ethics of clinical research. *N Engl J Med*. 1987;317:141–145.

6. Royall RM. Ethics and statistics in randomized clinical trials. *Statist Sci*. 1991;6:52–88.

7. Temple R, Ellenberg SS. Placebo-controlled trials and active-controlled trials in the evaluation of new treatments. Part 1: ethical and scientific issues. *Ann Intern Med*. 2000;133:456–464.

8. Ellenberg SS, Temple R. Placebo-controlled trials and active-controlled trials in the evaluation of new treatments. Part 2: practical issues and specific cases. *Ann Intern Med*. 2000;133:464–470.

9. Durrleman S, Simon R. When to randomize? *J Clin Oncol*. 1991;9:116–122.

10. Matthay KK, Villablanca JG, Seeger RC, et al. Treatment of high-risk neuroblastoma with intensive chemotherapy, radiotherapy, autologous bone marrow transplantation, and 13-*cis*-retinoic acid. *N Engl J Med*. 1999;341:1165–1173.

11. Sposto R, Krailo MD. Use of unequal allocation in survival trials. *Statist Med*. 1987;6:119–125.

12. Pocock SJ. Allocation of patients to treatment in clinical trials. *Biometrics*. 1979;35:183–197.

13. Rosenberger WF, Lachin JM. *Randomization in Clinical Trials: Theory and Practice*. New York, NY; Chichester: John Wiley & Sons. 2002.

14. Kalish LA, Begg CB. Treatment allocation methods in clinical trials: a review. *Statist Med*. 1985;4:129–144.

15. Efron B. Forcing a sequential experiment to be balanced. *Biometrika*. 1971;58:403–417.

16. Zelen M. Play the winner rule and the controlled clinical trial. *J Amer Statis Assoc*. 1969;64:131–146.

17. Simon R. Adaptive treatment assignment methods and clinical trials. *Biometrics*. 1977;33:743–749.

18. Hey SP, Kimmelman J. Are outcome-adaptive allocation trials ethical? *Clin Trials*. 2015;12:102–106.

19. Buyse M. Commentary on Hey and Kimmelman. *Clin Trials*. 2015;12:119–121.

20. Korn EL, Freidlin B. Commentary on Hey and Kimmelman. *Clin Trials*. 2015;12:122–124.

21. Cornfeld J. Randomization by group: a formal analysis. *Am J Epidemiol*. 1978;108:100–102.

22. Campbell MJ, Donner A, Klar N. Developments in cluster randomized trials and *Statistics in Medicine*. *Statist Med*. 2007;26:2–19.

23. Campbell MJ, Donner A, Elbourne DR, eds. Design and analysis of cluster randomized trials. *Statist Med*. 2001;20(theme issue):329–496.

24. Klar N, Donner A. Current and future in the design and analysis of cluster randomization trials. *Statist Med*. 2001;20:3729–3740.

25. Donner A, Klar N. Pitfalls of and controversies in cluster randomization trials. *Am J Public Health*. 2004;94:416–422.

26. Crespi CM. Improved designs for cluster randomized trials. *Annu Rev Public Health*. 2016;37:1–16.

27. Brown BW Jr. Statistical controversies in the design of clinical trials some personal views. *Cont Clin Trials*. 1980;1:13–27.

28. Taves DR. Minimization: a new method of assigning patients to treatment and control groups. *Clin Pharmacol Ther*. 1974;15:443–453.

29. Pocock SJ, Simon R. Sequential treatment assignment with balancing for prognostic factors in the controlled clinical trial. *Biometrics*. 1975;31:103–115.

22

Case Report Form Development

Susan Barry

During the development of a new clinical trial much attention is devoted to the design of the trial and the protocol document, leaving the case report forms (CRFs) to be created at the last minute. However, principal investigators (PIs) should realize that the quality of the data collected will ultimately determine the success of the trial (1). As such, considerable thought should be devoted to planning and designing the CRFs.

This chapter describes:

- Timing of CRF development
- The CRF development team
- Common methods of data collection
- Frequently used CRFs
- Design and testing of CRFs

CRF DEVELOPMENT TIMELINE

The timing of CRF development is an important consideration in the study development process. Some institutions or sponsors prefer to delay the form development process until the protocol is near final while others are successful in developing the protocol and CRFs concurrently. There are advantages to both methods. Delaying the CRFs until the protocol is complete usually eliminates the need for multiple changes to the forms as most protocols undergo several revisions before being finalized. This may be especially important to note if the CRFs will be collected electronically as electronic data capture (eDC) systems require a significant effort to modify.

On the other hand, planning and developing the CRFs alongside the protocol can reduce the total study development time and lead to a quicker study activation. Many oncology clinical trials collect the same basic data elements and the development of standard forms can be done early in the process. Study-specific elements can be added after the protocol document is finalized. Additionally, the form development team may uncover inconsistencies or deficiencies in the protocol while developing the CRFs. For example, developing the chemotherapy dose form for a study in which treatment dose is based on body surface area (BSA) may lead to the realization that the preferred method of calculating BSA has not been stipulated in the protocol. In addition, if the protocol finalization takes longer than expected the form development may be rushed, which can lead to missing required data elements or errors on the forms that will require time-consuming changes later. Therefore, study teams must find a balance between the protocol and CRFs to ensure both are developed in an accurate and timely manner.

PLANNING FOR DATA COLLECTION

Careful planning for CRF development is essential to the success of the trial. Poorly designed CRFs can lead to the collection of insufficient or incorrect data or may involve unnecessary study team effort, either in collecting unnecessary data, difficulty in completing the forms due to unclear questions, or in modifying the CRFs. The PI should consider the following areas when planning CRF development: the form development team, method of collection, required data elements, and data submission time points.

Form Development Team

An important step in CRF development is determining who should be involved in the process of designing and testing the forms. There are many roles in the form development and data collection process and each of these should be involved in the initial development of the forms. While the PI and statistician are responsible for providing medical and scientific expertise to identify the data elements required to meet the study objectives, other roles such as research nurses, research coordinators, and study monitors can provide practical input about the clarity and ordering of questions, the availability of requested data, the feasibility of data submission timelines, and the monitoring effort required. CALGB 80101 included a clinical economics component, which involved collecting the institution's Medicare ID number. During the form development process not much thought was given to this seemingly innocuous data point but several sites had difficulty in obtaining this information as it was considered highly confidential information. The study team eventually stopped requiring this field to be completed and obtained these data through other methods. Had these forms been properly vetted by research nurses and study coordinators, the study team would have been aware of this issue prior to releasing the forms (2). Therefore, in addition to being involved in the CRF development, these research nurses, coordinators, and monitors should be heavily involved in the testing of forms prior to study activation. If the data will be collected electronically, involving someone with knowledge of the eDC system to be used is also key.

Methods of Data Collection

Before determining which data elements are required for a study, the study team should determine how the data will be collected. There are two basic CRF formats: paper and electronic. Each of these has several options for submission, data entry, and quality control. Understanding the advantages and limitations of each option is important in designing CRFs that are efficient and accurate.

Paper CRFs are relatively inexpensive and easy to develop, while the systems that can be used to collect data electronically are typically expensive and usually require a form builder with training in the specific eDC system (3). There are some eDC systems, such as REDCap that are less expensive and do not require special training (4). Modifying paper CRFs can be done quickly and with relatively little effort while amending electronic CRFs (eCRFs) is rather complicated and time-consuming.

Another point to consider is access to the CRFs. Paper forms must be distributed to each site by the study monitor during a site visit, by mail, or posted on a website. It may be difficult to control who has access to the forms or even to determine who has completed the forms. Most eDC systems require a unique login for each user, which allows for more access control and also tracks all changes made to the data, which is a requirement for 21 CFR Part 11 compliance (5). While there are advantages to restricting user access, a member of the study team will have to be responsible for managing user access, which can become quite cumbersome on a trial with many participating sites.

Despite the extra effort required by eDC systems, most eCRFs provide many time- and effort-saving benefits that cannot be accomplished with traditional paper forms including built-in edit checks to catch erroneous or missing data and prompts to submit data based on the study-specific time points. In addition, while eDC systems may be expensive, they do eliminate some costs associated with paper forms, such as postage for mailing paper CRFs, data entry staff, the need for filing space and personnel. These systems also guide research coordinators through the forms and, when built correctly, allow the user to enter only data required for each specific visit. These systems will greatly reduce the number of errors submitted on CRFs, which should reduce monitoring time and costs as well.

One of the most beneficial attributes of an eDC system is the ability to error-proof data before the forms are submitted. Most systems allow the study team to implement edit checks on data points to ensure data validity, such as acceptable ranges for laboratory values, correctly formatted dates, and compliance with eligibility criteria. While programming the system to run checks for every possible error may be tempting, these edit checks can be time-consuming to set up and must be thoroughly tested before releasing the forms for use. In addition, including too many edit checks can make navigating the system and submitting the data very difficult and frustrating. Certainly, the study team should use this functionality but should find a balance between ensuring clean data are submitted and the effort required to include edit checks in the CRFs.

While there are many benefits to using an eDC system, the PI should be aware of a few additional restrictions on these systems. Most systems require users to complete a system training before using the system to submit or review data. With the implementation of electronic medical records, having two computer monitors, so the user can view the medical records and eDC system simultaneously, is almost essential. Most pharmaceutical sponsors and major academic sites have determined the benefits of eCRFs outweigh the challenges and have transitioned to eDC systems, almost completely eliminating the use of paper forms. PIs should determine which data collection methods are available at their academic institution or within the pharmaceutical company sponsoring the trial.

REQUIRED DATA ELEMENTS

Most oncology clinical trials involve collecting similar data with each trial requiring study-specific and disease-specific data points. The commonly collected data elements can be grouped into three categories: baseline/eligibility, treatment, and follow-up. Table 22.1 summarizes the CRFs associated with each category and the frequency with which these should be collected. Each of these categories is discussed in detail. Not all trials necessitate the collection of every form listed in Table 22.1 and there may be some additional data that

TABLE 22.1 Frequently Collected Forms on Oncology Trials

Baseline and Eligibility Data		
On-Study Form	Key eligibility and disease diagnosis and staging data	Collect at baseline; prior to beginning therapy
Prior Treatment Form	Collect *relevant* treatment history	
Baseline Disease Status/Tumor Measurements	Collect for trials involving disease response or progression endpoints	
Preexisting Conditions Form	Collection allows distinction of AEs from preexisting conditions; confirm absence of specific conditions listed in exclusion criteria	
Concomitant Medications Form	Documents medications that may affect treatment response or AEs, or may be prohibited in the study exclusion criteria	
Treatment Data		
Treatment Form	Dosing information for all agents or therapies (e.g., radiotherapy) required per protocol	Each cycle or treatment period
AE Form	Record of AEs occurring during active treatment	AEs should be assessed at each clinic visit; AE form should be collected at least once per cycle
Disease Status/Tumor Measurements	Disease response and status updates	Collect only as often as disease assessments are performed, which may be less frequent than every cycle
Concomitant Medications Form	Documents medications that may affect treatment response or AEs, or have been prescribed to alleviate AEs	Concomitant medications should be evaluated at each clinic visit; the form should be collected/updated at least once per cycle
Nonprotocol Therapy Form	Record of any nonprotocol cancer therapy given to patient	Collect only if nonprotocol therapy is received
End-of-Treatment Form	Documents the reason for ending therapy	Collect at the end of all protocol therapy
Follow-Up/Survival Data		
Survival Data Form	Documents date last known alive and data and cause of death	At each follow-up clinic visit
AE Form	Record of AEs occurring during active treatment	AEs should be assessed until all treatment-related AEs have resolved or until nonprotocol therapy begins
Disease Status/Tumor Measurements	Disease response and status updates	Collect only as often as disease assessments are performed during the follow-up period
Nonprotocol Therapy Form	Record of any nonprotocol cancer therapy given to patient	Collect only if nonprotocol therapy is received

AE, adverse event.

is required to meet regulatory and sponsor requirements but is not needed to meet the objectives of the trials. For example, trials funded by the Cancer Therapy Evaluation Program (CTEP) may be required to collect preexisting conditions and a prior therapy form using CTEP-specific codes. These data may not be used for the trial but will be required for study reports to CTEP (6).

Baseline and Eligibility Data

Collection of baseline or on-study data is an opportunity to confirm eligibility and gather prestudy information about the trial participants, such as patient demographics, diagnosis information, disease stage and status, medical history, prognostic indicators, and prior treatment information (1). For patients with measurable disease a tumor measurement form should also be collected particularly if the endpoint of the trial is disease response. In addition, the collection of any stratification factors used during randomization is recommended. Some stratification factors, such as performance status, can change between randomization and treatment start. Collecting these data at registration and at treatment start can be useful during analysis.

While the baseline data forms may collect some key eligibility data, documentation of every eligibility criterion in a study database is not necessary. Study monitors should confirm eligibility for patients using source documentation, not the CRFs, so the collection of much of this data would be a wasted effort. PIs should work with the study statistician to determine the baseline data needed for the study analysis.

Some sponsors provide, or even require, an eligibility checklist and many institutions allow this checklist to be used as source documentation to confirm eligibility. Allowing the use of an eligibility checklist as source documentation is useful in documenting inclusion and exclusion criteria that are frequently not documented in a physician note. Examples of such criteria include patient life expectancy, such as "life expectancy of at least 6 months," or confirming that the patient is not taking certain prohibited medications (7).

Treatment Data

The data collected during the treatment phase of the study includes information about adverse events (AEs), disease assessments, and protocol treatment, which is information about any study-assigned interventions the patient may have received, such as chemotherapy (including oral agents), radiotherapy, or surgery. The details of protocol treatment data that is collected can vary widely based on the needs of the study. Commonly collected data elements include:

- Date treatment received: This may be a range (e.g., day 1 of the cycle to the last day of the cycle) if agents are taken several times throughout a cycle or on a daily basis. For some trials it may be necessary to collect the date each treatment is given.
- Cycle number: If the study divides treatments into cycles it is helpful to collect cycle numbers as dates can be difficult to track, especially if multiple dose delays are implemented.
- Dose received: This may be collected as total dose for an entire cycle, entire treatment regimen, or individual doses for each treatment received. If any agents are self-administered, such as oral agents, the use of a drug diary to document compliance is recommended.
- Dose modifications: Any variations from the protocol-prescribed treatment regimen should be documented on the CRFs. Dose modifications include dose delays (deferring a dose until a later date, but still receiving the dose), dose skips (omitting a dose from the treatment regimen), and dose reductions (decreasing the amount of the drug given). Most protocols do not allow dose reescalations after a dose reduction, but if permitted, then dose reescalation should also be included as a possible dose modification.
- Treatment continuation: This element is particularly important for electronic forms as this will serve as an indicator to the system which forms should be completed next for the particular patient. If the participant continues on protocol treatment another cycle of treatment data will required; if the participant discontinues therapy, the first posttreatment follow-up data will be required. Although not absolutely necessary, this question is useful to data managers collecting paper CRFs as well.
- Off-treatment reason and date: If the patient has discontinued therapy for any reason, it is important to collect the reason and date of last treatment. Certain sponsors, such as CTEP, require the use of standardized choices for this question, but frequently used reasons include: completed protocol therapy, disease progression, AE, patient death, patient/physician decision, and receiving nonprotocol therapy (5).

AE reporting is usually divided into two categories: routine and serious (or expedited). Routine AE reporting is accomplished using the study CRFs. Serious adverse events (SAEs) require special reporting to the Food and Drug Administration (FDA) and trial sponsors 21 CFR 312.32 (8). SAEs are usually reported to the FDA using the MedWatch form; however, National Cancer Institute (NCI) cooperative groups require SAEs to be reported via the CTEP AERS application (9). Additional events that are not SAEs but are "events of special interest" may also require expedited reporting to the sponsor. Any events of special interest and the reporting requirements for such events should be clearly defined in the protocol. As SAE reporting is done on

FDA- or CTEP-regulated forms, this section focuses on collection of routine events.

The collection of AE data is relatively standardized as it is very important to be able to merge data from multiple sets to create a complete toxicity profile. The use of a common dictionary of AE terms and grades, such as the Common Terminology Criteria for Adverse Events (CTCAE) is strongly encouraged (10). Along with the CTCAE a standard coding system, such as MedDRA, that has been mapped to the CTCAE is very useful in the collection and analysis of AEs as well. The common elements used in collecting AEs are:

- Name of event: This information should come from a list of standardized events, such as the CTCAE.
- Grade: The severity of the event is needed to meet various reporting requirements such as annual reports to the FDA and continuing reviews of an IRB. The collection of all grades is not necessary for all trials. Phase III trials may only collect grade 3 or higher events whereas a phase I trial may collect all events regardless of grade. Many trials also require only the most severe grade to be reported. If a particular event does not exist in the CTCAE, the study team can define the grading criteria for that event in the protocol.
- Attribution: This information may be collected in various ways, such as a yes/no indicator of attribution to the protocol therapy. It may also be collected as a range of causality, as is done on CTEP trials, by providing the choices: *unrelated*, *unlikely*, *possible*, *probable*, and *definite*. It is important to note on the AE form which agents the attribution assessment includes. If a treatment regimen includes both investigational and noninvestigational agents, it may be necessary to collect a separate attribution for each or specify that the requested information is only for the investigational agent. If very specific attribution information is required, a study may even require the attribution assessment to include the patient's disease, concomitant medications, and preexisting conditions.
- Start and stop dates and times of AEs: This information may be necessary to collect if very detailed information is needed for reporting or data analysis. These dates and times are difficult to document as patients do not always remember the exact date or times that symptoms began or subsided.

Many AEs are noted during the review of laboratory reports. It is very time-consuming for research staff to grade each event noted in laboratory results. An alternative to collecting out-of-range lab values as AEs is to collect the lab values themselves, which can be systematically graded during the study analysis. Institutional upper and lower limits of normal may be required to

perform such an assessment. Other options include reporting of lab values only if they are of a certain grade, lead to a dose modification, or if they are of a particular interest to the study team. While reporting requirements of AEs are quite standardized, for the sake of the time and effort of the study team members, careful consideration should be given to which events and grades are necessary for each study.

The third type of data collected during the treatment phase of a study is the response and disease assessment data. Depending on the trial objectives or the length of the treatment phase this type of data may not be collected during protocol treatment. For trials requiring disease assessment during treatment the response or disease assessment form usually includes questions about the disease status or the disease response to protocol therapy and the date of the last disease assessment. Collection of the method of assessment, such as CT or physical exam, may also be necessary for ensuring a consistent method is used for a participant throughout the trial.

Response, best response, or overall response is one of the questions most frequently answered incorrectly in oncology trials. The CRF question should be very clear as to what the requested information is. It is a common practice in oncology trials to collect *best response* or *best overall response*, meaning the best response the patient has had to therapy over the duration of the trial. For example, if a patient achieves a partial response and then later progresses, the best response is still recorded as "partial response." This is frequently misunderstood on CRFs. A study team could collect "response during this assessment" instead of "best overall response," but this too poses problems. If a patient achieves a partial response and then remains stable (i.e., no further decrease in the size of their disease is noted), it may be unclear if the correct answer to "response during this assessment" is "partial response" or "stable disease." CRF training, clear instructions on the forms, and vigilant data monitoring can help mitigate these issues.

An additional question that may be needed on a solid tumor response form is whether the response has been confirmed. As per Response Evaluation Criteria in Solid Tumors (RECIST) 1.1, confirmation of response is required for studies where objective response is the primary objective (11). Confirmation of response may also be a useful field to collect in other circumstances as determined by the study team.

In addition to response, some studies require the collection of tumor measurements. The structure and inconsistency of tumor measurement data pose many issues for study teams attempting to enter these data into a database. Common issues include categorization of target and nontarget lesions, tumors that are not measurable or visible at every evaluation, and variations in measurements among those reviewing the scans. Trials with response as a primary endpoint may require central review of images to ensure consistent and accurate measurements. (12–13). Trials with progression-free survival may only require tumor measurements at the time of progression.

Follow-up and Survival Data

Depending on the objectives of the study, follow-up data collection may not be required at all (e.g., a phase I dose escalation trial) or may be collected for many years. The PI and the statistician should determine which data are necessary, the frequency of data collection, and the amount of time the trial participants must be followed for each trial. Most phase II and III oncology trials will collect disease status, survival, nonprotocol treatment, and long-term AE data. Disease status data will be similar to the disease data collected during active treatment but will usually not include "best response" as response to treatment would normally have been noted during active treatment and not during the follow-up phase. Collection of specific survival information is also important. When analyzing the study data, one cannot assume that a patient is alive because a death notification has not been received or because the patient is not yet listed in a publicly available death record, such as the Social Security Death Index. A specific field on the follow-up form should collect the date the patient was last known to be alive. In addition, it is important to collect the date and the cause of death. CTEP standard choices for the cause of death are protocol-treatment-related, disease-related, and other causes (5). These general categories enable easy tabulation of cause of death and additional questions may be added to collect an exact cause of death.

Any long-term AEs, events that are still present at the time of discontinuation of protocol therapy, should continue to be reported during the follow-up period if they still meet the protocol-specific criteria for reporting. For example, if the protocol requires the reporting of grade 3 or higher events, grade 3 neuropathy should continue to be reported during follow-up until it has improved to a grade 2 or less. The CRFs should also collect any nonprotocol treatments received during the follow-up period. Nonprotocol treatments may not only affect the study endpoints, but may also allay the need to report long-term AEs.

Data collection requirements will differ across studies and will depend on the disease being studied, the objective(s) of the trial, and sponsor and regulatory requirements. The PI and statistician should work with the study sponsor to determine the appropriate detail and frequency of data needed for regulatory submissions and the analysis of the trial data. In addition, the timing of the collection of these data should coincide with the clinic visits and assessments. For example, a tumor response form should not be collected every three cycles if disease assessments are required every four cycles. A careful comparison of the data submission schedule and the required tests and procedures should be performed before activating the trial.

DETERMINING APPROPRIATE AMOUNT AND FREQUENCY OF DATA COLLECTION

Many sources on form development will instruct the study team to collect only the data that is needed for that particular trial. However, it is sometime reasonable to collect additional data that may be used in a meta-analysis or to justify a future study (1,14–15). Collecting more data than is necessary is a common practice, so it is important to review the reasons for limiting the data collected and to review what data is essential. Collecting more than the necessary data is primarily an issue for the research coordinators completing the CRFs. CRF completion is a time-consuming task that requires attention to detail. Requiring completion of data elements that are likely to not be used detracts from time that could have been spent on collecting data points that are essential to the study. Research coordinators may end up rushing to meet submission timelines and will not have time to enter the important data carefully. In addition, the extra data that are collected will require additional time to build and test in an eDC system. Significant monitor and PI review effort may also be required after the data are submitted. A PI should also check with the study statistician about the usability of any extra data collected. The study may not even be designed or powered appropriately to use that data in a secondary analysis. There may be circumstances that warrant the collection of data that will not be used for the trial in which it is collected, such as a very large trial that provides the opportunity to collect a previously unstudied data set. With limited resources available for clinical trials using any opportunity to collect data that *might* be used is tempting, but PIs need to consider the downside of the extra effort required to do so and ensure appropriate resources are available for data collection and management.

In addition to considering how much data is collected, consideration should also be given to the frequency of collection. When determining the data submission schedule it is a useful exercise to calculate the number of forms expected throughout the trial. Performing this exercise may bring to light unnecessary collection time points and help the study team determine the resources needed to complete the CRFs. When developing forms for CALGB 80702, it was noted that the follow-up forms were scheduled to be collected every 3 months, which would result in the submission of 10,000 forms in the first year of follow-up of 2,500 patients. The PI and the statistician determined that the frequency of collection could be reduced to every 6 months, which reduced the number of forms to be completed by half (16).

USE OF DEVELOPMENT OF CRF TEMPLATES

Whether using paper or eCRFs, thoroughly vetted CRF templates can be a useful place to start when developing forms. The use of templates decreases the amount of time and effort needed to create forms either on paper or in an electronic format (17). Most eDC systems allow users to copy previously used forms and the edit checks associated with those forms to a new study. Research coordinators become accustomed to the general layout and functionality of templated forms, which makes completing them easier. Collecting data in a similar manner across trials also decreases the chance of missing critical data points and allows for the use of standard error reports and data analysis by the statisticians. For example, if all studies use the same format and field names to collect AEs, developing a standardized program to summarize AE data will be much more feasible. Standardized data collection also facilitates meta-analyses across studies (18). Institutions and sponsors may have templates or forms previously used on a similar study that can be used as templates. Many templates and previously used CRFs can be found using the Common Data Element (CDE) Browser, which allows users to search the contents of the NCI cancer Standard Data Repository (caDSR) (19).

CRF DESIGN AND LAYOUT

Another important element of CRF development is the design and format of the forms themselves. As stated previously, there are two options for CRFs: paper and electronic. Elements necessary for both methods and elements unique to each are discussed.

Whether using paper CRFs or eCRFs the inclusion of participant identifiers on each CRF is mandatory. At least the participant initials (or name, if required by the sponsor) and two other identifiers should be collected on the CRFs, such as the institutional medical record number and the participant trial number that was assigned at enrollment. In addition to participant identifiers, fields identifying which visit or cycle the form refers to are necessary. This may be a cycle or visit number field, a date field, a choice field (e.g., Baseline, Induction, Consolidation, Maintenance, Follow-up) or a combination of these fields. When using paper forms, it is very important to include participant identifiers and cycle and visit identifiers on every page of multipage forms as pages may be separated. Most eCRF systems can be set up to autocomplete the identifiers on all pages but the study team should ensure that these fields are included on every form and are easily visible to the person entering data. It is also necessary to ensure that forms that are collected multiple times include a field to distinguish it from other forms of the same kind. For example, if a study requires the collection of a pain

score assessment form four times in one cycle, collecting the cycle number alone would not suffice. In this case it would be necessary to collect the date of the assessment or an assessment number to distinguish between the four assessments that were done in the same cycle.

The fields on the forms should be organized in a natural flow and like items should be grouped together to ease data entry. Font style and size should be easy to read and the entry fields on paper forms should be large enough to write text clearly. While it may be tempting to crowd as many fields as possible on a paper form to keep it to one page, crowding the form will make completing it more difficult and increase the likelihood of research coordinators missing a question. Paper forms should also include a field to indicate that the form has been amended. This will be very helpful in distinguishing the original from subsequently submitted versions.

One common functionality of eCRFs is dynamic forms, meaning that fields or entire forms may be hidden or visible based on answers to trigger questions. For example, instead of including several detailed questions about prior surgery, radiotherapy, and chemotherapy on a baseline form, answering "Yes" to the question "Has the patient received any prior therapy?" can trigger the addition of a prior therapy form. If the patient has not received any prior therapy, (i.e., the trigger question is answered "No") the form will not be added to the required form list for this patient. This functionality can be very helpful in reducing the number of forms that a research coordinator must see and complete but it should be used carefully. Ensure that *all* of the information collected in a dynamic field or form should only be accessed if the trigger question is answered in a certain way. If the study requires an answer to a question for all participants it should most likely not be a dynamic field.

Another formatting decision to make is the length of the forms. For most eDC systems it is recommended to limit forms to one page or what a user can see on the computer screen without scrolling. This will result in more overall pages but with the appropriate cues set up in the eDC system, research coordinators should be able to easily track which forms are required. The opposite of this tends to be true when using paper forms. Generally, it is better to have fewer but longer paper forms, so there are less actual forms for coordinators to remember to complete and submit.

EDIT CHECKS AND QUERIES

For a data manager or monitor one of the most useful features of an eDC system is the ability to build in edit checks and automatic queries. These can be immensely helpful in ensuring the appropriate forms are completed in a timely and accurate manner. Systems vary in the depth of their functionality but the more robust systems can be programmed to remind users about overdue and upcoming forms and prevent the submission of incomplete forms or discrepant data. However, careful planning and testing should be performed on all edit checks and queries prior to releasing the eCRFs. While the use of this functionality will conserve resources during data collection, setting up and testing the edits check and queries during form development are time-consuming. Also, one should ensure that the edit check will apply to all situations or that there is a way to bypass the edit if necessary. For example, a laboratory value form should *not* require all of the values to be completed in order to submit the form. Even if the lab values are required per protocol, there is always a chance that one or some of the values will not be available. Some eDC systems will also alert the user the field is blank but will not prevent the user from submitting the forms. A form builder may also include a separate "not available" field for each lab value, that, when checked, prevents the edit check from appearing.

REVIEW AND TESTING OF FORMS

During the form development process CRFs should be distributed to the form development team for review a few times. Including all members of the study team in the form review and testing process is extremely important as each member will focus on a different aspect of the forms. The research coordinator or research nurse should field-test the forms by completing each form using actual patient data. This is more likely to bring to light missing answer choices, incorrect lab values, or field formats. Data can be anonymized during this type of testing by changing the patient identifiers. When using an eDC system the dynamic forms and fields and any edit checks must also be thoroughly tested. Below is a brief form review checklist for reviewing CRFs. The study team should ensure:

- Collection of data to meet study endpoints including response and progression data, survival data, safety and feasibility data, or other specific data listed in the statistical analysis plan
- Frequency of data collection is appropriate, but not excessive, for meeting study objectives and consistent with the study calendar
- Questions and answer choices are consistent with analysis plan, medically accurate, mutually exclusive and exhaustive, and the correct units are provided
- "Other" and "Not applicable" choices are used appropriately
- Questions are in a logical order and not repetitive
- Required forms applicable to all participants and dynamic forms and fields are triggered correctly

SUMMARY

Careful planning and development of CRFs is essential to gathering usable data from a clinical trial. The objectives of the study, the study calendar, and the method of data collection, paper or electronic, strongly influence the content and format of the CRFs. Involving various study team member roles in the form development process, using form templates, and thorough testing of the forms will ensure the CRFs collect the necessary data for analysis and regulatory purposes while also being as user-friendly and as resource-conserving as possible.

There is arguably no more important document than the instrument that is used to acquire the data from the clinical trial, with the exception of the protocol, which specifies the conduct of that trial. The quality of the data collected relies first and foremost on the quality of that instrument. No matter how much time and effort go into conducting the trial, if the correct data points were not collected, a meaningful analysis may not be possible. It follows, therefore, that the design, development and quality assurance of such an instrument must be given the utmost attention. (20)

REFERENCES

1. Cook TD, DeMets DL. *Introduction to Statistical Methods for Clinical Trials*. Boca Raton, FL: CRC Press; 2007:171–199.
2. Fuchs CS, Tepper JE, Niedzwiecki D, et al. Postoperative adjuvant chemoradiation for gastric or gastroesophageal junction (GEJ) adenocarcinoma using epirubicin, cisplatin, and infusional (CI) 5-FU (ECF) before and after CI 5-FU and radiotherapy (CRT) compared with bolus 5-FU/LV before and after CRT: Intergroup trial CALGB 80101. *ASCO Ann Meet Proceed*. 2011;29(Suppl 15):4003.
3. Le Jeannic A, Quelen C, Corrine A, et al. Comparison of two data collection processes in clinical studies: electronic and paper case report forms. *BMC Med Res Methodol*. 2014;14(1):1.
4. Harris PA, Taylor R, Thielke R, et al. Research electronic data capture (REDCap): a metadata-driven methodology and workflow process for providing translational research informatics support. *J Biomed Inform*. 2009;42(2):377–381.
5. Food and Drug Administration. *Guidance for Industry: Part 11, Electronic Records; Electronic Signatures—Scope and Application*. FDA; 2003.
6. National Cancer Institute Cancer Therapy Evaluation Program. Clinical Data Update System (CDUS)- Instructions and Guidelines Version 3.0. CTIS; 2011.
7. Penel N, Clisant S, Lefebvre JL, et al. Sufficient life expectancy: an amazing inclusion criterion in cancer phase II-III trials. *J Clin Oncol*. 2009;27(26):e105.
8. US Food and Drug Administration. Code of Federal Regulations (21CFR312.32). *Invest New Drug App*. 2014.
9. National Cancer Institute. NCI Guidelines for Investigators: Adverse Event Reporting Requirements for DCTD (CTEP and CIP) and DCP INDs and IDEs; 2012. https://ctep.cancer.gov/protocolDevelopment/electronic_applications/docs/aeguidelines.pdf
10. National Cancer Institute. Common Terminology Criteria for Adverse Events v4.0. NCI, NIH, DHHS; 2009.

11. Eisenhauer E, Therasse P, Bogaerts J, et al. New response evaluation criteria in solid tumours: revised RECIST guideline (version 1.1). *Eur J Cancer*. 2009;45(2):228–247.

12. Food Drug Administration Center for Drugs Evaluation and Research. Clinical Trial Imaging Endpoint Process Standards Guidance for Industry (Draft Guidance); 2015. http://www.fda.gov/downloads/drugs/guidancecompliance regulatoryinformation/guidances/ucm268555.pdf

13. Erickson BJ, Buckner JC. Imaging in clinical trials. *Cancer Infor*. 2007;4:13–18.

14. EMA ICH Topic E 6 (R1) Guideline for good clinical practice. CPMP/ICH/135/95. 59; 2002. http://www.ema.europa.eu

15. CDISC CDASH Team. Clinical Data Acquisition Standards Harmonization (CDASH). CDISC; 2011. http://www.cdisc.org

16. Alliance for Clinical Trials in Oncology. Oxaliplatin, leucovorin calcium, and fluorouracil with or without celecoxib in treating patients with stage III colon cancer previously treated with surgery. In *ClinicalTrials.gov* [Internet]. Bethesda, MD: National Library of Medicine; 2000. http://clinicaltrials.gov/ct2/show/NCT01150045

17. Souza T, Kush R, Evans JP. Global clinical data interchange standards are here! Drug Discov Today. 2007;12:174–181.

18. Richesson RL, Nadkarni P. Data standards for clinical research data collection forms: current status and challenges. *JAMA*. 2011;18(3):341–346. doi:10.1136/amiajnl-2011-000107

19. caDSR Database and Tools. https://wiki.nci.nih.gov/display/caDSR/caDSR+Database+and+Tools

20. Good Clinical Data Management Practices. Version 4, Society for Clinical Data Management; 2005.

Monitoring, Assessing, and Reporting Adverse Events

Amy Callahan, Elizabeth Ness, and Helen Chen

An essential component in the development of cancer therapeutics is documentation and reporting of adverse events (AEs) during clinical trials. Accurate and timely assessment, documentation, and reporting of AEs are crucial components of good clinical practice (GCP), and are critical to protecting research participants, while ensuring data integrity (1). All physicians who sign the Food and Drug Administration (FDA) 1572 investigator registration form commit to accurate reporting (2). Information gained from AE reporting such as cumulative rates of events and details of specific major events could significantly impact ongoing and future trials utilizing the study agent, particularly with regard to patient inclusion criteria, safety monitoring plans, prophylaxis, and management of toxicities. The institutional review boards (IRBs) and ethics committees (ECs) are interested in accurate reporting of AEs to assist them in ensuring human subject protection.

The research team involved in AE investigation during execution of the study intervention has a responsibility to participate in activities that comprehensively evaluate and contribute to the development of the AE and toxicity profile of the drug. This extensive process is the culmination of incorporating the patient and clinician interaction, the surveillance and recording of signs and symptoms, and appropriate reporting of AEs.

This chapter is divided into four major sections: terminology associated with AEs, AE assessment and documentation, reporting of AEs for investigational new drug (IND) studies, and guidelines for Cancer Therapy Evaluation Program (CTEP) sponsored clinical trials under INDs. Reporting of AEs to the IRB is addressed in a prior Chapter 3.

TERMINOLOGY ASSOCIATED WITH ADVERSE EVENTS

Numerous terms have been used to convey AEs, including: toxicity, side effect, acute or late effect, complication, and adverse drug reaction. The aforementioned implies that an intervention caused the event, which is not the definition of an AE. The FDA, the Office for Human Research Protections (OHRP), and the International Council for Harmonisation Good Clinical Practice (ICH-GCP) guidelines provide various definitions associated with AEs. Table 23.1 (6) compares AE-related terminology used by these organizations.

A summary definition for an AE is any unwanted sign, symptom, or disease that was not seen before the individual's research participation, or worsening of baseline symptom, regardless of expectedness or relationship to research. It is instrumental to recognize that though an event or a certain response may be expected, it is still considered an AE. The expectedness is used to assess the causal relationship, which is discussed later in this chapter.

Standard terminology for AE collection in oncology clinical trials dates back over 35 years. Common terminology to describe toxicities and publication of clinical trial results helps to ensure patient safety. Awareness of the various terms and definitions associated with AEs, mentioned previously, is the first step in understanding what an AE is and how it is delineated.

Medical Dictionary for Regulatory Activities (MedDRA)

MedDRA® is a dictionary of medically valid terminology used by the biopharmaceutical industry and regulatory

The content of this chapter does not necessarily reflect the views or policies of the Department of Health and Human Services, nor does it mention trade names, commercial products, or organizations that imply endorsement by the U.S. government.

TABLE 23.1 Comparison of Adverse Event Terminology Among Regulatory Bodies

Term	OHRP (3)	FDA	ICH (4)
Adverse event	Any untoward or unfavorable medical occurrence in a human subject, including any abnormal sign (for example, abnormal physical exam or laboratory finding), symptom, or disease, temporally associated with the subject's participation in the research, whether or not considered related to the subject's participation in the research (modified from the definition of adverse events in the 1996 International Conference on Harmonisation E-6 Guidelines for Good Clinical Practice). AEs encompass both physical and psychological harms. They occur most commonly in the context of biomedical research, although on occasion, they can occur in the context of social and behavioral research.	Any untoward medical occurrence associated with the use of a drug in humans, whether or not considered drug related (5).	Any untoward medical occurrence in a patient or clinical investigation subject administered a pharmaceutical product and which does not necessarily have a causal relationship with this treatment. An AE can therefore be any unfavorable and unintended sign (including an abnormal laboratory finding), symptom, or disease temporally associated with the use of a medicinal (investigational) product, whether or not related to the medicinal (investigational) product.
Serious adverse event	Any AE temporally associated with the subject's participation in research that meets any of the following criteria: • Results in death • Is life-threatening (places the subject at immediate risk of death from the event as it occurred) • Requires inpatient hospitalization or prolongation of existing hospitalization • Results in a persistent or significant disability/incapacity • Results in a congenital anomaly/ birth defect; or • Any other AE that, based upon appropriate medical judgment, may jeopardize the subject's health and may require medical or surgical intervention to prevent one of the other outcomes listed in this definition	An AE or suspected adverse reaction is considered "serious" if, in the view of either the investigator or sponsor, it results in any of the following outcomes: death, a life-threatening AE, inpatient hospitalization or prolongation of existing hospitalization, a persistent or significant incapacity or substantial disruption of the ability to conduct normal life functions, or a congenital anomaly/ birth defect. Important medical events that may not result in death, be life-threatening, or require hospitalization may be considered serious when, based upon appropriate medical judgment, they may jeopardize the patient or subject and may require medical or surgical intervention to prevent one of the outcomes listed in this definition (5).	Any untoward medical occurrence that at any dose: • Results in death • Is life-threatening • Requires inpatient hospitalization or prolongation of existing hospitalization • Results in persistent or significant disability/ incapacity, or • Is a congenital anomaly/ birth defect
Life-threatening	See the preceding serious adverse event definition	An AE or SAR is considered "life-threatening" if, in the view of either the investigator or sponsor, its occurrence places the patient or subject at immediate risk of death. It does not include an AE or SAR that, had it occurred in a more severe form, might have caused death (5).	N/A

(continued)

TABLE 23.1 Comparison of Adverse Event Terminology Among Regulatory Bodies (*continued*)

Term	OHRP (3)	FDA	ICH (4)
Unexpected	Any AE occurring in one or more subjects participating in a research protocol, the nature, severity, or frequency of which is **not** consistent with either: 1. The known or foreseeable risk of AEs associated with the procedures involved in the research that are described in (a) the protocol-related documents, such as the IRB-approved research protocol, any applicable Investigator's Brochure, and the current IRB-approved informed consent document, and (b) other relevant sources of information, such as product labeling and package inserts; or 2. The expected natural progression of any underlying disease, disorder, or condition of the subject(s) experiencing the AE and the subject's predisposing risk factor profile for the AE.	An AE or SAR is considered "unexpected" if it is not listed in the Investigator's Brochure or is not listed at the specificity or severity that has been observed; or, if an Investigator's Brochure is not required or available, is not consistent with the risk information described in the general investigational plan or elsewhere in the current application, as amended (5).	An adverse reaction, the nature or severity of which is not consistent with the applicable product information (e.g., Investigator's Brochure for an unapproved investigational product or package insert/summary of product characteristics for an approved product).
Suspected adverse reaction	N/A	Any AE for which there is a reasonable possibility that the drug caused the AE. For the purposes of IND safety reporting, "reasonable possibility" means there is evidence to suggest a causal relationship between the drug and the AE. SAR implies a lesser degree of certainty about causality than AE, which means any AE caused by a drug (5).	N/A

AE, adverse event; FDA, Food and Drug Administration; ICH, International Council for Harmonisation; IND, investigational new drug; IRB, institutional review board; OHRP, Office for Human Research Protections; SAE, serious adverse event; SAR, suspected adverse reaction.

authorities for sharing of regulatory information (e.g., AE terms) and data between regulators and the sponsors (7). It is available in multiple translations of the original English version and includes the use of standard terminology to communicate, share, and compare AE data between trials, especially trials that have multiple international sites. MedDRA is a hierarchal structure arranged into five levels, general terminology to very specific terminology: System Organ Class (SOC), High Level Group Term (HLGT), High Level Term (HLT), Preferred Term (PT), and Lowest Level Term (LLT). See Figure 23.1 for example of nausea. MedDRA is reviewed

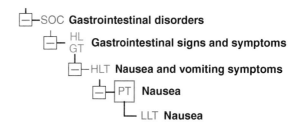

FIGURE 23.1 MedDRA version 20.0 hierarchy for nausea.

Acknowledgment statement: MedDRA® trademark is owned by IFPMA on behalf of ICH.

twice a year, which lends support to the incorporation of new and or unique AE-related terms.

ICH, International Council for Harmonisation; IFPMA, *International Federation of Pharmaceutical Manufacturers & Associations;* MedDRA, Medical Dictionary for Regulatory Activities. Advantages of MedDRA include the level of detail of its terminology and numerous terms to choose from. When appropriate, MedDRA includes combination terms, which combine a medical concept with additional medical wording that provide important information on pathophysiology or etiology. Some examples include: febrile neutropenia, eosinophilic pneumonia, and diabetic retinopathy. When using MedDRA there are some terms that fall under more than one SOC. This is referred to as multiaxiality. An example of this is for the diagnosis of metastatic malignant melanoma, which is found under two SOCs: Neoplasms benign, malignant and unspecified (incl cysts and polyps) and Skin and subcutaneous tissue disorders (Figure 23.2). This distinction is particularly important for data coding.

National Cancer Institute (NCI) Common Terminology Criteria for Adverse Events (CTCAE)

There is a need to describe the severity of AEs in clinical trials. Severity as well as nature of AEs is the basis for comparison of safety profiles between drugs, and determination of dose-limiting toxicities/maximum tolerated doses and treatment/dose modification. As a means to standardize AE assessment and reporting across oncology clinical trials and sites, the NCI CTEP developed the Common Toxicity Criteria (CTC) in 1984 (8). AE collection should include all AEs regardless of their cause. Since toxicity implied a relationship between intervention and the AE, the term CTC was changed to Common Terminology Criteria for Adverse Events (CTCAE). The most recently released version 4 of CTCAE had undergone significant revisions to harmonize with MedDRA (9).

NCI CTCAE combines MedDRA terms and a severity rating scale, and is a lexicon of commonly seen AEs in cancer clinical trials that includes a 5-point severity rating scale of general proportionality: 0 = no event, within normal limits, grade 1 = mild AE, 2 = moderate event, 3 = severe and undesirable, 4 = life-threatening or disabling, and 5 = death. The NCI CTCAE has been utilized as the worldwide standard dictionary for reporting AEs in cancer clinical trials and in scientific journals. See Table 23.2 for examples. CTCAE represents a synthesis of terminology fundamentally agreed upon and used by experts in oncology research for the designation, reporting, and grading of specific interest in oncology. As NCI CTCAE is revised, it is important for the protocol to note the version used.

ADVERSE EVENT ASSESSMENT AND DOCUMENTATION

Proper monitoring and reporting of AEs starts with proper assessment and documentation of the AEs encountered on trials. Once an AE is identified through clinical or laboratory evaluation, it must be properly assessed and characterized for proper documentation

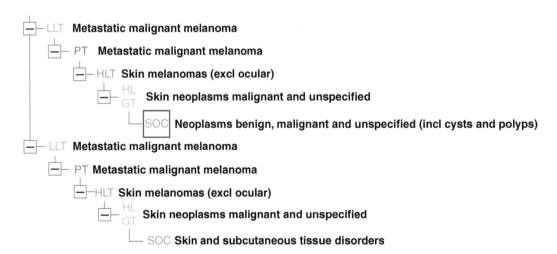

FIGURE 23.2 Multiaxial Preferred Term *Metastatic malignant melanoma.*

Acknowledgment statement: MedDRA® trademark is owned by IFPMA on behalf of ICH.
ICH, International Council for Harmonisation; IFPMA, International Federation of Pharmaceutical Manufacturers & Associations; MedDRA, Medical Dictionary for Regulatory Activities.

Source: From Medical Dictionary for Regulatory Activities Maintenance and Support Services Organization Maintenance and Support Services Organization (MedDRA® MSSO). http://www.meddra.org.

TABLE 23.2 CTCAE Grading Scale Examples

		Example	
Grade	Description	Nausea	Neutrophils/ Granulocytes
0	No AE or within normal limits		
1	Mild; asymptomatic or mild symptoms; clinical or diagnostic observations only; intervention not indicated	Loss of appetite without alteration in eating habits	<LLN—1,500/mm³ <LLN—1.5 x 10⁹/L
2	Moderate; minimal, local or noninvasive intervention indicated; limiting age-appropriate instrumental ADL*	Oral intake decreased without significant weight loss, dehydration, or malnutrition; IV fluids indicated for <24 hours	<1,500—1,000/mm³ <1.5—1.0 x 10⁹/L
3	Severe or medically significant but not immediately life-threatening; hospitalization or prolongation of hospitalization indicated; disabling; limiting self-care ADL**	Inadequate oral caloric or fluid intake; IV fluids, tube feedings, or TPN indicated for ≥24 hours	<1,000—500/mm³ <1.0—0.5 x 10⁹/L
4	Life-threatening consequences; urgent intervention indicated	Life-threatening consequences	<500/mm³ <0.5 x 10⁹/L
5	Death related to AE		

*Instrumental ADL refers to preparing meals, shopping for groceries or clothes, using the telephone, managing money, etc.
**Self care ADL refers to bathing, dressing and undressing, feeding self, using the toilet, taking medications, and not bedridden.

ADL, activities of daily living; AE, adverse event; CTCAE, common terminology criteria for adverse events; IV, intravenous; LLN, lower limit of normal; TPN, total parenteral nutrition.

and reporting. Essential attributes of an AE characterization include: CTCAE term for the AE, grade, and attribution.

AE Collection

The most common way to collect AEs is for a member of the clinical trial team (usually a physician or nurse or their assignees) to interview a patient and to identify AEs based upon discussions, the physical exam, and additional laboratory and radiological test findings. Sometimes the AE collection process is concurrent with the standard medical care; other times it is done independently. Typically, during the normal clinic visit, AE data will be elicited from the patient and documented in the medical record. Subsequent to that, the AE data will be extracted from the medical record by clinical trial personnel, such as data managers, at the clinical site and entered onto a patient case report form (CRF; paper or electronic).

Collection of AE information typically begins at the initiation of study intervention (drug/procedure), though this may vary from sponsor to sponsor. AE information should also be collected from the start of a placebo lead-in period or another observational period intended to establish a baseline status for the patient if applicable. The collection period and the data to be collected must be specified in the clinical protocol. For study drugs with potential for delayed AEs (e.g., delayed excretion of the parent or active metabolites), a longer follow-up period may be warranted to allow collection of these AEs, laboratory tests, and other assessments. AEs should be followed to resolution or stabilization. Follow-up also is required for AEs that cause interruption or discontinuation of the study drug, or those that are present at the end of study treatment as appropriate.

Selection of the AE Term and Grade

Selection of the term and grade of an AE is based on the CTCAE or another grading scale as indicated in the protocol. In addition to locating the right terms using CTCAE, appropriate selection of the AE terms also requires appropriate understanding of the clinical picture. If known, the AE term best representing the underlying cause of the symptom(s) should be selected. For example, if a patient was admitted to the hospital for severe shortness of breath and clinical evaluation revealed findings consistent with a diagnosis of congestive heart failure, simply reporting grade 4 dyspnea would be inadequate. Unfortunately, it is not uncommon to include nonspecific symptoms even if the definitive diagnoses are available in CTCAE. Sometimes, etiology may not be known at the time of initial AE assessment; once known, the AE terms and grades should be updated.

On the other hand, if a presumed diagnosis or etiology does not adequately explain the clinical picture, the AE terms should retain the major clinical presentations. The investigators should use their best clinical judgment to decide which AE terms would best capture the events experienced by the patient. One example may include a patient who developed bilateral pulmonary interstitial infiltrates with a low-grade fever, and was diagnosed with infection even though microbiological studies were not obtained or were negative. In this case, despite the working diagnosis of infection (pneumonia), the clinician cannot ascertain whether the pulmonary findings are truly due to infection or protocol therapy. To capture the potential diagnosis of drug-induced pneumonitis for future analysis, it would be more prudent to report "pulmonary infiltrate" (rather than "lung infection") with infection and treatment listed as possible causes.

Determination of Attribution

The attribution of the AE is a determination of the relatedness of the AE to the medical intervention(s) investigated in the trial. Terms used to describe attribution include definite, probable, and possible and are used to define when the investigator has identified that there is a relationship; while unlikely and unrelated are used where there is no clear relationship (see Table 23.3). The principal investigator (PI) or delegated member assigns attribution. Patient's prior treatments, comorbidities, and current medication profile may all have an impact on the complex task of determining attribution. Examples of questions to consider when determining attribution are provided in Table 23.4.

For AEs that are unique to drug effects (e.g., neutropenia, hand–foot syndrome, infusion reaction) or those

TABLE 23.4 Questions to Ask When Assessing Adverse Event Attribution

Is the AE a previously known reaction of the study drug?
Has the AE occurred before during this study?
Does the AE improve or stop when the intervention is discontinued?
Does it reoccur with retest?
Does a temporal relationship exist between the AE and the study therapy?
Was the AE present at the baseline assessment or is the AE a worsening of baseline symptoms?
Can the participants underlying clinical disease state explain the AE?
Are there any other potential causes for the AE?

AE, adverse event.

that wax and wane with each treatment cycle, attribution to the drug is usually obvious. For AEs that overlap with common noncancer diagnoses (e.g., myocardial infarction) or tumor-related complications (e.g., perforation or bleeding at the tumor site), the precise contribution by the study drug often cannot be ascertained within an individual patient, and the investigator must use his or her judgment based on the patient's underlying risk factors for the specific events, other agents in the protocol regimen, concomitant medications, as well as the temporal relationship to the study regimen.

Documentation

All AEs including attribution should be documented in the patient's medical record. The description of the AE should be detailed to provide the appropriate CTCAE grade and include: date the AE began, treatment for the AE, and date the AE improves, worsens, or resolves. Some sponsors or institutions may require an AE log to also be maintained.

AE REPORTING GUIDELINES

All clinical trials conducted in the United States must comply with regulatory requirements as set forth by the FDA. Clinical trials that include sites outside the United States must also comply with the rules of the local regulatory authorities. FDA regulations outline reporting requirements by the PI to the sponsor and the sponsor to the FDA (2). In general, AEs are reported by two mechanisms: routine reporting through submission of CRFs for all AEs as required by the protocol at fixed intervals, and expedited reporting of serious adverse events (SAEs) through dedicated report form or electronic system. The protocol should ideally define what events are reported via routine or expedited mechanisms.

TABLE 23.3 Numeric Coding Used to Describe the Attribution of AE Based on Relatedness to the Treatment

Attribution	Code	Definition
Unrelated	1	The AE is clearly not related to the study treatment.
Unlikely	2	The AE is doubtfully related to the study treatment.
Possible	3	The AE may be related to the study treatment.
Probable	4	The AE is likely related to the study treatment.
Definite	5	The AE is clearly related to the study treatment.

AE, adverse event.

Reporting by PI to IND Sponsor

Routine AE Reporting Through CRFs

The PI is to report all non-SAEs via an AE CRF. The timing is sponsor-dependent and the protocol needs to specify how to record and report non-SAEs. A typical AE CRF contains the following data elements for each AE: CTCAE term, grade, start date, stop date, attribution, if treatment was indicated, and if any action was taken with the study therapy (e.g., dose reduction or discontinuation).

Expedited Reporting

As per the FDA regulations, all SAEs are to be reported to the sponsor immediately unless the protocol has exceptions noted for reporting of SAEs (10). Most sponsors interpret this to be within 24 hours of the PI becoming aware of the AE. How the SAE is reported will be sponsor-dependent (i.e., electronic system, paper SAE form, MedWatch form). The protocol should define the types of AEs requiring expedited reporting and the procedures for reporting. In addition to SAEs, there may be adverse events of special interest (AESI) that the sponsor wants to be notified of in an expedited manner. An AESI may be serious or nonserious but is one of scientific and medical concern specific to the IND product (11). It is worth noting that all AEs reported via the expedited reporting mechanism also need to be collected on the routine AE CRF.

Key Elements of an SAE/AESI Report

An accurate and adequately informative SAE report is essential to independent assessment by the sponsor, as he or she does not have firsthand knowledge of the patient and yet must make timely judgment concerning conduct of the trial and administration of the agent. As with the CRFs in routine reporting, the key components of the SAE report are the AE terms, grades, and attributions, and these should be reported upon careful assessment of the AE with all available information.

A high-quality narrative summary can considerably facilitate the reviewer's assessment of the seriousness and attribution of the SAE/AESI and reduce subsequent queries for additional information. Depending on the nature of the events, the narratives may include the context of the SAE/AESI (e.g., patient's baseline conditions and relevant comorbidities), diagnostic studies, medical interventions, as well as the patient's current status. A narrative that simply repeats the AE terms (e.g., "The patient was admitted for confusion") is not acceptable for adequate assessment of the event. The purpose of such information is to enable the sponsor to ensure accurate coding and grading of the AEs and to independently assess the attributions and determine if the sponsor is to report the SAE to the FDA. In order to meet the sponsor's reporting timeline, not all information about the AE may be available for the investigator. As additional information becomes available, every effort should be made to update the report in a timely manner.

The extent of supplemental documentation with an SAE report depends on the complexity and nature of the event. It is generally recommended that the site submit the admission and discharge notes if the patient was admitted for the SAE. For those SAEs possibly related to tumor progression (e.g., severe fatigue or liver function abnormalities), documentation of the extent of tumor involvement would be critical to the accurate assessment of whether the event was a consequence of the therapy or of the cancer.

Reporting by IND Sponsor to the FDA

Routine Reporting

For trials performed under an IND, the FDA requires the sponsor to submit IND annual reports, which should include a comprehensive list of all AEs reported in association with the agent over the year. For clinical trials that are used to support approval in a therapeutic indication, a comprehensive toxicity profile should also be provided at the time a new drug application (NDA) or biologic license application (BLA), or supplemental NDA/BLA is completed.

Expedited Reporting

The sponsor must notify the FDA <u>and</u> participating investigators (i.e., any investigator who uses the IND agent in a clinical trial) as soon as possible, but no later than **15 calendar** days for the following events:

- All suspected, unexpected, serious adverse reaction (SUSAR)
- Findings from animal or in vitro testing
- Findings from other studies
- Increased rate of occurrence of serious suspected adverse reactions.

These reports are referred to as an IND safety report (ISR; see Table 23.5) (10).

Any unexpected AE that is life-threatening or fatal and is associated with the use of the IND agent must also be reported to the FDA by telephone or facsimile no later than 7 calendar days after the sponsor first learns of the event (10). The FDA defines the phrase associated with the use of the IND agent as a reasonable possibility that the event may have been due to the investigational agent (12).

The following are all acceptable formats for the sponsor to notify the FDA and investigators:

- Mandatory MedWatch: FDA Form 3500a
- Narrative summary indicating that the report is an ISR

TABLE 23.5 Events for IND Safety Reporting

Event	Definition/Reporting

SUSAR	• Report only if there is *evidence to suggest a causal relationship* between the drug and the AE, such as:
	  • Single occurrence
	  • One or more occurrences of an event
	  • Aggregate analysis of specific events
	• FDA considers these as *unanticipated problems* and reportable by the investigator to the IRB

Findings from animal or in vitro testing	Findings from animal or in vitro testing, whether or not conducted by the sponsor, that suggest a significant risk in humans exposed to the drug: • Mutagenicity • Teratogenicity • Carcinogenicity • Significant organ toxicity at or near the expected human exposure
Findings from other studies	• Includes findings from clinical, epidemiological, or pooled analysis of multiple studies • Reports are required for studies from any source, regardless of whether they are conducted under the IND or by the sponsor
Increased occurrence of serious SARs	• Sponsor must report any clinically important increase in the rate of a serious SAR over that listed in the protocol or Investigator's Brochure

AE, adverse event; FDA, Food and Drug Administration; IND, investigational new drug; IRB, institutional review board; SAR, suspected adverse reaction; SUSAR, suspected, unexpected, serious adverse reaction.

Source: IND Safety Reporting, 21 C.F.R. 312.32; 2016. Retrieved from http://www.accessdata.fda.gov/scripts/cdrh/cfdocs/cfcfr/CFRSearch.cfm?fr=312.32

• Council for International Organizations of Medical Sciences (CIOMS) I Form

See Figure 23.3 for how the PI is to handle an ISR or other information that indicates a new or increased risk, or a safety issue.

NCI/CTEP REPORTING GUIDELINES

To provide an example of how to follow AE reporting guidelines and operating procedures to monitor safety and meet regulatory requirements in the context of clinical trials, we describe here the experience at the CTEP of NCI as the sponsor of multiple cancer therapeutics trials. CTEP provides funding and infrastructure for a large portfolio of clinical trials through extensive networks of community practices and academic centers in the U.S. and ex-U.S. sites. These may involve investigational or commercial cancer drugs and can be conducted under CTEP- or investigator-held INDs. *The guidelines described next are specific to CTEP-sponsored trials using investigational agents under CTEP-held INDs.*

Consistent with the general practice of clinical trials, AE reporting for CTEP-sponsored trials is also divided into routine periodic reporting and expedited reporting. Therefore, after an AE has been identified, graded, and assigned an attribution, the investigator must then decide if the AE qualifies for expedited reporting to CTEP. While all AEs require reporting according to a given protocol as per the CRF with periodic submission to the data center, those that meet CTEP's requirement for expedited reporting should also be submitted to CTEP's Adverse Event Reporting System (AERS) (13). For complete guidelines for Adverse Event Reporting Requirements for Division of Cancer Treatment and Diagnosis (DCTD; CTEP and Cancer Imaging Program [CIP]) INDs, refer to the CTEP website: https://ctep.cancer.gov/protocolDevelopment/adverse_effects.htm.

Routine AE Reporting to NCI

Routine AEs (all AEs required reporting as defined by protocol, including SAEs) should be submitted to the Clinical Data Update System (CDUS) or the Clinical Trials Monitoring System (CTMS) for phase I and phase II trials. The frequency of routine AE reporting depends on the phase of the trial and the experience with the study regimen, and can range from every 2 weeks for phase I trials to every month or every quarter for phase II trials. For phase III trials, routine AE reports are submitted to the groups' data center as per protocol-specific requirements.

Expedited AE Reporting to NCI

SAEs as defined by the expedited reporting guidelines are reported to CTEP through the CTEP-AERS. AERS is

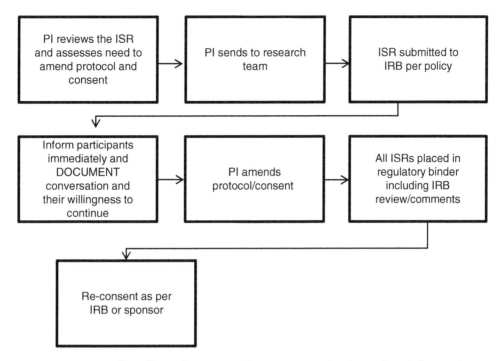

FIGURE 23.3 PI handling of an IND safety report and other safety information.

IND, investigational new drug; IRB, institutional review board; ISR, IND safety report; PI, principal investigator.

a web-based reporting system that in May 2014 replaced its predecessor Adverse Event Expedited Reporting System (AdEERS). CTEP uses this mechanism, in conjunction with routine AE monitoring, to ensure compliance with the FDA regulation for SAE reporting and to identify unexpected safety signals that may impact the safety and conduct of the trial.

For trials utilizing investigational agents, the SAE reporting guidelines for phase I or phase II/III trials are described in Tables 23.6 and 23.7, respectively (13). The timeline for AERS submission is defined to ensure timely review by CTEP drug monitors and (when indicated) subsequent reports to the FDA within the FDA-defined reporting timeline. Since the CTEP's guidelines for expedited reporting via AERS are subject to change to accommodate new regulatory requirements and/or emerging drug development needs, investigators should refer to the CTEP website given earlier for most updated reporting guidelines.

In addition to the general criteria for expedited reporting, individual trials may also add protocol-specific or agent-specific exceptions to the general guidelines. For example, if an AE is of specific interest and has potentially significant consequence to patients or the trial, the protocol may require expedited reporting even if it does not meet the general criteria (e.g., grade 2 left ventricular ejection fraction [LVEF] decrease in pediatric trials). On the other hand, if an AE and its severity is expected and well known to be associated with the agent (e.g., grade 3 neutropenia with cytotoxic agents),

the agent-specific guidelines may exempt this grade 3 AE from expedited reporting.

SAE Review and Processing by the Sponsor (NCI)

All submitted AERS reports are reviewed by a designated NCI/CTEP medical officer. Additional data or source documents may be requested for CTEP to fully assess the event. NCI/CTEP's assessment may differ from that of the submitting investigator in certain AE attributes such as the AE term, grade, IND agent attribution, and other causal factors. The independent assessment by CTEP (sponsor) is the basis for a decision regarding whether a given SAE meets the criteria for expedited reporting to the FDA (i.e., AEs that are serious, unexpected, and attributable to the investigational agent).

CTEP as the sponsor is responsible for notifying the FDA and all participating investigators in a written ISR, as specified in FDA 21 CFR 312.32. CTEP/ NCI is also responsible for submitting summaries of all AEs reported through routine reporting as well as SAEs through expedited reporting, in the Annual Report to the IND. NCI/CTEP's assessments of all SAE reports are communicated to the investigators. Investigators should then determine if the AE data (term, grade, and attribution) should be modified in both the SAE and routine AE database.

The process for CTEP-sponsored trials from submission of an AERS report to CTEP assessment and ending

TABLE 23.6 Phase 1 and Early Phase 2 Studies: Expedited Reporting Requirements for Adverse Events That Occur on Studies Under an IND/IDE within 30 Days of the Last Administration of the Investigational Agent/Intervention[1, 2]

FDA REPORTING REQUIREMENTS FOR SERIOUS ADVERSE EVENTS (21 CFR Part 312)

NOTE: Investigators **MUST** immediately report to the sponsor (NCI) **ANY** Serious Adverse Events, whether or not they are considered related to the investigational agent(s)/intervention (21 CFR 312.64).

An adverse event is considered serious if it results in **ANY** of the following outcomes:

1) Death
2) A life-threatening adverse event
3) An adverse event that results in inpatient hospitalization or prolongation of existing hospitalization for ≥24 hours
4) A persistent or significant incapacity or substantial disruption of the ability to conduct normal life functions
5) A congenital anomaly/birth defect.
6) IME that may not result in death, be life-threatening, or require hospitalization may be considered serious when, based upon medical judgment, they may jeopardize the patient or subject and may require medical or surgical intervention to prevent one of the outcomes listed in this definition. (FDA, 21 CFR 312.32; ICH E2A and ICH E6).

ALL SERIOUS adverse events that meet the preceding criteria MUST be immediately reported to the NCI via electronic submission within the time frames detailed in the following table.

Hospitalization	Grade 1 and Grade 2 Time Frames	Grades 3–5 Time Frames
Resulting in hospitalization ≥24 hr	10 calendar days	24-hour 5 calendar days
Not resulting in hospitalization ≥24 hr	Not required	

NOTE: Protocol-specific exceptions to expedited reporting of serious adverse events are found in the SPEER portion of the CAEPR.

Expedited AE reporting timelines are defined as:
o "24-hour; 5 calendar days": The AE must initially be submitted electronically within 24 hours of learning of the AE, followed by a complete expedited report within 5 calendar days of the initial 24-hour report.
o "10 calendar days": A complete expedited report on the AE must be submitted electronically within 10 calendar days of learning of the AE.

---

[1]Serious adverse events that occur more than 30 days after the last administration of investigational agent/intervention and have an attribution of possible, probable, or definite require reporting as follows:

Expedited 24-hour notification followed by complete report within 5 calendar days for:
• All grade 3, 4, and grade 5 AEs

Expedited 10 calendar day reports for:
• Grade 2 AEs resulting in hospitalization or prolongation of hospitalization

[2]For studies using PET or SPECT IND agents, the AE reporting period is limited to 10 radioactive half-lives, rounded UP to the nearest whole day, after the agent/intervention was last administered. Footnote 1 applies after this reporting period.

Effective Date: May 5, 2011

AE, adverse event; CAEPR, Comprehensive Adverse Events and Potential Risks; CFR, Code of Federal Regulations; FDA, Food and Drug Administration; ICH, International Council for Harmonisation; IDE, investigational device exemption; IME, important medical events; IND, investigational new drug; NCI, National Cancer Institute; SPECT, single-photon emission computed tomography; SPEER, Specific Protocol Exceptions to Expedited Reporting.

Source: Office for Human Research Protections. Guidance on reviewing and reporting unanticipated problems involving risks to subjects or others and adverse events; 2007. Retrieved from http://www.hhs.gov/ohrp/policy/advevntguid.html; IND Safety Reporting, 21 C.F.R. 312.32; 2016. Retrieved from http://www.accessdata.fda.gov/scripts/cdrh/cfdocs/cfcfr/ CFRSearch.cfm?fr=312.32

with a report to the FDA and communication with the investigators is depicted in Figure 23.4.

Comprehensive Adverse Events and Potential Risks (CAEPR) list for CTEP-held IND

A unique aspect of CTEP SAE reporting mechanisms is the inclusion of a CAEPR list for the investigational agents (13). CAEPR is compiled by CTEP based on the Investigator's Brochure and Prescription Information (if the investigational drug is available commercially), as well as manufacturer ISRs, peer-reviewed publications, and AEs reported through CTEP-AERS. CTEP updates the CAEPR at least annually, and any time as needed depending on the nature of the safety information. The

TABLE 23.7 Late Phase 2 and Phase 3 Studies: Expedited Reporting Requirements for Adverse Events That Occur on Studies Under an IND/IDE within 30 Days of the Last Administration of the Investigational Agent/Intervention[1, 2]

FDA REPORTING REQUIREMENTS FOR SERIOUS ADVERSE EVENTS (21 CFR Part 312)

NOTE: Investigators **MUST** immediately report to the sponsor (NCI) **ANY** Serious Adverse Events, whether or not they are considered related to the investigational agent(s)/intervention (21 CFR 312.64).

An adverse event is considered serious if it results in **ANY** of the following outcomes:

1) Death
2) A life-threatening adverse event
3) An adverse event that results in inpatient hospitalization or prolongation of existing hospitalization for ≥24 hours
4) A persistent or significant incapacity or substantial disruption of the ability to conduct normal life functions
5) A congenital anomaly/birth defect.
6) IME that may not result in death, be life-threatening, or require hospitalization may be considered serious when, based upon medical judgment, they may jeopardize the patient or subject and may require medical or surgical intervention to prevent one of the outcomes listed in this definition. (FDA, 21 CFR 312.32; ICH E2A and ICH E6).

ALL SERIOUS adverse events that meet the preceding criteria **MUST** be immediately reported to the NCI via electronic submission within the time frames detailed in the following table.

Hospitalization	Grade 1 Time Frames	Grade 2 Time Frames	Grade 3 Time Frames	Grade 4 and 5 Time Frames
Resulting in hospitalization ≥24 hr	10 calendar days			24-hour 5 calendar days
Not resulting in hospitalization ≥24 hr	Not required		10 calendar days	

NOTE: Protocol-specific exceptions to expedited reporting of serious adverse events are found in the SPEER portion of the CAEPR.

Expedited AE reporting timelines are defined as:
- "24-hour; 5 calendar days": The AE must initially be submitted electronically within 24 hours of learning of the AE, followed by a complete expedited report within 5 calendar days of the initial 24-hour report.
- "10 calendar days": A complete expedited report on the AE must be submitted electronically within 10 calendar days of learning of the AE.

[1]Serious adverse events that occur more than 30 days after the last administration of investigational agent/intervention and have an attribution of possible, probable, or definite require reporting as follows:

Expedited 24-hour notification followed by complete report within 5 calendar days for:
- All grade 4, and grade 5 AEs

Expedited 10 calendar day reports for:
- Grade 2 adverse events resulting in hospitalization or prolongation of hospitalization

1) Grade 3 adverse events

[2]For studies using PET or SPECT IND agents, the AE reporting period is limited to 10 radioactive half-lives, rounded UP to the nearest whole day, after the agent/intervention was last administered. Footnote 1 applies after this reporting period.

Effective Date: May 5, 2011

AE, adverse event; CAEPR, Comprehensive Adverse Events and Potential Risks; CFR, Code of Federal Regulations; FDA, Food and Drug Administration; ICH, International Council for Harmonisation; IDE, investigational device exemption; IME, important medical events; IND, investigational new drug; NCI, National Cancer Institute; SPECT, single-photon emission computed tomography; SPEER, Specific Protocol Exceptions to Expedited Reporting.

Source: Office for Human Research Protections. Guidance on reviewing and reporting unanticipated problems involving risks to subjects or others and adverse events; 2007. Retrieved from http://www.hhs.gov/ohrp/policy/advevntguid.html; IND Safety Reporting, 21 C.F.R. 312.32; 2016. Retrieved from http://www.accessdata.fda.gov/scripts/cdrh/cfdocs/cfcfr/ CFRSearch.cfm?fr=312.32

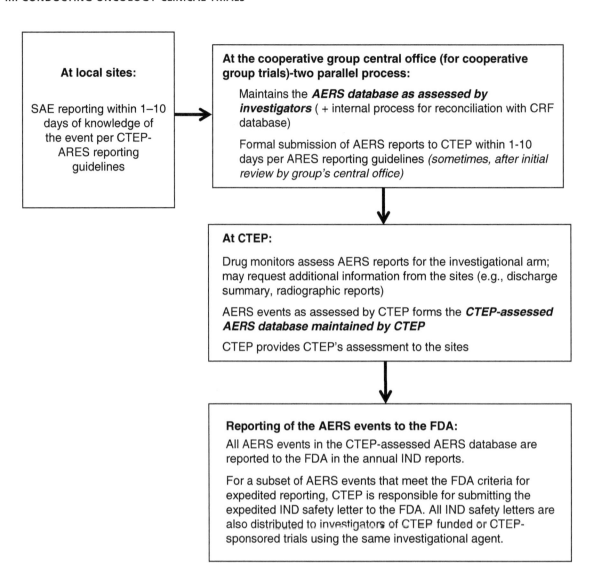

FIGURE 23.4 Process of AERS reports from submission, to CTEP assessment, and to reporting to regulatory authorities.

AERS, Adverse Event Reporting System; CRF, case report form; CTEP, Cancer Therapy Evaluation Program; FDA, Food and Drug Administration; IND, investigational new drug; SAE, serious adverse event.

purpose of CAEPR is to serve as a centrally developed, uniform document of the safety profile for all CTEP-sponsored trials using the same agent. Investigators use this agent-specific document to develop the risk list in the informed consent documents and to triage AEs for routine or expedited reporting (in conjunction with the generic AE reporting guidelines).

The CAEPR list contains three components (see Table 23.8 as an example): (a) a list of all AEs with possible relationship to the IND agent (expected events or identified risks)—AEs under this list should be included in the informed consent document, (b) a list of AEs that have been reported in clinical trials with the agent but there is insufficient evidence to suggest a possible causal relationship with the drug, and (c) a separate column Specific Protocol Exceptions to Expedited Reporting (SPEER). The SPEER lists is a subset of identified AEs

for which expedited reporting is required only if the grade exceeds the grade listed under SPEER (e.g., while general guideline would require AERS reporting for all grade 3 events or grade 2 events requiring hospitalization, for Drug X in Table 23.8, grade 2 hemolysis would require expedited reporting but grade 3 neutropenia would not).

Overall, although the specific reporting mechanics may be unique to CTEP-sponsored trials, all principles described in the previous sections (AE assessment and documentation; regulatory requirements) are applicable to CTEP investigators, and the current Good Clinical Practice (cGCP) guidelines should be followed. For complete and updated guidelines for Adverse Event Reporting Requirements for DCTD (CTEP and CIP) INDs, refer to CTEP website https://ctep.cancer.gov/protocolDevelopment/adverse_effects.htm.

TABLE 23.8 Sample of CAEPR list for Drug X

The CAEPR list provides a single list of reported and/or potential AEs associated with an agent using a uniform presentation of events by body system. In addition to the comprehensive list, a subset, the SPEER, appears in a separate column and is identified with bold and italicized text. This subset of AEs (SPEER) is a list of events that are protocol-specific exceptions to expedited reporting to NCI (except as noted in the following). Refer to "CTEP, NCI Guidelines: Adverse Event Reporting Requirements" http://ctep.cancer.gov/protocolDevelopment/electronic_applications/docs/aeguidelines.pdf for further clarification. *Frequency is provided based on 389 patients.* Following is the CAEPR for Drug X.

NOTE: Report AEs on the SPEER **ONLY IF** they exceed the grade noted in parentheses next to the AE in the SPEER. If this CAEPR is part of a combination protocol using multiple investigational agents and has an AE listed on different SPEERs, use the lower of the grades to determine if expedited reporting is required.

AEs With Possible Relationship to Drug X (CTCAE 4.0 Term); n = 389			SPEER
Likely (>20%)	Less Likely (≤20%)	Rare but Serious (<3%)	
Blood and Lymphatic System Disorders			
Anemia			*Anemia (Gr 3)*
	Hemolysis		*Hemolysis (Gr 1)*
	Disseminated intravascular coagulation		
	Febrile neutropenia		*Febrile neutropenia (Gr 3)*
Cardiac Disorder			
	Atrial fibrillation		
	Sinus tachycardia		Sinus tachycardia (Gr 3)
		Ventricular tachycardia	Ventricular tachycardia (Gr 1)
	Ejection fraction decrease		
	....		

Adverse events reported on Drug X trials, but for which there is insufficient evidence to suggest that there was a reasonable possibility that Drug X caused the adverse event:

GASTROINTESTINAL DISORDERS—Ascites

INFECTIONS AND INFESTATIONS—Infections and infestations—Other (oral candidiasis)

NERVOUS SYSTEM DISORDERS—Cognitive disturbance

RESPIRATORY, THORACIC, AND MEDIASTINAL DISORDERS—Pneumonitis

VASCULAR DISORDERS—Thromboembolic event

AE, adverse event; CAEPR, Comprehensive Adverse Events and Potential Risks; CTCAE, Common Terminology Criteria for Adverse Events; NCI, National Cancer Institute; SPEER, Specific Protocol Exceptions to Expedited Reporting.

CONCLUSION

In summary, accurate assessment, documentation of AEs, and timely reporting is necessary from the investigators and sponsors involved in clinical trials. Investigators must be familiar with their responsibilities for AE reporting to the IND sponsors and/or the regulatory authorities. To ensure accurate documentation of the AEs, investigators should be closely involved in the process of translating clinical symptoms/signs or laboratory abnormalities into the appropriate AE terms, grades, and attributions. Finally, to compile a comprehensive AE profile for safety monitoring, analysis, and publication, all collected AE data should be thoughtfully considered and integrated, including information from routine and expedited AE databases.

REFERENCES

1. Ness EA, Clark AM. (2016). Adverse events. In: Klimaszewski AD, Bacon MA, Ness EA, Westendorp JG, & Willingberg K, eds. *Manual for Clinical Trials Nursing 3rd edition*. Pittsburgh, PA: Oncology Nursing Society; 2016:271–290.

2. U.S. Food and Drug Administration. *Guidance for clinical investigators, sponsors, and IRBs: Adverse event reporting to IRBs—Improving human subject protection*; 2009. Retrieved from http://www.fda.gov/downloads/RegulatoryInformation/Guidances/UCM126572.pdf

3. Office for Human Research Protections. *Guidance on reviewing and reporting unanticipated problems involving risks to subjects or others and adverse events*; 2007. Retrieved from http://www.hhs.gov/ohrp/policy/advevntguid.html

4. International Council for Harmonisation of Technical Requirements for Registration of Pharmaceuticals for Human Use. *Guideline for Good Clinical Practice*; 2016. Retrieved from http://www.ich.org/fileadmin/Public_Web_Site/ICH_Products/Guidelines/Efficacy/E6/E6_R2__Step_4.pdf

5. IND Safety Reporting, 21 C.F.R. 312.32; 2016. Retrieved from http://www.accessdata.fda.gov/scripts/cdrh/cfdocs/cfcfr/CFRSearch.cfm?fr=312.32

6. Klimaszewski AD, Bacon M, Eggert JA, et al., eds. *Manual for Clinical Trials Nursing*, 3rd ed. Pittsburgh, PA; Oncology Nursing Society; 2015:272–273.

7. Medical Dictionary for Regulatory Activities Maintenance and Support Services Organization Maintenance and Support Services Organization (MedDRA® MSSO). http://www.meddra.org

8. Trotti A, Colevas AD, Setser A, et al. CTCAE v3.0: Development of a comprehensive grading system for the adverse effects of cancer treatment. *Semin Radiat Oncol.* 2003;13:175–181. doi:10.1016/S1053-4296(03)00031-6

9. National Cancer Institute Cancer Therapy Evaluation Program. *Common Terminology Criteria for Adverse Events* [v4.03]; 2010. Retrieved from http://evs.nci.nih.gov/ftp1/CTCAE/About.html

10. IND Safety Reporting, 21 C.F.R. 312.32; 2016. Retrieved from http://www.accessdata.fda.gov/scripts/cdrh/cfdocs/cfcfr/CFRSearch.cfm?fr=312.32 FDA

11. U.S. Food and Drug Administration. *Guidance for clinical investigators, sponsors, and IRBs adverse event reporting to IRBs—Improving human subject protection*; 2009. Retrieved from http://www.fda.gov/downloads/RegulatoryInformation/Guidances/UCM126572.pdf

12. National Cancer Institute. *NCI Guidelines for Investigators: Adverse Event Reporting Requirements for DCTD (CTEP and CIP) and DCP INDs and IDEs*; 2013. Retrieved from https://ctep.cancer.gov/protocolDevelopment/electronic_applications/docs/aeguidelines.pdf

13. International Council for Harmonisation of Technical Requirements for Registration of Pharmaceuticals for Human Use. *Guideline for Good Clinical Practice*; 2016. Retrieved from http://www.ich.org/fileadmin/Public_Web_Site/ICH_Products/Guidelines/Efficacy/E6/E6_R2__Step_4.pdf

Dose Modification and Use of Ancillary Treatments in Investigational Studies in Clinical Trials

Yoshihito David Saito, Pamela Harris, Ming Poi, and Robert Wesolowski

INTRODUCTION

Ensuring patient safety on clinical trials testing investigational therapies, with no or incomplete understanding of risk–benefit ratio in humans, is an absolute necessity. This is particularly important in "first-in-human" (FIH) trials for which there is only preclinical safety information. Preclinical animal studies may hint at potential toxicities but serious and nonserious toxicity can occur unexpectedly in humans. This requires clinical trials to focus on strict monitoring of patient safety and filing of adverse events to the regulatory authorities. Furthermore, management of emerging toxicities with clear criteria for treatment interruptions, dose modifications, and appropriate supportive care is necessary and should be delineated in the protocols for all clinical trials. To minimize excessive risks of unexpected and serious toxicities, early-phase oncology clinical trials typically enroll the smallest possible number of patients with good organ function and performance status. In addition, patients with treatment-refractory, incurable malignancies are typically recruited to FIH trials as these clinical trials, by definition, have unproven benefit and unknown safety profile. Once the safety profile of a particular investigational therapy is better defined, larger, clinical trials are undertaken with more emphasis on efficacy measures.

Expedited reporting of serious, investigational agent-related and unexpected, adverse events are especially important since it can alert other investigators and study participants of a clinically significant safety concern that could change the risk–benefit ratio. Safety information from clinical trials is commonly overseen and periodically reviewed by a Data and Safety Monitoring Committee (DSMC) that consists of independent experts and investigators in the field who are not directly involved in the study conduct but have access to the study results in real time to ensure that there are no excessive risks to the study participants. If such concern is found, the committee may recommend terminating the study or amending the existing study plan. Alternatively, the committee can recommend continuing the study but amending the informed consent and notifying the study participants of a new safety concern. The recommendation depends on the clinical significance of the safety concern and how it affects risk–benefit ratio of the investigational therapy.

GENERAL RULES OF MANAGING TOXICITIES IN CLINICAL TRIALS

Pharmacologic Class of Investigational Therapy Guides Toxicity Management in Clinical Trials

Antineoplastic agents are often classified based on their mechanism of action. Knowledge of the class-specific toxicities is useful in projecting the toxicities of new agents of the same class. This knowledge commonly guides the protocol-mandated dose modifications and supportive care measures in clinical trials. For example, studies that pointed to a possible risk of pneumonitis associated with a class of immune modulating agents called PD-1 inhibitors led to protocol-mandated monitoring for signs and symptoms of pneumonitis in trials testing other PD-1 inhibitors (1). This also led to protocol-mandated stipulations for dose modifications/dose delays and specific recommendation for ancillary care in patients who develop pneumonitis. Clinical observation of hypertension associated with early vascular endothelial growth factor (VEGF) inhibitors is another example of how experience with one agent from a particular class led to mandated monitoring of blood pressure (BP), dose modifications/delays for various levels of hypertension and therapeutic management of hypertension for subjects on clinical trials with newer VEGF inhibitors (2).

Understanding the class-specific toxicities of investigational therapy is a good starting point for incorporating safety parameters and supportive care guidelines for clinical trial protocols. Nonetheless, it is important to keep in mind that each agent may also have produced a unique set of toxicities that need to be accounted for in the protocol. Such problem is addressed by clear delineation of dose modification and delays of study treatment for any clinically significant drug-related toxicities. General principles of dose modifications and commonly employed supportive care measures for clinically significant adverse events are discussed for each general class of agents in the sections below.

Identifying, Grading, and Assigning Attributions to Study Emergent Adverse Events

Adverse Events that develop in patients participating in clinical trials are generally coded using the Medical Dictionary for Regulatory Activities (MedDRA®) and the severity of specific types of adverse events is graded according to the most recent version of National Cancer Institute's Common Terminology Criteria for Adverse Events (CTCAE). Table 24.1 summarizes general criteria used for grading based on the most recent version of CTCAE. When a patient develops a symptom or disorder that is not listed in the CTCAE, general criteria listed in Table 24.1 should be used.

All toxicities must be attributed to the investigational test article, study procedures, underlying disease, or other causes (for example, concomitant medications or concurrent medical illness). Attribution of the adverse event to the test article is further described as (a) not related, (b) unlikely related, (c) possibly related, (d) probably related, or (e) definitively related.

If the toxicity is deemed to be at least possibly related to an investigational therapy, it must be deemed to be either expected or unexpected as described in the Investigator's Brochure. Unexpected toxicities may require expedited reporting to the regulatory authorities.

General Guidelines Used to Modify Doses of Study Therapy Due to Toxicities

Protocols provide separate guidelines for management of specific hematologic and nonhematologic toxicities. These can also be further divided into management of specific toxicities that are more commonly encountered with the class of agents tested. These will be specifically reviewed in the subsequent section. Tables 24.2A to 24.2C give examples of management guidelines for the investigational agent when hematologic (excluding neutropenia), neutropenia, and nonhematologic toxicities occur respectively. Of note, most protocols typically stipulate that test subjects who require a dose delay of greater than 2 to 3 weeks should come off protocol specified therapy. Since each patient is unique and it is impossible to predict the risks of each individual case, the purpose of these guidelines is to provide a framework for dose modifications and should not replace the physician's experience and clinical judgment.

DOSE MODIFICATIONS BASED ON TYPE OF INVESTIGATIONAL THERAPY

In this section, we briefly discuss the most common and unique adverse events associated with three broad types of therapy, namely: cytotoxic therapy, targeted therapy, and immune therapies. Dose adjustments based on the severity and grade of toxicity are generalizable with typical examples shown in Tables 24.2A to 24.2C.

TABLE 24.1 CTCAE Version 4.03 Grading Criteria

Grade	Definition
1	Mild; asymptomatic or mild symptoms; clinical or diagnostic observations only; intervention not indicated
2	Moderate; minimal, local or noninvasive intervention indicated; limiting age-appropriate instrumental ADL*
3	Severe or medically significant but not immediately life-threatening; hospitalization or prolongation of hospitalization indicated; disabling; limiting self-care ADL†
4	Life-threatening consequences; urgent intervention indicated
5	Death related to AE‡

*Instrumental ADL refer to preparing meals, shopping for groceries or clothes, using telephone, managing money, etc.
†Self-care ADL refer to bathing, dressing and undressing, feeding self, using the toilet, taking medications, and not bedridden.
‡Grade 5 (death) is not appropriate for some AEs and therefore is not an option.
ADL, activities of daily living; AE, adverse event; CTCAE, Common Terminology Criteria for Adverse Events.

TABLE 24.2A   Example of Dose Modification Rules for Treatment-Related Hematologic Toxicities

Neutropenia	Management/Next Dose for Study Drug
≤Grade 2	No change in dose.
Grade 3 (first occurrence)	Hold* until grade ≤2. Resume at same dose level. For neutropenia, consideration may be given for starting growth factor support with G-CSF. If the toxicity does not recover to ≤grade 2 within 7 days, reduce dose by 1 dose level†.
Grade 3 (second occurrence)	Hold* until grade ≤1. Resume dose by one dose level†. Provide growth factor support with G-CSF.
Grade 4	Off protocol therapy.

*Patients requiring a delay of >2 weeks should go off protocol therapy.
†Patients requiring >two dose reductions should go off protocol therapy.
G-CSF, granulocyte colony stimulating factor.

TABLE 24.2B   Example of Dose Modification Guidelines for Treatment-Related Febrile Neutropenia

Febrile Neutropenia	Management/Next Dose for Study Drug
Grade 3 or 4 (first and second occurrences)	Hold until grade ≤2.* Resume at same dose level. If neutrophil count does not recover to grade ≤2 within 7 days, reduce dose by 1 dose level†. Provide growth factor support with G-CSF.
Grade 3 or 4 (second occurrence)	Hold until grade ≤2. Resume once neutropenia improves to grade ≤2; reduce dose by 1 dose level†. Provide growth factor support with G-CSF.
Grade 3 or 4 (third occurrence)	Off protocol therapy.

*Patients requiring a delay of >2 weeks should go off protocol therapy.
†Patients requiring >two dose reductions should go off protocol therapy.
G-CSF, granulocyte colony stimulating factor.

TABLE 24.2C   Example of Dose Modification Guidelines for Treatment-Related Nonhematologic Toxicity

Nonhematologic Toxicities	Management/Next Dose of Study Therapy
Grade ≤2	No change in dose
Grade 3 (first and second occurrence)*	Hold‡ until grade ≤1†. Reduce the dose by 1 dose level.
Grade 3 (third occurrence)*	Off protocol therapy.
Grade 4	Off protocol therapy.

*Patients who develop grade 3 fatigue may continue treatment without dose reduction as per discretion of treating physician.
†Patients requiring a delay of >2 weeks should go off protocol therapy.

Exceptions to this are addressed individually in the following sub-sections.

Cytotoxic Therapy

For the purposes of this discussion, cytotoxic therapy will be defined as agents that nonspecifically interfere with the function of cells that undergo rapid cell division and interfere with specific phases of cell cycle (G1, S, G2, or M phases). These agents include alkylating agents, topoisomerase inhibitors, certain antibiotics (i.e., bleomycin), platinum-containing compounds, purine/pyrimidine analogs, inhibitors of microtubule formation or disassembly, and other agents.

Hematologic Toxicities

Myelosuppression is the most common toxicity of most cytotoxic agents and the period of time needed to resolve them often dictates the interval between dosing. Phase 1 to 3 study protocols provide guidance for dose delays and dose modifications for grade ≥3 (absolute neutrophil count ≤1.0/mm³) neutropenia as well as for grade 2 to 4 thrombocytopenia (platelet count <75,000/mm³). The next dose is generally delayed until the hematologic toxicity resolves to grade 1 or 2. Unlike grade 3 neutropenia or thrombocytopenia, decreases in hemoglobin can be monitored closely while the patient continues to receive study therapy and most protocols will permit use of red blood cell transfusion to treat patients with severe, symptomatic anemia. Occasionally, it is stated in the protocol that the dose or interval between doses does not have to be modified unless the adverse event recurs. For example, patients may be rechallenged with the original dose but must have the dose reduced upon experiencing the second episode of grade ≥3 neutropenia or thrombocytopenia. The protocol also indicates when and what kind of supportive care measures should be administered, such as of granulocyte colony stimulating factor (G-CSF; filgrastim, pegfilgrastim), granulocyte–macrophage colony stimulating factor (GM-CSF; sargramostim), erythropoietin analogs, and platelet and/or red blood cell transfusions (3). Occasionally, in phase I clinical trials, growth factors or transfusions may not be permitted until the dose-limiting toxicity (DLT) period has been completed.

Nonhematologic Toxicities

Oropharyngeal mucositis is a common and treatment-limiting toxicity most often seen with antimetabolite agents (i.e., fluorouracil, methotrexate, purine antagonists), anthracyclines, and taxanes. Supportive care includes the use of topical analgesics such as 2% topical lidocaine or Magic Mouthwash (viscous lidocaine with bicarbonate and diphenhydramine) solutions. The duration of mucositis is highly variable although 7 to 10 days is typical and thus standard dose modification guidelines in Table 24.2C are usually sufficient. Preventive measures include oral cryotherapy (typically with ice chips) during the infusion that results in vasoconstriction and reduced chemotherapy exposure of the oral mucosa (4). Cryotherapy is contraindicated in regimens with agents that can instigate cold-induced neuropathic pain such as oxaliplatin.

Chemotherapy-induced peripheral neuropathy (CIPN) is a common adverse event of cytotoxic therapy and most frequently observed with platinum drugs, taxanes, vinca alkaloids, and proteasome inhibitors. This adverse event may be long-lasting and eligibility for most trials testing agents that can potentially cause neuropathy may be limited to patients without significant baseline neuropathy (typically grade 1 or less). Given the long-lasting effects of chronic CIPN, it is reasonable to recommend decreasing the offending agent by 1 dose level with the first observation of a new grade 2 neuropathy. With the exception of a single trial that demonstrated modest improvement in patients with CIPN with duloxetine treatment, there is no other evidence-based study to guide management of neuropathy (5). Nevertheless, patients who develop CIPN are often treated with gamma-aminobutyric acid (GABA) analogs (such as gabapentin or pregabalin) or tricyclic antidepressants (such as amitriptyline, nortriptyline) based on extrapolation of trial results testing these agents for the treatment of diabetic neuropathy (6). A study protocol should provide adequate guidance on the use of such agents as prevention and/or treatment for CIPN taking into consideration that some of the antidepressants used for CIPN may elicit potential cytochrome P450-based drug–drug interactions.

Gastrointestinal (GI) toxicities occur commonly in patients treated with cytotoxic agents. Chemotherapy-induced diarrhea (CID) is a major source of morbidity in patients undergoing cytotoxic chemotherapy. Chemotherapeutic agents that are commonly associated with diarrhea include 5-fluorouracil, capecitabine, and irinotecan. With proper supportive care (i.e., fluid management), and pharmacological (i.e., antidiarrheal medications) and nonpharmacological (i.e., diet modification) interventions, CID is usually reversible and therefore no significant modifications to the general dose modification guidelines are necessary as long as diarrhea improves to grade 1 or better with aggressive supportive care. Grade 3 diarrhea that responds to supportive care measures within 1 to 2 days can also be excluded from the definition of DLTs. Similarly, chemotherapy-induced nausea and vomiting (CINV) are treated with use of preventive antiemetics as per standard guidelines, which include use of corticosteroids, neurokinin-1 receptor inhibitors, 5-HT$_3$ receptor blockers, and antidopaminergic agents (depending on the anticipated emetogenic risk of the study treatment) (7). Therapeutic guidelines with antiemetics to treat acute, delayed, or anticipatory nausea/vomiting (despite preventive measures) are also available (8). In phase I clinical trials, grade 3 or 4 nausea/vomiting is commonly excluded from the DLT definitions, if it improves to grade 1 or better within 24–48 hours following adjustments in the supportive care.

The management of treatment-related toxicity in clinical trials testing investigational therapy for hematologic malignancies involves challenges that are unique from toxicities related to treatment of solid malignancies. Profound cytopenias are characteristically seen in hematologic malignancies even in the absence of treatment. In particular, patients with myelodysplastic syndrome and leukemia often have preexisting neutropenia or thrombocytopenia related to their disease process. When neutropenia, thrombocytopenia, and anemia preexist at baseline in patients with hematologic malignancies, dose delays and dose modifications are not desirable as the full-dose treatment may remedy, rather than worsen these cytopenias.

Tumor lysis syndrome (TLS) occurs when antineoplastics cause rapid killing of malignant cells leading to the release of intracellular materials into the extracellular space. This syndrome is characterized by electrolyte imbalances (hyperkalemia, hyperphosphatemia, hypocalcemia) and high levels of uric acid. The electrolyte abnormalities may result in cardiac conduction abnormalities and high uric acid levels can lead to renal failure. TLS occurs most commonly in patients with acute leukemia and high-grade non-Hodgkin's lymphoma but can occasionally occur in patients with other hematologic malignancies. TLS is uncommon in patients with solid tumors but is occasionally seen in malignancies that respond rapidly to chemotherapy such as small-cell lung cancer or germ cell testicular cancers (9). TLS is generally managed with intensive electrolytes and uric acid level monitoring, aggressive electrolyte replacement, and hyperuricemia management. Allopurinol, a xanthine oxidase inhibitor that inhibits synthesis of uric acid from hypoxanthine and xanthine, is commonly used for the prevention and treatment of TLS-associated hyperuricemia. However, rasburicase (a recombinant urate oxidase that oxidizes uric acid to allantoin) is given in cases of severe hyperuricemia or as prophylaxis to patients with significant risk of TLS (i.e., high malignant cell burden) (10). The risk of TLS is highest with the initial cycle of chemotherapy and it decreases with subsequent cycles of treatment.

Targeted Therapy

In contrast to conventional cytotoxic chemotherapy, which disrupts all rapidly dividing cells (malignant and nonmalignant), targeted therapy refers to the use of agents that block or bind to a specific molecular target such as intracellular signaling proteins or surface receptors that are mutated or overexpressed in malignant cells relative to normal cells and which are vital for carcinogenesis and tumor growth. There are various classes of targeted therapies including small molecules, monoclonal antibodies (mAbs), and antibody–drug conjugates (ADCs), which will herein be collectively referred to as inhibitors. Small molecule inhibitors primarily consist of tyrosine kinase inhibitors (TKI) while serine–threonine kinase inhibitors (STKI) such as BRAF and mTOR inhibitors account for most of the remainder.

Toxicities seen in targeted therapy tend to be different from the toxicities associated with cytotoxic chemotherapy with common adverse reactions including rash, diarrhea, and fatigue. Toxicity of a targeted agent is mainly related to on-target activity of the inhibitor due to inhibition of intended molecular target found in normal, nonmalignant tissue. An example of on-target

toxicity is the typical rash seen with epidermal growth factor receptor (EGFR) inhibitor therapy. EGFR activation serves essential functions in the skin, such as promotion of keratinocyte proliferation, survival, motility, as well as regulation of differentiation and keratinization. On-target inhibition of EGFR on normal keratinocytes is what is believed to drive the rash observed with EGFR inhibitors (11). Similarly, trastuzumab, an mAb, can cause reversible cardiomyopathy in a small subset of patients because its target, HER2, is expressed by cardiac myocardium. Toxicities due to interactions with other unintended molecular targets can also occur but are less common. Off-target toxicities occur because many inhibitors (in particular, small molecule kinase inhibitors) inhibit other kinases albeit often at significantly higher concentration than the intended target. An example of such toxicity is hypertension induced by BCR-ABL TKI ponatinib, which also causes hypertension by inhibiting vascular endothelial growth factor receptor (VEGFR) (12). Similarly, ibrutinib (Bruton's tyrosine kinase [BTK] inhibitor) causes atrial fibrillation that is thought to involve BTK (on-target) and TEC kinase (off-target) inhibition in the myocardium, henceforth downregulating the PI3K-Akt activity, which has been shown to be an essential regulator of cardiac protection during stress conditions (13). The following are selected toxicities seen with targeted therapy and recommended dose modifications.

Toxicities of Selected Targeted Therapies

EGFR inhibitors including small molecule TKIs such as erlotinib, gefitinib, and afatinib, and mAbs such as cetuximab and panitumumab are particularly well known for significant dermatologic toxicity because of on-target effects on EGFR in the skin. The typical rash is an acneiform rash, characterized by an eruption of papules and pustules that often appear on the face, scalp, upper chest, and back (14–15). Guidelines for the management of dermatologic toxicity associated with EGFR inhibition are available from the National Comprehensive Cancer Network (NCCN) task force (16). VEGF inhibitors (TKIs and mAbs) are also notable for a host of dermatologic toxicities, most commonly palmar–plantar erythrodysesthesia (PPE) (17). BRAF and MEK STKIs also commonly cause a variety of dermatologic toxicities including maculopapular rash, xerosis, and PPE (18). Standard dose modifications are recommended for grade ≥3 rash although provisions for dose reductions may often be required for grade 2 rash given that rash is cumulative and can be symptomatic.

Diarrhea is very common with targeted therapy particularly with EGFR inhibitors. Diarrhea also commonly occurs after administration of VEGF, mTOR, and multikinase inhibitors as well as other various small molecule inhibitors such as imatinib, trametinib, and crizotinib (19). Other causes of diarrhea such as iatrogenic diarrhea from laxative use and infectious diarrhea need to be considered in the differential. Management of targeted-therapy-induced diarrhea is identical to management of CID as discussed previously, which includes adequate fluid hydration, avoiding foods that exacerbated symptoms, and antidiarrheal medications such as loperamide if needed (19). Diarrhea is typically reversible with such supportive care measures. For grade 3 or higher diarrhea that does not improve despite the previously noted measures can be usually managed with treatment interruptions and dose modifications as detailed in Table 24.2C (20).

VEGF and VEGFR-R inhibitors are often associated with hypertension. In general, the Eighth Joint National Committee (JNC 8) guidelines should be followed for hypertension management (21). If there is need to initiate antihypertensive therapy, a reasonable choice would be angiotensin-converting enzyme inhibitors as they are effective in mild hypertension and can also decrease proteinuria, which is another relatively common toxicity of VEGF/VEGF-R inhibitors (22). The nondihydropyridine calcium channel blockers (CCBs) verapamil and diltiazem are CYP3A4 inhibitors and should therefore be avoided in patients on VEGF TKIs (23). Although grade 2 hypertension (systolic BP 140–159 mmHg or diastolic BP 90–99 mmHg) is commonly controlled with BP medications, 1 dose level reduction is recommended if the test subject's BP does not improve to grade 1. Likewise, for grade 3 hypertension, the investigative drug should be held until it improves to grade 2 or better and restarted with 1 level dose reduction. If the patient requires hospitalization for management of symptomatic systolic BP >180 or diastolic BP >110 mmHg, permanent discontinuation of investigative drug is recommended.

VEGF inhibitors, particularly bevacizumab, are also associated with increased bleeding events. Most bleeding events are relatively limited and are nonserious episodes of epistaxis or GI bleeding (24). Fatal hemorrhaging events have occurred however, particularly in the GI, respiratory, urinary tracts, and brain (25). Bleeding events are typically grade 1 to 2 and reversible with no or minimal medical intervention. For grade 2 or greater central nervous system (CNS) or pulmonary hemorrhage, VEGF TKI should be discontinued.

Increased thromboembolic events have been described in various targeted therapies including VEGF inhibitors and to a lesser extent EGFR targeting mAbs (26). Venous thromboembolism (VTE) can typically be managed with standard anticoagulation and the study drug can often be reinstituted without dose modification once the test subject has therapeutic levels of anticoagulation. Provisions to repeat Doppler studies to ensure clot stability can be considered given that progression of a VTE while on treatment is worrisome and should warrant consideration for discontinuation of the study drug. VEGF inhibitors are also associated with arterial thromboembolic events and events of any grade should prompt immediate discontinuation of the offending drug (27).

Metabolic derangements such as hyperglycemia or hyperlipidemia (elevation of low-density lipoprotein [LDL] and triglyceridemia) have been observed in several classes of targeted therapy including STKI of mammalian target of rapamycin (mTOR) and insulin growth factor receptor 1 (IGF-1R) and to a lesser extent STKIs of PI3K and AKT as well as EGFR inhibitors (28). These effects are managed by close monitoring (fasting glucose and fasting lipid panel) and institution of appropriate medical therapy for grade 2 or greater events. Interruption or dose reduction of antineoplastic targeted therapy is generally not necessary unless severe events develop or progressive metabolic derangements persist despite maximal therapeutic interventions for an extended period of time. Guidelines for management of metabolic abnormalities related to anticancer therapies exist (29).

Some other grade 3 toxicities may not necessarily warrant the standard 1 dose level reduction. An example of this includes noninfectious pyrexia that is fairly common with BRAF-MEK TKIs and can be seen in up to half of patients treated with both dabrafenib and trametinib (30). Another example includes cancer-related fatigue that has been noted in 36% to 85% of patients on VEGF inhibitors for renal cell carcinoma (31). The decision to include a provision to continue the same dose level despite a grade 3 toxicity should be made on a case-by-case basis taking into consideration the target patient population, cancer specific prognosis, and factors related to the particular toxicity such as related comorbidities, natural history of the malignancy, and medical management options.

Hematologic toxicities are less common with targeted therapy as compared to cytotoxic therapy (32). Cyclin-dependent kinase 4 and 6 inhibitors are associated with neutropenia and thrombocytopenia (which led to dose reductions in more than a third of patients treated with palbociclib) (33,34). Rituximab (anti-CD20 mAb) and alemtuzumab (anti-CD52 mAb) are also associated with dose-related neutropenia. In clinical trials, the incidence of all-grade neutropenia was noted to be 50% with alemtuzumab although this was typically reversible with cessation of treatment (35–37). Regarding dose modifications for hematological toxicity, standard dose interruptions and reductions utilized in hematologic toxicity associated with cytotoxic therapy shown in Tables 24.2A and 24.2B are typically followed.

Additional Considerations for Monoclonal Antibody Therapy

mAbs are generally well tolerated due to their high-specificity minimizing off-target effects. An additional consideration with mAb therapy is the common occurrence of infusion reactions. Acute infusion reactions can be observed with any mAb although much more commonly with chimeric mAbs than with humanized or fully human mAbs (38). Acute infusion reactions present with a wide spectrum of symptoms including flushing, fever, chills, rigors, bronchospasm, and hypotension and, if severe, may include generalized urticaria, severe wheezing, severe hypotension, and angioedema (39). Depending on the agent, mild reactions are fairly common and thought to be cytokine-mediated (40). Acute infusion reactions typically develop between initiation of the drug and 30 to 90 minutes after drug infusion and most often occur with either the first or second exposure of the agent. Given this phenomenon, rate titration was commonly instituted in early-phase clinical trials testing mAb therapy. The fixed rate was instituted in later phase clinical trials only after safety was established at a given rate in early-phase trials. Guidelines on how to manage acute infusion reactions exist in most protocols testing mAbs. Most grade 1 reactions are treated with slowing down the infusion by 50% and subsequent reescalation if the reaction resolves. If a grade 2 reaction occurs, stopping the infusion and administration of antihistamines with or without steroids or antipyretics is recommended. The infusion can be restarted at 50% of the original rate if the reaction resolves and if tolerated, the rate can be reescalated. Consideration may be given to instituting premedications with antihistamines and corticosteroids prior to infusions. Grade 3 or 4 infusion reactions are considered medical emergencies and are managed aggressively with intravenous (IV) antihistamines, antipyretics, glucocorticoids, epinephrine, bronchodilators, oxygen, and possibly admission to the intensive care unit for close monitoring. Rechallenging of patients with grade 3 or 4 acute infusion reactions is discouraged. Primary prophylaxis against infusion reactions may be recommended for some agents that are expected to have a high rate of such toxicities.

Antibody–Drug Conjugates (ADC)

ADC toxicity can be mediated by either the cytotoxic or mAb moieties of the drug (41). ADC therapy is generally better tolerated than cytotoxic therapy because the antibody portion of the molecule ensures specificity toward malignant cells that express the intended target and minimize the unintended exposure of the cytotoxic payload to normal tissues. However, spontaneous hydrolysis of the ADC can occur and this produces some undesirable effects (albeit to a lesser extent than the cytotoxic payload administered alone). Currently, there are two Food and Drug Administration (FDA) approved ADCs: brentuximab vedotin and trastuzumab emtansine. Mertansine, the parent molecule of emtansine, causes GI toxicity, hepatocellular injury, thrombocytopenia, and neutropenia (42). Consequently, the most significant toxicities observed in EMILIA, a phase 3 study of ADC trastuzumab emtansine in patients with HER2 positive breast cancers, were transaminitis (22.4%), nausea (39.2%), diarrhea (23.3%), and thrombocytopenia (28.0%) (43). Similarly, in clinical trials with brentuximab vedotin, the most common toxicities were driven by the cytotoxic

moiety (monomethyl auristatin E; an antitubular agent) including fatigue (40%), peripheral neuropathy (26%), neutropenia (37%), diarrhea (31%), and vomiting (23%) (44). These adverse events can be managed in the same manner as adverse events encountered with mAbs and cytotoxic chemotherapy using dose modification guidelines presented in Tables 24.2A to 24.2C.

Immune Therapy

Immunotherapy is intended to stimulate or block some immune functions. Cancer immunotherapy refers to the use of cancer vaccines, cytokine therapy, oncolytic viruses, and inhibitors of tumor-induced immune suppression mechanisms such as blockade of inhibitory immune checkpoints or tumor-associated macrophages. Immune-based therapies are associated with toxicities that are distinct from those that are associated with cytotoxic or targeted therapy. Immunotherapy can lead to toxicities related to immune overactivation (systemic cytokine release) and can also result in autoimmune phenomena, which most commonly occur with immune checkpoint inhibitors and are called immune-related adverse events (irAEs). The most common irAEs include dermatitis, colitis, hepatitis, and endocrine abnormalities (hypophysitis, thyroiditis, adrenalitis) although autoimmune toxicities of many other organ systems have been reported (45). Unlike toxicities encountered with cytotoxic or targeted therapies, immune therapy can induce these effects at any dose. Dose modifications for toxicities encountered in clinical trials of selected classes of immunotherapies are briefly discussed as follows.

Vaccine Therapy

Currently, the only FDA-approved therapeutic cancer vaccine is sipuleucel-T (Provenge) for the treatment of metastatic, hormone-refractory prostate cancer although many others are currently in development (46). Early-stage clinical trials of sipuleucel-T did not identify DLTs (47). Administration of sipuleucel-T consists of infusion of ≥50 million autologous dendritic cells (obtained through leukapheresis) activated by treatment with prostatic acid phosphatase (PAP) linked to GM-CSF and cultured for ~40 hours. Treatment is administered at ~2-week intervals for a total of three doses. Acute infusion reactions with symptoms that included nausea, fever, rigor or chills, respiratory distress/failure were fairly common in phase 3 trials of sipuleucel-T (48). Supportive care measures are similar to those described with acute infusions seen with mAb therapies and premedication with oral antihistamine and acetaminophen prior to each infusion is recommended.

Oncolytic Viruses

At this time, talimogene laherparepvec (Imylgic) is FDA-approved for the treatment of unresectable melanoma (49). Early-phase clinical trials testing safety of oncolytic viruses showed no autoimmune toxicities or DLTs and the most common reactions were grade 1 fever, fatigue, constitutional symptoms, nausea, anorexia, and injection site reactions (50,51). However, a number of promising genetically modified oncolytic viruses are in clinical development. Standard dose modifications for treatment-related toxicities as listed in Tables 24.2A to 24.2C are satisfactory.

Cytokine Therapy

Therapy with cytokines is associated with significant systemic toxicities but continues to be an active area for clinical research. Currently FDA-approved antineoplastic cytokine therapies include interferon (IFN) a-2b and interleukin 2 (IL-2). High-dose IFNa-2b is in general very poorly tolerated and fatigue, fevers, myalgias, nausea, vomiting, transaminitis, and myelosuppression occur in over 50% of patients. Neuropsychiatric symptoms are also a concern in patients receiving IFNa-2b. In the E1684 phase 3 trial for melanoma, the incidence of neuropsychiatric symptoms and signs were seen in 40% of patients and grade 3 and 4 neuropsychiatric symptoms were seen in 2% to 10% of patients (52). IL-2 therapy is highly toxic and is associated with capillary leak syndrome. Capillary leak syndrome is thought to be cytokine-mediated and results in fluid accumulation in the extravascular space causing peripheral edema, rash, transaminase elevations, circulatory collapse/shock, cardiac arrhythmia, metabolic acidosis, fevers/chills, renal failure, and neurotoxicity, often necessitating treatment or monitoring in intensive care units (53–55). Specific guidelines regarding management of these events are discussed elsewhere (56).

Immune Checkpoint Inhibitors

A subset of therapeutic mAbs includes those that primarily target molecules that cause suppression of effector T cells. In particular, inhibitors of immune checkpoint regulation have recently proven to be effective in the management of various malignancies (57,58). FDA-approved immune checkpoint inhibitors include anti-PD-1 receptor antibodies nivolumab, a human IgG4 antibody, and pembrolizumab, a fully humanized, engineered mAb of IgG4 isotype. Atezolizumab is also FDA-approved and is a fully humanized, engineered monoclonal antibody of IgG1 isotype against the protein programmed cell death-ligand 1 (PD-L1). Other PD-1 and PD-L1 inhibitors are under development. Ipilimumab and tremelimumab, which inhibit cytotoxic T-lymphocyte-associated protein 4 (CTLA-4), are also being tested. Ipilimumab is FDA-approved for treatment of patients with metastatic melanoma and as adjuvant treatment for completely excised melanoma and involvement of lymph nodes.

IrAEs related to checkpoint inhibition can have various manifestations. The most common irAE is dermatologic toxicity seen in half of patients treated with ipilimumab (59). A typical rash is reticular and maculopapular located primarily on the trunk or extremities. Diarrhea and hepatotoxicity, with rises in aspartate aminotransferase (AST) and alanine aminotransferase (ALT), are also common. In addition, endocrinopathies such as hypophysitis, adrenal insufficiency, hypo- and hyperthyroidism are also occasionally seen. For ipilimumab, the average time to symptom onset for irAEs is 2 to 3 weeks for dermatologic toxicity, 6 to 7 weeks for GI and hepatic toxicities, and 9 weeks for endocrine toxicity (60). In general, toxicities are seen more commonly with CTLA-4 mAbs than they are with PD-1 or PD-L1 mAbs (61). However, PD-1/PD-L1 inhibitors are associated with an increase in the risk of autoimmune pneumonitis with a rate of grade 3 to 4 toxicity developing in approximately 2% to 6% (with higher rates seen in patients with lung cancer and when these agents were combined with other agents known to also increase risk of pneumonitis). Severe pneumonitis led to three treatment-related deaths in an early-phase study of nivolumab (62). The symptoms include shortness of breath, cough, fever, or chest pain. Excellent reviews on specific algorithms to manage irAEs have been published (63). IrAEs may initially be subtle yet progressive despite cessation of the offending agent. Therefore, DLT definitions should not be limited to grade 3 to 4 events. In general, management of grade 2 irAEs results in holding treatment. If there is no resolution of the event within a week, systemic corticosteroids equivalent to prednisone 0.5 to 1.0 mg/kg/day may be started. Furthermore, patients with a prior history of grade 4 irAE or grade 3 irAE requiring steroid treatment with prednisone at doses greater than 10 mg/day for more than 12 weeks should not receive immune checkpoint inhibitors (64).

There are exceptions that can be considered to these guidelines; however, in general, the approach to these adverse events should be conservative. Further details regarding management of specific toxicities are available via the FDA Risk Evaluation and Mitigation Strategy (REMS) program (65).

PROHIBITED THERAPY

The use of concomitant medications in patients who enroll in phase 1 clinical trials is common, ranging from 90.9% to 99.6% in single-institution retrospective reviews (66–67). Fifty-four percent of trials have one or more medication-related exclusion criteria (68). Trial protocols should include general guidelines for the use of concomitant agents while on trial. A pharmacist should review all concomitant medications for potential interactions with investigational drugs. In addition, inclusion or exclusion of patients with prior exposure to therapies of the same class or therapies with similar mechanisms of action to the investigative drug should be addressed as they have the potential to confound the assessment of the investigative drug. The concurrent use of other

TABLE 24.3 Strong Inhibitors and Inducers of Cytochrome P450 (CYP)*

Strong Inhibitors	Strong Inducers
1A2: fluvoxamine, ciprofloxacin **2C8:** gemfibrozil **2C9:** fluconazole **2D6:** bupropion, cinacalcet, fluoxetine, paroxetine, quinidine **3A3, 5, 7:** HIV antivirals (indinavir, nelfinavir, ritonavir, saquinavir), clarithromycin, itraconazole, ketoconazole, nefazodone, Suboxone, telithromycin	**1A2:** carbamazepine, phenobarbital, rifampin, tobacco **2C9:** carbamazepine, phenobarbital, phenytoin, rifampin **2C19:** carbamazepine, phenytoin, rifampin **3A4, 5:** carbamazepine, *Hypericum perforatum* (St. John's wort), phenobarbital, phenytoin, rifampin

*This is not an exhaustive list and the strength assignment of inhibitor/induction may vary between references.

investigational therapies or other antineoplastic therapies while participating in a therapeutic clinical trial is almost always prohibited.

An investigational drug that is a substrate of phase I and/or phase II metabolizing enzymes responsible for ≥25% of its systemic clearance requires additional assessment and monitoring of concomitant medications for drug–drug interaction risks. Of the more than 30 human cytochrome P450 (CYP) isoenzymes (phase I enzymes) identified to date, CYP3A4, CYP2D6, CYP1A2, and the CYP2C subfamily are the major ones responsible for drug metabolism (69). Concomitant medications that are inducers or inhibitors of CYPs should be avoided as they may either decrease or increase exposure to the investigative drug, respectively. Similarly, the investigational agent could be an inhibitor or inducer of CYPs (Table 24.3). The Flockhart Table™ is an extensive list of CYP inducers and inhibitors available online and can be reviewed prior to trial initiation. In addition, the most relevant cytochrome P450 inducers and inhibitors should explicitly be listed in the clinical trial protocol document (70). Another useful reference with regular updates is the Pharmacist's Letter/Prescriber's Letter "Cytochrome P450 Drug Interactions" table (71).

Investigational therapies that demonstrate a risk of prolonging QTc require close monitoring with frequent and serial ECGs. Most FIH trials will prohibit QTc prolonging medications and commonly will mandate triplicate ECGs to measure change in QTc while on study therapy. Patients with a history of QT interval prolongation or who are receiving antiarrhythmic drugs are excluded or if not excluded may require closer monitoring of ECGs. Table 24.4 lists medications most commonly associated with QTc prolongation. In addition, the Arizona CERT QT Drug Lists by Risk Groups provides an online list of medications known or suspected to prolong QTc and can provide a framework for outlining medications that should be avoided in investigative therapies suspected of prolonging QTc (72).

Instructions for use of concomitant medications are included in clinical trial protocols. Study drug metabolism may be affected by concomitant medications, particularly compounds that are characterized as CYP-450 inhibitors and inducers, as well as those proven or suspected to impact drug transporters and efflux proteins. Drugs that may interfere with the study drug metabolism are often prohibited or should be avoided and this is often specified in the protocol.

While a study protocol typically contains recommendations and prohibitions for use of concomitant medications (prescription and over the counter), guidelines for concomitant use of herbal medications and specific food that may also impact the study drug metabolism should also be included. There are many herbal medications that may impact drug metabolism and are reviewed elsewhere (73,74). Prominent examples

TABLE 24.4 Common QTc Prolonging Agents*

Antiarrhythmics	Antimicrobials	Antidepressants	Antipsychotics	Others
amiodarone	levofloxacin	amitriptyline	haloperidol	cisapride
sotalol	gatifloxacin	desipramine	droperidol	sumatriptan
quinidine	moxifloxacin	imipramine	quetiapine	zolmitriptan
procainamide	ciprofloxacin	doxepin	thioridazine	arsenic
dofetilide	clarithromycin	fluoxetine	ziprasidone	dolasetron
ibutilide	erythromycin	sertraline		methadone
	ketoconazole	venlafaxine		
	itraconazole			

*This is not an exhaustive list.

include the herbal remedy St. John's Wort, which is a potent inducer of CYP3A4 and depending on the dose and route of administration, may be an inducer or inhibitor of other CYP isoenzymes and the drug efflux pump P-glycoprotein (Pgp) (75,76). Grapefruit juice is also a potent CYP3A4 inhibitor as well as an inhibitor of a member of the influx transporter protein family (organic anion transporter polypeptide [OATP]) (77). Ginseng root (*Panax ginseng*) has the potential to affect CYP2C9, 2C19, 2D6, and 3A4 although studies are conflicting as to the degree of inhibition or induction of these enzymes (78,79). Licorice root (*Glycyrrhiza glabra*) is an inhibitor of CYP2B6, 2C9, and 3A4 (80). As it is currently impossible to develop a comprehensive list of known herbal supplements to avoid, most early trial protocols typically will prohibit their use and will require careful monitoring of such use in study subjects. The Natural Medicines Comprehensive Database is accessible online and may serve as a useful reference for potential interactions (81).

CONCLUSION

The management of treatment-related toxicities that occur in clinical trials are generally well articulated in protocols. First, patients who are eligible to participate in clinical trials are selected based on factors such as good performance status, normal organ function (with the exception of organ dysfunction trials), reasonable life expectancy, resolution of prior treatment related toxicity to grade 1 or less, and ability to understand and sign an informed consent. These patients are different than the general patient population with a given disease. Therefore toxicity profile of the agent in study patients may differ when used in routine clinical practice. In fact, examples of differences in the toxicity profile of treatment regimens between clinical trials and when the treatment entered routine practice are abundant. An example of this is the relatively low rate of febrile neutropenia of 5% observed in clinical trials using docetaxel with cyclophosphamide in early-stage breast cancer (82). Subsequently, several groups reported single-institution experiences of much higher rates of febrile neutropenia ranging from 23% to 46% (83–86). This may have been the result of strict patient selection for the trials and differences in the use of prophylactic antibiotics to prevent neutropenic fever among patients treated on the trial compared to standard practice.

In addition, there are times when a rare but clinically important toxicity is not detected in early clinical trials but noted later as the clinical development proceeds in subsequent large, phase III or phase IV clinical studies. Given the low frequency of the toxicity, the event may simply not occur in trials enrolling a small number of patients. It is also possible that a rare toxic effect, even if it occurs, is initially not attributed to study therapy but rather to underlying disease or a patient's comorbid condition. Cardiotoxicity associated with a mAb against HER2 (trastuzumab) in patients with HER2 positive breast cancer was not detected until a large, registration phase III trial was conducted. Twenty-seven percent of patients treated with trastuzumab and anthracycline-containing chemotherapy (doxorubicin and cyclophosphamide) developed heart failure (16% had severe cardiac dysfunction) (87).

In conclusion, monitoring patient safety in clinical trials testing therapies without a completely known toxicity profile is of critical importance. Minimizing enrollment of patients who are at unacceptable risk of complications from study therapy, applying strict parameters for dose interruptions and modifications due to treatment emergent toxicities as well as guidelines in regard to monitoring parameters, supportive care measures, and prohibited therapies are vital components of all well-designed clinical trial protocols. However, even the best protocols cannot account for all possible risks and how to best manage them. Therefore, the principal investigator's, study team's, and DSMC's attention to detail and experience with conducting and monitoring clinical trials are the key requirements.

REFERENCES

1. Topalian SL, Hodi FS, Brahmer JR, et al. Safety, activity, and immune correlates of anti–PD-1 antibody in cancer. *N Engl J Med*. 2012;366:2443–2454.
2. Kain RK, Duda DG, Clark JW, et al. Lessons from phase III clinical trials on anti-VEGF therapy for cancer. *Nat Clin Pract Oncol*. 2006;3(1):23–40.
3. Crawford J, Armitage J, Balducci L, et al. Myeloid growth factors. *J Nat Compr Cancer Netw*. 2013;11(10):1266–1290.
4. Rubenstein EB, Peterson DE, Schubert M, et al. Clinical practice guidelines for the prevention and treatment of cancer therapy–induced oral and gastrointestinal mucositis. *Cancer*. 2004;100(S9):2026–2046.
5. Smith EM, Pang H, Cirrincione C, et al. Effect of duloxetine on pain, function, and quality of life among patients with chemotherapy-induced painful peripheral neuropathy: a randomized clinical trial, *J Am Med Assoc*. 2013;309(13):1359–1367.
6. Hershman DL, Lacchetti C, Dworkin RH, et al. Prevention and management of chemotherapy-induced peripheral neuropathy in survivors of adult cancers: American Society of Clinical Oncology Clinical Practice Guideline. *J Clin Oncol*. 2014;32(18):1941–1967.
7. National Comprehensive Cancer Network. Antiemesis. (Version 2.2016). http://www.nccn.org/professionals/physician_gls/pdf/antiemesis.pdf
8. Basch E, Prestrud AA, Hesketh PJ, et al. Antiemetics: American society of clinical oncology clinical practice guideline update. *J Clin Oncol*. 2011;29(31):4189–4198.
9. Kalemkerian GP, Darwish B, Varterasian ML. Tumor lysis syndrome in small cell carcinoma and other solid tumors. *Am J Med*. 1997;103(5):363–367.
10. Coiffier B, Altman A, Pui CH, et al. Guidelines for the management of pediatric and adult tumor lysis syndrome: an evidence-based review. *J Clin Oncol*. 2008;26(16):2767–2778.

11. Lynch Jr. TJ, Kim ES, Eaby B, et al. Symptom management and supportive care. *Oncologist.* 2007;12(5):610–621.

12. Moslehi JJ, Deininger M. Tyrosine kinase inhibitor-associated cardiovascular toxicity in chronic myelogenous leukemia. *J Clin Oncol.* 2015;33(35):4208–4210.

13. McMullen JR, Boey EJ, Ooi JY, et al. Ibrutinib increases the risk of atrial fibrillation, potentially through inhibition of cardiac PI3K-Akt signaling. *Blood.* 2014;124(25):3829–3830.

14. Balagula L, Lacouture ME, Cotliar JA. Dermatologic toxicities of targeted anticancer therapies. *J Support Oncol.* 2010;8(4):149–161.

15. Peuvrel L, Dréno B. Dermatological toxicity associated with targeted therapies in cancer: optimal management. *Am J Clin Dermatol.* 2014;15(5):425–444.

16. Burtness B, Anadkat M, Bastl S, et al. NCCN Task Force report: management of dermatologic and other toxicities associated with EGFR inhibition in patients with cancer. *J Nat Compr Cancer Netw.* 2009;7(S1):5–21.

17. Eskens, FA, Vereweji J. The clinical toxicity profile of vascular endothelial growth factor (VEGF) and vascular endothelial growth factor receptor (VEGFR) targeting angiogenesis inhibitors; A review. *Europ J Cancer.* 2006;42(18):3127–3139.

18. Welsh SJ, Corrie PG. Management of BRAF and MEK inhibitor toxicities in patients with metastatic melanoma. *Therap Advan Med Oncol.* 2015;7(2):122–136.

19. Pessi MA, Zilembo N, Haspinger E, et al. Targeted therapy-induced diarrhea: a review of the literature. *CritRev Oncol/Hematol.* 2014;90(2):165–179.

20. Hirsh V, Blais N, Brukes R, et al. Management of diarrhea induced by epidermal growth factor receptor tyrosine kinase inhibitors. *Curr Oncol.* 2014;21(6):329–336.

21. James PA, Oparil S, Carter BL, et al. 2014 Evidence-based guideline for the management of high blood pressure in adults. *J Am Med Assoc.* 2014;311(5):507–520.

22. Herrmann J, Yang EH, Iliescu CA, et al. Vascular toxicities of cancer therapies. *Circulation.* 2016;133(13):1272–1289.

23. Izzedine H, Ederhy S, Goldwasser F, et al. Management of hypertension in angiogenesis inhibitor-treated patients. *Ann Oncol.* 2009;20(5):807–815.

24. Kamba T, McDonald DM. Mechanisms of adverse effects of anti-VEGF therapy for cancer. *Br J Cancer.* 2007;96(12):1788–1795.

25. Ranpura V, Hapani S, Wu S. Treatment-related mortality with bevacizumab in cancer patients. *J Am Med Assoc.* 2011;305(5):487–494.

26. Ferroni P, Formica V, Roselli M, et al. Thromboembolic events in patients treated with anti-angiogenic drugs. *Curr Vascul Pharmacol.* 2010;8(1):102–113.

27. Zhang D, Zhang X, Zhao C. Risk of venous and arterial thromboembolic events associated with anti-VEGF agents in advanced non-small-cell lung cancer: a meta-anaysis and systemiatic review. *Onco Target Therapy.* 2016;9:3695–3704.

28. Goldman JW, Mendenhall MA, Rettinger SR. Hyperglycemia associated with targeted oncologic treatment: mechanisms and management. *Oncologist.* 2016;21(12):1326–1336.

29. Busaidy NL, Farooki A, Dowlati A, et al. Management of metabolic effects associated with anticancer agents targeting the PI3K-Akt-mTOR pathway. *J Clin Oncol.* 2012;30(23):2919–2928.

30. Menzies Am, Ashworth MT, Swann S, et al. Characteristics of pyrexia in BRAFV600E/K metastatic melanoma patients treated with combined dabrafenib and trametinib in a phase I/II clinical trial. *Ann Oncol.* 2015;26(2):415–421.

31. Anand D, Escalante CP. Ongoing screening and treatment to potentially reduce tyrosine kinase inhibitor-related fatigue in renal cell carcinoma. *J Sympt Pain Manage.* 2015;50(1):108–117.

32. Everds NE, Tarrant JM. Unexpected hematologic effects of biotherapeutics in nonclinical species and in humans. *Toxicol Pathol.* 2013;41(2):280–302.

33. Turner NC, Jungsil R, André F, et al. Palbociclib in hormone receptor-positive advanced breast cancer. *New Engl J Med.* 2015;373(3):209–219.

34. Finn, RS, Crown JP, Lang I, et al. The cyclin-dependent kinase 4/6 inhibitor palbociclib in combination with letrozole versus letrozole alone as first-line treatment of oestrogen receptor-positive, HER2-negative, advanced breast cancer (PALOMA-1/TRIO-18): a randomised phase 2 study. *Lancet Oncol.* 2016;16(1):25–35.

35. Gibbs SD, Westerman DA, McCormack C, et al. Severe and prolonged myeloid haematopoietic toxicity with myelodysplastic features following alemtuzumab therapy in patients with peripheral T-cell lymphoproliferative disorders. *Br J Haematol.* 2005;130(1):87–91.

36. Elter T, Hallek M, Montillo M. Alemtuzumab: What is the secret to safe therapy? *Clin Advance Hematol Oncol.* 2011;9(5):364–373.

37. Enblad, G, Hagberg H, Erlanson M, et al. A pilot study of alemtuzumab (anti-CD52 monoclonal antibody) therapy for patients with relapsed or chemotherapy-refractory peripheral T-cell lymphomas. *Blood.* 2004;103(8):2920–2924.

38. Maggi E, Vultaggio A, Matucci A. Acute infusion reactions induced by monoclonal antibody therapy. *Exp Rev Clin Immunol.* 2011;7(1):55–63.

39. LaCasce AS, Castells MC, Burstein H, et al. Infusion reactions to therapeutic monoclonal antibodies used for cancer therapy. In: Post TW, ed, *UpToDate.* Waltham, MA.

40. Dillman RO, Hendrix CS. Unique aspects of supportive care using monoclonal antibodies in cancer treatment. *Supportive Cancer Therapy.* 2003;1(1):38–48.

41. Donaghy H. Effects of antibody, drug and linker on the preclinical and clinical toxicities of antibody-drug conjugates. *mAbs,* 2016;8(4):659–671.

42. Blum RH, Kahlert T. Maytansine: A phase 1 study of an ansa macrolide with antitumor activity. *Cancer Treat Rep.* 1978;62(3):435–438.

43. Verma S, Miles D, Gianni L, et al. Trastuzumab emtansine for HER2-positive advanced breast cancer. *Engl J Med.* 2012;367(19):1783–1791.

44. Younes A, Bartlett NL, Leonard JP, et al. Brentuximab vedotin (SGN-35) for relapsed CD30-positive lymphomas. *Engl J Med.* 2010;363(19):1812–1821.

45. Postow MA, Wolchok JD. Ipilimumab: developmental history, clinical considerations and future perspectives. *Melanoma Lett.* 2012;30(1):1–4.

46. Melief CJM, van Hall T, Arens R, et al. Therapeutic cancer vaccines. *J Clin Invest.* 2015;125(9):3401–3412.

47. Small EJ, Fratesi P, Reese DM, et al. Immunotherapy of hormone-refractory prostate cancer with antigen-loaded dendritic cells, *J Clin Oncol.* 2000;18(23):3894–3903.

48. Small EJ, Schellhammer PF, Higano CS, et al. Placebo-controlled phase III trial of immunologic therapy with sipuleucel-T (APC8015) in patients with metastatic, asymptomatic hormone refractory prostate cancer. *J Clin Oncol.* 2006;24(19):3089–3094.

49. Ott PA, Hodi FS. Talimogene laherparepvec for the treatment of advanced melanoma. *Clin Cancer Res.* 2016;22(13):3127–3131.

50. Hu JC, Coffin RS, Davis CJ, et al. A phase I study of OncoVEXGM-CSF, a second-generation oncolytic herpes simplex virus expressing granulocyte macrophage colony-stimulating factor. *Clin Cancer Res.* 2006;12(22):6737–6747.

51. Senzer NN, Kaufman HL, Amatruda T, et al. Phase II clinical trial of a granulocyte-macrophage colony-stimulating factor-encoding, second-generation oncolytic herpesvirus in patients with unresectable metastatic melanoma. *J Clin Oncol.* 2009;27(34):5763–5771.

52. Kirkwood JM, Strawderman MH, Ernstaff MS, et al. Interferon alfa-2b adjuvant therapy of high-risk resected cutaneous melanoma: the Eastern Cooperative Oncology Grout trial EST 1684. *J Clin Oncol.* 2002;14(1):7–17.

53. Numerof RP, Aronson FR, Mier JW. IL-2 stimulates the production of IL-1 alpha and IL-1 beta by human peripheral blood mononuclear cells. *J Immunol*. 1988;141(12):4250.

54. Mier JW, Vachino G, can der Meer JW, et al. Induction of circulating tumor necrosis factor (TNF alpha) as the mechanism for the febrile response to interleukin-2 (IL-2) in cancer patients. *J Clin Immunol*. 1988;8(6):426–436.

55. Lotze MT, Matory YL, Ettinghausen SE, et al. In vivo administration of purified human interleukin 2. II. Half life, immunologic effects, and expansion of peripheral lymphoid cells in vivo with recombinant IL-2. *J Immunol*. 1985;135(4):2865–2875.

56. Schawrtzentruber, DJ. Guidelines for the safe administration of high-dose interleukin-2. *J Immunother*. 2001;24(4):287–293.

57. Sharma P, Allison JP. The future of immune checkpoint therapy. *Science*. 2015;348(6230), 56–61.

58. Pardoll DM, The blockade of immune checkpoints in cancer immunotherapy. *Nat Rev Cancer*. 2012;12(4):252–264.

59. Weber JS, Dummer R, de Pril V, et al. Patterns of onset and resolution of immune-related adverse events of special interest with ipilimumab. *Cancer*. 2013;119(9):1675–1682.

60. Assi H, Wilson KS. Immune toxicities and long remission duration after ipilimumab therapy for metastatic melanoma: two illustrative cases. *Curr Oncol*. 2013;20(2):165–169.

61. Villadodid J, Amin A. Immune checkpoint inhibitors in clinical practice: update on management of immune-related toxicities. *Trans Lung Cancer Res*. 2015;4(5):560–575.

62. Nishino M, Sholl LM, Hatabu H, et al. Anti-PD-1-related pneumonitis during cancer immunotherapy. *New Engl J Med*. 2015;373(3):288–290.

63. Naidoo J, Page DB, Li BT, et al. Toxicities of the anti-PD-1 and anti-DL-L1 immune checkpoint antibodies. *Ann Oncol*. 2015;26(12):2375–2391.

64. Postel-Vinay S, Aspeslagh S, Lanoy E, et al. Challenges of phase 1 clinical trials evaluating immune checkpoint-targeted antibodies. *Ann Oncol*. 2016;27(2):214–224.

65. Bristol-Myers Squibb Company. BLA125377 Yervoy (ipilimumab) injection, for intravenous infusion, risk evaluation and mitigation strategy (REMS). http://www.accessdata.fda.gov/drugsatfda_docs/label/2011/125377_REMS.pdf

66. Borad MJ, Curtis KK, Babiker HM, et al. The impact of concomitant medication use on patient eligibility for phase I cancer clinical trials. *J Cancer*. 2012;3:345–353.

67. Genre D, Viens P, Von Hoff DD, et al. Patients who are receiving concomitant medications should not systematically be excluded from phase I studies. *Anti-cancer Drugs*. 1999;10(1):1–17.

68. Van Spall, HG, Toren A, Kiss A, et al. Eligibility criteria of randomized controlled trials published in high-impact general medical journals: a systematic sampling review. *J Am Med Assoc*. 2007;297(11):1233–1240.

69. Michalets EL. Update: clinically significant cytochrome P-450 drug interactions. *Pharmacotherapy*. 1998;18(1):84–112.

70. Indiana University School of Medicine. P450 drug interactions table, http://medicine.iupui.edu/clinpharm/ddis/main-table

71. Cytochrome P450 drug interactions, *The Pharmacist's Letter*. http://pharmacistsletter.therapeuticresearch.com/cat4978-Cardiology-Charts/Browse.aspx?cs=&s=PL

72. Woosley, RL, Heise, CW, Romero, KA. Combined QTdrugs Lists. *CredibleMeds*, https://crediblemeds.org/index.php/new-drug-list

73. Fasinu PS, Bouic PJ, Rosenkranz B. An overview of the evidence and mechanisms of herb–drug interactions. *Front Pharmacol*. 2012;3:69. doi:10.3389/fphar.2012.00069

74. Wanwimolruk S, Phopin K, Prachayasittikul V. Cytochrome P450 enzyme mediated herbal drug interactions (Part 2). *EXCLI J*. 2014;13:869–896.

75. Roby CA, Anderson GD, Kantor E, et al. St. John's Wort: effect on CYP3A4 activity. *Clin Pharcol Therap*. 2000;67(5):451–457.

76. Markowitz JS, Donovan JL, DeVane CL, et al. Effect of St John's Wort on drug metabolism by induction of cytochrome P450 3A4 Enzyme. *J Am Med Assoc*. 2003;290(11):1500–1504.

77. Pirmohamed M. Drug-grapefruit juice interactions: two mechanisms are clear but individual responses vary. *Br Med J*. 2013;346:f1.

78. Gurley BJ, Gadner SF, Hubbard MA, et al. Clinical assessment of effects of botanical supplementation on cytochromone P450 phenotypes in the elderly. *Drugs Aging*. 2005;22(6):525–539.

79. Malati CY, Robertson SM, Hunt JD, et al. Influence of Panax ginseng on cytochrome P450 (CYP)3A and P-glycoprotein (P-gp) activity in healthy participants. *J Clin Pharmacol*. 2012;52(6):932–939.

80. Kent UM, Aviram M, Rosenblat M, et al. The licorice root derived isoflavan glabridin inhibits the activities of human cytochrome P450S 3A4, 2B6, and 2C9. *Drug Metabol Disposit*. 2002;30(6):709–715.

81. Natural Medicine Comprehensive Database. http://naturaldatabase.therapeuticresearch.com

82. Jones S, Holmes FA, O'Shaughnessy J, et al. Docetaxel with cyclophosphamide is associated with an overall survival benefit compared with doxorubicin and cyclophosphamide: 7-year follow-up of US Oncology Research Trial 9735. *J Clin Oncol*. 2009;27(8):1177–1183.

83. Younis T, Rayson D, Thompson K, et al. Primary G-CSF prophylaxis for adjuvant TC or FEC-D chemotherapy outside of clinical trial settings: a systematic review and meta-analysis. *Support Care Cancer*. 2012;20(10):2523–2530.

84. Ngamphaiboon N, O'Connor TL, Advani PP, et al. Febrile neutropenia in adjuvant docetaxel and cyclophosphamide (TC) with prophylactic pegfilgrastim in breast cancer patients: a retrospective analysis. *Med Oncol*. 2012;29(3):1495–1501.

85. Vandenberg T, Younus J, Al-Khayat S. Febrile neutropenia rates with adjuvant docetaxel and cyclophosphamide chemotherapy in early breast cancer: discrepancy between published reports and community practice—a retrospective analysis. *Curr Oncol*. 2010;17(2):2–3.

86. Myers R, Higgins B, Myers J, et al. Chemotherapy induced febrile neutropenia of docetaxel with cyclophosphamide (TC) for adjuvant therapy of breast cancer in the community—reality check. The 32nd Annual San Antonio Breast Cancer Symposium. *Cancer Res*. 2009;69(24 Suppl):Abstract#2092.

87. Hudis C, Seidman A, Paton V, et al. Characterization of cardiac dysfunction observed in the Herceptin (trastuzumab) clinical trials [abstract 24]. 21st Annual San Antonio Breast Cancer Symposium. Dec. 12–15, 1998, San Antonio, TX. *Breast Cancer Res Treat*. 1998;50(3):232.

Assessment of Patient-Reported Outcomes in Industry-Sponsored Clinical Trials

Ari Gnanasakthy and Ethan Basch

INTRODUCTION

Symptoms are common in many cancers, although they may not be noticeable during early stages of disease. While fatigue, fever, and pain are common in many cancers, many symptoms are cancer-specific. For example, long-term constipation, diarrhea, or a change in stool size may be a sign of colon cancer; and pain when passing urine, blood in the urine, or a change in bladder function could be related to bladder or prostate cancer. While some patients with brain cancer may experience increasing hearing difficulties, others may show cognitive impairments. Decline in physical functioning and sexual functioning is also common among many cancer sufferers. When treatment is no longer possible, symptom control becomes the focus of cancer care.

Patients with cancer not only experience symptoms of their disease but experience symptoms as a result of the treatment they receive. Symptoms caused by treatment are often referred to as side effects or toxicity. The impact of the symptoms attributable to cancer and its treatment often result in secondary symptoms such as worry, depression, anger, and grief. Patients with cancer experience physical and psychological problems for long periods, even long after the cancer is cured (1–3).

Historically, treatment benefit in oncology trials was largely measured by endpoints related to survival and tumor reduction. Until recently, assessment of treatment benefit that can be reported only by patients has not been prominent in cancer research. Patients may even accept death as a preferred alternative to treatments that result in unacceptable side effects. The need to consider the patient perspective has become a prominent aspect of drug development.

The Food and Drug Administration (FDA) has included the patient perspective in advisory committee meetings since 1991, and the recent FDA Patient-Focused Drug Development initiative encourages the systematic approach to conducting benefit–risk assessment for new drugs by considering disease severity and unmet medical needs (4). This initiative further supports the goals of the 21st Century Cures Act to "incorporate patient perspectives into the regulatory process and help address their unmet needs" (5).

As a result of these initiatives and due to the increasing need to demonstrate the value of new products in the market, an increasing number of cancer clinical trials now include patients' input to generate evidence of treatment benefit (6). Treatment benefit in clinical trials, based on efficacy or safety or both, is demonstrated by evidence that the treatment has a positive impact on how long a patient lives and how a patient feels and functions in daily life (7).

CLINICAL OUTCOME ASSESSMENTS

As advancement in cancer therapies improves the longevity of patients, the focus of the effectiveness of new cancer treatments has begun to shift from survival alone to clinical outcome assessments (COAs) such as progression-free survival (PFS), disease-free survival, and various measures of responses such as complete responder and partial responder (8).

A COA is any assessment that may be influenced by human choices, judgment, or motivation and may support either direct or indirect evidence of treatment benefit. Unlike biomarkers that rely completely on an automated process or algorithm, COAs depend on implementation, interpretation, and reporting from a patient, clinician, or observer (9). The four types of COAs are clinician-reported outcomes (ClinROs), observer-reported outcomes (ObsROs), performance outcomes (PerfOs), and patient-reported outcomes (PROs).

Clinician-Reported Outcomes

ClinRO is a report that comes from a trained healthcare professional after observation of a patient's health condition. A ClinRO involves a judgment (based on professional training or experience) or interpretation of the observable signs, behaviors, or other physical manifestations thought to be related to a disease or condition. ClinRO measures cannot directly assess symptoms that are known only to the patient (e.g., pain intensity). Typical ClinROs in cancer clinical trials are PFS, complete responder, and adverse events (AEs).

A recent review of cancer drugs newly approved by the FDA between 2011 and 2015 shows that endpoints of 36% of the pivotal studies relied on survival as an endpoint. This compares to 76% of endpoints that relied on a ClinRO as a primary endpoint (10).

Observer-Reported Outcomes

When a patient is too ill, perhaps during advanced stages of cancer or in pediatric settings, outcomes may be captured by an observer such as a parent, spouse, or another nonclinical caregiver who is regularly in a position to observe and report on a specific aspect of the patient's health. An ObsRO includes only events or behaviors that can be observed and does not include medical judgment or interpretation. Examples of ObsROs include a parent report of a child's vomiting episodes or perceived cognition function reported by parents of children with brain tumors.

Performance Outcomes

Assessment of physical performance is commonly used during cancer treatment as an indirect measure of treatment benefit (2,11). A PerfO is a measurement based on a task or tasks performed by a patient according to instructions and that is administered by a healthcare professional. PerfOs require patient cooperation and motivation. They include measures of gait speed (e.g., timed 25-foot walk test) or cognitive testing (e.g., digit symbol substitution test).

Patient-Reported Outcomes

A PRO is a measurement based on a report that comes from the patient (i.e., study subject) about the status of the patient's health condition without amendment or interpretation of the patient's report by a clinician or anyone else. A PRO can be measured by self-report or by interview, provided that the interviewer records only the patient's response. Symptoms or other unobservable concepts known only to the patient can be measured only by PRO instruments. PROs can also assess the patient perspective on functioning or activities that may also be observable by others.

PROs encompass symptoms related to the disease such as pain and the impact of treatment-related toxicity, as well as distal concepts such as anxiety, depression, performance functioning, and health-related quality of life (HRQOL). PROs are often a prognostic indicator for PFS and overall survival (OS), suggesting that tumor responses are associated with patients' expression of feelings and function (12–14).

Traditionally, industry-sponsored cancer studies included endpoints related to HRQOL. While HRQOL is a key outcome of interest in chronic or poorly curable diseases, where the aim of the interventions is to keep patients symptom free or to reduce the distress of the disease, the focus of the rest of this chapter is on all PROs that include symptoms, physical functioning, HRQOL, treatment satisfaction, and compliance.

PRO MEASURES IN CANCER STUDIES

Data to support PRO-related endpoints in clinical trials are collected using standardized questionnaires. These may be referred to as instruments, diaries, scales, checklists, or event logs. Collectively, they are referred to as PRO measures (PROMs). PROMs must be valid, reliable, and have the ability to detect change (responsiveness). Further, PROMs in clinical trials must be easily understood and ideally present a minimal burden to patients and clinical research staff for effective use in the clinical trial setting.

Many PROMs are available to assess the impact of new treatments in cancer clinical trials. The most commonly used measures are the European Organization for Research and Treatment of Cancer (EORTC) core questionnaire, the QLQ-C30, and the Functional Assessment of Cancer Therapy-General (FACT-G). In addition, researchers can use the MD Anderson Cancer Center's Symptom Index (MDASI), the Patient-Reported Outcomes version of the Common Terminology Criteria for Adverse Events (PRO-CTCAE), and the Patient-Reported Outcomes Measurement Information System (PROMIS). Short descriptions of these measures are given in the following.

EORTC QLQ-C30 AND FACT-G

The EORTC core questionnaire, QLQ-C30, and the FACT-G are the two most widely used cancer-specific questionnaires to assess PROs. They constitute the core questionnaires of the EORTC and the Functional Assessment of Chronic Illness Therapy (FACIT) measurement systems. Both are modular systems, such that the issues related to HRQOL are covered by QLQ-C30 and FACT-G and can be further complemented by site- and/or treatment-specific modules. Normative data are available for both measures to aid interpretation of findings.

Although there is considerable overlap between QLQ-C30 and FACT-G, there are differences between the two.

In a study of patients with breast cancer or Hodgkin's disease, both the QLQ-C30 and the FACT-G were found to measure markedly different aspects of HRQOL (15). When deciding to select an appropriate PROM for a study, the measures used in past studies may be confusing. For example, studies related to mesothelioma may include the Lung Cancer Symptom Scale adapted for patients with mesothelioma (LCSS-Meso), or QLQ-LC13, or FACT-L. It is important to note that there may have been multiple reasons for the choice of a PROM for a specific study that was carried out in the past. Duplicating someone else's strategy in a blinded fashion may provide the answers to the research question, but odds are it will not. Lockett and colleagues provide a guide for choosing between EORTC QLQ-C30 and FACT-G (16).

The MD Anderson Symptom Inventory

Both EORTC QLQ-C30 and FACT-G were based on the conceptual model to assess HRQOL. Although the disease-specific modules include items related to symptoms, neither measure was developed to measure symptoms in a comprehensive manner. The MDASI was designed to assess the severity of common cancer-related and treatment-related symptoms that may better reflect the symptom experience of the cancer population. The MDASI's 13 core symptom items include those found to have the highest frequency and/or severity in patients with various cancers and treatment types. It assesses not only the intensity of cancer-related symptoms but the level of symptom interference with daily functioning. The instructions and the response options are easily understood by patients, and the measure is available in many languages and modes of administration (17,18).

MDASI modules augment the 19 core MDASI symptom and interference items with additional items identified as unique to a particular patient population. MDASI modules may be disease specific, disease site specific, or treatment specific.

PRO-CTCAE

Cancer therapies are often associated with significant symptomatic AEs, and rigorous collection of information about these AEs is an essential component of understanding treatment characteristics and impact on patients (19). However, clinician assessment of AEs is relatively unreliable, meaning that if two different clinicians evaluate the same patient, they often disagree with each other's assessments (19–21). Patient reporting is substantially more reliable, and numerous studies have shown it to be feasible (22).

PRO-CTCAE is a library of 78 symptomatic AEs represented by 124 items for patients to directly report the frequency, severity, and impact of AEs during clinical trials. Patients can complete specific items selected from the library but based on prior knowledge of the expected AE profile of the drugs within the context of the clinical trial (23). Data provided by patients via PRO-CTCAE can be useful for illustrating the time course of AEs and the impact of the AEs of new treatments.

PROMIS

PROMIS is a set of person-centered measures that evaluate and monitor physical, social, and emotional health in adults and children. It can be used with the general population and with individuals living with chronic conditions. Similar to PRO-CTCAE, the PROMIS system can be considered an item bank from which the domains (e.g., physical functioning) and the items within the domain can be selected based on prior knowledge and the study requirements.

Other Measures

Apart from the PROMs mentioned previously, various disease-specific or generic measures are available to assess PROs in cancer clinical trials. For example, the LCSS is a disease- and site-specific PROM with both patient and an observer (healthcare professional) forms. Studies related to skin cancer often include the Dermatology Life Quality Index or Skindex. Breast reconstruction studies may use the BreastQ. There are many other examples of context-specific PROMs used in oncology.

In summary, the choice of PROMs to be included in clinical trials should be based on the strategy driven by the conceptual model and the research question. Validity of the measure(s) should be appropriate for the study population, and care should be taken to avoid patient burden.

FORMULATING PRO STRATEGY

Unlike clinical trials related to many other diseases, cancer clinical trials are different. Not only is the primary focus of most cancer trials to improve survival, they are far more likely than noncancer trials to be single arm and open label and far less likely to be double-blind, randomized, controlled trials. Further, chemotherapy used for treating cancer, often as intravenous injection, results in many unwanted side effects such as fatigue, hair loss, and anemia.

However, newer treatments for treating cancer include combination therapies, immunotherapy, targeted therapies, antibodies, and small molecules targeting various pathways. These treatments have different side-effect profiles than the chemotherapies of yesteryear. Future treatment options that include nanotechnology and robotic surgeries will further improve treatment options and patient experience during treatment.

Formulating PRO strategy for cancer studies therefore requires understanding the characteristics of newer therapies. This will not only influence the concepts that need to be measured but also when the concepts are assessed (i.e., frequency and timing of assessment), how they are assessed (e.g., data provided at patients' convenience at home), and the method of analysis (e.g., dose interruptions of orally administered treatments due to low-grade toxicity may influence the method of analysis).

The strategic purposes of including PRO-related endpoints in industry-sponsored cancer clinical trials are to satisfy regulatory authorities or payers or for the purpose of publication as part of product promotion. Although PROs are seldom used as primary endpoints in cancer clinical trials, they are often used as secondary endpoints to provide vital information to regulators to assess the overall risk and benefits associated with new treatments. For example, PROs assessed in clinical trials related to metastatic renal cell carcinoma and metastatic castration-resistant prostate cancer treatments provided valuable information for regulators to assess the treatment benefit of recent therapeutic agents (12,24). The inclusion of disease-specific symptoms reported as a secondary endpoint by patients in pivotal clinical trials was key in facilitating the approval of ruxolitinib for the treatment of myelofibrosis (25). In palliative or maintenance settings, PROs can be the primary endpoint. For example, in reviewing the use of olaparib in the management of ovarian cancer, PROs were recommended to be a primary endpoint along with PFS and OS (26).

Formulating a PRO strategy for clinical trials consists of the following seven broad steps (Figure 25.1). These steps should not be necessarily considered to be in sequence. Rather, they should be considered as steps in an iterative process.

Developing a Conceptual Model

Formulating a rationale for PRO assessment in cancer clinical trials and specifying how that would add value to the overall objective of the study is the first important step when planning a study. The concepts of interest should be driven by a conceptual model based on patient insight, expert input, and information gleaned from the literature.

A conceptual model can be useful to understand the impact of the disease and treatment in terms of outcomes. A conceptual model should provide the rationale for and specification of the PRO outcome of interest in a specific population. For example, a conceptual model developed for lung cancer suggests that the physical and functional dimensions are important predictors of quality of life

Develop a conceptual model	Conceptual model depicting concepts of interest should typically bo based on patient insight, expert input, and information gleaned from the literature. A conceptual model helps in defining appropriate value messages.
Define value messages	Value messages highlighting product characteristics should also resonate with key stakeholders. Value messages drive the PRO related research questions, and thus the choice of study endpoints and PROMs.
Develop an endpoint model	An endpoint model demonstrating the hypothesized relationships among all measures, including PROMs, to support the overall study objective.
Choose appropriate PROMs	PROMs should be based on the conceptual model and the endpoint model that satisfy the overall strategy. If not readily available, study specific PROMs may be modified from an existing measure or created from scratch.
Measurement strategy	Measurement strategy defines the respondent (who?), the assessment schedule (when?), location of data entry (where?), and any exceptions (e.g. time windows).
Data capture strategy	Data capture should minimize patient and study burden while also minimizing missing data. Data capture using e-devices will minimize missing values and increase overall operational efficiency.
Analysis and reporting	Analysis should address the research question(s) to support the generation of predefined value messages. Reporting of findings based on PROs should follow the recommendations of the CONSORT PRO statement.

FIGURE 25.1 Key components of PRO strategy.

(27). Similarly, for a conceptual model relating to breast cancer survivors, only physical and social factors were found to be significantly related to HRQOL (28). Given that impact of biological and targeted therapies is not yet fully known, careful consideration must be given to the concepts that need to be considered.

Concepts can be simple (pain) or complex (depression or HRQOL). Simple concepts such as pain may be easier to measure with single-item questions, whereas concepts that are distal to the disease may require multidimensional questionnaires.

Defining a Value Message

Having understood the treatment benefit to patients from the conceptual model, the next step is to decide on the value messages that would resonate with key stakeholders. As such, value messaging should not be secondary to other components of PRO research but should be the main objective of an optimal PRO strategy. Formulation of appropriate value messages should be based on a thorough understanding of the disease or condition, identification of PRO-related treatment benefit, and understanding of the competitive landscape—a key component of assessing the commercial potential of a value message.

The selected value messages drive the selection of endpoints. For example, a value message "Treatment X improves pain intensity by 6 weeks" will be based on the endpoint "time to improvement in pain intensity." Similarly, value messages can be based on various endpoints, such as the difference between group means, event-free time, time to deterioration of specific symptoms, or the percentage of responders.

Value messages crafted following these steps should be explicit in the target product profile and should drive an appropriate program-specific strategy, including the development of an endpoint model and the selection of the appropriate PROMs.

Developing an Endpoint Model

An endpoint model for a specific study describes the various measurable concepts for a specific disease state. Additional treatment-specific concepts relevant to the patient population may be included in the model. A hierarchy of endpoints, including PRO endpoints, can then be defined to support hypothesized relationships among all measures to support the overall study objective. Typically, an endpoint model takes account of the natural history of the disease, treatment goals, and the PROMs intended to demonstrate treatment benefit. Patrick and colleagues provide a hypothesized endpoint model for head and neck cancer (29).

Choosing an Appropriate PRO Measure

It is possible that no single PROM will address all the concepts identified in the conceptual model. In such instances, study teams may need to use multiple PROMs. PROMs may have to be modified or developed from scratch. Selection of PROMs should be based on the conceptual model and the endpoint model that satisfy the overall strategy (30,31).

It is noteworthy that cancer is one of the few disease areas with the luxury of having access to readily available PROMs to be used in a variety of indications. While having a battery of readily available PROMs can reduce the time and resources to formulate an appropriate measurement strategy, it can also give a false sense of security and encourage study teams to formulate an appropriate PRO strategy around the available PROMS—the proverbial tail wagging the dog.

The preference for the choice between the measures must be driven by the research question, as well as the strength and weakness between PROMs considered. For example, the two most commonly used PROMS in ovarian cancer trials (QLQ-OV28 and FACT-O) were not developed and validated in patients with platinum-resistant recurrent ovarian cancer (32). However, both PROMs have been widely used in ovarian cancer clinical trials, including in studies relating to recurrent ovarian cancer where the symptom burden may be high, and studies have rarely reported any differences between treatments. Use of inappropriate PROMS in pivotal cancer studies has also been noted by the FDA during recent approvals of cabazitaxel and olaparib (33). Care should also be taken when investigating the impact of newer therapies such as cancer immunotherapies or immunocellular therapies. For example, cancer immunotherapy agents attempt to use activated T lymphocyte responses (directly or indirectly) to kill the malignant cells. So in addition to the typical disease manifestations, patients' experience related to immune activation—problems like cytokine release syndrome, generalized edema, and so on—may not be captured by PROMs that were developed to study the impact of chemotherapies.

New translations of PROMs are often required for trials carried out in multiple countries. PROM translations, also called cultural adaptations, must adhere to strict methodology and may take 6 to 9 months to develop (34).

Study teams may be tempted to change various aspects of an existing PROM to suit their specific study. However, any changes to wording, sequence, response options, instructions, and administration method may invalidate a PROM. Permission must be obtained from the authors of the PROM (or authors of translation) and documented before any changes are made. Changes may also warrant validation studies. These issues are important when a PROM developed for paper administration is considered for use in electronic data capture (electronic patient-reported outcome [ePRO]) (35).

Measurement Strategy

Consideration should also be given to the assessment of PROs as this can impact the choice of PROMs as well as the overall strategy. For example, studies involving adults and children may include PROMs for adults only but not for children, as appropriate PROMs may not be available for children or the burden of completing PROMS by children may be considered to be unreasonable. Although age-appropriate PROMs may be available for children with severe cancers, such as those with relapsed and refractory B-cell acute lymphoblastic leukemia who may go through long-term treatment, not all may be at age-appropriate development stages to be able to comprehend and respond to PROMs. Reports from parents or caregivers are most appropriate in studies involving very young children or patients with cognitive or physical impairment.

PRO assessments should be mandatory before the start of treatment. Baseline administration is required not only to be able to make intergroup comparison for changes in PRO-related endpoints before and after treatment but also to assess patients' baseline symptom characteristics. Since the first day of clinical trials tend to be hectic for the study staff and the patients the baseline PRO data can be captured the day before (or the morning of the visit day) the patients come to their baseline visit.

The timing is very important for administering PROMs in relation to the expected outcomes as well as the research question. For example, when assessing two chemotherapy regimens PRO assessments should be made at least at baseline and at the beginning of every cycle until disease progression, end of study, or death. Frequent assessment of symptoms may be required for an analysis of time to symptom reductions. The analysis of the PRODIGE 4/ACCORD 11 study showed significantly long OS but increased toxicity with the experimental treatment (gemcitabine). Since PROs were assessed every 2 weeks until progression, a detailed analysis enabled to demonstrate symptom benefit and impact of treatment on various aspects of HRQOL in favor of the treatment (14). Long-term data may be necessary because some side effects of treatments can occur after the last treatment (36). To improve study compliance acceptable time widows for completing the PROMs may be considered. For example, in studies that compare two chemotherapy regimens patients may complete their PROMs up to 2 days before their study visit.

Patients experience the impact of immunotherapies much earlier during the treatment than patients receiving chemotherapies. Consideration to the assessment schedule of PROs would be important in such settings in order to be able to make optimal comparison between treatments. Frequent assessments (e.g., daily assessment of symptoms) or assessments that require spontaneous reporting (e.g., episodes of pain, seizures) may require patients to enter data via e-devices outside study visits.

Data-Capture Strategy

Having decided on the PROMs to be used in a study and the appropriate measurement strategy, adequate thought should be given to the method of data capture. A good data-capture strategy is necessary to minimize missing data and limit variation in data. The two most important aspects of a data-capture strategy are patient burden and mode of data capture.

The following aspects of patient burden must be considered:

- Number of questions/questionnaires: As a general rule, the data quality may be adversely impacted if patients need more than 20 minutes to provide PRO data because completion of long or numerous instruments can become tiresome. Patient burden can be managed by creating a manageable administration schedule that allows appropriate data collection and limits patient burden. For example, not all parts of the study questionnaire may need to be repeated at each study visit.
- Ability of patients to provide PRO data: Younger patients, patients with severe disease status, or physically or cognitively impaired patients may not be able to provide data accurately. Proxy collection or interview administration may be considered.

The advantages of e-devices for the collection of PRO data are well documented (35). In addition to gaining significant operational efficiencies, researchers benefit from valuable scientific improvements that e-devices offer. By capturing PRO data in real time, e-devices overcome the recall biases associated with back-filled paper diaries. By also gathering multiple data points, e-device data can provide a more detailed and more reliable understanding of the drug's effects.

Collection of PRO data may be considered a day or two before the day of the scheduled visit. This may ease the patient burden and study burden, especially during the baseline visit when patients and study staff are preoccupied with administrative matters and various procedures such as physical examination, biopsies, laboratory, and imaging procedures.

Also, given that many new cancer therapies are now taken orally and at home, patients may be advised by their physicians to temporarily interrupt or even discontinue their medication in the event of serious AEs such as diarrhea. Patients may themselves stop taking their medication temporarily if their daily lives are adversely impacted due to low-grade toxicity. It is vital to capture details of dose interruptions (start and end date) and reasons for treatment continuation (e.g., "patient was too ill to provide data," "patient refused") to appropriately analyze the PRO data.

Whereas frequent administration of multidimensional questionnaires is unusual in cancer studies, capturing data relating to toxicity using PRO-CTCAE via e-devices would increase operational efficiency because patients can provide data in real time from the comfort of their homes (37).

Analysis and Reporting

A combination of efficacy, toxicity, and PRO endpoints consisting of symptoms and aspects of HRQOL can play a major role in assessing the effectiveness of a new cancer therapy (38). Simply reporting changes in overall scores of PROMs consisting of multiple domains may mask important differences in treatment efficacy.

For example, a recent review showed no differences relating to overall HRQOL between cancer regimens in trials relating to advanced breast cancer. While this may be true, to conclude that PROs therefore should not be assessed in future advanced breast cancer trials would be misleading because important differences may be hidden among the domain or item level scores (39). For example, there was no difference found in the overall score in HRQOL data based on EORTC QLQ-C30 and EORTC QLQ-BR23 between treatment groups in a study comparing eribulin mesylate with capecitabine in patients with metastatic breast cancer who had been previously treated with anthracyclines and taxanes. However, findings based on detailed post hoc analysis showed that each treatment performed better in different aspects of HRQOL assessed by the PROMs. The post hoc analysis showed that eribulin performed significantly better than capecitabine in assessments of cognitive functioning, nausea and vomiting, and diarrhea. In comparison, capecitabine performed significantly better compared to eribulin in evaluations of emotional functioning, systemic side effects, and upset by hair loss (40,41).

Overall scores may mask important domain-based differences in three ways:

1. A treatment may affect domains of a PROM differently, such that it may change one domain directly, which in turn affects another domain. Thus understanding treatment effects may be more complex than simply comparing overall change on a given domain.
2. There may be subgroups within treatment arms that respond to treatment differentially, and this may vary by treatment arm. Combining those subgroups and comparing treatment arms on mean change or differences at posttreatment may mask this differential change and thus differential treatment effects.
3. Missing data may mask differences in treatment effects. Differences in treatment efficacy or AEs by treatment arm may result in differential dropout. Use of the last observation carried forward is often based on untenable assumptions (data missing at random) and will not aid in understanding whether dropout at different points in a trial makes a difference in the overall outcome. More rigorous tests and analytic methods are available to evaluate the effects of (differential) dropout on endpoints, including survival.

Reporting the proportion of patients reaching a specified threshold of PROs or change from baseline may be informative to stakeholders. As seen in the analysis of ruxolitinib for the treatment of myelofibrosis, cumulative distribution of changes in PROs can be a simple but powerful way of depicting differences between two treatments (42). PRO data from the SQUIRE trial used various methods of depicting individual and overall symptom scores. The analysis included examination of OS by baseline symptom severity and by maximum severity score recorded during treatment (43).

Since a typical data set would include patients who responded as well as those who did not, innovative analytic methods can be employed to identify subsets of differential responders (44). Specifically, these analyses identify subgroups of patients who respond differently (i.e., show different trajectories of change) in outcomes of interest. Once identified, these subsets of patients can be analyzed specifically to understand how they differed in treatment response (e.g., nonresponder, responder, hyperresponder) and the characteristics of each subgroup that may help explain why they respond differently (e.g., duration or stage of disease, comorbidities, concomitant medication use, prior therapies). Three main advantages of these analytic methods are:

1. They use individual patient-level data rather than mean group changes.
2. They use all available data (i.e., assessments) rather than a focus on baseline and end-of-treatment or efficacy time point. Sometimes the interim time points can be informative about a patient's progression.
3. They are efficient at identifying subgroups of differential responders to treatment if they exist.

PRO data can be very much influenced by the impact of treatment toxicity. Therefore, the impact of treatment toxicity leading to dose interruptions (for orally administered treatments) or delay in treatment cycles (for regimens involving chemotherapies) should be taken into consideration during the analysis of the data.

Another challenge that needs attention is the multiregional aspect of contemporary clinical trials. Most clinical trials sponsored by pharmaceutical companies are carried out in multiple countries that cover many cultures. Caution needs to be exercised when interpreting the findings from multiregional studies. Symptoms reported for some cancers, such as gastric cancer, may vary between regions (45). Moreover, even after following a rigorous development process of PROMs, PROs from multiregional trials can be impacted by cultural aspects such as attitude and taboos associated with specific cancers (46). Feelings of shame, anger, fear, and fatalism as well as the literacy levels of those taking part in a clinical trial can also impact PROs from multiregional clinical trials (47,48).

For example, an analysis of PRO data from a study comparing imatinib or interferon alfa plus low-dose cytarabine (IRIS study) showed that 18 of the 27 items from FACT-BRM collected in 1,049 patients may have been impacted by cultural differences (English vs. French, and English vs. German). Based on the analysis, the magnitude of the treatment differences was adjusted, although the findings did not make any difference to the direction or the magnitude of the treatment difference (49). Similarly, differential response patterns based on cultural groups were also identified for many items within the scales of the EORTC QLQ-C30 (50). While such systematic measurement variability due to the impact of culture in a multiregional study would be minimal in the interpretation of PRO findings based on data from a large comparative setting, caution should be exercised when interpreting PRO findings of data from a small number of patients from multiple cultures.

Reporting of findings based on PROs should follow the recommendations of the Consolidated Standards of Reporting Clinical Trials (CONSORT) PRO statement. The aim of this extension is to improve the reporting of PROs in clinical trials to facilitate the use of findings to inform clinical practice and health policy (51). The statement recommends the following five checklist items: (a) that the PRO(s) be identified as a primary or secondary outcome(s) in the abstract; (b) the hypothesis related to PROs should be stated and the relevant domains (if applicable) identified; (c) evidence for the validity and reliability of the PROMs as well as the person completing the PROM and the method of data collection; (d) statistical approaches for dealing with missing data be explicitly stated; and (e) that the PRO-specific limitations of the study findings and generalizability of results to other populations and clinical practice be discussed.

While a detailed discussion on the analysis of data is beyond the scope of this chapter, an analysis can only be good as the quality of data. Data quality depends on many factors, including study conduct, processes being in place to ensure data quality, acceptable patient burden, and the dedication of study staff to ensure timely and complete data collection. Further discussion relating to the analyses of PROs is found elsewhere (52–54).

In summary, an appropriate strategy should be based on a conceptual model, an endpoint strategy that addresses the research question, utilization of appropriate PROMs and, assessments and subsequently the analysis to maximize the value messages of a new treatment. Inappropriate or flawed strategy often leads to lack of enthusiasm among study teams, cascades into data collection and quality control, and leads to missing values and unanalyzable data—a waste of time all around.

CHALLENGES FACING STUDY TEAMS

Study teams in pharmaceutical companies face multiple challenges when it comes to capturing PROs in cancer-related clinical trials because cancer trials are likely to follow regulatory pathways designed to accelerate the development and regulatory process and study teams may not have adequate time to formulate an optimal PRO strategy. Study teams may also be discouraged from including PRO-related endpoints in clinical trials because the vast majority of contemporary cancer studies are carried out in noncomparative settings with small numbers of patients (55).

A recent study showed that, based on a sample of the 160 new cancer drug approvals between 2011 and 2014, cancer trials were far more likely than noncancer trials to be single arm (37.5% vs. 8.3%) and open label (67.5% vs. 8.3%) and far less likely to be double-blind, randomized, controlled trials (35% vs. 87.5%). Furthermore, 35% of the oncology trials had fewer than 200 patients in registration trials versus 15.8% of non oncology products (33). The study also shows that, of the 40 new oncology drugs approved by FDA's Office of Hematology and Oncology Products between January 2010 and December 2014, only 3 (7.5%) included PRO-related labeling (33).

The design features of cancer trials also make it difficult to include validated PROMs because of the risk of bias. Although bias in open-label studies may be a cause of concern, conclusions based on robust analysis, even if based on data from open-label studies, can be of value to providers and patients. For example, the PROFILE study, an open-label study comparing crizotinib and chemotherapy in patients with anaplastic lymphoma kinase-positive advanced non–small-cell lung cancer, was the first study to demonstrate improvement in lung cancer symptoms, HRQOL, and the general health status of a targeted agent compared to second-line chemotherapy (56).

PRO findings from single-arm, open-label studies can also provide useful data to patients and physicians who may want to compare experience to supportive care or standard of care. These studies can be useful for reviewers who may want to study the experience of patients during PFS. Such realization led to one of the reviewers for brentuximab to comment that "progression-free survival alone is a pyrrhic victory" (57).

IMPLEMENTATION OF PROS IN CANCER STUDIES

A carefully crafted strategy is only of value if it is implemented with the required rigor. PRO data should be treated as any other data in clinical trials. While this is true, the collection of PRO data, especially in severe diseases such as cancer with the challenges outlined previously, is not like any other data from a typical cancer trial. For patients to provide information about various aspects of their health and illness, they should have the motivation, willingness, and necessary support from the study staff and the study sponsor.

Protocol Specifications

The study protocol should describe in detail the plan for conducting the clinical trial and explain the purpose and function of the study and how to implement it. It should include pertinent information such as PRO objectives, rationale for the assessment, the assessment schedule, the modality of data capture, and an analysis plan.

The protocol should also include the names of the PROMs to be used in the study along with their version numbers or citations of original publication. Wherever possible, the protocol should also include citations of validation and cultural adaptation.

Procedures should also be specified when data are expected from "special" populations (e.g., caregivers of elderly patients, parents of young children).

Obtaining Appropriate PRO Measures

Once a PROM has been identified for use, the following three criteria must be met before the PROM is integrated in a clinical study: (a) the PROM must be the latest version available (there may be exceptions if the drug development program requires maintaining consistency between studies), (b) permission to use the PROM must be obtained from the appropriate authorities, and (c) all necessary validated language versions should be available at the time of institutional ethics committee or institutional review board (IEC/IRB) submissions.

Translations of PROMs

The translations of PROMs required for a clinical trial are governed not only by the official languages of the country but by the languages spoken by minority populations in that country.

Knowledge of ethnic mix and the locations of study centers may also help identify the language versions required. For example, there are more than 20 officially recognized languages in India with thousands of dialects. Knowing the locations of study centers would be a key factor to decide the language versions of PROMs required for use in India. Recognizing such factors, Swedish ethics committees often request that PROMs be available both in Swedish and Danish when study centers are located near the Swedish/Danish border. Additionally, linguistic similarities of a language spoken in different countries may differ significantly. For example, separate translations of French may be required for France, Belgium, and Canada.

Companies that provide translation services also provide certificates of translation. Certificates for existing translations can be obtained from the authors of the instruments; it is important to have the corresponding certificates of translation in time for IRB/IEC submissions.

Vendor Management

The efficiency of integrating all language versions of PROMs in a clinical trial depends on seamless interaction among the sponsoring company, the translation vendor, the company that manages the data-capture device (ePRO), and the PROM developer. Since a typical study may include multiple PROMs, the roles, responsibilities, and lines of communication should be defined as early as possible following the completion of necessary legal obligations among all parties.

Investigator Meetings

Investigator meetings are key opportunities to provide information and training materials related to the assessment of PROs. These meetings should cover topics such as the purpose of the PRO assessments, brief background to each PROM, including the number of questions in each PROM, and details of response scales (Figure 25.2) (58).

Written instructions such as training manuals or data completion guidelines are strongly recommended, and having training materials available at the site may help refresh training or train new staff for longer trials. Documentation of this training should be included in the PRO evidence dossiers submitted to the regulatory agencies.

Preparing the Site

Preparing the study sites is the key to successful study execution. Because field monitors are the main contacts with the participating sites, it is essential that both field monitors and clinical sites are informed and trained on the objectives, requirements, and methods of PRO data collection. In addition, it is crucial that the following steps have been taken:

1. The center has received approval for specific IRB requirements.

- Purpose of inclusion of each PRO measure

- Number of questions and the time required to complete each PRO measure

- Details of response scales (e.g., descriptors of response anchors)

- Domains covered (e.g., physical functioning, social functioning, etc.)

- Recall period related to the questions or the domains

- Assessment schedule of each PRO measure by the way of a schematic diagram of the study design highlighting the visits and order in which the PROMs will be administered

- Language versions of PRO measures for use in each participating country

- Aspects related to how the required materials (e.g., PRO measures, ePRO devices, training materials, storage of devices) will be distributed to the study centers

- Ways of dealing with patients with special needs such as visual impairment or movement disorders

- Responsibilities of the study coordinator and investigator before, during, and after the PRO measures are completed

FIGURE 25.2 Recommended topics to be covered at investigator meetings when PROs are included in clinical trials.

ePRO, electronic patient-reported outcome; PRO, patient-reported outcome; PROMS, PRO measures.

Source: With permission from Gnanasakthy A, DeMuro, C. Logistical considerations for integrating patient-reported outcomes in multiregional clinical trials, *Clin Research* 2014;44 18.

2. Study coordinators and investigators are trained for their duties and responsibilities before, during, and after data-collection activities.
3. The site is aware that PROMs are integral to the study and not separate from the protocol. A person dedicated to the trial (e.g., study coordinator) should be designated as the person responsible for administering the PROM, and he or she should have the interpersonal skills necessary to assist patients without influencing their responses.
4. Whenever PROMs are included as part of a trial design—especially in serious conditions such as cancer—patients may have a heightened expectation of access to support services. For this reason, in disease areas where this may be a concern, study coordinators should identify a short list of social services and mental health, counseling, or pastoral resources that may be available to address patients' emotional needs. It may also be important for study staff to have the name and contact number for someone to call in case a patient becomes upset. For protocols using PROMs with especially sensitive questions,

it is also important to note that some IRBs require researchers to state how psychosocial distress will be identified and addressed.
5. The site needs to agree on resources and guidelines for storage, protection, and access restriction of source documentation.

Site Training

The field monitor is the key liaison between the sites and the trial sponsor during the course of a clinical study. Although initial site training may be done at the investigator meetings, most interaction will occur between the field monitor, site coordinators, and investigators. Therefore, field monitors' acceptance of the importance of PRO assessments is crucial to ensuring that the correct message is transmitted to participating sites.

Data collection for PROMs needs special consideration not only because patients are involved but also because the quality of data depends on the training and the predefined responsibilities of the study coordinator, investigator, and field monitor.

The training of study coordinators is essential for improving data quality, minimizing inconsistencies, and satisfying regulatory guidance (7). Training considerations must consider the possibility of inexperienced study staff administering questionnaires and the burden on both staff and patients of administering and completing multiple questionnaires. Documentation of appropriate site and patient training is part of a PRO evidence dossier submission to support label claims, so care should be taken in documenting this training.

Field monitor and site personnel training should not be confined to investigator meetings or site initiation visits. Ongoing dialog should be encouraged among site coordinators and field monitors, who may in turn communicate issues or concerns directly to the study trial leader (Figure 25.3) (58).

PROS AND REGULATORS (FDA AND EMA)

The FDA and the European Medicines Agency (EMA) acknowledge the importance of PROs in assessing the effectiveness of new medicines. However, there are differences in the ways PRO-related evidence is assessed.

The FDA issued a formal guidance in 2009 that set standards for the use of PROMs in support of product labeling (7). This guidance was intended to

increase efficiency of discussions with the FDA during the medical product development process, streamline the FDA's review of PRO instrument adequacy and resultant PRO data collected during a clinical trial, and provide optimal information about the patient perspective for use in making conclusions about treatment effect at the time of medical product approval. (p. 1)

Drug manufacturers utilize FDA-approved labeling to make claims about their products in marketing and promotional activities in the United States.

Related to this effort, a second initiative for drug development tools including PROs was created by the Center for Drug Evaluation and Research as part of the FDA's Critical Path Initiative. The purpose of this initiative was to provide a framework to facilitate the development and regulatory acceptance of scientific tools utilized in drug development programs. The guidance is intended to encompass multiple levels of instrumentation including PROs, biomarkers, animal models, and other COAs.

Unlike the FDA, the EMA has not issued formal guidelines specific to PROs but instead published a reflection paper (59) to provide broad recommendations on HRQOL in the context of clinical trials, which is being updated currently. Additionally, the EMA has developed the Biomarkers Qualification program (60)

- All sites and field monitors should be encouraged to watch the presentation given at the investigator meeting. Sites should be encouraged to communicate any changes in site coordinators to allow for communication of training materials to new personnel.

- A specific section of clinical trial newsletters should be established to deal with any PRO-related issues.

- Positive feedback should be given to sites to encourage compliance and keep their focus on the PRO section of the protocol.

- A regular question-and-answer letter may be circulated by the study teams to site field monitors to ensure resolution of any questions that arise.

- Site field monitors should be encouraged to address their questions directly to study leaders to ensure consistency of solutions.

- A feedback questionnaire may be collected from site coordinators and patients to obtain their comments on the PRO assessment process.

- "Webinars" or training modules should be offered to centers that join the study late.

FIGURE 25.3 Recommendations for study site training when PROs are included in clinical trials.

PRO, patient-reported outcome.

Source: With permission from Gnanasakthy A, DeMuro, C. Logistical considerations for integrating patient-reported outcomes in multiregional clinical trials, *Clin Research.* 2014;44–48.

that is somewhat similar to the drug development tool guidance in the United States. This qualification program provides a formal mechanism for ratifying clinical trial endpoints, including new or existing PROMs (60).

Whereas the EMA relies on subject matter experts from member countries for expertise relating to PROs, the FDA has access to an in-house, dedicated group of experts specializing in COAs that includes PROs. Expertise relating to COAs—including the development and validation of PROMs and interpretation of clinical benefit based on PRO endpoints during the review process for FDA reviewers—may be provided by Clinical Outcome Assessment Staff (COA Staff) from the Office of New Drugs. Importantly, although the COA Staff when consulted may provide input regarding the PROMs for a specific context of use and the interpretation of clinical findings, the decision regarding drug approval and, if approved, the final labeling language is entirely that of the individual reviewing divisions.

In general, the FDA's guidelines regarding PRO development and validation are more stringent than those of the EMA, although both agencies note the role and value of these measures in bringing the patient's perspective to the assessment of therapeutics. A review of products approved both in Europe and the United States shows that the EMA is more likely to grant product labeling based on PRO-related endpoints than the FDA is and is more likely to grant claims for higher order constructs such as HRQOL and functioning. This discrepancy in product labeling may necessitate that pharmaceutical manufacturers develop agency-specific PRO strategies, adding strain to limited resources and time required for drug development programs. In terms of similarities between the EMA and the FDA, both offer sponsors the opportunity to consult during the various stages of product development. Guidance documents specific to cancer drug development by both agencies acknowledge the importance of symptom assessments. Recent publications by the Office of Hematological and Oncology Products and COA Staff further emphasize the need to assess PROs related to disease-specific symptoms, physical functioning, and symptomatic AEs (61). Key differences between the two agencies are summarized elsewhere (62).

BEYOND LABELING

Much of the recent focus on PROs has been on product labeling. U.S. regulators tend to prefer proximal concepts such as pain and fatigue for product labeling. However, patients with cancer are often interested in more distal concepts, as well, including disease-related symptoms they may experience, the impact of their treatment, the available treatment options and evidence for each, and the outcomes they can expect.

Given these factors, product labeling should not be the only goal for including PROs in oncology clinical trials. A more comprehensive evaluation of study participants' experiences can provide useful information for patients on the impact of the new therapy. Such use of PROs can also aid regulators, as well as healthcare providers, caregivers, and payers who need to choose among competing therapies (63).

PROs captured during disease progression could assist in the development of improved diagnostic tools or potentially even new interventions, including new targets for drug development (64).

Recent evidence has shown that oncologists learn about PRO-related value messages primarily through peer-reviewed publications (65). Publication of findings based on PRO-related endpoints that demonstrate the benefits of a new treatment may have greater impact than PRO labeling based on concepts that may be irrelevant to stakeholders. These value messages are of interest to both patients and patient advocacy groups, and are more likely to be presented on patient websites. Additionally, these messages are the data that patient advocacy groups need in order to lobby payers and politicians for greater access to newer, often more expensive cancer treatments (66).

REFERENCES

1. Hoffman MC, Mulrooney DA, Steinberger J, et al. Deficits in physical function among young childhood cancer survivors. *J Clin Oncol*. 2013;31(22):2799–2805.
2. Knols RH, de Bruin ED, Uebelhart D, et al. Effects of an outpatient physical exercise program on hematopoietic stem-cell transplantation recipients: a randomized clinical trial. *Bone Marrow Transplant*. 2011;46(9):1245–1255.
3. Shahrokni A, Wu AJ, Carter J, Lichtman SM. Long-term toxicity of cancer treatment in older patients. *Clin Geriatr Med*. 2016;32(1):63–80.
4. Perfetto EM, Burke L, Oehrlein EM, Epstein RS. Patient-focused drug development a new direction for collaboration. *Med Care*. 2015;53(1):9–17.
5. Avorn J, Kesselheim AS. The 21st century cures act–will it take us back in time? *N Engl J Med*. 2015;372(26):2473–2475.
6. Vodicka E, Kim K, Devine EB, et al. Inclusion of patient-reported outcome measures in registered clinical trials: evidence from ClinicalTrials.gov (2007–2013). *Contemp Clin Trial*. 2015;43:1–9.
7. US Department of Health and Human Services FaDA, Center for Drug Evaluation and Reserach, Center for Biologics Evaluation and Research, & Center for Devices and Radiological Health. *Guidance for Industry: Patient-Reported Outcomes Measures: Use in Medical Product Development to Support Labeling Claims*; 2009.
8. Kluetz PG, Pazdur R. Looking to the future in an unprecedented time for cancer drug development. *Semin Oncol*. 2016;43(1):2–3.
9. Administration USFaD. Clinical Outcome Assessment (COA): Glossary of Terms. http://www.fda.gov/Drugs/DevelopmentApprovalProcess/DrugDevelopmentToolsQualificationProgram/ucm370262.htm
10. Gnanasakthy A, DeMuro C. Outcome assessment of primary endpoints of new drugs approved by the FDA (2011–2015). *Value Health*. 2016;19(3):A275.

11. Kilgour RD, Vigano A, Trutschnigg B, et al. Handgrip strength predicts survival and is associated with markers of clinical and functional outcomes in advanced cancer patients. *Support Care Cancer.* 2013;21(12):3261–3270.

12. Cella D. Quality of life in patients with metastatic renal cell carcinoma: the importance of patient-reported outcomes. *Cancer Treat Rev.* 2009;35(8):733–737.

13. Cella D, Cappelleri JC, Bushmakin A, et al. Quality of life predicts progression-free survival in patients with metastatic renal cell carcinoma treated with sunitinib versus interferon alfa. *J Oncol Pract.* 2009;5(2):66–70.

14. Gourgou-Bourgade S, Bascoul-Mollevi C, Desseigne F, et al. Impact of FOLFIRINOX compared with gemcitabine on quality of life in patients with metastatic pancreatic cancer: results from the PRODIGE 4/ACCORD 11 randomized trial. *J Clin Oncol.* 2013;31(1):23–29.

15. Kemmler G, Holzner B, Kopp M, et al. Comparison of two quality-of-life instruments for cancer patients: the functional assessment of cancer therapy-general and the European Organization for Research and Treatment of Cancer Quality of Life Questionnaire-C30. *J Clin Oncol.* 1999;17(9):2932–2940.

16. Luckett T, King MT, Butow PN, et al. Choosing between the EORTC QLQ-C30 and FACT-G for measuring health-related quality of life in cancer clinical research: issues, evidence and recommendations. *Ann Oncol.* 2011;22(10):2179–2190.

17. Kirkova J, Davis MP, Walsh D, et al. Cancer symptom assessment instruments: a systematic review. *J Clin Oncol.* 2006;24(9):1459–1473.

18. Cleeland CS, Mendoza TR, Wang XS, et al. Assessing symptom distress in cancer patients: the M.D. Anderson Symptom Inventory. *Cancer.* 2000;89(7):1634–1646.

19. Basch E. The missing voice of patients in drug-safety reporting. *New Engl J Med.* 2010;362(10):865–869.

20. Atkinson TM, Li Y, Coffey CW, et al. Reliability of adverse symptom event reporting by clinicians. *Qual Life Res.* 2012;21(7):1159–1164.

21. Xiao C, Polomano R, Bruner DW. Comparison between patient-reported and clinician-observed symptoms in oncology. *Cancer Nurs.* 2013;36(6):E1–E16.

22. Lipscomb J, Reeve BB, Clauser SB, et al. Patient-reported outcomes assessment in cancer trials: Taking stock, moving forward. *J Clin Oncol.* 2007;25(32):5133–5140.

23. Basch E, Rogak LJ, Dueck AC. Methods for Implementing and Reporting Patient-reported Outcome (PRO) Measures of Symptomatic Adverse Events in Cancer Clinical Trials. *Clin Ther.* 2016;38(4):821–830.

24. Clark MJ, Harris N, Griebsch I, et al. Patient-reported outcome labeling claims and measurement approach for metastatic castration-resistant prostate cancer treatments in the United States and European Union. *Health Qual Life Outcomes.* 2014;12:104.

25. Moran N. Incyte comes of age with JAK inhibitor approval. *Nat Biotechnol.* 2012;30:3–5.

26. Bixel K, Hays JL. Olaparib in the management of ovarian cancer. *Pharmgenomics Pers Med.* 2015;8:127–135.

27. Hollen PJ, Gralla RJ, Kris MG, Cox C. Quality of life during clinical trials: conceptual model for the Lung Cancer Symptom Scale (LCSS). *Support Care Cancer.* 1994;2(4):213–222.

28. Paskett ED, Herndon JE, 2nd, Day JM, et al. Applying a conceptual model for examining health-related quality of life in long-term breast cancer survivors: CALGB study 79804. *Psychooncology.* 2008;17(11):1108–1120.

29. Patrick DL, Burke LB, Powers JH, et al. Patient-reported outcomes to support medical product labeling claims: FDA perspective. *Value Health.* 2007;10(Suppl 2):S125–S137.

30. Patrick DL, Burke LB, Gwaltney CJ, et al. Content validity–establishing and reporting the evidence in newly developed patient-reported outcomes (PRO) instruments for medical product evaluation: ISPOR PRO Good Research Practices Task Force report: part 2–assessing respondent understanding. *Value Health.* 2011;14(8):978–988.

31. Patrick DL, Burke LB, Gwaltney CJ, et al. Content validity–establishing and reporting the evidence in newly developed patient-reported outcomes (PRO) instruments for medical product evaluation: ISPOR PRO good research practices task force report: part 1–eliciting concepts for a new PRO instrument. *Value Health.* 2011;14(8):967–977.

32. Friedlander ML, King MT. Patient-reported outcomes in ovarian cancer clinical trials. *Ann Oncol.* 2013;24(Suppl 10):x64–x68.

33. Gnanasakthy A, DeMuro C, Clark M, et al. Patient-reported outcomes labeling for products approved by the office of hematology and oncology products of the US Food and Drug Administration (2010–2014). *J Clin Oncol.* 2016;34(16):1928–1934.

34. Wild D, Eremenco S, Mear I, et al. Multinational trials-recommendations on the translations required, approaches to using the same language in different countries, and the approaches to support pooling the data: the ISPOR Patient-Reported Outcomes Translation and Linguistic Validation Good Research Practices Task Force report. *Value Health.* 2009;12(4):430–440.

35. Coons SJ, Eremenco S, Lundy JJ, et al. Capturing Patient-Reported Outcome (PRO) data electronically: the past, present, and promise of ePRO measurement in clinical trials. *Patient.* 2015;8(4):301–309.

36. Gralla RJ. Quality-of-life evaluation in cancer: the past and the future. *Cancer.* 2015;121(24):4276–4278.

37. Farnell DJ, Routledge J, Hannon R, et al. Efficacy of data capture for patient-reported toxicity following radiotherapy for prostate or cervical cancer. *Eur J Cancer.* 2010;46(3):534–540.

38. Ellis LM, Bernstein DS, Voest EE, et al. American Society of Clinical Oncology perspective: raising the bar for clinical trials by defining clinically meaningful outcomes. *J Clin Oncol.* 2014;32(12):1277–1280.

39. Adamowicz K, Jassem J, Katz A, Saad ED. Assessment of quality of life in advanced breast cancer. An overview of randomized phase III trials. *Cancer Treat Rev.* 2012;38(5):554–558.

40. Cortes J, Hudgens S, Twelves C, et al. Health-related quality of life in patients with locally advanced or metastatic breast cancer treated with eribulin mesylate or capecitabine in an open-label randomized phase 3 trial. *Breast Cancer Res Treat.* 2015;154(3):509–520.

41. Kaufman PA, Awada A, Twelves C, et al. Phase III open-label randomized study of eribulin mesylate versus capecitabine in patients with locally advanced or metastatic breast cancer previously treated with an anthracycline and a taxane. *J Clin Oncol.* 2015;33(6):594–601.

42. Verstovsek S, Mesa RA, Gotlib J, et al. A double-blind, placebo-controlled trial of ruxolitinib for myelofibrosis. *N Engl J Med.* 2012;366(9):799–807.

43. Reck M, Socinski MA, Luft A, et al. The effect of necitumumab in combination with gemcitabine plus cisplatin on tolerability and on quality of life: results from the Phase 3 SQUIRE trial. *J Thorac Oncol.* 2016;11(6):808–818.

44. Stull DE, Houghton K. Identifying differential responders and their characteristics in clinical trials: innovative methods for analyzing longitudinal data. *Value Health.* 2013;16(1):164–176.

45. Xu J, Evans TJ, Coon C, et al. Measuring patient-reported outcomes in advanced gastric cancer. *Ecancermedicalscience.* 2013;7:351.

46. Sriram N, Mills J, Lang E, et al. Attitudes and stereotypes in lung cancer versus breast cancer. *PLoS One.* 2015;10(12):e0145715.

47. Vrinten C, Wardle J, Marlow LA. Cancer fear and fatalism among ethnic minority women in the United Kingdom. *Br J Cancer.* 2016;114(5):597–604.

48. Gnanasakthy A, DeMuro C, Boulton C. Integration of patient-reported outcomes in multiregional confirmatory clinical trials. *Contemp Clin Trials.* 2013;35(1):62–69.

49. Hahn EA, Bode RK, Du H, Cella D. Evaluating linguistic equivalence of patient-reported outcomes in a cancer clinical trial. *Clin Trials.* 2006;3(3):280–290.

50. Scott NW, Fayers PM, Aaronson NK, et al. The relationship between overall quality of life and its subdimensions was influenced by culture: analysis of an international database. *J Clin Epidemiol.* 2008;61(8):788–795.

51. Calvert M, Brundage M, Jacobsen PB, et al. The CONSORT Patient-Reported Outcome (PRO) extension: implications for clinical trials and practice. *Health Qual Life Outcomes.* 2013;11:184.

52. Bell ML, Fairclough DL. Practical and statistical issues in missing data for longitudinal patient-reported outcomes. *Stat Methods Med Res.* 2014;23(5):440–459.

53. Cappelleri JC, Zou KH, Bushmakin AG, et al. *Patient-Reported Outcomes: Measurement, Implementation and Interpretation.* Florida: Chapman & Hall/CRC Biostatistics Series; 2014.

54. Fairclough DL. Design and analysis of quality of life studies in clinical trials. Florida: Chapman & Hall; 2010.

55. Gnanasakthy A, DeMuro C. Overcoming organizational challenges of integrating patient-reported outcomes in oncology clinical trials. *Therapeut Innov Regulat Sci.* 2015;49(6): 822–830.

56. Blackhall F, Kim DW, Besse B, et al. Patient-reported outcomes and quality of life in PROFILE 1007: a randomized trial of crizotinib compared with chemotherapy in previously treated patients with ALK-positive advanced non-small-cell lung cancer. *J Thorac Oncol.* 2014;9(11):1625–1633.

57. Dombrowski C. *Adcetris review add some clarity to principles for accelerated approvals.* The Pink Sheet; 2011.

58. Gnanasakthy A, DeMuro, C. Logistical considerations for integrating patient-reported outcomes in multiregional clinical trials, *Clin Research.* 2014;44–48.

59. European Medicines Agency. Reflection paper on the regulatory guidance for the use of health-related quality of life (HRQL) measures in the evaluation of medicinal products; 2005. https://www.ispor.org/workpaper/emea-hrql-guidance.pdf

60. European Medicines Agency. Qualification of novel methodologies for drug development: guidance to applicants; 2014. http://www.ema.europa.eu/docs/en_GB/document_library/Regulatory_and_procedural_guideline/2009/10/WC500004201.pdf

61. Kluetz PG, Slagle A, Papadopoulos EJ, et al. Focusing on core patient-reported outcomes in cancer clinical trials: symptomatic adverse events, physical function, and disease-related symptoms. *Clin Cancer Res.* 2016;22(7):1553–1558.

62. Hao Y. Patient-reported outcomes in support of oncology product labeling claims: regulatory context and challenges. *Expert Rev Pharmacoecon Outcomes Res.* 2010;10(4):407–420.

63. Hao Y, Krohe M, Yaworsky A, et al. Clinical trial patient-reported outcomes data: going beyond the label in oncology. *Clin Therapeut.* 2016;38(4):811–820.

64. Strong LE. The past, present, and future of patient-reported outcomes in oncology. *Am Soc Clin Oncol Educ Book.* 2015;e616–e620.

65. Meldahl ML, Acaster S, Hayes RP. Exploration of oncologists' attitudes toward and perceived value of patient-reported outcomes. *Qual Life Res.* 2013;22(4):725–731.

66. Doward LC, Gnanasakthy A, Baker MG. Patient reported outcomes: looking beyond the label claim. *Health and Quality of Life Outcomes.* 2010;8.

Recruitment of Research Participants

Christopher Gantz

"The best way to find yourself is to lose yourself in the service of others."

—*Ghandi*

INTRODUCTION

If asked, most research study team members would list participant enrollment and retention as the biggest barriers to successful project completion. According to a Tufts University report from 2013, 37% of sites are underenrolled and 11% failed to enroll a single patient (1).

GARNERING PUBLIC SUPPORT FOR RESEARCH

While new technologies and social media are creating new ways in which study teams are able to interact with participants, they alone will not address the challenges of getting people involved in research. The research community must also work to educate the public about the need for their involvement in clinical trials. At the Children's Hospital of Philadelphia, researchers often promote the idea that "today's discoveries are tomorrow's treatments," but the reality is that many discoveries and breakthroughs would not be possible without the support and involvement of the public.

Following are a few valuable insights about some of the major barriers to participation that have been gathered from clinical trial coordinators and study participants about how researchers can reduce, and in some cases eliminate, recruitment and retention obstacles. See Figure 26.1 for more information.

Barrier 1: Research Participants Do Not Feel As If Their Efforts Make A Difference

Many research teams do not have a mechanism in place to convey study results to their past participants. It is easy to understand the effect this lack of communication

has on individuals who agree to volunteer their time and energy as a participant but never know the results of the project. Building in a communication plan using readily available tools such as email blasts and newsletters can be a fantastic way to stay in touch and should be considered a standard practice for all research studies.

Barrier 2: Research Participants Do Not Feel Welcomed

A common complaint from participants is that they have trouble finding the location of their clinical study visit and encounter staff who are unable to direct them. This is a problem faced by most, if not all, large research institutions. With multiple studies being conducted in a number of different locations, people are bound to encounter challenges getting to their appointments. A number of research coordinators have come up with novel solutions to these challenges.

Some have sent reminder letters/emails with a photograph of the building and the meeting location, including their cell phone numbers. Others have taken the time to walk across the campus to meet a participant who arrived at the wrong location. In addition to those strategies, researchers should ensure that they are giving nonstudy staff such as security guards and information desk attendants the tools and information they need to help direct participants.

Barrier 3: Potential Research Participants Lack a Background In Volunteering

Many of the people who are contacted about participating in a study will not have had previous experience with how research projects are conducted. Teams need to ensure that their recruitment materials and outreach activities take this into account and make an effort to clearly define what is being asked of the potential participant.

Additionally, 95% of people who do participate in a clinical trial indicate that they would be willing to do

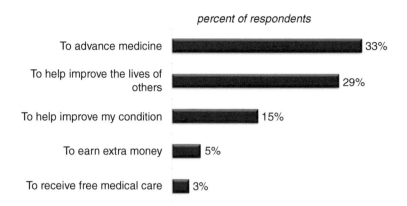

FIGURE 26.1 Top reasons people choose to participate in clinical trials.

Source: CISCRP. Perceptions & Insights Study – Report on Study Participant Experiences. https://www.ciscrp.org/download/our-full-set-of-graphs-and-tables-in-pdf-format/?wpdmdl=4951 (pp. 19, 34, 38); https://www.ciscrp.org/our-programs/research-services/charts-and-statistics. Published 2013.

so again if they were asked (2). Participant registries, if used correctly, can be a great resource for engaging with people who have expressed a continued desire to help move research forward. These registries should not just be used to repeatedly ask individuals to participate in research but should also provide information and resources that people will find useful and keep them engaged.

Barrier 4: Volunteer Tasks Are Too Routine

Most people lead incredibly busy lives and have many demands on their time. Teams often run into challenges with enrollment and retention when the study tasks are seen as being boring or requiring too much of a time commitment. During feasibility planning discussions, study teams should address these realities, and if possible, offer inventive solutions. Some teams have held weekend appointments, conducted offsite visits, converted paper questionnaires into forms that can be completed online, and provided packaging so that study equipment can be returned by mail rather than having the participant return to the site.

When designing a new study, we ask investigators and other study staff to be mindful of any potential barriers to participation (Figure 26.2). Often the study design does not take into account the demands the study might place on the time and resources of potential participants. We ask that the study team place themselves in the position of being a participant and evaluate whether they would enroll in the study if approached. When looked at through that filter, the answer is often no. Frequently this leads teams to think through the potential barriers and come up with solutions that increase the likelihood that an individual will enroll and complete the study.

Barrier 5: Efforts of Study Participants Are Not Recognized

It is an undeniable fact that without the generosity and dedication of members of the public who take the time

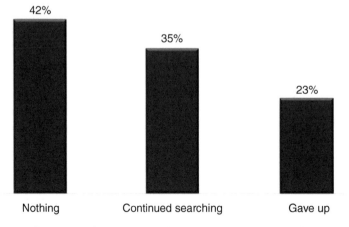

FIGURE 26.2 Most volunteers who are ineligible for a clinical trial do not search for another

Source: CISCRP. Perceptions & Insights Study – Report on Study Participant Experiences. https://www.ciscrp.org/download/our-full-set-of-graphs-and-tables-in-pdf-format/?wpdmdl=4951 (pp. 19, 34, 38); https://www.ciscrp.org/our-programs/research-services/charts-and-statistics. Published 2013.

to be a part of research study, many trials would not succeed. This message needs to be communicated broadly and over and over again. Some organizations have begun referring to their participants as medical or research heroes. These terms capture the importance of their participation perfectly and should be more widely adopted.

Even though there are many research groups that do an excellent job connecting with people, the overall research community can, and must, do more to raise awareness of the importance of public support for research to address the issues listed previously.

GENERALIZABLE BEST PRACTICES

There is no magic bullet when it comes to enrolling participants, and each study will have its own set of challenges that will need to be addressed. Listed below are some best practices to keep in mind when developing recruitment and outreach strategies.

Community Outreach

Engaging the community in the discussion is vital to the continued success of research. Teams have pursued several avenues of engagement, with strategies ranging from speaking at community events and attending health fairs to incorporating information about clinical trials into the existing marketing materials distributed to the patient population. The approach a group chooses to take will depend on the design of the study and the enrollment population sought. As a first step, teams can evaluate what strategies other studies have used in the past and are in current use. Often there will be opportunities to learn from what has already been done by others working in the same space.

Study Letters/Emails

If sending out a letter or email is part of the recruitment strategy, teams will want to create a document that is:

- Personalized. Introduce the principal investigator and why he or she is contacting the potential participant.
- Concise. Consider the communication an invitation to a conversation. The letter should give enough information so that individuals can gauge their interest without overwhelming readers with details that you will provide to them when they contact you.
- Framed accurately. Study teams often craft letters that present the study as an exciting opportunity in which the recipient might be eligible to participate. The communication is more compelling if it highlights the importance of the individual's contribution and the key role that he or she will play in moving research forward.

Teams should also consider additional details such as the return address being used and any additional materials that will be included in the mailing. Study teams have had success with mailings that have the flyer on one side of the page and the letter on the other. With the flyer facing out when the letter is opened, the recipient can glean the key points of the study quickly.

Rapid Response To Inquiries

When working with study teams on their recruitment plans, the need for responding to phone calls and emails from interested individuals in a timely manner should be considered a high priority. The time frame for responding to a contact is 24 to 48 hours. Study teams generally agree to this approach, but they often find it challenging to implement unless they have identified staff responsible for the contact and carved out dedicated time for responding to messages.

Social Media Plan

The Internet is the number one way that people report finding out about clinical trials (Figure 26.3). Having a well-thought-out plan for the use of social media and

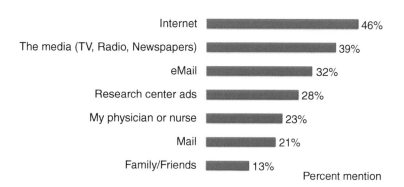

FIGURE 26.3 Top ways that people report finding out about clinical trials.

Source: CISCRP. Perceptions & Insights Study – Report on Study Participant Experiences. https://www.ciscrp.org/download/our-full-set-of-graphs-and-tables-in-pdf-format/?wpdmdl=4951 (pp. 19, 34, 38); https://www.ciscrp.org/our-programs/research-services/charts-and-statistics. Published 2013.

websites will increase the effectiveness of any campaign a clinician chooses to initiate. Researchers will need to:

- Identify which platform has the highest likelihood of connecting with your target demographic (e.g., Facebook, Twitter, Instagram, Pinterest).
- Determine the budget for the campaign.
- Have a plan for driving traffic to the website or landing page with additional study information.
- Keep information on the website accurate and current.

When it comes to the frequency of times a potential participant might need to be exposed to study-related messaging, one can look to the world of marketing as many of their best practices can be applied to the research world. Herbert E. Krugman, speaking about television advertising, wrote that it could take three exposures before someone would act. Following is his description of the types of responses associate with each exposure (3):

Exposure No. 1 is . . . a "What is it?" type of . . . response. Anything new or novel no matter how uninteresting on second exposure has to elicit some response the first time . . . if only to discard the object as of no further interest . . . The second exposure . . . response . . . is "What of it?" . . . whether or not [the message] has personal relevance . . .

By the third exposure the viewer knows he's been through his "What is it's?" and "What of it's?," and the third, then, becomes the true reminder . . . The importance of this view . . . is that it positions advertising as powerful only when the viewer . . . is

interested in the [product message] . . . Secondly, it positions the viewer as . . . reacting to the commercial—very quickly . . . when the proper time comes round.

CONCLUSIONS

The information in this chapter will be helpful as teams formulate recruitment plans, but many challenges will still need to be overcome as they work to meet recruitment goals. As mentioned previously, team members should explore the landscape and learn from others who have had success with engaging the public. A simple Google search will also help identify like-minded people working within research groups across the county and around the world. As new approaches and strategies are developed, study staff should seek out opportunities to share them with the research community so that others can benefit from what is learned.

REFERENCES

1. Analysis and Insight into Critical Drug Development Issues. Tufts Center for the Study of Drug Development. Vol. 15, No. 1 Jan/Feb 2013. http://csdd.tufts.edu/files/uploads/jan-feb_2013_ir_summary.pdf
2. CISCRP. *Perceptions & Insights Study – Report on Study Participant Experiences.* https://www.ciscrp.org/download/our-full-set-of-graphs-and-tables-in-pdf-format/?wpdmdl=4951 (pp. 19, 34, 38); https://www.ciscrp.org/our-programs/research-services/charts-and-statistics. Published 2013.
3. Wikipedia, The Free Encyclopedia. Effective Frequency. https://en.wikipedia.org/w/index.php?title=Effective_frequency&oldid=742599769

Barriers to Oncology Clinical Trials

Chethan Ramamurthy and Yu-Ning Wong

Since the first randomized cancer clinical trial in 1955, there has been a rapid proliferation of oncology clinical trials. While in the 1950s there were only a few trials being conducted in a small set of designated centers, in 2016 there were over 200,000 clinical trials listed on clinicaltrials.gov. Yet, despite this increase in studies, unfortunately nearly 40% of National Cancer Institute (NCI) sponsored cooperative group trials and 20% of phase II and III cancer clinical trials fail to complete accrual or have long delays in accrual. Estimates of cancer clinical trial accrual rates range from 2% to 7%, which have not changed for over 40 years (1–3). The barriers to clinical trial accrual can be traced to a complex network of patient-related, provider-related, and organizational factors (Figure 27.1) (4,5).

PATIENT FACTORS

Patient factors are often divided into logistical barriers or attitudinal and knowledge barriers.

Logistical Issues

Several factors from the patient side of the equation can pose as barriers to trial enrollment. The simple issue of the logistics of trial participation can prohibit patients from participating. In a systematic review of publications that describe barriers to accrual, 65 cancer-related studies (including 46 treatment trials) noted that cost, transportation, and time commitment were the highest patient-reported logistical barriers to acceptance of clinical trials (4). A qualitative study with focus groups of clinical research associates (CRAs) at six tertiary cancer centers in Ontario, Canada, investigated barriers to clinical trials. The CRAs reported that patients worry participating in a trial will carry greater burdens compared to standard care in these respects, not just for themselves, but also for their caregivers and families. In addition, patients are sometimes caregivers for family members, and these responsibilities can make trial participation feel too cumbersome (5). Efforts to accommodate patients' schedules, provide transportation support, and address financial concerns are therefore extremely important to improving trial enrollment. As discussed in the section Geography/Location, the use of community sites to facilitate enrollment reduces some, but not all, barriers.

Knowledge and Attitudinal Barriers

Although both population-based and elderly patient specific studies have indicated positive attitudes and willingness to participate in cancer clinical trials, the low actual rate of participation demonstrates that there is a rift between how individuals respond to general statements regarding the value and benefit of clinical trials and how they make personal choices (6,7). The challenge of the choice patients encounter when considering clinical trial enrollment is fed by interrelated factors of lack of knowledge, fears, negative attitudes or expectations, and poor self-efficacy (8).

Cancer patients endorse several fears and negative attitudes toward clinical trials. As described by focus groups of CRAs, one of the most commonly reported fears is that of potentially greater toxicity with study medications (5). Studies show that this fear is often underestimated by treating oncologists, indicating that there may be benefit to increased discussion of this when recruiting patients (9). Another major fear is that of being experimented upon or being "treated like a guinea pig" (5,6). This fear can stem from a mistrust of medical research in general, misunderstanding a protocol, or discomfort with personally being the subject of experimentation and randomization. A systematic review and meta-analysis of 21 quantitative studies on barriers to clinical trial enrollment found that 38% of patients dislike randomization, 53% dislike the possibility of a placebo, and 19% dislike being experimented upon (10). These concerns are particularly pronounced

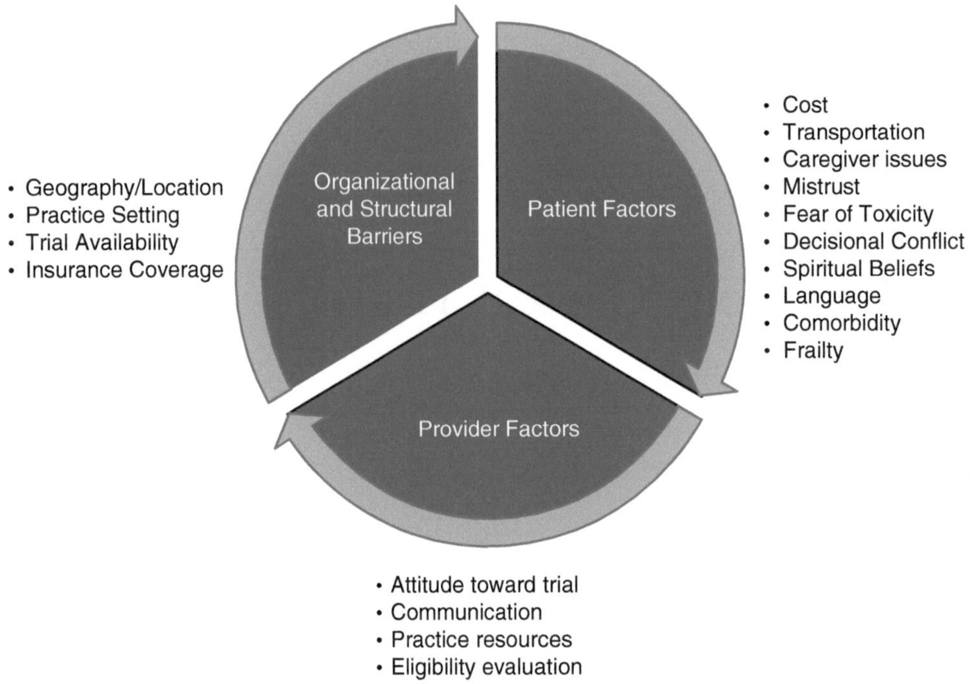

- Geography/Location
- Practice Setting
- Trial Availability
- Insurance Coverage

Organizational and Structural Barriers

Patient Factors

- Cost
- Transportation
- Caregiver issues
- Mistrust
- Fear of Toxicity
- Decisional Conflict
- Spiritual Beliefs
- Language
- Comorbidity
- Frailty

Provider Factors

- Attitude toward trial
- Communication
- Practice resources
- Eligibility evaluation

FIGURE 27.1 Barriers to clinical trial enrollment.

in minority populations, which are discussed in a later section.

These fears, potential misconceptions about clinical trials, and knowledge barriers have a large effect on a patient's decision making. Not having sufficient knowledge or having negative preconceptions about clinical trial participation are factors that can influence self-efficacy, a patient's confidence or belief in his or her decision-making ability. In addition, many patients need assistance with clarifying their own personal values and preferences to inform their decision making and promote self-efficacy (11).

Communication

The nature of the doctor–patient relationship and communication style can affect a patient's decision to enroll in a clinical trial. One study at two urban cancer centers of video and audio recordings of outpatient encounters between cancer patients eligible for a clinical trial and their providers aimed to determine the influence of communication on patients' decision making about participation in clinical trials. Investigators noted that the extent of shared conversation control (defined as the "extent to which the physician and patient share talk time and speak on the same level to one another") positively correlated with clinical trial enrollment. Patients with greater alliances (defined as a "trusting, cordial relationship" with the physician) were less influenced by cost or family opinions. Reassurance that the decision regarding clinical trial enrollment would not affect

the patients' care at the center was associated with a lower influence of cost and adverse events on clinical trial enrollment (12).

Decision Aids

Decision aids have been identified as potential tools to help increase knowledge about clinical trials, and have been used in other settings to help patients make treatment decisions across a variety of disease settings where decision making can be complex (13).

Preparatory Education About Clinical Trials (PRE-ACT;www.cancer.net/preact) is one potential decision aid for patients considering enrolling in a clinical trial. It was developed to improve patients' preparation for considering a clinical trial as a treatment option. It initially assesses patients' knowledge about clinical trials, attitudinal barriers, and preparedness for decision making. Patients are then given a tailored set of videos based on their responses to these questions to address knowledge gaps or attitudinal barriers. In a multi-institutional clinical trial where patients seeing a medical oncologist for their first visit were randomized to either PRE-ACT or standard text from the NCI, both improved knowledge, attitudes, and preparation for decision making about clinical trials. However the PRE-ACT videos were more effective in reducing attitudinal barriers and improving knowledge (14).

Another web-based decision aid was developed to address knowledge, empowerment, and value clarifications. Its sections included "Introduction," "About

Studies," "Common Questions," "Talking to your Doctor," "What's Important to You," "Research Terms," and "Additional Resources." It was studied in an urban academic medical center in which 200 patients were randomized to either the decision aid or the cancer center's website. It showed improvement in knowledge, self-efficacy, certainty about choice, and value clarity among the decision aid group (15).

SPECIAL POPULATIONS

While the preceding factors apply to all patients, there are specific challenges faced by particular populations, such as ethnic/racial minorities, non-English speakers, and older adults.

Ethnic/Racial Minorities

Ethnic and racial minorities in this country are underrepresented in cancer clinical trials, with large studies demonstrating that less than 15% of trial participants are non-White. Among the minority populations represented, African American patients account for 9% and Hispanic patients for 3% (2). This is despite the African American and Hispanic populations accounting for 13% and 16% of the national population, respectively (16). Awareness appears to be a substantial barrier in these patients, as surveys indicate that non-White patients are far less likely to have heard of clinical trials than White patients (2). Several patient- and provider-related factors contribute to lack of trial awareness, and these barriers are amplified in minority populations with lower median socioeconomic status and lower median educational levels.

Yet, the disparity persists beyond awareness. Evidence from multiple studies shows that African Americans are less willing to participate in clinical trials compared to White counterparts (17–21). This association holds true even when controlling for socioeconomic status and geography. Multiple factors contribute to this trend. In a survey of 218 patients (72 African American, 146 White) examining a variety of factors contributing to willingness to participate in clinical trials, spiritual and cultural beliefs were demonstrated to have an effect. Those who believe that "God will determine the course of one's cancer" are less likely to participate in clinical trials (17). This belief is held more often in the African American population and likely contributes to a relatively reduced rate of clinical trial participation. Psychosocial barriers such as this prevent proportional representation of racial and ethnic minorities in cancer clinical trials (22).

There is also a long history of unethical treatment of African American patients in the United States dating to the antebellum past. From experimental surgeries on slaves to the infamous Tuskegee Syphilis study where lifesaving therapy was withheld from African American

patients to study the natural history of syphilis, there is a troubling legacy in American medical science (23). For many African Americans, this history poses a deep-seated barrier to trusting in the ethical conduct of clinical trials (17,24).

Overcoming these barriers requires a multifaceted approach. A review of 50 clinical trials conducted at an inner city research hospital identified challenges and strategies. They noted that field-based approaches for recruiting were the most effective, including going into the communities to work with and build trust with potential patients. The most common barrier was distrust, followed by low compensation for time and effort. To overcome barriers, they recommended educating the African American community about clinical trials through engagement activities and treating them with respect. The authors also noted that the presence of multiracial staff can be a facilitator to enrollment of minority patients (25).

As with all populations, giving patients the time to explore their concerns about trials with a provider who can provide reassurance and extra information is associated with an increased willingness to participate in clinical trials (25,26). The focus of conversations may be different depending on the population; a focus group of 67 African American patients noted that men preferred to know more about trial funding mechanisms, financial benefits, and the impact of research, while women noted that treatment as an individual rather than as a study subject was most important (27).

Tailored educational tools along with the ones described previously may also be helpful. An educational video developed at an urban cancer center that included narratives of African American patients discussing their clinical trial experience, as well as commentaries from physicians, ethicists, and staff was designed to impact attitudes toward clinical trials in African American patients. In a study of 108 African American patients, this tool was successful in effecting positive changes in attitudinal barriers and intention to enroll in a clinical trial (28).

Larger scale systemic efforts have also shown promise in improving minority recruitment. The Minority-Based Community Clinical Oncology Program (MB-CCOP) was developed by the NCI to foster enrollment to clinical trials in hospitals that provide care to a patient population with at least 40% representation of minority groups (29). By creating the infrastructure and bringing trials to locations where minority patients are treated, MB-CCOPs have been able to recruit up to 67% minority patients, drastically higher than other cooperative group members (30).

Non-English Speakers

Language barriers can also limit enrollment for several reasons. Some trials may have language-specific eligibility criteria, for example. An analysis of clinicaltrials.gov found an increased number of trials requiring English fluency from 1.7% before 2000 to 9% after 2010. This language restriction was associated with trial- and community-related factors. For example, trials opening in zip codes with more residents self-identifying as African American or Asian were more likely to have language requirements, while those with larger Hispanic populations were less likely. Higher poverty rates were also associated with more language restrictions on clinical trials (31).

Apart from formal eligibility criteria, the logistics of enrolling patients who do not speak English requires additional effort on the part of the research staff. The Department of Health and Human Services regulations for protection of human subjects require that informed consent be presented in a language understandable to the subject, either with a complete consent document (preferred) or a witnessed oral presentation with a short form written consent (32). In addition, adequate interpreting services, multilingual materials, and family member involvement can be protective factors against language as a barrier to trial enrollment in ethnic minorities (5).

Older Adults

Although cancer risk increases with age, elderly patients have historically been underrepresented in therapeutic cancer clinical trials. An analysis of the package inserts of the 24 drugs approved from 2007 to 2010, found that only 33% of the patients in the registration trials were 65 or older, compared to the 59% of the cancer population that is 65 or older. Only 10% were 75 or older (33). This low level of participation limits the generalizability of clinical trial findings in terms of both safety and efficacy.

There are several reasons this occurs. While some barriers (insurance concerns, travel distance) may affect all patients, some may disproportionately affect elderly patients. Most trials exclude patients with decreased performance status or comorbid conditions such as renal insufficiency; these criteria exclude many patients. In addition, certain studies may specifically exclude elderly patients. A review of phase 1 to 3 studies focusing on hematologic malignancies listed on July 1, 2013 found that 27% of these trials had age-based exclusion criteria (34,35).

In recent years, there has been increased attention on developing geriatric-specific studies whose eligibility criteria reflect this population. In addition, these studies may focus on elderly patient specific endpoints, include older patients (>75), make use of geriatric assessments, and characterize frailty. In designing these studies, investigators may propose risk-adapted dosing and toxicity management guidelines (35). Therefore, elderly patient specific trials may help to address the bias both patients and physicians may have regarding clinical trials of novel agents by focusing on toxicity reduction in this population.

PROVIDER FACTORS

Providers, as gatekeepers, hold a central role in clinical trial enrollment. As such, their concerns can contribute to why patients may not be offered clinical trials. Various studies, both prospective survey-based and retrospective analyses that have reported trial enrollment rates, have found that 20% to 50% of the time in which a patient is seen and is eligible for an available clinical trial, a provider does not discuss it or present it as an option (26,36–38).

One of the ways in which providers' subjectivity can affect trial enrollment is through eligibility evaluation. Though inclusion and exclusion criteria are often very specific, there remains room for providers' assessment. Performance status is a prime example, as even this standardized scale that is crucial to determining trial eligibility demonstrates significant interobserver variability (39). This highlights a possible rift between provider-deemed suitability and criteria-guided eligibility for clinical trials.

Apart from determination of eligibility, physicians may carry beliefs about a patient's preferences regarding trials or a patient's ability to handle the logistics of trial participation that lead to not disclosing trial options (5,40). Physicians' attitudes about particular trials and the effectiveness of the trial intervention can also negatively impact the discussion with the patient regarding whether to enroll in a clinical trial. Though a physician may agree to take part in a study as an investigator, he or she may not favor trial participation for certain patients depending on patient allocation to trial arms or perceived likelihood of intervention success (5,41).

As discussed earlier, physicians' communication styles, alliance building, and trust in the therapeutic relationship can strongly influence patients' decisions (26). A survey of 1,107 patients who were presented cancer clinical trials found that those reporting physician-controlled decisions regarding trial enrollment were much less likely than those reporting shared decisions to participate in a trial (37). As noted earlier, encouraging greater patient conversational control can improve patient attitudes toward trials. Explicitly discussing possible adverse effects promotes patient involvement in the conversation and decision making, while also giving providers an opportunity to reassure patients that there are plans for managing toxicity (26). These communication techniques are learned behaviors, and are prime targets for coaching interventions to improve trial enrollment.

Practice resources and time are frequently reported by physicians as barriers to trial enrollment as well. Providers cite challenges such as lack of time, abundant paperwork, and difficulty remembering active protocols (1,42). In a survey of 221 medical oncologists among 11 health plans funded by the NCI across the United States, more than 50% reported lack of adequate support staff for enrollment and data management, and described effort and time for informed consent and learning trial eligibility as large barriers to trial enrollment. These factors were found to be strong predictors of decreased trial enrollment (43).

ORGANIZATIONAL BARRIERS

Trial Availability

On a system level, one of the largest barriers to clinical trial accrual is a mismatch between available clinical trials and the pool of eligible patients. This problem is multifaceted and manifests differently across practice settings.

With 85% of patients being treated in the community setting, the availability of appropriate trials in this setting is paramount (44). However, analyses of clinical trials in the community show that in up to 60% of cases, no trials are available for a patient's stage and type of cancer. Another 8% to 20% of the time, a patient is found to be ineligible for an available study, further decrementing trial enrollment (1,45).

Academic settings face different challenges. Physicians in academic centers are more likely to enroll patients and have more active clinical trials available (9). However, an analysis of the clinical trial database of the Pancreatic Cancer Action Network found that in academic settings often the issue is not the number of trials offered but the types of trials and whether they are appropriate for the patient populations. The study found that for the trials opened in 2011 nationally 83% of resectable pancreatic cancer patients and 26% of metastatic pancreatic cancer patients would need to have enrolled for the studies to have completed accrual. These estimates far exceed the usual estimate that only 20% of patients are eligible for clinical trials, and led the authors to estimate that at those rates, it would take nearly 7 years for pancreatic cancer trials opened in 2011 to complete accrual (45). Similar statistics hold for other tumor types and demonstrate a mismatch between trial offerings at academic centers and the available potential participant pool.

Geography/Location

Among the important structural barriers to trial participation is the location of trials. Academic centers that offer the greatest number of clinical trials are largely found in urban areas. Patients rate travel/commute concerns as strongly influential factors in the decision to participate in cancer clinical trials, and rural patients in particular cite these as a barrier (46).

Given the limited access many patients have to academic centers, the NCI has funded initiatives to increase access to clinical trials in community settings. This includes the NCI Community Clinical Oncology Program (CCOP), NCI Community Cancer Centers Program (NCCCP), and most recently, the NCI Community Oncology Research Program (NCORP).

These efforts have increased accrual in the community setting. The CCOP collaborative network has contributed to various practice-changing trials, including for example, NSABP-B31, which led to the discovery of recurrence-free and survival benefit to trastuzumab in early-stage breast cancer. In this study, 40% of patients came from the CCOP network. The network grew to enroll a third of NCI treatment trials and a vast majority of prevention and control trials (47). An analysis of NCCCP pilot hospital sites showed that those that already had established research programs increased their enrollment in year 1 and maintained this, as well as increased the number of phase I and II clinical trials. Programs with less developed programs showed more gradual enrollment, with expansion of phase 3 clinical trials. Overall, accrual to NCI-sponsored trials increased 27% during the 3-year period. In addition, the number of minority and elderly patients enrolled increased (48). In a participating center in Nebraska, clinical trial staff at this center increased over threefold, and total accruals over 5 years increased from 83 to 640 (49). In 2014, these two programs were replaced by NCORP, which includes 7 research bases, 334 community sites, and 12 minority/underserved community sites (50).

Insurance

Many patients cite insurance concerns when making a decision to enroll in a clinical trial (51). This is a structural barrier to clinical trial enrollment. A retrospective study examined the insurance coverage clearance rates of 4,617 cancer patients at Johns Hopkins University who signed consent for cancer treatment trials. Of these, 628 (13.6%) were denied enrollment in a therapeutic cancer trial. Seventy-eight percent of this group had insurance policies that provided some coverage for clinical trials, but were denied due to clinical trial characteristics (such as study phase). The remaining patients did not have clinical trial benefits in their insurance policies (52).

Policy changes have been implemented to reduce insurance barriers to clinical trials. In 2000, President Clinton signed a National Coverage Decision that requires Medicare to cover routine costs associated with clinical trials (53). An analysis of Southwest Oncology Group studies found that this was associated with an increase in enrollment of patients with supplemental private coverage (54).

Prior to 2014, coverage for patients with commercial insurance was regulated by state laws that vary widely (55). While some states required coverage for routine costs associated with all clinical trials, some had no protections, while others excluded phase 1 clinical trials or had other restrictions (56). Analyses of state mandates and agreements have noted increased enrollment for clinical trial coverage in certain circumstances (56–58). Making this even more complicated for patients and providers was that patients covered by employer self-insured plans were regulated by federal law (which did not require coverage of clinical trials). Therefore, state laws with greater protections did not apply to those patients.

To address this disparity among states, starting January 1, 2014, Section 2709 of the Affordable Care Act (ACA) established a national minimum coverage standard for clinical trials (59). It mandates that commercial insurers cover the routine costs of clinical trials for patients participating in phases I to IV clinical trials for the prevention, detection, or treatment of cancer or other life-threatening illnesses.

Studies must be federally funded and conducted under an investigational new drug (IND) application, or be drug trials that are exempt from the IND application requirements. However, despite the broad language of the ACA, many questions still remain, including enforcement of the law, the definition of routine costs of clinical trials, and access to care for patients whose narrow network and lack of out-of-network benefits may not provide access to clinical trials (60).

CONCLUSION

Clinical trials are the backbone of advancing cancer therapy, yet trial accrual rates remain at dismal levels. A variety of interrelated patient, provider, and systemic factors are associated with low accrual rates. A multi-faceted approach that addresses each of these barriers is vital to improving cancer clinical trial enrollment. Several interventions aimed at different level barriers have demonstrated success. Decision aids can improve patient's knowledge and self-efficacy in decision making, provider training can improve communication, legislation can improve insurance coverage for clinical trials, and federally funded programs can improve trial availability in the community. Further studies and public interventions to improve trial accrual are necessary to advance the enterprise of cancer clinical trials.

REFERENCES

1. Go RS, Frisby KA, Lee JA, et al. Clinical trial accrual among new cancer patients at a community-based cancer center. *Cancer.* 2006;106(2):426–433. doi:10.1002/cncr.21597
2. Murthy VH, Krumholz HM, Gross CP. Participation in cancer clinical trials: race-, sex-, and age-based disparities. *JAMA.* 2004;291(22):2720–2726.
3. Nass SJ, Moses HL, Mendelsohn J. *A National Cancer Clinical Trials System for the 21st Century: Reinvigorating the NCI Cooperative Group Program.* Washington, DC: National Academies Press; 2010.
4. Ford JG, Howerton MW, Lai GY, et al. Barriers to recruiting underrepresented populations to cancer clinical trials: a systematic review. *Cancer.* 2008;112(2):228–242.
5. Grunfeld E, Zitzelsberger L, Coristine M, Aspelund F. Barriers and facilitators to enrollment in cancer clinical trials. *Cancer.* 2002;95(7):1577–1583.
6. Comis RL, Miller JD, Aldigé CR, et al. Public attitudes toward participation in cancer clinical trials. *J Clin Oncol.* 2003;21(5):830–835.
7. Townsley CA, Selby R, Siu LL. Systematic review of barriers to the recruitment of older patients with cancer onto clinical trials. *J Clin Oncol.* 2005;23(13):3112–3124.
8. Manne S, Kashy D, Albrecht T, et al. Knowledge, attitudes, and self-efficacy as predictors of preparedness for oncology clinical trials: a mediational model. *Med Decis Making.* 2014;34(4):454–463.
9. Meropol NJ, Buzaglo JS, Millard J, et al. Barriers to clinical trial participation as perceived by oncologists and patients. *J Natl Compr Canc Netw.* 2007;5(8):753–762.
10. Mills EJ, Seely D, Rachlis B, et al. Barriers to participation in clinical trials of cancer: a meta-analysis and systematic review of patient-reported factors. *Lancet Oncol.* 2006;7(2):141–148.
11. Hamilton JG, Lillie SE, Alden DL, et al. What is a good medical decision? A research agenda guided by perspectives from multiple stakeholders. *J Behav Med.* 2016;40:52–68.
12. Albrecht TL, Eggly SS, Gleason MEJ, et al. Influence of clinical communication on patients' decision making on participation in clinical trials. *J Clin Oncol.* 2008;26(16):2666–2673. doi:10.1200/JCO.2007.14.8114
13. Gillies K, Cotton SC, Brehaut JC, et al. Decision aids for people considering taking part in clinical trials. *Cochrane Database Syst Rev.* 2015;(11):CD009736.
14. Meropol NJ, Wong YN, Albrecht T, et al. Randomized trial of a web-based intervention to address barriers to clinical trials. *J Clin Oncol.* 2016;34(5):469–478. doi:10.1200/JCO.2015.63.2257
15. Politi MC, Kuzemchak MD, Kaphingst KA, et al. Decision aids can support cancer clinical trials decisions: results of a randomized trial. *Oncologist.* 2016;21(12):1461–1470.
16. DeNavas-Walt C, Proctor BD, Smith JC. *Income, Poverty, and Health Insurance Coverage in the United States: 2009* (U.S. Census Bureau, current population reports, P60–238). Washington, DC: U.S. Government Printing Office; 2010.
17. Advani AS, Atkeson B, Brown CL, et al. Barriers to the participation of African-American patients with cancer in clinical trials: a pilot study. *Cancer.* 2003;97(6):1499–1506.
18. Farmer DF, Jackson SA, Camacho F, Hall MA. Attitudes of African American and low socioeconomic status white women toward medical research. *J Health Care Poor Underserved.* 2007;18(1):85–99.
19. Holcombe RF, Jacobson J, Li A, Moinpour CM. Inclusion of black Americans in oncology clinical trials: the Louisiana State University Medical Center experience. *Am J Clin Oncol.* 1999;22(1):18–21.
20. Harris Y, Gorelick PB, Samuels P, Bempong I. Why African Americans may not be participating in clinical trials. *J Natl Med Assoc.* 1996;88(10):630.
21. Linden HM, Reisch LM, Hart A, et al. Attitudes toward participation in breast cancer randomized clinical trials in the African American community: a focus group study. *Cancer Nurs.* 2007;30(4):261–269.
22. Wells AA, Zebrack B. Psychosocial barriers contributing to the under-representation of racial/ethnic minorities in cancer clinical trials. *Soc Work Health Care.* 2008;46(2):1–14.
23. Washington HA. *Medical Apartheid: The Dark History of Medical Experimentation on Black Americans From Colonial Times to the Present.* New York, NY: Doubleday Books; 2006.
24. Swanson GM, Ward AJ. Recruiting minorities into clinical trials: toward a participant-friendly system. *J Natl Cancer Inst.* 1995;87(23):1747–1759.
25. Otado J, Kwagyan J, Edwards D, et al. Culturally competent strategies for recruitment and retention of African American populations into clinical trials. *Clin Transl Sci.* 2015;8(5):460–466.
26. Albrecht TL, Eggly SS, Gleason ME, et al. Influence of clinical communication on patients' decision making on participation in clinical trials. *J Clin Oncol.* 2008;26(16):2666–2673.

27. Belue R, Taylor-Richardson KD, Lin J, et al. African Americans and participation in clinical trials: differences in beliefs and attitudes by gender. *Contemp Clin Trials.* 2006;27(6): 498–505.

28. Banda DR, Libin AV, Wang H, Swain SM. A pilot study of a culturally targeted video intervention to increase participation of African American patients in cancer clinical trials. *Oncologist.* 2012;17(5):708–714.

29. Wieder R, Teal R, Saunders T, Weiner BJ. Establishing a minority-based community clinical oncology program: the University of Medicine and Dentistry of New Jersey, New Jersey Medical School-university Hospital Cancer Center experience. *J Oncol Pract.* 2013;9(2):e48–e54.

30. Mccaskill-Stevens W, Mckinney MM, Whitman CG, Minasian LM. Increasing minority participation in cancer clinical trials: the minority-based community clinical oncology program experience. *J Clin Oncol.* 2005;23(22):5247–5254.

31. Egleston BL, Pedraza O, Wong YN, et al. Characteristics of clinical trials that require participants to be fluent in English. *Clin Trials.* 2015;12(6):618–626.

32. Code of Federal Regulations. Title 45: Public Welfare—Department of Health and Human Services (Part 46, Protection of Human Subjects); 2009. https://www.hhs.gov/ohrp/regulations-and-policy/regulations/45-cfr-46/index.html

33. Scher KS, Hurria A. Under-representation of older adults in cancer registration trials: known problem, little progress. *J Clin Oncol.* 2012;30(17):2036–2038.

34. Hamaker ME, Stauder R, van Munster BC. Exclusion of older patients from ongoing clinical trials for hematological malignancies: an evaluation of the National Institutes of Health Clinical Trial Registry. *Oncologist.* 2014;19(10):1069–1075.

35. Hurria A, Dale W, Mooney M, et al.; Cancer and Aging Research Group. Designing therapeutic clinical trials for older and frail adults with cancer: U13 conference recommendations. *J Clin Oncol.* 2014;32(24):2587–2594.

36. Lara PN, Higdon R, Lim N, et al. Prospective evaluation of cancer clinical trial accrual patterns: identifying potential barriers to enrollment. *J Clin Oncol.* 2001;19(6):1728–1733.

37. Kehl KL, Arora NK, Schrag D, et al. Discussions about clinical trials among patients with newly diagnosed lung and colorectal cancer. *J Natl Cancer Inst.* 2014;106(10). doi:10.1093/jnci/dju216

38. Unger JM, Hershman DL, Albain KS, et al. Patient income level and cancer clinical trial participation. *J Clin Oncol.* 2013;31(5):536–542.

39. Sørensen JB, Klee M, Palshof T, Hansen HH. Performance status assessment in cancer patients. An inter-observer variability study. *Br J Cancer.* 1993;67(4):773–775.

40. Antman K, Amato D, Wood W, et al. Selection bias in clinical trials. *J Clin Oncol.* 1985;3(8):1142–1147.

41. Somkin CP, Ackerson L, Husson G, et al. Effect of medical oncologists' attitudes on accrual to clinical trials in a community setting. *J Oncol Pract.* 2013;9:e275–e283.

42. Schroen AT, Brenin DR. Clinical trial priorities among surgeons caring for breast cancer patients. *Am J Surg.* 2008;195(4):474–480.

43. Somkin CP, Altschuler A, Ackerson L, et al. Organizational barriers to physician participation in cancer clinical trials. *Am J Manag Care.* 2005;11(7):413–421.

44. Copur MS, Ramaekers R, Gönen M, et al. Impact of the National Cancer Institute Community Cancer Centers program on clinical trial and related activities at a community cancer center in rural Nebraska. *J Oncol Pract.* 2016;12(1):67–68.

45. Hoos WA, James PM, Rahib L, et al. Pancreatic cancer clinical trials and accrual in the United States. *J Clin Oncol.* 2013;31(27):3432–3438.

46. Virani S, Burke L, Remick SC, Abraham J. Barriers to recruitment of rural patients in cancer clinical trials. *J Oncol Pract.* 2011;7(3):172–177.

47. Minasian LM, Carpenter WR, Weiner BJ, et al. Translating research into evidence-based practice. *Cancer.* 2010;116(19):4440–4449.

48. Hirsch BR, Locke SC, Abernethy AP. Experience of the National Cancer Institute Community Cancer Centers Program on community-based cancer clinical trials activity. *J Oncol Pract.* 2016;12(4):e350–e358. doi:10.1200/JOP.2015.005090

49. Dimond EP, St Germain D, Nacpil LM, et al. Creating a "culture of research" in a community hospital: Strategies and tools from the National Cancer Institute Community Cancer Centers Program. *Clin Trials.* 2015;12(3):246–256.

50. Printz C. NCI launches program for community-based clinical research: NCORP replaces 2 previous programs. *Cancer.* 2014;120(20):3097–3098. doi:10.1002/cncr.29067

51. Wong YN, Schluchter MD, Albrecht TL, et al. Financial concerns about participation in clinical trials among patients with cancer. *J Clin Oncol.* 2016;34(5):479–487.

52. Klamerus JF, Bruinooge SS, Ye X, et al. The impact of insurance on access to cancer clinical trials at a comprehensive cancer center. *Clin Cancer Res.* 2010;16(24):5997–6003.

53. Centers for Medicare and Medicaid Services. Medicare Clinical Trial Policies. https://www.cms.gov/Medicare/Coverage/ClinicalTrialPolicies/index.html

54. Unger JM, Coltman CA, Crowley JJ, et al. Impact of the year 2000 Medicare policy change on older patient enrollment to cancer clinical trials. *J Clin Oncol.* 2006;24(1):141–144. doi:10.1200/JCO.2005.02.8928

55. Kircher SM, Benson AB, Farber M, Nimeiri HS. Effect of the accountable care act of 2010 on clinical trial insurance coverage. *J Clin Oncol.* 2012;30(5):548–553.

56. Gross CP, Murthy V, Li Y, et al. Cancer trial enrollment after state-mandated reimbursement. *J Natl Cancer Inst.* 2004;96(14):1063–1069.

57. Mcbride G. More states mandate coverage of clinical trial costs, but does it make a difference? *J Natl Cancer Inst.* 2003;95(17):1268–1269.

58. Martel CL, Li Y, Beckett L, et al. An evaluation of barriers to accrual in the era of legislation requiring insurance coverage of cancer clinical trial costs in California. *Cancer J.* 2004;10(5):294–300.

59. Protection P. Act AC, No PL. Public Law 111-148 Stat. 124. *STAT.* 2014;894.

60. Martin PJ, Davenport-Ennis N, Petrelli NJ, et al. Responsibility for costs associated with clinical trials. *J Clin Oncol.* 2014;32(30):3357–3359.

28

The Role of Novel Imaging Techniques in Clinical Trials

Binsheng Zhao and Lawrence H. Schwartz

Radiographic imaging has been increasingly incorporated into all phases of oncological clinical trials, particularly early-phase trials, for various purposes including (but not limited to) patient selection, evidence of biologic activity, and as surrogate biomarkers for clinical outcomes (1). Early-phase clinical trials are designed to assess the safety and preliminary efficacy of drugs with small numbers of patients. Oncological endpoints, measurement precision of the endpoints, and response assessment criteria can have a significant impact on the study duration, cost, and success. In addition to clinical and/or physical assessments, medical imaging allows us to visibly depict disease extension and quantify drug-induced morphological and/or functional changes of diseases, which will play an important role in further drug development.

A REVIEW OF THE IMAGING MODALITIES USED

Conventional CT and MRI have been generally considered as the best (currently) available, most accurate, and most reproducible imaging modalities. They allow the clinician to identify target lesions from baseline scans performed prior to the onset of therapy, to measure and follow up size change of the target lesions, and to identify new lesions on subsequent scans for monitoring and assessment of response to therapy. These modalities can provide sectional images showing detailed (both normal and abnormal) anatomical structures inside the body, allowing tumor detection and tumor size measurement as well as follow-up. Over recent years, our understanding of drug mechanisms of action has been increased drastically. As a result, drug designs have shifted away from traditional cytotoxic agents (which typically shrink tumors) to cytostatic agents (which usually inhibit tumor growth, resulting in tumor consolidation rather than shrinkage). Meanwhile, quantitative imaging technologies have evolved from the anatomical to the

functional to better coincide with the advances in drug discovery. Being able to both noninvasively and in vivo characterize and measure cancer's biological processes at a molecular level, the functional imaging techniques such as PET with fluorine-18-fluorodeoxyglucose ([18F-FDG) and dynamic contrast-enhanced (DCE) MRI have shown great promises in early response assessment and are being utilized more and more in early-phase clinical trials testing molecular-targeted anticancer agents.

Conventional CT and MRI

CT scans are well suited for imaging the neck, chest, abdomen, and pelvis, where anatomical and pathological structures can be differentiated by their relative attenuation. Intravenous, oral, and rectal CT contrast media are often administered to emphasize specific vascular structures, organs, and tissues so that the presence of an abnormality can be better depicted and identified. More advanced CT imaging techniques such as multiphase imaging protocols are applied to some specific studies (e.g., hepatocellular carcinoma treated with hepatic artery embolization) to better differentiate vasculature, live tumor components, necrosis, and surrounding parenchyma (Figure 28.1). With the remarkable advances of multidetector (MD) CT technology, CT scans can be acquired at an *ultra* fast speed with isotropic submillimeter image spatial resolution. The new generation MDCT offers more accurate tumor measurements, particularly tumor volume, which may provide more accurate and early assessment of therapeutic response compared to conventional measurements.

MRI also provides high-quality anatomical information. It is, however, less frequently used than CT in oncology studies because of its cost, complexity, scan duration, and limitation in imaging the chest, a frequent site of metastatic spread. However, in some regions of the body, MRI is the preferred method (i.e., the head, for assessing brain tumors). Moreover, MRI should be

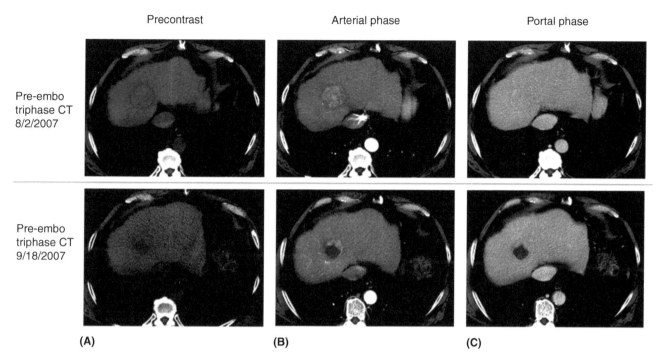

FIGURE 28.1 Triphasic CT imaging of HCC. Upper row shows an HCC before onset of hepatic embolization, and lower row is the same HCC 6 weeks after the treatment. (A) Precontrast. (B) Arterial phase. (C) Portal phase.

HCC, hepatocellular carcinoma.

used where CT is medically contraindicated. Due to the multiple sequences that can be produced during a single MRI study, it is important that lesions must be measured at the same anatomical levels on the same sequence in both baseline and subsequent follow-up examinations.

In clinical trials, both CT and MRI are widely used for identification of target lesions on the baseline study, monitoring of (target) lesion size change during the course of therapy, and detection of new lesions on follow-up examinations.

PET

PET scanners capture signals emitted from a radiopharmaceutical (e.g., ^{18}F-FDG) that contains a radionuclide and is injected into the patient. Studies have found that the uptake of ^{18}F-FDG signals on PET is associated with cellular growth rate and proliferation capacity (2,3). As cancer cells are more metabolically active, their FDG uptakes on the PET images are more intense than those of normal tissues. A decrease in the FDG uptake of a tumor indicates decay of the tumor activity and thus possible death of viable tumor cells. These findings allow the use of changes in tumor glucose metabolism during therapy to assess tumor response. There are a number of semiquantitative or quantitative parameters derived from the ^{18}F-FDG PET that are used to quantify tumor glucose metabolism. Since metabolic alterations precede anatomic changes after the onset of therapy, the ability to measure viable cancer cells by imaging metabolic activity of tumors has placed PET imaging as the cutting-edge functional technology for early response

assessment in clinical trials testing new anticancer medication.

^{18}F-FDG PET has already added special value to the accuracy of response assessment in lymphoma, in which a residual mass after completion of therapy often contains fibrosis or necrosis that is indistinguishable from viable tumor on CT scans. This scenario particularly limits the use of CT to categorize complete remission and partial response (PR) of tumors involving the lymph nodes. Functional PET imaging, however, can differentiate viable tumor components from fibrosis and necrosis by identifying focal areas of increased metabolic activity. One of the shortcomings of the PET imaging is the lack of anatomical information, which has been resolved with the advent of hybrid PET/CT scanners.

To enhance the ability to differentiate tumor cells from healthy tissue, more effective tumor-specific radiotracers are under intensive investigation. Among the numerous tracers being studied, the thymidine analog 3'-deoxy-3'-[F18]fluorothymidine (^{18}F-FLT) shows promise as a potential biomarker for quantifying tumor proliferation in several different cancers (4–6).

Dynamic Contrast-Enhanced MRI

Tumor survival requires oxygen, which is delivered by the blood. Angiogenesis, the formation of new capillaries from existing blood vessels, is an important process that is necessary for the growth of malignant tumors and the development of metastasis. Angiogenesis can be inhibited by antiangiogenic agents and existing blood vessels can be interrupted by vascular disrupting compounds. By tracking the pass of an injected intravenous bolus of contrast agent (e.g., the low molecular weight paramagnetic gadolinium) through the tumor vasculature, intensity change of the repeatedly acquired T1-weighted DCE-MRI can be converted into contrast agent concentration data upon which kinetic modeling can be applied. The modeled parameters produced are sensitive to physiological processes including tissue microvessel perfusion, permeability, and extracellular extravascular leakage space (EES) (7). Changes in these parameters with therapy can thus be used to evaluate antiangiogenic effects of cancer treatments. Since alteration in tumor vascularity occurs earlier than alteration in tumor size after initiation of therapy (8), DCE-MRI is being increasingly used as a surrogate biomarker in early clinical trials testing new antiangiogenics and vascular disrupting compounds.

WHAT CAN THESE MODALITIES BE USED FOR?

With more and more anticancer drugs available and under evaluation, clinicians/radiologists can be faced with more than one choice in treating cancer patients and monitoring tumor changes with therapy. Many factors, including (but not limited to) patient clinical characteristics, cancer type and stage, specific medication, and available imaging equipment will jointly influence determination of the treatment plan and methodology for assessing response to therapy. Personalized medicine will play a central role in future clinical trials testing novel anticancer agents.

Imaging modalities can play different roles at different stages of clinical trials. For instance, they can be used to stratify patients to appropriate clinical trials (e.g., PET) (9), serve as early surrogate biomarkers for prediction of survival (e.g., PET and DCE-MRI) (10), and assess time to progression (TTP; e.g., CT). In the following subsections, the use of imaging modalities to quantify tumor changes (as surrogate biomarkers), identify target lesions in baseline studies, detect new lesions in follow-up studies, and confirm tumor response after completion of therapy will be discussed.

Surrogate Imaging Biomarkers

In clinical trials, especially in phase II trials, endpoints are likely to be surrogate endpoints such as biomarkers of the disease. A biomarker is defined as a characteristic that is objectively measured and evaluated as an indicator of normal biologic processes, pathogenic processes, or pharmacologic responses to a therapeutic intervention (11). Biomarkers should be relevant to drug mechanisms of action so that they can be used to evaluate treatment efficacy. Quantitative imaging biomarkers can thus be, for example, changes in tumor size measured on CT or MRI, uptake of ^{18}F-FDG on PET, and modeled parameters derived from DCE-MRI during the course of therapy.

Tumor should eventually shrink if a drug is effective. Change in tumor size measured between baseline and follow-up scans has been widely used to quantify tumor response and progression in clinical trials as well as routine clinical practice. To date, tumor mass has been typically approximated by the greatest diameter (unidimensional measurement) or the product of the two greatest perpendicular diameters (bidimensional measurement) of the tumor in a transverse image plane. However, contemporary CT scanners can produce submillimeter isotropic image data that allows accurate estimation of tumor volume/volume change, and evidence is beginning to show the potential of earlier detection of tumor change by volume rather than by conventional diameters (Figure 28.2) (12). Despite this, unidimensional and bidimensional response assessment criteria are still widely used in clinical trials partially due to historical reasons. Lack of efficient and robust computer-aided measurement tools also hinders the volumetric response assessment from being thoroughly validated and widely accepted by clinical trials.

FDG uptake on PET is a measure of glucose metabolism, which is proven to be associated with growth rate and proliferation capacity (3,13,14). Glucose metabolism is higher in tumor cells than in healthy cells. Therefore, a decrease in tumor uptake after the initiation of therapy indicates possible tumor cell death and therefore efficacy of the treatment. A number of methods have been developed to assess FDG uptake of tumors on PET, including visual interpretation (e.g., visual comparison of metabolic activities between tumor and background tissues such as mediastinal blood pool on ^{18}F-FDG PET), semiquantitative measurements (e.g., standard uptake value [SUV]), and analytical kinetic techniques (e.g., rate of glucose metabolism) (15,16). The SUV is defined as the attenuation-corrected ^{18}F-FDG accumulation in a lesion normalized to the injected dose and the patient's body weight, body surface area, or lean body mass. Although the SUV is a single snapshot of a dynamic process, it has been widely used in response assessment because of its simplicity and ability to quantify the number of viable tumor cells (Figure 28.3) (17). Full kinetic quantitative analysis can provide an absolute rate of ^{18}F-FDG uptake over the measurement duration. However, complexity of the dynamic data acquisition and the need for arterial blood sampling make kinetic analysis difficult to implement in clinical settings.

A number of semiquantitative and quantitative methods are being applied to DCE-MRI data to assess tissue physiology and contrast agent kinetics (18). Semiquantitative parameters include simple features that characterize the signal intensity–time curve such as the gradient, initial area under the time–signal curve (area under the curve [AUC]), and time to maximum enhancement. These parameters are readily computed from the T1-weighted sequentially acquired MRI. However, they do not accurately reflect contrast agent

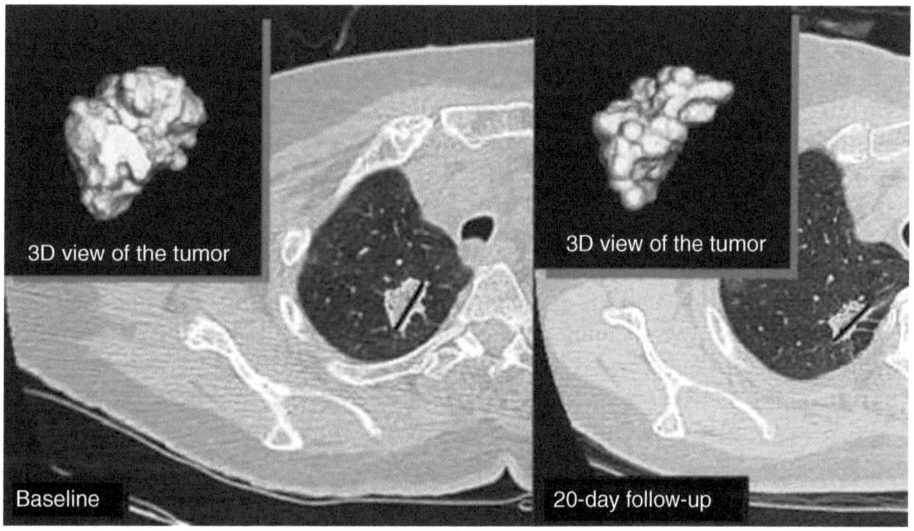

FIGURE 28.2 Detection of tumor change on CT, comparing volumetric and unidimensional measurement, for an EGFR mutant tumor at baseline (A) and at 20-day follow-up (B). Computer delineated tumor contours and diameter lines are superimposed on one image from each study date. Three-dimensional view of each segmented tumor is displayed at the upper-left corner of each panel. For this case, a significant change is detected using volume measurement (−52.4%), but not using unidimensional measurement (−4.4%).

EGFR, epidermal growth factor receptor.

Source: From Zhao B, Oxnard GR, Moskowitz CS, et al. A pilot study of volume measurement as a method of tumor response evaluation to aid biomarker development. *Clin Cancer Res.* 2010;16:4647–4653.

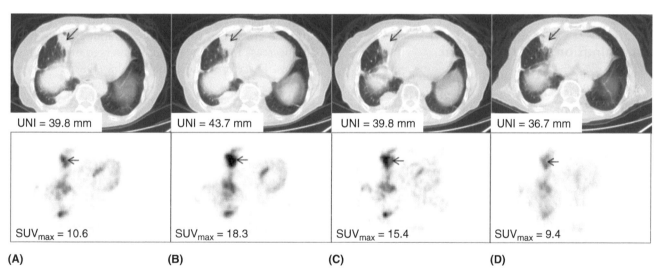

FIGURE 28.3 ¹⁸F-FDG PET/CT in the monitoring of tumor size and metabolic changes with therapies. (A) Baseline CT (upper row) and PET (lower row) (obtained from a hybrid PET/CT scanner) taken in an NSCLC patient who had discontinued treatment with gefitinib. One target lesion (arrow) in right lung is indicated on CT and on corresponding PET. (B) PET/CT after 3 weeks without receiving gefitinib. Both tumor size (i.e., unidimensional maximal tumor diameter) measured on CT and tumor SUV measured on ¹⁸F-FDG PET increased. The patient then resumed treatment with gefitinib. (C) PET/CT 3 weeks after resumption of the gefitinib treatment. Both tumor size and SUV_{max} deceased. At this time point daily everolimus was added. (D) PET/CT 3 weeks after the combined treatment with gefitinib and everolimus. Tumor size and SUV_{max} continued to decrease.

¹⁸F-FDG, fluorine-18-fluorodeoxyglucose; NSCLC, non–small-cell lung cancer; SUV, standard uptake value.

Source: From Riely GJ, Kris MG, Zhao B, et al. Prospective assessment of discontinuation and re-initiation of erlotinib or gefitinib in patients with acquired resistance to erlotinib or gefitinib followed by the addition of everolimus. *Clin Cancer Res.* 2007;13:5150–5155.

concentration and they present considerable variability due to different scanner settings and individual examinations. Difficulties in direct comparisons between different studies and within individual studies render the semiquantitative methods less useful in the evaluation of responses to therapy. Quantitative parameters, derived from pharmacokinetic modeling of contrast agent concentration data representing a nonlinear conversion of MRI signal intensity changes observed during the dynamic acquisition, allow more robust study on contrast agent kinetics including vessel permeability, perfusion/flow, blood volume, and EES volume (7). The two parameters of most interest in the vascular response assessment are the initial area under the contrast agent concentration–time curve (initial area under the curve [IAUC]) and the volume transfer constant of contrast agent between the blood plasma and the EES (K^{Trans}). The former is a model-free parameter that is robust and easy to compute. However, its relationship with the underlying physiology is complex and undefined. The latter is a parameter derived from relatively simple, compartmental kinetic models and reflects a nonlinear composite of various physiologic processes including blood flow, endothelial surface, and endothelial permeability. A decrease in K^{Trans} indicates that a drug is active. The quantitative parameters are independent of acquisition protocol, but complicated to derive. Interpretation of a parameter change during the course of therapy needs to take into consideration the specific model used for analysis.

Determination of Target Lesion

Anatomical imaging, particularly CT, remains the modality of choice for cancer detection, diagnosis, treatment planning, response assessment, and disease recurrence monitoring. CT has the ability to accurately and reproducibly depict both normal and abnormal anatomical structures inside the body. Furthermore, CT is widely available, relatively inexpensive, and easy to operate. Because of these, CT scan is often the first choice for baseline studies (i.e., studies performed shortly before the onset of a therapy). If the date of diagnosis and the date of therapy initiation are close enough, the diagnostic CT scan can be used as the baseline CT study in which target lesions (as well as nontarget lesions) residing in different body sites will be determined and their sizes quantitatively measured for monitoring tumor changes in the follow-up studies.

Identification of Response

Objective response rate (ORR) is the most widely used quantitative measure to categorize tumor response to therapeutic agents and to assess efficacy of the new agents in clinical trials. The ORR is defined as the percentage change in tumor size (or other response parameters) between baseline and follow-up studies. Methodology

used to assess tumor response is vitally important, as a trial's outcome may provide support for the drug's approval by regulatory agencies and thus determine the fate of the experimental drug under investigation. Drug mechanism of action along with cancer type will play a critical role in the selection of imaging technique and response assessment methodology for both clinical trials and routine clinical practice.

Traditional cytotoxic drugs were designed to halt the division of rapidly dividing cells. It is anticipated that the tumor will shrink considerably and ultimately suffer damage over a certain time period after the onset of therapy. In addition, the available imaging modalities have been primarily anatomical modalities until the recent emergence of functional imaging technologies. Tumor size change measured through serial imaging examinations has therefore been used as a surrogate marker for evaluation of clinical benefits in the development and use of various therapies.

Development of the newer generation of molecular-targeted agents, however, is aiming at identifying and selectively inhibiting molecular targets that play certain roles in tumor cell growth and differentiation. Two promising targets are the vascular endothelial growth factor (VEGF) pathway, a key mediator of tumor angiogenesis, and the epidermal growth factor receptor (EGFR), the cell-surface receptor for members of the epidermal growth factor family of extracellular protein ligands. The molecular-targeted agents are usually cytostatic rather than cytotoxic. They may slow down or stop the growth of cancer cells without causing tumor size decrease that can be readily observed on anatomical images. Therefore, traditional size-based response methodologies may no longer be appropriate for recognizing tumor changes, as they may only be able to detect tumor response (by size) well after the initiation of therapy. If molecular-targeted drugs inhibit the proliferation of cancer cells, treatment-induced metabolic change can be detected by the reduction of FDG uptake, the metabolic biomarker for measuring the efficacy of targeted molecular therapies. For the emerging vascular-targeted compounds that prevent blood flow to and from the tumors, DCE-MRI is a more appropriate biomarker for measuring efficacy of the antiangiogenics and vascular disrupting agents because of its high spatial resolution and ability to quantify metabolic changes such as the rate of tumor blood flow.

In comparison with the tumor size change, the functional biomarkers allow the metabolic and/or vascular alterations of tumor to be detected at a much earlier time point. Therefore, these functional biomarkers are increasingly used in early clinical trials testing new anticancer agents. Being able to provide both metabolic and anatomic information with fused images, the hybrid ^{18}F-FDG PET/CT is requested more and more after set time periods following treatment completion to both confirm treatment results and to monitor for disease recurrence.

Assessment of Time to Progression

Survival prolongation is the ultimate goal for cancer treatments. However, such clinical outcomes usually take very long to attain and may be complicated by other factors such as noncancer-related death or multiple treatments given to a single patient. In addition to the ORR, another surrogate endpoint that was proven to be predictive of mortality in metastatic colorectal cancer and non–small-cell lung cancer (NSCLC) was TTP (19). The TTP is defined as the time from a patient's entry into the clinical trial to the date when progression of disease or death is documented. Disease progression is usually assessed based on the radiological changes of tumors and the established response evaluation criteria (20). To obtain the necessary information for TTP, a number of follow-up examinations need to be performed every 6 to 8 weeks during treatment. The presence of new lesions on follow-up imaging studies is also a sign of disease progression.

RESPONSE ASSESSMENT CRITERIA

Uniform interpretation and valid comparison of the outcomes among clinical trials, particularly among multicenter trials, demand at least the use of consistent imaging acquisition technique/protocol and standardized response assessment criteria. Guidelines regarding appropriate imaging procedures and protocols to optimally visualize and reliably measure tumors on serial examinations for evaluating therapeutic response should be recommended based upon our best understanding of drug mechanisms of action and on previous pertinent experiences.

Historically, tumor response to therapy has been assessed by measuring tumor size on serial radiographic examinations using the criteria known as the World Health Organization (WHO) criteria (21,22) or the Response Evaluation Criteria in Solid Tumors (RECIST) (23,24). The latter was a simplification and an extension of the former criteria. With recent innovations in discovering molecular-targeted agents and functional imaging technologies, the evaluation of tumor response to therapy has opened a new window by measuring tumor metabolism/vasculature at the molecular level. The guidelines for functional/molecular response assessment were proposed for ^{18}F-FDG PET (25,26) and DCE-MRI (27–29), and functional imaging biomarkers are being intensively investigated and validated in early-phase clinical trials worldwide.

WHO Criteria

The WHO response assessment criteria were proposed in the late 1970s and early 1980s, after recognizing a need to standardize reporting of clinical outcomes from cancer treatment trials (21,22). The guideline suggested to use bidimensional measurement (i.e., cross product of the greatest diameter of the tumor and its greatest perpendicular diameter on a transverse image) to approximate target lesion tumor burden and to use the sum of the cross products to quantify tumor change on serial examinations. Based upon the change of these sums, the WHO recommended reporting the result of cancer response to therapy using the following four categories: complete response (CR), partial response (PR), stable disease (SD), and progressive disease (PD) (Tables 28.1). A size reduction of 50% or more from the baseline study was considered as response (PR), whereas a size increase of 25% or more was deemed to be progressive (PD). The presence of any new disease would be considered PD and any *substantial* enlargement in tumor size that was not easily measured would also be considered progression.

RECIST 1.0 and 1.1 Criteria

Since the inception of the WHO criteria, several variations of the response assessment criteria had been used in clinical trials. In 1994, the European Organization for Research and Treatment of Cancer (EORTC), the National Cancer Institute (NCI) of the United States, and the NCI of Canada trials group set up a task force to review the existing criteria used in the evaluation of

TABLE 28.1 WHO and RECIST Response Criteria

Response Category	WHO Definition	RECIST Definition
CR	Disappearance of all disease, as confirmed at 4-week follow-up	Disappearance of all disease, as confirmed at 4-week follow-up
PR	50% decrease or more in the sum of the cross products of measurable disease, as confirmed at 4 weeks	30% decrease or more in the sum of the maximal diameters of measurable disease, as confirmed at 4 weeks
SD	Neither PR nor PD	Neither PR nor PD
PD	25% increase or more in the sum of the cross products or in a single lesion, or presence of new disease	20% increase or more in the sum of the maximal diameters of measurable disease, or presence of new disease

CR, complete response; PR, partial response; SD, stable disease; PD, progressive disease; RECIST, Response Evaluation Criteria in Solid Tumors; WHO, World Health Organization.

response to treatment. The committee then published a new guideline for the response assessment in solid tumors based on a thorough, retrospective review of collaborative studies in 2000 (23). Their recommendations included simplifying tumor size measurement by only measuring the greatest diameter (unidimensional measurement) and then using of the sum of the greatest diameters rather than the sum of the cross products to quantify tumor change on serial examinations. These new criteria became known as RECIST 1.0 (Table 28.1) and were guided by several important principles: (a) the need to maintain the standard four categories of response assessment (CR, PR, SD, PD), (b) the goal of maintaining constancy of results such that no major discrepancy in the meaning of partial response would exist between the older WHO criteria and the new criteria, (c) the recognition of both the arbitrary nature of the cutoff for PR and the need to maintain this cutoff until other potentially more reliable or powerful surrogates could be developed, (d) concern about categorizing patients as PD too easily, and (e) recognition that cytostatic agents may not have the same measurement *activity* and that other serum markers and specific tumors may present unique challenges.

After about a decade's practice, partially based on the analyses of data collected from 16 clinical trials, the RECIST Working Group published a revised version of RECIST 1.0 (i.e., RECIST 1.1) in 2009 (24). The significant changes in RECIST 1.1 guidelines include (a) reduction in the maximal number of target lesions (up to five lesions per patient and two lesions per organ), (b) new rules for measuring lymph nodes, (c) an extended definition of PD, (d) new criteria for selecting bone lesions and cysts as target lesions, and (e) inclusion of PET findings for assessing tumor response.

Lugano and Lyric Criteria for Lymphoma

Lymphoma, unlike the most solid tumors, is a type of cancer that usually resides in the normal structure of the lymph nodes. Conventional response criteria, when applied to lymphoma clinical trials, have encountered difficulties, particularly in classifying CR and PR, because of the size variation of the *normal* lymph nodes and posttreatment residual masses that often consist of nontumor components such as fibrosis, necrosis, or inflammation, which can be indistinguishable from tumors. A study showed that changing definitions of the normal node size from 1 cm × 1 cm to 1.5 cm × 1.5 cm (the same as to 2 cm × 2 cm) had significantly affected the CR rates in a rituximab trial (30).

The initial published response assessment criteria for both non-Hodgkin's lymphoma (NHL) and Hodgkin's lymphoma (HL) were published in 1999 by the National Cancer Institute Working Group (31), which were updated in 2007 by the International Working Group (IWG) to incorporate PET as well as bone marrow immunohistochemistry and flow cytometry in response assessment (Table 28.2)(32). Subsequent to working with these

criteria for a number of years and with more experience in imaging, the criteria were further refined into the Lugano criteria. The Lugano criteria use a five-point scale for assessing PET–CT scans in both an interim analysis and end-of-treatment assessment. A score of 1 or 2 is a complete metabolic response at interim and end of treatment. An interpretation of a score of 3 is somewhat variable depending upon the timing of assessment, the clinical context, and the treatment. A score of 4 or 5 at interim suggests chemotherapy-sensitive disease only if uptake has reduced from baseline, and is considered to represent partial metabolic response. At the end of treatment, however, a score of 4 or 5 represents treatment failure even if uptake has reduced from baseline. Finally, a score of 4 or 5 with intensity that does not change or increases compared to baseline represents treatment failure both at interim and at the end-of-treatment assessment (33).

18F-FDG PET Response Criteria

To ensure the quality of tumor PET imaging and compare PET findings reported from multicenter trials, a standardization was necessary regarding ^{18}F-FDG PET imaging technique/protocol and response criteria for clinical trials. Such standardization is imperative given the number of factors associated with this technology that can influence FDG uptake measurement and thus response assessment. In 1999, after having reviewed the status of the technique, the EORTC PET study group proposed and published the first recommendation for common measurement standards and criteria while reporting changes in ^{18}F-FDG uptake to assess clinical and subclinical responses to anticancer treatment (25). The guidelines made recommendations on patient preparation, timing of PET scan, attenuation correction, ^{18}F-FDG dose, ^{18}F-FDG uptake measurement methodology, tumor sampling, measurement reproducibility, and definition of a metabolic response. In parallel to the RECIST criteria, the EORTC criteria also use four categories (i.e., metabolic progressive disease, stable disease, partial response, and complete response) to define the metabolic response and progression based on percentage change of the ^{18}F-FDG uptake (Table 28.3). The EORTC criteria have served as the guidelines for monitoring tumor response in early-phase clinical trials using ^{18}F-FDG PET as a surrogate biomarker.

With increasing use of ^{18}F-FDG PET in oncology practice over recent years, significantly more experience has been gained with the modality. In 2005, the Cancer Imaging Program of the NCI of the United States convened a workshop and reviewed the latest progress regarding ^{18}F-FDG PET in both diagnosis and response assessment. Out of the workshop came revised and refined consensus recommendations, which were published in 2006 (26). These recommendations will be used to design and guide the ever-growing number of NCI-sponsored clinical trials utilizing ^{18}F-FDG PET as an indicator of therapeutic response (34).

TABLE 28.2 Response Criteria for Lymphoma

Response	Definition	Nodal Masses	Spleen Liver
Complete Response (CR)	Disappearance of all disease	1. PET positive prior to therapy; mass of any size permitted if PET negative 2. Variably positive or PET negative; regression to normal size on CT	Not Palpable, not disappeared
Partial Response (PR)	Regression of measurable disease and no new disease	1. ≥50% decrease in SPD of up to 6 largest masses; no increase in size of the other nodes 2. PET positive prior to therapy; one or more PET positive at previously involved site 3. Variably positive or PET negative; regression on CT	≥50% decrease in SPD of nodules; no increase in size of liver or spleen
Stable Disease (SD)	No evidence of CR/PR and no PD	1. FDG-avid or PET positive prior to therapy; PET positive at prior sites of disease and no new sites on CT or PET 2. Variably FDG-avid or PET negative, no change in size of previous lesions on CT	
Relapsed Disease (PD)	Any new lesion or increase by ≥50% of previously involved lesions from nadir	Appearance of a new lesion >1.5 cm, ≥50% increase in SPD of more than one node, or ≥50% increase in longest diameter of a previously identified node >1 cm in short axis Lesions PET positive if PET-avid lymphoma or PET positive prior to therapy	≥50% increase from nadir in the SPD of any previous lesions

FDG, [18F]fluorodeoxyglucose; SPD, sum of the product of the diameters.

TABLE 28.3 EORTC Response Criteria

Response Category	Definition
PMD	25% increase or more in tumor 18F-FDG SUV, visible increase in the extent of 18F-FDG tumor uptake (20% or more in the longest diameter) or appearance of new 18F-FDG uptake in metastatic lesions
SMD	Neither PMR nor PMD
PMR	15% reduction or more in tumor 18F-FDG SUV after one cycle of chemotherapy and 25% reduction or more after more than one treatment cycle
CMR	Complete resolution of 18F-FDG uptake within the tumor volume

CMR, complete metabolic response; 18F-FDG, fluorine-18-fluorodeoxyglucose; PMD, progressive metabolic disease; PMR, partial metabolic response; SMD, stable metabolic disease; SUV, standard uptake value.

Source: From Young H, Baum R, Cremerius U, et al. Measurement of clinical and subclinical tumour response using [18F]-fluorodeoxyglucose and positron emission tomography: review and 1999 EORTC recommendations. *Eur J Cancer.* 1999;35:1773–1782. Copyright 1999, with permission from Elsevier.

PERCIST

It has been recognized that PET assessment of response with 18F-FDG has true biologic meaning when obtained at the end of a patient's treatment, in the middle of treatment, and sometimes even soon after treatment is initiated. To further clarify PET response criteria, a new set of rules were devised known as Positron Emission tomography Response Criteria In Solid Tumors (PERCIST) (35). In PERCIST, a response to therapy is assessed as a continuous variable and recorded as percentage change in SUL (SUV corrected for lean body mass) peak between the pre- and posttreatment scans. A complete PERCIST metabolic response is considered the visual disappearance of all metabolically active tumors. A partial PERCIST response is defined by a greater than 30% and 0.8-unit decline in SUL peak between the most intense lesion before treatment and the most intense lesion after treatment. More than a 30% and 0.8-unit increase in SUL peak or the appearance of new lesions, if confirmed, is classified as PD. A greater than 75% increase in total lesion glycolysis is also considered another quantitative measure of disease progression.

DCE-MRI Response Criteria

In recent years, DCE-MRI parameters are increasingly being used as endpoints in assessing vascular response in early-phase clinical trials evaluating antiangiogenic and antivascular agents. Because of the technical complexity, disease heterogeneity, and nonlinear relationships between the derived response parameters (e.g., K^{trans}) and physiological processes, DCE-MRI readouts can have considerable variability among studies and need to be interpreted carefully. Over the past several years, consensus recommendations for the design and analysis of clinical trials that incorporate DCE-MRI investigations have been outlined by specialist panels in the United Kingdom and the United States and are being increasingly used for the development and validation of the DCE-MRI technique as a surrogate imaging biomarker in early clinical trials (27–29). The recommendations have mainly focused on the following issues: imaging protocol, measurement methodology, primary and secondary endpoints, trial design, pharmacokinetic models, data analysis, measurement reproducibility, and future developments. The parameter K^{trans} is commonly used as the primary endpoint in early-phase clinical trials and a change (i.e., decrease) in K^{trans} >40% is considered as response (36,37). DCE-MRI as used in the assessment of therapy response is still in its infancy and intensive investigations are under way.

RADIOMICS—AN EMERGING TECHNOLOGY

Recently, radiogenomics/radiomics has emerged as an exciting field of cancer research. Radiogenomics refers to the relationship between the imaging characteristics of a tumor (a.k.a. its imaging phenotype) and its gene expression profile, gene mutation profile, and other genome-related characteristics (38,39). Radiomics refers to the determination of tumor phenotypes by analysis of a large number of quantitative image features (radiomic features) (40–42). Unlike molecular- and tissue-based analyses, radiomics characterizes differences in tumor phenotype based on noninvasive radiographic imaging that can be obtained from clinical practice and clinical trials at almost no additional cost. Radiomics can capture the heterogeneity of a whole tumor and of tumor metastases in multiple body sites, and can be used to characterize tumor heterogeneity before treatment initiation and monitor changes in tumor biology (e.g., in mutation status) over time. Preliminary data shows the potential of radiomics-based phenotypes to improve the stratification and response assessment between EGFR positive and wild-type patient populations in NSCLC (43). Radiomics is expected to add a new dimension to the precision medicine paradigm by developing image-based textural and morphologic biomarkers to advance cancer diagnosis and prognosis, and for the prediction and assessment of response to therapy.

SOURCES OF VARIABILITY

Quantitative imaging response assessments are based on measured changes in tumor size, metabolism, or vascularity on serial examinations. A measured tumor change, however, consists of the real tumor change (if the tumor has in fact changed) and measurement variations. Although each type of imaging modality has its own sources of variability, in general, variations arise during the procedures of image acquisition and tumor measurement. In addition, patient weight loss/tumor change during therapy can also introduce measurement variation.

Variations in tumor size measurement on serial CT scans can be caused by nonuniform imaging techniques (e.g., contrast-enhanced images acquired at different phases), inconsistent imaging parameters (e.g., slice thickness, image reconstruction algorithm), repeat CT scans, and different measurement tools (e.g., manual measurement, computer software). Over the past few years a number of studies have begun to reveal the magnitude of variability in the measurement of tumor diameter and volume, as well as the resulting variability in radiomic feature output (Figure 28.4) (44–52). Such information is vitally important in guiding not only the reevaluation of conventional response assessment criteria but also in establishing response guidelines for new imaging biomarkers such as tumor volume.

Change in ^{18}F-FDG uptake measured on PET represents a complex biological process, though it is linked to the alteration of tumor's proliferative activity. Sources of variability in the uptake measurement include chemosensitivity of the tumor to the drug, blood glucose level of patient, overall body weight and tumor size, fasting time before the PET scan, the dose of ^{18}F-FDG injected, time between tracer injection and the start of scanning, image reconstruction algorithm, data analysis software, chosen method for measurement of ^{18}F-FDG uptake, and selection of tumor regions of interest (ROIs) (25,26).

Interpretation of tumor perfusion through pharmacokinetic analyses of DCE-MRI is complicated and subject to variations because of the dynamic acquisition procedure, different kinetic models, and data analysis based on a human defined ROI (or volume of interest [VOI]). There are a number of other factors as well that can bring variations into the measurement of response parameters and affect the DCE-MRI outcomes. These factors include, but are not limited to, imaging technique/protocol, injection of contrast medium bolus, heterogeneous physiologies of tumors and their reactions to agents, selection of the kinetic models, measurement of arterial input function (AIF), and tumor ROI placement (28,29).

COMPUTER-AIDED RESPONSE ASSESSMENT

Quantitative imaging biomarkers can be either manually measured by the radiologist (e.g., tumor diameter)

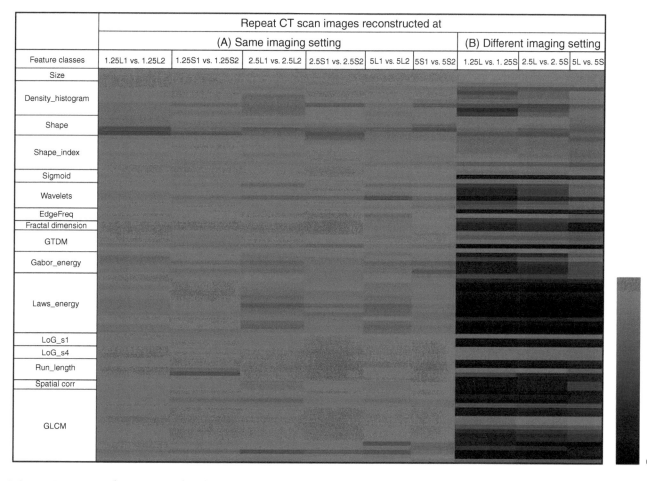

FIGURE 28.4 CCC heat map of radiomic features. The CCCs (0–1) of the studied radiomic features were computed from the same-day repeat CT images reconstructed at (**a**) six identical imaging settings or (**b**) three different imaging settings. There were 89 quantitative features grouped into 15 feature classes. The brighter the red color, the higher the CCC value (i.e., the more reproducibility) of a feature computed for the repeat scans. The label of "1.25L1 vs 1.25L2" means both first and second scans were reconstructed at 1.25 mm slice thickness using the lung algorithm. "2.5L vs 2.5S" means both scans were reconstructed at 2.5 mm slice thickness but using different algorithms (i.e., lung vs. standard algorithms).

CCC, concordance correlation coeefficient.

Source: From Zhao B, Tan, Y, Qi J, et al. Reproducibility of radiomics for deciphering tumor phenotype with imaging. *Nat Sci Rep.* 2016;6;23428.

or calculated with the help of computer modeling (e.g., K^{trans}). Manual measurement is prone to subject error and oftentimes a lack of reproducibility. Moreover, tumor volume—an accurate measure of tumor burden—will be extremely time-consuming and impractical if obtained manually. Computer algorithms, as anticipated, will play an important role in providing accurate and reproducible measurements of radiomic features including volume measurements.

Contemporary imaging viewing workstations with powerful manipulation, measurement, and analysis tools provided by either medical imaging equipment companies or software application vendors have been assisting radiologists and other physicians in efficient and accurate image interpretations for more than a decade. In the field of quantitative imaging response assessment, increasing numbers of diversified and robust

image processing methods are expected to be developed for automated/semiautomated segmentation, quantification, and change analysis. Such software packages can be used either in a stand-alone mode, as additional modules to be integrated into the existing diagnostic workstations, or as a web-based system. Successful development of computer software tools would ensure the successful development and qualification of both new and preexisting quantitative imaging metrics as surrogate imaging biomarkers for the prediction and assessment of tumor therapeutic response for an ever-increasing number of future clinical trials as well as routine clinical practice.

SUMMARY

Drug mechanisms of action and cancer type and staging are playing a key role in the selection of appropriate imaging modality or combination of multiple imaging modalities for the prediction and assessment of tumor response to therapy in clinical trials. Image acquisition protocol needs to be defined before a trial starts and followed strictly throughout the trial in order to minimize possible measurement inconsistency caused by varying image acquisition techniques and parameters. A general principle to follow in the imaging of response assessment is that any subsequent follow-up examinations should be performed with the same modality and either the same or equivalent imaging technique and parameters. In this manner, accurate comparison of tumor changes over time is possible and significantly more meaningful. The introduction of new modalities or imaging of new body sites should be performed, however, if there are questions left unanswered by the initial imaging, or if new clinical symptoms should manifest. Increasingly, radiologists are also asked to participate in clinical investigations or trials involving novel imaging or therapeutic agents in order to assess their efficacy. In the years to come, advanced computer software for automated or semiautomated quantification of baseline tumor phenotype as well as phenotypic changes with therapy are expected to be developed, validated, and applied to further clinical trials. New software will assist in the development and qualification of advanced imaging biomarkers as predictors for response to targeted therapies and as surrogate endpoints during treatment for clinical trials, especially early-phase clinical trials evaluating novel anticancer agents. General guidelines regarding good clinical practice are appropriate in these investigations as well, and at present the greatest differences lie in the degree of quantification for clinical investigational studies as well as in documentation of the findings. Several consensus recommendations with regard to trial design, response assessment methodology and criteria, quality control, and outcome analysis have been proposed for different imaging modalities to guide ongoing and future clinical trials. Ultimately, individual patient care and overall accurate interpretation of the imaging findings is paramount, whether in a routine case or in one involving a clinical investigation.

REFERENCES

1. Ollivier L, Husband JE, Leclere J. Chapter 6. Assessment of response to treatment. In: Husband JH Reznek RH, eds. *Imaging in Oncology*. 3rd edn. P50-61. Taylor and Francis; 2009.
2. Higashi K, Clavo AC, Wahl RL. Does FDG uptake measure proliferative activity of human cancer cells? *In vitro* comparison with DNA flow cytometry and tritiated thymidine uptake. *J Nucl Med*. 1993;34:414–419.
3. Minn H, Joensuu H, Ahonen A, et al. Fluorodeoxyglucose imaging: a method to assess the proliferative activity of human cancer in vivo. *Cancer*. 1988;61:1776–1781.
4. Vesselle H, Grierson J, Muzi M, et al. In vivo validation of 3'deoxy-3'-[(18)F]fluorothymidine ([(18)F]FLT) as a proliferation imaging tracer in humans: correlation of [(18)F]FLT uptake by positron emission tomography with Ki-67 immunohistochemistry and flow cytometry in human lung tumors. *Clin Cancer Res*. 2002;8:3315–3323.
5. van Westreenen HL, Cobben DC, Jager PL, et al. Comparison of 18F-FLT PET and 18F-FDG PET in esophageal cancer. *J Nucl Med*. 2005;46:400–404.
6. Chen W, Cloughesy T, Kamdar N, et al. Imaging proliferation in brain tumors with 18F-FLT PET: comparison with 18F-FDG. *J Nucl Med*. 2005;46:945–952.
7. Tofts PS, Brix G, Buckley DL, et al. Estimating kinetic parameters from dynamic contrast-enhanced T(1)-weighted MRI of a diffusible tracer: standardized quantities and symbols. *J Magn Reson Imaging*. 1999;10:223–232.
8. Morgan B, Thomas AL, Drevs J, et al. Dynamic contrast-enhanced magnetic resonance imaging as a biomarker for the pharmacological response of PTK787/ZK222584, an inhibitor of the vascular endothelial growth factor receptor tyrosine kinases, in patients with advanced colorectal cancer and liver metastases. *J Clin Oncol*. 2003;21:3955–3964.
9. Lordick F, Ott K, Krause B, et al. PET to assess early metabolic response and to guide treatment of adenocarcinoma of the oesophagogastric junction: the MUNICON Phase II trial. *Lancet Oncol*. 2007;8:797–805.
10. de Geus-Oei LF, van der Heijden HFM, Corstens FHM, et al. Predictive and prognostic value of FDG-PET in NSCLC: a systematic review. *Cancer*. 2007;110:1654–1664.
11. Biomarkers Definitions Working Group. Biomarkers and surrogate endpoints: preferred definitions and conceptual frame work. *Clin Pharmacol Ther*. 2001;69:90–95.
12. Zhao B, Oxnard GR, Moskowitz CS, et al. A pilot study of volume measurement as a method of tumor response evaluation to aid biomarker development. *Clin Cancer Res*. 2010;16:4647–4653.
13. Herhole K, Rudolf J, Heiss WD. FDG transport and phosphorylation in human gliomas measured with dynamic PET. *J Neuro Oncol*. 1992;12:159–165.
14. Duhaylongsod FG, Lowe VJ, Patz EF, et al. Lung tumor growth with glucose metabolism measured by fluoride-18 fluorodeoxyglucose positron emission tomography. *Ann Thorac Surg*. 1995;60:1348–1352.
15. Larson SM, Erdi Y, Akhurst T, et al. Tumor treatment response based on visual and quantitative changes in global tumor glycolysis using PET-FDG imaging. The visual response score and the change in total lesion glycolysis. *Clin Positron Imaging*. 1999;2:159–171.
16. Hoekstra CJ, Paglianiti I, Hoekstra OS, et al. Monitoring response to therapy in cancer using [18F]-2-fluoro-2-deoxy-D- glucose and positron emission tomography: an overview of different analytical methods. *Eur J Nucl Med*. 2000;27:731–743.
17. Riely GJ, Kris MG, Zhao B, et al. Prospective assessment of discontinuation and re-initiation of erlotinib or gefitinib in patients with acquired resistance to erlotinib or gefitinib followed by the addition of everolimus. *Clin Cancer Res*. 2007;13:5150–5155.
18. Collins DJ, Padhani AR. Dynamic magnetic resonance imaging of tumour perfusion. *IEEE Eng Med Biol Mag*. 2004;23: 65–83.
19. Johnson KR, Ringland C, Stokes BJ, et al. Response rate or time to progression as predictors of survival in trials of metastatic colorectal cancer or non-small-cell lung cancer: a meta-analysis. *Lancet Oncol*. 2006;7:741–746.
20. Sullivan D, Schwartz L, Zhao B. Progression-free survival as an endpoint in solid tumors. The imaging viewpoint: how imaging affects determination of progression-free survival. *Clin Cancer Res*. 2013;19(10):2621–2628.
21. World Health Organization. WHO handbook for reporting results of cancer treatment. Geneva, Switzerland: Author; 1979.
22. Miller AB, Hogestraeten B, Staquet M, et al: Reporting results of cancer treatment. *Cancer*. 1081;47:207–214.

23. Therasse P, Arbuck SG, Eisenhauer EA, et al. New guidelines to evaluate response to treatment in solid tumors. *J Natl Cancer Inst.* 2000;92:205–216.

24. Eisenhauer EA, Therasse P, Boqaerts J, et al. New response evaluation criteria in solid tumours: revised RECIST guideline (version 1.1). *Eur J Cancer.* 2009; 45:228–247.

25. Young H, Baum R, Cremerius U, et al. Measurement of clinical and subclinical tumour response using [18F]-fluorodeoxyglucose and positron emission tomography: review and 1999 EORTC recommendations. *Eur J Cancer.* 1999;35:1773–1782.

26. Shankar LK, Hoffman JM, Bacharach S, et al. Guidelines for the use of 18FDG-PET as an indicator of therapeutic response in patients in National Cancer Institute trials. *J Nucl Med.* 2006;47:1059–1066.

27. Leach MO, Brindle KM, Evelhoch JL, et al. Assessment of antiangiogenic and antivascular therapeutics using MRI: recommendations for appropriate methodology for clinical trials. *Br J Radiol.* 2003;76(Suppl 1):S87–S91.

28. Leach MO, Brindle KM, Evelhoch J, et al. The assessment of antiangiogenic and antivascular therapies in early-stage clinical trials using magnetic resonance imaging: issues and recommendations. *Br J Cancer.* 2005;92:1599–1610.

29. Evelhoch J, Garwood M, Vigneron D, et al. Expandingthe use of magnetic resonance in the assessment of tumor response to therapy: workshop report. *Cancer Res.* 2005;65:7041–7044.

30. Grillo-Lopez AJ, Cheson BD, Horning SJ, et al. Response criteria for NHL: importance of "normal" lymph node size and correlations with response rates. *Ann Oncol.* 2000;11:399–408.

31. Cheson BD, Horning SJ, Coiffier B, et al. Report of an International Workshop to standardize response criteria for non-Hodgkin's lymphomas: NCI Sponsored International Working Group. *J Clin Oncol.* 1999;17:1244–1253.

32. Cheson BD, Pfistner B, Juweid ME, et al. Revised response criteria for malignant lymphoma. *J Clin Oncol.* 2007;25:579–586.

33. Cheson BD, Fisher RI, Barrington SF, et al. Recommendations for initial evaluation, staging, and response assessment of Hodgkin and non-Hodgkin lymphoma: the Lugano classification. *J Clin Oncol.* 2014;20;3059–3068.

34. Larson SM, Schwartz L. 18F-FDG PET as a candidate for "qualified biomarker": functional assessment of treatment response in oncology. *J Nucl Med.* 2006;47:901–903.

35. Wahl RL, Jacene H, Kasamon Y, et al. From RECIST to PERCIST: evolving Considerations for PET response criteria in solid tumors. *J Nucl Med.* 2009;50(Suppl 1):122S–125OS.

36. Galbraith SM, Lodge MA, Taylor NJ, et al. Reproducibility of dynamic contrast-enhanced MRI in human muscle and tumors: comparison of quantitative and semi-quantitative analysis. *NMR Biomed.* 2002;15:132–142.

37. Padhani AR, Hayes C, Landau S, et al. Reproducibility of quan-titative dynamic MRI of normal human tissues. *NMR Biomed.* 2002;15:143–153.

38. Rutman AM, Kuo MD. Radiogenomics: creating a link between molecular diagnostics and diagnostic imaging. *Eur J Radiol.* 2009;70:232–241.

39. Kuo MD, Jamshidi N. Behind the numbers: decoding molecular phenotypes with radiogenomics—guiding principles and technical considerations. *Radiology.* 2014; 270:320–325.

40. Lambin P, Rios-Velazquez E, Leijenaar R, et al. Radiomics: extracting more information from medical images using advanced feature analysis. *Eur J Cancer.* 2012; 48:441–446.

41. Kumar V, Gu Y, Basu S, et al. Radiomics: the process and the challenges. *Magn Reson Imaging.* 2012;30:1234–1248.

42. Aerts HJ, Velazquez ER, Leijenaar RT, et al. Decoding tumour phenotype by noninvasive imaging using a quantitative radiomics approach. *Nat Commun.* 2014;5:4006.

43. Aerts HJ, Grossmann P, Tan Y, et al. Defining a Radiomic Response Phenotype: A Pilot Study using TKI therapy in NSCLC. *Nat Sci Rep.* 2016;6;33860.

44. Erasmus JJ, Gladish GW, Broemeling L, et al. Interobserver and intraobserver variability in measurement of non-small-cell carcinoma lung lesions: implications for assessment of tumor response. *J Clin Oncol.* 2003;21:2574–2582.

45. Wormanns D, Kohl G, Klotz E, et al. Volumetric measurements of pulmonary nodules at multi-row detector CT: in vivo reproducibility. *Eur Radiol.* 2004;14:86–92.

46. Goodman LR, Gulsun M, Washington L, et al. Inherent variability of CT lung nodule measurements in vivo using semiautomated volumetric measurements. *Am J Roentgenol.* 2006;186:989–994.

47. Zhao B, James LP, Moskowitz C, et al. Evaluating variability in tumor measurements from same-day repeat CT scans in patients with non-small cell lung cancer. *Radiology.* 2009;252:263–272.

48. Oxnard GR, Zhao B, Sima CS, et al. Variability of lung tumor measurements on repeat computed tomography (CT) scans taken within 15 minutes: implications for care and clinical research. *J Clin Oncol.* 2011;29:3114-9.

49. Tan Y, Mann H, Guo P, et al. Assessing the effect of computed tomographic (CT) slice thickness on unidimensional (1D), bidimensional (2D) and volumetric measurements of solid tumors. *Cancer Imaging.* 2012;12:497–505.

50. Zhao B, Tan Y, Bell DJ, et al. Exploring manual and computer-aided intra- and inter-reader variability in tumor unidimensional (1D), bidimensional (2D) and volumetric measurements. *Eur J Radiology.* 2013;82:959–968.

51. Zhao B, Lee S, Lee HJ, et al. Variability in assessing treatment response: metastatic colorectal cancer as a paradigm. *Clin Cancer Res.* 2014; 20:3560–3568.

52. Zhao B, Tan, Y, Qi J, et al. Reproducibility of radiomics for deciphering tumor phenotype with imaging. *Nat Sci Rep.* 2016;6;23428.

29

Practical Issues With Correlative Studies

David McConkey and Woonyoung Choi

As genomics are more widely integrated into clinical trials and the routine clinical management of patients with cancer, the practical issues related to genomics platforms are taking on more significance. Formalin-fixed, paraffin-embedded (FFPE) tissues represent both the greatest opportunity but also the greatest challenge in integrating sophisticated analyses into clinical trials. Advances in next-generation sequencing technology have made DNA panel and whole-exome sequencing (WES) highly feasible, but the accuracy of tumor exome sequencing is greatly enhanced by the availability of germ-line data, which requires special consent that needs to be integrated prospectively into clinical protocols. Isolated ribonucleic acid (RNA) from FFPE tissues is too fragmented for the conventional RNA sequencing platforms that are used on high-quality flash-frozen tissues (such as those utilized by The Cancer Genome Atlas [TCGA]), but several new platforms have been developed that can generate high-quality RNA expression data from this material. Each is associated with distinct strengths and weaknesses that make each more or less appropriate for particular applications, but few cross-platform comparisons have been performed to determine the level of concordance in the results generated by them. In this chapter, we discuss these and other practical issues associated with correlative studies in cancer clinical trials.

As next-generation sequencing technologies have become more and more accessible and affordable, the number of opportunities to perform high-quality correlative studies within the context of cancer clinical trials has increased dramatically. The National Clinical Trials Network (NCTN) has established a process to broaden access to tissues whereby investigators can submit proposals to use archived tissue collected within the context of completed NCTN clinical trials to study validated biomarkers and biomarker panels (https://cgb.cancer.gov/access/scientific.review.html), and the National Cancer Institute (NCI) has established the Biomarker, Imaging and Quality of Life Studies Funding Program (BIQSFP), which can be used to offset the costs of integral or integrated translational medicine studies within ongoing NCTN trials (www.cancer.gov/about-nci/organization/ccct/funding/biqsfp). Even though high-throughput technologies have created increases in the number and quality of companion biomarker studies in clinical trials, they have also helped to underscore some very important practical issues that can pose challenges for the quality and robustness of the data obtained in these studies and the biological conclusions that are based on these data. The overall purpose of this chapter is to highlight some of the more important among these challenges and to provide possible solutions to them. However, the field is moving rapidly, so every year brings with it a new set of specific opportunities and challenges. In particular, methods for measuring various endpoints in metabolism and for quantifying protein expression on microscope slides or in fixed tissue extracts are being developed particularly aggressively, and they will bring new sets of challenges that can mostly only be identified by more widespread use of them. Therefore, this chapter focuses on nucleic acid (and particularly RNA-based) measurements, where enough experience is already available to generate some fairly firm conclusions.

CHALLENGE #1: TUMOR HETEROGENEITY

The idea that cancers are highly heterogeneous has been popular for decades, but whole-genome approaches have made it possible to visualize heterogeneity with very high resolution. Recent studies employing conventional and single-cell next-generation DNA sequencing approaches on different regions (1) and/or cellular subpopulations (2,3) within primary tumors and metastases (4,5) have provided particularly strong experimental support for the concept. Although these studies have generally inferred the existence of a clonal progenitor, subsequent genomic changes cause biologically significant tumor subclones with different properties to emerge. Conventional systemic therapies (4,6) and immunotherapies (7,8) also have important effects, driving both clonal evolution and reversible (mRNA-level) changes in tumor biology. Stromal cells, including immune cells and fibroblasts, play critical roles in tumor progression and response to therapy (8,9), but their presence or absence is not necessarily a stable property of tumors, and their relative abundances can change dramatically in response to signals from the tumor microenvironment. Finally, evidence is emerging to support the widely held view that even localized cancer is a systemic disease that is influenced by physiological signals controlled by metabolism and the microbiome (10). Therefore, it is challenging to ascribe specific biological characteristics to bulk tumor populations, since rates of tumor progression (tied to prognosis) and therapeutic outcomes can be more tightly linked to specific tumor subclones that represent minor fractions of the primary tumor and variable effects of the host and tumor microenvironment. In situ techniques such as immunohistochemistry and RNA in situ hybridization (11,12) have the power to visualize heterogeneity at the single-cell level, albeit at the cost of high content. Ultimately noninvasive imaging strategies with single-cell resolution could potentially be developed to comprehensively visualize heterogeneity at the whole-organism level, but these technologies are obviously not available at present.

It is envisioned that robust methods for performing single-cell whole-exome DNA or whole-transcriptome RNA sequencing on conventional FFPE tissues will emerge in the next few years. For now, these methods require sorting and capturing single cells or nuclei isolated from fresh tissues (3), and they possess some technical limitations, particularly for detecting poly(A)-negative and low abundance transcripts (13,14), which makes it very challenging to incorporate these technologies into clinical trials, especially those performed at multiple centers. Feasibility could be increased by using circulating tumor cells rather than disaggregated fresh primary tumors as the starting material, but assumptions about molecular phenotypes must be made in capturing circulating tumor cells and/or identifying them. There is also a tendency to assume that systemic tumor heterogeneity is comprehensively captured in circulating tumor cells, which may or may not be true. Similarly, mutations and fusions can be measured in the cell-free/circulating tumor (cf/ctDNA) that can be collected from the peripheral blood, urine, and other body fluids (15,16), but whether or not all of the important DNA alterations that drive tumor progression and response/resistance to therapy are present in these fluids is still unclear, and although they are improving, there are limits to the sensitivities of these assays to detect rare variants. In addition, it is not possible to determine which of the observed DNA alterations occur together in tumor subclones, which could have very important implications for deploying targeted agents that possess synergistic antitumor activities. It is possible that methods for sorting extracellular vesicles (exosomes) could be developed and applied for this purpose, but these methods are not available at present.

Immunotherapies bring the issue of stromal instability and intertumoral heterogeneity to the forefront because they are designed to target stromal cells. Studies have consistently demonstrated that the levels of PD-1 and PD-L1 on tumor and/or tumor-infiltrating stromal cells correlate significantly with clinical benefit from blocking anti-PD1 or –PDL1 antibodies (8), but the predictive power of PD-1 or PD-L1 expression is limited, presumably because their expression is dynamic and the cells that express them enter or exit tumors in response to environmental cues. Likewise, although DNA mutational load, which is at least temporarily hardwired into tumors, is associated with response (8), many tumors with high mutation loads fail to respond and some tumors with low mutation loads do, indicating that other mechanisms contribute to sensitivity and resistance. Finally, although RNA sequencing studies have demonstrated that specific immune signatures are associated with response or resistance to immunotherapy (17), these signatures are often linked to the actions of cytokines (IFNs) or other signal transduction pathways (Wnt, etc.) (18) that are controlled by dynamic tumor–stromal interactions, reinforcing the idea that environmental signals play important roles. Protein biomarkers associated with activated signal transduction pathways (i.e., phosphorylated signal transduction intermediates), hypoxia/angiogenesis, and proliferation can also display marked locoregional heterogeneity. For example, past studies have established that biomarkers associated with proliferation and angiogenesis are expressed at higher levels in the tumor periphery as compared with the tumor core (19,20). Aside from locoregional effects, these "reversible" biomarkers also tend to be particularly sensitive to different tissue handling conditions. Overall, biomarkers that measure tumor–stromal interactions and other biological properties that are regulated by the tumor microenvironment are by their very natures likely to be relatively unstable, and dynamic assays are probably necessary to accurately monitor them.

Solutions

There is no way to completely avoid the caveats that are introduced by tumor heterogeneity at present. However, one approach that can be used to minimize its effects is to focus biomarker studies on tumor properties that are more stable. These properties can be identified using bioinformatics tools (i.e., silhouette score analyses), by performing longitudinal studies (i.e., measurements in primary tumors, recurrences, and metastases), and by sampling multiple independent regions of tumors. They include "truncal" driver mutations and copy number variations, the RNA-based gene expression signatures that are associated with them, and tumor molecular subtype membership. These biomarkers are mathematically more stable as compared to biomarkers that change as a function of tumor–stromal interactions and reversible cytoprotective phenotypes associated with responses to stress (i.e., different systemic therapies). Biomarkers that are expressed by the lesion(s) that are clearly linked to disease aggressiveness (i.e., highest grade and/or stage, distant metastasis) are also more likely to be more closely associated with clinical outcomes, but it is expected that effective control of one tumor subclone or phenotype could lead to the evolution and emergence of another. Finally, biomarker panels that measure very general properties (the "hallmarks") of cancers (i.e., proliferation, DNA damage repair, epithelial-to-mesenchymal transition, "stemness," and/or differentiation) are expected to be prognostic and/or predictive regardless of the specific molecular mechanisms that drive cancer initiation and progression. These types of "pan-cancer" biomarkers tend to serve as the foundations for biomarker panels that have survived large validation studies, including the OncotypeDx test for breast cancer and many other panels that were developed to inform cancer prognostication.

CHALLENGE #2: FFPE TISSUES

One of the keys to the success of TCGA projects was that strict metrics were adopted to ensure that the tissues that were used as the starting materials were of optimal quality for nucleic acid and protein extraction. All tumor tissues were flash-frozen within minutes of surgical excision, and tissue sections were carefully reviewed by expert pathologists so that tumors with excessive stromal content or content of variant histopathological features were excluded from downstream analyses. Standard workflows were established for nucleic acid isolation and purification, and isolates that were not of exceptional quality and/or purity were excluded from subsequent analyses. Finally, the sequencing, direct hybridization array, and reverse phase protein array (RPPA) platforms that were included in the projects were selected to be the best available, the assays were run by international experts, and they were changed when better platforms emerged. This attention to quality control produced unsurpassed results.

Unfortunately, it is very difficult, if not impossible, to apply such strict standards to routine clinical tissue collection, in part because pathological assessments are made on FFPE tissue sections, and FFPE blocks are the universal medium for tissue storage. Alternatives to FFPE can be built into clinical trials and other prospective studies as long as these collections do not interfere with clinical management, which now must include preservation of sentinel lesion(s) for future DNA sequencing and/or other CLIA biomarker companion diagnostic tests that would make patients eligible for treatment with certain targeted agents. Many institutions are becoming more protective of blocks as an increasing

number of targeted therapeutic approaches are allocated based on DNA sequencing. Therefore, by definition, studies on flash-frozen or other research-grade tissues are typically not performed on the same tissues that are used for clinical diagnosis and treatment planning and are therefore subject to the caveats introduced by tumor heterogeneity that were discussed earlier. The challenges and costs associated with collecting fresh or flash-frozen tissues are magnified in studies that involve multiple institutions, such as those performed within the context of NCTN trials.

Study feasibility can therefore be increased markedly if tests can be performed on routinely collected tissues, including FFPE tissue and minimally processed blood or urine. For multi-institutional studies feasibility can be increased further if tests can be performed on FFPE slides, scrolls, or cores as opposed to blocks, which enables host institutions to maintain possession of the blocks for future clinical management purposes. Measurements of protein expression by conventional immunohistochemistry or immunofluorescence can be done relatively easily, although these methods are subject to high interoperator and interobserver variability even when they are performed by experts. With the use of locked down protocols and modern image analysis tools, the quantitative robustness of marker measurements can be optimized, although intrinsic vulnerabilities related to nonspecific and background staining and problems with the stability of certain target antigens (particularly posttranslationally modified proteins) present unique challenges for these FFPE-tissue-based studies. Quantification of biomarkers in "liquid biopsies" (serum, plasma, or urine) can also be highly feasible, although each assay usually has its own protocol for preservation of the target molecule(s) that can introduce complexity into the handling of these otherwise routinely collected tissues.

Solutions

Fortunately, methods have been developed that enable whole-exome or -transcriptome analyses to be performed using FFPE tissues as the starting material, and they yield fairly robust results. With regard to DNA analyses, panel exome sequencing of genes that are commonly mutated, amplified, deleted, or fused to other genes has entered CLIA and is now used for routine clinical management, and whole-exome sequencing (with parallel germ-line sequencing of whole-blood DNA) is also highly feasible (21,22). The most important practical issues associated with tumor DNA exome sequencing studies are obtaining adequate consent for parallel germ-line sequencing (required for optimal accuracy) and the fact that different downstream bioinformatics approaches can produce divergent final results. Sharing the raw data for subsequent independent reanalyses by other investigators is therefore critically important so that results can be independently cross-compared by other investigators.

However, obtaining robust RNA expression data is much more challenging because RNA that is isolated from FFPE tissues is highly fragmented. Therefore, quantitative approaches must be capable of producing accurate results from short RNA fragments. Quantitative reverse transcriptase *polymerase chain reaction* (PCR) is usually feasible and sensitive if primer pairs are designed to amplify short transcript segments, but throughput is low, and if conventional (as opposed to digital droplet) PCR is used, it requires a relatively large amount of RNA per target. The NanoString platform is a better alternative (23) if higher data density is desired—off-the-shelf or custom panels can accommodate up to 800 different targets in a single reaction. Precisely what amount of input RNA is required to produce robust results is still a matter of debate among investigators using the platform, but the amount recommended by the manufacturer (100–300 ng, based on RNA quality) is probably higher than necessary. Likewise, even though the manufacturer recommends that RNA integrity be fairly high (>50% of RNA fragments longer than 300 bp; see the following), in unpublished work we and others have found that the platform can generate good results with more highly fragmented samples (<30% greater than 200 bp). The cost per sample (about $300 per sample) and input amount of RNA definitely beats real-time *polymerase chain reaction* (RT-PCR) for larger transcript panels, making NanoString ideal for measuring the expression of genes that are already known to be associated with a particular biological or clinical phenotype. However, if generating data for unbiased discovery purposes is desirable, then even 800 target genes may not be sufficient.

Fortunately, whole-transcriptome expression profiling using FFPE RNA as the starting material is now feasible. The first whole-transcriptome and whole-genome RNA expression profiling platforms that could accommodate highly degraded FFPE RNA were Illumina's cDNA-mediated Annealing, Selection, Extension and Ligation (DASL) platform (24) and the Affymetrix GeneChip array (25). Illumina has since discontinued DASL, but the Affymetrix arrays and the hardware required to analyze them are still available (from Thermo Fisher) and are being used by GenomeDx, ALMAC, and other clinical diagnostic companies to profile tumor transcriptomes in a CLIA environment. More recently, Illumina and Ion Torrent have developed whole-transcriptome RNA sequencing platforms that are compatible with FFPE-derived and other degraded DNA samples (26,27). Illumina's platform, called TruSeq RNA Access, has become the industry standard, and it is now being routinely incorporated into multicenter clinical trials. Ion Torrent's platform, called Ampliseq, is not as popular but possesses some advantages that may make it a better choice in some situations. We have

performed (limited) head-to-head comparisons of RNA Access versus DASL, RNA Access versus Ampliseq, and Ampliseq versus NanoString, and we have observed concordance in the results ($r = 0.5$–0.7), with good agreement in detecting biologically relevant biomarkers.

Historically, RNA quality has been estimated using 28S to 18S ribosomal RNA ratios (an older method) or by quantifying RNA integrity numbers (RINs) using an Agilent Bioanalyzer. However, because FFPE samples are highly fragmented, isolated FFPE RNA is characterized by very low RIN numbers that are not predictive of success when using the NanoString, RNA Access, or Ampliseq platforms. Instead, the relative quality of FFPE-derived RNA is now usually estimated by calculating the fraction of RNA fragments longer than 200 base pairs in length, and the target value for this fraction is usually 30% to 50% (known as the DV_{200}) (28). Like the RIN, this fraction is determined by capillary electrophoresis with an Agilent Bioanalyzer. The 200-base-pair cutoff is important because the total read lengths for Ampliseq and RNA Access are ≥100 base pairs, so shorter fragments cannot be sequenced. Importantly, in our experience the DV_{200} value is not a great predictor of success; we have generated high-quality NanoString and RNAseq data from samples with low DV_{200} values (10%–20%), and we have also had failures with samples that have DV_{200} values above 30%. Low RNA yields (and associated RNA purities) seem to be more closely associated with failures, so the combination of a good yield and a higher DV_{200} value may be a better predictor of outcome.

As introduced earlier, if an RNA-based project is focused on a discrete number of biomarkers, the NanoString platform possesses significant advantages over RNAseq and Affymetrix arrays (23). First and foremost, the platform involves no enzymatic amplification step(s) and can be performed on very crude RNA extracts, so it may be less dependent on RNA purity and artifacts caused by the fixations and handling-associated chemical modifications of RNA. The company still recommends that investigators use pure RNA (an A260/280 ratio of 1.7–2.3 and an A260/230 ratio of 1.8–2.3). Although the company's protocol recommends using 100 to 300 ng of input RNA, investigators have generated excellent results with input levels as low as 10 ng. Finally, the platform requires almost no hands-on preparation time, and the few sample manipulations are extremely simple, so it is easy to imagine how NanoString's biomarker panels could be incorporated into a CLIA environment for routine clinical testing.

Fixation and storage conditions can vary markedly within and especially across institutions. In our experience, the quality of RNA expression results varies more by institution rather than by the age of the source blocks, suggesting that interinstitutional differences in tissue handling contribute substantially to "batch effects." It appears that the time between tissue harvest and fixation in formalin is the most important variable contributing to differences in RNA quality, although surgical ischemic time and other factors probably play important roles as well. In addition, the quality of the RNA that is isolated from FFPE tissues deteriorates as blocks and unstained slides age. This decay seems to be most pronounced within the first few weeks after blocks are cored or cut and then seems to stabilize. Nevertheless, we have performed DASL and RNAseq successfully on RNA harvested from blocks that were over 20 years old, although the quality of the data we generated from these older blocks was significantly lower than we routinely obtain with "younger" samples. Unstained slides may be the most vulnerable, perhaps because they expose nucleic acids to more oxidative damage; once blocks have been cut, it is best to harvest the DNA and RNA as soon as possible, preferably within 1 to 2 weeks, and if this is not possible, slides should be stored in a refrigerator or –20°C freezer. Tissue cores that are left within the coring device and stored at 4°C or –20°C are probably even more stable, but coring blocks is less routine and usually adds cost to a project.

Tissue gene expression patterns in tumors are the sum of gene expression patterns in tumor, stromal, and adjacent normal cells. Therefore, relative tumor cell content should always be evaluated in hematoxylin and eosin (H&E) sections by an expert pathologist, and tumor areas should be marked so that the H&Es can be used as templates for macrodissection of tumor areas from the unstained slides. Ideally, a second H&E should be generated after the unstained slides have been cut to confirm that the bottom of the section still contains tumor. Scanned images of the H&Es should be generated so that independent pathological review can be performed in the future.

Methods are now available to sequentially extract RNA and DNA from the same FFPE tissues. The approach exploits the fact that DNA is more stable than RNA. After tissue deparaffinization, FFPE tissues are incubated in a proteinase K solution; in our experience, the optimal balance between optimization of RNA quality and yield is obtained when tissues are incubated in this solution for 3 hours. Samples are then centrifuged and the supernatants are used in subsequent steps for RNA purification. The pellets still contain significant amounts of DNA, and they can either be stored at –20°C or processed immediately for DNA purification. Our protocol is based on one that was developed jointly by the Southwest Oncology Group's Tissue Bank and Nationwide Children's Hospital and TCGA, and we are happy to provide it to other investigators upon request.

CHALLENGE #3: ASSAY REPRODUCIBILITY AND ROBUSTNESS

Ultimately a biomarker or biomarker panel is only useful as a prognostic and/or predictive tool if multiple replicates of the assay used to measure it generate almost

exactly the same result and it is not particularly sensitive to variability in tissue handling. Even though immuno-histochemistry is a core component of diagnostic pathology, few would argue that it is highly quantitative, and it is surprising how much variation can be generated when a given clinical biomarker test is performed at different institutions and evaluated by different expert pathologists, even when they employ modern quantitative image analyses. The quantitative accuracies of next-generation DNA sequencing technologies tend to be very robust, but the mutation calls generated by them depend on downstream bioinformatics analyses that can vary markedly, and the quality of these calls falls off markedly in tumors with high stromal contents. Furthermore, there is no set standard for what relative fraction of tumor cells that contain the mutation (1,4) (now usually estimated by mutant allele frequencies) is clinically significant. Most of the current clinically available mRNA-based biomarker panels were determined empirically (29), so even the best ones can only estimate risk based on previous experience with large populations of heterogeneous cancers from the same organ site, making single-tumor predictions imperfect. They also tend to be proprietary and tied to a specific measurement platform, making it difficult or impossible to perform independent studies to evaluate their reproducibility.

Solutions

The solutions to this problem are quite straightforward. First, when a new candidate biomarker or biomarker panel is discovered, it helps if the discoverer performs mechanistic studies to determine the biological basis for its association with a given phenotype. A good example of this is the discovery that inactivating ERCC2 mutations are associated with clinical benefit from neoadjuvant cisplatin-based combination chemotherapy in bladder cancer (30); after observing the connection between ERCC2 mutations and cisplatin sensitivity in a retrospective cohort of primary tumors, the group that made the discovery performed mechanistic studies, which demonstrated that the same ERCC2 mutations caused resistance to cisplatin-induced cell death in human bladder cancer cell lines. Second, the robustness of the assay used to measure the biomarker should be evaluated. This can be done by comparing the results obtained with "technical replicates" of the sample (e.g., multiple sections or extracts produced at the same time from the same section of the tumor). The reproducibility of the results should then be determined by having an independent investigator in another laboratory run the same test on the same samples, and positive and negative controls should be incorporated into the workflow. Finally, limits in terms of tissue quality and sample amount must be determined. A truly robust biomarker or biomarker panel should perform well with any reliable assay used to measure it.

The tissues that are collected within the context of clinical trials are precious and should not be used to analyze biomarkers or biomarker panels that are not reproducible and robust. Biomarkers discovered in one retrospective cohort should be validated and locked down in at least one independent cohort prior to being taken forward for the next level of validation in clinical trials. Prior to integrating them into clinical practice, biomarkers should be validated prospectively in a clinical trial—an example of this can be found in the Southwest Oncology Group's CoXEN (S1314) Phase II trial (31), which will prospectively validate the predictive performance of several retrospectively validated biomarkers of response and resistance (including *ERCC2* mutations) in patients receiving neoadjuvant cisplatin-based combination chemotherapy. The mindset in these investigations should be to make every effort to show that the biomarker in question does *not* perform well enough to integrate it into clinical practice—"killing" a biomarker early is the best way to prevent wasting clinical and financial resources (and more importantly, patient lives).

CHALLENGE #4: UNEVEN QUALITY OF CLINICAL ANNOTATION

By definition, correlative studies relate biomarker expression with one or more clinical endpoint(s). Therefore, the final results are equally influenced by the robustness of the biomarker and the quality of the clinical data it is being related to. Generally speaking, the clinical data that are collected within the context of clinical trials (and in particular, Food and Drug Administration [FDA] registration trials) are highly robust, although there are challenges to maintaining the evenness of data quality across institutions in multicenter trials. However, the retrospective studies that biomarker discovery is typically dependent on are extremely vulnerable to inadequate or inaccurate clinical data collection. Unfortunately, even though the quality of tissues and platforms was outstanding, the quality of the clinical data collected within TCGA's projects was not ideal (32). The implementation of electronic medical records should increase the quality of routinely collected clinical data, but the data elements that are routinely collected for clinical management are usually only a minor fraction of what are desired for comprehensive clinical annotation in a research study.

Solution

The best way to ensure robust clinical annotation for future biomarker studies is to collect research data prospectively. Here at Johns Hopkins we have launched a precision medicine initiative in bladder cancer that will involve comprehensive, prospective collection of clinical and genomic data on every patient at every hospital visit. The clinical data are being collected in a REDCap database with fields that were selected in a joint effort between Johns Hopkins and MD Anderson, and tissue derivatives are being logged in OpenSpecimen. The intent is to make all of our data-collection platforms as "industry standard" as possible to allow for open access data sharing with other investigators and institutions. Clearly comprehensive clinical data collection is a moving target; what is considered comprehensive today will probably not be tomorrow. (Similarly, genomic platforms and the quality of the data they produce are also constantly changing.) Therefore, clinical research databases (and technology platforms) must be reevaluated regularly and updated when necessary to ensure that the most robust correlative analyses can be performed.

CONCLUSIONS AND FUTURE DIRECTIONS

Increasingly, high-quality research and biology-based biomarkers are entering our clinical trials, creating more demand for the precious tissues that are collected within them. Therefore, we must devote more effort to defining the technical limits of our measurements and to validating their performance and potential clinical impact prior to incorporating them into these trials. High-quality whole-genome platforms that generate data sets that can subsequently be leveraged by other investigators with different hypotheses are in concept most attractive, but they are also associated with practical issues, including heterogeneity, suboptimal quality of the starting materials, and reproducibility and robustness that must be addressed prior to implementing them. We must also work aggressively to improve the quality of the clinical data we are collecting from patients on- and off-trial, and this effort is challenged by the fact that we may not even be aware of clinical variables that will become highly relevant in the future. Overall, we should be constantly investing effort to improve our technologies and data-collection systems to keep pace with their rapid evolution. We should also continue to work to create data storage platforms that enable more widespread data sharing while preserving the anonymity of the information that is collected.

Looking to the future, it seems clear that the feasibility of incorporating additional high-throughput measurements into our clinical studies is on the near horizon. Examples include proteomics, metabolomics, and analyses of systemic immunity and the microbiome, and approaches need to be developed to make sense of all of these "big" data sets and integrate them with clinical databases. Many institutions and private companies are interested in using supercomputing and machine learning to address this upcoming issue. An important corollary to this exciting opportunity is that it will require massive data storage capacities beyond what we have today; indeed, even the storage of raw next-generation DNA and RNA sequencing data has already become challenging for academic institutions. Government funding for research has become more uncertain, so alternative strategies to raise money for these efforts should be developed. An underappreciated downstream benefit of these "big data" initiatives is that they are already strengthening "team science" collaborative relationships that will create synergies that are not possible when independent investigators work in isolation.

REFERENCES

1. Gerlinger M, Rowan AJ, Horswell S, et al. Intratumor heterogeneity and branched evolution revealed by multiregion sequencing. *N Engl J Med*. 2012;366(10):883–892.
2. Navin N, Kendall J, Troge J, et al. Tumour evolution inferred by single-cell sequencing. *Nature*. 2011;472(7341):90–94.
3. Wang Y, Waters J, Leung ML, et al. Clonal evolution in breast cancer revealed by single nucleus genome sequencing. *Nature*. 2014;512(7513):155–160.
4. Faltas BM, Prandi D, Tagawa ST, et al. Clonal evolution of chemotherapy-resistant urothelial carcinoma. *Nat Genet*. 2016;48(12):1490–1499.
5. Robinson D, Van Allen EM, Wu YM, et al. Integrative clinical genomics of advanced prostate cancer. *Cell*. 2015;161(5):1215–1228.
6. Choi W, Porten S, Kim S, et al. Identification of distinct basal and luminal subtypes of muscle-invasive bladder cancer with different sensitivities to frontline chemotherapy. *Cancer Cell*. 2014;25(2):152–165.
7. Gao J, Shi LZ, Zhao H, et al. Loss of IFN-gamma pathway genes in tumor cells as a mechanism of resistance to anti-CTLA-4 therapy. *Cell*. 2016;167(2):397–404.e9.
8. Sharma P, Hu-Lieskovan S, Wargo JA, Ribas A. Primary, adaptive, and acquired resistance to cancer immunotherapy. *Cell*. 2017;168(4):707–723.
9. Kalluri R. The biology and function of fibroblasts in cancer. *Nat Rev Cancer*. 2016;16(9):582–598.
10. Honda K, Littman DR. The microbiota in adaptive immune homeostasis and disease. *Nature*. 2016;535(7610):75–84.
11. Bingham V, Ong CW, James J, et al. PTEN mRNA detection by chromogenic, RNA in situ technologies: a reliable alternative to PTEN immunohistochemistry. *Hum Pathol*. 2016;47(1):95–103.
12. Yu X, Guo S, Song W, et al. Estrogen receptor alpha (ERalpha) status evaluation using RNAscope in situ hybridization: a reliable and complementary method for IHC in breast cancer tissues. *Hum Pathol*. 2017;61:121–129.
13. Combs PA, Eisen MB. Low-cost, low-input RNA-seq protocols perform nearly as well as high-input protocols. *PeerJ*. 2015;3:e869.
14. Picelli S, Faridani OR, Bjorklund AK, et al. Full-length RNA-seq from single cells using Smart-seq2. *Nat Protoc*. 2014;9(1):171–181.
15. Christensen E, Birkenkamp-Demtroder K, Nordentoft I, et al. Liquid biopsy analysis of FGFR3 and PIK3CA hotspot mutations for disease surveillance in bladder cancer. *Eur Urol*. 2017;71(6):961–969.
16. Birkenkamp-Demtroder K, Nordentoft I, Christensen E, et al. Genomic alterations in Liquid Biopsies from patients with bladder cancer. *Eur Urol*. 2016;70(1):75–82.
17. Rosenberg JE, Hoffman-Censits J, Powles T, et al. Atezolizumab in patients with locally advanced and metastatic urothelial carcinoma who have progressed following treatment with platinum-based chemotherapy: a single-arm, multicentre, Phase 2 trial. *Lancet*. 2016;387(10031):1909–1920.
18. Spranger S, Bao R, Gajewski TF. Melanoma-intrinsic beta-catenin signalling prevents anti-tumour immunity. *Nature*. 2015;523(7559):231–235.
19. Slaton JW, Inoue K, Perrotte P, et al. Expression levels of genes that regulate metastasis and angiogenesis correlate with advanced pathological stage of renal cell carcinoma. *Am J Pathol*. 2001;158(2):735–743.
20. Scheel C, Eaton EN, Li SH, et al. Paracrine and autocrine signals induce and maintain mesenchymal and stem cell states in the breast. *Cell*. 2011;145(6):926–940.
21. Bonfiglio S, Vanni I, Rossella V, et al. Performance comparison of two commercial human whole-exome capture systems on formalin-fixed paraffin-embedded lung adenocarcinoma samples. *BMC Cancer*. 2016;16:692.
22. Carrick DM, Mehaffey MG, Sachs MC, et al. Robustness of next generation sequencing on older formalin-fixed paraffin-embedded tissue. *PLoS One*. 2015;10(7):e0127353.
23. Veldman-Jones MH, Brant R, Rooney C, et al. Evaluating robustness and sensitivity of the NanoString Technologies nCounter platform to enable multiplexed gene expression analysis of clinical samples. *Cancer Res*. 2015;75(13):2587–2593.
24. Mittempergher L, de Ronde JJ, Nieuwland M, et al. Gene expression profiles from formalin fixed paraffin embedded breast cancer tissue are largely comparable to fresh frozen matched tissue. *PLoS One*. 2011;6(2):e17163.
25. Linton K, Hey Y, Dibben S, et al. Methods comparison for high-resolution transcriptional analysis of archival material on Affymetrix Plus 2.0 and Exon 1.0 microarrays. *Biotechniques*. 2009;47(1):587–596.
26. Schuierer S, Carbone W, Knehr J, et al. A comprehensive assessment of RNA-seq protocols for degraded and low-quantity samples. *BMC Genomics*. 2017;18(1):442.
27. Li W, Turner A, Aggarwal P, et al. Comprehensive evaluation of AmpliSeq transcriptome, a novel targeted whole transcriptome RNA sequencing methodology for global gene expression analysis. *BMC Genomics*. 2015;16:1069.
28. Landolt L, Marti HP, Beisland C, et al. RNA extraction for RNA sequencing of archival renal tissues. *Scand J Clin Lab Invest*. 2016;76(5):426–434.
29. Prat A, Ellis MJ, Perou CM. Practical implications of gene-expression-based assays for breast oncologists. *Nat Rev Clin Oncol*. 2011;9(1):48–57.
30. Van Allen EM, Mouw KW, Kim P, et al. Somatic ERCC2 mutations correlate with cisplatin sensitivity in muscle-invasive urothelial carcinoma. *Cancer Discov*. 2014;4(10):1140–1153.
31. Dinney CP, Hansel D, McConkey D, et al. Novel neoadjuvant therapy paradigms for bladder cancer: results from the National Cancer Center Institute Forum. *Urol Oncol*. 2014;32(8):1108–1115.
32. Cancer Genome Atlas Research Network; Weinstein JN, Collisson EA, Mills GB, et al. The cancer genome atlas pan-cancer analysis project. *Nat Genet*. 2013;45(10):1113–1120.

The Development of Companion Diagnostics in Oncology Clinical Trials

Zixuan Wang and Stephen C. Peiper

"Variability is the law of life, and as no two faces are the same, so no two bodies are alike, and no two individuals react alike and behave alike under the abnormal conditions which we know as disease." (1)
—Sir William Osler

OVERVIEW

The current paradigm of personalized medicine is dependent upon precision diagnostics that help to program individualized therapeutic interventions. Simply stated, the goal of personalized medicine is therapy with the highest efficacy and safety. In the past, the goal of accurately characterizing human diseases, perhaps best exemplified in human malignancies, to explain differences in clinical outcomes has been restricted by limitations in the power of resolution of the available tools. The genomic age has provided an armamentarium of powerful technologies that have identified gain-of-function changes in oncogenes that can serve as driver mutations in human tumors and can be used for the interrogation of routinely processed diagnostic tissues in the surgical pathology archive. The abundance of antagonists for activated kinases, notably tyrosine kinase inhibitors (TKI), has led to the importance of molecular diagnostics to detect mutations that sensitize tumors to specific pharmacologic antagonists of activated driver mutations. Precision diagnostics are now positioned to extend from determining the status of signal transduction elements in the tumor to the immunologic context of the tumor and the microenvironment.

The first formally recognized successful molecular target of the "age of molecular medicine" was the amplified HER2 gene, which occurs in up to 30% of breast cancer cases. The finding that a monoclonal antibody to the HER2 receptor inhibited the growth of breast cancer cell lines in vitro led to the development of trastuzumab, a humanized monoclonal antibody for the therapy of patients with metastatic breast cancer overexpressing the HER2 protein. The addition of trastuzumab was found to enhance clinical response rates to cisplatin chemotherapy and to increase the survival of these patients as a single agent (2). These clinical trials were all performed in patients whose tumors had overexpression of HER2, as determined by immunohistochemical (IHC) analysis. Trastuzumab was approved by the Food and Drug Administration (FDA) for the therapy of patients with metastatic breast cancer overexpressing the HER2 protein in September 1998, and the companion diagnostic (CDx) for detection of this status by IHC (Dako) was approved on the same day (3) This is the first FDA-approved CDx test. In the latter clinical trial, patients without amplification of the HER2 gene, determined by fluorescence in situ hybridization (FISH), lacked a response to trastuzumab therapy. The detection of HER2 amplification by FISH (Abbott) was approved by the FDA as a CDx in 1999. Thus, the HER2 amplification that began as a prognostic indicator for a poor clinical outcome evolved to be predictive of responsiveness to a therapeutic agent.

The advent of companion diagnostics represents a critical milestone in the spectrum of precision diagnostics for personalized medicine. A CDx is defined by the FDA as "a medical device that provides information that is essential for the safe and effective use of a corresponding therapeutic product" (4). Companion diagnostics are paired with targeted therapies as tests that are predictive of a clinical response that enhances clinical outcome.

In this chapter multiple clinical trials are presented to illustrate the critical role of CDx in the validation of targeted therapy and provide examples of pitfalls that occur when CDx is not included in clinical trial design. This approach provides a conceptual framework for the coordinated development of novel targeted therapies, informative biomarkers, and, ultimately CDx, as shown in Figure 30.1.

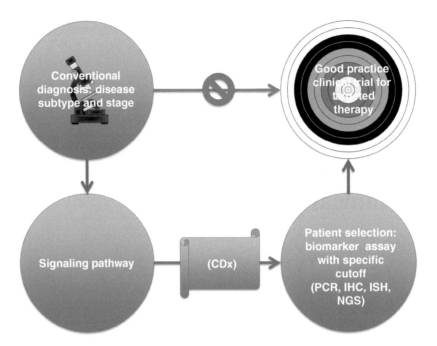

FIGURE 30.1 The critical role of CDx analysis in eligibility for targeted therapy. The power of resolution of histopathologic analysis in precision diagnostics is not sufficient to identify patients who will benefit from molecularly targeted therapies. Molecular analysis using companion diagnostic tests is required to determine eligibility for therapy with these agents.

CDx companion diagnostic; IHC immunohistochemistry; ISH in situ hybridization; NGS next-generation sequencing; PCR polymerase chain reaction.

DEVELOPING A COMPANION DIAGNOSTIC (CDX)

At this time a total of 32 companion diagnostic applications (CDx PMA) have been approved by the FDA for 18 therapeutic agents, among which 17 are antitumor drugs. (5) A summarized list is shown in Table 30.1.

In order to understand the spectrum ranging from therapeutic target identification to biomarker development to the establishment of a prototype laboratory test that serves as a CDx precursor to a mature companion diagnostic approved CDx (or cleared) by the FDA, it is helpful to describe important features of each step in some detail. While a detailed analysis of therapeutic target identification is beyond the scope of this chapter, it is clear that this involves the discovery of cellular pathways that are required to maintain the transformed behavior and viability of malignant cells.

Biomarkers can be generically described as an indicator of a disease process. They are typically the consequence of a fundamental molecular change in cell biology and are measurable. Biomarkers can have multiple applications, including: (a) diagnostic; (b) predictive; (c) prognostic; (d) monitoring disease progression, evolution, relapse/recurrence; (e) monitoring therapy; (f) screening and susceptibility; and (g) prevention. Candidates for use as a CDx should be predictive of the outcome of response to a therapeutic agent. Biomarker identification is the first step of developing a CDx.

As illustrated later in this chapter, CDx candidates may be the precise molecular change that defines the therapeutic target (i.e., amplification of the HER2 gene in breast cancer treated with trastuzumab, tyrosine kinase domain mutations in epidermal growth factor receptor [EGFR] in non–small-cell lung cancer [NSCLC] treated with EGFR TKIs), a (downstream) component of the signaling pathway activated by a target (i.e., RAS wild-type status in colorectal carcinoma treated with monoclonal antibodies to EGFR), or to a molecular change involved in oncogenesis that makes tumor cells sensitive to a therapy (i.e., mutations in BRCA2 that impair DNA repair and render cells vulnerable to poly(ADP-ribose) polymerase [PARP] inhibition). While the CDx for trastuzumab, the first FDA-approved molecular-targeted therapy, measured the consequences of HER2 gene amplification, the presupposition that molecular changes that provide therapeutic targets are the default candidates for CDx has not been productive in therapies targeting high-level EGFR expression in colorectal carcinoma and NSCLC, but instead lack of mutation of the KRAS/NRAS in the signaling pathway downstream of EGFR and activating mutations in the TK domain of EGFR, respectively.

The process of biomarker identification and development of prototype laboratory assays has been revolutionized by the availability of powerful technologies for the interrogation of tumor tissues, importantly routinely processed tissues from diagnostic archives. This

TABLE 30.1 Companion Diagnostic Assays Cleared by the FDA (April 2017), Grouped by Malignancy Type.

(A) MAMMARY CARCINOMA

Dx	Rx Target	CDx Target	PMA	Drug	Specimen	CDx	CDx Co/ Date Appr
BRCA	HER2	HER2 >express	P980018 S001-018	trastuzumab	FFPE	IHC	Dako 09/25/1998
BRCA			P980018 S015	pertuzumab			Dako 06/18/2015
BRCA			P980018 S016	ado-trastuzumab emtansine			Dako 02/22/2013
GACA			P980018 S018	trastuzumab			Dako 11/26/2013
BRCA	HER2	HER2 amp	P040005 S001-010	trastuzumab	FFPE	FISH	Dako 09/23/2005
BRCA GACA			P040005 S006	pertuzumab trastuzumab			Dako 06/08/2012
BRCA			P04005 S009	ado-trastuzumab emtansine			Dako 02/22/2013
BRCA	HER2	HER2 amp	P100024 S001-005	trastuzumab	FFPE	CISH	Dako 02/09/2011
BRCA	HER2	HER2 amp	P940004	trastuzumab	FFPE	FISH	Roche/V 08/01/2000
		HER2 >express	P990081 S001-028	trastuzumab	FFPE	IHC	Roche/V 12/12/2000 05/06/2014
		HER2 amp	P100027 S001-017	trastuzumab	FFPE	dual ISH	Roche/V 06/15/2011 05/06/2014
		HER2 amp	P980024 S001-012	trastuzumab	FFPE	FISH	Abbott 01/20/1999 12/20/2013
		HER2 >express	P040030	trastuzumab	FFPE	IHC	Biogenex 04/02/2005
		HER2 amp	P050040 S001-003	trastuzumab	FFPE	CISH	Lifetech 07/06/2012
		HER2 >express	P090015	trastuzumab	FFPE	IHC	Leica 04/25/2012

(B) NON–SMALL-CELL LUNG CANCER

NSCLC	EGFR	Δ-ex19, L858R T790M; G719X, ins-ex20, S768I, L861Q	P120022	afatinib	FFPE	PCR	Qiagen 07/15/2013 07/10/15

(continued)

(B) NON–SMALL-CELL LUNG CANCER (*CONTINUED*)

Dx	Rx Target	CDx Target	PMA	Drug	Specimen	CDx	CDx Co/ Date Appr
NSCLC	EGFR	Δ-ex19, L858R T790M; G719X, ins-ex20, S768I, L861Q	P120022 S001	gefitinib	FFPE	PCR	Qiagen 07/10/2015
	EGFR	Δ-ex19, L858R	P120019 S001-004	erlotinib	FFPE	PCR	Roche 05/14/2013 11/30/2015 06/06/2016 10/10/2016
		Δ-ex19, L858R T790M; G719X, ins-ex20, S768I, L861Q	P120019 S007	osimertinib			
		Δ-ex19, L858R T790M; G719X, ins-ex20, S768I, L861Q	P15047	erlotinib	FFPE and plasma		
		Δ-ex19, L858R T790M; G719X, ins-ex20, S768I, L861Q	P15044	osimertinib			
NSCLC	ALK	Rearrange	P110012S	crizotinib	FFPE	FISH	Abbott 04/17/13
	ALK	Expression	P140025	crizotinib	FFPE	IHC	Roche/V 07/10/15
	PD-L1	TPS ≥ 50%	P150013	pembrolizumab	FFPE	IHC	Dako 11/02/15
	PD-L1	TPS ≥ 1% TPS ≥ 50% (high)	P150013 S001	pembrolizumab			10/24/16

(C) COLORECTAL ADENOCARCINOMA

CRC	EGFR	Expression	P030044 S001-02	cetuximab panitumumab	FFPE	IHC	Dako 09/27/06
	KRAS	Mut codons 12,13	P110030 P110027	cetuximab panitumumab	FFPE	PCR	Qiagen 07/16/12 06/10/14
	KRAS	Mut codons 12,13,61	P140023	cetuximab panitumumab	FFPE	PCR	Roche 05/18/15

(*continued*)

(C) COLORECTAL ADENOCARCINOMA (*CONTINUED*)

Dx	Rx Target	CDx Target	PMA	Drug	Specimen	CDx	CDx Co/ Date Appr
GIST	KIT	Expression	P040011	imatinib mesylate	FFPE	IHC	Dako 11/02/12
GC/ GEJC (met)	HER2	Amp	P040005 S001-10	trastuzumab pertuzumab ado-trastuzumab emtansine	FFPE	FISH	Dako 06/08/12
		>> Expression	P980018 S001-18	trastuzumab pertuzumab ado-trastuzumab emtansine	FFPE	IHC	Dako 12/26/13

(D) VARIOUS MALIGNANCIES

Melanoma	BRAF	V600E	P110020 S001-010	vemurafenib	FFPE	PCR	Roche 08/19/11
Melanoma	BRAF	V600E V600K	P120014	trametinib dabrafenib	FFPE	PCR	bioMerieux 06/14/13
OvCa	PARP	BRCA1,2 (germ line)	P140020	olaparib	Blood	PCR and SS	Myriad 12/30/14
OvCa	PARP	BRCA1,2 (somatic)	P160018	rucaparib	FFPE-T	NGS	Foundation 12/19/16
B-CLL	BCL2	Del TP53	P150041	venetoclax	Blood	FISH	Abbott 05/11/16
Systemic Masto	KIT	D816V	H140006	imatinib mesylate	BM (fr)	PCR	ARUP 01/14/16
MDS/MPD	PDGFRB	Rearr	H14005	imatinib mesylate	Blood BM (fr)	FISH	ARUP 01/14/16

CDx, companion diagnostic; CISH, chromogenic in situ hybridization; Dx, diagnostic; FFPE, formalin-fixed, paraffin-embedded; FISH, fluorescence in situ hybridization; IHC, immunohistochemical; ISH, in situ hybridization; NGS, next-generation sequencing; NSCLC, non–small-cell lung cancer; PCR, polymerase chain reaction; PMA, premarket approval; Rx, drug; TPS, tumor proportion score.

armamentarium includes IHC analysis to detect protein expression, in situ hybridization (ISH; fluorescent: FISH, chromogenic: CISH) to detect gene amplification, rearrangements, and translocations, real-time polymerase chain reaction (PCR) to detect mutations, next-generation sequencing (NGS) to detect mutations and possibly copy number abnormalities and gene fusions, and multiple techniques for detection of RNA expression and gene fusions. It has been noted that CDx and genetic tests approved by the FDA have used each of these technologies.

The initial step in the development of a prototypic laboratory test is the transition from a research setting biomarker testing to a format that can be performed in a Clinical Laboratory Improvement Amendments (CLIA) certified clinical laboratory, including assessment of available specimen types and workflow in clinical settings to analysis and optimization of test performance characteristics, standardization. The goal of the prototype is to create a test with analytical accuracy and precision. This represents the starting point for adapting the laboratory assay to a CDx, in which the endpoint is a binary result predictive of clinical outcome—will benefit from therapy or will not benefit from therapy. Thus, the final steps in the creation of a CDx from a laboratory assay is the establishment of a cutoff value of the assay that uses the results of the clinical trial to calibrate the numerical results and convert them to reflecting the clinical outcome of the therapy in question. Assignment of a cutoff value that is too low will expand the test population and run the risk of diluting the statistical power to identify a significant outcome from the therapy. It will not, however, deny any patient access to the drug, nor will it protect patients who may not receive therapeutic benefit from adverse reactions. Conversely, assignment of a cutoff value that is too high will not threaten the statistical analysis of the clinical trial, but will limit access to the treatment of patients who may benefit. The limitation of patients receiving the therapy is predicted to present financial challenges, either a high cost of the treatment or lack of financial feasibility to this project.

To date, all companion diagnostics for oncology therapeutics approved by the FDA use standard archival tissues except three that require fresh blood (germ-line testing) or bone marrow (hematological malignancies). It is required for the laboratory to adhere to the specimen type and procedures specified by the FDA approval and listed in the package insert. There are, however, several considerations for "good molecular and genomic practice" that have been recommended by the College of American Pathologists (CAP), Association for Molecular Pathology (AMP), and American Society of Clinical Oncology (ASCO) (6,7) These guidelines call for review of samples submitted for analysis by CDx by a pathologist in order to optimize characterization of viable tumor, avoiding areas of necrosis and infiltration of inflammatory cells, which dilutes the absolute and relative content of tumor cells. Additional guidelines provide time thresholds from the diagnosis of a malignancy to test results of a biomarker for performing CDx tests in-house or submitting them to an external reference laboratory.

CDX PLAYS A CRITICAL ROLE TO THE SUCCESS OF CLINICAL TRIALS AND DRUG DEVELOPMENT

The spectrum of experience in the development of therapy with targeted agents in NSCLC provides excellent insight into the role of CDx in clinical trials. The finding that EGFR is overexpressed in many epithelial malignancies led to the development of monoclonal antibodies and TKIs as candidates for therapy. Since EGFR was found to be frequently overexpressed in NSCLC, this receptor was explored as a candidate for targeted therapy, using TKIs in this disease. Two antagonists were studied in randomized clinical trials, gefitinib and erlotinib. None of the initial clinical trials with oral TKIs in patients with NSCLC employed a biomarker for screening, stratification, or eligibility (8–13).

Two large phase II trials, designated IDEAL-1 and IDEAL-2, were performed to test gefitinib as a single agent in patients with advanced NSCLC (8,9). No biomarker was used for stratification. The objective response rates (ORRs) in IDEAL-1 and IDEAL-2 were 18% and 10%, respectively, and the 1-year overall survival was

similar to that observed with standard chemotherapy. Despite the limited findings, a small subgroup of patients experienced dramatic responses, which provided a rationale for FDA approval of gefitinib for salvage therapy. Statistical analysis revealed that the response rates were significantly higher in Japanese patients (27% versus 10%), in females, nonsmokers, and in patients with adenocarcinoma histopathology (8,9). Gefitinib was then examined in combination with standard chemotherapy in the INTACT trials, which included more than 2,000 patients with NSCLC. The two INTACT clinical studies failed to demonstrate a benefit of gefitinib for overall survival (14,15). Subsequently, gefitinib was evaluated as a second-line therapy in 1,692 patients with NSCLC refractory to chemotherapy, but found to not provide a survival benefit, resulting in the restriction of its clinical use (16).

The evaluation of erlotinib went through a similar process to that described for gefitinib. A phase II study of 57 patients with NSCLC treated with erlotinib as a single agent showed response rates and 1-year survivals similar to results obtained with salvage chemotherapy (12). Erlotinib in combination with chemotherapy was not found to be superior to chemotherapy alone in the TRIBUTE and TALENT clinical trials in 1,059 and 1,159 patients with advanced NSCLC, respectively (15). The BR.21 trial demonstrated a survival advantage in patients treated with second-line erlotinib versus placebo in 731 patients, 6.7 months versus 4.7 months, respectively, resulting in FDA approval for second- and third-line treatment of NSCLC (13).

After the take-all-comers clinical trials, an association between the presence of mutations in the EGFR tyrosine kinase domain and clinical responsiveness of NSCLC to gefitinib was demonstrated in two separate laboratories (17,18). After this observation was reproduced by multiple groups, the analysis of tumor specimens from the IDEAL and INTACT trials revealed the presence of EGFR TK domain mutations in 18% and 10%, respectively (19). These mutations were more commonly observed in patients with adenocarcinoma histopathology, nonsmokers, females, and Asians. In the IDEAL clinical trial, the response rate to gefitinib was higher in patients with an EGFR TK domain mutation (46%) than in patients with wild-type sequences (10%), but no advantage in survival was detected (19). Analysis of samples from the TRIBUTE study showed similar clinical outcomes (20). Analysis of samples from the BR.21 study failed to demonstrate a survival advantage in patients with tumors containing EGFR exon 19 deletions or L858R mutations (21). The subgroup of 12% of patients in the ISEL trial with mutations in EGFR had a response rate of 37.5% in comparison to patients with wild-type EGFR (2.6%) (22).

The collective experience of "take-all-comers" clinical trials for gefitinib and erlotinib therapy in patients with advanced NSCLC provides multiple lessons. These clinical trials were designed with large groups of subjects in order to achieve statistical power to test the hypothesis that antagonism of EGFR with a TKI could provide therapeutic benefit. However, despite the analysis of large groups of patients, it was not possible to demonstrate a significant benefit because of the limited number of patients with EGFR activating mutations that sensitize patients to this therapeutic mechanism. Since sensitizing mutations occur more frequently in NSCLC in Asian patients (~30% vs. 10% incidence in the United States) and women, a study inclusion typical of the U.S. population would be biased against the optimal clinical cohort for testing this hypothesis. Prescreening candidates for eligibility with a CDx would have enriched the content of patients who could have benefitted from TKI therapy.

While the frequency of patients with NSCLC harboring sensitizing mutations in the anaplastic lymphoma kinase (ALK) gene (~5%) is actually lower than the population of NSCLC patients with mutations associated with eligibility for EGFR TKIs, the clinical trials for FDA approval of crizotinib were conducted in a fashion to avoid the pitfalls encountered with gefitinib and erlotinib. Crizotinib received accelerated approval for the therapy of patients with NSCLC with ALK gene rearrangements in August 2011, along with the paired CDx. This FISH assay, which used a break-apart probe from adjacent regions of the ALK gene separated by the rearrangement, was used to screen patients with locally advanced or metastatic NSCLC for eligibility for Study A and Study B in a single-arm crizotinib trial. The population of 255 patients (Study A: n = 136; Study B: n = 119) with ALK rearrangements included 30% Asians, 48% males, <3% smokers, 96% with adenocarcinoma histopathology, and 95% with metastatic disease. ORRs for Study A and B were 50% and 61%, respectively and the median durations of the response were 42 and 48 weeks, respectively (23).

Crizotinib received regular approval by the FDA on Nov 20, 2013 after fulfilling the FDA's requirement of a successful postmarket phase 3 clinical trial. An open-label, multinational randomized trial was performed on a cohort of 347 patients with metastatic NSCLC positive for ALK rearrangement by the FDA-approved FISH assay. Progression-free survival in patients receiving crizotinib (n = 173) versus those treated with chemotherapy (n = 174) was 7.7 versus 3.0 months, respectively. Similarly, the overall response rate in patients in the crizotinib arm was 65% compared to 20% who received chemotherapy. The median duration of response was also higher in the crizotinib group (7.4 vs. 5.6 months) (24). Crizotinib demonstrated a superior clinical outcome than platinum-based chemotherapy.

The codevelopment of crizotinib with the CDx for ALK rearrangement facilitated the FDA approval when compared to the analogous process for gefitinib and erlotinib. Despite the lower frequency of ALK rearrangements (approximately 5%) than EGFR sensitizing mutations (approximately 10%) in NSCLC in the United States, the key clinical trials for crizotinib included approximately 600 patients in contrast to a combined total of almost 10-fold greater for gefitinib and erlotinib. Consequently, the costs associated with the crizotinib trials were significantly less.

The use of a CDx in the crizotinib clinical trials also illustrates an important contribution to patient safety. A minimum of 25% of patients in the study for accelerated approval experienced adverse reaction, which was severe pneumonitis in 1.6% (25). Serious adverse events were reported in 37% of the 172 patients in the clinical trial for regular FDA approval, nine of which were fatal (24). Thus, in the absence of a CDx to prescreen patients for eligibility for crizotinib therapy, a population of NSCLC patients similar to that in the gefitinib or erlotinib studies would have been subjected to the possibility of severe adverse reactions.

FDA RECOMMENDATION OF CODEVELOPMENT OF TARGETED AGENTS WITH CDX

To date, at least three companion diagnostics have been established concurrently with the novel therapeutic agent, (a) Herceptin and IHC analysis for HER2 overexpression, (b) crizotinib and FISH for ALK rearrangement, and (c) vemurafenib and PCR analysis for BRAF V600 mutation. In each of these examples, the biomarker that provided predictive data was the direct analysis of the precise molecular target for the therapy. It is clear that CDx tests have both clinical and financial value. The clinical value involves selection of a therapy that will be effective and safe in the patient while avoiding unnecessary toxicities and side effects in patients who will not receive a benefit. The financial considerations include the ability to avoid the cost of expensive therapies in patients who will not benefit, as well as the impact to pharmaceutical companies of limiting the number of patients and influencing (both positively and negatively) the advancement of drugs into clinical use.

The FDA and the Institute of Medicine have recommended that the process of biomarker discovery for a disease be closely followed by the development of a diagnostic test and the evaluation of clinical utility (26). It is anticipated that the FDA may require a CDx when the action of a drug is on a specific genetic or biologic target that is only present in a subpopulation of patients, based on FDA's draft guidance "Principles for Codevelopment of an In Vitro Companion Diagnostic Device with a Therapeutic Product," released on July 15, 2016 (4).

In the strategy of codevelopment of therapy and diagnostic, the two processes are pursued in parallel. The ultimate success of this approach is dependent upon the durability of therapeutic hypothesis and its relevance to clinical behavior (i.e., the contribution of the targeted abnormality or mechanism to tumor cell biology, the connection between the selected biomarker and the target, etc.). Biomarker selection, determination of feasibility, and the development of pilot assays occur during early phases of discovery, testing of preclinical models, and phase I clinical studies. Analytical and clinical validations occur during phase II and phase III clinical trials, respectively. More specifically, the use of the biomarker assay designed to serve as a CDx evolves from the detection of biologic events to clinical endpoints and outcomes. This process determines whether the candidate CDx has sufficient predictive ability to identify patients who will benefit from therapy.

Three types of clinical trial designs have been used for the codevelopment of therapeutics and diagnostics: (a) open accrual in which all patients are enrolled, independent of CDx results; (b) enrichment in which only patients positive for the CDx are enrolled; and (c) stratified, in which patients positive and negative for the CDx are enrolled in both arms and are randomized. Enrichment trials, such as the BRAF mutant melanoma—vemurafenib trial (Roche), ALK rearranged NSCLC—crizotinib, and breast cancer—ado-trastuzumab emtansine trial (Roche), offer the advantage of requiring fewer patients for the clinical trial that can be completed rapidly and with less expense than other types that require a higher number of patients. In addition to these examples, it has been demonstrated by a comprehensive study that clinical trials with a suitable biomarker or a CDx used for patient selection have a significantly higher success rate in comparison to ones without using a biomarker (27). The study analyzed all drug development clinical trials for NSCLC between 1998 and January 2012, including 676 clinical trials and 199 unique compounds. The cumulative clinical trial success rate for stage IIIb–IV NSCLC trials that did not include a biomarker in the inclusion criteria was 11%. In contrast, the success rate for trials using a biomarker indication was 62%, about a sixfold increase by using a biomarker (27).

CHALLENGES FOR DEVELOPING CDX

Even when armed with strong preclinical data, it is not always possible to formulate a strong therapeutic hypothesis that reflects the genuine mechanism driving the malignancy or to select the optimal biomarker to use as a predictive test. Perhaps the best example of this is the evolution of CDx testing for cetuximab in colorectal carcinoma. Since many colorectal carcinomas express high levels of EGFR (28), the initial CDx approved by the FDA was IHC analysis to detect high-level expression of EGFR. Clinical trials revealed limitations in the predictive ability of this test, but retrospective analysis of specimens demonstrated that detection of activation of a key downstream component of the EGFR signaling pathway, KRAS somatic mutation status, provided superior predictive ability for clinical responsiveness to cetuximab (29). A second instance of focusing insight into fundamental mechanisms of normal homeostasis and oncogenesis for the development of novel therapeutics and a CDx is the use of inhibitors of PARP for the therapy of ovarian cancer associated with germ-line mutations or somatic mutations of BRCA1 and BRCA2. It was demonstrated by Farmer and coworkers (30) that in the context of malfunction of BRCA1 or BRCA2, cells are dramatically sensitized to PARP inhibitors, with subsequent chromosomal instability, cell-cycle arrest, and ultimately programmed cell death. Since BRCA1/2 play an important role in homologous recombination and DNA repair and PARP is involved in multiple mechanisms in cellular repair (30), it is interpreted that PARP inhibition results in the perpetuation of DNA damage normally repaired by homologous recombination. This illustrates the importance of targeting of overlapping mechanisms that may be compromised in tumor cells in the development of novel therapeutics and companion diagnostics.

CDX AND TYPES OF LABORATORY TESTS

It is noted that among the cadre of CDx tests approved by the FDA, there are significant omissions. Two hematopoietic malignancies with signature genetic abnormalities, chronic myeloid leukemia and acute promyelocytic leukemia, have FDA-approved therapies directed against the molecular targets created by these translocations. All-trans retinoic acid was approved by the FDA in 1995 for the treatment of acute promyelocytic leukemia (31), which is associated with the t(15;17) translocation (molecularly cloned in 1991 [(32)]) that disrupts the retinoic acid receptor on chromosome 17 and imatinib was approved by the FDA in 2001 for treatment of chronic myeloid leukemia (33), which is characterized by the t(9;22) translocation that results in activation of the ABL tyrosine kinase (34). Since no FDA-approved or -cleared (CDx) tests are available for the detection of the active molecular targets in CML and APL, the ABL kinase and retinoic acid receptor, respectively, laboratory developed tests (LDTs) are employed. Of note, the diagnostic genomic signature for both of these hematologic malignancies coincides with the molecular target for therapy and, therefore, the CDx.

The CLIA of 1988 provides a regulatory framework for laboratory tests that are used clinically in the care of patients. These tests fall into two categories: (a) approved or cleared by the FDA and (b) laboratory developed.

The FDA has two mechanisms for the evaluation of in vitro diagnostics (35). The most stringent is the evaluation for "premarket approval" (PMA). This application requires extensive documentation of design, manufacturing, and preclinical and clinical studies to demonstrate the safety and clinical utility of the diagnostic "device." This is a very expensive process because it requires a clinical trial. The utility of the diagnostic device is correlated with clinical performance and the prediction of clinical endpoints to achieve "approval." Many of FDA-approved CDx belong to this category.

An alternative mechanism is the 510(k) or "premarket notification" (PMN), which requires that the manufacturer of the diagnostic test inform the FDA at least 90 days before they intend to market the assay. The FDA investigation consists of determining whether the test has the same performance as a device already categorized into one of the three classes: Class I devices do not require PMA or clearance, but production must be controlled (i.e., dental floss); Class II tests/devices must be shown to have similar performance to a previously existing "predicate device"; and Class III devices, which provide critical functions and have an evaluation analogous to a "New Drug Application." Evaluation through the 510(k)/PMN pathway results in a test that has been "cleared" by the FDA.

In contrast to a diagnostic assay approved or cleared by the FDA, a "laboratory developed test" (LDT) is one that has been designed, developed, manufactured, and used within an individual laboratory. While this type of test requires significant analytical validation using panel samples with known results, the validation process does not require demonstration of clinical utility. Therefore, the endpoints are not based on clinical outcomes, as is the case for a PMA, or even a 510(k) evaluation, but rather on analytical accuracy and sensitivity. Recently, the FDA has raised concerns regarding LDTs that include the lack of (a) clinical validation based on outcomes, (b) adverse event reporting, (c) withdrawal of unsafe tests from clinical use, (d) assessment of quality manufacturing, and (e) informed consent and a regulatory framework for the validation trials. The FDA has elected to undertake a phased approach to the regulation of LDTs in order to maintain continuity in the testing market and avoid disruption of access to specific types of tests for which there are limited FDA-approved/cleared options (i.e., no NGS panels for somatic mutations in malignant diseases have been approved by FDA other than FDA-approved CDx limited for BRCA 1 and BRCA 2 genes). At this time, LDTs continue to play a major role in the mainstream of standard of care in oncology molecular diagnostics. Although FDA-approved tests dominate the CDx field, guidelines established by ASCO, AMP, and CAP recommend analysis of some biomarkers for which only LDTs are available (i.e., extended RAS analysis, BCR-ABL1 fusion, PML–RARA fusion).

UTILITY OF CDX IN CLINICAL PRACTICE AFTER CLINICAL TRIALS

Of the 31 FDA-approved CDx PMA applications for anticancer agents, commercial kits are available for 27

and 4 are proprietary tests performed exclusively by reference laboratories (Table 30.1D). Among the four most common cancers in Europe and the Americas, only prostate cancer stands without an FDA-approved CDx for the spectrum of therapies. In contrast, breast, lung, and colorectal carcinomas have formal CDx tests to determine eligibility for targeted therapies.

Lung Cancer

NSCLC has FDA-approved companion diagnostics for three classes of therapy: TKIs for (a) EGFR and (b) ALK, and (c) an immunologic modifier, PD-L1. The analysis of EGFR and ALK represents predictive tests that directly determine the presence of an activating mutation present in tumor cells. The interpretation of the IHC analysis for PD-L1 may well be more complex, but is based upon the intensity of staining of tumor cells.

The ASCO has endorsed guidelines for genomic analysis of EGFR and ALK in patients with lung cancer recommended by CAP, the International Association for the Study of Lung Cancer, and the AMP (6). It is emphasized that pathologic examination of the tissue to be tested represents an important part of both the preanalytical process and interpretation. Other recommendations include the following:

- Clinical features should not influence the selection of patients with adenocarcinoma of the lung for EGFR and ALK testing.
- Testing is recommended for adenocarcinomas and tumors with both adeno- and squamous carcinoma components.
- Testing is recommended in (limited) biopsy specimens in which an adenocarcinoma component cannot be excluded.
- Testing is not recommended in excision specimens that have only squamous, small-cell, or large-cell histopathology features.
- It is acceptable to test primary tumor or metastases.
- In the context of multiple tumors that appear to be separate, it is acceptable to test all, but multiple sampling of a single tumor is not recommended.
- EGFR and ALK testing is recommended in advanced-stage disease, but encouraged in early-stage disease.
- The turnaround time for EGFR and ALK testing should be within 10 working days of histopathologic diagnosis.
- Following histopathologic diagnosis, specimens should be submitted for analysis within 24 hours if testing is performed in-house and within 3 days if referred to an outside laboratory.
- Routinely processed surgical pathology (formalin-fixed, paraffin-embedded [FFPE]) and cytopathology samples are acceptable for analysis; specialized fixation and decalcification should be avoided.

- Pathologists should determine the adequacy of tissue for analysis.
- Each laboratory should determine a lower threshold of tumor cell content for analysis.
- Laboratories may use any validated EGFR testing method with sufficient performance characteristics.
- While the requirement is for the detection of EGFR mutations in ≥50% tumor cells, a sensitivity of ≥10% tumor cells is recommended.
- EGFR testing should detect all mutations with a frequency of ≥1% in EGFR mutated lung cancer.
- IHC analysis for EGFR expression is not recommended.
- Analysis of EGFR copy number is not recommended.
- Testing for KRAS mutations is not a surrogate for EGFR TKI therapy.
- If testing for TKI resistance is performed, a sensitivity of 5% tumor cells is recommended.
- ALK testing with a dual labeled break-apart probe is recommended.
- IHC analysis may be used as a screening test (*note*: these recommendations were submitted before the ALK IHC analysis test was approved by the FDA).
- PCR-based tests are not recommended for detection of ALK rearrangement.
- Testing for mutations associated with TKI resistance is not required for clinical management.
- Testing for EGFR and ALK mutations should be prioritized over other genomic analyses.

Gastrointestinal Cancer

The finding that the EGFR, a receptor tyrosine kinase, is overexpressed in a significant number of colorectal carcinomas led to exploration of the EGFR signaling pathway for candidates for targeted therapy. Monoclonal antibodies to EGFR that inhibit ligand binding and EGFR signaling were found to influence clinical outcomes in a subset of patients with metastatic colorectal carcinoma in clinical trials. Since the primary molecular abnormality targeted was overexpression of EGFR, the initial CDx evaluated in clinical trials was immunohistochemical staining for semiquantification of EGFR expression. This approach was not found to have optimal predictive value and it was subsequently recognized that patients whose tumors had activation of signaling downstream of EGFR via a mutated KRAS gene (exon 2, codons 12 and 13) lacked responsiveness to therapy with cetuximab and panitumumab, but those with wild-type KRAS had increased overall survival. Further clinical trials have refined our insight into RAS mutants that activate signaling downstream of EGFR, and are associated with lack of responsiveness to cetuximab and panitumumab therapy. This "extended RAS analysis," which includes codons 12 and 13 (exon 2), 59 and 61 (exon 3), and 117 and 146 (exon 4) of KRAS and the same set of codons in the NRAS gene, has been found to identify mutations in approximately 20% of patients with colorectal carcinoma with wild-type KRAS codons 12 and 13. Mutational analysis of other intermediates in the EGFR/RAS signaling pathway, including BRAF, PTEN, and PIK3CA, has not been found to be predictive of a lack of clinical response to anti-EGFR therapy.

The American Society of Clinical Pathology, CAP, AMP, and ASCO have established guidelines for the use of molecular biomarkers to guide therapy for advanced-stage colorectal carcinoma (7). These recommendations include the following:

- Patients with colorectal carcinoma who are candidates for anti-EGFR antibody therapy, such as cetuximab and panitumumab, must have molecular extended RAS gene analysis of their tumor that includes codons 12, 13, 59, 61, 117, and 146 of both KRAS and NRAS genes.
- While metastatic or recurrent colorectal carcinoma are the optimal tissues for extended RAS analysis for predictive testing, primary tumor specimens may be used if the latter is insufficient or not available.
- Results of predictive testing should be available with a maximum turnaround time of 10 working days.
- The assay for extended RAS analysis should have a sensitivity of 5% mutant allele.
- Analysis of the BRAF V600 mutation status, which is associated with a poor prognosis, should be performed in colorectal carcinoma for prognostic value for stratification for therapy. There is insufficient evidence to use BRAF V600 mutation status as a predictive marker indicative of lack of response to anti-EGFR antibody therapy.
- There is insufficient evidence to recommend the mutational analysis of BRAF (V600), PIK3CA, and PTEN be performed as a predictive marker indicative of lack of response to anti-EGFR antibody therapy

At this time two diagnostic kits have been approved by the FDA for analysis of KRAS mutations. The therascreen KRAS RGQ PCR kit (Qiagen) detects mutations in exon 2, and codons 12 and 13. The cobas® KRAS mutation kit (Roche) detects mutations in exon 2 (codons 12 and 13) and codon 61 in exon 3, but not codon 59 or codons in 117 or 146 in exon 4. No assays for mutational analysis of the NRAS gene have been approved by the FDA for diagnostic use. Thus, there is a gap between available FDA-approved companion diagnostics and the guidelines for extended RAS analysis established by the relevant professional societies.

CONCLUDING REMARKS

Clinical trials underwent a transformation in 1998 with the simultaneous FDA approval of trastuzumab and a companion (diagnostic) test designed to identify patients who will benefit from this therapy and to determine eligibility for the drug. Dramatic advances in genomic technology have armed oncology scientists with insights into somatic genetic changes in malignant diseases that can serve as molecular targets as well as diagnostic tools to detect them in routinely processed tissues from the pathology archives.

It is clear that the active adoption of CDx testing provides significant advantages to efficacy of therapy, patient safety, efficiency of clinical trials, and advancement of novel therapies into the clinic. The FDA has encouraged the codevelopment of biomarkers with preclinical and early phases of drug development and planning of clinical trials and has provided recommendations for this process. It is emphasized that in contrast to LDTs, CDx approved by the FDA have cutoff values that are established based on patient outcomes in clinical trials, and have additional important features, including reporting of adverse events and transparency of performance through a formal reporting process. As the "precision diagnostics guiding personalized medicine" paradigm is refined and is reconciled with the demand for a higher level of quality and efficiency in medicine, CDx will continue to occupy center stage in standard-of-care oncology therapy and the development of novel therapeutics.

REFERENCES

1. New Haven Medical Association. On the educational value of the medical society. *Yale Med J.* 1903;9(10):325.
2. Pegram MD, Lipton A, Hayes DF, et al. Phase II study of receptor-enhanced chemosensitivity using recombinant humanized anti-p185HER2/neu monoclonal antibody plus cisplatin in patients with HER2/neu-overexpressing metastatic breast cancer refractory to chemotherapy treatment. *J Clin Oncol.* 1998;16(8):2659–2671.
3. Graziano C. HER-2 breast assay, linked to Herceptin, wins FDA's okay. *CAP Today.* 1998;12(10):14–16.
4. U.S. Food and Drug Administration. Companion diagnostics. https://www.fda.gov/MedicalDevices/Products andMedicalProcedures/InVitroDiagnostics/ucm407297.htm
5. U.S. Food and Drug Administration. List of cleared or approved companion diagnostic devices (in vitro and imaging tools). https://www.fda.gov/MedicalDevices/ProductsandMedicalProcedures/InVitroDiagnostics/ucm301431.htm (accessed on 04/12/2017)
6. Leighl NB, Rekhtman N, Biermann WA, et al. Molecular testing for selection of patients with lung cancer for epidermal growth factor receptor and anaplastic lymphoma kinase tyrosine kinase inhibitors: American Society of Clinical Oncology endorsement of the College of American Pathologists/International Association for the study of lung cancer/association for molecular pathology guideline. *J Clin Oncol.* 2014;32(32):3673–3679.
7. Sepulveda AR, Hamilton SR, Allegra CJ, et al. Molecular biomarkers for the evaluation of colorectal cancer: guideline from the American Society for Clinical Pathology, College of American Pathologists, Association for Molecular Pathology, and the American Society of Clinical Oncology. *J Clin Oncol.* 2017;35(13):1453–1486.
8. Fukuoka M, Yano S, Giaccone G, et al. Multi-institutional randomized phase II trial of gefitinib for previously treated patients with advanced non-small-cell lung cancer (The IDEAL 1 Trial) [corrected]. *J Clin Oncol.* 2003;21(12):2237–2246.
9. Kris MG, Natale RB, Herbst RS, et al. Efficacy of gefitinib, an inhibitor of the epidermal growth factor receptor tyrosine kinase, in symptomatic patients with non-small cell lung cancer: a randomized trial. *JAMA.* 2003;290(16):2149–2158.
10. Pérez-Soler R, Chachoua A, Hammond LA, et al. Determinants of tumor response and survival with erlotinib in patients with non-small-cell lung cancer. *J Clin Oncol.* 2004;22(16):3238–3247.
11. Herbst RS, Prager D, Hermann R, et al.; TRIBUTE Investigator Group. TRIBUTE: a phase III trial of erlotinib hydrochloride (OSI-774) combined with carboplatin and paclitaxel chemotherapy in advanced non-small-cell lung cancer. *J Clin Oncol.* 2005;23(25):5892–5899.
12. Perez-Soler R. The role of erlotinib (Tarceva, OSI 774) in the treatment of non-small cell lung cancer. *Clin Cancer Res.* 2004;10(12, Pt 2):4238s–4240s.
13. Shepherd FA, Rodrigues Pereira J, Ciuleanu T, et al.; National Cancer Institute of Canada Clinical Trials Group. Erlotinib in previously treated non-small-cell lung cancer. *N Engl J Med.* 2005;353(2):123–132.
14. Giaccone G, Herbst RS, Manegold C, et al. Gefitinib in combination with gemcitabine and cisplatin in advanced non-small-cell lung cancer: a Phase III trial—INTACT 1. *J Clin Oncol.* 2004;22(5):777–784.
15. Herbst RS, Giaccone G, Schiller JH, et al. Gefitinib in combination with paclitaxel and carboplatin in advanced non-small-cell lung cancer: a phase III trial—INTACT 2. *J Clin Oncol.* 2004;22(5):785–794.
16. Thatcher N, Chang A, Parikh P, et al. Gefitinib plus best supportive care in previously treated patients with refractory advanced non-small-cell lung cancer: results from a randomised, placebo-controlled, multicentre study (Iressa Survival Evaluation in Lung Cancer). *Lancet.* 2005;366(9496):1527–1537.
17. Lynch TJ, Bell DW, Sordella R, et al. Activating mutations in the epidermal growth factor receptor underlying responsiveness of non-small-cell lung cancer to gefitinib. *N Engl J Med.* 2004;350(21):2129–2139.
18. Paez JG, Jänne PA, Lee JC, et al. EGFR mutations in lung cancer: correlation with clinical response to gefitinib therapy. *Science.* 2004;304(5676):1497–1500.
19. Bell DW, Lynch TJ, Haserlat SM, et al. Epidermal growth factor receptor mutations and gene amplification in non-small-cell lung cancer: molecular analysis of the IDEAL/INTACT gefitinib trials. *J Clin Oncol.* 2005;23(31):8081–8092.
20. Eberhard DA, Johnson BE, Amler LC, et al. Mutations in the epidermal growth factor receptor and in KRAS are predictive and prognostic indicators in patients with non-small-cell lung cancer treated with chemotherapy alone and in combination with erlotinib. *J Clin Oncol.* 2005;23(25):5900–5909.
21. Tsao MS, Sakurada A, Cutz JC, et al. Erlotinib in lung cancer—molecular and clinical predictors of outcome. *N Engl J Med.* 2005;353(2):133–144.
22. Hirsch FR, Varella-Garcia M, Bunn PA Jr, et al. Molecular predictors of outcome with gefitinib in a Phase III placebo-controlled study in advanced non-small-cell lung cancer. *J Clin Oncol.* 2006;24(31):5034–5042.
23. Kwak EL, Bang YJ, Camidge DR, et al. Anaplastic lymphoma kinase inhibition in non-small-cell lung cancer. *N Engl J Med.* 2010;363(18):1693–1703.
24. Kazandjian D, Blumenthal GM, Chen HY, et al. FDA approval summary: crizotinib for the treatment of metastatic non-small cell lung cancer with anaplastic lymphoma kinase rearrangements. *Oncologist.* 2014;19(10):e5–e11
25. Camidge DR, Bang YJ, Kwak EL, et al. Activity and safety of crizotinib in patients with ALK-positive non-small-cell lung cancer: updated results from a phase 1 study. *Lancet Oncol.* 2012;13(10):1011–1019.
26. Graig LA, Phillips JK, Moses HL, eds. Committee on Policy Issues in the Clinical Development and Use of Biomarkers for Molecularly Targeted Therapies. In: *Biomarker Tests for Molecularly Targeted Therapies: Key to Unlocking Precision Medicine.* Washington, DC: National Academies Press; 2016.

27. Falconi A, Lopes G, Parker JL. Biomarkers and receptor targeted therapies reduce clinical trial risk in non-small-cell lung cancer. *J Thorac Oncol.* 2014;9(2):163–169.

28. Porebska I, Harlozińska A, Bojarowski T. Expression of the tyrosine kinase activity growth factor receptors (EGFR, ERB B2, ERB B3) in colorectal adenocarcinomas and adenomas. *Tumour Biol.* 2000;21(2):105–115.

29. Linardou H, Dahabreh IJ, Kanaloupiti D, et al. Assessment of somatic k-RAS mutations as a mechanism associated with resistance to EGFR-targeted agents: a systematic review and meta-analysis of studies in advanced non-small-cell lung cancer and metastatic colorectal cancer. *Lancet Oncol.* 2008;9(10):962–972.

30. Farmer H, McCabe N, Lord CJ, et al. Targeting the DNA repair defect in BRCA mutant cells as a therapeutic strategy. *Nature.* 2005;434(7035):917–921.

31. FDA approves all-trans retinoic acid for treating a rare leukemia. https://archive.hhs.gov/news/press/1995pres/951128a.html

32. de Thé H, Chomienne C, Lanotte M, et al. The t(15;17) translocation of acute promyelocytic leukaemia fuses the retinoic acid receptor alpha gene to a novel transcribed locus. *Nature.* 1990;347(6293):558–561.

33. Center for Drug Evaluation and Research. https://www.accessdata.fda.gov/drugsatfda_docs/nda/2001/21-335_Gleevec_Approv.pdf

34. Salesse S, Verfaillie CM. BCR/ABL: from molecular mechanisms of leukemia induction to treatment of chronic myelogenous leukemia. *Oncogene.* 2002;21(56):8547–8559.

35. U.S. Food and Drug Administration. Overview of IVD Regulation https://www.fda.gov/MedicalDevices/DeviceRegulationandGuidance/IVDRegulatoryAssistance/ucm123682.htm

IV

Analyzing Results of Oncology Clinical Trials

31

Interim Analysis and Data Monitoring

Scott R. Evans and William T. Barry

INTRODUCTION

Interim data monitoring is an important part of a clinical trial. Data monitoring is conducted to evaluate the safety and tolerability of interventions given to the trial participants. Monitoring activities also include evaluation of accrual, baseline characteristics, patient disposition, data quality and timeliness, and design assumptions. Activities may include formal testing of the primary hypotheses with rules to define early termination and reporting of study results. Interim testing has: (a) an ethical attractiveness as it can result in fewer patients being exposed to potentially harmful or inefficacious interventions, (b) economic advantages in that research questions may be able to be answered sooner, and (c) a public health impact since trial results may be communicated to the medical community faster. Careful thought should be given to how a trial should be monitored. Here we describe interim data monitoring methodologies and data monitoring committees (DMCs).

INTERIM MONITORING METHODS

Interim monitoring plans can include repeated evaluations of the primary objective of a trial. For this activity, it is considered good clinical practice (1) to include formal analysis plans to define guidelines for early termination of the study for strong evidence of superiority/noninferiority of an intervention. Guidelines for early termination may also be specified if the probability of reaching statistical significance at the end of the study is too low or important effects can be ruled out with reasonable confidence, that is, "futility." In these cases, the statistical methods that are applied during the interim and final analyses need to consider the trial-wide error rates of the hypothesis testing procedure.

When interim analysis plans include testing of the hypothesis associated with the primary objective, one must be aware of the consequences of multiplicity and the probability of a false-positive result over the course of the trial. To illustrate the increased risk of trial-wide error, Armitage et al. (2) calculated the probability of at least one false-positive result when conducting a series of hypothesis tests at the significance level of 0.05. They showed that a series of four tests would result in an inflated trial-wide error of 0.126, and that increasing to a series of 10 tests would result in an inflated error of 0.193. This numerical example illustrates the need to implement *group-sequential testing* methods, which control the overall error rate of the trial.

Group-Sequential Tests

Early Stopping for Efficacy

For definitive phase III studies, there are several ethical and public health interests to allow early termination of a study for strong evidence of efficacy in either a superiority trial or a noninferiority trial. In order to implement early termination procedures into the analysis plans of a study, methods for group-sequential testing have been developed for randomized controlled trials, which follow the frequentist paradigm for hypothesis testing. In brief, one defines a null hypothesis of no difference (for superiority trials) or a noninferiority margin (for noninferiority trials), and a test statistic to indicate whether any observed results would occur by chance, for example, if there was truly no difference in a superiority trial. In a single-stage test, one derives a boundary to the test statistic, which controls the probability of making an (type I) error under the null at a prespecified level, a. Next, a sample size, N, is selected to control the probability of making an (type II) error under an alternative hypothesis. For group-sequential tests, a series of stopping boundaries are selected to control the overall type I error at a, and sample size may be recalculated in order to maintain power at $1 - \beta$. Using the same relationship between multiple comparisons and trial-wide error noted previously, Pocock (3) derived boundaries for conducting sequential tests at a constant nominal a_k. For example, if there were $K = 4$ equally sized tests, for example, three interim tests and a final analyses, then one could use $a_k = 0.0194$ in order for the type I error under the null to be 0.05. However, this method has been criticized as being inconsistent with the goal of only stopping early for "overwhelming" evidence, including by Pocock and White (4). Further, with the small alpha-sized test at final analysis, sample size requirements are greater in order to have the same level of power as a trial without early stopping (here, 17% larger when designing a trial to have 90% power). In contrast to the Pocock method, Haybittle (5) and Peto et al. (6) suggested applying a nonconstant set of (a_k), using more conservative boundaries for the early interim tests so that the nominal level at the final analysis is closest to the overall a. For instance, with $a_k = 0.001, k = 1 \ldots 3$, the stopping boundary at final analysis is close to nominal a; as such, only a 0.8% increase in sample size over a single-stage test is needed to maintain power. An alternative strategy was proposed by O'Brien and Fleming (7), where the boundaries for early stopping are chosen to be gradually more conservative with each interim analysis, using a functional form that keeps the nominal level at final analysis close to the overall a. Figure 31.1 displays the stopping boundaries for each of the three methods when planning three interims and one final.

For each of the group-sequential test procedures discussed previously, the timing of the interim analysis was assumed to be fixed and conducted after enrolling and evaluating equally sized groups of patients. When the clinical outcome is a discrete or continuous measure, then scheduling of interim analyses can be straightforward and correspond to the fraction of total patients enrolled. However, if one is evaluating the relative efficiency and expected sample sizes of a test, it is important to consider the impact of any lag time from study entry to ascertainment of the primary endpoint unless the enrollment is suspended, which is rarely done. Furthermore, in oncology trials the primary outcome for efficacy is often a time-to-event endpoint (e.g. overall survival, disease-free survival), and the power to detect target hazard ratios (HRs) is defined by the total number of events that are observed rather than sample size. Thus, for a group-sequential test, the timing of interim analysis is based on the cumulative number of events. In order to accommodate flexibility in the timing of interim monitoring, Lan and DeMets (8) extended the methods for group-sequential testing from being equally spaced to being defined as occurring at levels of "percent information" relative to the final analysis. One can then use an error-spending function to control the type I error used at each interim and final analysis. In order to compute a total sample size, the timing of the interim analyses is prespecified. Once the overall a, N, and the spending function are set, the number and spacing of interim analyses can be updated over the course of the trial to accommodate periodic monitoring. The use of error-spending functions also provided a framework for deriving boundaries under the framework of stochastic curtailment (9), where early stopping is allowed when a final decision is highly likely to occur given the current data. Then, investigators can define rules using meaningful scales for what is considered highly likely, such as the conditional or predictive power observed at an interim analysis. As a graphical illustration, Figure 31.1 displays stopping bounds for a study with $K = 4$ equally spaced tests based on stochastic curtailment with a 99% predicted probability of concluding efficacy at final analysis.

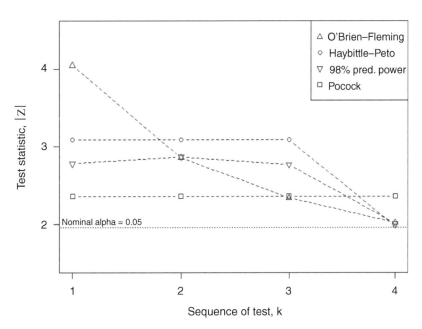

FIGURE 31.1 Stopping boundaries to control the overall type I error at $a = 0.05$ with $K = 4$ tests (three interim and one final) using the methods of Pocock, Haybittle–Peto and O'Brien–Fleming, and 98% predicted power using Lan–DeMets error-spending functions.

Early Stopping for Futility

In addition to early stopping of a phase III trial for overwhelming evidence of efficacy, some of the ethical considerations in participating in a randomized controlled trial and costs extend to early stopping for "futility." Futility can be defined as scenarios where the likelihood of a trial reaching an inconclusive result or of failing to reject the null hypothesis reaches a level that continuation of the trial is no longer appropriate. Futility may also mean that the alternative hypothesis can be rejected with reasonable confidence. It is important to distinguish between futility and overwhelming evidence of inferiority. Group-sequential testing methods can be used to define formal stopping boundaries for futility, using methods similar to efficacy analysis. For instance, error-spending functions, including those related to the O'Brien–Fleming method, can be applied to the β probability of a false-negative test under the targeted alternative hypothesis. Likewise, unacceptably low levels of conditional or predictive power could be defined at each interim analysis. For instance, a common heuristic in randomized phase II trials is to conduct a single interim for futility halfway through the study (i.e., 50% information) and stop if greater activity is seen in the control arm. This boundary corresponds to a predictive power less than or equal to the alpha level of a one-sided test. Another approach is to base futility boundaries on testing the alternative hypothesis (10) with less aggressive rules (e.g., one-sided 0.005) to reach desired properties for early stopping (11). Finally, it is important to distinguish whether the early-stopping rules for futility will be binding. Although this would allow for a slight retention of power if the error-spending functions account for the probabilities of early stopping, this may not be consistent with the process and charter for review of the study by the independent DMC and recommendation to sponsor.

Example Phase III Trial With Efficacy and Futility Bounds

Cancer and Leukemia Group B (CALGB) 40502 was a three-arm randomized phase III trial comparing two experimental agents, nab-paclitaxel and ixabepilone, against a control of paclitaxel when given as first-line chemotherapy concurrent with bevacizumab for locally recurrent or metastatic breast cancer. Each experimental agent was separately evaluated against paclitaxel with a primary endpoint of progression-free survival (PFS), using stratified log-rank tests with a one-sided $a = 0.0135$ to control trial-wide error rates for the multi-arm study (12). Final analysis was targeted to occur after 716 (476 events per contrast) events to have 88% power to see improvements in PFS from 11 to 15 months (HR of 0.73). Interim analysis for superiority and futility was performed using Lan–DeMets error-spending functions that corresponded to 99% predictive probability of significance at final analysis and using the test of the alternative hypothesis proposed by Freidlin and Korn (11).

As reported by Rugo et al. (13), at the first interim analysis for efficacy at 165 PFS events, ixabepilone crossed the futility boundary and the arm was closed per the Data and Safety Monitoring Board (DSMB) recommendation. Study results were not released, and CALGB 40502 reopened as a two-arm randomized study of nab-paclitaxel versus paclitaxel. At the second planned interim analysis, the nab-paclitaxel arm also crossed the futility boundary and accrual to the study was closed. The primary manuscript was later published with 18 months of additional follow-up. Therein, a post hoc analysis of ixabepilone was determined to be inferior to paclitaxel with an HR for PFS of 1.59 (95% CI: 1.31–1.93, $p < .0001$). Nab-paclitaxel results failed to reach statistical significance with an HR of 1.20 (95% CI: 1.00–1.45, log rank $p = .054$), but with greater toxicity observed than with the standard arm of weekly paclitaxel.

Prediction for Interim Data Monitoring

Traditional group-sequential methods preserve statistical error rates (a and β) through error-spending and sample size adjustments. However, while these methods consider the statistical significance of effects, they have limitations. The methods generally do not: (a) consider information regarding the effect size (clinical relevance) and associated precision, and (b) convey information regarding potential effect size estimates and associated precision with trial continuation.

Jennison and Turnbull (14) proposed use of repeated confidence intervals (RCIs) for monitoring trials to address the first limitation. RCIs are a sequence of confidence intervals (CIs) (one at each interim analysis) with specified simultaneous (joint) coverage probability, constructed such that the confidence of each sequential CI varies using principles of group-sequential a-spending. The attractive features of RCIs are that they provide an estimate of effect, the width and the location of the CIs explicitly convey the precision of the estimate, and they provide flexibility in decision making. The stochastic curtailment approach addresses the second limitation by defining the criterion for early stopping for futility based on a measure of the probability of rejecting the null hypothesis at the final analysis (9,15). However, these methods do not evaluate the potential gain in precision and power with trial continuation to give the investigators a better understanding of the pros and cons associated with the decision to continue versus terminating the trial.

Motivated by these limitations, Evans et al. (16) proposed using prediction and predicted intervals to augment traditional methods when monitoring a clinical trial. The concept of predicted intervals is intuitive. One simply predicts the CI that would be observed at the end of the trial if it were to continue, conditional upon: (a) data observed to date, and (b) assumptions regarding data yet to be collected. Reasonable assumptions regarding data yet to be collected include: (a) that the observed trend continues, (b) the alternative hypothesis is true, (c) the null hypothesis is true, and (d) best or worst case scenarios are true. Predicted intervals can be used with repeated CIs when monitoring to control error rates. One can use a model to simulate future data and produce predicted interval plots (PIPs) (17), a concise, intuitive graphical summary that can be used by DMCs for evaluation. The methods can be implemented using modern software: www.cytel.com/software-solutions/east/predict.

Predicted intervals convey information regarding the effect size, thus providing a quantitative assessment in addition to qualitative assessment of the effect. Modest p values (and low estimates of conditional power) from traditional methods of interim data monitoring, may imply: (a) no effect, (b) larger variation than expected, or (c) not enough data. Predicted intervals can help distinguish between these. Low p values (and high estimates of conditional power) imply statistical significance but do not convey information regarding clinical relevance of the effect. Predicted intervals allow assessment of clinical significance as well as statistical significance.

One may also assess the potential improvement in precision with continued enrollment by comparing the width of the current CI (based on interim data) to the width of the predicted interval. If the width of the predicted interval is not sufficiently narrower than the CI, then the cost of trial continuation may outweigh the benefit of the minimal improvement in precision. Conditional power can be obtained directly from the plot as the percentage of predicted intervals excluding the null value.

One-Sample Designs

Sequential testing strategies have also been implemented in oncology trials that are earlier in the drug development process, including the use of two-stage designs for single-arm phase II studies. Clinical trials will often begin to explore the clinical activity of a drug when given at or near the maximum tolerated dose established from phase I trials as this is thought to deliver the maximum effect. Smaller single-arm trials can gain efficiency from stopping early for futility and minimizing cost and the number of patients exposed to ineffective treatments. To accomplish this goal, an exact two-stage inference plan for binary data was introduced by Fleming (18) and further developed by Simon (19) and others. The general idea is to enroll a small number (n_1) of trial participants and evaluate them for response (stage 1). If the number of responses (r_1) is not promising enough for further study, then the trial is stopped. Otherwise, the trial continues to enroll additional (n_2) participants in stage 2. Exact tests are constructed to test $H_0: p \leq p_0$ for a predefined "maximum unacceptable response rate" (p_0) and under the alternative target a certain response rate as sufficient to warrant further investigation, $p = p_1$, to determine a sample size that controls the type II

error, β. With the understanding that different sample sizes and tests can control (α, β), Simon (19) proposed maximizing the efficiency of the trial under two scenarios, which are referred to as "optimal" and "minimax" designs. Once p_0, p_1, α, and β, have been selected, the "optimal" design identifies n_1, n_2, and r_1, which minimizes the expected sample size under the null (EN_0). Alternatively, the "minimax" design uses the smallest possible $N = n_1 + n_2$, which generally results in more efficient trials when the targeted level of clinical activity is true. Jung et al. expanded the framework to consider "admissible" designs that are optimal for some combination of the two parameters defined by the weight, $w * N + (1 - w) * EN_0$. Figure 31.2 gives an illustration of the utility of an admissible design for $(p_0, p_1, \alpha, $ and $\beta) = (0.1, 0.2, 0.1, 0.1)$. The admissible design with $N = 90$ patients is nine patients smaller in total sample size than the optimal design, but only modestly increases EN_0 from 63.7 to 64.0 patients.

The framework has been extended to construct exact tests for binary data in three-stage designs (18,20), but are generally found to have minimal gains in efficiency over Simon two-stage designs. The principle of sequential testing can be taken to its limit with continuous monitoring with each patient enrolled. While this could negatively impact power when evaluating clinical activity, Ivanova et al. (21) suggested a continuous monitoring plan for toxicity in small phase II trials where the safety profile of a compound may not be fully developed. Pocock-style stopping boundaries are applied to the discrete binomial distribution to control study-wide probability of early termination with an acceptable toxicity rate.

After completion of a multistage trial, it is important to consider the impact of the design on interval estimates for the parameter of interest. Several methods have been proposed for binary data (22,23).

Example Phase II Trial With a Two-Stage Design

Evans et al. (24) describes a phase II trial evaluating low-dose oral etoposide for the treatment of relapsed or progressed AIDS-related Kaposi's sarcoma after systemic chemotherapy. The primary endpoint was tumor response defined as at least a 50% decrease in the number or size of existing lesions without the development of new lesions. A two-stage design was employed with the plan for enrolling 41 total participants. However, if there were no objective responses $(r_1 = 0)$ after the first $n_1 = 14$ participants have been evaluated (stage I), then the trial would be discontinued for futility. Notably, responses were observed in the first 14 participants, the trial continued, and etoposide was shown to be effective.

Adaptive Designs

In clinical trials, adaptive procedures have been considered in a number of different manners as a means of

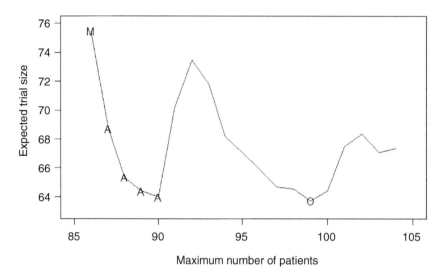

FIGURE 31.2 Different two-stage designs that satisfy the parameters (p_0, p_1, a, and β) = (0.1, 0.2, 0.1, 0.1). The line shows for a range of total sample sizes (x-axis) the smallest expected sample size under the null (y-axis) among all possible two-stage tests. Designs that satisfy the minimax ("M"), optimal ("O"), and admissible ("A") criteria are labeled accordingly.

improving efficiency of a study in answering the research question. Adaptive designs can be broadly categorized as studies that are updated iteratively over the course of the trial, in some characteristic of the design, whether it is patient eligibility and enrollment, study procedures, or analysis plans. In oncology, this includes the majority of phase I trials, where the initial dose of a patient is dependent on the dose levels and observed toxicities of earlier participants. In phase II and III studies, group sequential testing is generally not considered to be adaptive since early termination of the study is the only consideration in the decision rule. Rather adaptive methods include (a) reestimate sample size requirements, (b) population enrichment, (c) dose selection, and more controversially, (d) to modify randomization ratios according to patient outcomes (25). Here, we explore sample size reestimation in the context of group-sequential tests.

A motivation for sample size reestimation is when a clinically meaningful treatment effect cannot be targeted in an initial sample size and power calculation for a study, due to lack of prior knowledge of outcomes in the study population or operational constraints. With the accumulation of information in a group-sequential test, one considers adjustment of the final sample size (potentially either up or down) to modify the probability of rejecting the null hypothesis under effect sizes of interest. In order to maintain the integrity of the trial, the overall type I error must be controlled while performing the adaptations. This can be achieved by changing the test statistic with any change in sample size to one that partitions the data before and after the event, and then apply weights to each component such that a is preserved (26). A popular approach to formulating the new sample size is to divide the conditional power into three zones: Favorable, Promising, and Unfavorable. If

results fall in the Favorable or Unfavorable zone, sample size is unchanged; conversely if they fall within the Promising zone, one adjusts the sample size to bring the conditional power of target effects up to a more acceptable level (27). It is important to acknowledge that the adaptive method will be less efficient than a standard group-sequential design powered for the target effect, but does not negate the utility of the design when a trial of that size is not viable at study onset (28). Adaptive methods are becoming increasingly common in oncology trials, and the sample size reestimation plan noted previously is embedded in the international phase III trial of the addition of palbociclib to standard adjuvant endocrine therapy in early-stage breast cancer (PALLAS, NCT02513394) (29).

When implementing adaptive procedures, trial integrity can be threatened if trial results can be inferred as a result of the adaptation, for example, if people can backcalculate the observed treatment effect based on a revised sample size or randomization ratio. For example the VALOR trial evaluated vosaroxin for the treatment of acute myeloid leukemia. The sample size was increased by 225 patients following a recommendation by the DMC based on the Promising zone strategy described previously. While the study team was blinded to the details of the interim analysis results, the decision on whether or not to increase the sample size had to be announced creating speculation of survival benefit. This announcement had effects on investors and could have an impact on the patient characteristics or conduct of the study. It is possible that the study conduct, for example, patient population, might be different before and after the interim analysis. In fact, VALOR concluded with a negative, albeit borderline result (30). A mechanism to prevent this should be developed, for example, keeping the details regarding sample size methodology and recalculated sample size in very limited distribution.

DATA MONITORING COMMITTEES

DMCs/DSMBs

Considerations when monitoring the conduct of clinical trials include the potential use of DMCs, which are also frequently called DSMBs in National Institutes of Health (NIH) sponsored trials. DMCs are a group of individuals who review accumulating trial data by treatment arm in order to monitor patient safety and efficacy, ensure the validity and integrity of the trial, and make a benefit–risk assessment (31). Use of DMCs may enhance the credibility of trials. In 2016, the Clinical Trials Transformative Initiative (CTTI) provided a set of recommendations on best practices for DMCs.

DMCs traditionally monitor blinded trials that evaluate interventions intended to reduce major morbidity or mortality, where the trial may be sponsored by industry, government, or other organizations. DMCs then make recommendations to the trial sponsor regarding future trial conduct. DMCs typically oversee the conduct of a single trial but they are occasionally asked to review multiple related trials, for example, all late-phase trials from a pharmaceutical development program, a NIH-funded cooperative group, or an academic institution. We discuss the importance that DMC members are independent of the trial sponsor. Useful references regarding issues with DMCs include DeMets et al. (32), Ellenberg et al. (33), and Herson (34).

When Are DMCs Needed?

There are several considerations when determining whether a DMC is needed. The NIH has required DSMB oversight for all phase III multicenter trials since 1979. DMCs are more likely to be necessary in trials with:

- High-risk interventions or when very little is known about the safety and efficacy profile of the intervention (e.g., novel interventions)
- Invasive interventions or procedures (e.g., requiring surgery)
- Conditions that are life-threatening or have a high mortality or morbidity (e.g., oncology)
- Ethical dilemmas
- Long duration as accumulating medical information can influence the utility and ethics of ongoing trials
- A requirement of a "waiver of informed consent" (e.g., emergency treatment trials; or psychiatric conditions)
- Vulnerable populations (e.g., pediatric, elderly, pregnant women, mentally ill, people of poverty)

Composition

DMC membership is multidisciplinary with generally three to seven members. Essential members include clinicians who have expertise in the disease and intervention area and statisticians who are knowledgeable in clinical trials and statistical methods for data monitoring. Additional members may include bioethicists, patient advocates, pharmacologists, or others as needed.

DMC members should be free from conflict of interest so that recommendations are objective. Conflicts can be financial, intellectual, professional, or regulatory-based. Members are often paid, but the payment is not linked to trial outcome and does not include company stock. DMC conflicts should be reviewed before each DMC activity during the course of a trial. Contracts with DMC members now often include indemnification clauses for the protection from liability claims.

An ongoing concern in clinical trials has been the paucity of experienced DMC members. Although there are many people who are clearly experts in various disease areas, many are not experienced with DMC service and processes, and may not fully appreciate the consequences of DMC actions and recommendations.

Roles

DMCs have a unique role in trial oversight, and while responsibilities may vary somewhat according to the clinical trial setting, some fundamental principles apply broadly. DMCs are used to periodically review the accumulating unmasked safety and efficacy data by treatment arm, and advise the trial sponsor on whether to continue, modify, or terminate a trial based on benefit–risk assessment.

The role of the DMC may be described as proactive trial stewardship, preserving the scientific integrity of the trial while monitoring participant safety. The DMC mission consists of: (a) protecting patients and evaluating equipoise (e.g., is it still ethical to randomize or follow trial participants on current interventions?); (b) protecting credibility of the trial by preserving the blind, confidentiality, protecting statistical error rates, minimizing operational bias, and maintaining consistency with the protocol; (c) ensuring that the research objectives can be appropriately addressed; and (d) ensuring that reliable results are available to the medical community in a timely fashion (this role is not universally viewed as necessary in industry-sponsored trials).

DMCs evaluate safety and may recommend stopping any arm of a trial if an intervention is unacceptably toxic. DMCs need to be aware of multiplicity and the role of chance when evaluating safety using between-arm comparisons of many adverse events (AEs) or laboratory abnormalities. Statistical significance is neither necessary nor sufficient for the DMC to take action. Clinical relevance and the severity of events are carefully considered. Safety is often interpreted within the context of observed or hypothesized efficacy.

DMCs may evaluate efficacy and recommend stopping early according to the principles of group-sequential testing described previously. With early stopping for efficacy, a DMC should still consider whether a positive trial should continue to collect important safety data. Conversely, when evaluating futility DMCs should carefully consider the importance of continuing in order to obtain a conclusive result (i.e., that relevant effects can be ruled out with reasonable confidence).

Responsibilities

Prior to the trial, the DMC carefully reviews the trial protocol, and may offer feedback to the trial sponsor on elements that would enhance the ability of the DMC to carry out its responsibilities.

During trial conduct, a DMC reviews trial data that may not yet be clean or adjudicated. Evaluation consists of the primary and secondary outcome measures, deaths, patient disposition, other serious and nonserious AEs, benefit–risk assessment, consistency of effect for different outcomes, and the consistency of outcomes across important subgroups. DMCs also consider recruitment progress and feasibility, representativeness of enrolled participants, continued relevance of the trial objective, data quality and timeliness (e.g., missing endpoint data and accuracy of important measurements), protocol adherence, the prevalence of missing data, length of follow-up, whether results could change with trial continuation, external consistency of results with other studies, comparability of the intervention groups with respect to baseline factors, concomitant therapy use, and the impact of external information (e.g., results from other studies) on trial conduct.

The DMC provides recommendations to the sponsor steering committee (a committee not involved in trial operations) in a timely fashion, in writing and perhaps verbally. DMCs may request additional unplanned analyses or unscheduled DMC meetings without notifying the sponsor or investigators.

It is recommended that DMCs not adjudicate study endpoints, review all AEs individually (but may review specific AEs of interest as necessary), or have a role in redesigning the trial after reviewing data.

Organization and Operations

The DMC process is a design feature to be planned during protocol development and before trial initiation. A typical organization flow includes the DMC, a statistical and data analysis center (SDAC), the sponsor, and a steering committee associated with the sponsor. A modern industry model is displayed in Figure 31.3. For NIH-funded trials, the steering committee often consists of NIH personnel. In industry-sponsored trials, the steering committee may consist of members of senior management and possibly academic consultants with expertise in the disease area.

The DMC receives the protocol from the sponsor and interim reports from the SDAC. The DMC does not generally receive raw electronic data or conduct the statistical analyses. After reviewing and discussing the data, the DMC makes a recommendation to the steering committee.

Food and Drug Administration (FDA) guidance suggests that an "independent statistician" from the SDAC prepare the DMC reports and present the data during closed sessions of DMC meeting to protect the blind and avoid potential bias. Thus, this is the general practice in industry-sponsored trials. The independent

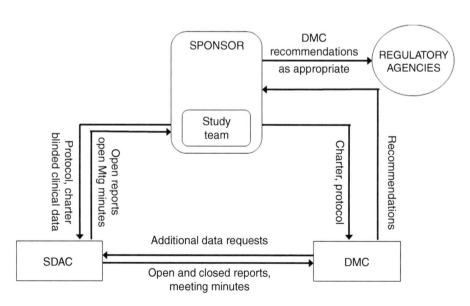

FIGURE 31.3 Organizational flow for a data monitoring committee.

statistician role is often contracted to contract research organizations (CROs). Although the independent statistician is paid by the sponsor, it is advantageous to view the independent statistician as working at the behest of the DMC. The independent statistician may iteratively interact with the DMC to ensure that appropriate data summaries for effective DMC evaluation are prepared and to ensure that the analyses are truly independent. The protocol statistician remains blinded in this model.

One concern that can arise with the independent statistician model is that an independent statistician may not be knowledgeable enough about the trial to prepare a high-quality report that will be adequate for quality DMC evaluation. The DMC also frequently asks questions about the data and trial conduct. Thus, some clinical trial networks funded by the NIH do not utilize the independent statistician model. Instead the protocol statistician prepares the DMC reports.

Given the concerns with creating a quality DMC report and the ability to address DMC questions, it is important that the independent statistician be very engaged and knowledgeable about the trial design and conduct, knowledgeable regarding the disease and interventions being studied, and capable of answering questions and discussing issues. Good independent statisticians understand the roles and needs of the DMC. They anticipate potential DMC questions/concerns arising from the data even if not a part of preplanned analyses and proactively addresses them. The independent statistician may lead the DMC through the closed report during the closed session.

Charter
The roles, responsibilities, and operational processes of the DMC should be outlined in a DMC charter. The charter should be concise, well organized, and written in plain language. The charter is not a legal document and language should reflect this so as not to handicap the DMC. The charter is designed to empower the DMC, allowing flexibility in operations and recommendations but also ensures that the sponsor perspectives are represented. The charter is reviewed and discussed at the first DMC meeting and finalized by the sponsor and the DMC prior to patient enrollment. A suggested outline for a DMC charter is provided in Table 31.1.

Meetings
The first meeting of a DMC is generally an organizational meeting prior to patient recruitment to review the trial protocol, DMC charter, monitoring plan, and the proposed data summaries that will be presented as part of the DMC reports. It is advised that this meeting is face to face given the depth of the meeting agenda.

Subsequent DMC meetings typically consist of two or three sessions. The first session is a limited open session where often a summary of baseline data and trial issues are presented by leaders of the study team to the DMC.

Blinded data are not discussed. The second session is closed with only the DMC members and the independent statistician attending. The independent statistician may present highlights from the DMC report, and the DMC members discuss the blinded results. Questions or recommendations are prepared by the DMC. The third session is generally reserved for the DMC to provide recommendations to the steering committee. Recently the third session has been eliminated to allow a period for written comments from the sponsor to the DMC.

DMCs may meet a prespecified number of times per year (e.g., 1–4) or may meet based upon a trigger (e.g., enrolling a particular number of participants, a particular number of participants having reached a specific time point, or a specific number of events having been observed). The DMC should meet face to face at least annually at a neutral location. Additional meetings may be held by telecom/webinar.

Occasionally, an unscheduled DMC meeting may be held. For example, if an unexpected death occurs potentially indicating an immediate safety concern or if other data has become available that may influence the ethics or science associated with the trial.

Two sets of DMC meeting minutes are prepared: one set of minutes for the open session, which can be distributed to team members, and another set of minutes for the closed session, which is not distributed but is archived in case it is needed as part of a regulatory submission.

Reports
Data Monitoring Plan. It is often useful for a project team, led by the project statistician, to develop a data monitoring plan (DMP). A DMP may be viewed as an analog to a statistical analysis plan (SAP) that describes how the trial data will be monitored. The project statistician and the medical monitor interact with DMC members regarding particular safety concerns and generate a plan regarding when and how often reports need to be constructed and what they will contain. Typical elements of a DMP include: a description of the reports that will be generated during trial conduct, what the reports will contain (e.g., analyses that will be performed), the rationale for the report, who prepares the report, who receives the report, when the reports will be generated and their frequency, and whether the report contains blinded data. The DMP can be reviewed and discussed at the first DMC meeting.

Preparation. Preparation for a DMC meeting begins several months prior to the meeting and may include time for some data cleaning, endpoint adjudication, a rehearsal meeting, and allowance for review time. An example timeline is provided in Table 31.2.

Good planning is an essential part of DMC report generation. The SDAC should receive a scheduled transfer of accumulating data rather than only at regularly scheduled DMC reviews, to ensure they can meet

TABLE 31.1 Suggested Outline for a DMC Charter

- **Introduction**
  - Title, objectives, interventions, and trial schema
  - DMC charter scope
- **DMC Roles and Responsibilities**
- **DMC Composition**
  - COI disclosure and procedure for ongoing evaluation
  - Replacing members
- **Governance and Relationships With Other Trial Committees**
- **Independence**
  - Affirm the independence of DMC members from the trial sponsor and investigators
  - Indicate flexibility for DMC to request additional analyses and conduct unscheduled DMC meetings
- **Prior to the First Interim Analysis**
  - Describe the DMC involvement in the protocol review process
  - Describe DMC meetings prior to the first interim analysis including the DMC charter review
- **Organization of DMC Meetings**
  - Expected frequency of DMC meetings including flexibility to have ad hoc meetings
  - Meeting format (e.g., face to face, teleconference)
  - Meeting sessions (e.g., open, closed) including the attendees
- **Documentation, Confidentiality, and Communication**
  - Outline the material available in the open and closed sessions
  - Indicate to whom the DMC communicates recommendations and the process
  - Describe data security procedures and the flow of information (i.e., how reports will be distributed to DMC members; collection or destroying of DMC reports after the meeting)
- **Decision Making**
  - Define a DMC quorum, voting process, and how recommendations will be achieved
  - Outline potential DMC recommendations, reference statistical methods for decision making and whether methods are binding or nonbinding for recommendations
- **Reporting**
  - Process for recording, archiving, and distributing DMC minutes
  - Describe how DMC recommendations and sponsor responses are communicated to stakeholders (e.g., IRBs, investigators) and how to resolve disagreements between the DMC and sponsor
- **After Study is Completed**
  - Plan for acknowledgment of the DMC in publications
- **Appendix**
  - Research design synopsis/figure
  - DMC contact information including the SDAC
  - Figure: relationship between DMC, trial committees, and other stakeholders (e.g., IRBs, investigators, regulatory agencies)
  - DMC report contents: tables, listings, and figures
  - Process for executing revisions to the charter
  - List of abbreviations

COI, conflict of interest; DMC, data monitoring committee; IRB, institutional review board; SDAC, statistical and data analysis center.

charter-driven responsibilities. A specific yet flexible schedule for transfer of accumulating data should be described in the charter. To create a DMC report, typically, clean formatted/labeled SAS data sets are sent to the SDAC with other important information (e.g., protocol, case report forms [CRFs]). There has been debate as to whether canned programs that produce standard output should also be provided to the independent statistician. The advantage of doing so is that the preplanning provides efficiency and eliminates surprises and analyses that the sponsor views as undesirable. The disadvantage is that the independent statistician and the resulting report that he or she generates is not truly independent of the sponsor and that such preplanned

analyses may not address issues raised by review of the data itself (e.g., additional data may be needed to understand an unexpected result or event such as a participant death).

Planning to have important endpoints adjudicated, batching participant samples for analyses in a timely fashion so that lab data are available, data entry, and the potential cleaning important endpoint data, help to ensure that the DMC has the most complete and up-to-date data as possible. Reporting of important data (e.g., deaths, serious adverse events [SAEs]) can lag resulting in underreporting. *Sweeping* can be performed whereby each investigator contacts each participant at a particular time point prior to a DMC meeting, essentially

TABLE 31.2 Example Timeline for DMC Review Preparation

Key Task	Relative to DMC
Memo sent to sites alerting of DMC review	13 weeks before
First clinical endpoint review*	12 weeks before
Last date of clinic visits/specimens included in the review	9 weeks before
Second clinical endpoint review*	8 weeks before
All CRFs up through the last date of clinic visits keyed	7 weeks before
Final data delinquency report run	7 weeks before
Final queries/discrepancies to sites	6 weeks before
Deadline for last corrections from sites	5 weeks before
Analysis files frozen	5 weeks before
Draft reports due	3.5 weeks before
Rehearsal meeting	3 weeks before
Final DMC reports due	2 weeks before
Reports distributed to DMC members	2 weeks before
DMC meeting	Day 0

*Materials for review are provided 1 week in advance of the scheduled meeting.

CRF, case report form; DMC, data monitoring committee.

fast-tracking important data into the database and ultimately the DMC report. A data freeze is typically conducted as recently as possible (e.g., 4 weeks) prior to the DMC meeting. Reports should be delivered to DMC members 1 to 2 weeks prior to the meeting to allow time for a thorough review. DMC reports are generally collected at the end of the meeting and are destroyed to protect trial integrity. Interim data and DMC discussion must remain confidential as leaks can create operational bias by affecting recruitment, adherence, follow-up, or participant/clinician outcome assessment.

Reports. The format of the report should be agreed upon prior to the first DMC interim analysis meeting. DMC reports should be informative, thoughtful, and efficient. The goal of the report is to inform the DMC members regarding the status and health of the trial participants and summarize the intervention effects. A DMC report should begin with a brief schema that reminds the DMC members of the trial design. A summary of the trial history including minutes from prior DMC meetings

is helpful. Historically, there have been issues with the quality of DMC reports. Many are too voluminous (i.e., several hundred or even thousands of pages) and difficult to digest with hundreds of tables and AE listings that span many pages. Examples of poor report preparation are provided in Table 31.3. Tables with zeros in most of the cells, too many decimal places in summaries, or case summaries of all patients are also generally undesirable although patient case summaries may be helpful in very small trials. Creative graphics such as a CONSORT chart, Kaplan–Meier plots, forest plots, and side-by-side boxplots are useful displays that are easy to interpret. Special cases (e.g., deaths, unexpected outcomes) should be investigated and reported in patient narratives. Long listings and other voluminous information can be put into appendices. Although preprogramming a report is likely necessary, it is often not sufficient. DMC reports should include text summaries of important findings (facts and not opinions). Suggestions for preparing DMC reports are summarized in Table 31.3.

DMC reports may include by-treatment summaries of accrual, important baseline variables and demographics, study status and duration of follow-up, participants off-study with reasons, participants off-treatment with reasons, protocol violations, adherence, concomitant medication use, deaths and AEs, endpoint evaluability and data completeness for important variables, and possibly efficacy endpoint summaries. Whether efficacy endpoint summaries are provided to DMCs when there is no formal efficacy analysis planned has been an issue of debate. Recent guidelines have suggested that efficacy data be available to the DMC since even evaluation of safety should be interpreted within the context of efficacy.

Open versions of the DMC report are often provided to project team members. Open reports typically contain aggregate summaries (i.e., not by intervention). However, aggregate summaries of efficacy data can be informative regarding treatment effects and should only be reviewed by DMC members. Thus, many independent statisticians limit the open report to only baseline and possibly safety summaries.

When preparing DMC reports, only the independent statistician is unblinded. It is also not necessary to blind a DMC. The DMC may need to be unblinded in order to make a thorough evaluation and an informed recommendation. Some independent statisticians mask treatment with arbitrary labels (e.g., "Treatment A") but may provide a sealed envelope to DMC members with the DMC report to be opened at their discretion (i.e., when DMC members feel that they need to know the identity of the treatment groups).

Communication and Recommendations

Communication processes between the DMC and trial sponsor should be carefully specified in the charter. The DMC should have minimal interactions with the

TABLE 31.3 Real Examples of Poor DMC Report Preparation and Suggestions for Preparing Reports

- Examples of Poor Preparation.
  - Example 1: One day prior to a scheduled DMC meeting for a large pharmaceutical company, DMC members are delivered a disk with the report. The disk contained 49 files. The first file contained 1,600 pages of tables.
    - Lesson: Reports should be delivered 1–2 weeks prior to a meeting. Reports should not be so voluminous such that it cannot be digested. Text is needed to highlight important results. A table of contents should map the report so that results are easy to find.
  - Example 2: DMC members receive a 300-page report but only four participants had been randomized.
    - Lesson: Automated programming cannot replace critical thinking. A case summary of each participant may be more helpful here.
- Suggestions for DMC report preparation.
  - Protect the blind and trial integrity; minimize access to data to only DMC members.
  - Use data as recent as possible. Updates to important results can be brought to a face-to-face meeting.
  - Use a table of contents so that results are easy to find.
  - Construct text to highlight important results (facts but not opinions).
  - Strive to answer important questions rather than provide extensive listings.
  - Be aware of the length of the report (strive for quality over quantity).
  - Use graphics to display the data (visual summaries are often easier to digest than lots of tables).
  - Use appendices for long data summaries (e.g., AE listings).
  - Predict DMC questions and address them in advance.
  - Use rehearsal meetings.
  - Prepare slides to present important results at DMC meetings.

AE, adverse event; DMC, data monitoring committee.

sponsor outside the formal DMC open session of the meeting.

DMC trial recommendations and proposed modifications should be provided to a steering committee authorized to act on those recommendations, and not to those directly involved with implementation of the trial. DMCs may recommend a protocol modification, early trial termination, or a temporary hold until issues have been resolved. The most common DMC recommendation is to simply continue the trial as planned. However, the role of the DMC is advisory. The steering committee can filter the recommendation before providing the trial team with a recommendation. The sponsor then must decide to accept or reject the recommendation. This can be a difficult decision because the recommendations may conflict with the interests of the sponsor. Recommendations can have significant implications in terms of the future of the trial or intervention development as well as regulatory activities. Most DMC recommendations are carried forward, however. Some steering committees (frequently with NIH-sponsored trials) prefer not to filter the recommendation and have the DMC make recommendations directly to the project team.

Recommendations from the DMC to the trial sponsor should be conveyed with the minimal amount of information necessary to provide clarity and constructed so that operational bias is not induced, and that blinding is maintained. Operational bias can be induced when participants, clinicians, or others involved in the trial change their actions due to the leaking of trial results such that inferences regarding trial results can be made. Such actions may be intentional or unintentional. For

example, the integrity of the Immunotherapy for Prostate Adenocarcinoma Treatment (IMPACT) trial was jeopardized (35) when a press release was issued during trial conduct indicating that Provenge reduced mortality in castration-resistant prostate cancer. Operational bias may manifest in participants dropping out of the trial or not adhering to the protocol or investigators choosing not to enroll participants or rating patient responses differently. Thus, extreme care must be taken when making recommendations. The DMC recommendation should be limited to a recommendation and is not necessarily a statement of the results particularly if the trial is to continue. Statements such as "the DMC recommends that the trial continue as planned" are generally sufficient. DMC members should not have discussions about the trial outside of DMC meetings to prevent operational bias from occurring.

The charter should specify how disagreements between the sponsor and the DMC are to be managed. If the sponsor agrees with the DMC recommendations, then the sponsor should report the major DMC recommendations to regulatory bodies and institutional review boards (IRBs) within an appropriate time period. Minor operational recommendations need not be reported. If the sponsor does not agree with the DMC recommendations, the sponsor and DMC should first try to come to resolution. However, the sponsor makes the ultimate decision. That decision, along with supporting rationale and the DMC's written recommendations, should be provided to regulatory bodies and IRBs within an appropriate time period. Since 1999, the NIH has required that local IRBs be notified of the outcome of all DSMB reviews, even when no major change has been recommended, to document that appropriate data and safety monitoring is occurring as expected. IRBs and regulatory bodies may act independently based on their assessment of the disputed information.

Other Issues

The increasing use of adaptive designs has also generated discussion regarding how such trials affect the roles and operations of DMCs. Given the statistical complexity of adaptive trials and the experience of some expert statisticians, it is worth considering to have more than one statistician on these DMCs and having a statistician serve as the DMC chair. Care should be taken when drafting a DMC charter in an adaptive trial. It is important to carefully consider the role of the DMC in such trials as some adaptations should be made independent of the observed treatment effects in the trial. In this case, the DMC is not the appropriate body to make decisions regarding or implementing adaptations as they see these data. Other adaptations can only be made after observing the interim treatment effects. In this case, the DMC may be an appropriate body to review these data and recommend or implement an adaptation. For example, in a recent randomized controlled trial evaluating a treatment of lymphoma, a plan was made to calculate the conditional power during the interim analyses. A prespecified sample size (actually the required number of events given the event-time primary endpoint) rule was developed (i.e., if very low then stop trial for futility; if very high then continue as scheduled; but if in the middle then adjust the number of required events based on the observed effect size). Details of the rule were put into a "closed protocol" and made available only to the DMC but not primary members of the protocol team. To protect trial integrity from operational bias induced back-calculation if a revised number of required events are announced to the project team, the DMC did not reveal the results of the calculation. Instead the DMC was kept apprised of the number of events, and indicated "stop" when the required number of events was observed.

DISCUSSION

Interim data monitoring is a fundamental aspect of clinical trials. It can help protect the welfare of trial participants and improve efficiency. However, interim data monitoring also carries risks including inflation of statistical error rates associated with multiple testing and the introduction of operational bias that can jeopardize trial integrity. We have described statistical methods that have been developed to control statistical error rates when interim evaluations of trial hypotheses are conducted. We have also described DMCs that help to preserve trial integrity and reduce the risk of operational bias that can occur with interim evaluation of data. The integrity of a clinical trial can be threatened if a trial is not designed or conducted with appropriate data monitoring processes and interim analysis methods.

Concerns have arisen that DMC decisions are often not truly independent but are driven by marketing considerations rather than the health of trial participants and the public. An example where DMC actions have been questioned occurred in a randomized placebo-controlled trial evaluating Zytiga for the treatment of prostate cancer. The study had coprimary endpoints of radiographic PFS and overall survival, with the type I error split to 0.04 and 0.01, respectively, with group-sequential testing procedures for each. At the first interim analysis, a highly significant 57% reduction in the risk of progression crossed the boundary for superiority ($p < .0001$); however, a trend in improvement in overall survival failed to cross the prespecified boundary ($p = .01$ vs. $p = .008$) (36). Nevertheless, the independent DMC recommended terminating the study early, unblinding results, and allowing patients on placebo to receive Zytiga. As a consequence, a statistically significant improvement in overall survival was never demonstrated. Yet, based on the observed treatment benefit, there was a high likelihood that results would have crossed the O'Brien–Fleming boundary at the next interim, and led to a statistically significant improvement in survival. Since the initial randomized version of the trial was stopped, there is a perception that the DMC decision was motivated by business rather than scientific and ethical concerns. This illustrates the careful balance of ethical considerations when monitoring clinical trials. The independence of the DMC is critical in maintaining trial integrity during trial monitoring and methodologies that rigorously control trial-wide error when making inferences regarding treatment effects should be utilized.

REFERENCES

1. Food and Drug Administration. *Guidance for Industry: E9 Statistical Principles for Clinical Trials.* Rockville, MD: Food and Drug Administration; 1998.
2. Armitage P, McPherson C, Rowe B. Repeated significance tests on accumulating data. *J R Stat Soc Series A.* 1969;132:235–244.
3. Pocock SJ. Group sequential methods in the design and analysis of clinical trials. *Biometrika.* 1977;64(2):191–199.
4. Pocock S, White I. Trials stopped early: too good to be true? *Lancet.* 1999;353(9157):943–944.
5. Haybittle J. Repeated assessment of results in clinical trials of cancer treatment. *Br J Radiol.* 1971;44(526):793–797.
6. Peto R, Pike M, Armitage P, et al. Design and analysis of randomized clinical trials requiring prolonged observation of each patient. I. Introduction and design. *Br J Cancer.* 1976;34(6):585.
7. O'Brien PC, Fleming TR. A multiple testing procedure for clinical trials. *Biometrics.* 1979;35(3):549–556.
8. Lan KKG, DeMets DL. Discrete sequential boundaries for clinical-trials. *Biometrika.* 1983;70(3):659–663.
9. Lan K, Simon R, Halperin M. Stochastically curtailed tests in long–term clinical trials. *Sequential Analysis.* 1982;1(3):207–219.

10. Fleming TR, Harrington DP, O'Brien PC. Designs for group sequential tests. *Control Clin Trials*. 1984;5(4):348–361.

11. Freidlin B, Korn EL. A comment on futility monitoring. *Control Clin Trials*. 2002;23(4):355–366.

12. Jung SH, Kim C, Chow SC. Sample size calculation for the log-rank tests for multi-arm trials with a control. *J Korean Stat Soc*. 2008;37(1):11–22.

13. Rugo HS, Barry WT, Moreno-Aspitia A, et al. Randomized Phase III trial of paclitaxel once per week compared with nanoparticle albumin-bound nab-paclitaxel once per week or ixabepilone with bevacizumab as first-line chemotherapy for locally recurrent or metastatic breast cancer: CALGB 40502/ NCCTG N063H (Alliance). *J Clin Oncol*. 2015;33(21):2361–2369.

14. Jennison C, Turnbull BW. Repeated confidence intervals for group sequential clinical trials. *Control Clin Trials*. 1984;5(1):33–45.

15. Choi SC, Smith PJ, Becker DP. Early decision in clinical trials when the treatment differences are small: experience of a controlled trial in head trauma. *Control Clin Trials*. 1985;6(4):280–288.

16. Evans SR, Li L, Wei L. Data monitoring in clinical trials using prediction. *Drug Inf J*. 2007;41(6):733–742.

17. Li, L, Evans SR, Uno H, et al., Predicted interval plots (PIPS): a graphical tool for data monitoring of clinical trials. *Stat Biopharm Res*. 2009;1(4):348–355.

18. Fleming TR. One-sample multiple testing procedure for Phase II clinical trials. *Biometrics*. 1982;38(1):143–151.

19. Simon R. Optimal 2-stage designs for Phase-II clinical-trials. *Control Clin Trials*. 1989;10(1):1–10.

20. Chen TT. Optimal three-stage designs for Phase II cancer clinical trials. *Stat Med*. 1997;16(23):2701–11.

21. Ivanova A, Qaqish BF, Schell MJ, Continuous toxicity monitoring in Phase II trials in oncology. *Biometrics*. 2005;61(2):540–545.

22. Atkinson EN, Brown BW. Confidence limits for probability of response in multistage Phase II clinical-trials. *Biometrics*. 1985;41(3):741–744.

23. Koyama T, Chen H. Proper inference from Simon's two-stage designs. *Stat Med*. 2008;27(16):3145–3154.

24. Evans SR, Krown SE, Testa MA, et al. Phase II evaluation of low-dose oral etoposide for the treatment of relapsed or progressive AIDS-related Kaposi's sarcoma: an AIDS Clinical Trials Group clinical study. *J Clin Oncol.*, 2002;20(15):3236–3241.

25. Korn EL, Freidlin B. Outcome—adaptive randomization: is it useful? *J Clin Oncol.*, 2011;29(6):771–776.

26. Chi L, Hung H, Wang SJ. Modification of sample size in group sequential clinical trials. *Biometrics*. 1999;55(3):853–857.

27. Gao P, Ware JH, Mehta C. Sample size re-estimation for adaptive sequential design in clinical trials. *J Biopharm Stat*. 2008;18(6):1184–1196.

28. Mehta CR, Pocock SJ. Adaptive increase in sample size when interim results are promising: a practical guide with examples. *Stat Med*. 2011;30(28):3267–3284.

29. Mayer E, DeMichele A, Dubsky P, et al. Abstract OT1-03-21: PALLAS: PAlbociclib Collaborative Adjuvant Study: a randomized Phase 3 trial of palbociclib with adjuvant endocrine therapy versus endocrine therapy alone for HR+/HER2- early breast cancer. *Cancer Res*. 2016;76(4, Suppl):OT1-03-21-OT1-03-21.

30. Ravandi F, Ritchie EK, Sayar H, et al. Vosaroxin plus cytarabine versus placebo plus cytarabine in patients with first relapsed or refractory acute myeloid leukaemia (VALOR): a randomised, controlled, double-blind, multinational, Phase 3 study. *Lancet Oncol*. 2015;16(9):1025–1036.

31. DeMets DL, Ellenberg SS. Data monitoring committees—expect the Unexpected. *N Engl J Med*. 2016;375(14):1365–1371.

32. DeMets DL, Friedman LM, Furberg CD. *Data Monitoring in Clinical Trials*. New York, NY: Springer Publishing; 2006.

33. Ellenberg SS, Fleming TR, DeMets DL. *Data Monitoring Committees in Clinical Trials: A Practical Perspective*. Chichester, West Sussex, UK: John Wiley & Sons; 2003.

34. Herson J. *Data and Safety Monitoring Committees in Clinical Trials*. Boca Raton, FL: Chapman & Hall/CRC Press; 2009.

35. Kantoff PW, Higano CS, Shore ND, et al. Sipuleucel-T immunotherapy for castration-resistant prostate cancer. *N Engl J Med*. 2010;363:411–422.

36. Ryan CJ, Smith MR, de Bono JS, et al. Abiraterone in metastatic prostate cancer without previous chemotherapy. *N Engl J Med*. 2013;368(2):138–148. doi:10.1056/nejmoa1209096

Reporting of Results: Data Analysis and Interpretation

Donna Niedzwiecki

The clinical trial process culminates with the reporting of study results. These reports may be prepared in many ways including via scientific presentations and through published journal articles. The reporting of clinical trial results has evolved over time, particularly with respect to the use and presentation of statistical methods. Standardization of reporting has been promoted including uniformity of study endpoints; elements of data capture; content; format; and the use of graphics to allow clearer comparisons and interpretation of results across reported trials in the same disease site.

Momentum toward the goal of standardization in the design, conduct, and reporting of randomized clinical trials was provided by the pharmaceutical industry. In the 1980s, the European community pioneered the harmonization of regulatory requirements across Europe with the goal of minimizing the length of time necessary to bring safe and effective treatments to the market. Japan and the United States became engaged in the process expanding the international effort. The International Conference on Harmonisation, comprising representatives from regulatory agencies and industries from the participating countries, was formed in April 1990. Expert working groups have been formed to make recommendations on specific topics related to the goals of the organization. In November 1995 the International Conference on Harmonisation Steering Committee approved and recommended guidelines on the structure and content of clinical study reports for adoption by the participating regulatory agencies (1–3). In October 2015 the group reorganized as the International Council for Harmonisation (ICH) (4). Another group consisting of clinical trial experts, medical journal editors, and epidemiologists first published the Consolidated Standards of Reporting Clinical Trials (CONSORT) statement in the *Journal of the American Medical Association* in 1996. The CONSORT statement addresses the issue of inadequate reporting of clinical trial results and is considered an evolving document (5,6). The CONSORT statement was updated in 2010; details about CONSORT (6) can be obtained on the CONSORT website (7).

Methods of data analysis and results reporting from clinical trials depend closely on the trial design and statistical analyses and, as much as possible, should be conducted according to the statistical considerations presented in the protocol document. This dependence reemphasizes the need for careful trial planning at the outset. However, not all events can be anticipated and unexpected events that occur during the conduct of the trial must also be addressed. For example, the targeted accrual of the trial may not be met; unexpected toxicity may be observed or statistical assumptions made at the design stage may not hold. Such occurrences potentially impact the analytic methods used and the reporting and interpretation of results. Results of data analyses are also heavily dependent on the quality of the data captured. Thus, an organized mechanism for data collection and review is essential.

In this chapter, aspects of the final data analysis and how to report results are discussed according to their relevance to specific sections of the final research publication. Illustrative examples are provided.

MANUSCRIPT STRUCTURE AND CONTENT

Manuscripts reporting the results from a clinical trial contain the following general elements: a title, authorship, an abstract, an introduction (background and significance), a description of clinical and statistical methods, the presentation of results, a discussion, and references. Each of these elements is described in the following in the context of providing a clear and valid representation of the design and conduct of the trial and its outcomes.

Title and Authorship

The title should identify the main elements of the study and include relevant key words with respect to search queries. Authors should be listed generally in order of the magnitude of their contributions to the study and to the development of the manuscript with the primary (first) author being responsible for the manuscript composition. A senior (last) author is often named; senior authorship acknowledges the role of the individual as a mentor. The roles of other authors can be determined according to their degrees and affiliations. Many journals include a specific listing of author contributions to each publication, which include activities such as concept and trial design, data collection, manuscript writing, review, and approval.

Abstract

The abstract is a brief summary of the background, primary goals of the trial, the methods employed in trial conduct, key results, and conclusions. The full manuscript content should be distilled to only the most important aspects of the study. Contents of the abstract should be consistent with the details provided in the manuscript. Based on the abstract a reader should be able to understand the significance of the trial in the broader area of research for the disease under study, how the trial was conducted, the primary endpoints studied, and what was learned.

Introduction

The introduction provides the background and significance of the trial and contains information regarding the patient population under study, prior treatment approaches, and justification for the treatment studied in the trial. Results from previous trials in the same or similar patient populations are referenced. Authors should provide a clear rationale for the conduct of the trial consistent with the prior data.

Methods

Detailed information regarding the study population, patient eligibility, treatment administration, clinical and laboratory methods of patient evaluation, and a general description of the study conducted are provided in the methods section. Often, the statistical methods are included in the general methods section though they may also appear separately as Statistical Considerations, Statistical Plan, or Statistical Analysis. The information provided in this section, again, should reflect all the specifications in the protocol and any other methods used.

Study Population

The explicit disease type and established cancer staging criteria used in the protocol, for example, the staging system proposed by the American Joint Committee on Cancer (AJCC), should be included to define the study population (8). Staging is specific to the particular disease and classifies the severity of the disease at presentation. Uniform classification of tumors allows, at minimum, descriptive comparisons of efficacy and toxicity across studies and the potential for meta-analyses. Other nonstandard staging systems are used in describing leukemia (9).

Disease state may further be defined using known prognostic factors that depend on the cancer type, for example, Gleason score and prostate-specific antigen (PSA) level in prostate cancer and Breslow depth in melanoma. Validated prognostic indices incorporating multiple prognostic factors into one assessment are also often used to classify or stratify patients by risk. Examples include the Halabi nomogram used to classify patients with prostate cancer and the Follicular Lymphoma International Prognostic Index (FLIPI) for patients with follicular lymphoma (10,11).

With the move to targeted therapy, based on the identification of molecular markers and pharmacogenomic characterization of tumors, patients may be increasingly identified as candidates for tumor-specific treatment strategies.

Additional eligibility, inclusion, and exclusion criteria should be listed. In addition to disease type and stage, examples of eligibility criteria include patient age, performance status (e.g., Karnofsky and Eastern Cooperative Oncology Group [ECOG]), numbers of prior treatment regimens, laboratory values, resection margins, and for biomarkers, patient's status on the molecular marker (12,13).

Understanding the patient population is critical to the interpretation of results. In 2002, results of a study on the use of hormone replacement therapy (HRT) among postmenopausal women indicated that the use of HRT was associated with a higher risk of certain cancers in this patient group (14). This finding led to an observed reduction in the use of HRT over the following years. In 2007 and 2008, reanalyses of the data stratifying women by time since onset of menopause showed no increased cancer risk when time past onset of menopause was considered (15,16).

Treatment and Administration

For treatment trials, the treatment under investigation is described as per protocol including the scheduling and dosing of each agent and methods of administration. The length of each treatment cycle and the duration of treatment should be specified. For example, treatment may be administered for a fixed number of cycles or until a specified event such as progression of disease. Sufficient details should be provided so that the treatment strategy can be replicated. Differences in dosing and administration of the same agent can greatly impact results in terms of efficacy or toxicity, which may require early reporting.

As an example, consider the use of irinotecan in the treatment of colon cancer. Irinotecan is a topoisomerase I inhibitor with demonstrated efficacy in the treatment of metastatic colon cancer in both the first-line and second-line settings. Based on the prior evidence of efficacy in patients with metastatic disease, the Cancer and Leukemia Group B (CALGB) activated a randomized phase III trial of irinotecan, fluorouracil plus leucovorin (IFL) versus fluorouracil plus leucovorin (FL), among patients with resectable stage III disease (C89803). In the IFL regimen, fluorouracil is given by bolus administration (17). A North Central Cancer Treatment Group (NCCTG) trial that was running simultaneously randomized patients with metastatic colorectal cancer to treatment with combinations of fluorouracil, irinotecan, and oxaliplatin and included an IFL treatment arm (N9741) (18). During the conduct of these trials, a higher than expected early (within 60 days of starting therapy) death rate was observed in the irinotecan-containing treatment arms relative to the FL control on C89803 and the oxaliplatin, fluorouracil plus leucovorin and oxaliplatin plus irinotecan treatment arms on N9471, resulting in temporary suspension of accrual on both trials. The 60-day all-cause death rates were 4.8% versus 1.8% on N9741 (Fisher exact $p = .06$) and 2.2% versus 0.8% on C89803 (Fisher exact $p = .06$). The lethal toxicity was reported in a letter to the editor of the *New England Journal of Medicine* in July 2001 (19). An independent group of investigators that was subsequently assembled to review the adverse events identified two syndromes associated with the bolus administration of irinotecan (20). (This toxicity is in contrast to the toxicity profile observed for the administration of irinotecan in combination with intravenously administered fluorouracil plus leucovorin, the FOLFIRI regimen, though the two regimens have not been directly compared in a single trial [(21)].) Treatment modifications were made as necessary to both trials. The clinical report for C89803 describes the toxicity experience (17). Though mentioned in the clinical report for N9741, the toxicity experience was more fully reported in a separate article (22).

Disclosure of the complete trial conduct is essential in reporting to allow the proper interpretation of results. For nontreatment trials, details regarding the intervention(s) should be presented.

Biomarker Studies

Tumor biomarker studies are often incorporated into clinical trials. When tumor biomarkers are used in defining the trial population they are described as integral. Biomarkers are also described as integral if they are needed for disease monitoring or the definition of study endpoints. Hypotheses based on biomarker status may also be included in a study as part of the scientific investigation; in this case the biomarkers are described as integrated. McShane and Hayes describe three main types of reporting bias associated with tumor marker research (23). These are publication bias, which arises due to a failure to submit or publish manuscripts reporting negative study results; selective reporting within a publication whereby only selected results are presented, for example, results that are statistically significant; and incomplete study reporting, lack of full details of study design, conduct, and analysis. The authors propose strategies to address these bias issues. To address publication bias they suggest creation of a registry of tumor marker studies. Their strategies to address selective and incomplete reporting are described under the Study Conduct and Results sections.

Study Conduct

Study conduct is described according to the study design given in the protocol. Studies can be classified as pilot or exploratory, safety trials, efficacy trials, or comparative trials. Other design features should be given such as whether a crossover was employed, whether blinding was used, if subjects were matched on prognostic factors, or whether the design was single stage or multistage. Details regarding the standard study designs used in clinical trials in cancer (e.g., phase I, phase II, phase III) are presented in earlier chapters. The individuals or organizations responsible for trial design and analysis, data capture, and monitoring should be identified. Ethical aspects, including institutional review board (IRB) approval for the protocol, patient informed consent, and monitoring by a formal data monitoring committee (if applicable), should be described.

For biomarker studies, adhering to the Biospecimen Reporting for Improved Study Quality (BRISQ) guidelines is recommended (23). These guidelines relate to the reporting of specimen collection, storage and handling, and details regarding laboratory assays and analyses (24).

Statistical Methods

The trial design and statistical considerations of the trial are provided in this section. Statistical methods should include the details of the trial design from the protocol: definitions of the primary and secondary endpoints; identification of patient subsets to be considered; stratification factors; estimation goals (precision); trial hypotheses; operating characteristics for tests of hypotheses (significance level, power); success criteria; targeted sample size; planned length of accrual and follow-up periods; planned interim analyses; and design modifications, if applicable. Detailed lists of recommended items for inclusion in reports of clinical trial results are provided by the Asilomar working group and the revised CONSORT statement (6,25).

The goal of the trial should be stated, for example, specify if the trial is hypothesis-testing, hypothesis-generating, or a screening trial. Data analysis methods are also presented. These should include all statistical tests used including those that are not specified in the protocol. Examples are the chi-square, Wilcoxon, or *t*-test to compare patient characteristics between treatment arms or subgroups based on sociodemographic and disease characteristics.

Define statistical estimates, in particular, time-to-event endpoints, where a lack of consistency exists in definition. Time-to-event endpoints in clinical trials include overall survival (OS), progression-free survival (PFS), time to progression (TTP), time to treatment failure (TTF), disease-free survival (DFS), and others. The starting time from which the time-to-event endpoint is measured (e.g., study entry or time of randomization) and the outcomes included as events (e.g., death or progression) should be provided. Patients who do not experience an event are considered as "censored," that is, observed only to a known time point prior to an event. For example, PFS is often measured from the time of study entry until documented progression of disease or death from any cause but is sometimes defined as the time from study entry until documented progression or death with documented progression. Under the first definition, censored patients consist of the group alive without progression at the last observed follow-up time. Under the second definition, censored patients consist of the group alive without progression or dead without documented progression at the last observed follow-up time. To reduce confusion, one naming convention might be to include the term "survival" in the name when all-cause mortality (e.g., DFS) is an event and to omit the term "survival" in the name when death is either not considered as an event or is considered as an event only if certain conditions exist, such as death with documented progression (e.g., TTP). The inclusion of death from any cause as an event is more conservative and is preferred in cases where it is difficult to determine if progression has occurred. In general, clearly defined estimates given in an article are potentially useful to other investigators for future study development in the same disease area.

Follow-up time can also be estimated in several ways and is important in the interpretation of long-term results. Estimates based on data at time points well beyond the median follow-up may be imprecise. Schemper and Smith describe and compare several methods of quantifying follow-up. They conclude that the Kaplan–Meier estimate of potential follow-up, obtained by reversing the role of the censoring variable in a Kaplan–Meier analysis, is the preferred method (26). Other authors recommend use of median follow-up among subjects who are alive at the time of analysis (27). Whatever method is used to estimate follow-up, it should be described in the statistical methods and the estimate reported under Results. The median follow-up time is also often used as a measure of data completeness though its interpretation is limited in this context. A more useful method for quantifying data completeness, proposed by Clark, et al. is discussed under the Results section (28).

Often analyses are conducted and reported in more than one patient subgroup. The group or subgroup of patients in which the primary endpoint is studied should be clearly defined. For example, specify if an analysis is intent to treat (ITT). In an ITT analysis all patients are included in the statistical analysis according to randomization assignment regardless of the treatment received (29). Primary and planned analyses should be distinguished from secondary or unplanned analyses.

Results

The Results section relates the actual experience of the clinical trial and the results of the statistical analyses. Results associated with the primary hypothesis are the main focus; results associated with secondary endpoints or unplanned analyses must be clarified as such. The appropriate test statistics must be used. Only facts relating to the conduct of the trial and the analytic results should be presented in this section. Qualifying and descriptive statements can be made in the Discussion section. Describe whether the trial successfully completed its research goals. For example, a trial may conclude early due to lack of efficacy according to protocol or unexpectedly due to unanticipated toxicity or relevant information obtained from external trials. If difficulties were encountered in the conduct of the trial these events and their impact on the trial should be provided in an administrative summary.

Patient Characteristics

State the actual number of patients enrolled on each stratum or randomized to each treatment arm at the outset, specifying the time period between activation (or first patient enrolled) and end of accrual (last patient enrolled). Patient flow can be illustrated in a diagram of study subjects and is required by some journals (30). The patient flow diagram provides the numbers of enrolled patients, eligible patients, patients who withdrew or who received protocol therapy, and patients included in the primary statistical analyses. Other information such as numbers of patients completing treatment by treatment arm may also be summarized in this chart. A flow diagram, as recommended by CONSORT (7), of study subjects from C89803 is provided in Figure 32.1.

For trials with a time-to-event endpoint and longer median time to event, such as OS in an adjuvant trial, a determination of data completeness is useful in interpreting results. More complete data are generally associated with greater reliability. Clark, Altman, and De Stavola proposed a simple measure of completeness of follow-up (C) based on the observed and potential person-time of follow-up (28). To adjust for the effect of unobserved patient deaths when computing the potential person-time of follow-up, this concept was modified by Wu et al. (C*) (31). To illustrate the level of data completeness in January 2014, these quantities were

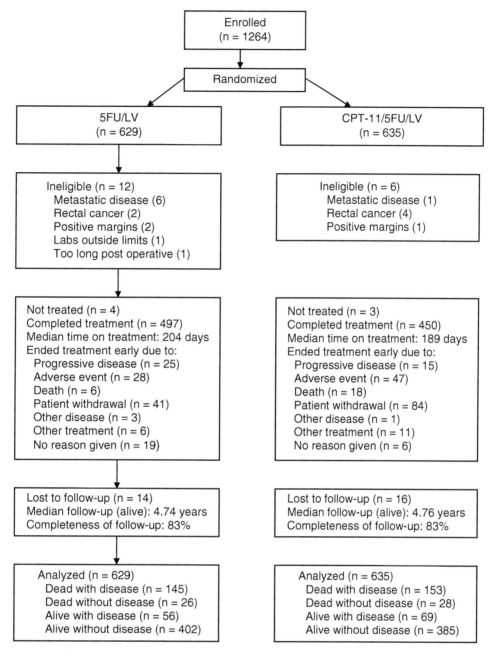

FIGURE 32.1 CONSORT flow diagram illustration of patient experience by treatment arm for patients randomized on CALGB 89803.

computed for the survival data from CALGB 80405, a phase III study of treatment with chemotherapy plus the monoclonal antibody, bevacizumab versus chemotherapy plus the monoclonal antibody, cetuximab among patients with untreated metastatic adenocarcinoma of the colon or rectum (32). Table 32.1 provides the values of the measures, C and C*, and other descriptive measures of follow-up. Enrollment on C80405 occurred between September 2005 and March 2012. The trial was amended in November 2008 restricting enrollment to patients with KRAS wild-type tumors; 1,137 patients met study criteria for the primary test of hypothesis. Assuming a maximum potential follow-up

from the date of first enrollment until March 2015 the unadjusted potential follow-up was approximately 9.0 years. A graphical illustration of completeness, observed survival time by time from study entry, is provided in Figure 32.2. Due to suspension of the trial while under amendment no patient registrations were made between June 16, 2008 and January 21, 2009 resulting in a gap in the plot.

Describe the patient population with respect to demographic attributes, disease and tumor characteristics, and data captured at study entry and treatment, if there is more than one treatment stratum or arm. Statistical comparisons of patient characteristics should

TABLE 32.1 Measures of Follow-up and Completeness of Overall Survival for Patients Studied on CALGB (Alliance) 80405

Sample size	1,137
Number of events	746
Accrual period (dates of first and last patient enrolled	11/17/2005–2/29/2012
Study termination date (assumed)	03/15/2015
Median follow-up (range) in years**	
Maximum follow-up	4.9 (3.0, 9.3)
Potential follow-up (T2)	2.6 (0.03, 9.1)
Observed follow-up (T1)	2.0 (0.0, 7.1)
Reverse Kaplan–Meier (95% CI)	3.5 (3.3, 3.6)
Median among patients still alive	2.6 (31.7 months)
Complete individuals (survival, current to within 6 months)	1,050 (92.3%)
Clark's completeness measure (C)1	79.0%
R (death rate: number dead/number of patients/mean T1)2	0.29
Wu's completeness measure (C^)2	85.0%

**Maximum follow-up is defined as the time from study entry to the end of the study whether or not an event occurred; potential follow-up (T2) is defined as the time from study entry to an event time or to study termination; observed follow-up (T1) is defined as the time from study entry to the date of last contact whether or not an event occurred.
CALGB, Cancer and Leukemia Group B; CI, confidence interval.

be made if sample sizes are adequate. These results are best presented in table format.

Adverse Events

The toxicity experience should be reported by treatment arm or stratum. Adverse events should be reported by treatment actually received. Usually toxicity of grade 3 or greater is reported but lower grade toxicity may be reported as relevant.

Efficacy

Describe the number of interim analyses conducted and the impact of these analyses on the trial, if applicable. For example, a trial may be stopped at an interim analysis due to efficacy or futility, which may affect the interpretation of the results. The final analysis of a trial is impacted when interim analyses are conducted and, in particular, when a trial is stopped early due to crossing

an interim boundary. The interim looks must be considered in the reporting of the final results (33,34). Montori et al. provide a review of randomized trials stopped early for benefit and conclude that information about the decision to stop the trial early is not adequately presented by authors and that such results should be viewed with caution (35).

Be explicit about the test of hypothesis associated with each reported p value. One way to accomplish this is to specify the test statistic with the p value in parentheses. Footnotes and text may also be used to convey this information.

For time-to-event endpoints, estimated proportions of patients free of the event are often given at a landmark time such as 1, 3, or 5 years. Clarify whether estimates are binomial proportions or Kaplan–Meier estimates and also clarify whether the test of hypothesis compares the proportions of patients event-free at the specified number of years (binomial test of proportion) or are associated with a survival analysis such as the log-rank test or Cox regression. When estimating the binomial proportion of patients surviving to a landmark time point, only patients who have achieved the endpoint prior to the landmark time or have follow-up greater than the landmark time should be included in the analysis.

In trial design, stratified randomization or dynamic allocation is often used to control the distribution of factors, between the treatment arms being compared, that are known prognostic variables. If patients are stratified at randomization, a stratified analysis of the endpoint should be presented (36). That is, the stratification factors must be considered in the comparison. The p value associated with an unstratified test should be less extreme.

Multivariable analyses are often presented. For example, if a treatment difference is observed it might be of interest to show that the treatment difference is not explained by other prognostic factors that were not considered in the primary analysis as stratification factors. In conducting such analyses the size of the data set and the relationships among the explanatory factors must be considered.

When multiple hypothesis testing is conducted on the same data set the probability of finding a significant result is increased. If the overall type I error rate is not controlled, caution should be used in interpreting the significance of results.

Example

CALGB 9481 was a phase III randomized trial of hepatic arterial infusion (HAI) versus systemic therapy for patients with hepatic metastasis from colorectal cancer (37). The trial enrolled 135 patients between January 1996 and December 2000. Patients were randomized with equal probability to treatment with HAI or systemic therapy and were stratified at randomization by

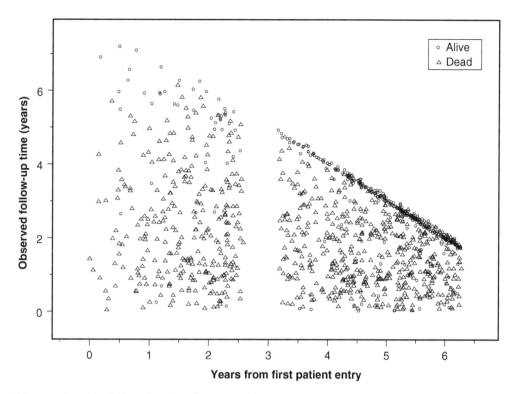

FIGURE 32.2 Observed survival time by time from study entry for 1,137 patients enrolled on CALGB 80405. Open circles indicate patients who are alive and open triangles indicate patients who are deceased. Completeness is illustrated by the cluster about the line representing the maximum potential follow-up time. The Clark completeness measure for these data is 79.0%. See Table 32.1.

percent liver involvement, presence of synchronous disease, and prior chemotherapy.

The trial was designed to detect a hazard ratio of 0.667 for OS in favor of HAI with 90% power (two-sided α = .05). The original targeted sample size was 340 patients to be enrolled over 4.5 years with a 1.5-year follow-up period and 262 deaths expected at the time of the final analysis. The results from this trial illustrate some of the issues that may be encountered in the analysis and reporting of data from clinical trials.

Poor Accrual. Patient accrual to this trial was slower than expected, 29 actual versus 75 projected patients per year. The slower rate of accrual was attributed to physician prejudice with respect to randomizing patients to treatment with HAI. In August 1999, the trial was amended to decrease the targeted sample size from 340 to 147 patients (262 to 112 expected deaths) and increase the follow-up time from 1.5 to 3 years. (The National Cancer Institute [NCI] now requires that the accrual rate be monitored for all NCI-funded trials and, if possible, that the statistical considerations be amended to address slow accrual.) No formal interim analyses of the primary endpoint were conducted prior to the amendment. This amendment was reviewed and approved by the CALGB Data and Safety Monitoring Board (DSMB). However, due to continued lagging accrual the trial was closed by the DSMB in December

2000 with 135 patients enrolled. Data monitoring by the CALGB DSMB continued until November 2001 according to the prespecified monitoring plan for OS. Due to size limitations, information regarding the slow accrual and the consequent amendment to the protocol were not presented in the paper. However, reporting the difficulty in patient enrollment to this trial may have been helpful to investigators planning a similar study.

Stratified Analysis. Stratified randomization can be useful in small trials when prognostic factors are known and in large trials with planned interim monitoring (38). However, misinterpreted and poorly chosen stratification factors can adversely impact the ability to capture these data and their usefulness in the final analysis. In C9481, 20.5% of patients classified at randomization as <30% liver involvement and 4.4% of patients classified as ≥30% liver involvement, respectively, were misclassified as determined by comparison with the actual percent liver involvement reported independently. Similarly, 21% of patients classified at randomization as 'no synchronous disease' were misclassified. Finally, 97% of patients enrolled (n = 123) had received no prior chemotherapy and this stratification variable could, therefore, not be considered in a stratified analysis. Because of these discrepancies, in the paper, results of the unstratified log-rank test for OS were reported as the primary analysis (log-rank p = .0034).

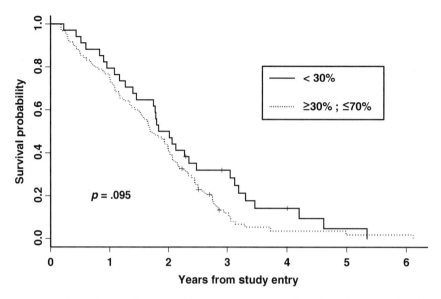

FIGURE 32.3 Kaplan–Meier plot of overall survival by actual percent liver involvement (<30%; ≥30% and ≤70%) for 135 patients randomized on CALGB 9481.

Under the proportional hazards model, an unstratified test, comparing OS by treatment arm for these data, results in a p value of .0038. Using the actual values for percent liver involvement and synchronous disease in place of the stratification factors, there was a trend toward improved OS with limited percent liver involvement defined as percent liver involvement <30% or ≥30% and <70% (Figure 32.3; $p = .095$). The presence of synchronous disease was not associated with OS. The p value associated with the treatment arm decreases when both variables, synchronous disease and percent liver involvement, are considered as covariates ($p = .0021$) primarily due to the association between percent liver involvement and OS. This outcome also illustrates how misclassification can bias results toward the null since the adjusted p value for the treatment arm based on the two stratification factors as reported is $p = .006$ (39).

Multivariable Analyses. Multivariable analyses are often conducted to determine if the significance of treatment arm can be explained by other factors potentially associated with outcome. In C9481, the following factors were considered in multivariable analyses: age at study entry, performance status (0: 1, 2), location of primary (colon; rectum), number of liver lesions (<5; ≥5), weight loss within 3 months of trial entry (no; yes), nonprotocol therapy postprogression (no; yes), lactate dehydrogenase (LDH; continuous measurement), baseline carcinoembryonic antigen (continuous measurement), white blood cell (WBC; <10,000, ≥10,000 K/μL), alkaline phosphatase (<300; ≥300 U/L), and albumin (<4; ≥4 g/dL). Two issues must be considered in the interpretation of these results: first, the sample size ("overfitting")

and, second, potential collinearity among the covariates. To avoid "overfitting," Harrell et al. recommend that the number of degrees of freedom in the model, p, should not exceed $m/10$, where m denotes the number of uncensored observations (40). Including the stratification factors, this rule of thumb is not met in C9481 ($p = 13 > m/10 = 125/10 = 12.5$). The authors further recommend that if p exceeds $m/10$, data reduction methods should be employed. However, added complexity exists in this data set as strong associations were observed among many of the covariates under study. These associations, particularly those between percent liver involvement and the laboratory values, can be anticipated based on the science. Thus, only the two-factor models including treatment arm and each of the covariates were considered. In the interpretation of results, the goal and methods of conducting the multivariable analysis must be considered. Most reported results will require validation.

Discussion and Study References

The discussion should put the study results in context, comparing and contrasting with data available from other trials. Qualifying statements can be made with respect to study results indicating the strengths and weaknesses of the research. Suggestions for extending the research can also be made. References should be provided for all nonoriginal work.

Reporting Recommendations for Tumor Marker Prognostic Studies (REMARK)

Paralleling the CONSORT statement for clinical trials, REMARK provides guidelines for the reporting of results from tumor biomarker studies (41). A checklist of

20 reporting elements related to the background, methods, results, and discussion sections of a manuscript is provided by the authors. Following these guidelines will raise the quality of study reporting and impact the ability of the scientific community to interpret results and effectively direct future research.

SUMMARY

In summary, the goal of reporting results from clinical trials and associated biomarker studies should be the clear and precise dissemination of scientific knowledge. Sufficient details should be provided to allow reproducibility and appropriate interpretation of study results for both clinical trials and biomarker studies within the context of current scientific evidence and provide a solid basis for future scientific discovery.

REFERENCES

1. Lewis JA. Statistical principles for clinical trials (ICH E9) an introductory note on an international guideline. *Statist Med.* 1999;18:1903–1904.
2. ICH Topic E3: Structure and content of clinical study reports. MCA EuroDirect Publication No. 137/95, EuroDirect Publications Office. London, UK; 1995.
3. ICH Expert Working Group. Statistical principles for clinical trials. *Statist Med.* 1999;18:1905–1942.
4. International Council for Harmonisation (ICH). ICH for technical requirements for pharmaceuticals for human. http://www.ich.org
5. Moher D, Schulz KF, Altman DG. The CONSORT statement: revised recommendations for improving the quality of reports of parallel-group randomised trials. *Lancet.* 2001;357(9263):1191–1194.
6. Schulz KF, Altman DG, Moher D, for the CONSORT Group. CONSORT 2010 Statement: updated guidelines for reporting parallel group randomised trials. *Trials.* 2010;11:32.
7. Consolidated Standards of Reporting Trials (CONSORT). CONSORT statement home page for transparent reporting of trials. http://www.consort-statement.org
8. American Joint Committee on Cancer. AJCC Staging Manual Sixth Edition. New York, NY: Springer Science + Business Media, Inc; 2002.
9. O'Brien S, Keating MJ. Chronic lymphoid leukemias. In: DeVita VT, Hellman S, Rosenberg SA, eds. *Cancer: Principles and Practice of Oncology.* 7th ed. Philadelphia, PA: Lippincott Williams & Wilkins; 2005:2121–2143.
10. Halabi S, Small EJ, Kantoff PW, et al. Prognostic model for predicting survival in men with hormone-refractory metastatic prostate cancer. *J Clin Oncol.* 2003;21:1232–1237.
11. Leonard JP. The "FLIPI" is no "FLOPI". *Blood.* 2004;104:1233–1234.
12. Schag CC, Heinrich RL, Ganz PA. Karnofsky performance status revisited: reliability, validity, and guidelines. *J Clin Oncol.* 1984;2:187–193.
13. Oken MM, Creech RH, Tormey DC, et al. Toxicity and response criteria of the Eastern Cooperative Oncology Group. *Am J Clin Oncol.* 1982;5:649–655.
14. Rossouw JE, Anderson GL, Prentice RL, et al. Writing group for the women's health initiative investigators. Risks and benefits of estrogen plus progestin for healthy postmenopausal women. *JAMA.* 2002;288:321–333.
15. Rossouw JE, Prentice RL, Manson JE, et al. Postmenopausal haormone therapy and risk of cardiovascular disease by age and years since menopause. *JAMA.* 2007;297(13):1465–1477.
16. Grodstein F, Manson JE, Stampfer MJ, Rexrode K. Postmenopausal hormone therapy and stroke Role of time since menopause and age at initiation of hormone therapy. *Arch Intern Med.* 2008;168:861–866.
17. Saltz LB, Niedzwiecki D, Hollis D, et al. Irinotecan fluorouracil plus leucovorin is not superior to fluorouracil plus leucovorin alone as adjuvant treatment for stage III colon cancer: results of CALGB 89803. *J Clin Oncol.* 2007;25:3456–3461.
18. Goldberg RM, Sargent DJ, Moron RF, et al. A randomized controlled trial of fluorouracil plus leucovorin, irinotecan, and oxaliplatin combinations in patients with previously untreated metastatic colorectal cancer. *J Clin Oncol.* 2004;22:23–30.
19. Sargent D, Niedzwiecki D, O'Connell MJ, Schilsky R. Recommendation for caution with irinotecan fluorouracil and leucovorin for colorectal cancer. *N Engl J Med.* 2001;345(2):144–145.
20. Rothenberg ML, Meropol NJ, Poplin EA, et al. Mortality associated with irinotecan plus bolus fluorouracil/leucovorin: summary findings of an independent panel. *J Clin Oncol.* 2001;19:3801–3807.
21. de Gramont A, Bosser JF, Milan C, et al. Randomized trial comparing monthly low-dose leucovorin and fluorouracil bolus with bimonthly high-dose leucovorin and fluorouracil bolus plus continuous infusion for advanced colorectal cancer. *J Clin Oncol.* 1997;15:808–815.
22. Goldberg RM, Sargent DJ, Morton RF, et al. Randomized controlled trial of reduced-dose bolus fluorouracil plus leucovorin and irinotecan or infused fluorouracil plus leucovorin and oxaliplatin in patients with previously untreated metastatic colorectal cancer: a North American Intergroup Trial. *J Clin Oncol.* 2006;24(21):3347–3353.
23. McShane LM, Hayes DF. Publication of tumore marker research results: the necessity for complete and transparent reporting. *J Clin Oncol.* 2012;30(34):4223–4232.
24. Moore HM, Kelly AB, Jewell SD, et al. Biospecimen reporting for improved study quality (BRISQ). *Cancer Cytopathol.* 2011;119:92–101.
25. The Asilomar Working Group on Recommendations for Reporting of Clinical Trials in the Biomedical Literature. Checklist of information for inclusion in reports of clinical trials. *Ann Int Med.* 1996;124(8):741–743.
26. Schemper M, Smith T. A note on quantifying follow-up in studies of failure time. *Control Clin Trials.* 1996;17:343–346.
27. Green S, Benedetti J, Crowley J. *Clinical Trials in Oncology.* Boca Raton, FL: CRC Press; 2002.
28. Clark TG, Altman DG, De Stavola BL. Quantification of the completeness of follow-up. *Lancet.* 2002;359:1309–1310.
29. Lachin JM. Statistical considerations in the intent-to-treat principle. *Control Clin Trials.* 200;21:167–189.
30. Simon R, Wittes RE. Methodologic guidelines for reports of clinical trials. *Cancer Treat Reports.* 1985;69(1):1–3.
31. Wu Y, Takkenberg JM, Grunkemeier GL. Measuring follow-up completeness. *Ann Thorac Surg.* 2008;85:1155–1157.
32. Venook AP, Niedzwiecki D, Lenz H-J, et. al. CALGB/SWOG 80405: Phase III trial of irinotecan/5-FU/leucovorin (FOLFIRI) or oxaliplatin/5-FU/leucovorin (mFOLFOX6) with bevacizumab (BV) or cetuximab (CET) for patients (pts) with KRAS wild-type (wt) untreated metastatic adenocarcinoma of the colon or rectum (MCRC). *J Clin Oncol.* 2014;32:5s(suppl; abstr LBA3).
33. Todd S, Whitehead A, Stallard N, Whitehead J. Interim analyses and sequential designs in phase III studies. *Br J Clin Pharmacol.* 2001;51:394–399.
34. Whitehead J. The design and analysis of sequential clinical trials. New York, NY: Halsted Press: a division of John Wiley & Sons. 1983;121–123.

35. Montori VM, Devereaux PJ, Adhikari NKJ, et al. Randomized trials stopped early for benefit: a systematic review. *JAMA.* 2005;294:2203–2209.

36. Peto R, Pike MC, Armitage P, et al. Design and analysis of randomized clinical trials requiring prolonged observation of each patient. I. Introduction and Design. *Br J Cancer.* 1976 34:585–612.

37. Kemeny NE, Niedzwiecki D, Hollis D, et al. Hepatic arterial infusion versus systemic therapy for hepatic metastases from colorectal concer: a randomized trial of efficacy, quality of life, and molecular markers (CALGB 9481). *J Clin Oncol.* 2006;24:1395–1403.

38. Kernan WN, Viscoli CM, Makuch RW, et al. Stratified randomization for clinical trials. *J Clin Epidemiol.* 1999;52: 19–26.

39. Greenland S. The effect of misclassification in the presence of covariates. *Am J Epidemiol.* 1980;112:564–569.

40. Harrell FE, Lee KL, Mark DB. Tutorial in biostatistics, multivariable prognostic models: issues in developing models, evaluating assumptions and adequacy, and measuring and reducing errors. *Statist Med.* 1996;15:361–387.

41. McShane LM, Altman DG, Sauerbrei W, et al. Reporting recommendations for tumour MARKer prognostic studies (REMARK). *J Natl Cancer Inst.* 2005;93:387–391.

Statistical Considerations for Developing and Validating Prognostic Models of Clinical Outcomes

Susan Halabi and Lira Pi

Prognostic models will continue to play a fundamental role in medical decision making and patient management. The assessment of prognostic factors, which relate baseline clinical and experimental variables to outcomes, independent of treatment, is one of the major objectives in clinical research in oncology. In contrast, predictive factors describe the interaction between a factor and the treatment in predicting outcome, and it is implicit that the treatment is effective. In oncology, the variability in outcome may be related to prognostic factors rather than to differences in treatments. Historically, the impetus for the identification of prognostic factors has been the need to accurately estimate the effect of treatment adjusting for these variables.

This chapter begins with a brief review of prognostic factors, and subsequently offers a general discussion of the importance of prognostic factors. Within this context, it summarizes the types of prognostic factors and describes the significance of study design. It then presents various modeling methods for identifying these factors. Finally, the relative values of different validation approaches are presented and discussed.

IMPORTANCE OF PROGNOSTIC FACTOR STUDIES

There are several reasons why prognostic factors are important (1,2). First, by determining which variables are prognostic of outcomes, insights are gained on the biology and the natural history of cancer. Second, patients and their families are informed about the risk of recurrence or death. Third, appropriate treatment strategies may be optimized based on the prognostic factors of an individual patient (1,2). Finally, prognostic factors play an important role in the design, conduct, and analysis of future clinical trials.

Criteria for evaluating prognostic models have been developed and published by the Precision Medicine Core (PMC) of the American Joint Committee on Cancer (AJCC) (3). Although the AJCC criteria were developed independently by the PMC, they corresponded fully to the guidelines recently developed by the Transparent Reporting of a Multivariable Prediction Model for Individual Prognosis Or Diagnosis (TRIPOD) and the Critical Appraisal and Data Extraction for Systematic Reviews of Prediction Modelling Studies (CHARMS) (4,5). In following these guidelines, rigorous development, validation, and the overall quality of the prognostic models result in a larger number of tools that may become part of routine patient care, as well as decision making in trial design and conduct.

Regression models that relate baseline clinical and experimental factors (such as treatment) to endpoints, such as overall survival (OS), are called prognostic models. Although individual prognostic factors are useful in predicting outcomes, investigators may be interested in constructing classification schemes. Combining multiple prognostic variables to form a prognostic index or score is a powerful strategy that will allow for the identification of groups of patients with differing risks of progression or death. For this reason, prognostic models have been widely used and will continue to be utilized in the design, conduct, and analysis of controlled trials in cancer. Risk models are employed for screening patients for eligibility on recent trials (6). For example, in Cancer and Leukemia Group B 90203, which is a neoadjuvant phase III trial of 750 men who are at high risk were randomized to either radical prostatectomy or docetaxel plus hormones followed by radical prostatectomy. High-risk men are considered eligible to participate on this trial if their predicted probability of being disease free 5 years after surgery <60% on the basis of the Kattan nomogram (6).

In addition, researchers may employ prognostic models that are used in stratified randomized trials. As patient outcomes often depend on prognostic factors, randomization helps balance such factors by treatment assignments. Some imbalances may nevertheless occur by chance. One strategy to limit this effect is to use blocked randomization within predefined combinations of the prognostic factors (strata). In a recently designed trial by the Alliance for clinical Trials in Oncology (NCT01949337), randomization was prospectively stratified by the predicted survival probability based on a prognostic model. In CALGB 90401, a phase III trial that assigned 1,050 men with castration-resistant prostate cancer (CRPC) to receive either docetaxel or docetaxel plus bevacizumab, randomization was stratified by the predicted survival probability at 24 months: <10%, 10% to 29.9%, or ≥30% (7).

Adjusting on prognostic factors in order to avoid bias in estimating the treatment effect is important even if the baseline factors are balanced between treatment groups. The need though to adjust on prognostic factors is more critical when the randomization is unbalanced. In a randomized phase III trial, 127 asymptomatic men with CRPC were randomized in a 2:1 ratio to either sipuleucel-T or placebo. The primary and secondary endpoints were time to progression and OS, respectively. In the multivariable analysis of OS, Small et al. identified five clinical variables (lactate dehydrogenase [LDH] prostate-specific antigen [PSA], number of bone metastases, body weight, and localization of disease) that were highly prognostic of OS in this study cohort.

To correct for any potential imbalances in prognostic factors, the treatment effect of sipuleucel-T was adjusted using the preceding variables. The observed hazard ratio (HR) was estimated to be 2.12 (95% CI: 1.31–3.44) (8).

TYPES OF PROGNOSTIC FACTORS

According to Gospodarowicz et al. prognostic factors are classified as tumor-related, host, or environmental factors (9). Tumor-related factors are variables that are related to the presence of the tumor and reflect tumor pathology, anatomic disease extent, or tumor biology. Examples of tumor-related factors are histologic grade, TNM stage, tumor markers, and molecular markers (overexpression of p53). Host-related factors do not relate to the malignancy of the tumor but may influence outcomes. These factors may be demographic, comorbidity, performance status, and compliance. Environmental-related factors are external factors that may be related to an individual patient such as physician expertise, access to healthcare, education, and availability of cancer control programs. All these factors are important as they have an impact on clinical outcomes. Figure 33.1 presents the relationship between host, tumor, environmental, and clinical outcomes. The reader is referred to Gospodarowicz et al. for a more detailed discussion on the different types of prognostic factors (9). The focus in this chapter is on factors that are relevant at the time of diagnosis or initial treatment.

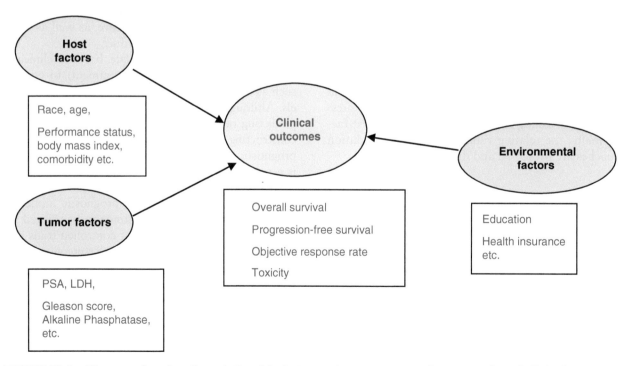

FIGURE 33.1 Diagram showing the relationship between host, tumor, environmental, and clinical outcomes.
LDH, lactate dehydrogenase; PSA, prostate-specific antigen.

STUDY DESIGN

The literature is rich in articles related to prognostic factors. Despite their abundance, however, results may conflict on the importance of certain markers in predicting outcomes. Accurate and reliable information based on the accessible literature with regard to prognostic factors needs to be consistent so that the two critical questions on "who to treat" and "how to treat each individual" can be addressed (10). General principles and methods related to the assessment and evaluation of prognostic factors are not as well developed as the clinical trial methodology. Recently, guidelines (Reporting Recommendations for Tumor Marker Prognostic Studies [REMARK]) have been developed to improve the quality of reporting of prognostic factors in cancer (11).

Most prognostic factor studies are based on retrospective data analysis that have a small sample size or sparse data and as a result have poor data quality (1). As with any scientific study, investigators planning a prognostic factor analysis should start with a primary hypothesis, the endpoint should be specified a priori and sample size or power computations should be justified. As suggested by Altman, the sample size should be large in order to account for the multitude of potential biases that may arise in conducting such trials (1). These issues are related to multiple comparisons of variables, selection of variables, comparisons of different models, and missing data of the variables or outcomes (1).

Several papers have considered the sample size required for prognostic studies (2,12). To examine the role of a prognostic factor, sample size needs to be justified. For example, investigators in a CALGB study were interested in determining whether the presence of autoimmunity at the beginning of therapy is associated with improved OS in metastatic renal cell carcinoma (mRCC) patients treated with interferon alpha with or without bevacizumab controlling for treatment arm (13). To design this study, the prevalence of positive autoimmunity needs to be known. In this case, it was considered that a subject is positive for autoimmunity if any of the antibody assays meet the definition of positive either at baseline or during their time on interferon alpha treatment. Five hundred eighty-nine patients of the 732 enrolled on CALGB 90206 had plasma samples collected at baseline. We used the sample size formula from Schmoor et al. (12) to compute the minimum HR that can be detected and is presented in Table 33.1. The following assumptions were made: OS follows exponential distribution, 80% power, a two-sided type I error rate of 0.05, positive autoimmunity decreases hazard of an event, prevalence of positive autoimmunity of 0.05 to 0.20, correlation of 0 to 0.6, and events rate of 75% to 90%.

As for model building, a general *ad hoc* rule of thumb is to use 10 subjects per variable for a binary endpoint (such as objective response) and 15 events (deaths) per variable for time-to-event endpoints (2). For predictive factor studies, sample size computation should be formally justified based on a test of interaction between the prognostic factor and the treatment (14). Usually, the sample size required for such studies is very large.

TABLE 33.1 Minimum Detectable HR Under a Range of Assumptions for the Prevalence of Positive Autoimmunity and Correlation With Two-Sided Type I Error Rate and 80% Power

Prevalence of Positive Autoimmunity	Correlation with Other Factors	Proportion of events observed among 589 patients with plasma available		
		75% Events	80% Events	90% Events
5%	0	0.542	0.553	0.572
	0.3	0.526	0.537	0.557
	0.6	0.465	0.477	0.497
10%	0	0.641	0.650	0.667
	0.3	0.627	0.637	0.653
	0.6	0.574	0.584	0.602
20%	0	0.716	0.724	0.737
	0.3	0.705	0.713	0.727
	0.6	0.659	0.668	0.683

HR, hazard ratio.

For more on this topic, see Simon and Altman, who provide a rigorous and thoughtful review of statistical aspects of prognostic factor studies in oncology (15).

IDENTIFICATION OF PROGNOSTIC FACTORS

Multiple strategies exist for the identification of prognostic factors. The modeling approaches described in the following sections are: logistic regression for binary endpoints (15), proportional hazards (PH) regression for time-to-event endpoints (16) (such as OS), and recursive partitioning for both binary and time-to-event endpoints (17,18).

LOGISTIC REGRESSION MODEL

Logistic regression is a statistical model that can be applied when the endpoint is dichotomous in nature. In addition, it can be used to describe the relationship of the independent prognostic factors (denoted as X_i) to the binary endpoint (denoted as D). Examples of binary endpoints are objective response, recurrence-free survival at 1 year, or OS at 5 years. The logistic model is popular because the logistic function relates the expected odds of an event to the explanatory variables and provides estimates of the event probabilities (16). The logistic function can be written as the expected probability of the event given z:

$$E[D = 1 | X1, X2,..., Xp] = 1/[1 + e^{-z}]$$

where $z = \beta_0 + \beta_1 X_1 + \beta_2 X_2 + \ldots + \beta_p X_p$ and is known as the prognostic index or score. β_0 is the intercept and β_i are the unknown regression coefficients where $i = 1, 2, \ldots p$.

The logit transformation is essential to the use of the logistic model and can be described as:

$$\log [P(D = 1 | X_1, X_2, \ldots X_p)/1\text{-}P(D = 1 | X_1, X_2, \ldots X_p)] = \beta_0 + \beta_1 X_1 + \beta_2 X_2 + \ldots + \beta_p X_p$$

where log is the natural logarithm (i.e., to the base e). The estimated regression coefficients can be used to estimate the predicted probability by inverting the regression model as demonstrated in the following example.

Example

Robain et al. used a logistic regression model to predict objective response in 1,426 women with metastatic breast cancer. Objective response was defined as either the presence of a partial or complete response (19). Fifteen baseline covariates were examined as potential predictors of objective response. These were: age, performance status (Karnofsky index [KI]), number of sites (1, ≥2), and location of metastases (bone, lung, pleura, liver, peritoneum, skin, lymph nodes), serum LDH, weight loss before treatment, menopausal status,

disease-free interval from primary tumor diagnosis to metastases, year of inclusion in a metastatic trial, serum alkaline phosphatase, γ glutamyl transferase (γ GT), aspartate aminotransferase (AST), serum albumin levels, and absolute lymphocyte count.

Forward stepwise regression was utilized to select the prognostic factors and the maximized log-likelihood was used for comparison of models based on selection of prognostic factors at each step. Prior chemotherapy (yes vs. no), low KI (<60 vs. ≥60), high LDH (>1 x N vs. ≤1 x N), presence of lung metastases (yes vs. no), and pleural metastases (yes vs. no) were combined to form a predictive score. The estimated score was: –1.32 + 0.54 (no prior adjuvant chemotherapy) + 0.80 (low KI) + 0.75 (elevated LDH) + 0.49 (lung metastases) + 0.51 (pleural metastases).

The estimated regression coefficients can be used to compute the predicted probability by inverting the regression model. For example, the predicted probability of not achieving objective response for a woman without prior adjuvant chemotherapy (coded as 0), low KI (coded as 1), high LDH (coded as 1), presence of lung (coded as 1), and pleural metastases (coded as 1) is calculated to be:

$$\exp(-1.32 + 0.54 \times (0) + 0.80 \times (1) + 0.75 \times (1) + 0.49 \times (1) + 0.51 \times (1)) = /$$

$$[1 + \exp(-1.32 + 0.54 \times (0) + 0.80 \times (1) + 0.75 \times (1) + 0.49 \times (1) + 0.51 \times (1))] = 0.774.$$

PROPORTIONAL HAZARDS MODEL

Often, an investigator seeks to assess the prognostic importance of several independent variables on the time-to-event endpoint. In phase III trials, time-to-event endpoints refer to outcomes where time is measured from randomization until occurrence of an event of interest. The time variable is referred to as the failure time and is measured in years, months, weeks, or days. The event may be death, death due to a specific cause, disease progression, or the development of metastases. In general, OS is the most common time-to-event endpoint in phase III trials in oncology. Most time-to-event endpoints must consider a basic analytical element known as censoring. Censoring arises when information about individual failure time is unknown and it occurs when patients either do not experience the event before the study ends or patients are lost during the follow-up period.

Two quantitative terms are fundamental in any survival analysis. These are survivor function, denoted by $S(t)$, and hazard function, denoted by $\lambda(t)$ (20). The survivor function is the probability that a person survives longer than some specified time t. The hazard function $\lambda(t)$ is the instantaneous potential per unit time for an event to occur, given that the individual survived until time t. There is a clearly defined relationship between these two functions, but it is simpler to mathematically model the hazard function than the survival function when an investigator is interested in assessing prognostic factors of time-to-event endpoints.

Perhaps one of the most common approaches in the medical literature is the use of the regression PH model (16). The PH model is used to analyze such time-to-event data and it is a powerful method because it can incorporate both baseline and time-varying factors. A PH model with a hazard function is given by:

$$\lambda(t|X_1, X_2, \ldots, X_p) = \lambda_0(t) \exp(\beta_1 X_1 + \beta_2 X_2 + \ldots + \beta_p X_p)$$

where $X_1, X_2, \ldots X_p$ represent the baseline covariates, and β are the regression or the log-HR parameters. $\lambda_0(t)$ is the baseline hazard, which is a function of time and is equal to the overall hazard function when all the values of covariates are zero. The PH model is semiparametric as it does not specify the form of $\lambda_0(t)$. The covariates are assumed to be linearly related to the log-hazard function. The parameter β can be estimated by maximizing the partial likelihood function as described by Cox (16). By estimating β it allows one to quantify the relative rate of failure for an individual with covariates x_1 compared to an individual with covariates x_2. From the PH model, the estimated HR for death and 95% confidence intervals are usually summarized.

The PH model specifies a multiplicative relationship between the underlying hazard function and the log-linear function of the covariates. This assumption is also known as the *proportional hazard assumption*. In other words, if we consider two subjects with different values for the covariates, the ratio of the hazard functions for those two subjects is independent of time. The PH model is a powerful tool as it can be extended to include time-dependent covariates and stratification. Time-varying covariates are factors whose values change over time.

The PH model can be extended to allow for different strata and is written as:

$$\lambda_{0s}(t) \exp(\beta_1 X_1 + \beta_2 X_2 + \ldots + \beta_p X_p)$$

where $\lambda_{0s}(t)$ is the baseline hazard function in the sth stratum, $s = 1, 2, \ldots, l$. The stratified PH model assumes that patients within each stratum satisfy the PH assumption but patients in different strata have a different baseline hazard function and thus are allowed to have non-PH. It is important to note that β do not depend on the strata.

Both graphical and test-based methods are used for assessing the PH assumption (20–22). Some of the graphical approaches include plotting the log $[-\log S(t)]$ versus time or using the stratified Cox model. There are several formal tests for assessing the PH assumption. These tests are either based against a specified alternative or a general alternative hypothesis. An omnibus test against a general alternative test developed by Schoenfeld is a common and effective approach for testing the PH assumption (22).

Example

Halabi et al. identified seven prognostic factors of OS in men with CRPC using clinical data from 1,100 patients enrolled on CALGB studies (7). The goal was to have at least 20 events per variable. The data were split into two: two thirds ($n = 760$) for the learning set and one third ($n = 341$) of the data to be used for the validation set. The prognostic variables were identified a priori based on the review of the literature. Schoenfeld residuals were used to check the PH assumption. In addition, PSA, LDH, and alkaline phosphatase were modeled using the log transformation as these variables were not normally distributed. The final model included the following factors: LDH, PSA, alkaline phosphatase, Gleason sum, Eastern Cooperative Oncology Group (ECOG) performance status, hemoglobin, and the presence of visceral disease.

The observed HR associated with Gleason sum can be computed as $exp(0.335)$, which is 1.40; see Table 3 (7). This means that men with high Gleason sum (8–10) had a 1.4-fold increased risk of death compared to men with Gleason sum <8 after adjustment for other covariates in the model.

CLASSIFICATION TREES

Recursive partitioning is another powerful approach to identify distinct groups. Its value lies in the fact that this approach is a powerful tool for model development and validation as it can be nonparametric and uses a linear combination of factors to determine splits (23). Furthermore, this method will estimate a regression relationship by binary recursive partitioning where the data is split into homogeneous subsets until it is not feasible to continue. Other advantages of recursive partitioning are: controls for the global type I error rate and can also be applied to both binary and time-to-event endpoints (24). In addition, it can handle missing covariate values, and is effective at modeling complex interactions.

One of the major disadvantages of tree models is that complicated structures may emerge making the interpretation of the data difficult. In addition, a failure to utilize continuous variables effectively may result in unstable tree structures or overfitting (24). Overfitting indicates that a model is fit with random noise and the associations between the outcomes and the covariables will be spurious (25). Simply put, overfitting refers to overestimation of the performance of the prediction rule. The reader is referred to Halabi et al. for an illustration for the concept of overfitting (25).

Example

Banjeeree et al. used data from 1,055 women with stage I–III breast cancer to identify recurrence-free survival (26). The primary endpoint was recurrence-free survival, which is defined as the time between diagnosis and documented recurrence (local, regional, or distant recurrence), excluding new primary breast cancer. The investigators considered 15 baseline variables, which were: age, race, socioeconomic status, marital status, obesity, tumor size, number of positive lymph nodes, progesterone receptor status, estrogen receptor status, tumor differentiation, hypertension, heart disease, diabetes, cholesterol level, and stroke. Using recursive partitioning, four distinct risk groups were identified based on the prognostic factors: race, marital status, tumor size, number of positive nodes, progesterone receptor status, and tumor differentiation.

VARIABLE SELECTION METHODS

Penalized procedures, such as the least absolute shrinkage and selection operator (LASSO) and adaptive LASSO (ALASSO), have been also used to develop prognostic models of clinical outcomes (27,28). Generally speaking, the penalized methods fit p predictors that constrain or shrink the unimportant coefficient estimates toward zero (29–32). By shrinking the coefficient estimates one can reduce the variance of the coefficient estimates, which should improve the model fitting accuracy. The LASSO estimates p predictors by minimizing the residual sum of squares while restricting the sum of absolute values of the coefficients to less than a tuning parameter. The L_1 penalty is used for the LASSO and it drives the unimportant coefficient estimates to be equal to 0 if a large tuning parameter has been chosen. Thus, selecting a tuning parameter is critical for the LASSO (30). However, the LASSO is likely to choose highly correlated predictors so that it could lead to wrong prediction (30). Moreover, there are situations where the LASSO coefficient estimates are inconsistent (30). The ALASSO is an improvement over the LASSO as it enjoys the oracle property (31,32). Specifically, the ALASSO can correctly identify the set of nonzero components of β, with probability tending to 1. Second, it estimates the nonzero components accurately (32). Consequently, the ALASSO tends to select fewer nonzero coefficients than the LASSO in spite of having smaller prediction error.

As an example, Halabi et al. updated the prognostic model of OS in men with CRPC using clinical data from 1,050 patients enrolled on CALGB 90401 trial (28). The data were split into two: two thirds ($n = 705$) for the learning set and one third ($n = 345$) of the data to be used for the validation set. The adaptive LASSO was used to select the final variables in the model among 22 potential predictors and to estimate the HR. The final model included the following factors: LDH, PSA, alkaline phosphatase, albumin, ECOG performance status, hemoglobin, metastatic site, and analgesic opioid use. The fitted model was used to plot the nomogram, which is a visual representation of the prognostic model; see

Figure 33.2 (28). The predicted probability of OS has been used as a stratification factor for several of the prostate cancer trials (33). This tool is also available online to facilitate computing of the predicted survival probability for an individual patient and for risk grouping. The tool is available online: https://www.cancer.duke.edu/Nomogram/firstlinechemotherapy.html. The risk group has been used as a stratification factor in the randomization in ongoing phase II (NCT02218606) and phase III metastatic castration-resistant prostate cancer (mCRPC) trials (NCT01949337).

Nonparametric procedures are worth considering when the nonlinearity of the covariates holds. The component selection and smoothing operator (COSSO) and adaptive COSSO could be options for variable selection, although there are many limitations as discussed in Lin and Halabi (34). Random forests (RF) is another nonparametric variable selection method that has been widely used in clinical study (35–37). For variable selection, the RF defines the variable importance (VIMP) score as a measurement of how important a variable is in explaining an outcome. A VIMP close to zero indicates no importance to the outcome, while a VIMP >0 represents moderate or strong importance. The VIMP of highly correlated variables is, however, likely to depart from zero although the true VIMP should be nearly zero. To improve on this limitation, conditional VIMP was introduced (37). Significance testing for either the VIMP or conditional VIMP is still open to question. Although the RF provides high accuracy on training samples, it has the main drawbacks of being computationally intensive and potentially may lead to overfitting.

SMALL *n*, LARGE *p*

With the advent of high-throughput technologies, several authors have focused on the development of a novel methodology relevant to the "small *n*, large *p*" problem (38,39). While it is not feasible to use the preceding variable selection approaches in ultra-high-dimensional space, there are several prescreening methods that can be useful. The prescreening procedures, such as the sure independence screening (SIS), the iterative version of the sure independence screening (ISIS), and principled sure independence screening (PSIS) focus on reducing the ultra-high-dimensional space (38,39). The prescreening procedures aim to select a number of predictors that is less than the sample size. The reduction in dimensionality makes the aforementioned variable selection methods perform more accurately in ultra-high-dimensional settings. Furthermore, the prescreening approaches are often adapted for ultra-high-dimensional problems in spite of two main limitations; computational intensity and high false discovery rate (FDR) (40). The FDR can be used as another prescreening approach as discussed

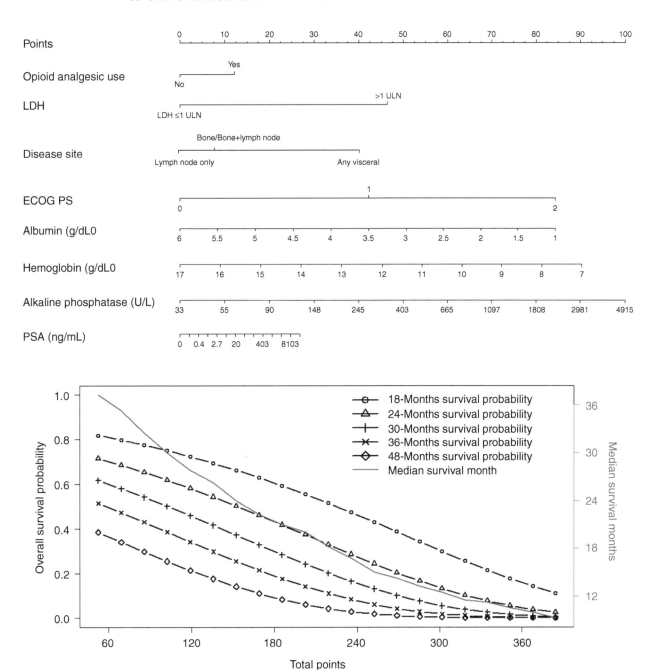

FIGURE 33.2 Pretreatment nomogram predicting probability of survival in men with CRPC.

CRPC, castration-resistant prostate cancer; ECOG, Eastern Cooperative Oncology Group; LDH, *lactate dehydrogenase*; PSA, prostate-specific antigen.

Source: Printed with permission from Halabi S, Lin CY, Kelly WK, et al. An updated prognostic model for predicting overall survival in first-line chemotherapy metastatic castration-resistant prostate cancer patients. *J Clin Oncol.* 2016;32(7):671–677. Copyright 2016, American Society of Clinical Oncology. All rights reserved.

by Kim and Halabi (40). Afterward, the FDR can also be controlled by using the aforementioned variable selection methods (40).

COMMON PROBLEMS WITH MODELING

In this section, common pitfalls in building models are discussed so that they can be avoided.

Categorizing a continuous prognostic factor as a binary variable based on the sample median is a common practice in the medical literature (1,2). In the PH model, it is assumed that continuous variables have a log-linear relation with the hazard function. While many researchers cannot make this assumption, dichotomizing a continuous variable may result in substantial loss of information. Altman suggested another alternative that is to use several categories for quantifying the relationship of a continuous variable to the hazard of death (41). Other approaches such as cubic splines or fractional polynomial have been applied in assessing the relationship between continuous variables and hazard function (42).

Identification of a prognostic factor based on the optimal cut point is often applied in prognostic studies, but this approach is based on identifying the cut point that yields the minimal p value (43). The approach is problematic as it does not correct for the multiplicity of comparisons and is rightly criticized due to the subjectivity and arbitrariness of the cut point. There are new algorithms that adjust for multiple comparisons, but even if this approach is employed, it should be considered only as exploratory. A confirmatory study of this prognostic factor should be undertaken and the sample size needs to be large in order to increase the precision of the estimate.

As an example, exploratory statistical methods were used to find different cut points for the association between vascular endothelial growth factor (VEGF) levels and OS in men with CRPC. Several cut points above and below the median showed an association between high VEGF levels and decreased duration of survival. At a cut point of 260 pg/ml, differences in median survival were 17 months (95% CI: 14–18) versus 11 months (95% CI: 6–13, $p < .0005$) for patients below and above the cut point, respectively (44). The multivariable HR associated with a VEGF level ≥260 pg/ml was 2.42, demonstrating the strongest association between VEGF levels and survival time (43). This analysis is deemed as exploratory and this cut point is being validated prospectively in an ongoing CALGB phase III trial.

Variable selection is a critical step of model building. Some investigators have used the stepwise method for selecting prognostic factors. This type of variable selection approach may produce overoptimistic regression estimates that will yield a low predictive ability (1,10).

As with any regression method, one needs to understand and verify the assumptions of the model. If these assumptions are not held, then accurate interpretation of the results of the fitted model may be difficult. Assessing the proportional hazards assumption in the PH model is often overlooked.

Example

In Smaletz et al. a proportional regression model was initially used to fit the baseline covariates (47). Several variables, however, violated the PH assumption of a constant hazard over time. Consequently, an accelerated failure time model was used.

The reader is referred to an excellent review of strategies involved in model building that is provided by Harrell (2).

MODEL VALIDATION

The primary goal of a prognostic model is to minimize uncertainty in predicting outcome in new patients (2). Validating a prognostic model is a critical step in developing a prognostic model. Assessing predictive accuracy is the next important step for model validation (1–2). As described by Harrell (2), calibration or reliability refers to the extent of the bias or match between forecast and outcome. Discrimination, on the other hand, measures a model or predictor's ability to classify or separate patients with different responses (2). Overfitting, or overlearning, will invalidate a model. Overfitting refers to a situation in which a model has been fit to random noise and the associations between the covariates and the outcomes will be spurious.

There are several useful and frequently employed measures of assessing the predictive accuracy of a model performance (2). Among them is the concordance index, a widely used measure of predictive accuracy. The c-index refers to the proportion of agreement between prediction and outcomes among all patients. An index of 0.5 indicates no discrimination while a value of 1 indicates perfect discrimination. On the other hand, Somers' D rank correlation is computed by calculating 2*(c-0.5). If the endpoint is binary, then the c-index is identical to the area under the receiver operating characteristic (ROC) curve. Both c and Somers' D can be obtained using standard statistical software (SAS, S-PLUS, or R).

Another measure for assessing a survival model is the time-dependent area under the receiver operating characteristic (tAUROC) curve. The tAUROC is a measure of predictive accuracy and is calculated for each time point. The tAUROCs at specific time points can be merged as an integrated area under the ROC curve (iAUROC). There are several methods in computing the tAUROC and calculating sensitivity and specificity (46–48), which would yield different results. The iAUROC is generated as a sum of weighted tAUROCs (46–48). In general, an iAUROC of 0.5 indicates no impact of finally chosen variables to predict a survival outcome while the iAUROC >0.7 is regarded as a meaningful model predicting a survival endpoint.

There are two types of validation: external and internal. External validation is the most rigorous approach where the *frozen* model is applied to an independent data set from the development data. Ideally, investigators would have an independent data set available for validation purposes, although this is rarely available. Other types of internal validation such as split sample, cross-validation, and bootstrapping are used to obtain an unbiased estimate of predictive accuracy (49).

In split-sample validation, the data set is randomly divided into two groups: a learning data set where the model is developed, and a testing set where the model performance is evaluated. This is a critical process as improperly distributed imbalances by outcomes or predictors may occur and produce an unreliable estimate of model performance.

Cross-validation is a generalization of data splitting. Similar to data splitting, with this approach one fits a prognostic model based on a random sample before subsequently testing it on the sample that was omitted. For example, in 10-fold cross-validation, 90% of the original sample is used to develop the model and 10% to test the sample. This procedure is repeated 10 times, such that all subjects have once served to test the model. To obtain accurate estimates using cross-validation, more than 200 models need to be fitted and tested with the results averaged over the 200 repetitions. The major advantage of cross-validation over data splitting is that the former reduces variability by not relying on a single sample split.

Bootstrapping is a very effective technique of deriving reliable estimates without making any assumptions about the distribution of the data (50). The bootstrap does with a computer what the experimenter would do in practice if it were possible: he or she would repeat the experiment. In bootstrap, the observations are randomly drawn with replacement and reassigned, and estimates are recomputed.

Bootstrapping reflects the process of sampling from the underlying population. Bootstrap samples are drawn with replacement from the original sample. They are of the same size as the original sample. For example, when 500 patients are available for model development, bootstrap samples also contain 500 patients, but some patients may not be included, others once, others twice, others three times, and so on. As with cross-validation, the drawing of bootstrap samples needs to be repeated many times to obtain stable estimates.

In summary, prognostic studies can address important questions that are relevant to patient outcomes; however, they must be rigorously and carefully designed to ensure accurate and reliable results. Such studies should begin with a hypothesis, defining a priori the endpoint, using appropriate variable selection approaches, testing the robustness of the models applied, and justifying the sample size. As the primary goal of such studies is to minimize uncertainty in predicting outcome in future patients, it is vital to validate such factors or models so that prognosis in patients is better understood.

REFERENCES

1. Altman DG. Studies investigating prognostic factors: conduct and evaluation. In Gospodarowicz MK, O'Sullivan B, Sobin H, eds. *Prognostic Factors in Cancer*. 3rd ed., Hoboken, NJ: Wiley-Liss; 2006: 39–54.
2. Harrell F Jr, *Regression Modeling Strategies: With Applications to Linear Models, Logistic Regression, and Survival Analysis*, 2nd ed. Switzerland: Springer International Publishing; 2015.
3. Kattan MW, Hess KR, Amin M, et al. American Joint Committee on Cancer acceptance criteria for inclusion of risk models for individualized prognosis in the practice of precision medicine. *CA: Cancer J Clin*. 2016;66(5):370–374. doi:10.3322/caac.21339
4. Moons KGM, de Groot JAH, Bouwmeester W, et al. Critical appraisal and data extraction for systematic reviews of prediction modeling studies: The CHARMS checklist. *PLoS Med*. 2014;11:1–12.
5. Moons KGM, Altman DG, Reitsma JB, et al. Transparent Reporting of a multivariable prediction model for Individual Prognosis Or Diagnosis (TRIPOD): Explanation and Elaboration The TRIPOD Statement: Explanation and Elaboration. *Ann Intern Med*. 2015;162(1):W1–W73.
6. Eastham JA, Kelly WK, Grossfeld GD, et al. Cancer and Leukemia Group B (CALGB) 90203: a randomized phase 3 study of radical prostatectomy alone versus estramustine and docetaxel before radical prostatectomy for patients with high-risk localized disease. *Urol*. 2003;62(supple 1):55–62.
7. Halabi S, Small EJ, Kantoff PW, et al. Prognostic model for predicting survival in men with hormone-refractory metastatic prostate cancer. *J Clin Oncol*. 2003;21:1232–1237.
8. Small EJ, Schllhammer PF, Higano CS, et al. Placebo-controlled phase III trial of immunologic therapy with sipuleucel-T (APC8015) in patients with metastatic, asymptomatic hormone refractory prostate cancer. *J Clin Oncol*. 2006;24:3089–3094.
9. Gospodarowicz MK, O'Sullivan B, Koh ES. Prognostic factors: principles and applications. In Gospodarowicz MK, O'Sullivan B, Sobin H, eds. *Prognostic Factors in Cancer*. 3rd ed., Hoboken, NJ: Wiley-Liss; 2006:23–34.
10. Altman DG, Royston P. What do we mean by validating a prognostic model? *Stat Med*. 2000;19:453–473.
11. McShane LM, Altman DG, Sauerbrei W, et al. Reporting recommendations for tumor marker prognostic studies (REMARK). *J Natl Cancer Inst*. 2005;97:1180–1184.
12. Schmoor CW, Sauerbrei W, Schumacher M. Sample size considerations for the evaluation of prognostic factors in survival analysis. *Stat Med*. 2000;19:441–452.
13. Rini BI, Halabi S, Rosenberg JE, et al. Bevacizumab plus interferon-alpha versus interferon-alpha monotherapy in patients with metastatic renal cell carcinoma: results of CALGB 90206. *J Clin Oncol*. 2008;26:5422–5428.
14. Simon R, Altman DG. Methodological challenges in the evaluation of prognostic factors in breast cancer. *Br J Cancer*. 1994;69:979–985.
15. Hosmer DW, Lemeshow S. *Applied Logistic Regression*. New York, NY: Wiley & Sons; 1989.
16. Cox DR. Regression models and life tables (with discussion). *J Royal Stat Soc B*. 1972;34:187–220.
17. Breiman L, Friedman JH, Olshen RA, Stone CJ. *Classification and Regression Trees*. Belmont, CA: Wadsworth; 1984.
18. LeBlanc M, Crowley J. Survival trees by goodness of split. *J Am Stat Assoc*. 1993;88:457–467.
19. Robain M, Pierga JY, Jouve M. Predictive factors of response to first-line chemotherapy in 1426 women with metastatic breast cancer. *Eur J Cancer*. 2000;36:2301–2312.
20. Kalbfleisch JD, Prentice RL. *The Statistical Analysis of Failure Time Data*. New York, NY: Wiley & Sons; 1980.
21. Grambsch P, Therneau TM. Proportional hazards tests and diagnostics based on weighted residuals. *Biometrika*. 1994;81:515–526.
22. Schoenfeld D. Partial residuals for the proportional hazards regression model. *Biometrika*. 1982;69:239.
23. Torsten H, Kurt H, Achim Z. Unbiased recursive partitioning: a conditional inference framework. *J Comp Graph Stat*. 2006;15:651–674.
24. McShane LM, Simon R. Statistical methods for the analysis of prognostic factor studies. In Gospodarowicz MK, Henson DE, Hutter RV, et al, eds. *Prognostic Factors in Cancer*. 2nd ed. New York, NY: Wiley-Liss; 2001: 37–48.

25. Halabi S, Owzar K. The importance of identifying and validating prognostic factors in oncology. *Semin Oncol.* 2010;37:e9–e18.

26. Banjeeree M, George J, Song EY, et al. Tree-based model for breast cancer prognostication. *J Clin Oncol.* 2004;22:2567–2575.

27. Halabi S, Lin CY, Small EJ, et al. Prognostic model for predicting overall survival in metastatic castration-resistant prostate cancer (mCRPC) men treated with second line chemotherapy. *J Natl Cancer Inst.* 2013;105(22):1729–1737.

28. Halabi S, Lin CY, Kelly WK, et al. An updated prognostic model for predicting overall survival in first-line chemotherapy metastatic castration-resistant prostate cancer patients. *J Clin Oncol.* 2016;32(7):671–677.

29. Tibshirani R. The lasso method for variable selection in the Cox model. *Stat Med.* 1997;16:385–395.

30. Hastie T, Tibshirani R, Friedman JH. *The Elements of Statistical Learning: Data Mining, Inference, and Prediction.* New York, NY: Springer Publishing; 2001.

31. Zhang HH, Lu W. Adaptive lasso for Cox's proportional hazards model. *Biometrika.* 2007;94:691–703.

32. Zou H. The adaptive Lasso and its oracle properties. *J Am Stat Assoc.* 2006;101:1418–1429.

33. Kelly WM, Halabi S, Carducci M, et al. Randomized, double-blind, placebo-controlled phase III trial comparing docetaxel and prednisone with or without bevacizumab in men with metastatic castration-resistant prostate cancer: CALGB 90401. *J Clin Oncol.* 2012;30:1534–1540.

34. Lin CY, Halabi S. On model specification and selection of the Cox proportional hazards model. Stat Med. 2013;32(26):4609–4623.

35. Ishwaran H, Kogalur UB, Blackstone EH, Lauer MS. Random survival forests. *Ann Appl Stat.* 2008;2:841–860.

36. Breiman L. Random forests. *Mach Learn.* 2001;45:5–32.

37. Strobl C, Boulesteix AL, Kneib T, et al. Conditional variable importance for random forests. *BMC Bioinformatics.* 2008;9:307.

38. Fan J, Feng Y, Wu Y. High-dimensional variable selection for Cox's proportional hazards model. In Berger JO, Cai T, Johnstone I, eds. Borrowing strength: theory powering applications–A Festschrift for Lawrence D. Brown. Beachwood, OH: Institute of Mathematical Statistics; 2010:70–86.

39. Zhao SD, Li Y. Principled sure independence screening for Cox models with ultra0high0dimensional covariates. *J Am Stat Assoc.* 2012;105:397–411.

40. Kim S, Halabi S. High dimensional variable selection with error control. Biomed Res Int. 2016:8209453.

41. Royston J, Altman DG, Sauerbrei W. Dichotomizing continuous predictors in multiple regression: a bad idea. *Stat Med.* 2006;25:127–141.

42. Durrleman S, Simon R. Flexible regression models with cubic splines. *Stat Med.* 1989;8:551–561.

43. Hilsenbeck SG, Clark GM. Practical p-value adjustment for optimally selected cutpoints. *Stat Med.* 1996;15:103–112.

44. George D, Halabi S, Shepard T, et al. Prognostic significance of plasma vascular endothelial growth factor (VEGF) levels in patients with hormone refractory prostate cancer: a CALGB study. *Clin Cancer Res.* 2001;7:1932–1936.

45. Smaletz O, Scher HI, Small EJ, et al. A nomogram for overall survival of patients with progressive metastatic prostate cancer following castration. *J Clin Oncol.* 2002;20:3972–3982.

46. Heagerty PJ, Zheng Y. Survival model predictive accuracy and ROC curves. *Biometrics.* 2005;61:92–105.

47. Uno H, Cai T, Tian L. Evaluating prediction rules for t-year survivors with censored regression models. *J Am Stat Assoc.* 2007;102:527–537.

48. Kamarudin AK, Cox T, Kolamunnage-Dona R. Time-dependent ROC curve analysis in medical research: current methods and applications *BMC Med Res Methodol.* 2017;17:53. doi:10.1186/s12874-017-0332-6

49. Steyerberg EW, Harrell FE Jr, Borsboom GJ, et al. Internal validation of predictive models: efficiency of some procedures for logistic regression analysis. *J Clin Epidemiol.* 2001;54:774–781.

50. Efron B, Gong G. A leisurely look at the bootstrap, the jackknife, and cross-validation. *Am Statist.* 1983;37:36.

Statistical Evaluation of Surrogate Endpoints in Cancer Clinical Trials

Marc Buyse, Geert Molenberghs, Xavier Paoletti, Koji Oba, Ariel Alonso, Wim Van der Elst, and Tomasz Burzykowski

A surrogate endpoint is intended to replace a clinical endpoint for the evaluation of new treatments when it can be measured more cheaply, more conveniently, more frequently, or earlier than that clinical endpoint. A surrogate endpoint is expected to predict clinical benefit, harm, or lack of these. Besides the biological plausibility of a surrogate, a quantitative assessment of the strength of evidence for surrogacy requires the demonstration of the prognostic value of the surrogate for the clinical outcome, and evidence that treatment effects on the surrogate reliably predict treatment effects on the clinical outcome. We focus on these two conditions, and outline the statistical approaches that have been proposed to assess the extent to which these conditions are fulfilled. When data are available from a single trial, one can assess the *individual-level association* between the surrogate and the true endpoint. When data are available from several trials, one can additionally assess the *trial-level association* between the treatment effect on the surrogate and the treatment effect on the true endpoint. In the latter case, the *surrogate threshold effect* (STE) can be estimated as the minimum effect on the surrogate endpoint that predicts a statistically significant effect on the clinical endpoint. All these concepts are discussed in the context of randomized clinical trials in oncology, and illustrated with two meta-analyses in gastric cancer. This chapter is aimed at a clinical audience, with all technical details omitted but provided in full in a parallel peer-reviewed publication aimed at a statistical readership (1). The methods described in this chapter are further detailed in (2), and SAS and R software to implement them in (3).

The development of new drugs is facing unprecedented challenges today, with more molecules than ever potentially available for clinical testing, a better targeting of the populations likely to respond, but a slow, costly, and inefficient clinical development process. A very important factor influencing the duration and complexity of this process is the choice of endpoint(s) used to assess drug efficacy. Often, the most clinically relevant endpoint is difficult to use in a trial. This happens if the measurement of this clinical endpoint (a) is costly to measure (e.g., cachexia, a condition associated with malnutrition and involving loss of muscle and fat tissue, is assessed using expensive equipment that measures the levels of nitrogen, potassium, and water in the patient's body); (b) is difficult to measure (e.g., quality-of-life assessments involve multidimensional instruments that are prone to missing data and difficult to validate); (c) requires a large sample size because of low incidence of the event of interest (e.g., cytotoxic drugs may have rare but serious side effects, such as leukemias induced by topoisomerase inhibitors); or (d) requires a long follow-up time (e.g., survival in early-stage cancers). A potential strategy in these cases is to look for surrogate endpoints or biomarkers that can be measured more cheaply, more conveniently, more frequently, or earlier than the true clinical endpoint of interest.

DEFINITIONS

The Biomarker Definitions Working Group proposed definitions that have since been widely adopted (4). A clinical endpoint is considered the most credible indicator of drug response and is defined as "a characteristic or variable that reflects how a patient feels, functions, or survives." In clinical trials aimed at establishing the worth of new therapies, clinically relevant endpoints should be used, unless a biomarker or another endpoint is available that has risen to the status of surrogate endpoint. A biomarker is defined as "a characteristic that can be objectively measured as an indicator of healthy or pathological biological processes, or pharmacological responses to therapeutic intervention." A surrogate endpoint is a biomarker that is intended for substituting a clinical endpoint, and as such is "expected to predict clinical benefit, harm, or lack of these."

Evaluation of a potential surrogate involves a host of considerations, ranging from statistical conditions to clinical and biological evidence (5). A surrogate endpoint can play different roles in different phases of drug development; hence it could conceivably be considered valid for one goal but not for another. Earlier ("intermediate") endpoints are already in common use in phase I or II trials. However very few of these earlier endpoints—mostly in cardiovascular disease, where blood pressure and cholesterol levels have been surrogates de facto for a long time—have reached the point where they can be used as substitutes for the clinical endpoint in pivotal phase III trials. For a biomarker to be used as a "valid" surrogate to establish the efficacy of new treatments, a number of conditions must be fulfilled. The International Council for Harmonisation (ICH) Guidelines on Statistical Principles for Clinical Trials state that:

> In practice, the strength of the evidence for surrogacy depends upon (i) the biological plausibility of the relationship, (ii) the demonstration in epidemiological studies of the prognostic value of the surrogate for the clinical outcome, and (iii) evidence from clinical trials that treatment effects on the surrogate correspond to effects on the clinical outcome. (6)

Here we focus on the latter two conditions, and we discuss statistical approaches that may be used to assess the extent to which these conditions are fulfilled.

EARLY FAILURES WITH POOR SURROGATES

Surrogate endpoints have been used in medical research for a long time (7). Despite the potential advantages of surrogates, their use has been surrounded by controversy (8). An unfortunate precedent set the stage for heightened skepticism about surrogates in general: the Food and Drug Administration (FDA) approved three antiarrhythmic drugs (encainide, flecainide, and moricizine) based on their major effects on the suppression of arrhythmias. It was believed that, because arrhythmias are associated with an almost fourfold increase in the rate of cardiac-complication-related death, drugs that reduced arrhythmic episodes would also reduce the death rate. However, postmarketing trials showed that the active-treatment death rate with antiarrhythmic drugs could be twice higher than the placebo rate. Another instance of a poorly validated surrogate came with the surge of the AIDS epidemic. The impressive early therapeutic results obtained with zidovudine, and the pressure for accelerated approval of new therapies, led to the use of CD4 blood count as a surrogate endpoint for time to clinical events and overall survival (OS) (9), in spite of concerns about its limitations as a reliable predictor for clinically

relevant endpoints (10). The main reason behind these historical failures was the incorrect assumption that surrogacy simply follows from the association between a potential surrogate endpoint and the corresponding clinical endpoint, the mere existence of which is insufficient for surrogacy (7). Even though the existence of an association between the potential surrogate and the clinical endpoint is a desirable property, what is required to replace the clinical endpoint by the surrogate is that the *effect* of the treatment on the surrogate endpoint reliably predicts the *effect* on the clinical endpoint. Owing to a lack of appropriate methodology, this condition was not checked in the early use of surrogates, which in turn led to negative opinions about the use of surrogates in the assessment of new treatment efficacy (11, 12).

THE NEED FOR SURROGATES

Nowadays, there is increasing public pressure for the fast approval of promising new drugs, which creates a need to shift the approval process, at least in part, to biomarkers rather than on long-term, costly clinical endpoints. This trend is especially clear in oncology, where the increased knowledge about the genetic mechanisms operating in cancer cells leads to a large number of novel therapies with specific molecular targets. These therapies may have larger effects than conventional cytotoxic agents, and if so, one would like to detect these effects (or lack thereof) as soon as possible. The ability to predict clinical benefits on long-term endpoints such as survival from benefits observed on earlier endpoints could be enormously useful, hence the acute interest in surrogate endpoints. Shortening the duration of clinical trials not only decreases the cost of the evaluation process; it may also limit potential problems with noncompliance and missing data, which are more likely in longer studies. Alongside the increased pressure for a speedier clinical development, the rapid advances in molecular biology, in particular the -omics revolution and the advent of new drugs with well-defined mechanisms of action at the molecular level, dramatically increase the number of biomarkers that can potentially define surrogate endpoints (13). Surrogate endpoints also hold potential for the earlier detection of safety signals that could point to toxic problems with new drugs. The duration and sample size of clinical trials aimed at evaluating the therapeutic efficacy of new drugs are often insufficient to detect rare or late adverse effects (14); using surrogate endpoints or biomarkers in this context might allow one to obtain information about such effects even during the clinical testing phase.

SURROGATES IN CANCER

The ultimate objective of new anticancer agents is their ability to prolong survival with acceptable toxicity. Phase III trials that compare these new agents to the standard of care typically use OS as their primary endpoint. OS is defined as the time from randomization to death from any cause or to the last date a patient was seen alive. This endpoint requires prolonged follow-up and treatment effects on OS are diluted by risks of death unrelated to the cancer or treatment toxicities. In addition, the evaluation of the effect of a new agent on survival is potentially confounded by the further lines of treatment a patient will receive after failing on the new agent. For all these reasons, endpoints have been used that are observed earlier and that more directly assess the antitumor effect of new agents, specifically disease-free-survival (DFS) in the adjuvant setting (for patients whose tumor can be surgically resected with a curative intent) and response rate or progression-free-survival (PFS) in the advanced disease setting (for patients whose tumor is locally advanced or metastatic and cannot be surgically removed). DFS is defined as the time from randomization to a cancer recurrence, second cancer, or death from any cause, while PFS is defined as the time from randomization to the time of cancer progression or death from any cause. Although DFS and PFS have commonly been used as primary endpoints of phase III trials, their value as surrogate endpoints for OS has been questioned. In advanced disease, in particular, PFS is a controversial endpoint because some new agents (e.g., antiangiogenic agents in breast cancer) were shown to have a marked effect on PFS, which led to their regulatory approval, but no sizable benefit on OS. Statistically, the question can be cast in terms of surrogacy: Can DFS (or PFS) be used as *surrogate* endpoints for OS? The question seems straightforward, but addressing it is fraught with conceptual difficulties.

STRUCTURE OF THIS CHAPTER

This chapter is structured as follows: the next two sections present methods for the evaluation of surrogacy, using data from a single trial (Evaluating Surrogacy in a Single Trial) or from a meta-analysis of trials (Evaluating Surrogacy in a Meta-Analysis of Multiple Trials). Implications for the prediction of the treatment effect in a new trial, and for designing studies based on surrogates, are discussed in Prediction of Treatment Effect. Two case studies with contrasting results are presented in Two Case Studies in Gastric Cancer, one in early (resectable) gastric cancer and the other in advanced (metastatic) gastric cancer.

EVALUATING SURROGACY IN A SINGLE TRIAL

Historically, the first attempts to define and evaluate surrogacy assumed data to be available from a single randomized clinical trial. Figure 34.1 schematically illustrates the general situation of interest to establish surrogacy: Z denotes a specific treatment (e.g., an experimental treatment, the effect of which is typically

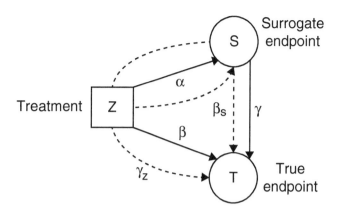

FIGURE 34.1 Schematic representation of the surrogacy problem: α represents the treatment effect on T, β represents the treatment effect on S, and γ represents the prognostic impact of S on T. In addition, β_s represents the treatment effect on T after adjustment for S, and γ_z represents the prognostic impact of S on T after adjustment for T.

compared against a standard of care in a randomized clinical trial), S denotes a tentative surrogate endpoint, and T denotes the "true" or "final" clinical endpoint that the surrogate is aimed at replacing.

Prentice's Definition and Criteria

In a landmark paper published in 1989, Ross Prentice proposed to define a surrogate endpoint as "a response variable for which a test of the null hypothesis of no relationship to the treatment groups under comparison is also a valid test of the corresponding null hypothesis based on the true endpoint" (15). Using the notation in Figure 34.1, this definition simply states that for the surrogate to be a valid surrogate for the true endpoint, α and β must simultaneously be equal to, or different from, zero. This definition cannot be operationalized if data are available from a single trial only, since it would require multiple estimates of α and β to be available, preferably from a large number of trials, some with treatment effects on both endpoints, and some without such effects. In the case of a single trial, Prentice suggested to use the following operational criteria (15):

1. The treatment has a significant impact on the surrogate endpoint ($\alpha \neq 0$).
2. The treatment has a significant impact on the true endpoint ($\beta \neq 0$).
3. The surrogate endpoint has a significant impact on the true endpoint ($\gamma \neq 0$).
4. The full effect of treatment upon the true endpoint is captured by the surrogate ($\beta_s = 0$).

The fourth criterion requires that the true endpoint does not depend on treatment, conditional on the surrogate value; in other words, the treatment effect on T is entirely captured by S (16). It has been noted that the

Prentice criteria are not equivalent to the definition (17). Yet Prentice's fourth criterion is very appealing, because it appears to provide a mathematical way of testing that there exists a biological mechanism through which the surrogate fully captures the effect of treatment on the true endpoint. In cancer trials, for example, if the surrogate (say, a change in prostate-specific antigen [PSA] levels) was the unique mechanism in the causal chain leading from treatment exposure to the final endpoint (say, death), then any treatment effect on the final endpoint could be *causally* explained by the treatment effect on the surrogate. This is a high bar that very few if any surrogates are likely to fulfill; for instance, it is a priori implausible to assume that changes in PSA levels can capture all events leading to death in patients with prostate cancer. Finally, the fulfillment of Prentice's fourth criterion does not support a claim of causality. Methods of causal inference have been used to implement this criterion through a so-called *mediation* analysis, which falls beyond the scope of the present chapter (18).

Related Statistical Approaches

Freedman et al. (19) pointed out that Prentice's fourth criterion raises a conceptual difficulty because it requires the treatment effect on the true endpoint be *non*-significant after adjustment for the surrogate. These authors argued that the non-significance of this test does not prove that the effect of treatment upon the true endpoint is *fully* captured by the surrogate, and instead they proposed to estimate the "proportion explained," defined as $1 - \beta_S/\beta$. If $\beta_S = 0$ the proportion explained is equal to 1, and if $\beta_S = \beta$ the proportion explained is equal to 0. A valid surrogate would be one for which the proportion explained is as close to 1 as possible.

Difficulties surrounding the proportion explained have been discussed in the literature (17, 20–22), so despite its intuitive appeal it cannot be considered a criterion of surrogacy. For normally distributed endpoints, the proportion explained is a simple function of two other statistics, the adjusted association between the surrogate and the true endpoint (γ_Z in Figure 34.1), and the relative effect β/α, that is, the treatment effect on the true endpoint relative to treatment effect on the surrogate. As we see in the section Evaluating Surrogacy in a Meta-Analysis of Multiple Trials, when data are available from multiple trials, these two statistics generalize respectively to the correlation between the true endpoint and the surrogate endpoint, and the slope of a regression line through the treatment effects on the true and surrogate endpoints.

Examples of Analyses Based on a Single Trial

There has been much research on using PSA to define surrogate endpoints for cancer-specific survival in locally advanced prostate cancer, or for OS in hormone-resistant advanced prostate cancer. Note that the surrogate endpoints can be binary (e.g., whether a patient achieved a PSA decline greater than 30% as compared to baseline), continuous (e.g., PSA doubling time), censored continuous (e.g., time to distant metastases), or longitudinal (e.g., repeated measurements of PSA over time). Table 34.1 shows some potential surrogate endpoints in prostate cancer that were evaluated using data from a single trial.

Some authors claimed surrogacy based on the Prentice criteria (24–26), while others made similar claims based on the proportion explained (27). More in-depth analyses of PSA-based endpoints suggest that, although PSA changes are prognostic in the sense that they predict survival in individual patients, treatment effects on PSA are poorly predictive of treatment effects on survival (30–32). The latter analyses were based on data from several trials, which is the topic of the section Evaluating Surrogacy in a Meta-Analysis of Multiple Trials.

EVALUATING SURROGACY IN A META-ANALYSIS OF MULTIPLE TRIALS

Bearing in mind the difficulties encountered when trying to evaluate a surrogate using data from a single randomized trial, several authors have proposed a meta-analytic

TABLE 34.1 Examples of Surrogate Evaluation in a Single Trial

Tumor Type	Tumor	Surrogate	Type	Final	Type	Refs
Locally advanced solid tumors	Prostate	PSA doubling time	Continuous	CSS	Time to event	23, 24
	Prostate	PSA nadir	Continuous	CSS	Time to event	25
	Prostate	TDM	Time to event	CSS	Time to event	26
Advanced solid tumors	Hormone-resistant prostate	PSA 30% reduction	Binary	OS	Time to event	27, 28
	Hormone-resistant prostate	Circulating tumor cells	Longitudinal	OS	Time to event	29

CSS, cancer-specific survival; OS, overall survival; PSA, prostate-specific antigen; TDM, time to distant metastases.

approach when data can be collected from several randomized clinical trials (33–35).

Normally Distributed Endpoints

A meta-analytic approach was originally formulated for the case where both the surrogate endpoint and the true endpoint are continuous, normally distributed outcomes (34). An example of such a situation was studied in ophthalmology, with the change in visual acuity at 3 months being evaluated as a surrogate for the change in visual acuity at 12 months. Similar situations are admittedly uncommon in cancer trials, but they are of interest because they lead to the simplest mathematical formulation (34).

A hierarchical two-level model can be used when the surrogate and the true endpoint are jointly normally distributed. At the first level, the association between the surrogate and the true endpoints is assessed using the variance–covariance matrix of their joint distribution. This association is called "individual level," because it measures the association between S and T at the level of the individual patient (adjusted for treatment). For normally distributed outcomes, the individual-level association can be quantified by a coefficient of determination denoted by R^2_{indiv}, or the familiar Pearson correlation coefficient, equal to R_{indiv}. This metric has the same interpretation as the adjusted association, that is, an R_{indiv} close to 1 indicates that an individual patient's true endpoint can be accurately predicted from this individual's surrogate endpoint.

At the second level, a linear mixed-effects model is defined for the treatment effects on the surrogate and on the true endpoint in all trials. The association between the treatment effects on S and T is assessed using the variance–covariance matrix of the random effects in this model. This association is called "trial level," because it measures the association between the treatment effects on S and T in all trials. The trial-level association can be quantified by a coefficient of determination denoted by R^2_{trial} or the correlation coefficient R_{trial}. An R^2_{trial} close to 1 indicates that the treatment effect on the true endpoint can be accurately predicted from the treatment effect on the surrogate endpoint.

The hierarchical model can be fitted to the data by using the linear mixed–models methodology. Depending on the number of trials available and their size, the variance–covariance matrix of the random effects may be ill-conditioned and/or nonpositive definite. Various simplified modeling strategies (36) or Bayesian models (37) have been suggested to address such situations. In particular, one can fit the model in two stages using the fixed–effects formulation (34). In the first stage, the individual–level association is evaluated by using a bivariate normal distribution for the surrogate and the true endpoints with trial–specific treatment effects regarded as fixed effects. In the second stage, the trial–level association is evaluated by using a linear regression model for the treatment effects estimated in the first stage.

It is worth noting that many publications use a naïve approach to estimate the trial-level association, and simply fit a linear regression line through the observed treatment effects on the surrogate and the true endpoints. This linear regression ignores the estimation error in the treatment effects on S and T, and as such it is likely to lead to biased estimates of the true association (38). To take the estimation error into account, methods related to the measurement–error models should be used (41). As these methods are numerically complex, an approximate solution is to fit a weighted linear regression line, with weights proportional to the trial sizes. This weighted linear regression does account for the heterogeneity in information content between trials of different sizes, though it does not properly account for the estimation error in the treatment effects on S and T (38).

Other Types of Endpoints

The two-stage modeling strategy in the section Normally Distributed Endpoints has been extended to other types of endpoint: binary, ordinal, time to event, or longitudinally measured. Renard et al. have addressed the situation of two binary endpoints with unobserved latent variables assumed to have a joint normal distribution. The observed binary endpoints are obtained by dichotomization of these latent variables (39). Burzykowski et al. have suggested copulas to model the association between the surrogate and the true endpoints when both are time-to-event endpoints, a common situation in cancer trials (40). Different copulas may be used, depending on assumptions made about the nature of the association between the surrogate and the true endpoint; in practice, several copulas are tried, and the best fitting copula is selected. Similar ideas have been proposed by Burzykowski et al. when one of the endpoints is categorical and the other is a time-to-event endpoint (41). In this case, one marginal distribution can be modelled by using a proportional odds logistic regression, while the other can be obtained from a proportional hazards model. This situation is relevant to cancer clinical trials, when the surrogate is a dichotomous endpoint indicating response to treatment, and the true endpoint OS or some other failure-time endpoint.

Perhaps the most complex situation occurs when the surrogate endpoint is based on longitudinal measurements of biomarkers and/or clinical measurements, while the true endpoint is a failure-time endpoint. In most forms of advanced cancer, for instance, the size of the tumor is measured repeatedly over time, with tumor shrinkage indicating treatment benefit, and tumor growth lack of responsiveness to treatment. In this case, endpoints that are defined using simple metrics based on the longitudinal measures, such as a binary indicator of response, may fail to be adequate surrogates. The question is whether use of the whole vector of tumor measurements over time might be a more promising alternative. Renard et al. (30) and Alonso et al. (42) have extended the aforementioned models to the longitudinal setting, which requires a nontrivial extension of these models. They argue that if treatment effect can be assumed constant over time, then R^2_{trial} can still be useful to evaluate surrogacy at the trial level. However, at the individual level, R^2_{indiv} becomes a function of time, and has a less straightforward interpretation.

Other Units of Analysis

We have assumed previously that several trials were available, in which case the meta-analytic method uses trial as the unit of analysis. If a single multicenter trial of sufficient size is available, it may also be reasonable to "split" this trial into smaller units of analysis, such as country, center, or investigator (43). This choice may depend on practical considerations, such as the information available in each unit, expert considerations about the most suitable unit for a specific problem, the amount of replication at a potential unit's level, and the number of patients per unit. From a technical point of view, the most desirable situation is when the number of units and the number of patients per unit are both sufficiently large (44).

Surrogacy Criteria Based on Several Trials

In the meta-analytic approach, a surrogate can be considered acceptable if R^2_{indiv} and R^2_{trial} are both sufficiently close to 1, with due allowance for the confidence intervals of these quantities. Some authors (45) and health authorities (e.g., the German Institute for Quality and Efficiency in Health Care) (46) have proposed thresholds that need to be met by these measures of association. While such thresholds provide useful guidance, there will always be clinical and other judgments involved in the decision to adopt a surrogate. In recent years, Ciani et al. have reviewed the statistical methods and results of surrogacy analyses, with a focus on advanced solid tumors (47). Based on their findings, they have proposed a validation framework for the use of surrogate endpoints for healthcare policy makers (48, 49).

Examples of Analyses Based on Several Trials

Table 34.2 shows examples of potential surrogate endpoints for various tumor types. These surrogates were evaluated using data from several trials or, when a single trial was available, after splitting the trial into several analysis units, as discussed in the section Other Units of Analysis. We illustrate the meta-analytic evaluation of surrogacy in detail in the section Two Case Studies in Gastric Cancer, using the two meta-analyses in gastric cancer patients shown in Table 34.2 (51, 61).

PREDICTION OF TREATMENT EFFECT

The key motivation for validating a surrogate endpoint is the ability to predict the effect of treatment on the true endpoint based on the observed effect of treatment on the surrogate endpoint. The meta-analytic approach provides a natural setup to do such a prediction. The trial-level association is obtained by fitting a linear regression through the treatment effects on the surrogate and on the true endpoint in all trials (see the section Normally Distributed Endpoints). Suppose a new trial is carried out, in which the treatment effect can already be estimated on the surrogate endpoint but not yet on the true endpoint. The regression analysis can be used to predict the effect the treatment is likely to have on the true endpoint, assuming constancy of all parameters, that is, assuming that the statistical associations seen in the meta-analysis of previous trials will still hold in the new trial.

Prediction Error

The prediction is, of course, subject to error. The prediction error has three distinct sources: (a) the regression line is estimated with error, which can be made small by increasing the size of the meta-analysis if possible, (b) the treatment effect on the surrogate is estimated with error, which can be made small by increasing the size of the new trial if possible, and (c) the association between the treatment effects is not perfect if R^2_{trial} is less than 1, and this source of error cannot be reduced. Hence, the prediction will always entail a loss of efficiency as compared with a direct estimation (35), though the prediction may still be worthwhile if it can be made much earlier and/or with fewer patients than a direct estimation of the treatment effect on the true endpoint.

The Surrogate Threshold Effect

Burzykowski and Buyse have proposed the *surrogate threshold effect* as a useful measure of surrogacy when interest focuses on predicting the treatment effect on the true endpoint, having observed the treatment effect on the surrogate (67). The STE is the smallest treatment effect on the surrogate that predicts a nonzero treatment effect on the true endpoint. In practical terms, one would like the STE to be realistically achievable, given the range of treatment effects on surrogates observed in previous clinical trials. If the STE was too large to be achievable, the surrogate would not be useful. If the STE was reasonably achievable, then it could be used to design a clinical trial aimed at showing an effect on the surrogate that exceeds the STE, which in turn is anticipated to predict a significant effect on the true endpoint.

TWO CASE STUDIES IN GASTRIC CANCER

To illustrate the concepts and difficulties inherent in the evaluation of surrogate endpoints, we use two meta-analyses of randomized clinical trials conducted by the Global Advanced/Adjuvant Stomach Tumor Research International Collaboration (GASTRIC) Group. The first meta-analysis was carried out using individual data from patients with curatively resected gastric cancer. It confirmed the benefit of adjuvant chemotherapy as compared

TABLE 34.2 Examples of Surrogate Evaluation in Multiple Trials

Tumor Type	Tumor	Surrogate	Type	Final	Type	Refs
Resectable solid tumors	Colon	DFS	Time to event	OS	Time to event	(50)
	Stomach	DFS	Time to event	OS	Time to event	(51)
	Melanoma	EFS	Time to event	OS	Time to event	(52)
	Breast	pCR	Binary	EFS	Time to event	(53)
Locally advanced solid tumors	Head and neck	EFS	Time to event	OS	Time to event	(54)
	Lung	EFS	Time to event	OS	Time to event	(55)
	Prostate	EFS	Time to event	OS	Time to event	(56)
Advanced solid tumors	Ovary	PFS	Time to event	OS	Time to event	(41)
	Colon	PFS	Time to event	OS	Time to event	(57, 58)
	Breast	PFS	Time to event	OS	Time to event	(59, 60)
	Lung	PFS	Time to event	OS	Time to event	(61)
	Stomach	PFS	Time to event	OS	Time to event	(62)
	Colon	ORR	Binary	OS	Time to event	(63)
	Breast	ORR	Binary	OS	Time to event	(59)
	HD Prostate	PSA repeated measures	Longitudinal	OS	Time to event	(31, 64)
	Hormone-resistant prostate	PSA 30% reduction	Binary	OS	Time to event	(32)
Hematologic malignancies	AML	LFS	Time to event	OS	Time to event	(65, 66)

AML, acute myeloid leukemia; DFS, disease free survival; EFS, event-free survival; HD, hormone dependent; LFS, leukemia-free survival; ORR, overall response rate; OS, overall survival; pCR, pathological complete response; PFS, progression-free survival; PSA, prostate-specific antigen.

with no adjuvant treatment in terms of both DFS and OS (51). The second meta-analysis was carried out using individual data from patients with advanced or recurrent gastric cancer. It confirmed the benefit of adding experimental agents to standard chemotherapy regimens in terms of both PFS and OS (62). We apply the methods described in the previous sections to investigate whether DFS and PFS are acceptable surrogates for OS. Even though both of these early endpoints are a priori plausible surrogates for OS, we will show that DFS can be used as a reasonable surrogate for OS in localized disease, while PFS cannot be used reliably as a surrogate for OS in advanced disease.

Resectable Gastric Cancer: Can DFS Be Used as a Surrogate for OS?

The meta-analysis of trials for patients with resected gastric cancer was used to evaluate DFS as a surrogate for OS. Data were available on 3,288 patients from 14 trials with documented OS and DFS (51).

At the individual level, a Plackett copula was fitted on the joint distribution of DFS and OS. The individual-level association, quantified by Spearman's rank correlation coefficient, was equal to 0.974 (95% CI: 0.971–0.976), indicating a very tight correlation between DFS and OS for a given patient. At the trial level, there was also a tight association between the treatment effects on DFS and on OS. With adjustment for the estimation error in treatment effects, $R^2_{trial} \approx 1$ (95% CI: 0.999–1.000). Caution is required to interpret an estimated R^2 value so close to the upper limit of 1, because the results can easily be influenced by numerical errors. The qualitative interpretation however remains that there is a tight association between the treatment effects. Figure 34.2 shows the regression line through the treatment effects in the 14 trials included in the analysis. Each trial is represented by a bubble whose size is proportional to the trial sample size. The 95% prediction limits indicate the range of effects on OS that can be expected for a given effect on DFS.

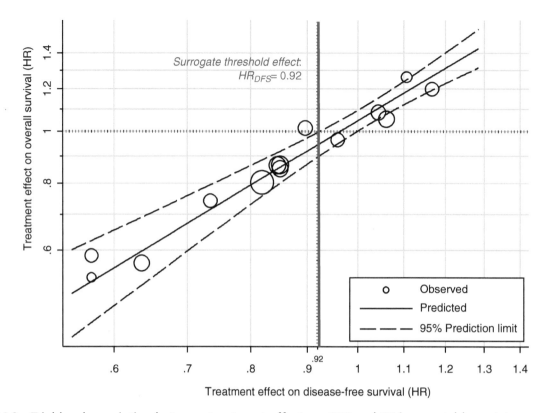

FIGURE 34.2 Trial-level association between treatment effects on DFS and OS in resectable gastric cancer (both axes on a log scale). Each trial is represented by a bubble whose size is proportional to the trial sample size.

DFS, disease-free survival; OS, overall survival.

The STE was equal to 0.92. Hence, in a future trial using similar treatment modalities as in the set of trials in the meta-analysis, a hazard ratio for DFS of less than 0.92 would predict a significant effect on OS. This fact can be used to design a trial based on the surrogate, rather than the true endpoint. The size of this new trial can be calculated so that the 95% confidence interval of the estimated hazard ratio for DFS lies entirely under 0.92. In other words, the null and alternative hypotheses of interest for DFS are H_0: $HR_{DFS} \geq 0.92$ versus H_A: $HR_{DFS} < 0.92$. The test of hypothesis for DFS is more stringent than the test of hypothesis for OS, which is based on the conventional null and alternative hypotheses H_0: $HR_{OS} \geq 1$ versus H_A: $HR_{OS} < 1.0$. Even so, the test of hypothesis for DFS may require less patients and less follow-up time to reach the same statistical power than the test of hypothesis for OS, since the treatment effect may be larger on DFS than on OS, and the events are observed earlier.

The results of our surrogate evaluation could be externally validated using six trials not included in the meta-analysis, three for which the treatment effects were extracted from reports published in the literature, and three for which individual patient data became available after the meta-analysis was completed. Table 34.3 shows the observed treatment effects on survival in these six trials, and the treatment effects on survival predicted from the treatment effects on the surrogate, along with

their 95% prediction intervals. There is excellent agreement between the observed and the predicted treatment effects, and in the four trials for which the predicted treatment effect on OS would be significant, the observed effects actually reached statistical significance, which confirmed the reliability of DFS as a surrogate for OS in gastric cancer (51).

Advanced Gastric Cancer: Can PFS be Used as a Surrogate for OS?

The meta-analysis of trials in advanced disease was used for the purposes of evaluating PFS as a surrogate for OS. Data were available on 4,069 patients from 20 eligible randomized trials with documented OS and PFS (62).

The individual-level association, quantified by Spearman's rank correlation coefficient, was equal to 0.853 (95% CI: 0.852–0.854), indicating substantial correlation between PFS and OS for a given patient. At the trial level, the association between the treatment effects on PFS and on OS was only moderate. With adjustment for the estimation error in treatment effects, $R^2_{trial} = 0.61$ (95% CI: 0.04–1.00). Note the very large confidence interval, which casts doubts on the usefulness of R^2 in this setting. Figure 34.3 shows the regression line through the treatment effects in the 20 trials included in the analysis. Each trial is represented by a bubble whose size is proportional to the

TABLE 34.3 Observed Treatment Effects (95% Confidence Intervals) on DFS and OS, and Predicted Treatment Effect on OS (95% Prediction Intervals) in Five Validation Trials in Resectable Gastric Cancer

Trial (51)	Observed HR$_{DFS}$	Observed HR$_{OS}$	Predicted HR$_{OS}$
Cirera	0.55 [0.36–0.85]*	0.60 [0.39–0.93]*	0.50 [0.28–0.87]*
CLASSIC	0.56 [0.44–0.72]*	0.72 [0.52–1.00]*	0.51 [0.36–0.73]*
ACTS-GC	0.65 [0.54–0.79]*	0.67 [0.54–0.83]*	0.61 [0.47–0.81]*
INT-1018	0.66 [0.53–0.82]*	0.75 [0.61–0.92]*	0.63 [0.46–0.84]*
GOIM-9602	0.88 [0.66–1.17]	0.91 [0.69–1.21]	0.89 [0.62–1.28]
GOIRC	0.92 [0.66–1.27]	0.90 [0.64–1.26]	0.94 [0.63–1.42]

*Significant treatment effects.
DFS, disease-free survival; OS, overall survival.

trial sample size. The 95% prediction limits indicate the range of effects on OS that can be expected for a given effect on PFS.

The moderate correlation at the trial level is reflected by an STE equal to 0.56: hence, in a future trial using similar treatment modalities as in the set of trials in the meta-analysis, it would take an HR$_{PFS}$ smaller than 0.56 to predict an HR$_{OS}$ smaller than 1.

The results of our surrogate evaluation could be externally validated using 12 trials not included in the meta-analysis, using treatment effects extracted from

reports published in the literature after the meta-analysis was completed. Table 34.4 shows the observed treatment effects on survival, and the treatment effects on survival predicted from the treatment effects on the surrogate, along with their 95% prediction intervals. The prediction intervals are wide and include one (no treatment effect on OS) in all trials, which means that the observed effects on PFS would not have allowed predicting an effect on OS in any of these 12 trials. Yet, 3 of the 12 trials showed a statistically significant effect of treatment on survival (62).

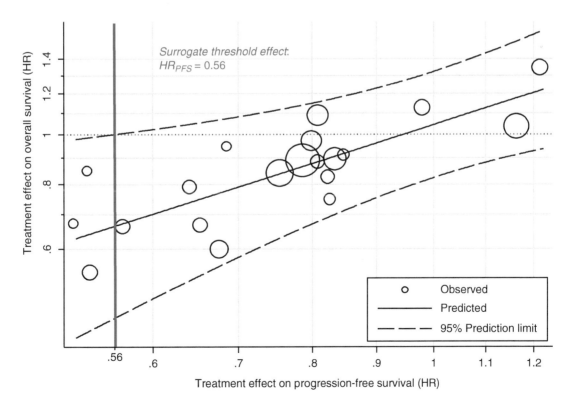

FIGURE 34.3 Trial-level association between treatment effects on PFS and OS in advanced gastric cancer (both axes on a log scale). Each trial is represented by a bubble whose size is proportional to the trial sample size.

PFS, progression-free survival; OS, overall survival.

TABLE 34.4 Observed Treatment Effects (95% Confidence Intervals) on PFS and OS, and Predicted Treatment Effect on OS (95% Prediction Intervals) in 12 Validation Trials in Advanced Gastric Cancer

Trial (62)	Observed HR$_{DFS}$	Observed HR$_{OS}$	Predicted HR$_{OS}$
Jeung	0.63 [0.38–1.05]	0.56 [0.35–0.88]*	0.73 [0.46–1.04]
AIO	0.67 [0.43–1.04]	0.82 [0.47–1.45]	0.76 [0.53–1.07]
ToGA	0.71 [0.59–0.85]*	0.74 [0.60–0.91]*	0.80 [0.58–1.09]
AVAGAST	0.80 [0.68–0.93]*	0.87 [0.73–1.03]	0.88 [0.76–1.14]
Kang	0.80 [0.63–1.03]	0.85 [0.64–1.13]	0.88 [0.76–1.14]
Park	0.86 [0.54–1.37]	0.96 [0.60–1.52]	0.93 [0.71–1.18]
REAL(a)	0.92 [0.80–1.04]	0.92 [0.80–1.10]	0.98 [0.77–1.22]
REAL(b)	0.92 [0.81–1.05]	0.86 [0.80–0.99]*	0.98 [0.77–1.22]
Ross	0.95 [0.80–1.08]	0.91 [0.76–1.04]	1.00 [0.79–1.29]
FLAGS	0.99 [0.86–1.14]	0.92 [0.80–1.05]	1.03 [0.81–1.31]
Rao	1.13 [0.63–2.01]	1.02 [0.61–1.70]	1.14 [0.89–1.46]
Moehler	1.14 [0.59–2.21]	0.77 [0.51–1.17]	1.15 [0.90–1.48]

*Significant treatments effects.
PFS, progression-free survival; OS, overall survival.

Contrasting Conclusions About DFS and PFS

The analyses shown in the section Resectable Gastric Cancer: Can DFS Be Used as a Surrogate for OS suggest that DFS is a good surrogate for OS in patients with gastric tumors that can be surgically resected or locally treated. These findings parallel those in resectable colon cancer and melanoma as well as operable or locally advanced head and neck and lung cancers (50,52,54,55). Taken together, these findings suggest that in early forms of cancer that are amenable to local treatment, DFS or event-free survival can be used as a reliable surrogate for OS.

In contrast, the analyses shown in the section Advanced Gastric Cancer: Can PFS be Used as a Surrogate for OS suggest that PFS is not a useful surrogate for OS in advanced gastric cancer. PFS was also found to be a poor surrogate for OS in advanced breast cancer (59). In contrast, PFS was a good surrogate in advanced ovarian cancer (41). PFS appeared to be a good surrogate for OS in advanced colorectal cancer treated with fluoropyrimidines (57), but not with more recent therapies (58). In advanced lung cancer, the value of PFS as a surrogate for OS is questionable (61). All in all, PFS tends to be an unreliable surrogate for OS in advanced solid tumors (68).

These contrasting findings for DFS and PFS may seem counterintuitive. If anything, one would expect PFS to be a better surrogate for OS than DFS, because the time between tumor progression and death is much shorter in advanced disease than after surgical resection of the tumor. However, from a biological standpoint, the reappearance of a tumor after a long disease-free period may be a far more consequential event than an increase in size of a measurable tumor mass.

CONCLUDING COMMENTS

Over the years, a variety of surrogate endpoint evaluation strategies have been proposed. The initial attempts to validate a surrogate endpoint using data from a single trial have been shown insufficient insofar as they focus solely on the individual-level association. Indeed none of these attempts has, to the best of our knowledge, successfully identified an acceptable surrogate endpoint for use in the clinic. Today, much of the attention has shifted to the meta-analytic setting in which data are available from several trials; hence investigation of the trial-level association is possible as well. Getting individual patient data from several trials is a tall order, but the reliable validation of a surrogate endpoint may come at that price. If the current climate of data sharing is any indication (69,70), access to individual patient data will hopefully become a less daunting task in the future.

In this chapter we have not discussed extensions of the meta-analytic evaluation framework using information theory, which provides an elegant unification that can be broadly applied (71,72). We have not discussed alternative methods for surrogate evaluation, especially those based on causal inference, which inform surrogacy using a completely different approach than the one presented here (73–75). Joffe and Green present a taxonomy of causal paradigms (76) while Alonso et al. establish a link between the causal-inference and meta-analytic paradigms for the validation of surrogate endpoints (77). Finally, we have not addressed all the complex issues that come into play when assessing potential surrogates. One key issue is the biological plausibility of a surrogate, which is a prerequisite to any statistical evaluation of surrogacy. A good surrogate ideally lies on the causal pathway of the treatment effect on the true endpoint. In reality, however, there is often a complex interplay between a potential surrogate and the true endpoint, since treatment decisions that affect the true endpoint are made after observing the surrogate. For instance, in most forms of advanced cancer, treatments are modified and/or intensified if possible when there is clinical, radiological, or biomarker-based evidence that the tumor is progressing. Hence the surrogate (PFS) is observed under first-line therapy, while the true endpoint (OS) is observed under subsequent-line therapies that may confound the effect of first-line therapy on the true endpoint. Such a situation may explain why PFS was an acceptable surrogate for OS in advanced colorectal cancer in an era of marginally effective fluoropyrimidine-based therapies (57) while it is a much less convincing surrogate today, because patients who are in progressive disease may receive many lines of active therapy that may further impact their survival (58).

Finally, perhaps the most challenging question is whether a surrogate that has been evaluated for a given class of drugs is still likely to be valid for different classes of drugs. Here again, a combination of biological reasoning and statistical evidence will be required for a surrogate to be used outside of the conditions in which it was initially evaluated. Statistical evidence favoring use of the surrogate will be most helpful for new drugs that are similar to the drugs used in the evaluation data sets. For new drugs having a substantially different mode of action, whether the surrogate can be used in confidence is an open question that may warrant another prospective evaluation. The more we understand about surrogates, the more we realize how difficult it is to formally "validate" them. A statistical evaluation using the methods described in this chapter can however be invaluable to inform the decision to rely on a surrogate, and for what purpose.

ACKNOWLEDGMENTS

The authors gratefully acknowledge support from IAP Research Network P7/06 of the Belgian Government (Belgian Science Policy). They thank the GASTRIC Group for permission to use their data. A full description of the methods discussed in this paper is available in (1).

REFERENCES

1. Buyse M, Molenberghs G, Paoletti X, et al. Statistical evaluation of surrogate endpoints with examples from cancer trials. *Biomet J.* 2016;58:104–132.
2. Burzykowski T, Molenberghs G, Buyse M. *The Evaluation of Surrogate Endpoints.* New York, NY: Springer Publications; 2005.
3. Alonso A, Bigirumurame T, Burzykowski T, et al. *Applied Surrogate Endpoint Evaluation Methods with SAS and R.* New York, NY: Chapman and Hall/CRC Press; 2017.
4. Biomarkers Definition Working Group. Biomarkers and surrogate endpoints: preferred definitions and conceptual framework. *Clin Pharmacol Therapeut.* 2001;69:89–95.
5. Schatzkin A, Gail M. The promise and peril of surrogate end points in cancer research. *Nature Reviews Cancer.* 2002;2:19–27.
6. International Conference on Harmonisation of Technical Requirements for Registration of Pharmaceuticals for Human use. ICH Harmonised Tripartite Guideline. Statistical principles for clinical trials; 1998. http://www.ich.org/pdfICH/e9.pdf), Federal Register 63, No. 179, 49583.
7. Cardiac Arrhythmia Suppression Trial (CAST) Investigators. Preliminary Report: effect of encainide and flecainide on mortality in a randomized trial of arrhythmia suppression after myocardial infraction. *New Engl J Med.* 1989;321:406–412.
8. Fleming TR, DeMets DL. Surrogate end points in clinical trials: are we being misled? *Annals of Internal Medicine.* 1996;125:605–613.
9. Lagakos SW, Hoth DF. Surrogate markers in AIDS: where are we? Where are we going? *Ann Inter Med.* 1992;116:599–601.
10. DeGruttola V, Fleming TR, Lin DY, Coombs R. Validating surrogate markers—are we being naive? *J Infect Dis.* 1997;175:237–246.
11. Ferentz AE. Integrating pharmacogenomics into drug development. *Pharmacogenomics.* 2002;3:453–467.
12. Fleming TR. Surrogate markers in AIDS and cancer trials. *Stat Med.* 1994;13:1423–1435.
13. Lesko LJ, Atkinson AJ. Use of biomarkers and surrogate endpoints in drug development and regulatory decision making: criteria, validation, strategies. *Ann Rev Pharmacol Toxicol.* 2001;41:347–366.
14. Jones TC. Call for a new approach to the process of clinical trials and drug registration. *Br Med J.* 2001;322:920–923.
15. Prentice RL. Surrogate endpoints in clinical trials: definitions and operational criteria. *Stat Med.* 1989;8:431–440.
16. Alonso A, Molenberghs G, Geys H, Buyse M. A unifying approach for surrogate marker validation based on Prentice's criteria. *Stat Med.* 2005;25:205–211.
17. Buyse M, Molenberghs G. Criteria for the validation of surrogate end-points in randomized experiments. *Biometrics.* 1998;54:1014–1029.
18. Vandenberghe S, Duchateau L, Slaets L, et al. Surrogate marker analysis in cancer clinical trials through time-to-event mediation techniques. *Stat Method Med Res.* 2017. doi:10.1177/0962280217702179
19. Freedman LS, Graubard BI, Schatzkin A. Statistical validation of intermediate endpoints for chronic diseases. *Stat Med.* 1992;11:167–178.
20. Flandre P, Saidi Y. Letter to the editor: estimating the proportion of treatment effect explained by a surrogate marker. *Stat Med.* 1999;18:107–115.
21. Begg C, Leung D. On the use of surrogate endpoints in randomized trials. *J Royal Stat Soc, Series A.* 2000;163:26–27.

22. Molenberghs G, Buyse M, Geys H, et al. Statistical challenges in the evaluation of surrogate endpoints in randomized trials. *Control Clin Trial.* 2002;23:607–625.
23. Valicenti RK, DeSilvio M, Hanks GE, et al. Posttreatment prostatic-specific antigen doubling time as a surrogate endpoint for prostate cancer-specific survival: an analysis of Radiation Therapy Oncology Group Protocol 92-02. *Inter J Radiat Oncol Biol Phys.* 2006;66:1064–1071.
24. Denham JW, Steigler A, Wilcox C, et al. Time to biochemical failure and prostate-specific antigen doubling time as surrogates for prostate cancer-specific mortality: evidence from the TROG 96.01 randomised controlled trial. *Lancet Oncol.* 2008;9:1058–1068.
25. D'Amico AV, Chen MH, de Castro M, et al. Surrogate endpoints for prostate cancer-specific mortality after radiotherapy and androgen suppression therapy in men with localized or locally advanced prostate cancer: an analysis of 2 randomized trials. *Lancet Oncol.* 2012;13:189–195.
26. Ray ME, Bae K, Hussain MH, et al. Potential surrogate endpoints for prostate cancer survival: analysis of a phase III randomized trial. *J Natl Cancer Inst.* 2009;101:228–236.
27. Petrylak DP, Ankerst DP, Jiang CS, et al. Evaluation of prostate-specific antigen declines for surrogacy in patients treated on SWOG 99-16. *J Natl Cancer Inst.* 2006;98:516–521.
28. Armstrong AJ, Garrett–Mayer E, Yang YCO, et al. Prostate-specific antigen and pain surrogacy analysis in metastatic hormone-refractory prostate cancer. *J Clin Oncol.* 2007;25:3965–3970.
29. Scher HI, Heller G, Molina A, et al. Circulating tumor cell biomarker panel as an individual level surrogate for survival in metastatic castration-resistant prostate cancer. *J Clin Oncol.* 2015;33:1348–1355.
30. Renard D, Geys H, Molenberghs G, et al. Validation of a longitudinally measured surrogate marker for a time-to-event endpoint. *J Appl Stat.* 2002;30:235–247.
31. Collette L, Burzykowski T, Carroll KJ, et al. Is prostate-specific antigen a valid surrogate end point for survival in hormonally treated patients with metastatic prostate cancer? *J Clin Oncol.* 2005;23:6139–6148
32. Halabi S, Armstrong AJ, Sartor O, et al. Prostate-specific antigen changes as surrogate for overall survival in men with castration resistant prostate cancer treated with second-line chemotherapy. *J Clin Oncol.* 2013;31:3944–3950.
33. Daniels MJ, Hughes MD. Meta-analysis for the evaluation of potential surrogate markers. *Stat Med.* 1997;16:1515–1527.
34. Buyse M, Molenberghs G, Burzykowski T, et al. The validation of surrogate endpoints in meta-analyses of randomized experiments. *Biostatistics.* 2000;1:49–68.
35. Gail MH, Pfeiffer R, van Houwelingen HC, Carroll RJ. On meta-analytic assessment of surrogate outcomes. *Biostatistics.* 2000;1:231–246.
36. Tibaldi FS, Cortinas Abrahantes J, Molenberghs G, et al. Simplified hierarchical linear models for the evaluation of surrogate endpoints. *J Stat Comput Simulat.* 2003;73:643–658.
37. Renfro LA, Shi Q, Sargent DJ, Carlin BP. Bayesian adjusted R^2 for the meta-analytic evaluation of surrogate time-to-event endpoints in clinical trials. *Stat Med.* 2012;31:743–761.
38. Shi Q, Renfro LA, Bot BM, et al. Comparative assessment of trial-level surrogacy measures for candidate time-to-event surrogate endpoints in clinical trials. *Computat Stat Data Anal.* 2011;55:2748–2757.
39. Renard D, Geys H, Molenberghs G, et al. Validation of surrogate endpoints in multiple randomized clinical trials with discrete outcomes. *Biometrics.* 2002;44:1–15.
40. Burzykowski T, Molenberghs G, Buyse, M. The validation of surrogate endpoints using data from randomized clinical trials: a case-study in advanced colorectal cancer. *J Royal Stat Soc, Series A.* 2004;167:103–124.
41. Burzykowski T, Molenberghs G, Buyse M, et al. Validation of surrogate endpoints in multiple randomized clinical trials with failure-time endpoints. *J Royal Stat Soc, Series C.* 2001;50:405–422.

42. Alonso A, Geys H, Molenberghs G, et al. Validation of surrogate markers in multiple randomized clinical trials with repeated measurements. *Biometrics.* 2003;45:931–945.
43. Renfro LA, Shi Q, Xue Y, et al. Center-within-trial versus trial-level evaluation of surrogate endpoints. *Computat Stat Data Anal.* 2014;78:1–20.
44. Cortinas Abrahantes J, Molenberghs G, Burzykowski T, et al. Choice of units of analysis and modeling strategies in multilevel hierarchical models. *Computat Stat Data Anal.* 2004;47:537–563.
45. Lassere M, Johnson K, Boers M, et al. Definitions and validation criteria for biomarkers and surrogate endpoints: development and testing of a quantitative hierarchical levels of evidence schema. *J Rheumatol.* 2007;34:607–615.
46. Institut für Qualität und Wirtschaftlichkeit im Gesundheitswesen. Validity of surrogate endpoints in oncology; 2011. https://www.iqwig.de/download/A10–05_Executive_Summary_v1–1_Surrogate_endpoints_in_oncology.pdf
47. Ciani O, Davis S, Tappenden P, et al. Validation of surrogate endpoints in advanced solid tumors: systematic review of statistical methods, results, and implications for policy makers. *Inter J Technol Assess Health Care.* 2014:30:1–13.
48. Ciani O, Buyse M, Drummond M, et al. Use of surrogate end points in health care policy: a proposal for adoption of a validation framework. *Nat Rev Drug Discov.* 2016;15:516.
49. Ciani O, Buyse M, Drummond M, et al. Time to review the role of surrogate end points in health policy: state of the art and the way forward. *Inter J Technol Assess Health Care.* 2017;30:1–13.
50. Sargent DJ, Wieand HS, Haller DG, et al. Disease free survival versus overall survival as a primary end point for adjuvant colon cancer studies: individual patient data from 20,898 patients on 18 randomized trials. *J Clin Oncol.* 2005;23:8664–8670.
51. Oba K, Paoletti X, Alberts S, et al. Disease-free survival as a surrogate for overall survival in adjuvant trials of gastric cancer: a meta-analysis. *J Natl Cancer Inst.* 2013;5:1600–1607.
52. Suciu S, Eggermont AMM, Lorigan P, et al. Relapse-free survival as a surrogate endpoint for overall survival in adjuvant Interferon trials in patients with resectable cutaneous melanoma: an individual patient data meta-analysis. *J Natl Cancer Inst.* 2017.
53. Cortazar P, Zhang L, Untch M, et al. Pathological complete response and long-term clinical benefit in breast cancer: the CTNeoBC pooled analysis. *Lancet.* 2014. doi:10.1016/S0140–6736(13)62422-8
54. Michiels S, Le Maître A, Buyse M, et al. Surrogate endpoints for overall survival in locally advanced head and neck cancer: meta analyses of individual patient data. *Lancet Oncol.* 2009;10;341–350.
55. Mauguen A, Pignon JP, Burdett S, et al. Surrogate endpoints for overall survival in chemotherapy and radiotherapy trials in operable and locally advanced lung cancer: a re-analysis of meta-analyses of individual patients'data. *Lancet Oncol.* 2013;14;619–626.
56. Intermediate Clinical Endpoints of Cancer of the Prostate (ICECaP) Working Group. Metastasis-free survival is a strong surrogate of prostate cancer overall Survival. *J Clin Oncol.* 2017.
57. Buyse M, Burzykowski T, Carroll K, et al. Progression-free survival is a surrogate for survival in advanced colorectal cancer. *J Clin Oncol.* 2007;25:5218–5224.
58. Shi Q, de Gramont A, Grothey A, et al. Individual patient data analysis of progression-free versus overall survival as a first-line endpoint for metastatic colorectal cancer in modern randomized trials: Findings from 16,700 patients from the ARCAD database. *J Clin Oncol.* 2014. 33(1):22–28. doi:10.1200/JCO.2014.56.5887
59. Burzykowski T, Buyse M, Piccart-Gebhart MJ, et al. Evaluation of tumor response, disease control, progression-free survival, and time to progression as potential surrogate endpoints in metastatic breast cancer. *J Clin Oncol.* 2008;26:1987–1992.

60. Michiels S, Pugliano L, Marguet S, et al. Progression-free survival as surrogate endpoint for overall survival in clinical trials of HER2-targeted agents in HER2-positive metastatic breast cancer: an individual patient data assessment. *Ann Oncol.* 2016;27:1029–1034.

61. Laporte S, Squifflet P, Baroux N, et al. Prediction of survival benefits from progression-free survival benefits in advanced nonsmall cell lung cancer: evidence from a pooled analysis of 2,334 patients randomized in 5 trials. *Br Med J Open.* 2013;3:3.03.

62. Paoletti X, Oba K, Bang YJ, et al. Progression-free survival as a surrogate for overall survival in patients with advanced/recurrent gastric cancer: a meta-analysis. *J Natl Cancer Inst.* 2013;5:1608–1612.

63. Buyse M, Thirion P, Carlson RW, et al. Relation between tumour response to first-line chemotherapy and survival in advanced colorectal cancer: a meta-analysis. *Lancet.* 2008;356:373–378.

64. Buyse M, Vangeneugden T, Bijnens L, et al. Validation of biomarkers as surrogates for clinical endpoints. In Bloom JC, Dean RA, eds. *Biomarkers in Clinical Drug Development.* New York, NY: Marcel Dekker; 2003:149–168.

65. Buyse M, Michiels S, Squifflet P, et al. Leukemia-free survival as a surrogate endpoint for overall survival in the evaluation of maintenance therapy for patients with acute myeloid leukemia in complete remission. *Haematologica.* 2011; 69:1106–1112.

66. Burzykowski T, Döhner H, Döhner K, et al. Event-free survival is a surrogate for overall survival in patients treated for acute myeloid leukemia: analysis of individual data of 1,811 patients from four randomized trials. *Leukemia.* 2017.

67. Burzykowski T, Buyse, M. Surrogate threshold effect: an alternative measure for meta-analytic surrogate endpoint validation. *Pharmaceut Stat.* 2006;5:173–186.

68. Prasad V, Kim C, Burotto M, Vandross A. The strength of association between surrogate end points and survival in oncology. A systematic review of trial-level meta-analyses. *J Am Med Assoc Inter Med.* 2015;175:1389–1398.

69. Nisen P, Rockhold F. Access to patient-level data from GlaxoSmithKline clinical trials. *New Engl J Med.* 2013;369:475–478.

70. Strom BL, Buyse M, Hughes J, Koppers BM. Data sharing, year 1–Access to data from industry-sponsored clinical trials. *New Engl J Med.* 2014;371:2052–2054.

71. Alonso A, Molenberghs, G. Surrogate marker evaluation from an information theoretic perspective. *Biometrics.* 2007;63:180–186.

72. Alonso A, Van der Elst W, Molenberghs G, et al. An information-theoretic approach for the evaluation of surrogate endpoints based on causal inference. *Biometrics.* 2016;72(3):669–677. doi:10.1111/biom.12483

73. Frangakis CE, Rubin DB. Principal stratification in causal inference. *Biometrics.* 2004;58:21–29.

74. Li Y, Taylor JMG, Elliott MR. A Bayesian approach to surrogacy assessment using principal stratification in clinical trials. *Biometrics.* 2010;58:21–29.

75. Li Y, Taylor JMG, Elliott MR, Sargent DR. Causal assessment of surrogacy in a meta-analysis of colorectal clinical trials. *Biostatistics.* 201112:478–492.

76. Joffe MM, Greene T. Related causal frameworks for surrogate outcomes. *Biometrics.* 2008;64:1–10.

77. Alonso A, Van der Elst W, Molenberghs G, et al. On the relationship between the causal-inference and meta-analytic paradigms for the validation of surrogate endpoints. *Biometrics.* 2014;71:15–24.

35

Development and Validation of Genomic Signatures

Stefan Michiels, Nils Ternès, and Federico Rotolo

PROGNOSTIC GENE SIGNATURES

The treatment effect estimated in randomized controlled trials is an average effect in a given patient population. Nevertheless, the patients have different prognoses according to their characteristics—demographical, clinical, or pathological ones. In addition to the general features of the patients (e.g., their age and sex) and of their disease (e.g., the stage and size of their tumor), biological markers are studied as possible factors explaining different levels of risk or of response to treatment. Among the wide class of biological markers, genomic features are being increasingly investigated and discussed for their possible clinical interest. In addition to single biomarkers, genomic signatures derived from several biomarkers are expected to characterize more precisely the subgroups of patients in terms of prognosis. A molecular signature is not only a set of biomarkers, but is also characterized by the set of their weights, used to combine their respective contributions into a unique prognostic score.

Similarly to biomarkers, a genomic signature is called prognostic if it discriminates well between patients with a good or bad prognosis in the absence of treatment or in the context of a standard therapy. This means that the likely natural course of the disease can be forecasted thanks to the signature values (1), but that, whatever the risk group, the relative effect of treatment is similar. Conversely, a biomarker or signature is called predictive (of the treatment effect) if the relative treatment benefit varies according to signature values. This means that the magnitude and possibly the direction of the treatment effect is different according to signature values, or in other words, the gene signature is a treatment modifier. The most appropriate way to identify a predictive gene signature is through an interaction test between the signature and the treatment using data from a trial (2) in which the treatment has been randomly allocated to patients. Results from randomized controlled trials

are often difficult to translate into predictions for individual patients, but estimated absolute risk reductions from large randomized trials do still provide the best guidance (2).

According to the biomedical literature, genomic signatures are becoming increasingly important for anticipating the prognosis of individual patients (i.e., prognostic signature) or for predicting how individual patients will respond to specific treatments (i.e., predictive signature). Nevertheless, even though more than 150,000 papers document thousands of claimed biomarkers, fewer than 100 have been validated for routine clinical practice (3). Indeed, less than 20 prognostic or predictive biomarkers are recognized with variable levels of evidence in the 2014 European Society of Medical Oncology (ESMO) clinical practice guidelines for lung, breast, colon, and prostate cancer (4).

The Case of Early Breast Cancer

Although we discuss general concepts that apply to genomics data in a wide panel of clinical situations, we focus along this chapter on prognostic and predictive gene expression signatures in early breast cancer (EBC) to highlight the difficult path from the laboratory to the clinic.

In EBC, while several clinical prediction models exist based on clinical and pathological (CP) characteristics such as age, tumor size, nodal status, tumor grade, and estrogen receptor (ER), at least six different gene signatures are commercially available: Oncotype DX (5), MammaPrint (6), Genomic Grade Index (7), PAM50 (8), Breast Cancer Index (9), and EndoPredict (10). The concordance of predicted risk categories of the different gene signatures for individual patients is moderate (11,12), as illustrated by the recent OPTIMA study (13), which evaluated among others the two well-known tests MammaPrint (low vs. high) and Oncotype DX (≤25 vs. >25). This study, which compared these two tests head to head on 302 patients, found a low level of agreement, with a kappa value of 0.40 (95% confidence interval [CI]: 0.30–0.49). Of course, even when repeating the same assay twice on a single tumor sample, some inherent degree of inaccuracy would be expected, but unlikely to this extent. This has led to a pretty awkward situation where the treatment decision for adjuvant chemotherapy in EBC does not depend anymore on the clinician but on the genomic test ordered. Furthermore, according to a European consensus panel, none of these tests reached the highest level of evidence (14) and, according to an Evaluation of Genomic Applications in Practice and Prevention (EGAPP) panel, there was only indirect evidence that Oncotype DX could predict benefit from chemotherapy (15). In contrast, an American Society of Clinical Oncology (ASCO) panel in the United States gave a strong recommendation with high level of evidence that Oncotype DX may be used to guide decisions on adjuvant systemic chemotherapy for node-negative, ER-positive, HER2-negative breast cancer (16). This divergence may result from the degree of subjectivity in evidence evaluation or from a different vision of what type of evidence is needed for a gene signature to be clinically useful.

Development of Prognostic Gene Signatures

One of the very first challenges in the development of a gene signature is finding out how to compute a risk score based on the biomarkers measured, while the number of biomarkers keeps on increasing with technology advances. Identifying a meaningful prognostic model through high-dimensional regression raises particular issues from a statistical point of view. One of the main statistical problems due to high-dimensional data is the nonidentifiability of the models, which means that the biomarker weights cannot even be estimated if their number approaches or exceeds the number of observed events in the data. The problem of nonidentifiability can be dealt with by selecting the biomarkers with the highest impact on the clinical endpoint. Nevertheless, statistical procedures for feature selection can suffer from instability of the list of selected biomarkers (17) and have to deal with sparse model selection, multiple testing (18), or even correlation between biomarkers. Several penalized methods exist to perform variable selection in this high-dimensional space (19). An issue for penalized regression is the selection of tuning parameters, consisting in weighting the risk of false-positive selection against the risk of a low power for detecting highly discriminating biomarkers. Ad hoc procedures have been proposed to improve the biomarker selection of penalized regression techniques, while limiting the risk of false positives (20).

In the EBC example considered in this chapter, a well-known prognostic signature is the MammaPrint, a microarray-based signature developed by the Netherlands Cancer Institute. This 70-gene signature was developed retrospectively in a small sample ($n = 78$) of patients with EBC, with the goal of predicting the occurrence of distant metastases. In a larger sample of patients ($n = 295$) treated at the same institution, patients with a poor prognosis MammaPrint signature were confirmed to have a much higher risk of distant metastases within 5 years, when compared with patients with a good-prognosis signature (6).

Validation of Prognostic Gene Signatures and the Path to Clinical Utility

Once a candidate signature has been identified, it must satisfy several criteria of robustness and of practical utility to demonstrate its actual interest in clinical practice. The EGAPP initiative has proposed general definitions of analytical and clinical validity, and of clinical utility (21) to evaluate when developing a signature from bench to bedside. Table 35.1 (22) transposes the EGAPP criteria to the context of gene signatures.

Issues related to the assessment of the **analytical validity** of gene signatures are beyond the scope of this chapter. The assessment of the generalizability (**clinical validity**) of a gene signature needs external validation of its prognostic value in multiple independent series (23–25). The external validation of a signature relies on several criteria including those pertaining to discrimination, calibration, reclassification, and clinical usefulness (26). An independent validation study of the MammaPrint signature was conducted involving independent samples contributed by several European centers, with results confirming that the signature adds prognostic information over the risk classifier based on known CP factors (27). It has been estimated (23) that the sensitivity, or probability that a patient who will relapse is classified as high risk, of the MammaPrint signature at 5 years is high (in the Amsterdam series [A]: 0.93, in the validation series [V]: 0.90) but its 5-year specificity, or probability that a patient who will not relapse is classified as low risk, is poor (A: 0.53, V: 0.42). The negative predictive value of the signature for distant-metastasis-free survival 5 years after diagnosis was high (A: 0.90, V: 0.84), meaning that 8 out of 10 patients with good-prognosis signature are expected to actually be alive and free from metastasis at 5 years. However, the positive predictive value of the signature was modest (A: 0.63, V: 0.30), meaning that only 3 out of 10 patients with poor-prognosis signature do actually have metastasis or are dead at 5 years. Hence, the MammaPrint signature could not be claimed sufficiently accurate to predict which patients would develop metastases as a basis for treatment decision. In the United States, the development of the commonly used signature Oncotype DX followed similar steps (28). In the EBC context, the clinical utility of a prognostic signature can be defined as 'the likelihood that using a gene expression profiling test to guide management in patients with diagnosed EBC will significantly

TABLE 35.1 Evidence-Based Criteria for a Prognostic Gene Signature to Be Validated

No.	Concept	Elaboration
1	Development	Do signature levels differ substantially between patients with and without outcome?
2	Analytical validity	Signature's ability to accurately and reliably measure the genotype of interest between and within laboratories.
3	Clinical validity	Does the signature predict risk of outcome in multiple external cohorts or nested case–control/case–cohort studies?
4	Incremental value	Does the signature add enough information to established clinical and pathological prognostic markers or provide a more reproducible measurement of one of them?
5	Clinical impact	Does the signature change predicted risk sufficiently to change recommended therapy?
6	Clinical utility	Does use of the signature improve clinical outcome, especially when prospectively used for treatment decisions in a randomized controlled trial?
7	Cost-effectiveness	Does use of the signature improve clinical outcome sufficiently to justify the additional costs of testing and treatment?

improve health-related outcomes" (15). All in all, the clinical utility of gene signatures remains to be evaluated in prospective trials (14).

Comparison of the Signature With Established Clinical and Pathological Factors

A key issue in assessing the added value of a prognostic signature is to study whether it adds independent prognostic information to the risk determined by a CP model (**incremental value**). A gene signature could also be of interest if it provides a more reproducible, cheaper, or more accurate measurement of an already existing biomarker that has proven clinical utility so that the CP rule could be updated (24). Specific statistical challenges concerning how to account for CP factors since the signature development stage are debated in the literature (29,30).

The Onco*type* DX assay is very successful in the United States with an estimated target market penetration of 50% (31). Probably, one of the main reasons for its success is that it consists in a proliferation-based signature measured by a single reference laboratory and that it outperforms the histological tumor grading, which has been plagued by perceived suboptimal between-laboratory reproducibility (32).

To illustrate how to evaluate incremental prognostic value, we used publicly available microarray data of 845 patients (189 pathological complete responses [pCRs]) from eight clinical studies that included patients treated by anthracycline-based chemotherapy (33). We computed two gene signatures: an approximate version of the MammaPrint signature (called proliferation signature) and an immune-based gene signature (33). Because the gene signatures are often derived on different microarray platforms from different laboratories

and heterogeneous retrospective patient cohorts, we computed the scores as a weighted average of the genes and scaled each signature within study so that the 2.5% and 97.5% quantiles equaled –1 and +1, respectively (33,34). The added value of the two gene signatures was evaluated in logistic regression models after adjustment for CP factors (Table 35.2). When using the likelihood-ratio test at a 5% significance level relative to the model with CP factors only (35,36), both signatures do add statistically significant prognostic information to the CP model and they both add information to each other. We also evaluated the discrimination, that is, the ability to distinguish patients who had a pCR from those who did not, through the area under the receiver operating characteristic (ROC) curve (area under the curve [AUC]), for the CP model with and without the gene signatures. The AUC of the CP model was high (0.78; 95% CI: 0.75–0.82; Figure 35.1, Table 35.2), illustrating the strong discrimination of the CP factors. Adding both the signatures provided only a slight increase (0.80; 95% CI: 0.77–0.83). Therefore, the added discrimination of the gene signatures for pCR is moderate in this neoadjuvant example in EBC and the proof of concept is debatable. This is often the case in applications as only very strong and very independent prognostic factors can lead to large increases in predictive accuracy. For survival outcomes, there exist different generalizations of the AUC (37–39) and alternative measures are R^2-type statistics comparing the extra variation in clinical outcome explained by the signature (40). Of note, also the batch and laboratory effects play a role in the lack of applicability of many gene signatures in the clinic, for which a fully specified algorithm is needed for a single patient from a random batch or laboratory.

TABLE 35.2 Evaluation of the Incremental Prognostic Value of a Proliferation and Immune Gene Signature to a Standard Clinical and Pathological Model for Pathological Complete Response in 845 Early Breast Cancer Patients Treated With Neoadjuvant Anthracycline-Based Chemotherapy

Comparison between models	Likelihood-ratio statistic	*p* value	AUC (95% CI)
CP versus null model	151.4	$<10^{-16}$	0.78 (0.75–0.82)
CP + proliferation versus CP	9.40	2.2×10^{-3}	0.79 (0.75–0.82)
CP + immune versus CP	13.82	2.0×10^{-4}	0.79 (0.76–0.83)
CP + immune + proliferation versus CP	26.05	2.2×10^{-6}	0.80 (0.77–0.83)
CP + immune + proliferation versus CP + immune	12.22	4.7×10^{-4}	0.80 (0.77–0.83)
CP + immune + proliferation versus CP + proliferation	16.64	4.5×10^{-5}	0.80 (0.77–0.83)

Note: CP, clinical and pathological model for pathological complete response including: treatment (anthracyclines vs. anthracyclines plus taxanes), age (≤ 50 vs. >50 years), clinical tumor size (cT0, 1, 2 vs. cT3, 4), clinical nodal status (negative vs. positive), histologic grade (1, 2 vs. 3), estrogen receptor status (negative vs. positive), and HER2 status (negative vs. positive), and study effect using publicly available gene expression data of neoadjuvant studies (845 patients, 189 pathological complete responses) as described in (33). Proliferation gives the approximate version of the MammaPrint gene signature immune, which is immune1 signature from (33).

AUC, area under the receiver operating characteristic curve of the first model in the comparison of each line.

In another example of 883 women treated with either tamoxifen or letrozole monotherapy in the Breast International Group 1–98 trial, one of the cited proliferation signatures in EBC, the Genomic Grade Index, was more prognostic of the distant recurrence-free interval than the CP model alone, as measured by the likelihood-ratio test (41). Nevertheless, similar results were obtained with centrally reviewed continuous Ki67 by an expert pathologist, which highlights the importance of including all known prognostic factors in the CP model. Similarly to new treatments, which have to be compared head to head to the standard of care, new candidate signatures have to be contrasted to the best of the available prognostic models.

In addition to the discrimination, it is also of importance to evaluate the calibration of prediction models that include gene signatures, that is, the agreement between predicted risk and clinical outcome frequencies (42). To the best of our knowledge, very little is known about the calibration of the commercially available gene signatures in EBC.

A further criterion to be met by a gene signature in order to be fully validated is its potential **clinical impact**. Indeed, the incremental value as measured by likelihood-ratio tests or the AUC consists in an evaluation of the *statistical* significance of the added value of the signature. Similarly to treatments that are required to provide a *statistically* and *clinically* significant benefit, also new candidate gene signatures must change the predicted risk of a clinically relevant amount. Adding the gene signature to an established model will only be of interest if the predicted risk of such patients changes sufficiently compared with the standard CP model to have consequences in terms of treatment decisions. Figure 35.2 shows that the use of the immune and proliferation signatures does not improve the pCR probability prediction in the EBC example discussed earlier. Useful summary measures and graphical displays to evaluate the subtle changes in prediction scores of patients can be found elsewhere (42–44).

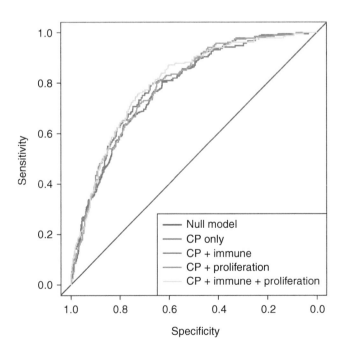

FIGURE 35.1 Receiver operating characteristics curves when adding a proliferation and immune gene signature to CP model for pathological complete response in 845 early breast cancer patients treated with neoadjuvant anthracycline-based chemotherapy.

CP, clinical and pathological.

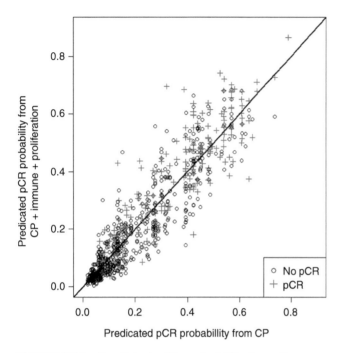

FIGURE 35.2 Predicted pCR probability from the CP model versus predicted pCR probability from the model including CP variables and the immune and proliferation signatures in 845 early breast cancer patients treated with neoadjuvant anthracycline-based chemotherapy.

CP, clinical and pathological; pCR, pathological complete response.

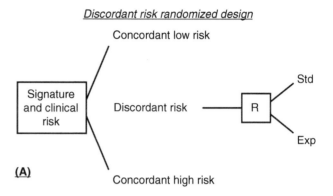

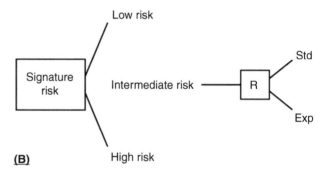

FIGURE 35.3 Clinical trial designs to evaluate the clinical utility of prognostic signatures. (A) Randomized design for discordant risk and (B) randomized design for intermediate risk (50).

Exp, experimental treatment; R, randomization; Std, standard treatment.

Clinical Trial Designs for Prognostic Signatures

As mentioned earlier, the ideal way to assess the readiness of genomics-based tests for guiding patient care is to validate it in an independent randomized clinical trial. The checklist developed by the U.S. National Cancer Institute (45) covers a broad range of issues related to the use of gene signatures in clinical trials. The issues related to the clinical trial design can be summarized as follows: clearly define the target population and the intended use of the signature; ensure that the expected benefit is clinically useful; determine whether the signature remains valid on stored specimens; establish to what extent the signature can be used in future trials for treatment decisions and to what extent randomization is required; include in the protocol full details on the validation of the signature; include the names of the people responsible for each aspect of the trial; establish a database with proper blinding between clinical and genomic data.

In practice, trial designs evaluating the clinical impact of patients being offered a prognostic gene signature are rather similar to available trial designs for diagnostic tests (46–49). The operating characteristics of some of the trial designs integrating gene signatures in breast cancer have been discussed previously (50). An example of the so-called discordant-risk randomized design (Figure 35.3A) is provided by the MINDACT study

(51,52), a randomized trial for women with EBC carried out in Europe under the auspices of the European Organization for Research and Treatment of Cancer. In this trial 1,550 out of 6,693 screened women (23.2%) were part of the discordant-risk population—based on a CP model and the gene signature—and were randomized between chemotherapy and control to evaluate the capacity of the MammaPrint signature to identify patients in whom chemotherapy can be avoided when the CP model says otherwise. The primary goal was to assess whether, among patients with high CP risk and a low signature risk in the control arm, the 5-year distant-metastasis-free survival rate was noninferior to 92%. At the end of the trial, 748 of the 1,550 patients (11.2% of the total) had been randomized to the control arm. In this primary-analysis subgroup, the 5-year distant-metastasis-free survival rate was 94.7% (95% CI: 92.5–96.2) (52). As this endpoint was not based on the randomization, a prospective cohort study would have been sufficient to answer this question. It has been shown that if the two prediction models (CP model and gene signature) disagree in 32% of the patients, and if the treatment reduces 10-year mortality in the overall population from 24% to 20%, then the absolute difference in mortality between the two strategies would be only 0.5%, and 50,000 patients would be necessary to identify this mortality difference in a statistically satisfactory manner (53). Note that this randomization in the discordant-risk population is exactly equivalent to randomizing patients between a group receiving chemotherapy or not based on CP characteristics, and a group receiving chemotherapy or not based on the signature. As such, the discordant-risk randomized design provides a head-to-head comparison between two decision-making strategies, one based on the CP model and one based on the signature.

A second type of design to evaluate the clinical utility of a prognostic signature is the so-called intermediate-signature-risk randomized design (Figure 35.3B). An example of a trial based on such a design is the TAILORx trial (54), carried out under the auspices of the U.S. National Cancer Institute in a similiar population as the MINDACT trial. In the TAILORx trial, women with intermediate Onco*type* DX risk score were randomized between adjuvant chemotherapy and not, and the primary objective is to evaluate the noninferiority of the control arm compared with the chemotherapy arm. It may seem peculiar to set up a noninferiority trial of standard chemotherapy of which the relative efficacy is already well known. Recently, the data and safety monitoring committee of the TAILORx trial recommended that the results of the unrandomized low-risk group defined by Onco*type* DX be released (55). After a median follow-up of 6.7 years, the estimated 5-year invasive disease-free survival was 93.8% (95% CI: 92.4–94.9) in this low-risk group. The question remains whether such a subgroup of patients could not have been identified with a solid CP model.

Independent of the specific design, the advantage of randomized trials including prospective collection of tumor samples and clinical outcomes from several thousands of patients selected and treated according to a well-defined protocol is that they allow the establishment of large bases of consistently measured data. The big hope behind these trials is that secondary analyses would reveal variation in relative efficacy according to fine-tuned modeling of CP factors and the gene signatures that were missed in prior analyses of historical trials by categorized CP risk groups. On the other hand, one could argue that, if the biological signal was really strong, even a less reliable measurement method (e.g., of ER and Ki67) with a different categorization would already have shown some variation. This may be a matter of subjective debate. In both the trials discussed earlier, since the annual rate of distant relapse or deaths is quite low in EBCs, a very long follow-up is required to answer the clinical questions (50). These examples illustrate that, in the context of a relatively good-prognosis population and a small absolute treatment benefit (of chemotherapy), developing a randomized controlled trial to demonstrate the clinical utility of a prognostic gene signature is quite challenging and that a cohort study may in several occasions be a more appropriate tool to develop and validate a fine-tuned prognostic CP plus gene signature model.

Cost-Effectiveness

The very last aspect in studying a gene signature is its cost-effectiveness: despite being more prognostic than the CP model alone, a signature could be of limited usefulness if its cost is too high. For illustration, in the population of node-negative breast cancer patients, the MammaPrint signature was deemed unlikely to be cost-effective from the French National Insurance perspective (56).

For EGAPP, the cost-effectiveness evaluation is only seen as a contextual factor (21), while for the National Institute for Health and Care Excellence in the United Kingdom, cost-effectiveness is one of the three main criteria—the two others being test accuracy and clinical effectiveness—on which the value of diagnostic technologies is based. Specific evidence requirements need to be defined for policy makers and reimbursement agencies to introduce gene signatures into clinical practice from a health economical perspective (4).

PREDICTIVE GENE SIGNATURES AS TREATMENT-EFFECT MODIFIERS

Treating broad populations of patients with large inclusion criteria in clinical trials relies on the assumption that treatment-by-subset interactions are unlikely on mortality endpoints (57). Nevertheless, increasing knowledge of biology suggests that such interactions are more likely than previously thought (58), with ER, HER2, KRAS, and EGFR mutations as well-known examples in cancer. Furthermore, ignoring strong treatment-by-biomarker interactions can substantially reduce the statistical power of trials aimed at showing the overall benefit of new treatments (59). Recently, some gene signatures have been proposed to predict a higher benefit of treatments, such as 8-gene and 14-gene signatures for trastuzumab benefit in EBC (60,61). The results of these studies are likely overoptimistic, since the former did not retest all the genes in each fold of the cross-validation (62) and the latter used data from another platform on a subset of the samples to prefilter the genes. Before outlying the approach to develop gene signatures that interact with relative treatment benefit, we discuss the possible predictive role of the prognostic signatures in EBC.

Can any of These Prognostic Signatures in Early Breast Cancer Also Predict the Magnitude of Treatment Effect?

None of the gene signatures in EBC discussed so far was developed for predicting the relative magnitude of a treatment effect: they were fitted only for prognosis purposes. Nevertheless, a study has claimed that the Oncotype DX signature predicts the magnitude of chemotherapy benefit (63), when including in a subtle manner the patients from the development series (23). The only truly independent evaluation of Oncotype DX was performed in a subset of 367 patients included in the S8814 trial for node-positive, ER-positive postmenopausal breast cancer women, in which the gene signature was tested for interaction with additional chemotherapy prior to tamoxifen (64). This study showed a significant treatment-by-signature interaction in the first 5 years after inclusion ($p = .03$). Nevertheless, when also including ER expression, the interaction was no longer statistically significant ($p = .15$), which suggests a possible confounding between the signature and ER expression. Furthermore, it is unclear whether the separate analysis before and after 5 years was preplanned. Finally, the small number of events in signature-defined subgroups makes treatment-effect estimates hardly reliable. The ongoing prospective randomized trial RxPonder tries to replicate this interaction, under the bold assumption of a qualitative interaction on invasive disease-free survival (65). To date, none of the prognostic signatures in EBC has been shown to be a sound predictor of the treatment effect.

Development of Predictive Gene Signatures

Testing multiple baseline biomarkers for a possible interaction with treatment effect is increasingly common in randomized controlled phase III trials. If the predictive signature is known beforehand, alternative procedures exist to test the effect of the treatment both in the overall trial population as well as in the signature-positive (or

-negative) subgroup of patients (50,66). Global interaction tests allow controlling the familywise type I error of a predictive set of biomarkers in a randomized controlled trial (34,67–69), by measuring the degree of differential treatment effect according to biomarker values, before developing any signature. To evaluate the statistical significance of global interaction signal, a permutation procedure is available (Figure 35.4), based on the idea that if the biomarkers are not predictive, they are exchangeable between patients in the same arm (34,67). In case of a significant interaction signal, a large number of events is needed to estimate the treatment-effect difference between signature-defined subgroups in order to determine its clinical importance.

There exist several strategies to identify and validate a signature in a randomized trial using cross-validation techniques to overcome a potential overfitting issue (50,70–72). The general scheme of cross-validation in this context can be depicted as follows: (a) the data are divided into K groups and, for each, the data from the remaining $K - 1$ groups are used to develop the predictive signature; (b) the data in the excluded group are used to evaluate the signature for left-out patients; (c) the entire procedure is iterated over the K folds to evaluate the capacity of the signature to predict the magnitude of treatment effect (Figure 35.5). The application of the gene signature building process to the full data set provides the signature to use for future patients (73). An application of this analysis strategy on trials of adjuvant anthracycline-based chemotherapy in EBC patients can be found in (34). Developing a gene signature requires selecting the biomarkers that are the most predictive and combining them efficiently in the

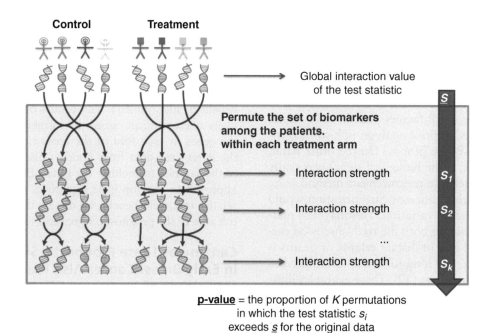

FIGURE 35.4 Permutation scheme for computing the p value of a global interaction test to evaluate the ability of a gene signature to be associated with the magnitude of treatment benefit.

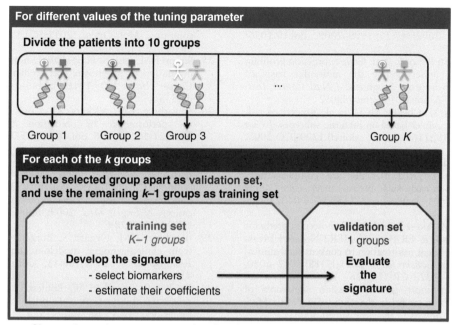

FIGURE 35.5 *K*-fold cross-validation process to develop a signature and to limit overfitting in the evaluation of the magnitude of treatment benefit according to gene signature values, when only one single randomized controlled clinical trial is available.

regression model. Those tasks get increasingly complex as the number of biomarkers at hand increases and recent statistical developments aim to extend existing selection methods to a higher dimensional setting (74). One of the major matters in this context is achieving the right balance between type I error and power. Once a predictive signature has been successfully identified in a phase III trial, its performances will need to be evaluated in a truly independent trial.

CONCLUSIONS

In this chapter, we have discussed the challenges that are met in developing a gene signature until its validation for routine clinical use, for which sound and clear evidence-based requirements are needed (4). Clinical trial designs originally proposed for diagnostic tests can be adopted for trials with prognostic gene signatures. Sometimes the prognostic and predictive roles of gene signatures are mixed up in the literature, with signature having a proved prognostic ability being used for therapeutic decision making. We stress the importance that predictive gene signatures should be specifically developed as treatment-effect modifiers and should be validated prospectively on randomized controlled trial data. We have previously proposed an approach consisting of first applying a global test that can give a green light to develop a treatment-modifying gene signature on the

trial data. We recommend a cross-validation scheme to estimate treatment effects within signature-defined subgroups. More research is ongoing on approaches to develop and validate gene signatures in randomized controlled trials. In the era of data sharing of clinical trials, a larger role for meta-analyses of individual patient data can be expected in this context. Last but not least, in clinical trials of gene signatures some of the strongest logistical challenges are to control confounding that can arise through the handling of the specimens, batch effects within and between laboratories, measurement error, and tumor heterogeneity.

REFERENCES

1. Buyse M, Michiels S, Sargent DJ, et al. Integrating biomarkers in clinical trials. *Expert Rev Mol Diagn.* 2011;11(2):171–182. doi:10.1586/erm.10.120
2. Rothwell PM. Subgroup analysis in randomised controlled trials: importance, indications, and interpretation. *Lancet.* 2005;365(9454):176–186. doi:10.1016/S0140-6736(05)17709-5
3. Poste G. Bring on the biomarkers. *Nature.* 2011;469(7329): 156–157. doi:10.1038/469156a
4. Schneider D, Bianchini G, Horgan D, et al. Establishing the evidence bar for molecular diagnostics in personalised cancer care. *Pub Health Genom.* 2015;18(6):349–358. doi:10.1159/000441556
5. Paik S, Shak S, Tang G, et al. A multigene assay to predict recurrence of tamoxifen-treated, node-negative breast cancer. *N Engl J Med.* 2004;351(27):2817–2826. doi:10.1056/NEJMoa041588

6. van de Vijver MJ, He YD, van't Veer LJ, et al. A Gene-Expression Signature as a Predictor of Survival in Breast Cancer. *N Engl J Med*. 2002;347(25):1999–2009. doi:10.1056/NEJMoa021967

7. Sotiriou C, Wirapati P, Loi S, et al. Gene expression profiling in breast cancer: understanding the molecular basis of histologic grade to improve prognosis. *J Natl Cancer Inst*. 2006;98(4):262–272. doi:10.1093/jnci/djj052

8. Parker JS, Mullins M, Cheang MCU, et al. Supervised risk predictor of breast cancer based on intrinsic subtypes. *J Clin Oncol*. 2009;27(8):1160–1167. doi:10.1200/JCO.2008.18.1370

9. Ma X-J, Salunga R, Dahiya S, et al. A five-gene molecular grade index and HOXB13:IL17BR are complementary prognostic factors in early stage breast cancer. *Clin Cancer Res*. 2008;14(9):2601–2608. doi:10.1158/1078-0432.CCR-07-5026

10. Filipits M, Rudas M, Jakesz R, et al. A new molecular predictor of distant recurrence in ER-Positive, HER2-Negative breast cancer adds independent information to conventional clinical risk factors. *Clin Cancer Res*. 2011;17(18):6012–6020. doi:10.1158/1078-0432.CCR-11-0926

11. Koscielny S. Why most gene expression signatures of tumors have not been useful in the clinic. *Sci Transl Med*. 2010;2(14):14ps2. doi:10.1126/scitranslmed.3000313

12. Dowsett M, Sestak I, Lopez-Knowles E, et al. Comparison of PAM50 risk of recurrence score with oncotype DX and IHC4 for predicting risk of distant recurrence after endocrine therapy. *J Clin Oncol*. 2013;31(22):2783–2790. doi:10.1200/JCO.2012.46.1558

13. Bartlett JMS, Bayani J, Marshall A, et al. Comparing breast cancer multiparameter tests in the OPTIMA prelim trial: no test is more equal than the others. *J Natl Cancer Inst*. 2016;108(9). doi:10.1093/jnci/djw050

14. Azim JA, Michiels S, Zagouri F, et al. Utility of prognostic genomic tests in breast cancer practice: The IMPAKT 2012 working group consensus statement. *Ann Oncol*. 2013;24(3):647–54. doi:10.1093/annonc/mds645

15. Evaluation of Genomic Applications in Practice and Prevention (EGAPP) Working Group. Recommendations from the EGAPP Working Group: does the use of Oncotype DX tumor gene expression profiling to guide treatment decisions improve outcomes in patients with breast cancer? *Genet Med*. 2016;18(8):770–779. doi:10.1038/gim.2015.173

16. Harris LN, Ismaila N, McShane LM, et al. Use of biomarkers to guide decisions on adjuvant systemic therapy for women with early-stage invasive breast cancer: American Society of Clinical Oncology Clinical Practice Guideline. *J Clin Oncol*. 2016;34(10):1134–1150. doi:10.1200/JCO.2015.65.2289

17. Michiels S, Koscielny S, Hill C. Prediction of cancer outcome with microarrays: a multiple random validation strategy. *Lancet*. 2005;365(9458):488–492. doi:10.1016/S0140-6736(05)17866-0

18. Goeman JJ., Solari A. Multiple hypothesis testing in genomics. *Stat Med*. 2014;33(11):1946–1978. doi:10.1002/sim.6082

19. Ternès N, Arnedos M, Koscielny S, et al. Statistical methods applied to omics data. *Curr Opin Oncol*. 2014;26(6):576–583. doi:10.1097/CCO.0000000000000134

20. Ternès N, Rotolo F, Michiels S. Empirical extensions of the lasso penalty to reduce the false discovery rate in high-dimensional Cox regression models. *Stat Med*. 2016;35(15):2561–2573. doi:10.1002/sim.6927

21. Teutsch SM, Bradley LA, Palomaki GE, et al. The Evaluation of Genomic Applications in Practice and Prevention (EGAPP) initiative: methods of the EGAPP Working Group. *Genet Med*. 2009;11(1):3–14. doi:10.1097/GIM.0b013e318184137c

22. Michiels S, Ternès N, Rotolo F. Statistical controversies in clinical research: prognostic gene signatures are not (yet) useful in clinical practice. *Ann Oncol*. 2016:mdw307. doi:10.1093/annonc/mdw307

23. Michiels S, Koscielny S, Hill C. Interpretation of microarray data in cancer. *Br J Cancer*. 2007;96(8):1155–1158. doi:10.1038/sj.bjc.6603673

24. Michiels S, Kramar A, Koscielny S. Multidimensionality of microarrays: statistical challenges and (im)possible solutions. *Mol Oncol*. 2011;5(2):190–196. doi:10.1016/j.molonc.2011.01.002

25. Simon RM, Paik S, Hayes DF. Use of archived specimens in evaluation of prognostic and predictive biomarkers. *J Natl Cancer Inst*. 2009;101(21):1446–1452. doi:10.1093/jnci/djp335

26. Steyerberg EW, Vickers AJ, Cook NR, et al. Assessing the performance of prediction models. *Epidemiology*. 2010;21(1):128–138. doi:10.1097/EDE.0b013e3181c30fb2

27. Buyse M, Loi S, van't Veer L, et al. Validation and clinical utility of a 70-Gene prognostic signature for women with node-negative breast cancer. *J Natl Cancer Inst*. 2006;98(17):1183–1192. doi:10.1093/jnci/djj329

28. Sotiriou C, Pusztai L. Gene-expression signatures in breast cancer. *N Engl J Med*. 2009;360(8):790–800. doi:10.1056/NEJMra0801289

29. Bøvelstad HM, Nygård S, Borgan O. Survival prediction from clinico-genomic models–a comparative study. *BMC Bioinformatics*. 2009;10:413. doi:10.1186/1471-2105-10-413

30. De Bin R, Sauerbrei W, Boulesteix A-L. Investigating the prediction ability of survival models based on both clinical and omics data: two case studies. *Stat Med*. 2014;33(30):5310–5329. doi:10.1002/sim.6246

31. Miller I, Ashton-Chess J, Spolders H, et al. Market access challenges in the EU for high medical value diagnostic tests. *Per Med*. 2011;8(2):137–148. doi:10.2217/pme.11.2

32. Rakha EA, Reis-Filho JS, Baehner F, et al. Breast cancer prognostic classification in the molecular era: the role of histological grade. *Breast Cancer Res*. 2010;12(4):207. doi:10.1186/bcr2607

33. Ignatiadis M, Singhal SK, Desmedt C, et al. Gene modules and response to neoadjuvant chemotherapy in breast cancer subtypes: a pooled analysis. *J Clin Oncol*. 2012;30(16):1996–2004. doi:10.1200/JCO.2011.39.5624

34. Michiels S, Rotolo F. Evaluation of clinical utility and validation of gene signatures in clinical trials. In: Matsui S, Buyse M, Simon R, eds. *Design and Analysis of Clinical Trials for Predictive Medicine*. CRC press; 2015: 396.

35. Vickers AJ, Cronin AM, Begg CB. One statistical test is sufficient for assessing new predictive markers. *BMC Med Res Methodol*. 2011;11(1):13. doi:10.1186/1471-2288-11-13

36. Pepe MS, Kerr KF, Longton G, Wang Z. Testing for improvement in prediction model performance. *Stat Med*. 2013;32(9):1467–1482. doi:10.1002/sim.5727

37. Pencina MJ, D'Agostino RB, Song L. Quantifying discrimination of Framingham risk functions with different survival C statistics. *Stat Med*. 2012;31(15):1543–1553. doi:10.1002/sim.4508

38. Heagerty PJ, Lumley T, Pepe MS. Time-dependent ROC curves for censored survival data and a diagnostic marker. *Biometrics*. 2000;56(2):337–344. doi:10.1111/j.0006-341X.2000.00337.x

39. Uno H, Cai T, Pencina MJ, et al. On the C-statistics for evaluating overall adequacy of risk prediction procedures with censored survival data. *Stat Med*. 2011;30(10):1105–1117. doi:10.1002/sim.4154

40. Dunkler D, Michiels S, Schemper M. Gene expression profiling: does it add predictive accuracy to clinical characteristics in cancer prognosis? *Eur J Cancer*. 2007;43(4):745–751. doi:10.1016/j.ejca.2006.11.018

41. Ignatiadis M, Azim HA, Desmedt C, et al. The genomic grade assay compared with Ki67 to determine risk of distant breast cancer recurrence. *JAMA Oncol*. 2016;2(2):217. doi:10.1001/jamaoncol.2015.4377

42. McGeechan K, Macaskill P, Irwig L, et al. Assessing new biomarkers and predictive models for use in clinical practice. *Arch Intern Med*. 2008;168(21):2304. doi:10.1001/archinte.168.21.2304

43. Steyerberg EW, Pencina MJ, Lingsma HF, et al. Assessing the incremental value of diagnostic and prognostic markers: a

review and illustration. *Eur J Clin Invest*. 2012;42(2):216–28. doi:10.1111/j.1365-2362.2011.02562.x

44. Steyerberg EW, Vedder MM, Leening MJG, et al. Graphical assessment of incremental value of novel markers in prediction models: from statistical to decision analytical perspectives. *Biometrical J*. 2015;57(4):556–570. doi:10.1002/bimj.201300260

45. McShane LM, Cavenagh MM, Lively TG, et al. Criteria for the use of omics-based predictors in clinical trials: explanation and elaboration. *BMC Med*. 2013;11(1):220. doi:10.1186/1741-7015-11-220

46. Bossuyt PM, Lijmer JG, Mol BW. Randomised comparisons of medical tests: sometimes invalid, not always efficient. *Lancet*. 2000;356(9244):1844–1847. doi:10.1016/S0140-6736(00)03246-3

47. de Graaff JC, Ubbink DT, Tijssen JGP, Legemate DA. The diagnostic randomized clinical trial is the best solution for management issues in critical limb ischemia. *J Clin Epidemiol*. 2004;57(11):1111–1118. doi:10.1016/j.jclinepi.2004.02.020

48. Lu B, Gatsonis C. Efficiency of study designs in diagnostic randomized clinical trials. *Stat Med*. 2013;32(9):1451–1466. doi:10.1002/sim.5655

49. Rodger M, Ramsay T, Fergusson D. Diagnostic randomized controlled trials: the final frontier. *Trials*. 2012;13(1):137. doi:10.1186/1745-6215-13-137

50. Buyse M, Michiels S. Omics-based clinical trial designs. *Curr Opin Oncol*. 2013:289–295. doi:10.1097/CCO.0b013e32835ff2fe

51. Bogaerts J, Cardoso F, Buyse M, et al. Gene signature evaluation as a prognostic tool: challenges in the design of the MINDACT trial. *Nat Clin Pract Oncol*. 2006;3(10):540–551. doi:10.1038/ncponc0591

52. Cardoso F, van't Veer LJ, Bogaerts J, et al. 70-Gene signature as an aid to treatment decisions in early-stage breast cancer. *N Engl J Med*. 2016;375(8):717–729. doi:10.1056/NEJMoa1602253

53. Hooper R, Díaz-Ordaz K, Takeda A, Khan K. Comparing diagnostic tests: trials in people with discordant test results. *Stat Med*. 2013;32(14):2443–2456. doi:10.1002/sim.5676

54. Sparano JA. TAILORx: Trial assigning individualized options for treatment (Rx). *Clin Breast Can*. 2006;7(4):347–50. doi:10.3816/CBC.2006.n.051

55. Sparano JA, Gray RJ, Makower DF, et al. Prospective validation of a 21-gene expression assay in breast cancer. *N Engl J Med*. 2015;373(21):2005–2014. doi:10.1056/NEJMoa1510764

56. Bonastre J, Marguet S, Lueza B, Michiels S, Delaloge S, Saghatchian M. Cost effectiveness of molecular profiling for adjuvant decision making in patients with node-negative breast cancer. *J Clin Oncol*. 2014;32(31):3513–3519. doi:10.1200/JCO.2013.54.9931

57. Yusuf S, Collins R, Peto R. Why do we need some large, simple randomized trials? *Stat Med*. 1984;3(4):409–420. doi:10.1002/sim.4780030421

58. Simon R. New challenges for 21st century clinical trials. *Clin Trials*. 2007;4(2):167–169. doi:10.1177/1740774507076800

59. Betensky RA, Louis DN, Cairncross JG. Influence of unrecognized molecular heterogeneity on randomized clinical trials. *J Clin Oncol*. 2002;20(10):2495–2499.

60. Pogue-Geile KL, Kim C, Jeong J-H, et al. Predicting degree of benefit from adjuvant trastuzumab in NSABP Trial B-31. *J Natl Cancer Inst*. 2013;105(23):1782–1788. doi:10.1093/jnci/djt321

61. Perez EA, Thompson EA, Ballman KV, et al. Genomic analysis reveals that immune function genes are strongly linked to clinical outcome in the North Central Cancer Treatment Group N9831 Adjuvant Trastuzumab Trial. *J Clin Oncol*. 2015;33(7):701–708. doi:10.1200/JCO.2014.57.6298

62. Dupuy A, Simon RM. Critical review of published microarray studies for cancer outcome and guidelines on statistical analysis and reporting. *J Natl Cancer Inst*. 2007;99(2):147–157. doi:10.1093/jnci/djk018

63. Paik S, Tang G, Shak S, et al. Gene expression and benefit of chemotherapy in women with node-negative, estrogen receptor-positive breast cancer. *J Clin Oncol*. 2006;24(23):3726–3734. doi:10.1200/JCO.2005.04.7985

64. Albain KS, Barlow WE, Shak S, et al. Prognostic and predictive value of the 21-gene recurrence score assay in postmenopausal women with node-positive, oestrogen-receptor-positive breast cancer on chemotherapy: a retrospective analysis of a randomised trial. *Lancet Oncol*. 2010;11(1):55–65. doi:10.1016/S1470-2045(09)70314-6

65. Barlow W. Design of a clinical trial for testing the ability of a continuous marker to predict therapy benefit. In: Crowley J, ed. *Handbook of Statistics in Clinical Oncology*. 3rd ed. CRC Press; 2012: 293–304.

66. Freidlin B, Korn EL. Biomarker enrichment strategies: matching trial design to biomarker credentials. *Nat Rev Clin Oncol*. 2013;11(2):81–90. doi:10.1038/nrclinonc.2013.218

67. Michiels S, Potthoff RF, George SL. Multiple testing of treatment-effect-modifying biomarkers in a randomized clinical trial with a survival endpoint. *Stat Med*. 2011;30(13):1502–1518. doi:10.1002/sim.4022

68. Wang R, Schoenfeld DA, Hoeppner B, Evins AE. Detecting treatment-covariate interactions using permutation methods. *Stat Med*. 2015;34(12):2035–2047. doi:10.1002/sim.6457

69. Callegaro A, Spiessens B, Dizier B, et al. Testing interaction between treatment and high-dimensional covariates in randomized clinical trials. *Biometrical J*. 2016. doi:10.1002/bimj.201500194

70. Matsui S, Simon R, Qu P, et al. Developing and validating continuous genomic signatures in randomized clinical trials for predictive medicine. *Clin Cancer Res*. 2012;18(21):6065–6073. doi:10.1158/1078-0432.CCR-12-1206

71. Polley M-YC, Polley EC, Huang EP, et al. Two-stage adaptive cutoff design for building and validating a prognostic biomarker signature. *Stat Med*. 2014;33(29):5097–5110. doi:10.1002/sim.6310

72. Freidlin B, Jiang W, Simon R. The cross-validated adaptive signature design. *Clin Cancer Res*. 2010;16(2):691–698. doi:10.1158/1078-0432.CCR-09-1357

73. Simon R. Clinical trials for predictive medicine. *Stat Med*. 2012;31(25):3031–3040. doi:10.1002/sim.5401

74. Ternès N, Rotolo F, Heinze G, Michiels S. Identification of biomarker-by-treatment interactions in randomized clinical trials with survival outcomes and high-dimensional spaces. *Biometrical J*. 2017. doi:10.1002/bimj.201500234

Competing Risks Analysis in Clinical Trials

Solange Bassale, Jeong Youn Lim, and Motomi Mori

INTRODUCTION

Survival analysis deals with the analysis of time to a certain event of interest (e.g., death), where the event of interest can only happen at most once to any subject. Such data are often censored; that is, the data are incomplete because we cannot follow all subjects until the event is observed. Common events of interest in oncology clinical trials include all-cause death, cancer-specific death, disease progression, local recurrence, distant metastasis, and relapse. In addition to censoring, time-to-event data are often highly skewed due to some subjects being followed for a long time with or without the event. Therefore, special statistical analysis methods, referred to as survival analysis methods, were developed to account for unique features of time to event data including censoring and non-normality.

Most common survival analysis methods are (a) the Kaplan-Meier method (1) to estimate a survival curve, (b) the log-rank test (2) to compare two survival curves, and (c) the Cox proportional hazards regression model (3) to evaluate the effects of covariates (subject characteristics or treatment assignment) on the event of interest. The Kaplan-Meier method and the log-rank test are nonparametric in that no assumptions are made with respect to the distribution of time-to-event data. In contrast, the Cox proportional hazards model is considered semiparametric because, although no assumption is made with respect to the baseline hazard (background event rate), the effect of covariates is assumed to follow a relative risk function, $\exp(\beta_1 x_1 + \beta_2 x_2 + \cdots + \beta_p x_p)$, where β represents the regression coefficients and x the covariate values (e.g., stage, age, and gender).

In a classical survival analysis, subjects are at risk for one event such as death. However, it is common for researchers to be interested in multiple types of events, such as different causes of death (e.g., cancer vs. non-cancer death). Gooley (4) defines a competing risk as "an event whose occurrence either precludes the occurrence of another event under examination or fundamentally alters the probability of occurrence of this other event." For instance, in a breast cancer trial, the primary endpoint may be breast cancer-specific mortality. In that case, death due to other causes is considered a competing risk, because death from other causes (e.g., cardiovascular disease) precludes the occurrence of death from breast cancer. Local recurrence and distant metastasis are also competing risks in that the incidence of one event may affect the other; thus, the two events are not independent. In the presence of competing risks, common survival analysis methods are inadequate and may lead to incorrect conclusions. In this chapter, we provide an overview of survival analysis methods developed to account for competing risks, illustrate the methods using simple and real data examples, and conclude with the practical analysis recommendations.

COMPETING RISKS IN ONCOLOGY CLINICAL TRIALS

Several common primary and secondary endpoints in oncology clinical trials involve competing risks (Table 36.1). In addition to the endpoints listed as follows, there are a number of disease-site–specific endpoints, such as biochemical recurrence in prostate cancer (defined in terms of prostatic-specific antigen values) and cytogenetic relapse in leukemia (defined in terms of abnormal cytogenetic findings) where death is considered a competing risk. Some endpoints may have multiple competing risks, such as time to the first infection in patients receiving a stem cell transplant. Potential competing risks include graft rejection, acute graft-versus-host disease, relapse, and death.

STATISTICAL METHODS FOR COMPETING RISKS

Basic Concepts and Notations

One of the key concepts in survival analysis is a hazard function defined as the instantaneous rate of failure at

TABLE 36.1 Examples of Typical Time-To-Event Endpoints in Oncology Clinical Trials

Endpoint	Definition	Event of Interest	Potential Competing Risks
Overall survival	Time from a study entry to death due to any causes	Death	None
Progression-free survival	Time from a study entry to disease progression or death	Disease progression or death	None
Time to progression	Time from a study entry to objective tumor progression	Objective tumor progression	Death
Time to treatment failure	Time from a study entry to discontinuation of treatment	Discontinuation of treatment for any reason	Death
Event-free survival	Time from a study entry to disease progression, death, or discontinuation of treatment	Disease progression, death, or discontinuation of treatment	None
Cause-specific mortality	Time from a study entry to death due to a specific cause	Death due to a specific cause	Death due to other causes
Time to relapse	Time from a study entry to relapse	Relapse	Death
Time to metastasis	Time from a study entry to metastasis	Metastasis	Death

time t (e.g., mortality rate at time t). A hazard function is denoted by $\lambda(t)$. When there are k types of failures, this concept can be extended to k cause-specific hazard functions, whose sum equals to the overall hazard:

$$\lambda(t) = \sum_{j=1}^{k} \lambda_j(t)$$

The overall survival function is given by:

$$S(t) = P(T > t) = exp\left[-\int_0^t \lambda(u)\,du\right]$$

The subdensity function for the time to a type j failure is:

$$f_j(t) = \lambda_j(t)S(t)$$

The density function of the time to failure is:

$$f(t) = \sum_{j=1}^{k} f_j(t)$$

Note that the subdensity function is a function not only of the cause specific hazard but also the overall survival that involves competing events.

To facilitate the presentation of competing risks analysis methods, we will use a simple numerical example (Table 36.2) of 10 subjects with two events: death

due to cancer and death due to noncancer. The following notations are used in this section:

- $S(t)$ represents the overall survival probability, and $1 - S(t)$ represents the probability of death due to any cause (cancer and noncancer).
- KM represents the Kaplan-Meier estimate of overall survival. $1 - KM$ represents the probability of death due to any cause.
- CI_c and CI_{nc} represent the cumulative incidence estimate of the probability of death due to cancer or noncancer, respectively.
- KM_c represents the Kaplan-Meier estimate of cancer-free survival obtained by censoring loss to follow-up and noncancer death (competing risk), and KM_{nc} represents the Kaplan-Meier estimate of noncancer-free survival obtained by censoring loss to follow-up and cancer death. Therefore, $1 - KM_c$ and $1 - KM_{nc}$ represent Kaplan-Meier estimates of cancer death and noncancer death, respectively.
- $\lambda(t)$ represents a hazard function of death due to any cause.
- $\lambda_c(t)$ represents a hazard function of cancer death, and $\lambda_{nc}(t)$ represents a hazard function of noncancer death. They are referred to as a cause-specific hazard.

Cumulative Incidence Function

Kalbfleisch and Prentice (5) introduced a concept of a cumulative incidence (CI) function as a measure of the

TABLE 36.2 Illustration of CI of Death Due to Cancer and Noncancer

ID	Time To Event in Months	Type of Event	KM(t): Any Event-Free Survival	1 − KM(t)	$CI_c(t)$	$CI_{nc}(t)$	1 − $KM_c(t)$	1 − $KM_{nc}(t)$
	0	—	1	0	0.0000	0.0000	1	0
1	20	Cancer	1−1/10 = 0.9000	0.1	1 × 1/10 = 0.1000	0.0000	1−1/10 = 0.9000	0.1
2	25	Noncancer	0.9000 (1−1/9) = 0.8000	0.2	0.1000 + 0.9000 × 0/9 = 0.1000	0.0000 + 0.9000 × 1/9 = 0.1000	0.9000 (1−0/9) = 0.9000	0.1
3	38	Cancer	0.8000 (1−1/8) = 0.7000	0.3	0.1000 + 0.8000 × 1/8 = 0.2000	0.1000 + 0.8000 × 0/8 = 0.1000	0.9000 (1−1/8) = 0.7875	0.2125
4	40+	Censored	0.7000	0.3	0.2000 + 0.7000 × 0/7 = 0.2000	0.1000 + 0.7000 × 0/7 = 0.1000	0.7875	0.2125
5	51	Noncancer	0.7000 (1−1/6) = 0.5833	0.4167	0.2000 + 0.7000 × 0/6 = 0.2000	0.1000 + 0.7000 × 1/6 = 0.2167	0.7875	0.2125
6	55	Cancer	0.5833 (1−1/5) = 0.4666	0.5334	0.2000 + 0.5833 × 1/5 = 0.3167	0.2167 + 0.5833 × 0/5 = 0.2167	0.7875 (1−1/5) = 0.6300	0.3700
7	75	Cancer	0.4666 (1−1/4) = 0.3500	0.6500	0.3167 + 0.4666 × 1/4 = 0.4333	0.2167 + 0.4666 × 0/4 = 0.2167	0.6300(1−1/4) = 0.4725	0.5275
8	83+	Censored	0.3500	0.6500	0.4333 + 0.3500 × 0/3 = 0.4333	0.2167 + 0.3500 × 0/3 = 0.2167	0.4725	0.5275
9	102	Cancer	0.3500 (1−1/2) = 0.1750	0.8250	0.4333 + 0.3500 × 1/2 = 0.6083	0.2167 + 0.3500 × 0/2 = 0.2167	0.4725 (1−1/2) = 0.2363	0.7637
10	115	Cancer	0.1750 (1−1/1) = 0.0000	1	0.6083 + 0.1750 x 1/1 = 0.7833	0.2167 + 0.1750 x 0/1 = 0.2167	0.2363 (1−1/1) = 0.0000	1

CI_c and CI_{nc}, cumulative incidence estimate of the probability of death due to cancer or noncancer, respectively; 1 − KM_c and 1 − KM_{nc} represent Kaplan-Meier estimates of cancer death and noncancer death, respectively.
+, censored event; CI, cumulative incidence.

probability of event of interest at time t in the presence of competing risks. The CI function is defined as:

$$CI(t) = P(T \le t, J = j) = \int_0^t f_j(u)\,du = \int_0^t \lambda_j(u)S(u)\,du$$

When competing risks are present, one should always use the CI function. The CI of each distinct type of event can be estimated, and the sum of the CIs,

$\sum CI_j(t)$, equals the probability of any of k events. For the example in Table 36.2, the sum of CI_c and CI_{nc} equals $1 − S(t)$. To be more precise, let d_{cj} denote the number of cancer deaths at time t_j and n_j be the number of patients at risk of cancer death at time j. Then 1 − KM_c and CI_c are estimated by:

$$1 - KM_c = \sum_{j=1}^{k} \frac{d_{cj}}{n_j} KM_c(t_{j-1})$$

$$\mathrm{CI}_c = \sum_{j=1}^{k} \frac{d_{cj}}{n_j} \mathrm{KM}\left(t_{j-1}\right)$$

Note that their mathematical expressions are very similar, with the only difference being a multiplier of d_{cj}/n_j. For $1 - \mathrm{KM}_c$, the multiplier is KM_c (KM obtained by censoring noncancer deaths), whereas for CI the multiplier is KM (overall survival). Table 36.2 illustrates how CI_c, CI_{nc}, $1 - \mathrm{KM}_c$, and $1 - \mathrm{KM}_{nc}$ are calculated, and Figure 36.1 shows a comparison of CI_c and $1 - \mathrm{KM}_c$ curves. From Table 36.2, the estimated probability that a patient dies before 75 months is $\mathrm{CI}_c(75) = 0.43$ due to cancer death and $\mathrm{CI}_{nc}(75) = 0.22$ due to noncancer death. The sum of $\mathrm{CI}_c(75)$ and $\mathrm{CI}_{nc}(75)$ equals $1 - \mathrm{KM}(75) = 0.65$. In contrast, $1 - \mathrm{KM}_c(75) = 0.47$ and $1 - \mathrm{KM}_{nc}(75) = 0.53$ are different and substantially higher than CI_c or CI_{nc}. Note that the sum of $1 - \mathrm{KM}_c(t)$ and $1 - \mathrm{KM}_{nc}(t)$ does not equal $1 - \mathrm{KM}$. Gooley (4) provides an alternative, more intuitive mathematical expression of CI, and KM in the presence of competing risks and shows that $1 - \mathrm{KM}_k \geq \mathrm{CI}_k$ for the event k, that is, $1 - \mathrm{KM}_k$ overestimates CI_k. The amount of discrepancy depends on the proportion of subjects experiencing competing events. When competing risks are present, $1 - \mathrm{KM}_c(t)$ and $1 - \mathrm{KM}_{nc}(t)$ do not have an appropriate probability interpretation. In the presence of competing risks, we should always use CI to describe the probability of event of interest.

We will illustrate CI using an example with real data. The B-04 study by the National Surgical Adjuvant Breast and Bowel Project (NSABP) is a phase III randomized clinical trial of breast cancer to compare the effect on traditional radical mastectomy versus less aggressive total mastectomy on overall survival (6). A total of 1,079 women with node-negative cancer and 586 women with node-positive cancer were assigned to one of the treatment arms. The trial had a long-term follow-up of more than 30 years; thus, some patients (about 30%) died due to non–breast cancer–related conditions such as heart disease. Because this study aimed to assess the effect of two different treatments only on death following the recurrence, non–breast cancer–related death needed to be considered as a competing risk. Figure 36.2 (7) depicts the two different estimates of cumulative incidence of death following the recurrence by nodal status. Estimates of $1 - \mathrm{KM}$ are always greater than ones from CI, and this discrepancy increases as the years from surgery increase. That is, the more competing risks occur as time goes by, the more biases will be created.

Comparison of Two Cumulative Incidence Functions

To test the equality of two cumulative incidence functions, Gray (8) proposed a test based on the weighted averages of difference of two CIs using a modified

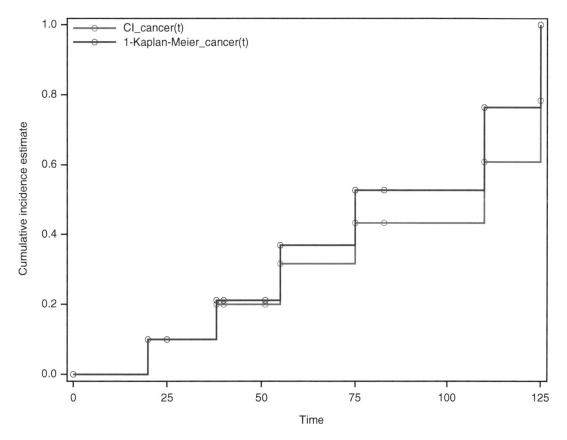

FIGURE 36.1 Cumulative incidence of cancer and noncancer using a simple data example.

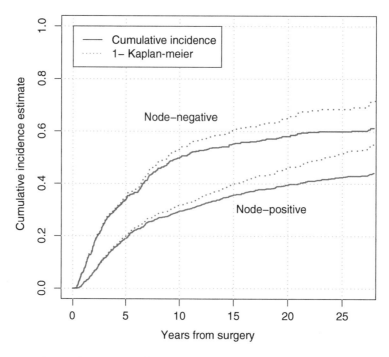

FIGURE 36.2 Cumulative incidence function and 1—Kaplan-Meier estimates based on the data from NSABP B-04 breast cancer trial.

chi-square test. This approach differs from the usual log-rank test in survival analysis, in which other event types (different from the main event of interest) are censored at the time they occur, and the competing risks are considered independent. No such assumption is made in Gray's test. To illustrate Gray's test, we will test the effect of stage (presence or absence of distant site involvement) on colon cancer death and death due to other causes in older colon cancer patients (9). Briefly, the data include 22,240 colon cancer cases diagnosed between 2000 and 2013 in the Surveillance, Epidemiology, and End Results (SEER) registry; patients were 75 or older at the time of the diagnosis. Approximately 12% of cases had distant site involvement at the time of diagnosis, 42% of the cases were still alive or lost to follow-up by November 2015, 29% of cases died of colon cancer, while 29% of cases died of other causes. Figures 36.3A and 36.3B show the cumulative incidence of colon cancer death and death due to other causes in those with or without distance site involvement at the time of diagnosis. Note that Gray's test and log-rank test provide consistent results with respect to colon cancer death, supporting the notion that distant site involvement is a significant risk factor for colon cancer death. In contrast, they give contradictory results with respect to non–colon cancer death. The log-rank test suggests that there is no significant difference in non–colon cancer mortality between those with or without distant site involvement. This makes biological sense. For example, we would not consider advanced cancer stage to affect cardiovascular mortality. On the other hand, because the majority of patients with distant site involvement die of colon cancer within 5 years, the proportion of subjects who die of other causes would be much smaller relative to those without distant site involvement. Gray's test picks up this difference in the cumulative incidence of noncancer deaths, suggesting that the majority of patients who do not die of colon cancer are those without distant site involvement.

Cumulative Incidence Regression

Fine and Gray (10) proposed a proportional hazards regression model that relates the cumulative incidence function to covariates in the presence of competing risks. We will refer to it as the cumulative incidence regression (CIR). Note that as with the CI, individuals that failed from an event other than j prior to t remain in the risk set. In other words, if an individual experiences a competing event instead of the event of interest, it is assumed that he or she remains at risk forever, and therefore the event time is infinite. Klein and Andersen (11) proposed a CIR model that does not assume proportional hazards. An example of CIR using SEER data for colon cancer death and other causes is shown in Table 36.3.

Note that the distant site involvement is significant for colon cancer death and non–colon cancer death with the hazard rate in opposite directions. Distant site involvement is a significant risk factor for colon cancer death (hazard ratio [HR] = 6.45; $p < .0001$), while it is protective of deaths from other causes (HR = 0.27; $p < .0001$). The Cox regression for overall survival shows an intermediate effect of distant site involvement (HR = 4.02; $p < .0001$).

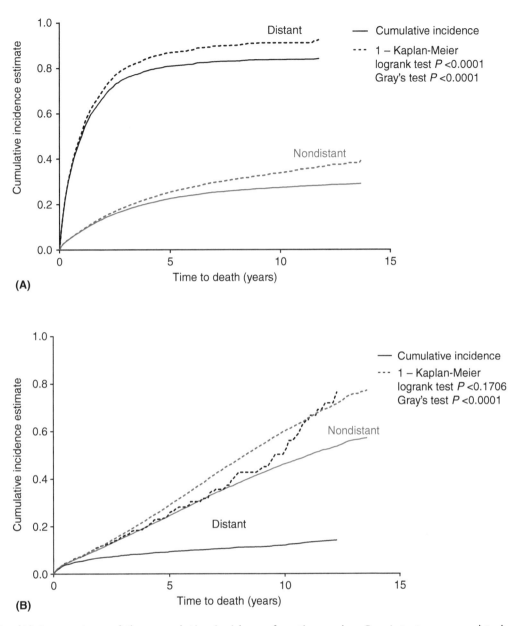

FIGURE 36.3 (A) Comparison of the cumulative incidence functions using Gray's test compared to log-rank test for colon cancer death. (B) Comparison of the cumulative incidence functions using Gray's test compared to log-rank test for other causes of death.

Cause-Specific Hazard Regression

The log-rank test and Cox proportional hazards regression test cause-specific hazards and do not take competing risks into account. However, this does not imply that the methods are invalid for the analysis of time-to-event data in the presence of competing risks. The methods ignore competing risks and focus only on the effect of covariate on a specific type of failure. Pintilie (12,13) provides insightful discussion and contrast between the CIR and Cox regression. The advantage of CIR is that it directly models the observed probabilities of events and does not assume independence in k failure types. In contrast, Cox regression, while assuming independence in k failure types, provides insight into the biological

mechanism ("pure effect") and is invariant to the size of competing risks. The main message is that CIR and cause-specific Cox regression test different hypotheses, and while both can be valid, their interpretations are different. For example, consider the effect of distant site involvement in noncancer death. Biologically we assume that advanced stage is only important to cancer death but not for death due to other causes. Cause-specific hazards Cox regression confirms this hypothesis. While a distant site involvement is significant for colon cancer death (HR = 7.05; p < .0001), it is not significant in non–colon cancer death (HR = 0.97; p = .64). This is in contrast to the CIR results. CIR shows that the distant site involvement is a significant factor for both colon

TABLE 36.3 Comparison of CIR and Cause-Specific HR

Covariate	Comparison	Cox Regression (All Causes)		CIR Colon Cancer		CIR Other Causes		Cox Regression Colon Cancer		Cox Regression (Other Causes)	
		HR	p value	HR	p value	HR	p value	HR	p value	HR	p value
Age	80 – 84 vs. 75 – 79	1.36	<.0001	1.16	<.0001	1.35	<.0001	1.23	<.0001	1.52	<.0001
	85+ vs. 75 – 79	2.09	<.0001	1.35	<.0001	2.03	<.0001	1.61	<.0001	2.76	<.0001
Gender	Male vs. Female	1.27	<.0001	1.08	0.0083	1.31	<.0001	1.14	<.0001	1.43	<.0001
Race	Black vs. White	1.20	<.0001	1.22	<.0001	1.03	0.4839	1.27	<.0001	1.11	0.0292
	Others vs. White	0.89	<.0001	0.98	0.5844	0.87	0.001	0.95	0.2684	0.84	<.0001
Marital status	Married/Living with Partner vs. Others	0.84	<.0001	0.90	0.0001	0.88	<.0001	0.86	<.0001	0.82	<.0001
Grade	2 vs. 1	1.08	0.0126	1.25	<.0001	0.92	0.0357	1.25	<.0001	0.99	0.8930
	3 vs. 1	1.40	<.0001	1.88	<.0001	0.81	<.0001	1.92	<.0001	1.04	0.3791
	4 vs. 1	1.62	<.0001	2.14	<.0001	0.66	<.0001	2.32	<.0001	1.07	0.5160
Stage	Distant Site(s) Involved vs. Non-Distant Site(s)	4.02	<.0001	6.45	<.0001	0.27	<.0001	7.05	<.0001	0.97	0.6383

CIR, cumulative incidence regression; HR, hazard regression.

cancer and non–colon cancer deaths, reflecting the fact that the majority of cases with the distant site involvement died of colon cancer, and therefore they contribute very little to the cumulative incidence of non–colon cancer death relative to those without the distant site involvement.

RESOURCES FOR COMPETING RISK SURVIVAL ANALYSIS

There are a number of excellent books and review articles on survival analysis in the presence of competing risks, including books by Kalbfleisch and Prentice (5) and Pintilie (12) and review articles by Pintilie (13), Bakoyannis and Touloumi (14), Putter et al. (15), Dignam et al. (16), Varadhan et al. (17), and Kim (18). Pintilie (13) has described the different use of CI regression and cause-specific hazard Cox regression depending on the study objectives and has illustrated them using real data examples. In addition, there are a few statistical programs available for competing risks analysis. R software has add-on packages such as *cmprsk*. The CI or each type of event can be estimated and tested across groups based on Gray's test using the *cuminc* function and be plotted using the *plot.cuminc*. It also has a function *crr* that fits Fine and Gray's regression modeling of subdistribution functions in competing risks. In the SAS software, macro %CIF estimates the CI for a specified type of event along with the CI curve and implements the Gray's test for testing difference between groups. The recent version of SAS 9.4 includes Fine and Gray's subdistribution hazard regression model using PROC PHREG by specifying the code for the type of event in a new option EVENTCODE (19).

DISCUSSION

In summary, when competing risks are present, CI should be used to describe the probability of event *k* over time. 1 – KM does not have a probabilistic interpretation. Gray's test should be used to compare two or more CIs. Fine and Gray's CIR should be used to evaluate the effects of covariates on the cumulative incidence of event k. It should be noted, however, that a log-rank test and cause-specific hazard regression are not necessarily invalid; rather, they test different hypotheses. When competing risks are present, one should examine not only the event of interest but also other events in order to gain a more comprehensive picture of the data. Although we did not discuss a sample size and power calculation in the presence of competing events, readers are encouraged to review the recent papers by Latouche and Porcher (20) and Tai et al. (21).

REFERENCES

1. Kaplan EL, Meier P. Nonparametric estimation from incomplete observation. *J Am Stat Ass*. 1958;53(282):457–481.
2. Bland JM, Altman DG. The logrank test. *BMJ*. 2004;328(7447):1073.
3. Cox DR. Regression models and life tables (with discussion). *J Royal Stat Soc*. 1972;34:187–220.
4. Gooley TA, Leisenring W, Storer BE. Estimation of failure probabilities in the presence of competing risks: new representations of old estimators. *Stat Med*. 1999;18:695–706.
5. Kalbfleisch JD, Prentice RL. *The Statistical Analysis of Failure Time Data*. Hoboken, NJ: Wiley; 2002.
6. Fisher B, Jeong J-H, Anderson S, et al. Twenty-five year findings from a randomized clinical trial comparing radical mastectomy with total mastectomy and with total mastectomy followed by radiation therapy. *N Engl J Med*. 2002;347:567–575.
7. Lim JY. Inference on censored survival data under competing risks. Ph.D. Dissertation, University of Pittsburgh. 2012.
8. Gray RJ. A class of K-sample tests for comparing the cumulative incidence of a competing risk. Ann Stat. 1988;16:1141–1154.
9. **SEER Research Data 1973–2013:** Surveillance, Epidemiology, and End Results (SEER) Program (www.seer.cancer.gov) Research Data (1973–2013), National Cancer Institute, DCCPS, Surveillance Research Program, Surveillance Systems Branch, released April 2016, based on the November 2015 submission.
10. Fine JP, Gray RJ. A proportional hazards model for the subdistribution of a competing risk. *J Am Stat Assoc*. 1999;94:496–509.
11. Klein JP, Andersen PK. Regression modeling of competing risks data based on Pseudovalues of the cumulative incidence function. *Biometrics*. 2005;61(1);223–229.
12. Pintilie M. Competing Risks: A Practical Perspective, Statistics in Practice. Chichester, UK: John Wiley & Sons; 2007.
13. Pintilie M. Analysis and interpreting competing risk data. *Stat Med*. 2007;26(6):1360–1367.
14. Bakoyannis G, Touloumi G. Practical methods for competing risks data: a review. *Stat Med Res*. 2012;21(3):157–172.
15. Putter H, Fiocco M, Geskus RB. Tutorial in biostatistics: competing risks and multi-state models. *Stat Med*. 2007;26(11):2389–2430.
16. Dignam JJ, Zhang Q, Kocherginsky M. The use of interpretation of competing risks regression models. *Clin Cancer Res*. 2012;18(8):2301–2308.
17. Varadhan R, Weiss CO, Segal JB, et al. Evaluating health outcomes in the presence of competing risks. *Med Care*. 2010;48(6 Suppl):S96–S105.
18. Kim HT. Cumulative incidence in competing risks data and competing risks regression analysis. *Clin Cancer Res*. 2007;13(2 Pt 1):559–565.
19. Lin G, So Y, Johnston G. Analyzing Survival Data with Competing Risks Using SAS Software, in Proceedings of the SAS Global Forum 2012 Conference; 2012.
20. Latouche A, Porcher R. Sample size calculations in the presence of competing risks. *Stat Med*. 2007;26(30):5370–5380.
21. Tai BC, Wee J, Machin D. Analysis and design of randomised clinical trials involving competing risks endpoints. *Trials*. 2011;12:127.

37

Systematic Reviews and Meta-Analysis

Claire Vale, Sarah Burdett, David Fisher, Larysa Rydzewska, and Jayne Tierney

Every year, hundreds of thousands of research articles are published in the biomedical literature, making it near impossible for clinicians, policy makers, and patients to stay abreast of the latest healthcare developments. Therefore, there is a clear need for summaries of research to advise clinical practice and policy, inform patient choice, and guide new research.

Traditional reviews are common in the medical literature, but can be problematic for summarizing research findings. They are usually narrative, which can make it difficult to make sense of studies with conflicting results. Also, they often lack clear aims and transparent methodology, which can prevent others from being able to reproduce or interpret their findings. They are commonly restricted to a particular group of studies, which may or may not be representative of the whole body of evidence. Moreover, they frequently present the opinion of individual authors, who, even with the best intentions, may not be wholly objective. Systematic reviews, in contrast (Table 37.1), aim to comprehensively identify and objectively appraise and collate all research studies relating to a specific research question, using explicit methodology. The methods used aim to minimize bias (1) and therefore provide reliable findings upon which decisions can be made.

Importantly, the objectives of the review and the nature of the trials to be included or excluded are well defined, to minimize the risk of basing the review on a selected group of trials (Table 37.1). The objectives and eligibility criteria are underpinned by a comprehensive search strategy to ensure that all the relevant studies are identified. Data from the eligible studies are then extracted in a consistent way to enable an assessment of the quality of each study to be made, and the results to be synthesized. Quantitative synthesis, in the form of a meta-analysis, aids interpretation of the results and informs the conclusions of the review. The methods relating to all of these systematic review features should be clearly set out, in advance, in a protocol or another plan (2), so that they are not unduly influenced by the results of the trials. Moreover, provided the protocol is made publicly available, this also allows others to appraise or even reproduce the approach taken. Finally, the review methods, characteristics and results of each trial, and the results and interpretation of the review are presented or reported in a structured and consistent way, ideally adhering to the Preferred Reporting Items for Systematic review and Meta-Analysis (PRISMA) guidelines (3,4).

Where new treatments only offer modest improvements in outcome compared to an existing standard, many trials lack power to detect such effects. This may be, for example, because trial sample size calculations assumed larger treatment effects, or simply because recruitment fell short of targets, but means that inconclusive or equivocal study results are relatively common, particularly in oncology. Hence, most systematic reviews include a meta-analysis, to quantitatively combine the results of included studies and obtain an overall estimate of the treatment effect, based on all relevant trials. As a meta-analysis is based on more participants than any of the individual trials, it provides greater power to establish whether a treatment effect exists, and greater confidence in any estimate of effect. A meta-analysis carried out within the context of a good-quality systematic review will together represent the most complete and reliable summary of the evidence available. Conversely, a meta-analysis that is not completed as part of a systematic review may encounter the sorts of problems that commonly affect traditional reviews (Table 37.1).

Systematic reviews and meta-analyses typically make use of summary or aggregate data extracted from study publications or obtained from trial investigators. However, there is also a long tradition in oncology of conducting systematic reviews based on the central collection and reanalysis of the original individual participant data (IPD) (5,6). Notable examples occur in breast (7), colorectal (8), head and neck (9), and lung cancer (10). Although the IPD approach can bring about substantial improvements to the data and analysis quality, which can sometimes lead to disparate results (11–14), much of the methodology is equally applicable to both

TABLE 37.1 Traditional Versus Systematic Reviews

	Traditional Review	**Systematic Review**
Protocol	No	Yes
Research objective	Unclear, nonspecific	Specific objective based on PICOS
Eligibility criteria for studies	Unclear, not specified or selective	Explicit inclusion and exclusion criteria based on PICOS
Search strategy	Unclear, not specified or limited	Systematic, multiple sources of studies and inclusive
Evidence synthesis	Usually narrative qualitative	Usually quantitative (meta-analysis)
Conclusions	Subjective and potentially biased or otherwise unreliable	More objective and reliable, based on results
Reproducibility	Difficult without transparent methodology	Use of transparent methodology and clear reporting enables reproducibility

PICOS, patients, interventions, comparisons, outcomes, and study type.

types of data. Therefore, in this chapter, we use examples of systematic reviews and meta-analysis based on aggregate data and IPD to illustrate the key principles and provide an overview of the methods for each.

Most commonly, systematic reviews and meta-analyses are used to investigate the effects of treatments or other interventions on a particular disease or condition. Such reviews, which use evidence from randomized controlled trials (RCTs) (15), have been widely used in oncology as well as other areas of medicine and the methods used in their conduct are well established. However, when randomized evidence is lacking, systematic reviews of other study designs (e.g., cohort or case control studies) can also provide evidence about treatment efficacy, albeit such reviews are not considered such a high level of evidence (16). Systematic reviews can also be used to synthesize results of prognostic or diagnostic test accuracy studies, with methods for each being developed accordingly (17–19). Largely irrespective of the nature of the research studies being synthesized, the underlying principles of systematic review methodology hold. Therefore, although the focus of this chapter is on systematic reviews of RCTs, much of it will be of relevance to systematic reviews of other study types.

It is now well recognized that systematic reviews are an optimal way to synthesize results of primary research and in particular, to resolve or confirm uncertainty around the effects of interventions. Therefore, before embarking on any review, it is worth establishing whether a preexisting systematic review provides a comprehensive, up-to-date, and robust evaluation of the question posed or at least whether one is planned, to avoid duplication of effort (20). Search strategies are available to locate reviews in the wider medical literature

(21). Additionally, the Cochrane Database of Systematic Reviews (22) and the International Prospective Register of Systematic Reviews (PROSPERO) (23), managed by the Centre for Reviews and Dissemination (CRD), maintain searchable records and protocols of planned and ongoing systematic reviews. There may be of course merit in duplicating a systematic review, for example if a prior one is substandard, or where substantial new information has become available.

Through the remainder of this chapter, using a variety of examples from the oncology literature, we describe the key features of a systematic review, namely:

- Clear objectives and eligibility criteria
- Search strategy to identify all relevant studies
- Consistent data collection across studies
- Assessment of study validity and risk of bias
- Synthesis of study characteristics and results (meta-analysis)
- Structured presentation of results

DEFINING THE OBJECTIVE AND ELIGIBILITY CRITERIA

First and foremost, a systematic review should have answerable and relevant objectives, which should provide a clear, precise statement about the nature of the review. This is further qualified by detailed and specific criteria that outline the studies that are to be included and excluded. Broad objectives and eligibility criteria can make for a comprehensive review that is widely generalizable, but perhaps one that is too large, labor-intensive, and hard to manage. If the scope is too broad, trials addressing quite different clinical questions may be combined, making interpretation difficult (15) or inappropriate. In contrast, a review with narrow objectives and eligibility criteria will likely include fewer trials and produce results that are easier to interpret and certainly more manageable. However, if the review comprises too few trials, there is a risk that the results will not reveal much more than the results of any individual trial, or that they will have very limited applicability (15).

The compromise is to define objectives and eligibility criteria that are inclusive, but at the same time minimize, as far as possible, the inevitable variability between studies, such as different treatment doses or scheduling, different participants, or different clinical settings. Trials that are sufficiently similar in design are more likely to have comparable results, making review results easier to interpret and more meaningful. In particular, ensuring that the interventions of interest are similar can help minimize potential statistical heterogeneity, which can blight the interpretation of meta-analysis results. One way to tackle a systematic review that is broad in scope is to subdivide it into a series of related narrower questions, to reduce inconsistencies and aid interpretation. For example, a broad systematic review of the effects of adding chemotherapy to standard care in participants with non–small-cell lung cancer (NSCLC) (10) was subdivided into a series of reviews with narrower objectives. These were defined by the type of standard treatment used, ranging from surgery and radical radiotherapy (24) through to best supportive care (25), and subsequently, how chemotherapy was given—either preoperatively (26) or as adjuvant treatment (27), which reflected the stage of disease of the included participants.

The PICOS tool (21) is a useful aid to defining clear objectives and eligibility criteria, as it sets out the population (P) of included participants; the new intervention (I) being tested; the comparison (C) against which the intervention is being compared; which outcomes (O) the intervention might affect; and the study designs (S)

that are eligible for the review. Note that for treatment efficacy reviews, RCTs will tend to be the default study type.

For an aggregate data systematic review in NSCLC (28), the objective was to assess whether the effect of preoperative chemotherapy (I) improved survival and reduced recurrence rates (O) when compared against standard of care (C) for patients with NSCLC (P). The eligibility criteria are shown in Table 37.2. Commonly, because systematic reviews aim to assess the effect of treatment on a number of outcomes, it would be too restrictive to use outcomes to define the eligibility criteria for trials to be included in a systematic review (Table 37.2).

IDENTIFYING ALL RELEVANT STUDIES

Searching for Trials

Although defining and applying specific eligibility criteria guards against study selection bias (Table 37.3), it cannot circumvent reporting biases. These occur when the characteristics of study results determine if, when, and where they are published. Therefore, the aim is to identify and include all relevant trials, irrespective of publication status, language, or the nature of the results, through systematic and comprehensive searches for trials across multiple sources, thereby reducing the risk of falling foul of such biases.

Bibliographic databases including MEDLINE, EMBASE, and the Cochrane Central Register of Controlled Trials (CENTRAL [(29)]), which are also populated by trial reports identified in other databases and through handsearching of journals, are important sources of (mainly) published RCTs. Validated search filters and exemplar strategies that use these filters have been developed to assist reviewers in the retrieval of RCTs for MEDLINE, CENTRAL, and EMBASE

TABLE 37.2 Example of Eligibility Criteria Based on PICOS

PICOS Elements	Definition	Eligibility Criteria for NSCLC Systematic Review (28)
Populations	Defines the included participants (e.g., by age, sex, condition under investigation)	Patients with NSCLC and no prior malignancy or chemotherapy
Interventions	The research or experimental treatment	Preoperative chemotherapy plus surgery with or without radiotherapy
Comparator (control)	The control (e.g., standard of care, placebo)	Surgery with or without radiotherapy
Outcomes	The review endpoints or outcomes of interest (e.g., survival, weight loss, quality of life)	NA
Study types	Types of studies eligible for inclusion in the review (e.g., RCTs, cohort studies, etc.)	Completed RCTs (S)

NSCLC, non–small-cell lung cancer; PICOS, patients, interventions, comparisons, outcomes, and study type; RCT, randomized controlled trial.

TABLE 37.3 Biases That Can Affect the Reliability of Systematic Review and Meta-Analysis Results

Type of Bias	Description
Biases associated with study selection, availability, or reporting	
Study selection bias (32)	Trials with clinically or statistically significant results are more likely to be selected for inclusion in the review
Data availability bias (32)	Data from trials with clinically or statistically significant results are more likely to be made available readily
Publication bias (33)	Trials with clinically or statistically significant results are more likely to be published
Time lag bias (34)	Trials with clinically or statistically significant results are more likely to be published quickly
Multiple publication bias (35)	Trials with clinically or statistically significant results are more likely to be published multiple times
Location bias (36)	Trials with clinically or statistically significant results are more likely to be published in readily accessible sources
Citation bias (37)	Trials with clinically or statistically significant results are more likely to be cited
Language bias (38)	Trials with clinically or statistically significant results are more likely to be published in the English language
Outcome reporting or availability bias (39)	Trial outcomes with clinically or statistically significant results are more likely to be published.
Biases associated with study design or analysis (40)	
Participant selection bias	Trial participants on the treatment arm of trials have more favorable characteristics or prognoses than participants on the control arm (prevented by random allocation and allocation concealment)
Performance and detection bias	Trial participants on the treatment arm receive additional care or are assessed more closely for positive outcomes than participants on the control arm
Attrition bias	Trial participants are followed up, or excluded from analyses, in such a way that results on the treatment arm appear more positive

(21,30). Although searching these three databases should be considered a minimum requirement for a systematic review (30), depending on the review topic, cancer- or region-specific databases may also be useful. A recent review of published systematic reviews indexed in MEDLINE (31) showed that a median of four electronic databases were searched by review authors. When devising search strategies and choosing search terms for these databases, again, the PICOS tool is helpful, with population, intervention, comparison, and study design being the most useful (21).

Although these databases are undoubtedly rich sources of reported trials, there are limitations. MEDLINE and EMBASE tend to include journals with higher impact factors, published in the English language, that cover more general medical than disease-specific theme topics. Added to this, there is now substantial empirical evidence that trials with more striking results are more likely to be published; published more quickly, in the English language, in more accessible sources and multiple times, compared to those with less striking results (Table 37.3). Thus, limiting searches to these major bibliographic databases potentially means including only those trials with the most striking results, leading to unrepresentative, biased, and very unreliable conclusions.

It has been estimated that around 10% of all trials included in Cochrane systematic reviews are identified in the gray literature (30), which includes conference proceedings, book chapters, theses, and reports. However, sources of unpublished trials are often overlooked in systematic reviews, with trial registries searched in only 19% and conference proceedings in only 16% of systematic reviews identified in a recent study (31). Given that results of many trials presented at conferences are never fully published (41), and others can take some time to be reported in full, conference proceedings, in particular should not be ignored. In oncology, searching the proceedings of both general cancer conferences, for example, the American Society of Clinical Oncology (ASCO) or European Society of Medical Oncology (ESMO), and cancer-specific conferences, for example, the World Conference on Lung Cancer (WCLC) or ASCO genitourinary cancers symposium can prove very useful. Finally, further trials can often be identified by handsearching the reference lists of the publications of eligible trials or related reviews, and by searching clinical trial registers, for example, U.S. National Institutes of Health ClinicalTrials.gov and by speaking to experts working in the field. For example, in a systematic review of preoperative chemotherapy for NSCLC (28), only half of the eligible trials identified were indexed in MEDLINE. The remainder of the trials were identified through searches of conference proceedings, CENTRAL, and by handsearching the reference lists of relevant articles.

Screening Search Results for Eligible Trials

Once all searches have been completed, the records retrieved must be screened for relevance and eligibility. Inevitably, any search strategy will pick up many irrelevant records that need to be removed, and searching multiple sources of trials can result in duplicate records. Often, scanning the titles and abstracts is enough to filter out obvious duplicates and irrelevant records. However, detailed checking of abstracts and full-text publications is needed to properly identify trials that fulfill the eligibility criteria and objectives of the review, and also to clarify and collate multiple reports arising from the results of a single trial. It is advisable for this process to be carried out by two reviewers, who should agree on eligibility (or otherwise) of the trials identified. A screening form listing questions relating to the eligibility criteria is very useful at this stage, both to aid the screening process and to document the decisions made. Reference management software can also facilitate the management of this stage of the review process. The flow of trial records though this process of screening search results is commonly recorded in a flow diagram, which is a mandatory requirement of the PRISMA reporting guidelines (4). An example from a systematic review and IPD meta-analysis of preoperative chemotherapy for NSCLC (26) is shown in Figure 37.1.

CONSISTENT DATA COLLECTION ACROSS STUDIES

Once a list of eligible trials has been established, key descriptive data and results need to be obtained for each included trial. Data items to be collected for each trial

should be outlined in advance in the systematic review protocol. Key data items often include, but are not limited to:

- Trial identifier/reference
- Lead investigator
- Details of study design, recruitment, and follow-up (**S**)
- Methods of analysis and number of patients randomized/analyzed
- Baseline characteristics (e.g., age, sex, stage) of participants (**P**)
- Planned treatment details (intervention and control arms) (**I/C**)
- Outcomes assessed and their definitions, and results for each (**O**)

Most systematic reviews rely on using aggregate summary data that has been extracted from trial reports, including journal articles, conference abstracts (or associated presentations), book chapters, theses, and pharmaceutical company reports. Developing a standardized data collection form helps to ensure that, as far as possible, results and other information are extracted consistently for each trial, and also provides a record of which data were available and which were not. Indeed one of the challenges for systematic reviewers is obtaining all of the necessary information needed for the systematic review. For example, trial reports may not describe the design of a trial in sufficient detail to determine the methods used or they may only provide results for some of the outcomes of interest or for a particular subgroup of participants. These problems can be magnified in conference abstracts. For example, for a systematic review of preoperative chemotherapy for NSCLC (28), data on survival were only available for 7 of the 12 eligible trials and for disease-free survival for 3 trials, representing only 75% and 35% of all participants randomized, respectively. Although the CONSORT (42) and CONSORT for abstracts (43) guidelines for trial reporting are no doubt helpful in this regard, information on unpublished trials can be even harder to establish. Trial protocols, which are increasingly available through trial institute websites or summarized in registers such as ClinicalTrials.gov, can provide information on treatments and comparators, inclusion and exclusion criteria of participants, and planned trial size and timelines. However, until such time as results become readily available, obtaining results for unpublished trials remains an issue.

Clearly, if the reporting of trials is related to results, it is important to include as much published and unpublished data as possible to limit the potential influence of reporting biases (Table 37.3). This may mean, for example, seeking results directly from trial investigators for any outcomes that were not reported. However,

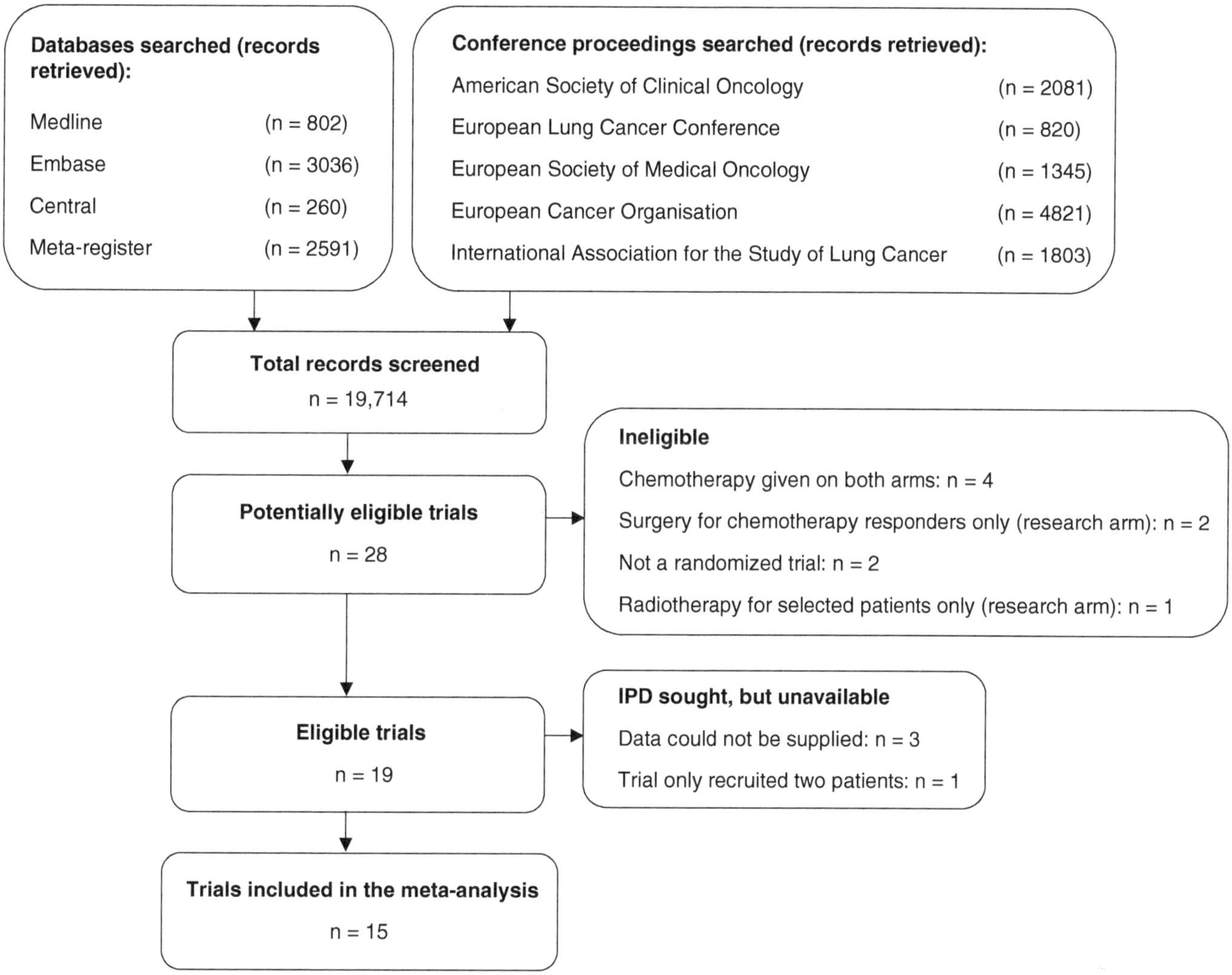

FIGURE 37.1 PRISMA flow diagram for systematic review of neoadjuvant chemotherapy for non–small-cell lung cancer.

IPD, individual participant data; PRISMA, Preferred Reporting Items for Systematic review and Meta-Analysis.

Source: Modified with permission from Elsevier. NSCLC Meta-analysis Collaborative Group. Preoperative chemotherapy for non-small cell lung cancer: a systematic review and meta-analysis of individual participant data. *Lancet.* 2014;383:1561–1571.

recent evidence (31) suggests that very few systematic reviewers do this. Similarly, additional information on, for example, the methods of randomization or concealment or reasons why participants were excluded from reported analyses can be sought from trial investigators to establish the quality of the included trials.

An alternative to extracting or obtaining aggregate data is the IPD approach, which involves the central collection of the raw data for each participant, from all the relevant trials worldwide. Although this may demand greater resources and be more time-consuming than a review of aggregate data, it can substantially improve both the quantity and quality of data available by virtue of including more trials (published and unpublished), participants, and outcomes (6,44,45). For example, a systematic review of preoperative chemotherapy for NSCLC based on IPD (26) included data on 15 trials,

representing 92% of all randomized patients for both survival and disease-free survival outcomes. All participants who had been excluded from the reported analyses for these trials were reinstated in the IPD review, the results of which were based on far more data than the aggregate data review conducted previously (28). The collection of IPD also enables standardization of outcomes such as disease-free survival across trials and allows for detailed data checking (6,44,45).

ASSESSING STUDY VALIDITY AND RISK OF BIAS

The validity and reliability of the results of any systematic review are determined not only by efforts undertaken to ensure that all (and only) eligible trials have been included, but also by the quality of the included studies. Although reporting biases (Table 37.3) can to some degree be circumvented by extensive searching, obtaining results based on all trials, participants, and outcomes, which may or may not require the collection and reanalysis of IPD, potential biases arising from inappropriate trial design, conduct, or analysis (participant selection bias, performance, and selection bias; Table 37.3) are harder to address. Therefore, assessments of the quality, or risk of bias, of included trials are now commonplace in systematic reviews, and are a requirement of the PRISMA reporting guidelines (4). One tool that is commonly used to assess the trial validity is the Cochrane Risk of Bias tool (46), in which reviewers assess whether the risk of various biases is low, high, or unclear for each of the included trials and ultimately, for the meta-analysis results overall. The tool does have some limitations. Reviewers are most often relying on information from trial reports to make judgments about the risk of bias. If the required information is scant or missing from trial reports, then assessments can be unreliable or limited (47,48). Contacting trial investigators for further details to inform the trial quality assessment may be important. Moreover, judgments are somewhat subjective, leading to differing assessments being made by independent reviewers (49,50) and can only ever highlight the potential for bias and not the actual validity of a trial and its results. The potential impact of observed biases within trials on the results of the systematic review should also be evaluated. This may be done qualitatively or through sensitivity analyses (51), if a meta-analysis is planned, but there is no standard approach (52).

SYNTHESIS OF STUDY CHARACTERISTICS AND RESULTS (META-ANALYSIS)

Results of a systematic review can be presented in a narrative way; indeed most reports of systematic reviews tabulate and summarize details of the eligible trials, including design, recruitment, treatments used, and characteristics of the included patients. However, systematic reviews of interventions will generally also incorporate a quantitative synthesis of trial results in the form of a meta-analysis.

Planning Meta-Analyses

If a meta-analysis is to be included in a systematic review, it is important that all aspects of the analysis are planned in advance and described in detail in the review protocol or analysis plan. This ensures that the analyses are guided by the objective(s), and not motivated and modified on the basis of known trial results or by the accumulating meta-analysis results, which could introduce bias. In addition, the planning stage can help, for example, to clarify definitions of outcomes to be assessed and the data items to be obtained.

Analysis plans should include the primary and secondary outcomes, their definitions; methods for analyses of efficacy, including those for exploring the impact of trial or participant characteristics; methods for measuring and accounting for heterogeneity; and methods for assessing risk of bias for included trials. Of course, developing a protocol and analysis plan does not preclude unplanned, additional exploratory analysis, which can inform or add to the main results or help generate new hypotheses. However, any post hoc analyses should be justified, and clearly described as such in any report of the results.

Outcomes and Effect Measures

How treatment effects are measured in individual trials and meta-analysis is largely dictated by the outcomes of interest in the review. For example, a hazard ratio (HR) would commonly be used to assess the effects of treatment on a time-to-event outcome such as survival, or an odds ratio (OR) or risk ratio (RR) (relative risk) for a dichotomous outcome such as toxicity (Table 37.4). In the case of an aggregate data review, the effects measures will either be extracted or

TABLE 37.4 Common Outcome Types and Effect Measures Used in Meta-Analysis

Outcome Type	Description	Examples of Outcome Type	Examples of Appropriate Statistics
Dichotomous outcome	Whether events do or do not happen	Mortality Adverse event	Risk ratio Odds ratio
Continuous outcome	Whether a disease or participant measure changes	Blood pressure Pain Weight loss	Mean difference Standardized mean difference
Time-to-event outcome	Whether events do or do not happen over a period of time	Survival Time to recurrence of disease Time to relief of symptoms	Hazard ratio

estimated from published results or obtained directly from trial investigators, whereas for IPD, they can be calculated directly from the reanalysis of the collated trial data, which also allows analytical assumptions to be checked and for the analysis methods to be kept consistent across trials.

How is a Meta-Analysis Done?

Meta-analyses are typically described as either "one-stage" or "two-stage" (53). The "two-stage" approach is more commonly used and applicable to aggregate data or IPD meta-analyses. In the first stage, an estimate of the treatment effect and its standard error (or variance) are obtained for each trial, and in the second stage, these are combined to obtain an overall estimate of effect, which is essentially a weighted average of the effects in each trial.

$$\text{Meta-analysis effect} = \frac{\text{Sum of (trial effect} \times \text{weight)}}{\text{Sum of weights}}$$

The weight applied to each trial determines how much influence each trial has on the meta-analysis effect estimate.

For IPD meta-analyses, although the two-stage approach remains common, so-called "one-stage" approaches (53) are being used increasingly (54) and typically involve analyzing the data all together in a single regression model, while also accounting for differences between trials. The model chosen will depend on the outcome(s) of interest (Table 37.4), for example, a logistic regression might be used for dichotomous outcomes, a Cox regression for time-to-event, or a linear regression for continuous outcomes. Theoretically, two-stage methods can be seen as special cases of one-stage models (55–57), and studies using both simulated (58,59) and real data (58–61) have shown that the results obtained will usually be similar, irrespective

of whichever is used. However, in particular scenarios, results from two-stage meta-analysis can be biased (58,59,62).

Visualizing Meta-Analysis Results

The results of two-stage meta-analyses are usually presented on forest plots. For example, the results of a meta-analysis of the effect of adding docetaxel to standard care on survival in metastatic hormone sensitive prostate cancer (63) are shown in Figure 37.2.

In Figure 37.2, the x-axis shows the range of effect sizes, in this case HRs, with the line running through 1 (or 0 on log HR scale) representing no effect of docetaxel (equivalence). The HR estimates of the effect of docetaxel for individual trials are represented by squares, and the 95% confidence intervals by the horizontal lines on either side. The size of each square is directly proportional to the amount of information (in this case events) contributed by the trial results, and the associated confidence interval shows the level of uncertainty in the estimation of the HRs. Those HRs less than 1, that is, lying to the left of the line of no effect, indicate a reduction in the risk of a death with docetaxel, and this is the case for all trials in Figure 37.2. However, results of individual trials are only conventionally significant (i.e., $p < .05$) if the 95% confidence intervals do not cross the line of no effect. Thus, only two of all the individual trials in Figure 37.2 show significantly improved survival with docetaxel. Note that for positive outcomes, such as resection rates, the conventions would be reversed, and beneficial effects of treatment would be represented by estimates of effect lying to the *right* of the line of equivalence.

The overall estimate for the meta-analysis is usually displayed as a diamond, with the center corresponding to the effect size, and the edges the 95% confidence interval. Again, a meta-analysis result is only

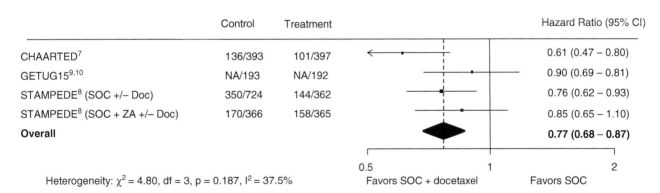

FIGURE 37.2 Effect of the addition of docetaxel to standard of care on overall survival of men with metastatic prostate cancer.

Source: Modified with permission from Elsevier. Vale CL, Burdett S, Rydzewska LH, et al. Addition of docetaxel or bisphosphonates to standard of care in men with localised or metastatic, hormone-sensitive prostate cancer: a systematic review and meta-analyses of aggregate data. *Lancet Oncol.* 2016;17(2):243–256.

conventionally statistically significant when the confidence interval does not overlap the line of equivalence. In Figure 37.2, the meta-analysis HR of 0.77 represents a 23% relative reduction in the risk of death with the addition of docetaxel, and is highly statistically significant (63) reflecting the gain in power from being able to include more patients and events. Also, as clearly seen in Figure 37.2, the confidence interval for the meta-analysis result (95% CI: 0.68–0.87) is much narrower than for any of the individual trials, reflecting the increased confidence in this estimate of effect.

Important to note is that as forest plots were designed for use with two-stage meta-analysis models, it remains a matter of debate how they might better be used in conjunction with one-stage models, which typically do not estimate treatment effects for the individual trials (38,54).

Measuring and Accounting for Heterogeneity

As described previously, effect estimates from individual trials are more likely to be similar if the populations, and particularly the interventions and comparisons of those trials are similar. Nevertheless, some variability in individual trial estimates is inevitable and expected, but where these are greater than expected by chance this is termed statistical heterogeneity (64). This is usually assessed using a chi-square test known as Cochran's Q (64). A p value of less than 0.05 or, because of the low power of the test, less than 0.10, for this test is considered suggestive of meaningful variation between effect estimates. An alternative measure is the inconsistency statistic, I^2, which describes the variability in the trial effect estimates that arise from heterogeneity rather than by chance (sampling error) alone (64). The I^2 statistic is presented as a percentage, with figures close to 0% suggestive of low heterogeneity and those close to 100% high heterogeneity (65).

Fixed-effects models for meta-analysis (66,67) assume that each trial estimates the same underlying treatment effect, and that variation in effects between trials occurs by chance alone. Trials in the meta-analysis are weighted directly by the amount of information they contribute to the meta-analysis. Larger trials, including more participants and with more events, have a larger weight than smaller trials and heterogeneity is not accounted for. Alternatively, a random-effects model, such as that proposed by DerSimonian and Laird (68), assumes that treatment effects will be normally distributed around a mean effect. Trials are weighted by a combination of their size, or amount of information provided, and by the underlying variability between the studies as estimated by the model. Where there is low heterogeneity, as assessed by Cochran's Q or the I^2 statistic, the results obtained will be very similar, or indeed, identical, regardless of whether a fixed-effects or random-effects model is employed.

Conversely, where there is evidence of heterogeneity, a fixed-effects model may provide an estimate of effect that is too precise (confidence intervals are too narrow), not appropriately reflecting the uncertainty associated with the meta-analysis estimate of treatment effect. Although a random-effects model will reflect the uncertainty, having wider confidence intervals, smaller trials will potentially influence the meta-analysis as much as larger, theoretically more reliable, trials.

In a systematic review of the effect of postoperative radiotherapy on survival in patients with NSCLC (69) there was some evidence of heterogeneity in the effect on survival (I^2 = 40%, p = .08). However, results from the fixed-effect (HR: 1.18, 95% CI: 1.07–1.31, p = .0001) and random-effects models (HR: 1.17, 95% CI: 1.02–1.34, p = .02) were similar, reassuringly demonstrating that the results were robust to the choice of model. By contrast, in an IPD meta-analysis of neoadjuvant chemotherapy prior to radiotherapy for cervical cancer (70) there was substantial evidence of heterogeneity in the effect on survival (p = .0003, I^2 = 62%), and the fixed-effects meta-analysis suggested no clear benefit of neoadjuvant chemotherapy (HR: 1.05, 95% CI: 0.93–1.19, p = .39). However, it is perhaps inappropriate to combine such variable results using a model that assumes the same effect across trials. Although the random-effects model better reflects the uncertainty of the result, with a much wider confidence interval (HR: 1.11, 95% CI: 0.90–1.36, p = .32), the estimate of effect is driven by a number of the small trials with extreme results (71). In fact, neither model provides an ideal synthesis of the trial results.

Exploring Heterogeneity and Robustness of Results

The presence of heterogeneity makes it more likely that a meta-analysis result will be nonsignificant and/or otherwise unclear, which inevitably hampers interpretation. Therefore, it is important to explore whether variability in characteristics of either the trials or of the included participants (so called "effect modifiers") may help to explain differences in treatment effects (71,72). Trial-level effect modifiers can be explored by grouping trials according to the characteristic(s) of interest, and performing separate meta-analyses within each group. Results are then compared using a test for interaction (subgroup differences) (64). Such analyses were useful in showing that the effects of neoadjuvant chemotherapy in cervical cancer (70) varied by chemotherapy cycle length (test for interaction p = .009), with a clear detriment from giving long-cycle neoadjuvant chemotherapy before radiotherapy (HR: 1.25, 95% CI: 1.07–1.46), but not short-cycle chemotherapy (HR: 0.83, 95% CI: 0.69–1.00), helping to explain the heterogeneity identified. Alternatively, metaregression (64) can be used to explore whether individual trial treatment effects change in response to changes in, for example, treatment doses or regimens.

The investigation of how treatment effects vary by patient characteristics is important not only in exploring heterogeneity, but also in determining which participants are more likely to benefit or are least likely to be harmed by particular treatments. However, using metaregression of aggregate data is usually inadequate for this purpose because it only allows investigation of interactions between trial treatment effects and summaries of patient characteristics, such as mean age or proportion of females, which may not reflect the genuine relationship between the effects and the age or sex of an individual participant (73). Therefore, full investigation of potential patient-level treatment effect modifiers is a common motivation for collecting IPD (6,74). For example, a systematic review and IPD meta-analysis showed that the benefits of tamoxifen or the survival of women with early breast cancer were limited to those with estrogen-receptor-positive tumors (75). Such findings would not have been possible without access to IPD. However, some methods of analyzing these interactions between patient characteristics and treatment effects are prone to ecological bias (73), so care must be taken to analyze these appropriately (76).

Another option for exploring variation in trial results is to conduct sensitivity analyses, whereby trials with particular characteristics are included (or excluded) from a meta-analysis, to determine their influence on the overall results. Candidates for sensitivity analyses might be trials with unusual designs, or with extreme results. However, it is possible that excluding trials in such a way can introduce bias, for example, if the analyses are driven by the results or trial effects vary for reasons other than those under consideration. Sensitivity analyses performed to exclude trials considered to be of poor quality (51), can also be problematic since quality judgments will always be somewhat subjective, and potentially unreliable if based on trial reports (47,48).

Ideally, the possible or likely sources of variation in treatment effects should be anticipated at an early stage in the systematic review process, and strategies to investigate or mitigate the effects of such heterogeneity described in detail in the protocol statistical analysis plan in advance of any analyses being conducted. Even if it transpires that there is little or moderate statistical heterogeneity, such analyses remain useful in exploring the robustness of the results to the variability that is inherent across trials in any meta-analysis. Conversely, the results of interaction tests or sensitivity analyses conducted post hoc should be interpreted cautiously, and regarded as hypothesis-generating rather than as conclusive.

Interpreting Meta-Analysis Results

When interpreting the results of a meta-analysis, examining just the direction of the effect and the significance level (p value) is insufficient. There is a need to also consider:

- The size of the effect (difference from the no-effect line), to assess if it is clinically worthwhile
- The strength of evidence for the effect (the number of eligible trials and amount of data included, and the width of the confidence interval)
- The consistency of the results of individual trials (visual inspection and heterogeneity statistics, and whether any variation can be explained by trial or patient characteristics)

Revisiting the aggregate data review of preoperative chemotherapy for NSCLC (28), the meta-analysis suggests an improvement in survival (HR: 0.82, 95% CI: 0.69–0.97), and results are consistent across trials (test for heterogeneity; $p = .98$). However, the p value is just conventionally significant ($p = .022$), and the upper limit of the confidence interval is close to 1, implying that the true effect may be very small. Perhaps most importantly, some key large trials, representing 25% of the randomized patients could not be included. As inclusion of these data could potentially alter either the size or direction of effect, the results can only be regarded as promising rather than conclusive. The potential impact of missing trials on the results of a meta-analysis can be indicated by the use of funnel plots. However, as reporting biases are one of a number of potential causes of funnel plot asymmetry, the interpretation of these plots is not always indicative of missing trials. Furthermore, funnel plots are not appropriate in situations where fewer than 10 trials have been included in the meta-analysis, where very few trials have statistically significant results, or where there is considerable heterogeneity (77,78).

For the aggregate data review of the effects of adding docetaxel to standard care on survival in metastatic prostate cancer (63) represented in Figure 37.2, we see that the HR is substantially smaller than 1, the confidence interval is narrow with an upper limit that is also much less than 1, and the effect estimate is highly statistically significant. Thus, the meta-analysis seems to provide reliable evidence of a large treatment effect. Heterogeneity across trial results is low (test for heterogeneity; $p = .187$; $I^2 = 37.5\%$) and unaffected by the choice of a fixed- or random-effects model providing further reassurance as to the robustness of the results. Although the meta-analysis is based on only three of the five eligible trials, it still represents 93% of all patients randomized. Thus, incorporation of data from the remaining two trials would have little impact. Taken together, this provides compelling evidence that adding docetaxel to standard care improves the survival of men with metastatic prostate cancer (79).

Is Meta-Analysis Always Appropriate?

Although most systematic reviews that set out to assess the effects of a treatment intervention do include a meta-analysis, there are occasions when it may not be feasible to formally synthesize the results of trials; for example, where data are sparse, either because very few trials have been conducted in the field of interest, or those that have are either still ongoing or have not reported results. In the latter circumstances, contact with the investigators can help establish if and when results may become available, allowing better planning of the timing of any meta-analysis. Alternatively, a request for the results or IPD can help make a meta-analysis feasible.

Another obvious circumstance in which meta-analysis may be inappropriate is where there is substantial heterogeneity across trial results that cannot be explained by differences in trial or patient characteristics. This could indicate that the included trials have assessed fundamentally different questions, such that combining them in meta-analysis could lead to erroneous or invalid conclusions.

A final consideration is whether it is appropriate to combine or include the results of trials (or trial analyses) that are clearly of "poor quality" or at high risk of bias in a meta-analysis at all, as it is likely that these biases will be further compounded. This was the approach taken in a systematic review of adjuvant chemotherapy for bladder cancer (80) in which there had been serious concerns raised about the quality of the design, conduct, and analysis of some of the eligible trials. If it is the analysis or reporting, rather than the conduct, of the trial that is at fault, then requesting results based on the intention-to-treat principle (that is, including all randomized participants), for all outcomes of interest, or with longer follow-up may mitigate the potential influence of these biases on the meta-analysis results. Indeed, a systematic review and meta-analysis based on IPD from many of these same trials of adjuvant chemotherapy in bladder cancer (81) was able to assess and resolve most of the issues affecting the aggregate data review. If time or resources are limited, this could be done only for those trials judged to be most at risk of bias.

Multivariate Meta-Analysis

Meta-analyses discussed in the bulk of this chapter are used to estimate the effect of a treatment on a specific outcome. However, multivariate meta-analysis is often used to estimate the overall effects of multiple outcomes simultaneously. For instance, in a meta-analysis in the field of cancer, a reviewer might be interested in both progression-free survival and in overall survival. The simplest approach would be to perform two independent meta-analyses, one for each outcome. However, if only the most significant outcome from each trial is reported (outcome reporting bias) then those meta-analyses will be biased. Importantly, though, outcomes such as progression-free survival and overall survival are often highly correlated; and

this correlation can be used in multivariate meta-analysis to permit so-called *borrowing of strength* from the effect in one outcome to assist in estimating the treatment effect on the other.

Network Meta-Analysis

Network meta-analysis is a similar concept to multivariate meta-analysis; however, in a network meta-analysis, multiple treatments may be assessed simultaneously (82). Each included trial compares two or more eligible treatments and trials should be as similar to each other as possible in terms of the included patients or settings to avoid or limit variability. The extent of available data can be presented as a web-like diagram called a network, showing where there are direct comparisons of treatment available from within one or more trials; and the relative strength of such evidence (using weighting similar to that as described for fixed- and random-effects models). A meta-analysis model is then fitted that allows information to "flow" through the network and borrowing of strength to occur between treatment comparisons, as well as providing information on any missing treatment comparisons. One common application of such a model is to rank multiple treatments in order of their efficacy compared with a common reference treatment.

STRUCTURED PRESENTATION OF RESULTS

Appropriately conducted systematic reviews provide a comprehensive and objective summary of all available evidence. However, to enable users to assess the validity of the methodology used, the assessments made, and the interpretation, structured and transparent reporting is vital. With this in mind, in 2005, a group of systematic reviewers, editors, clinicians, and others developed the PRISMA statement, which was first published in 2009 (3,4). The aim of the PRISMA statement and accompanying checklist was to improve the reporting of systematic reviews and meta-analyses. Published alongside the original statement was a paper giving further explanation to review authors on good practice in reporting, using a series of examples for each item on the checklist (83). The checklist details 27 items that should be included in every systematic review and meta-analysis report as well as a flow diagram that shows the flow of information through the review process (Figure 37.1). The statement has now been endorsed and taken up by a number of organizations including the Cochrane Collaboration, Council of Science Editors, and the World Association of Medical Editors, as well as several hundred journals that publish systematic reviews across healthcare. Since the launch of the original PRISMA statement, a number of extensions have been developed to facilitate the reporting of different types of systematic reviews (e.g. IPD meta-analyses [(84)]) as well as the reporting of abstracts (85) and protocols (86) of systematic reviews.

Impact of Systematic Reviews and Meta-Analyses

Clear and detailed reporting of results (4,86) allows for ease of understanding and facilitates the use of systematic reviews and meta-analysis. Because they are generally considered to be the highest level of evidence, and often resolve uncertainty about a particular healthcare intervention, systematic reviews have a key role in informing evidence-based clinical guideline recommendations and thus influencing clinical practice. In particular, systematic reviews based on IPD can often help guideline developers to make more nuanced recommendations by targeting particular treatments to those individuals who might benefit the most (87). However, the potential impact of

a systematic review can be further enhanced through timely publication. It should be noted that publication in medical journals alone may not maximize the potential impact of a systematic review, which may require making the publication freely available or engaging directly with guideline developers or patient advocacy organizations.

Systematic reviews and meta-analyses also have great potential to influence different stages of clinical research. Systematic reviews can inform the design (88), explain the rationale for (89–91), or directly influence new trials (90,91); for example, providing sufficient justification for the initiation of a new trial by identifying gaps in the existing evidence or informing the design and/or conduct of an ongoing trial by considering the external evidence. Because they often provide more detailed and reliable results, and a greater depth of understanding, well-conducted IPD meta-analyses thus have even greater potential to inform the design,

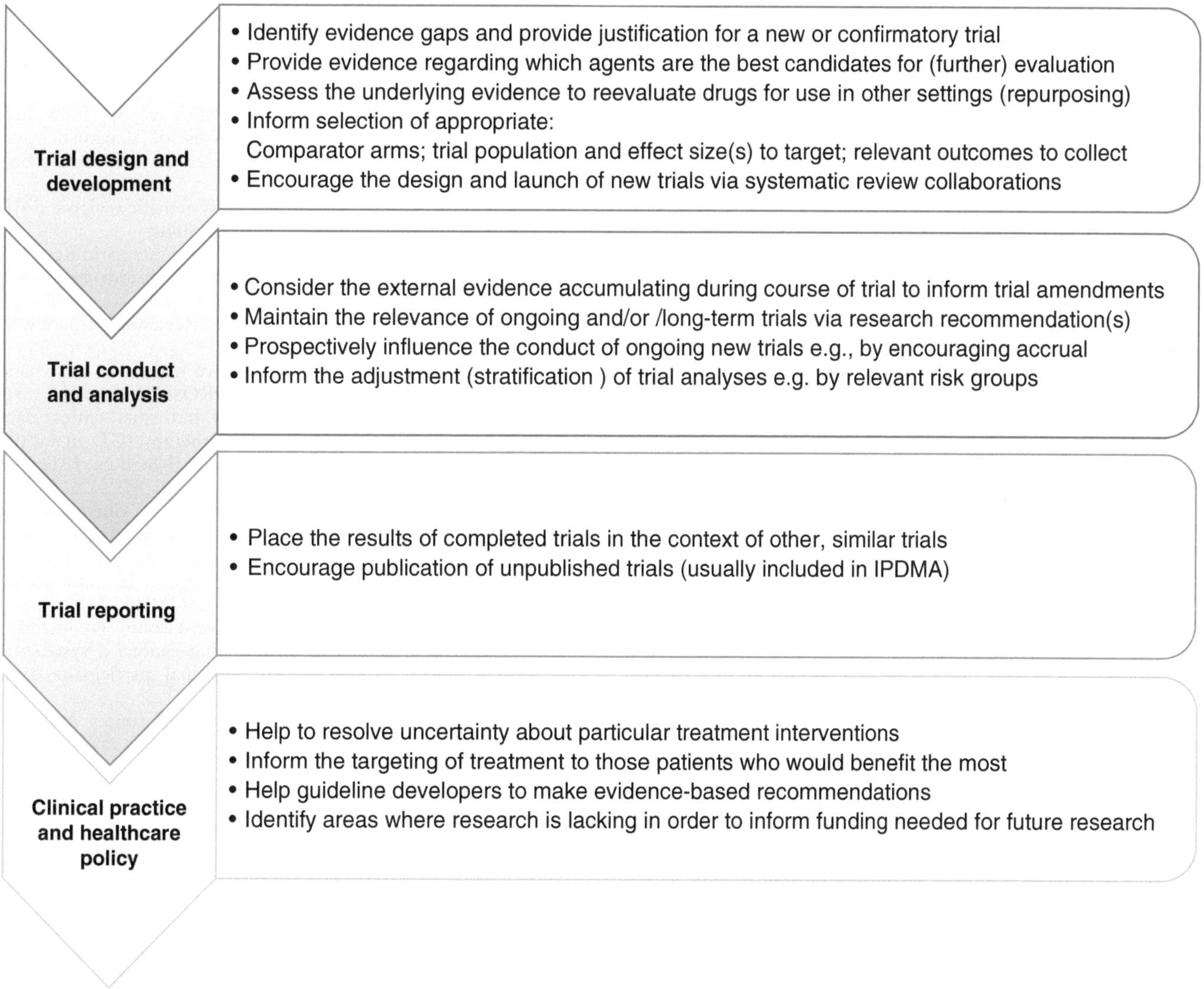

Trial design and development
- Identify evidence gaps and provide justification for a new or confirmatory trial
- Provide evidence regarding which agents are the best candidates for (further) evaluation
- Assess the underlying evidence to reevaluate drugs for use in other settings (repurposing)
- Inform selection of appropriate:
  Comparator arms; trial population and effect size(s) to target; relevant outcomes to collect
- Encourage the design and launch of new trials via systematic review collaborations

Trial conduct and analysis
- Consider the external evidence accumulating during course of trial to inform trial amendments
- Maintain the relevance of ongoing and/or /long-term trials via research recommendation(s)
- Prospectively influence the conduct of ongoing new trials e.g., by encouraging accrual
- Inform the adjustment (stratification) of trial analyses e.g. by relevant risk groups

Trial reporting
- Place the results of completed trials in the context of other, similar trials
- Encourage publication of unpublished trials (usually included in IPDMA)

Clinical practice and healthcare policy
- Help to resolve uncertainty about particular treatment interventions
- Inform the targeting of treatment to those patients who would benefit the most
- Help guideline developers to make evidence-based recommendations
- Identify areas where research is lacking in order to inform funding needed for future research

FIGURE 37.3 Impact of systematic reviews and meta-analysis throughout the clinical research process.

IPDMA, individual patient data meta-analysis.

conduct, analysis, and reporting of new or ongoing clinical trials (Figure 37.3) (92). The collective approach of systematic reviews based on IPD can also speed up the design and launch of new trials initiated by members of the collaborative group (63). Systematic reviews can also help place the results of a clinical trial in the context of the results of other related trials, and many journals now require this as part of the reporting standards for clinical trials (43).

SUMMARY

Systematic reviews and meta-analyses provide reliable and up-to-date evidence in oncology. Provided they are well designed, properly conducted, follow rigorous methodology, and are clearly reported, in accordance with appropriate guidelines, their results have the power and precision to guide clinical practice and policy. In addition, they can highlight where uncertainties about treatments persist, providing justification for further clinical research and informing future trials.

REFERENCES

1. Green S, Higgins JPT, Alderson P, et al. Introduction. In: Higgins JPT, Green S, eds. *Cochrane Handbook for Systematic Reviews of Interventions. Version 5.1.0.* The Cochrane Collaboration; 2011.
2. Green S, Higgins JPT. Preparing a cochrane review. In: Higgins JPT, Green S, eds. *Cochrane Handbook for Systematic Reviews of Interventions. Version 5.1.0.* The Cochrane Collaboration; 2011.
3. Preferred Reporting Items for Systematic Reviews and Meta-Analyses. http://prisma-statement.org
4. Moher D, Liberati A, Tetzlaff J, et al. Preferred reporting items for systematic reviews and meta-analyses: the PRISMA statement. *PLoS Med.* 2009;6(7):e1000097. doi:1000010.1001371/journal.pmed.1000097
5. Stewart LA, Clarke MJ, on behalf of the Cochrane Working Party Group on Meta-analysis using Individual Patient Data. Practical methodology of meta-analyses (overviews) using updated individual patient data. *Stat Med.* 1995;14:2057–2079.
6. Stewart LA, Tierney JF. To IPD or not to IPD? Advantages and disadvantages of systematic reviews using individual patient data. *Eval Health Prof.* 2002;25(1):76–97.
7. Early Breast Cancer Trialists Collaborative Group. Effects of adjuvant tamoxifen and of cytotoxic therapy on mortality in early breast cancer. *New Engl J Med.* 1988;319(26):1681–1692.
8. Meta-analysis Group in Cancer. Toxicity of fluorouracil in patients with advanced colorectal cancer: effect of administration scehdule and prognostic factors. *J Clin Oncol.* 1998;16(11):3537–3541.
9. Pignon JP, Bourhis J, Domenge C, Designé L, on behalf of the MACH-NC Collaborative Group. Chemotherapy added to locoregional treatment for head and neck squamous cell carcinoma: three meta-analyses of updated individual data. *Lancet.* 2000;355(9208):949–955.
10. Non-small Cell Lung Cancer Collaborative Group. Chemotherapy in non-small cell lung cancer: a meta-analysis using updated data on individual patients from 52 randomised clinical trials. *BMJ.* 1995;311:899–909.
11. Duchateau L, Pignon J-P, Bijnens L, et al. Individual patient-versus literature-based meta-analysis of survival data: time to event and event rate at a particular time can make a difference, an example based on head and neck cancer. *Control Clin Trials.* 2001;22(5):538–547.
12. Jeng GT, Scott JR, Burmeister LF. A comparison of meta-analytic results using literature versus individual patient data: paternal cell immunization for recurrent miscarriage. *J Am Med Assoc.* 1995;274:840–836.
13. Stewart LA, Parmar MKB. Meta-analysis of the literature or of individual patient data: is there a difference? *Lancet.* 1993;341:418–422.
14. Collaboration EHT. Value of updating a systematic review in surgery using individual patient data. *Br J Surgery.* 2004;91:495–499.
15. O'Connor D, Green S, Higgins JPT. Defining the review question and developing criteria for including studies. In: Higgins JPT, Green S, eds. *Cochrane Handbook of Systematic Reviews of Intervention. Version 5.1.0.* The Cochrane Collaboration; 2011.
16. Schünemann HJ, Oxman AD, Vist GE, et al. Interpreting results and drawing conclusions. In: Higgins JPT, Green S, eds. *Cochrane Handbook for Systematic Reviews of Interventions. Version 5.1.0.* The Cochrane Collaboration; 2011.
17. Altman DG. Systematic reviews of evaluations of prognostic variables. *BMJ.* 2001;323:224–228.
18. Leeflang MM, Deeks JJ, Gatsonis C, Bossuyt PM, Cochrane diagnostic test accuracy working group. Systematic reviews of diagnostic test accuracy. *Ann Internal Med.* 2008;149(12):889–897.
19. Debray TP, Riley RD, Rovers MM, et al. Individual participant data (IPD) meta-analyses of diagnostic and prognostic modeling studies: guidance on their use. *PLoS Med.* 2015;12(10):e1001886.
20. Moher D. The problem of duplicate systematic reviews. *BMJ.* 2013;347:f5040. doi:5010.1136/bmj.f5040
21. Centre for Reviews and Dissemination. Systematic Reviews: CRD's guidance for undertaking reviews in health care. York, UK: CRD, University of York; 2009.
22. Cochrane Database of Systematic Reviews. http://www.thecochranelibrary.com
23. PROSPERO: International prospective register of systematic reviews. http://www.crd.york.ac.uk/PROSPERO/prospero.asp
24. Le Pechoux C, Burdett S, Auperin A. Individual patient data (IPD) meta-analysis (MA) of chemotherapy (CT) in locally advanced non-small cell lung cancer (NSCLC). *J Thorac Oncol.* 2008;3(4, Suppl 1):S20, 35IN.
25. NSCLC Meta-analyses Collaborative Group. Chemotherapy in addition to supportive care improves survival in advanced non-small-cell lung cancer: a systematic review and meta-analysis of individual patient data from 16 randomized controlled trials. *J Clin Oncol.* 2008;26(28):4617–4625.
26. NSCLC Meta-analysis Collaborative Group. Preoperative chemotherapy for non-small cell lung cancer: a systematic review and meta-analysis of individual participant data. *Lancet.* 2014;383:1561–1571.
27. NSCLC Meta-analyses Collaborative Group. Adjuvant chemotherapy, with or without postoperative radiotherapy, in operable non-small cell lung cancer: two meta-analyses of individual patient data. *Lancet.* 2010;375(9722):1267–1277.
28. Burdett S, Stewart L, Rydzewska L. A systematic review and meta-analysis of the literature: chemotherapy and surgery versus surgery alone in non-small cell lung cancer. *J Thorac Oncol.* 2006;1(7):611–621.
29. Cochrane Central Register of Controlled Trials (CENTRAL). http://www.cochranelibrary.com/about/central-landing-page.html
30. Lefebvre C, Manheimer E, Glanville J. Searching for studies. In: Higgins JPT, Green S, eds. *Cochrane Handbook for*

Systematic Reviews of Interventions. Version 5.1.0. The Cochrane Collaboration; 2011.

31. Page MJ, Shamseer L, Altman DG, et al. Epidemiology and reporting charateristics of systematics reviews of biomedical research: a cross-sectional study. *PLoS Med.* 2016;13(5):e1002028.

32. Ahmed I, Sutton AJ, Riley RD. Assessment of publication bias, selection bias, and unavailable data in meta-analyses using individual participant data: a database survey. *BMJ.* 2012;344:d7762.

33. Dickersin K. Publication bias: recognising the problem, understanding its origins and scope, and preventing harm. In: Rothstein H, Sutton A, Borenstein M, eds. *Publication Bias in Meta-Analysis: Prevention, Assessment and Adjustments.* Chichester: John Wiley & Sons Ltd; 2005:261–286.

34. Hopewell S, Clarke M, Stewart L, Tierney J. Time to publication for results of clinical trials. *Cochrane Database Syst Rev.* 2007;(2):Art. No.: MR000011. doi:000010.001002/14651858.MR14000011.pub14651852

35. von Elm E, Poglia G, Walder B, Tramèr MR. Different patterns of duplicate publication: an analysis of articles used in systematic reviews. *JAMA.* 2004;291(8):974–980.

36. Easterbrook PJ, Berlin JA, Gopalan R, Matthews DR. Publication bias in clinical research. *Lancet.* 1991;337(8746):867–872.

37. Gøtzsche PC. Reference bias in reports of drug trials. *BMJ.* 1987;295:654–656.

38. Juni P, Holenstein F, Sterne J, et al. Direction and impact of language bias in meta-analyses of controlled trials: empirical study. *Inter J Epidemiol.* 2002;31(1):115–123.

39. Kirkham JJ, Dwan KM, Altman DG, et al. The impact of outcome reporting bias in randomised controlled trials on a cohort of systematic reviews. *BMJ.* 2010;340:c365.

40. Higgins JPT, Altman DG, Sterne JAC. Assessing risk of bias in included studies. In: Higgins JPT, Green S, eds. *Cochrane Handbook for Systematic Reviews of Interventions Version 5.1.0.* The Cochrane Collaboration; 2011.

41. Scherer RW, Langenberg P, von Elm E. Full publication of results initially presented in abstracts. *Cochrane Database Syst Rev.* 2007;(2):MR000005.

42. Altman DG. Better reporting of randomised controlled trials: the CONSORT statement. *BMJ.* 1996;313:570–571.

43. Hopewell S, Clarke M, Moher D, et al. CONSORT for reporting randomised trials in journal and conference abstracts. *Lancet.* 2008;371(9609):281–283.

44. Stewart L, Tierney J, Burdett S. Do systematic reviews based on individual patient data offer a means of circumventing biases associated with trial publications? In: Rothstein H, Sutton A, Borenstein M, eds. *Publication Bias in Meta-Analysis: Prevention, Assessment and Adjustments.* Chichester: John Wiley & Sons; 2005: 261–286.

45. Tierney JF, Vale CL, Riley R, et al. Individual participant data (IPD) meta-analyses of randomised controlled trials: guidance on their use. *PLoS Med.* 2015;12(7):e1001855.

46. Higgins JP, Altman DG, Gøtzsche PC, et al. The Cochrane Collaboration's tool for assessing risk of bias in randomised trials. *BMJ.* 2011;343:d5928.

47. Vale CL, Tierney JF, Burdett S. Can trial quality be reliably assessed from published reports of cancer trials: evaluation of risk of bias assessments in systematic reviews. *BMJ.* 2013;346: f1798.

48. Mhaskar R, Djulbegovic B, Magazin A, et al. Published methodological quality of randomized controlled trials does not reflect the actual quality assessed in protocols. *J Clin Epidemiol.* 2012;65(6):602–609.

49. Hartling L, Bond K, Vandermeer B, et al. Applying the risk of bias tool in a systematic review of combination long-acting beta-agonists and inhaled corticosteroids for persistent asthma. *PLoS One.* 2011;6(2):e17242.

50. Jordan VM, Lensen SF, Farquhar C. There were large discrepancies in risk of bias tool judgements when a randomized controlled trial appeared in more than one systematic review. *J Clin Epidemiol.* 2016.

51. Sterne JAC, Egger M, Moher D. Addressing reporting biases. In: Higgins JPT, Green S, eds. *Cochrane Handbook for Systematic Reviews of Intervention. Version 5.1.0.* The Cochrane Collaboration; 2011.

52. Jorgensen L, Paludan-Muller AS, Laursen DR, et al. Evaluation of the Cochrane tool for assessing risk of bias in randomized clinical trials: overview of published comments and analysis of user practice in Cochrane and non-Cochrane reviews. *Syst Rev.* 2016;5(80).

53. Simmonds MC, Higgins JPT, Stewart LA, et al. Meta-analysis of individual patient data from randomised trials - a review of methods used in practice. *Clin Trials.* 2005;2(3):209–217.

54. Simmonds M, Stewart G, Stewart L. A decade of individual participant data meta-analyses: a review of current practice. *Contemp Clin Trials.* 2015.

55. Olkin I, Sampson A. Comparison of meta-analysis versus analysis of variance of individual patient data. *Biometrics.* 1998;54:317–322.

56. Mathew T, Nordstrom K. On the equivalence of meta-analysis using literature and using individual patient data. *Biometrics.* 1999;55(4):1221–1223.

57. Mathew T, Nordstrom K. Comparison of one-step and two-step meta-analysis models using individual patient data. *Biom J.* 2010;52(2):271–287.

58. Tudur Smith C, Williamson PR. A comparison of methods for fixed effects meta-analysis of individual patient data with time to event outcomes. *Clin Trials.* 2007;4(6):621–630.

59. Bowden J, Tierney JF, Simmonds M, Copas AJ. Individual patient data meta-analysis of time-to-event outcomes: one-stage versus two-stage approaches for estimating the hazard ratio under a random effects model. *Res Synth Methods.* 2011;2(3):150–162.

60. Stewart GB, Altman DG, Askie LM, et al. Statistical analysis of individual participant data meta-analyses: a comparison of methods and recommendations for practice. *PLoS One.* 2012;7(10):e46042.

61. Koopman L, van der Heijden GJ, Hoes AW, et al. Empirical comparison of subgroup effects in conventional and individual patient data meta-analyses. *Inter J Technol Assess Health Care.* 2008;24(3):358–361.

62. Stijnen T, Hamza TH, Ozdemir P. Random effects meta-analysis of event outcome in the framework of the generalized linear mixed model with applications in sparse data. *Stat Med.* 2010;29(29):3046–3067.

63. Vale CL, Burdett S, Rydzewska LH, et al. Addition of docetaxel or bisphosphonates to standard of care in men with localised or metastatic, hormone-sensitive prostate cancer: a systematic review and meta-analyses of aggregate data. *Lancet Oncol.* 2016;17(2):243–256.

64. Deeks JJ, Higgins JPT, Altman DG. Analysing data and undertaking meta-analyses. In: Higgins JPT, Green S, eds. *Cochrane Handbook for Systematic Reviews of Interventions Version 5.1.0.* The Cochrane Collaboration; 2011.

65. Higgins JPT, Thompson SG, Deeks JJ, Altman DG. Measuring inconsistency in meta-analyses. *BMJ.* 2003;327:557–560.

66. Yusuf S, Peto R, Lewis J, et al. Beta blockade during and after myocardial infarction: an overview of the randomized trials. *Prog Cardiovasc Dis.* 1985;27:335–371.

67. Mantel N, Haenszel W. Statistical aspects of the analysis of data from retrospective studies of disease. *J Natl Cancer Inst.* 1959;22(4):719–748.

68. DerSimonian R, Laird N. Meta-analysis in clinical trials. *Control Clin Trials.* 1986;7;177–188.

69. PORT Meta-analysis Trialists Group. Postoperative radiotherapy for non-small cell lung cancer. *Cochrane Database Syst Rev.* 2005;(2):Art. No.: CD002142. doi:002110 .001002/14651858.CD14002142.pub14651852

70. Neoadjuvant Chemotherapy for Cervix Cancer Meta-analysis (NACCCMA) Collaboration. Neoadjuvant chemotherapy for locally advanced cervical cancer: a systematic review and meta-analysis of individual patient data from 21 randomised trials. *Eur J Cancer.* 2003;39(17):2470–2486.

71. Bowden J, Tierney JF, Copas AJ, Burdett S. Quantifying, displaying and accounting for heterogeneity in the meta-analysis of RCTs using standard and generalised Q statistics. *BMC Med Res Methodol.* 2011;11:41.

72. Higgins JPT, Thompson SG. Quantifying heterogeneity in a meta-analysis. *Stat Med.* 2002;21:1539–1558.

73. Berlin JA, Santanna J, Schmid CH, et al. Individual patient-versus group-level data meta-regressions for the investigation of treatment effect modifiers: ecological bias rears its ugly head. *Stat Med.* 2002;21(3):371–387.

74. Stewart LA, Tierney JF, Clarke M, on behalf of the Cochrane Individual Patient Data Meta-analysis Methods Group. Reviews of individual patient data. In: Higgins JPT, Green S, eds. *Cochrane Handbook for Systematic Reviews of Interventions Version 510 (updated March 2011).* Chichester, UK: Wiley-Blackwell; 2011: 547–558.

75. Early Breast Cancer Trialists' Collaborative Group (EBCTCG), Clarke M, Coates AS, et al. Adjuvant chemotherapy in oestrogen-receptor-poor breast cancer: patient-level meta-analysis of randomised trials. *Lancet.* 2008;371(9606):29–40.

76. Fisher DJ, Copas AJ, Tierney JF, Parmar MKB. A critical review of methods for the assessment of patient-level interactions in individual patient data (IPD) meta-analysis of randomised trials, and guidance for practitioners. *J Clin Epidemiol.* 2011;64:949–967.

77. Sterne JA, Sutton AJ, Ioannidis JP, et al. Recommendations for examining and interpreting funnel plot asymmetry in meta-analyses of randomised controlled trials. *BMJ.* 2011;343:d4002.

78. Ioannidis JP, Trikalinos TA. The appropriateness of asymmetry tests for publication bias in meta-analyses: a large survey. *CMAJ.* 2007;176(8):1091–1096.

79. National Health Service England. Clinical commissioning policy statement: docetaxel in combination with androgen deprivation therapy for the treatment of hormone naïve metastatic prostate cancer. https://www.england.nhs.uk/wp-content/uploads/2016/01/b15psa-docetaxel-policy-statement.pdf

80. Sylvester R, Sternberg C. The role of adjuvant combination chemotherapy after cystectomy in locally advanced bladder cancer: what we do not know and why. *Ann Oncol.* 2000;11:851–856.

81. Advanced Bladder Cancer (ABC) Meta-analysis Collaboration. Adjuvant chemotherapy in invasive bladder cancer: a systematic review and meta-analysis of individual patient data. *Eur Urol.* 2005;48(2):189–201.

82. Cipriani A, Higgins JP, Geddes JR, Salanti G. Conceptual and technical challenges in network meta-analysis. *Ann Inter Med.* 2013;159(2):130–137.

83. Liberati A, Altman DG, Tetzlaff J, et al. The PRISMA statement for reporting systematic reviews and meta-analyses of studies that evaluate healthcare interventions: explanation and elaboration. *BMJ.* 2009;339:b2700.

84. Stewart LA, Clarke M, Rovers M, et al. Preferred reporting items for a systematic review and meta-analysis of individual participant data: the PRISMA-IPD statement. *JAMA.* 2015;313(16):1657–1665.

85. Beller EM, Glasziou PP, Altman DG, et al. PRISMA for abstracts: reporting systematic reviews in journal and conference abstracts. *PLoS Med.* 2013;10(4):e1001419. doi:1001410.1001371/journal.pmed.1001419

86. Moher D, Shamseer L, Clarke M, et al. Preferred reporting items for systematic review and meta-analysis protocols (PRISMA-P) 2015 statement. *Syst Rev.* 2015;4:1.

87. Vale CL, Rydzewska LHM, Rovers MM, et al. Uptake of systematic reviews and meta-analyses based on individual participant data in clinical practice guidelines: descriptive study. *BMJ.* 2015;350:h1088.

88. Clarke M. Doing new research? Don't forget the old. *PLoS Med.* 2004;1(2):e35.

89. Cooper NJ, Jones DR, Sutton AJ. The use of systematic reviews when designing studies. *Clin Trials.* 2005;2(3):260–264.

90. Clarke M, Hopewell S, Chalmers I. Clinical trials should begin and end with systematic reviews of relevant evidence: 12 years and waiting. *Lancet.* 2010;376(9734):20–21.

91. Jones AP, Conroy E, Williamson PR, et al. The use of systematic reviews in the planning, design and conduct of randomised trials: a retrospective cohort of NIHR HTA funded trials. *BMC Med Res Methodol.* 2013;13:50.

92. Tierney JF, Pignon J-P, Gueffyier F, et al. How individual participant data meta-analyses can influence trial design and conduct *J Clin Epidemiol.* 2015;68(11):1325–1335.

Statistical Methods for Genomics-Driven Clinical Studies

Richard Simon

The application of high-throughput biotechnology to human tumors has led to improved understanding of tumor biology and is driving new strategies of drug development and clinical trial design. Tumors of the same primary site are often different with regard to the mutations and cellular programs that drive their invasion and also differ with regard to their sensitivity to treatments. Whole-genome assays can be used to characterize individual tumors and select appropriate treatments. The focus has changed to development of molecularly targeted treatments with companion diagnostic tests for guiding their use. The diagnostics can be based on "big data" genomic classifiers or on "small data" biomarkers indicating the genomic alteration status of the drug target. In this chapter we discuss the use of biomarkers in oncology therapeutics development, new clinical trial designs that are increasingly used, and statistical methods for development and validation of high-dimensional genomic classifiers.

KINDS OF BIOMARKERS

Traditionally a biomarker was thought of as a biological measurement that tracks the "pace" of a disease, increasing as the disease progresses and decreasing as the disease regresses. In clinical trials, such biomarkers are sometimes used as "endpoint biomarkers" or intermediate endpoints. Pharmacodynamic biomarkers are useful in phase I trials to determine whether the drug is having its intended biological effect. Intermediate endpoints are also generally used in phase II trials to evaluate whether the drug is having an effect on tumor proliferation or progression. It is more controversial to use an endpoint biomarker in phase III trials because it is very difficult to establish that an intermediate endpoint is a true surrogate for a clinical endpoint like survival (1,2).

The term biomarker is used today in many ways other than the original one. In discussing biomarkers, it is important to remember that the intended use of a biomarker is the key feature in determining how to develop and validate it as "fit for purpose."

Predictive Biomarkers

A predictive biomarker has come to mean a biological measurement made before treatment whose purpose is to enable prediction of whether the patient will benefit from a particular treatment. For example, in patients with metastatic breast cancer, estrogen receptor content of the tumor is a predictive biomarker for tamoxifen treatment. Amplification of the HER2 gene is a predictive biomarker for trastuzumab treatment in breast cancer (3) and the V600E point mutation in BRAF is a predictive biomarker for the effectiveness of vemurafenib in patients with melanoma (4). For drugs developed to inhibit an oncogene protein product that is activated by a genomic mutation, presence of the mutation often serves as a predictive biomarker for the effectiveness of the drug.

In some cases, finding the appropriate predictive biomarker to determine the effectiveness of a drug can be more difficult. For example, with anti-EGFR antibodies used in the treatment of advanced colorectal cancer, the presence of a RAS mutation turned out to be a predictive biomarker indicating the ineffectiveness of the antibodies (5). For drugs with more complicated mechanisms of action such as antiangiogenic agents and T lymphocyte checkpoint inhibitors identification of the appropriate predictive biomarker has been more difficult.

To evaluate a predictive biomarker when survival or disease-free survival (DFS) is the endpoint one needs a randomized study of the test treatment versus a control regimen. The curves for treated versus control patients should be separated in the biomarker positive patients but not separated for the biomarker negative patients.

Prognostic Biomarkers

Prognostic markers are baseline measurements that provide information about the likely long-term outcome of patients either untreated or with standard treatment. Prognostic biomarkers can be used to help determine whether a patient requires any systematic treatment or any beyond the standard treatment used for the patients in the study.

The oncology literature is replete with publications on prognostic factors but very few of these are used in clinical practice. Prognostic factors are rarely used unless they help with therapeutic decision making. Most prognostic factor studies are conducted using a convenience sample of patients whose tissues are available. Often these patients are too heterogeneous with regard to treatment, stage, and standard prognostic factors to support therapeutically relevant conclusions (6,7).

Many publications attempt to show that new factors are "independently prognostic" based on multivariate analysis. Usually this is done because the patients are too heterogeneous. A multivariate analysis, however, is an inadequate solution to the problem of case selection that is not therapeutically relevant. It is better to select patients for the study, prospective or retrospective, who are relevant based on stage and treatment for the intended use of the classifier. Then simply classify the patients using the new tool and determine whether the separation is useful for patient management. If there are established prognostic factors that can be used to classify the therapeutically homogeneous subsets of patients, it is much better to evaluate whether the new classifier is predictive of outcome within the levels of the standard factors than it is to do a multivariate analysis. A good example of a prognostic signature with clinical utility is the Oncotype DX breast cancer recurrence score (8). It is based on the expression levels of 21 genes and the developmental study was done in patients who had node-negative, ER-positive breast cancer treated only with local treatment and tamoxifen. A score was developed to identify women whose DFS was sufficiently good that they might elect to forgo cytotoxic therapy. Prognostic factors developed in such a focused manner can be relevant for therapeutic decisions. The score is often used as a classifier by introducing two cut points to distinguish patients with low, moderate, and high risks of tumor recurrence.

Prognostic classifiers can be therapeutically relevant if they identify a set of patients who have such a good prognosis without aggressive systemic therapy that they may choose to be spared the risks and inconvenience of such therapy and forgo the small potential benefit. Such a classifier needs to be independently validated before it is "ready for prime time." Validation can be ideally accomplished by prospectively applying the classifier to new patients who are considered to require systemic therapy by standard-of-care methods, identifying those considered low risk based on the new classifier and withholding intensive systemic therapy from them. This is the approach being used to validate Oncotype DX in the TAILORx study (9) and the Netherlands Cancer Institute 70-gene signature in the MINDACT study (10) for patients with node-negative primary breast cancer. Both studies involve up-front testing of all entered patients with node-negative breast cancer after local therapy and endocrine therapy for ER-positive patients. The primary analysis of both studies involves estimation of distant-metastasis-free survival in patients predicted to be low risk by the multigene signature for whom cytotoxic therapy is withheld. Such fully prospective studies are expensive and time-consuming however. In some cases, effective validation of a classifier predictive of low recurrence risk can be accomplished using a "prospective–retrospective" method using specimens archived from an appropriate clinical trial that withheld chemotherapy from such patients. Convincing results are only possible, however, if the number of patients is sufficiently large, if the proportion with available specimens adequate for testing is high, and if careful analytical and preanalytical validation provides assurance that assay results on archived samples are accurate predictors of assay results on fresh tissue (11).

A prognostic biomarker can also be used to identify patients whose outcome is very poor under standard chemotherapy. Such patients may be good candidates for experimental regimens. But unless there is a viable therapeutic option, such prognostic biomarkers may not be widely used in general practice.

CLINICAL TRIALS WITH PREDICTIVE BIOMARKERS

A predictive biomarker can substantially enhance the effectiveness of drug development. For example, approval of trastuzumab for treatment of metastatic breast cancer was based on a phase III randomized clinical trial that restricted entry to patients with overexpression of the HER2 protein or amplification of the gene (3). Approximately 25% of screened patients qualified for eligibility. The benefit of trastuzumab in the randomized trial of 469 patients was statistically significant, but not overwhelming. Had the biomarker not been measured and used to restrict eligibility, it is almost certain that the difference in outcome for the group as a whole would have been so diluted by lack of effectiveness of trastuzumab in patients who do not overexpress HER2 that the trial would have been negative.

Registration trials or trials that establish a new standard of care usually use an endpoint like overall survival (OS), DFS, or progression-free survival as the primary endpoint. Such trials are generally randomized comparing a regimen containing the new drug to a standard-of-care regimen. Usually such trials are preceded by phase II trials in which it is established that the biomarker is effective for identifying patients whose tumors cause tumor shrinkage.

Phase II Designs

In many cases there is sufficient biological evidence that the effectiveness of the test drug will be limited to "biomarker positive" patients; for example, those whose tumors contain the mutated oncogene for which the drug was developed. In such cases "biomarker negative" patients are excluded and a standard "Simon Optimal 2-Stage Design" is used (12).

When there is a question about whether one has the correct predictive biomarker, it is best not to exclude patients based on the candidate biomarker. Rather it is preferable to treat a broader selection of patients in phase II and to measure all relevant candidate biomarkers. In the case of a single binary candidate biomarker, Freidlin et al. have described a useful phase II design (13).

There are an increasing number of molecularly targeted drugs that have been approved for marketing for patients with a specified histologic type of cancer in which the tumor contains a specific genomic alteration. The question then becomes whether that same drug would be effective in patients whose tumors contain the same genomic alteration but in different histologic types of cancer than the one for which the drug was approved. The basket clinical trial was developed for this setting (14,15). Basket trials have become very popular. Generally they are not randomized clinical trials; all patients with the genomic alteration needed for eligibility are assigned the targeted therapy. Some multicenter or national basket trials are conducted with a large number of targeted drugs. Patients have their tumors tested for a panel of genomic alterations and are then triaged to the drug that targets the most prominent alteration in their tumors (16). Table 38.1 provides key characteristics of the basket design and some of the other recent biomarker-driven designs.

Phase III or II/III Designs

Enrichment Design

The objective of a phase III pivotal clinical trial is to evaluate whether a new drug, given in a defined manner, has medical utility for a defined set of patients. Pivotal trials test prespecified hypotheses about treatment effectiveness in specified patient population groups. The role of a predictive classifier is to prospectively specify the population of patients in whom the new treatment will be evaluated. By prospectively specifying the patient population in a manner defined in the protocol, one ensures that adequate numbers of such patients are available, and one avoids the problems of post hoc subset analysis. The process of classifier development may be exploratory and subjective based on data collected prior to the phase III trial, but the use of the classifier in the phase III trial should generally not be.

The enrichment design is a randomized phase III design in which eligibility is restricted to the patients who are "biomarker positive," that is, have the genomic alteration that makes their tumors more likely to respond to the test drug. This approach was used for the development of trastuzumab. Simon and Maitournam (17,18) studied the efficiency of this approach relative to the standard approach of randomizing all patients without measuring the diagnostic. They found that the efficiency of the enrichment design depended on the prevalence of test positive patients and on the effectiveness of the new treatment in test negative patients. For binary endpoint trials, they showed that the ratio of number of events (e.g., deaths) needed for the standard trial compared to the enrichment trial is approximately

$$E_{standard}/E_{enrichment} = \{(p_+\delta_+ + p_-\delta_-)/\delta_+\}^2 \qquad \text{(Eq. 38-1)}$$

where p_+ is the proportion of patients who are biomarker positive, p_- is the proportion biomarker negative, δ_+ is the log hazard ratio of treatment effect for biomarker positive patients, and δ_- is the log hazard ratio of treatment effect for biomarker negative patients In cases where the new treatment is completely ineffective in test negative patients, this formula simplifies to approximately $(1/p_+)^2$, which is 16 when only one quarter of the patients are biomarker

TABLE 38.1 Major Characteristics of Genomics-Driven Trial Designs

Design	Histology	Genomic Alteration	Phase	Randomized	Treatments Per Genomic Alteration
Basket	Multiple	One	II	No usually	1
Multidrug basket	Multiple	Multiple	II	No usually	1
Enrichment	One	One	III	Yes	1
Umbrella	One	Multiple	III usually	Yes usually	1

positive. If the new treatment is half as effective in biomarker negative patients as in biomarker positive patients, then the right-hand side of expression (Eq. 38-1) equals about 2.56 when 25% of the patients are test positive, indicating that the enrichment design reduces the number of required patients to randomize by a factor of 2.56.

When fewer than half of the patients are test positive and the new treatment is relatively ineffective in test negative patients, the number of randomized patients required for an enrichment design is often dramatically smaller than the number of randomized patients required for a standard design. This was the case for trastuzumab. The enrichment design that led to the approval of trastuzumab was conducted in 469 patients with metastatic breast cancer whose tumors overexpressed HER2 based on immunohistochemical analysis in a central laboratory. If benefit from the drug were limited to the 25% of patients expected to be test positive, then the overall improvement in 1-year survival rate would be only 3.375% for a standard design and a total of about 8,050 patients would be required for 90% power to detect such a small effect. This is 17.2 times as many patients as for the enrichment design, in good agreement with the ratio of 16 computed from the approximate form of equation (Eq. 38-1).

Focusing initial development on test positive patients can lead to clarity in determining who benefits from the drug. If the enrichment design establishes that the drug is effective in test positive patients, the drug could be later developed in test negative patients if the test was considered to have a substantial false-negative-error rate. This is preferable to testing new drugs in heterogeneous populations resulting in false-negative results for the overall population.

Umbrella Designs

Umbrella designs are multiple enrichment designs of the same histologic type conducted with a common infrastructure for characterization of the patients' tumors (Table 38.1). If the patient's tumor has a genomic alteration that makes him or her eligible for one of the enrichment designs, then he or she is triaged to that trial. Each clinical trial has additional eligibility considerations, which must be evaluated because the adverse effects of the drugs in the different enrichment designs are not the same. Once triaged, the patient will be asked to provide informed consent to that particular enrichment trial. Enrichment trials are generally randomized trials of patients with the same histologic type of cancer bearing the same genomic alteration. In an umbrella trial, all the patients have the same histologic type of cancer but different genomic alterations corresponding to the different component enrichment designs. Each enrichment design is sized independently. The enrichment designs may or may not use the same control treatment regimen but there is no pooling of information because patients with different genomic alterations must be analyzed

separately. Two recent examples of umbrella clinical trials are the Lung-MAP for patients with advanced squamous cell lung cancer (19) and FOCUS4 for patients with advanced colorectal cancer (20).

Including Both Test Positive and Test Negative Patients

When there is uncertainty about the appropriateness of the candidate biomarker, the biomarker can be measured on all patients but not used as an eligibility criterion; that is, both biomarker positive and biomarker negative patients are enrolled in the randomized phase III trial. A number of authors have introduced two-stage designs (21,22). An interim analysis is performed after the first stage of accrual. If the overall results are promising, accrual of both biomarker positive and negative patients continues. If the overall results are not promising but results for biomarker positive patients are, the accrual for biomarker positive patients continues but accrual of biomarker negative patients ceases. The accrual target for the biomarker positive patients may be increased by the reduced accrual of marker negative patients. If neither the overall results nor the results for marker positive patients are promising, then the trial may be terminated. Although only one significance test is conducted at the end of the second period, the critical level for declaring significance must be adjusted for the interim analysis.

MULTIVARIATE PROGNOSTIC CLASSIFIERS

Prognostic classifiers can be developed that combine the information from several biomarkers. Such classifiers are frequently developed based on genome-wide transcript expression profiling to predict survival risk groups based on combining the contributions for dozens of genes.

Many algorithms have been developed and used effectively with DNA microarray data to develop survival risk classifiers (23). One approach is penalized proportional hazards regression. This assumes that the logarithm of the hazard function depends on the gene expression only through the "predictive index." The predictive index is a weighted linear average of the expression values of the genes. The weights are the regression coefficients. The regression coefficients are determined to maximize the likelihood of the data subject to a penalty term used to avoid overfitting the data. This penalty results in reducing the magnitude of the regression coefficients; in many cases most of the regression coefficients are shrunken to zero. After fitting the model, one is left with a limited number of genes included in the model and the fitted regression coefficients for those genes. The "predictive index" for a patient with gene expression vector $(x_1, x_2, \ldots, x_p)$ is $PI = b_1x_1 + b_2x_2 + \ldots + b_px_p$, where the bs are the corresponding regression coefficients. One can calculate the predictive index for all of the cases in the training data set and select the median value as a cut point for survival risk classification. Those with *PI* values below the cut point have good survival risk relative to those *PI* values above the cut point.

Internal Validation of Multivariate Survival Risk Classifiers

There are special problems in evaluating whether classifiers based on high-dimensional genomic assays are promising using standard statistical methods (24). The difficulty derives from the fact that the number of candidate genes available for use in the classifier is much larger than the number of cases available for analysis. In such situations, it is always possible to find classifiers that accurately classify the data on which they were developed even if there is no relationship between expression of any of the genes and outcome. Consequently, even in developmental studies, some kind of validation on data not used for developing the model is necessary. This "internal validation" is usually accomplished either by splitting the data into two portions, one used for training the model and the other for testing the model, or some form of cross-validation based on repeated model development and testing on random data partitions.

The most straightforward method of estimating the prediction accuracy is the *split-sample* method of partitioning the set of samples into a training set and a test set. Rosenwald et al. (25) used this approach successfully in their international study of prognostic prediction for large B-cell lymphoma. They used two thirds of their samples as a training set. Multiple kinds of prognostic models were studied on the training set. They selected a single model for predicting survival risk as a function of selected gene expression measurements. The fitting and selection of the model used only data from the training set. For each gene expression vector the model provided a predictive index. Using the training data they also established a cut point to separate low-risk from high-risk expression profiles. When the collaborators of that study agreed on a single fully specified prognostic classifier, they accessed the test set for the first time. On the test set there was no adjustment of the model or fitting of parameters. They merely used the samples in the test set to classify the patients as either low risk or high risk for survival. They computed the survival curves for the low-risk patients and for the high-risk patients. The separation between the survival curves indicated the effectiveness of the survival risk classifier.

Complete cross-validation is an alternative to the split-sample method for estimating the accuracy of a prognostic risk classifier (26). One splits the data into, say, five approximately equal disjoint subsets. The first subset is withheld as the test set and the remaining four subsets are pooled into a training set. A multivariate prognostic two-risk group classifier is developed from scratch using the training set and the cases in the test set are classified using it; each case in the test set is classified

as high or low survival risk. Then the second subset is withheld as the test set and the remaining four subsets are pooled into a training set. A new multivariate prognostic two-risk group classifier is developed from scratch using this second training set and the cases in the second test set are classified using it. This process is iterated five times in the obvious way. At the end, all cases have been classified exactly once as either high or low survival risk. All of the classifications were accomplished using a model developed on a training set that the test patient was not a part of. Then using all of the patients, survival curves for the low- and high-risk patients are separately computed. The distance between these curves indicates the strength of the prognostic classification.

The so called *resubstitution* estimate, although commonly used, is very biased. With the *resubstitution* estimate you use all the samples to select the best features (genes) for inclusion in a prognostic model, fit the model, and select a classification cut point. Then you classify the same set of patients as low survival risk or high risk. Survival curves are then computed for the low-risk and high-risk cases. As shown by Subramanian and Simon (6), the separation between the survival curves is highly optimistic compared to what can be expected from independent data with that survival risk classifier. One needs to use either the split-sample method or complete cross-validation.

The methods used to develop these multivariate prognostic classifiers can also be used to develop classifiers that predict binary response to specific treatments. Ghidimi et al. (27) developed a classifier for predicting response to preoperative chemoradiotherapy for patients with rectal cancer and Hess et al. (28) have developed such a classifier for predicting response of patients with breast cancer to preoperative chemotherapy. As with survival data, using the resubstitution estimate of prediction accuracy is highly biased with high-dimensional data like gene expression profiles. That is, one should not use all of the data to fit the binary prediction classifier and then classify the same set of patients using that classifier. One should use either the split-sample method or complete cross-validation.

Although whole-genome transcript expression profiling is a powerful technology for developing prognostic and predictive classifiers, many studies do not use adequate statistical methods and present claims that may not be justified. Dupuy and Simon (7) reviewed 90 studies relating gene expression profiling to cancer outcomes. They found at least one serious problem in 50% of the publications and developed a list of "Dos and Don'ts" for such studies. The BRB-ArrayTools software provides extensive resources for development of a wide range of prognostic and predictive classifiers based on gene expression data for binary response or survival endpoints (29). It was developed for use by biomedical scientists. It provides an environment for developing a classifier on a training set and estimating the accuracy of the model on a test set of data or for using a wide range of valid complete cross-validation and bootstrap resampling methods for estimating the predictive accuracy of the model. BRB-ArrayTools is available for downloading online (http://brb.nci.nih.gov).

CONCLUSIONS

The genomics revolution is influencing clinical trials in fundamental ways. It has become increasingly clear that many of the entities currently treated in clinical trials are distinct molecularly and unlikely to be responsive to the same treatments. This has influenced clinical trial design and drug development strategies.

Predictive oncology based on patient genetics and disease genomics offers many benefits to patients and societies. Development and utilization of prognostic and predictive biomarkers, however, complicates the drug development process. Meeting the challenges and taking advantage of the opportunities for therapeutic progress will lead to the development of new paradigms and new kinds of partnerships among academia, industries, and government.

REFERENCES

1. Fleming TR, Demets DL. Surrogate end points in clinical trials: are we being misled? *Ann Intern Med.* 1996;125(7):605–613.
2. Buyse M, Molenberghs G, Burzykowski T, et al. The validation of surrogate endpoints in meta-analyses of randomized experiments. *Biostatistics.* 2000;1(1):49–67.
3. Slamon DJ, Leyland-Jones B, Shak S, et al. Use of chemotherapy plus a monoclonal antibody against HER2 for metastatic breast cancer that overexpresses HER2. *N Engl J Med.* 2001;344(11):783–792.
4. Chapman PB, Hauschild A, Robert C, et al. BRIM-3 Study Group. Improved survival with vemurafenib in melanoma with BRAF V600E mutation. *N Engl J Med.* 2011;364(26):2507–2516.
5. Amado RG, Wolf M, Peeters M, et al. Wild-type KRAS is required for panitumumab efficacy in patients with metastatic colorectal cancer. *J Clin Oncol.* 2008;26(10):1626–1634.
6. Subramanian J, Simon R. Gene expression-based prognostic signatures in lung cancer: ready for clinical use? *J Natl Cancer Inst.* 2010;102(7):464–474.
7. Dupuy A, Simon RM. Critical review of published microarray studies for cancer outcome and guidelines on statistical analysis and reporting. *J Natl Cancer Inst.* 2007;99(2):147–157.
8. Sparano JA, Paik S. Development of the 21-gene assay and its application in clinical practice and clinical trials. *J Clin Oncol.* 2008;26(5):721–728.
9. Sparano JA, Gray RJ, Makower DF, et al. Prospective trial of endocrine therapy alone in patients with estrogen receptor positive, HER2-negative, node-negative breast cancer: Results of the TAILORx low risk registry. Abstract P2-08-01, CTRC-AACR San Antonio Breast Cancer Symposium, 2015.
10. Bogaerts J, Cardoso F, Buyse M, et al. TRANSBIG consortium. Gene signature evaluation as a prognostic tool: challenges in the design of the MINDACT trial. *Nat Clin Pract Oncol.* 2006;3(10):540–551.
11. Simon RM, Paik S, Hayes DF. Use of archived specimens in evaluation of prognostic and predictive biomarkers. *J Natl Cancer Inst.* 2009;101(21):1446–1452.
12. Simon R. Optimal two-stage designs for phase II clinical trials. *Control Clin Trials.* 1989;10(1):1–10.
13. Freidlin B, Mcshane LM, Polley MY, Korn EL. Randomized Phase II trial designs with biomarkers. *J Clin Oncol.* 2012;30(26):3304–3309.
14. Simon R, Roychowdhury S. Implementing personalized cancer genomics in clinical trials. *Nat Rev Drug Discov.* 2013;12(5):358–369.
15. Simon R. Genomic driven clinical trials in oncology. *Ann Inter Med.* 2016;165:270–278.
16. Conley BA, Doroshow JH. Molecular analysis for therapy choice: NCI MATCH. *Semin Oncol.* 2014;41(3):297–299.
17. Simon R, Maitournam A. Evaluating the efficiency of targeted designs for randomized clinical trials. *Clin Cancer Res.* 2004;10(20):6759–6763.
18. Simon R, Maitournam A. Evaluating the efficiency of targeted designs for randomized clinical trials: supplement and correction. *Clin Cancer Res.* 2006;12:3229
19. Herbst RS, Gandara DR, Hirsch FR, et al. Lung Master Protocol (Lung-MAP)-A Biomarker-driven protocol for accelerating development of therapies for squamous cell lung cancer: SWOG S1400. *Clin Cancer Res.* 2015;21(7):1514–1524.
20. Kaplan R. The FOCUS4 design for biomarker stratified trials. *Chin Clin Oncol.* 2015;4(3):35.
21. Wang SJ, O'Neill RT, Hung HM. Approaches to evaluation of treatment effect in randomized clinical trials with genomic subset. *Pharm Stat.* 2007;6(3):227–244.
22. Brannath W, Zuber E, Branson M, et al. Confirmatory adaptive designs with Bayesian decision tools for a targeted therapy in oncology. *Stat Med.* 2009;28(10):1445–1463.
23. van Wieringen WN, Kun D, Hampel R, Boulesteix A-L. Survival prediction using gene expression data: a review and comparison. *Comput Stat Data Anal.* 2009;53(5):1590–1603.
24. Simon R, Radmacher MD, Dobbin K, Mcshane LM. Pitfalls in the use of DNA microarray data for diagnostic and prognostic classification. *J Natl Cancer Inst.* 2003;95(1):14–18.
25. Rosenwald A, Wright G, Chan WC, et al.; Lymphoma/Leukemia Molecular Profiling Project. The use of molecular profiling to predict survival after chemotherapy for diffuse large-B-cell lymphoma. *N Engl J Med.* 2002;346(25):1937–1947.
26. Simon RM, Subramanian J, Li MC, Menezes S. Using cross-validation to evaluate predictive accuracy of survival risk classifiers based on high-dimensional data. *Brief Bioinform.* 2011;12(3):203–214.
27. Ghadimi BM, Grade M, Difilippantonio MJ, et al. Effectiveness of gene expression profiling for response prediction of rectal adenocarcinomas to preoperative chemoradiotherapy. *J Clin Oncol.* 2005;23(9):1826–1838.
28. Hess KR, Anderson K, Symmans WF, et al. Pharmacogenomic predictor of sensitivity to preoperative chemotherapy with paclitaxel and fluorouracil, doxorubicin, and cyclophosphamide in breast cancer. *J Clin Oncol.* 2006;24(26):4236–4244.
29. Simon R, Lam A, Mc L, et al. Analysis of gene expression data using BRB-ArrayTools. *Cancer Informatics.* 2007;2:11–17.

Handling Missing Data in Oncology Clinical Trials

Xiaoyun (Nicole) Li, Cong Chen, and Xiaoyin (Frank) Fan

INTRODUCTION

The main purpose of clinical trials is to evaluate the safety and efficacy of experimental drugs of interest. Existence of missing data in clinical trials may introduce bias to the treatment effect estimate, make the study results less interpretable, and potentially decrease study power (1–5). Oncology clinical trials are no exception. Chan et al. have indicated that missing and inadequate data are a main concern in oncology drug application reviews by the Oncologic Drugs Advisory Committee (ODAC) (6). As indicated in the European Medicines Agency (EMA) guideline (4) on missing data, " . . . just ignoring missing data is not an acceptable option when planning, conducting or interpreting the analysis of a confirmatory clinical trial." General types of missing data will be discussed in this chapter. Compared to other disease areas, one unique situation in oncology clinical trials is that time-to-event endpoints such as progression-free survival (PFS) and overall survival (OS) are typical efficacy endpoints in randomized phase II or III trials. For a time-to-event endpoint, it is common that not all patients have an event at the time of the analysis; patients who did not have an event would be censored at some time point according to the statistical analysis plan. Common reasons for missing data and strategies to reduce such "missingness" in oncology clinical trials will be discussed. Statistical methodologies such as Cox regression analysis (7) for incorporating partial information (i.e., follow-up time) from patients into the analysis will also be considered. Furthermore, censoring methods and various sensitivity analyses in this regard will be discussed later in this chapter.

Types of Missing Data and Types of Censoring

Based on missing mechanisms, there are three types of missing data.

The first type is data missing completely at random (MCAR)—that is, the probability of data's being missing is independent of all observed and unobserved data. For example, some data become lost or unusable due to a random site procedure error or a patient missing a visit because of a traffic accident. This type of missing data would not create bias in the analysis. However, MCAR is a very stringent assumption and rarely happens in reality.

The second type is data missing at random (MAR)—that is, the "missing" is not completely at random but has a probability that can be fully explained by the observed data. For example, if females are more likely to miss radiology assessments than males (assuming gender is fully observed in the study), this is not MCAR because gender clearly affects the probability of "missingness." If the probability of whether the radiology assessment is missing is fully attributed to the patient gender, the missing data of radiology assessment is MAR. MAR is a more plausible missing data mechanism in reality.

The third type is data missing not at random (MNAR)—that is, the probability of missing data cannot be fully explained by the observed data. After taking into account of all of the observed data, the probability of missing data still depends on unobserved data. For example, patients who have progressed may be more likely to miss a clinic visit, which leads to missing the radiology assessment that documents the disease progression. The probability of missing radiology assessment data is directly tied to the unobserved events of whether the progression has occurred. As a result, these missing radiology assessment data will be MNAR. MNAR is the most common type of missing data in clinical trials. In both MAR and MNAR, the "missingness" cannot be simply ignored. In reality, it is difficult to verify if the missing mechanism in a specific study is truly MCAR, MAR, or MNAR.

Censored data are a special type of missing data and a standard feature in time-to-event analyses in oncology clinical trials. There are three types of censoring for a time-to-event endpoint: (1) right censoring, where an event is only observable if it occurs before a fixed time (e.g., the end of study follow-up period) but becomes censored after a recorded time (e.g., last contact date); (2) left censoring, where an event has occurred prior to a time point but it is unknown when it has occurred; and (3) interval censoring, where an event is only known to have occurred within a time interval. Right censoring is more common than left censoring because patients do not always experience an event during a clinical trial. Interval censoring is a more general type of censoring when patient events are not monitored continuously (e.g., time of disease progression). Similar to missing data for other endpoints, when censoring is related to outcome of the time-to-event endpoint, it is called informative censoring. Traditional survival analyses assume non-informative censoring (e.g., by the scheduled end of study visit). When study data violate the assumption of non-informative censoring (i.e., the censoring time is related to the treatment effect), the treatment effect estimate can be biased. Some analyses can provide clues about whether the censoring is informative; nevertheless, it is difficult to eliminate the bias resulting from informative censoring.

REASONS FOR MISSING DATA IN ONCOLOGY STUDIES

Efficacy endpoints used to evaluate the treatment effect in cancer clinical trials include those based on tumor assessments, such as objective response rate (ORR), PFS, time to progression (TTP), disease-free survival (DFS); those related to symptom assessments, such as patient-reported outcome of quality of life endpoint; and OS. Time-to-event endpoints based on tumor assessments (e.g., PFS, TTP) are unique in oncology. Because the overall constructions of PFS, TTP, and DFS are similar to each other in terms of data "missingness," which are all different from ORR, we will focus our discussion on PFS and ORR in this section.

Progression-Free Survival

PFS is defined as time from randomization to documented disease progression or death, whichever occurs first. Progressive disease (PD) is evaluated both quantitatively and qualitatively. For solid tumors, it is defined as at least a 20% increase in length in the sum of target lesions from nadir, or unequivocal PD in the non-target lesions, or appearance of new lesion per Response Evaluation Criteria in Solid Tumors (RECIST) 1.1 (8). Large PFS effect is generally predictive of OS benefit. PFS has gained in popularity in recent oncology drug development and is frequently used as a primary efficacy endpoint in randomized confirmatory clinical trials.

Compared to OS, PFS takes less time to observe, and the treatment effect may not be diluted by subsequent therapies. However, unlike in OS where an exact death date can be recorded, progression is determined by periodic tumor assessments. As a result, the exact date of progression is unknown. Rather, an interval in which the progression has occurred is recorded. PFS endpoints are more prone to be missing as compared to OS partly because of the complexity of the progression determination. For example, a patient may miss 1 or more scans, or technical difficulties may make the scans unreadable. Furthermore, progression events may be never observed when a patient starts a new anticancer therapy without disease progression or discontinues treatment and does not return for tumor assessments. Progression is more subjectively determined than death, and investigators may tend to call progression later for patients treated with an experimental drug likely beneficial to patients, which would introduce bias. This potential bias is especially a concern when the study is conducted as open labeled. When a study is double-blinded, the unique toxicity profile of each medicine sometimes reveals which group a patient is randomized to and therefore may still bias investigator's judgment on patient management.

Considering above potential biases, regulatory agencies have requested blinded independent central review (BICR) of tumor assessments, especially for open-label studies, which is meant to reduce the potential bias from investigator assessments on disease evaluation. However, the BICR approach has its own drawbacks, too. Due to operational and financial constraints, BICR is usually conducted after a patient has completed all the tumor assessments and is off the study, while with patient management based on investigator assessments of disease and toxicity. For example, if a patient is determined to have progressed by an investigator, the patient will be taken off study treatment without any more tumor assessments. In the case where BICR does not agree with the investigator's assessment of progressive disease, this patient's actual PD event will be missing and the PFS endpoint per BICR would be censored at the last tumor assessment time the investigator determined PD. The design of conducting BICR evaluation of tumor assessments at the end of the study while the local investigator is in charge of patient management may introduce informative censoring when estimating the treatment effect based on BICR evaluation, especially when there is large discordance in PD between the investigator and the BICR.

Although meta-analyses has not found much difference in the PFS effect between BICR and the investigator's assessment (9), regulatory agencies often require sponsors to evaluate the impact case by case (10). An ideal approach is to perform real-time BICR evaluation instead of reviewing scans after a patient has completed all of his or her tumor assessments. Real-time BICR is appealing in theory, but it is difficult to implement in reality because of logistic constraints and other operational issues. Cost of real-time BICR is also substantially higher because scans have to be reviewed from baseline to the most recent one every time a new scan is available.

For truly double-blinded studies, despite accidental unblinding due to different toxicity profiles, PFS analysis based on investigator's tumor assessments is generally considered acceptable to regulatory agencies. Different methods (11,12) have been proposed to audit investigator's assessments based on a random sample of patients. However, there is no consensus as to which method is appropriate and which criteria should be used for auditing.

Although it is impossible to completely eliminate the bias regardless of whether a study is open label or double blind, attention must be given to the potential informative censoring. One needs to make sure that the censoring is relatively balanced between treatment groups by comparing the censoring distribution using Kaplan-Meier curves. One example of informative censoring led to study bias is study C2325, a randomized, double-blind, placebo-controlled, multicenter phase III study in patients with advanced carcinoid tumor receiving Sandostatin LAR depot and everolimus or Sandostatin LAR depot and placebo (13). At the second interim analysis, the PFS hazard ratio by investigator assessment was 0.69 ($p = .003$), which crossed the efficacy boundary, while the PFS hazard ratio by BICR was 0.9 ($p = .233$), which crossed the futility boundary. The main reason for the contradicting PFS results between investigator and BICR evaluation is driven by the large discordance of PFS events between investigator and BICR induced by the informative censoring.

A possible mitigation strategy of the informative censoring is to continue tumor assessments after disease progression based on investigator's assessment. The immune-related response criteria (irRC) (14) and the recently published immune-related response criteria, which is a modified response criteria for immunotherapies in solid tumors, requires confirmation of progression at least 4 weeks after the initial progression. The requirement of subsequent tumor assessment beyond initial progressive disease such as irRC could substantially decrease the concern of informative censoring using BICR evaluation. Some immune-cancer therapies such as pembrolizumab (15) used irRC as the primary response evaluation criteria for patient management and anti-tumor assessments. The recently published modified response criteria 'iRECIST' (16) is a milestone of new response criteria for immuotherapies and will be used more frequently in new clinical trials.

Objective Response Rate

Similar to PFS, objective response is determined by RECIST 1.1 in solid tumors. In the metastatic disease setting, having measurable disease at the time of enrollment is usually a study inclusion criterion. However, at the time of enrollment, the baseline scan is evaluated only by the investigator. It is recommended by regulatory agencies to conduct BICR for evaluation of ORR if ORR is the primary efficacy endpoint. Due to financial and operational constraints, BICR evaluation is usually conducted when a patient is discontinued from the study or when the study is completed. BICR may not agree with the investigator's evaluation on baseline tumor assessment and rule that the patient does not have measurable disease at baseline. From the analysis standpoint, these patients do not have measurable disease at baseline in the analysis based on BICR evaluation. One approach is to conduct ORR analysis only in patients with measurable disease as evaluated by BICR. However, because of the missing data due to BICR, this approach deviates from the intent-to-treat (ITT) principle (17). Alternatively, real-time BICR evaluation of baseline scan for enrollment validation would eliminate these missing data, but this comes with a greater financial cost.

We have used solid tumors for illustration in this section. Similar missing data reasons apply to hematologic malignancies, too.

STUDY DESIGNS AND STRATEGIES TO REDUCE MISSING DATA

High-level suggestions on trial designs and strategies to reduce missing data in randomized clinical trials have been discussed (1). Good study designs and study strategies can substantially reduce the amount of missing data. In this section, we focus on the key sources of missing data in oncology clinical trials and provide suggestions on how to reduce missing data with a carefully planned study design.

One major source of missing data is the discontinuation of data collection when a patient is no longer participating in the study. Depending on the study endpoint, discontinuation of data collection may lead to considerable data loss and bias in the estimate of treatment effect. The common causes of lack of data collection beyond study treatment discontinuation are (1) the sponsor is unclear about what data need to be collected beyond treatment discontinuation, (2) the protocol or study flow chart does not clearly indicate what data collection is required beyond treatment discontinuation, and (3) site personnel and clinical research associates who work on data collection do not realize the importance of collecting data after a patient discontinues from study treatment. In oncology studies where the primary efficacy endpoint is PFS, it is crucial to continue tumor assessments until disease progression in order to prevent missing PFS data, regardless of whether patients are on study treatment. Cancer patients may discontinue study treatment due to unacceptable toxicity or symptomatic progressive disease. In addition, they may withdraw consent where progressive disease is not recorded at the time of treatment discontinuation. Following the ITT principle (17), every effort should be made to obtain the PD data on these patients after treatment discontinuation. When designing a study, follow-up visits should be clearly defined in the study flow chart with instructions on what data should be collected. For example, computed tomography/magnetic resonance imaging and corresponding tumor assessments for patients who have not progressed should be required at the follow-up visits for those who discontinued study treatment due to reasons other than PD. For studies where OS is the primary endpoint, survival status should be up-to-date for the analysis regardless of whether patients are on or off study treatment. To decrease a patient's burden of coming to the clinic and to increase the likelihood of obtaining survival data, survival follow-up visits can be designed as telephone follow-ups instead of in-person clinic visits. In addition to the protocol and flow chart, further clarification can be made in the informed consent form to include different levels of data collection for patients who elect to withdraw consent. Following the same idea as by the National Research Council (1), an example of language for withdrawal could be:

- I no longer wish to take trial XXX drug(s), but I am willing to attend follow-up clinic visits.
- I no longer wish to take trial XXX drug(s), and I do not wish to attend further follow-up clinic visits. I agree to be contacted via telephone for survival status follow-up and give my physician permission to use my medical records for survival status updates.
- I no longer wish to take trial XXX drug(s), and I do not wish to attend further follow-up clinic visits. I do not agree to be contacted via telephone for survival status follow-up and do not give my physician permission to use my medical records for survival status updates.

It is also important to collect reasons of missing data in the study (e.g., reasons of lost to follow-up on PFS and OS). Rothmann et al. (18) analyzed 24 oncology clinical trials submitted to the Food and Drug Administration (FDA) between August 2005 and October 2008. In the summary, Rothmann et al. found that clinical trials collecting reasons of lost to follow-up in terms of primary efficacy endpoint had lower percentages of missing data. The summary of lost to follow-up could facilitate further assessment of whether missing data is related to the treatment assignment. Table 39.1 presents a summary of reasons of lost to follow-up on PFS in a hypothetic phase III study. The definition of lost to follow-up used here is "no PFS event and missing more than one tumor assessment." In Table 39.1, the percentage of patients with missing PFS event due to treatment discontinuation from clinical progression is higher in the control

TABLE 39.1 Reason of Lost to Follow-up on Progression-Free Survival

Reasons	Experimental Arm n (%)	Control Arm n (%)
Off study treatment due to clinical progression	5 (10)	20 (40)
Off study treatment due to toxicity	20 (40)	20 (40)
In study treatment, scans not done for at least 2 scheduled assessments	20 (40)	5 (10)
Consent withdrawal	5 (10)	5 (10)

arm than in the experimental arm. If it is reasonable to believe that patients who clinically progressed are more likely to experience a PFS event, the imbalance in the reasons of missing PFS event shown in Table 39.1 suggests that missing data in PFS may bring in bias to the treatment effect estimate.

In addition to improving the protocol design and informed consent, another method to help reduce missing data is to provide proper training to the investigators and clinical research associates to ensure they understand the value of preventing missing data, especially after study treatment discontinuation.

Missing data may reduce study power or delay the timing of analyses. One should take into consideration the expected percentage of missing data during study design and planning. The expected percentage of lost to follow-up for primary efficacy endpoints should be pre-specified in the statistical analysis plan and monitored throughout the study to ensure data quality. Sample size and power calculation should always account for expected dropouts. For time-to-event endpoints, missing data would not necessarily reduce the study power. However, missing data can delay the timing of interim and final analyses. During study monitoring, the actual percentage of missing data should be evaluated against the target to check the quality of data completeness. It is also recommended that investigators provide a missing data summary to the data monitoring committee (DMC) as part of the DMC report to evaluate the data quality and reliability.

HANDLING MISSING DATA IN STATISTICAL ANALYSIS

Depending on the mechanism of missing data, statistical analyses often involve missing data imputation. In order to maintain the objectivity of the missing data handling approaches and related sensitivity analyses, we suggest that researchers prespecify sensitivity analyses in the statistical analysis plan before collecting any data, with the same rigor as in primary hypothesis testing of the study. In this section, we describe in detail how to handle missing data in statistical analysis for common efficacy endpoints in oncology studies.

The first critical question related to analysis and missing data is the analysis population (i.e., whether to include all randomized patients or a subgroup with complete data). The ITT population includes all randomized patients regardless of missing data. This analysis population maintains the benefits from the randomization and is the recommended analysis population by regulatory agencies. However, when there is a significant imbalance of missing data between treatment groups, data "missingness" may be confounded with treatment effect and sensitivity analyses with different imputation methods may be required to show the robustness of the results. The full analysis set population, which includes patients with baseline measurements and/or at least one postbaseline measurement, is often used as supportive or sensitivity analysis for demonstrating the robustness of the results.

In the following paragraphs, we list different efficacy endpoints and describe the respective statistical methods for missing data handling.

Progression-Free Survival

PFS is a composite endpoint defined by disease progression or death, whichever occurs first. The exact timing of the disease progression is usually unknown because disease evaluation is conducted periodically. Instead, an interval within which the disease progression occurred is provided. Because of the complexity of analyzing interval-censored data, it is a common practice to perform the PFS primary analysis at the time of detected disease progression, treating the data as right censored. Following the ITT principle, it is preferred to follow patients to documented disease progression regardless of treatment change, although new anticancer therapy following the study treatment may have altered the progress of the disease. Therefore, although the primary analysis considers following up until disease progression or death regardless of action of changes, sensitivity analyses should be performed to evaluate the impact of new anticancer therapy and other confounding factors that may lead to informative censoring (e.g., treatment discontinuation due to adverse events or clinical progression, missed at least two disease assessments). FDA guidance and Rothmann (17,18) provided examples of sensitivity analyses by censoring patients in various scenarios. Table 39.2 provides an example of censoring rules for primary and sensitivity PFS analyses. A similar version that covers both right censoring and interval censoring can be found in Sun, Chen, and Song (19). The censoring rule in the primary analysis strictly follows the ITT principle, which has been demonstrated to be reliable if not conservative (20) and has been strongly supported by the EMA (10). The censoring rules for the two sensitivity analyses are taken from the examples from the FDA guidance (17). In case there is an imbalance between the treatment groups on disease assessment schedules or censoring patterns, also as suggested by the FDA (17), an additional sensitivity analysis may be conducted using time to scheduled tumor assessment visit from randomization instead of time to actual tumor assessments. In addition, Finkelstein's likelihood-based score test for interval-censored data, which modifies the Cox proportional hazard model for interval-censored data, or other interval-censored methods may be used as a supportive analysis. The interval will be constructed so that the left endpoint is the date of the last disease assessment

TABLE 39.2 Censoring Rules for Primary and Sensitivity Analyses for PFS

Situation	Primary Analysis	Sensitivity Analysis 1	Sensitivity Analysis 2
No PD and no death; new anticancer treatment is not initiated	Censored at last disease assessment	Same as the primary analysis	Censored at last disease assessment if still on study therapy; progressed at treatment discontinuation otherwise
No PD and no death; new anticancer treatment is initiated	Censored at last disease assessment before new anticancer treatment	Same as the primary analysis	Progressed at date of new anticancer treatment
PD or death documented after ≤ 1 missed disease assessment	Progressed at date of documented PD or death	Same as the primary analysis	Same as the primary analysis
PD or death documented after ≥ 2 missed disease assessments	Progressed at date of documented PD or death	Censored at last disease assessment prior to the ≥ 2 missed disease assessments	Same as the primary analysis

PD, progressive disease; PFS, progression-free survival.

without documented PD and the right endpoint is the date of documented PD or death, whichever occurs first (21).

Informative censoring will introduce bias to the evaluation of treatment difference. Statistical analyses should be conducted to evaluate if censoring is informative and whether censoring is balanced between treatment arms. The most common analysis is the Kaplan-Meier analysis. It evaluates whether the missing data pattern is similar between treatment arms. Another common approach to evaluate whether there is informative censoring in the BICR evaluation is to analyze the discordance of progression between BICR and investigator assessments (22–25). For example, the early discrepancy rate and late discrepancy rate of the two evaluators should be compared between the treatment arms (10).

Objective Response Rate

Objective response is a direct method to evaluate tumor response and usually a key secondary endpoint in confirmatory clinical trials. Since a response can be observed as early as at the first post-baseline disease assessment (i.e., 1–3 months after enrollment, depending on the imaging schedule), it is usually used as a primary endpoint at the first interim analysis for early futility, or early efficacy as the basis for accelerated approval when there is compelling antitumor activity observed at the interim analysis. The most common way to analyze objective response is to categorize patients into responders and non-responders and treat them as categorical data. Patients who discontinued from the study early, or whose disease deteriorated rapidly, or died prior to the first postbaseline tumor assessment would not have any response assessment data. The most common approach is to treat all the patients with no post-baseline tumor assessment data as non-responders and include them in the denominator when estimating ORR. This approach is also recommended by regulatory agencies (e.g., FDA, EMA) because it tends to be more conservative and less biased.

Quality of Life

Quality of life (QoL) data have gained its importance in recent oncology confirmatory trials. QoL is a key endpoint in the health technology assessment to inform reimbursement decision. Missing QoL data during study or due to discontinuation from treatment is very common. Simply analyzing the complete cases will lead to bias of treatment difference. QoL data can be treated as a time-to-event endpoint (e.g., time to deterioration of certain symptom) or a longitudinal binary or continuous endpoint. When QoL data are analyzed as time-to-event endpoints, they change similar characteristics regarding missing data with PFS, which has been discussed in the previous section. When QoL data are treated as longitudinal data, statistical methods such as

mixed-effect models that assume missing data is MAR can be carried out. In addition, sensitivity analyses including multiple imputations (26) or translating QoL endpoint into a time-to-event endpoint could be conducted. General readings on missing data in QoL analyses can be found in several sources (27–29). The goal is to compare results between the primary and sensitivity analyses. If all analyses lead to the same conclusion, the analysis results are robust in presence of missing data.

EXAMPLES OF CLINICAL TRIALS

The first example in this section is from a phase II clinical trial with PFS as the primary efficacy endpoint. This clinical study is an open-label study of advanced melanoma. The study randomized a total of 360 subjects with 1:1 ratio into the control group and the experimental group. PFS is the primary efficacy endpoint of this study. Table 39.3 displays the summary of patients lost to follow-up on the PFS endpoint (i.e., patients who did not experience PFS events while no longer in follow-up at the time of the analysis). Approximately 17% to 26% patients were lost to follow-up on the PFS events, depending on the treatment groups and the tumor assessment method. Overall, percentage of lost to follow-up is balanced between the two treatment groups. There are more patients missing PFS events due to discontinuation from the study in the control arm compared to that in the experimental arm when evaluating PFS by BICR. On the other hand, the number of patients missing PFS events due to discontinuation from study is comparable between the two treatment groups when evaluating PFS by local investigators. Even though this is an open-label study, this study does not have informative censoring where PFS per BICR is censored at the last time when progression is called by the investigators. The main reason is that this study

TABLE 39.3 Summary of Lost-to Follow-up on PFS

Reasons of Lost to Follow-up on PFS	Experimental Arm N (%)	Control Arm N
	N = 181	N = 179
PFS assessed by BICR		
Discontinued from study	28 (15)	42 (23)
New anticancer therapy	5 (2)	6 (3)
PFS assessed by investigator		
Discontinued from study	34 (19)	37 (21)
New anticancer therapy	5 (2)	5 (3)

BICR, blinded independent central review; PFS, progression-free survival.

TABLE 39.4 Primary and Sensitivity PFS Analyses Results

	N	Number of Events	Median (Months)	Hazard Ratio (95% CI)	p Value (one-sided)
PFS Primary Analysis					
Experimental	181	126	2.9	0.50 (0.39, 0.64)	<.0001
Control	179	155	2.7		
PFS Sensitivity Analysis 1					
Experimental	181	123	2.9	0.51 (0.40, 0.65)	<.0001
Control	179	151	2.7		
PFS Sensitivity Analysis 2					
Experimental	181	135	2.9	0.49 (0.39, 0.62)	<.0001
Control	179	170	2.7		

CI, confidence interval; PFS, progression-free survival.

requires a consecutive scan at least 4 weeks after the initial progression scan to confirm the progressive disease prior to treatment discontinuation. In addition to lost to follow-up on PFS, 3 patients in the experimental arm and 4 patients in the control arm missed at least two scheduled disease evaluations.

Table 39.4 shows the primary PFS analysis results and the sensitivity PFS results with different censoring rules as outlined in Table 39.2. Because missing data are minimal and the missing data and lost to follow-up (censoring) are relatively balanced between the two treatment groups, sensitivity analyses results are consistent with the primary analysis results. Table 39.5 summarizes the concordance and discordance of PD between investigator assessment and BICR evaluation. The concordance rate is relatively high and the discordance is balanced between two treatment arms, indicating that the likelihood of informative censoring is low. Figure 39.1 displays the censoring distribution based on Kaplan-Meier estimates between two treatment groups. The censoring distribution is similar between two treatment groups, indicating informative censoring is less of a concern.

The second example is trial E2100 for locally recurrent or metastatic breast cancer (30). The E2100 study is an open-label, randomized study in patients who had not received prior chemotherapy for their locally recurrent or metastatic breast cancer. The study randomized 722 patients with 1:1 ratio into paclitaxel plus bevacizumab versus paclitaxel alone. The primary efficacy endpoint was PFS. In the original study design, PFS was evaluated by investigators only. Because this was an open-label study and investigator assessment of PFS may incur bias, the FDA requested to have the PFS endpoint adjudicated by BICR. Scans were sent for independent radiologist adjudication after the study was completed. Even though the median PFS had a 5.5-month increase when adding bevacizumab, the quality of the study was called into question. In particular, the amount of missing imaging data made the validity of the PFS results

TABLE 39.5 Concordance of PD Between Investigator and BICR

	Control	Experimental
Number of Patients in Population	179	181
Investigator Assessment—PD	135	90
BICR agreed	127(94.1%)	84(93.3%)
BICR and site agreed on time	95(70.4%)	59(65.6%)
BICR has earlier time	17(12.6%)	20(22.2%)
IRO has later time	15(11.1%)	5(5.6%)
BICR disagreed	8(5.9%)	5(5.6%)
No BICR time point assessment	0(0.0%)	1(1.1%)
Investigator Assessment—Non-PD	20	75
BICR agreed	14(70.0%)	53(70.7%)
BICR disagreed	6(30.0%)	22(29.3%)

PD, progressive disease; BICR, blinded independent central review.

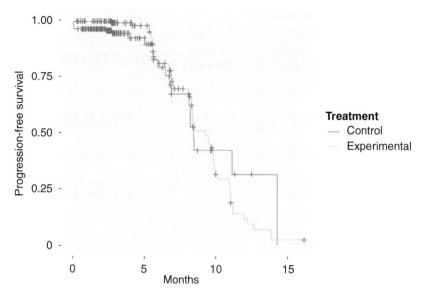

FIGURE 39.1 Kaplan-Meier estimates of censoring distribution.

questionable. For example, a total of 10% of patients did not have any radiographic images submitted for BICR evaluation. In addition, 3.0% to 8.8% of patients had at least one missing scan at scheduled tumor assessments (e.g., cycle 3, 6) up to 1 year when evaluating by cycle (in those who expected to have a scan visit). Consequently, two double-blinded studies were conducted several years later, but these were not able to substantiate the PFS results in E2100.

SUMMARY

Missing data have always been a challenge in clinical trials, whether controlled or uncontrolled, and this is not just unique in oncology. Missing data are more likely to result from less controllable aspects of the trial in which the missing mechanism is usually uncertain. As a consequence, missing data can cause serious problems from biased results to questionable trial validity.

The best weapon against missing data is prevention. However, in practice even with careful planning and execution, the missing data problem is usually unavoidable in oncology trials given the generally poor prognostics of the study populations. Because of the unknowns behind the "missingness," no single method is most appropriate under all circumstances. It is always desirable to check missing patterns and perform sensitivity analyses to evaluate the robustness of the study results. A small percentage of missing or lost–to–follow-up data in the primary efficacy, say 5% or less, may not have a big impact on the treatment estimate, and different sensitivity analyses tend to yield consistent results. Nonetheless, it is important to note that appropriate handling of missing data does not simply involve making up data to replace the unknown ones, but rather taking advantage of those available data and appropriate statistical models to make inferences about the unknown information.

REFERENCES

1. National Research Council. *The Prevention and Treatment of Missing Data in Clinical Trials.* Washington, DC: National Academies Press; 2010.
2. O'Neill RT, Temple R. The prevention and treatment of missing data in clinical trials: an FDA perspective on the importance of dealing with it. *Clin Pharmacol Ther.* 2012;91:550–554.
3. Statistical principles for clinical trials; step 5: note for guidance on statistical principles for clinical trials: International Conference on Harmonisation, Topic E9. London, UK: European Medicines Agency; 1998.
4. Committee for Medical Products for Human Use. *Guideline On Missing Data in Confirmatory Clinical Trials.* London, UK: European Medicines Evaluation Agency; 2010.
5. Little RJ, D'Agostino R, Cohen ML, et al. The prevention and treatment of missing data in clinical trials. *New Engl J Med.* 2012;367(14):1355–1360.
6. Chan JK, Kiet TK, Monk BJ, et al. Applications for oncologic drugs: a descriptive analysis of the oncologic drugs advisory committee reviews. *Oncologist.* 2014;19(3):299–304.
7. Cox D. Regression models and life-tables. *J Royal Stat Soc, Series B.* 1972;34(2):187–220.
8. Eisenhauer E, Therasse P, Bogaerts J, et al. New response evaluation criteria in solid tumours: revised RECIST guideline (version 1.1). *Euro J Cancer.* 2009;45(2):228–247.
9. Amit O, Mannino F, Stone AM, et al. Blinded independent central review of progression in cancer clinical trials: results from a meta-analysis. *Euro J Cancer.* 2011;47(12):1772–1778.
10. Committee for Medicinal Products for Human Use (CHMP). EMA/CHMP/205/95/Rev.4. Guideline on the Evaluation of Anticancer Medicinal Products in Man. London, UK. http://www.ema.europa.eu/docs/en_GB/document_library/Scientific_guideline/2013/01/WC500137128.pdf

11. Dodd LE, Korn EL, Freidlin B, et al. An audit strategy for progression-free survival. *Biometrics*. 2011;67(3):1092–1099.

12. Amit O, Bushnell W, Dodd L, et al. Blinded independent central review of the progression-free survival endpoint. *Oncologist*. 2010;15(5):492–495.

13. FDA Briefing Document Oncology Drug Advisory Committee Meeting April 12, 2011 BLA STN 22334 Afinitor (everolimus). http://www.fda.gov/downloads/advisorycommittees/committeesmeetingmaterials/drugs/oncologicdrugsadvisorycommittee/ucm250378.pdf

14. Wolchok JD, Hoos A, O'Day S, et al. Guidelines for the evaluation of immune therapy activity in solid tumors: immune-related response criteria. *Clin Cancer Res*. 2009;15(23):7412–7420.

15. Hamid O, Robert C, Daud A, et al. Safety and tumor responses with lambrolizumab (anti–PD-1) in melanoma. *New Engl J Med*. 2013;369(2):134–144.

16. Seymour L, Bogaerts J, Perrone A, et al. iRECIST: guidelines for response criteria for use in trials testing immunotherapeutics. *Lancet Oncol*. 2017;18(3):e143–152.

17. Guidance for Industry. *Clinical Trial Endpoints for the Approval of Cancer Drugs and Biologics.*. Rockville, MD: US Department of Health and Human Services, Food and Drug Administration, Center for Drug Evaluation and Research, Center for Biologics Evaluation and Research. 2007. http://www.fda.gov/downloads/Drugs/.../Guidances/ucm071590.pdf

18. Rothmann MD, Koti K, Lee KY, et al. Missing data in biologic oncology products. *J Biopharm Stat*. 2009;19(6):1074–1084.

19. Sun X, Chen C, Li X, Song Y. A review of statistical issues with progression-free survival as an interval-censored time-to-event endpoint. *J Biopharm Stat*. 2013;23(5):986–1003.

20. Stone AM, Bushnell W, Denne J, et al. Research outcomes and recommendations for the assessment of progression in cancer clinical trials from a PhRMA working group. *Euro J Cancer*. 2011;1763–1771.

21. Sun X, Chen C. Comparison of Finkelstein's method with the conventional approach for interval-censored data analysis. *Stat Biopharm Res*. 2010;2(1):97–108.

22. Thomas RF, Mark DR, Hong LL. Issues in using progression-free survival when evaluating oncology products. *J Clin Oncol*. 2009;27:2874–2880.

23. Dodd LE, Korn EL, Freidlin B, et al. Blinded independent central review of progression-free survival in phase III clinical trials: important design element or unnecessary expense? *J Clin Oncol*. 2008;26(22):3791–3796.

24. Sridhara R, Mandrekar SJ, Dodd LE. Missing data and measurement variability in assessing progression-free survival endpoint in randomized clinical trials. *Clin Cancer Res*. 2013;19(10):2613–2620.

25. Sridhara R, Johnson JR, Justice R, et al. Review of oncology and hematology drug product approvals at the US Food and Drug Administration between July 2005 and December 2007. *J Natl Cancer Inst*. 2010;102(4):230–243.

26. Rubin DB, Schenker N. Multiple imputation for interval estimation from simple random samples with ignorable nonresponse. *J Am Stat Assoc*. 1986;81(394):366–374.

27. Crowley J, Hoering A, editors. Handbook of statistics in clinical oncology. CRC Press; 2012. https://www.crcpress.com/Handbook-of-Statistics-in-Clinical-Oncology-Third-Edition/Crowley-Hoering/p/book/9781138199491

28. Simes RJ, Greatorex V, Gebski VJ. Practical approaches to minimize problems with missing quality of life data. *Stat Med*. 1998;17:725–737.

29. Huntington JL, Dueck A. Handling missing data. *Curr Prob Cancer*. 2005;29(6):317–325.

30. FDA Briefing Document Oncology Drug Advisory Committee Meeting December 5, 2007 BLA STN 125085/91.018 Avastin (bevacizumab). http://www.fda.gov/ohrms/dockets/ac/07/briefing/2007-4332b1-01-FDA.pdf

Special Considerations in Oncology
Clinical Trials

40

Health-Related Quality of Life Studies in International Randomized Controlled Oncology Clinical Trials

Andrew Bottomley, Corneel Coens, Murielle Mauer, Madeline Pe, and Francesca Martinelli

INTRODUCTION

Cancer is one of the leading causes of death (1). However, thanks to clinical research, new discoveries and therapies become available every year. As a consequence, more people are either fully treated or living longer despite having cancer.

However, survival is not the only purpose of anticancer treatments. For patients who have been fully treated, it is important to know that their treatment did not have long-term side effects. Also, for those who are living longer despite having cancer, it becomes critical that their health-related quality of life (HRQoL), at the very least, does not deteriorate as they live their lives with cancer.

HRQoL, which is often assessed as a patient-reported outcome, is defined as a multidimensional concept that refers to the patient's subjective perception of the impact of the disease and treatment(s) on the physical, psychologic, and social aspects of daily life (2,3).

For decades, clinicians have asked cancer patients about their feelings and experiences. In the past, this was done informally and often with no direct treatment consequences. These days, however, with the recognition of patient-centeredness as a critical component of quality health care (4) and the availability of reliable and validated instruments to measure HRQoL (2), these informal questions are now considered to be important data that can influence clinical trials and treatment decisions. In fact, HRQoL is now recognized as an important criterion in assessing the clinical benefit of anticancer treatments (European Society for Medical Oncology [ESMO] guidelines). These developments make it possible to reliably assess HRQoL in cancer clinical trials and allow the possibility to

evaluate the risks and benefits of cancer therapies from a patient's perspective.

This chapter explains (1) how to design a randomized controlled trial (RCT) with an HRQoL endpoint and (2) how to analyze and interpret results of these HRQoL trials. Some examples of trials are presented, outlining lessons learned from the early RCTs using HRQoLs as clinical endpoints. Hopefully, this chapter will not only guide researchers about how to include HRQoL endpoints in their trials but also encourage more researchers to include HRQoL endpoints in future trials.

DESIGNING TRIALS USING HRQOL ENDPOINTS

HRQoL application ranges from individual cancer care planning and patient monitoring to population-wide surveillance programs. The primary research area remains within RCTs where different interventions can be directly compared in terms of patient benefit.

Implementing HRQoL into clinical trials is very similar to the methodology used for the classical clinical endpoints of, for example, survival and disease control. However, some specific issues arise, mainly due to the inherent nature of patient involvement.

Including an HRQoL in a Randomized Controlled Trial

Any RCT must have a well-defined purpose, and so must HRQoL research: The HRQoL element must be based on a sound and detailed research objective. All too often, HRQoL is added to a clinical trial without a clear hypothesis to justify its inclusion. Vague statements such as "the objective is to measure HRQoL over time" or "we are interested in evaluating changes in HRQoL" are inadequate. A well-formulated objective includes:

- Having a specific research question
- Selecting relevant HRQoL domains
- Choosing validated reliable instruments to assess these HRQoL domains
- Identifying the time period of interest
- Noting the direction, magnitude, and duration of the hypothesized treatment effect

The objective of the RCT will affect all stages of the further design, analysis, and reporting (Table 40.1) (5).

If no clear objective can be specified, all resulting analyses will be exploratory in nature. In this case, an overall description of HRQoL in the study population can be established for future hypothesis-generating initiatives. Any exploratory analysis is, however, intrinsically limited and needs to be confirmed in an independent setting to be conclusive.

For some HRQoL assessment instruments, reference data for cancer patients (6) and sometimes also for the healthy individuals (7–10) are available. These data can be used to provide context for both exploratory and confirmatory analyses. Another option is to compare the obtained exploratory findings with findings obtained by other researchers in studies where instruments and populations are similar. In this case, a stratification by clinical and sociodemographic variables will be needed in order to avoid bias.

Instruments

Once the objective has been established, an appropriate and validated instrument needs to be selected (11). Many HRQoL instruments are composed of a simple, static questionnaire. Although it is often tempting for an investigator to construct a questionnaire from scratch to specifically tailor it to the proposed study, this is by far the worst choice possible if it is done without guidance. If more specific items than the ones addressed by a validated questionnaire are necessary, using validated items from an item library is a better alternative approach. For example, the European Organization for Research and Treatment of Cancer (EORTC) Item Library (12) is a repository of all the existing items from all EORTC questionnaires, with their available translations. It can be used to create tailored instruments if no existing instrument satisfies the study requirements. An item library allows personalization of instruments while maintaining important characteristics such as validity and reliability.

In general, a good HRQoL instrument needs to be tested for reliability and validity in order to be useful for clinical application. Many tools, designed for generic, cancer-specific, cancer site–specific, or even cancer symptom–specific applications, exist. When making a selection, keep in mind the method of administration and the intended RCT population. For example, in elderly patients, shorter questionnaires (e.g., the EORTC measure for the elderly, the QLQ-ELD13 [(13)]) are preferred in order to reduce noncompliance. When setting up an international study, verify whether validated translations exist. Make sure that the information needed is assessed by the questionnaire. For example, if pain is a major issue, the instrument (e.g., brief pain inventory) should have questions related to pain and its impact on quality of life.

The method of data gathering and scoring should be clear for the instrument. That is, it should be clear how patients' answers translate into the numbers used in the analysis.

Finally, there is interpretation of the results. Ideally, a minimal clinical important difference (MCID) should be defined for the tool. This is the smallest difference in an outcome that is considered to be clinically relevant. Such a difference is instrument-specific and cannot be easily substituted. One might, in this respect, prefer to choose a questionnaire that is already widely used in the research to allow for easier comparison with other RCTs. When using the EORTC QLQ-C30, for example,

TABLE 40.1 Key Issues in Designing a Trial

Objectives
  Research question
  Health-related quality of life domains
  Timing
  Expected differences
Instrument selection
  Validity and translations
  Ability to assess the selected domains
  Guidelines
  Method of administration
  Data scoring
    Interpretation
Trial schedule
  Assessment plan
  Time windows
  Alternative methods of instrument completion
Analysis
  Compliance and "missingness" mechanism
  Main analysis
  Sensitivity analyses
  Interpretation of results
Reporting*
  Hypothesis
  Compliance
  Main results
  Reliability: missing data and multiple testing
  Validity: clinical significance
  Context
  Conclusions

*For a full list of reporting guidelines, please consult the CONSORT-PRO (5).

a change of at least 10 points in an HRQoL parameter is considered to be of minimal clinical importance to the patients (14). Although work by Cocks et al validated the original cutoffs, the researchers advocated a smaller effect size of 4 points for treatment group comparisons in randomized clinical trials (15).

Scoring

HRQoL instruments make use of different scoring systems. In general, for the EORTC QLQ-C30 this consists of grouping and transforming the individual items into single 0-100 ranged outcomes (standardized scores) via linear transformation. For the QLQ-C30, for scales assessing functioning, higher scores represent a higher level of functioning (which is better for the patient), whereas for scales assessing symptoms, higher scores represent a higher degree of symptom burden (which is debilitating for the patient). The scoring for the EORTC QLQ-C30 (16) questionnaire is detailed in the EORTC QLQ-C30 scoring manual, and the scoring for the supplementary EORTC QLQ modules can be obtained through the Quality of Life department of the EORTC.

Time Schedule

A next important step in the design is the choice of time schedule for the HRQoL assessment in the RCT. Individual patient HRQoL values usually change over time; the interest lies in evaluating whether such evolution differs between treatment arms. The choice of the timing of the assessment should make the assessment schedule possible to follow and to be linked to the objective. In addition, it should minimize the total patient burden.

It is unrealistic to expect all patients to complete their questionnaire on a specific day. Therefore, time windows (i.e., extended periods of time) are often used to construct an assessment schedule rather than time points. Upper and lower limits around a target date should be defined so that HRQoL data obtained within the corresponding time window are considered valid assessments. Preferably this should be done a priori. Attention must be paid to minimize bias when choosing the time windows by avoiding differences between the treatment arms, having overlapping time windows, or having time windows that include treatment interventions (e.g., surgery, start of a chemotherapy cycle). Finally, the instrument recall time should be taken into account. Instruments can gauge patient HRQoL at a specific time point or during a determined period (e.g., the QLQ-C30 has a recall time of 2 weeks). Always exercise care to avoid overlapping recall windows or the occurrence of major interventions at the edge of the recall window.

The choice of the day of the assessment is also very important. It is unreasonable to expect patients to go to the hospital just to fill out the HRQoL questionnaire. In order to maximize compliance, it is advised to schedule HRQoL assessments to coincide with study-specific visits. Another option is to ask patients to complete questionnaires outside of the hospital setting. Questionnaires can then be retrieved at the next visit, by post or by electronic device. These options offer less control over the actual completion date and need to be in line with the stated objectives.

Sample Size

A final design step is checking if the RCT sample size is sufficient to address the objective. If HRQoL is only a secondary endpoint, the study sample size still needs to justify the HRQoL research. Sample size evaluation should take into account rates of attrition, noncompliance, and the ability to detect clinically relevant differences.

ANALYSIS OF TRIALS WITH HRQOL DATA

Missing Data

Missing data is a common problem in cancer clinical trials. This occurs when on-study patients do not complete questionnaires (missing forms) or some questionnaire items (missing items) at the time of a scheduled HRQoL assessment. When HRQoL data are collected up to progression or at the end of the period of clinical follow-up, missing data can also occur because patients drop out of the HRQoL assessment because of death or progression.

Missing data may seriously bias the results; patients who experience rapid deterioration are less likely to fill out the questionnaires than healthier patients. Also, if patients progress or die more rapidly in one arm compared with the other arm, the collection of HRQoL data will be stopped earlier in one group compared with the other. Consequently, differences in patient HRQoL at latter time points may simply reflect a more severe selection of patients in one arm compared with the other.

Therefore, missing HRQoL data must be handled very carefully. The baseline characteristics and efficacy outcomes should be compared between patients who were included and excluded for the HRQoL analyses. Reasons for missing HRQoL data should be collected and presented. If the proportion of missing data is nontrivial, the "missingness" mechanism should be further examined.

Compliance

To assess the amount of missing data, compliance rates are calculated for every treatment group. HRQoL compliance is defined as the number of valid (or completed) forms at a particular time point divided by the number of expected forms at that time point. HRQoL forms are expected for each patient (who is alive or whose disease has not progressed) within the HRQoL assessment schedule according to the trial design. Comparative tests can be used to determine whether there are significant differences in compliance between treatment arms that could bias treatment comparison results.

Even if a completed HRQoL form is returned, some questions might have been left blank or have nonvalid answers. Therefore, the scale compliance for each specific scale of interest should be presented. Scale compliance is defined as the ratio of the number of valid HRQoL forms for which the scale could be successfully scored over the number of total valid forms.

Based on the compliance results, only data from valid HRQoL forms should be included in the analyses. Preferably, analyses should be done on all patients with at least one valid HRQoL form according to the intention-to-treat principle, unless this is not feasible.

Methods of Analysis

Before starting any HRQoL analysis, its feasibility needs to be assessed by checking the amount of available data, compliance rates, and the overall design. If too few data are available, or the compliance rates are too low, then no confirmatory analyses should be performed. These important criteria stress the significance of designing and implementing a trial that limits the problem of missing data and biased comparisons of HRQoL data; the findings that result from any analysis of HRQoL data depend on the quality and quantity of data that is collected.

Different techniques may be used to analyze HRQoL data collected over time: cross-sectional analysis (analysis of the patient HRQoL scores at a specific time point) and the use of summary statistics (reduction of the total HRQoL data into a single patient result), longitudinal modeling using linear mixed models, and time-to-event models.

Cross-sectional analysis and the use of summary statistics allow the application of simpler analysis techniques. The reduction in complexity is achieved by either selecting a specific time point for the treatment comparison or reducing HRQoL data over time to a single measure, such as maximum increase or decrease from baseline or the proportion of patients experiencing an increase or decrease on a preset number of points from baseline (usually derived from the MCIDs) over time. Cross-sectional analysis considers data from a single time point and is therefore simple and easy to understand. However, it does not take into account evolution over time, and the resulting comparison may be biased because selection effects will undo the balance achieved by randomization.

Longitudinal modeling using linear mixed models has the advantage of making use of all longitudinal HRQoL data and providing estimates for the evolution of HRQoL data over the entire assessment period in the different study arms. This methodology can also allow adjustment for missing data under certain assumptions.

Recently, time-to-event based summaries, whereby an event is based on a patient's reported HRQoL outcomes, have been proposed as a way to analyze longitudinal HRQoL data. This methodology also uses all longitudinal HRQoL data, takes into account the MCIDs, and can deal with missing data by making assumptions about whether missing data reflect a deterioration in a patient's health status or not. Because findings are reported using Kaplan-Meier curves and hazard ratios, it has the advantage of being familiar to clinicians and thus may be easier to interpret (17).

All these methods may provide biased results in the presence of informative missing data (18). Moreover, group changes are not always representative of individual patient changes. The mean scores will appear stable over time if half of the patients improve and half of the patients deteriorate. Therefore, it is important to supplement a longitudinal analysis that models the evolution of mean scores over time with the proportion of patients experiencing a severe worsening or a considerable improvement from baseline during follow-up.

Because missing HRQoL data may seriously bias results, it is strongly advisable to produce sensitivity analyses to check the robustness of the main result (11,18). These additional sensitivity analyses may consist of analyzing HRQoL scales other than the primary selected scales, selecting patient subgroups, using different analysis techniques, or using imputation techniques for missing data.

There are various ways of dealing with and analyzing HRQoL data. However, these different possible statistical methods lead to findings that are difficult to compare across clinical trials. To address this issue, the Setting International Standards in Analyzing Patient-Reported Outcomes and Quality of Life Endpoints Data (SISAQOL) initiative has been established, with the goal of recommending guidelines and best practices for the analysis of patient-reported outcome endpoints in randomized cancer clinical trials (19).

Interpretation of Results

When interpreting results, both statistical significance and the clinical relevance of the HRQoL scores should be considered; it is possible to find statistically significant findings with a nonclinically relevant difference, especially if the sample is large. At this point, the instrument-specific and predefined MCID should be used as a benchmark for interpreting the magnitude and relevance of the treatment comparison.

When interpreting scores over time, researchers need to be careful not to conclude that global trends are the same as absolute individual patient changes. Patients vary in how their HRQoL scores change over time, and global trends use this information to estimate the average of these individual patient changes. This implies that the changes observed for each individual patient's data will not necessarily be the same as what is estimated by the global trend.

CHALLENGING TRIALS—A VIEW FROM THE PAST

A Brief History, and Why We Have to be Rigorous

One may ask why HRQoL researchers have to be so prescriptive in guidance and design, analysis, and interpretation. Over many years, particularly in the early 1980s when HRQoL really began to take a more significant role in RCTs, we learned that many HRQoL measures failed for a number of reasons. Although researchers had undertaken HRQoL measurements for years, there was a lack of internationally validated and translated measures, such as the EORTC tool, and many studies used ad hoc measures or measures lacking validation. Therefore, RCTs with such suboptimal HRQoL measures could not be robust or compared across trials.

Furthermore, as noted above, the analysis of HRQoL data is complex, and in the 1980s, limited attention was given to identifying the more effective methodology to use. Simple issues such as clinical significance, that is, the ability to understand trial effects on patients, was neither understood nor addressed (14). EORTC had several aborted RCTs in genitourinary and leukemia cancer simply because there was no policy about ensuring that HRQoL be a mandatory part of the protocols, and no necessary and resource intensive steps to monitor HRQoL data were undertaken. This lack of adherence resulted in low compliance, with one trial having less than 40% baseline compliance. This changed in the 1990s. Since then, EORTC and other groups have made significant gains in methodology, practice, and policy (20). In EORTC RCTs, baseline HRQoL is now an eligibility criterion, demonstrating the value of this measure to both patients and investigators from day one of the study. The fact that the American Society of Clinical Oncology (ASCO), ESMO, and European Medicines Agency (EMA) now support HRQoL as a valid clinical RCT endpoint illustrates the progress the field of HRQoL has made over the years (21).

Some Examples of Successful Trials

Example 1
EORTC (22) examined the HRQoL of patients with advanced breast cancer treated with a standard anthracycline-based chemotherapy regimen versus a dose-intensified anthracycline regimen (EORTC trial 10921). HRQoL assessments were carried out before random assignment, then once a month for the first 3 months, and then every 6 months to month 54. Four hundred forty-eight patients were entered onto this trial, of whom 384 (86%) completed the baseline HRQoL questionnaire.

The clinical results demonstrated no differences in survival between the two groups. The shorter but more intensified treatment resulted in significantly poorer HRQoL outcomes during the first 3 months of follow-up. However, thereafter, the HRQoL scores returned to baseline levels, and at 12 months no significant differences were observed between the treatment arms. During the remainder of the follow-up, the HRQoL levels were comparable between the study arms. The combined clinical and HRQoL results from this trial suggest that the shorter, dose-intensive therapy achieves similar survival outcomes without sacrificing patient HRQoL. This trial gave patients a choice. If, for example, the patient has a busy working life, with children involved, and a lifestyle demanding rapid treatment, regardless of toxicity, they can choose the more aggressive, but shorter, treatment duration option. If the patient is elderly and/or does not have a demanding lifestyle, the choice may be the less aggressive therapy. Clearly, if survival opportunity is basically equal, HRQoL can help a practicing clinician give patients a choice.

Example 2
Taphoorn et al. (23) reported on the HRQoL component of a phase III RCT for glioblastoma patients conducted by the EORTC brain cancer and radiotherapy groups in collaboration with the National Cancer Institute of Canada. In this study, 573 newly diagnosed glioblastoma multiforme (GBM) patients were randomly assigned to radiotherapy alone or radiotherapy and concomitant adjuvant temozolomide. Overall survival was the primary endpoint, with HRQoL examined at baseline and during treatment, at 3-month intervals, until progression. Changes from baseline on 7 selected HRQoL domains were measured: fatigue, overall health, social functioning, emotional functioning, future uncertainty, insomnia, and communication deficit. The clinical results showed a significant 3-month median overall survival benefit for the temozolomide arm. Baseline HRQoL questionnaires were available for 89.7% of patients (n = 514). Significant differences ($p = .005$) were observed at the end of radiotherapy for only one of the seven HRQoL domains, social functioning, in favor of standard treatment with radiotherapy. However, during follow-up, significant clinically meaningful differences were no longer observed between the standard arm and the temozolomide arm. The addition of temozolomide during and after external-beam radiotherapy for newly diagnosed GBM significantly improved survival and, importantly, without any negative long-term impact on HRQoL. These data contributed to setting a new standard of care. The US Food and Drug Administration approved temozolomide for the treatment of GBM based on the results of this trial.

REPORTING AND EVALUATING PUBLISHED STUDIES OF HRQOL IN CANCER CLINICAL TRIALS

Work Done So Far

With the aim of providing guidance on how to improve the quality of reporting of HRQoL endpoints in cancer clinical trials, there has been a growing amount of work that systematically evaluates the quality of reporting of HRQoL in RCTs in different disease sites over the years. Findings indicated that the quality of reporting of several RCTs with an HRQoL element were poor and diverse, and often the standard would not allow researchers to make comprehensible interpretations of the data. A series of systematic reviews in non–small cell lung cancer (24), breast cancer (25), prostate cancer (26), and other disease sites clearly showed this. We have issued guidance on how to draft a robust RCT HRQoL paper, published in the *Journal of Clinical Oncology*, along with others, trying to set standards for publishing high-quality trials (27). These guidelines specify much of what we have mentioned previously: the importance of having a hypothesis, the specification and use of reliable tools, undertaking and reporting good analysis of data, and presenting the data with clinical significance in a way that is easy for clinicians to interpret. Recently, guidance on how to improve the reporting of HRQoL data was published by CONSORT-PRO (19), with the hope that these guidelines will be of greater value to clinicians and help continue to guide treatment decisions.

CONCLUSIONS

As noted in this chapter, clinicians have assessed HRQoL for decades, although in the beginning this was often done informally. More recently, RCTs have been formalized using evidence-based guidance and robust tools. These robust, scientifically valid HRQoL tools can be added into almost any RCT. It is our hope that some of the practical, applied design and analysis approaches mentioned in this chapter will be helpful to investigators in the designing and planning of RCTs with an HRQoL endpoint.

REFERENCES

1. World Health Organisation. Cancer Fact sheet. 2015. http://www.who.int/mediacentre/factsheets/fs297/en
2. European Medicines Agency. Appendix 2 to the guideline on the evaluation of anticancer medicinal products in man: The use of patient-reported outcome (PRO) measures in oncology studies. 2016. http://www.ema.europa.eu/docs/en_GB/document_library/Other/2016/04/WC500205159.pdf
3. US Dep Heal Hum Serv Food Drug Adm. Guidance for Industry Patient Reported Outcome Measures: Use in Medical Product Development to Support Labeling Claims. 2009. http://www.fda.gov/downloads/Drugs/Guidances/UCM193282.pdf
4. Institute of Medicine. Crossing the Quality Chasm: A New Health System for the 21st Century. Washington, DC: National Academy Press; 2001.
5. Calvert M, Blazeby J, Altman DG, et al. Reporting of patient-reported outcomes in randomized trials. *JAMA*. 2013;309:814–822.
6. Scott NW, Fayers PM, Aaronson NK, et al. EORTC QLQ-C30 Reference Values. Brussels, Belgium: Quality of Life Department, EORTC Headquarters; 2008.
7. Derogar M, van der Schaaf M, Lagergren P. Reference values for the EORTC QLQ-C30 quality of life questionnaire in a random sample of the Swedish population. *Acta Oncologica*. 2012;51(1):10–16.
8. Schwarz R, Hinz A. Reference data for the quality of life questionnaire EORTC QLQ-C30 in the general German population. *Euro J Cancer*. 2001;37(11):1345–1351.
9. Hjermstad MJ, Fayers PM, Bjordal K, Kaasa S. Health-related quality of life in the general Norwegian population assessed by the European Organization for Research and Treatment of Cancer Core Quality-of-Life Questionnaire: the QLQ = C30 (+ 3). *J Clin Oncol*. 1998;16(3):1188–1196.
10. van de Poll-Franse LV, Mols F, Gundy CM, et al. Normative data for the EORTC QLQ-C30 and EORTC-sexuality items in the general Dutch population. *Europ J Cancer*. 2011;47(5):667–675.
11. Fayers P, Machin D. Quality of Life – assessment, analysis and interpretation. Chicester: John Wiley & Sons Ltd; 2000.
12. EORTC Quality of Life Group Item Bank. http://www.eortc.be/ItemBank
13. Wheelwright S, Darlington AS, Fitzsimmons D, et al. International validation of the EORTC QLQ-ELD14 questionnaire for assessment of health-related quality of life elderly patients with cancer. *Br J Cancer*. 2013;109(4):852–858.
14. Osoba D, Rodrigues G, Myles J, et al. Interpreting the significance of changes in health-related quality-of-life scores. *J Clin Oncol*. 1998;16:139–144.
15. Cocks K, King MT, Velikova G, et al. Evidence-based guidelines for determination of sample size and interpretation of the European Organisation for the Research and Treatment of Cancer Quality of Life Questionnaire Core 30. *J Clin Oncol*. 2011;29:89–96.
16. Aaronson NK, Ahmedzai S, Bergman B, et al. The European Organization for Research and Treatment of Cancer QLQ-C30: a quality-of-life instrument for use in international clinical trials in oncology. *J Natl Cancer Inst*. 1993;85:365–376.
17. Anota A, Hamidou Z, Paget-Bailly S, et al. Time to health-related quality of life score deterioration as a modality of longitudinal analysis for health-related quality of life studies in oncology: do we need RECIST for quality of life to achieve standardization? *Qual Life Res*. 2015;24(1):5–18.
18. Fairclough, DL. Patient reported outcomes as endpoints in medical research. *Stat Method Med Res*. 2004;13(2):115–138.
19. Bottomley A, Pe M, Sloan J, et al. Analysing data from patient-reported outcome and quality of life endpoints for cancer clinical trials: a start in setting international standards. *Lancet Oncol*. 2016. doi:10.1016/PII
20. Bottomley A, Aaronson NK. International perspective on health related quality of life research in cancer clinical trials: The European Organisation for Research and Treatment of Cancer Experience. *J Clin Oncol*. 2007;25(32):5082–5086.
21. Cherny NI, Sullivan R, Dafni U, et al. A standardised, generic, validated approach to stratify the magnitude of clinical benefit that can be anticipated from anti-cancer therapies: the European Society for Medical Oncology Magnitude of Clinical Benefit Scale (ESMO-MCBS). *Ann Oncol*. 2015;mdv249.

22. Bottomley A, Therasse P, Piccart MJ, et al. Health-related quality of life in survivors of locally advanced breast cancer: an international randomized controlled phase III trial. *Lancet Oncol.* 2005;6:287–294.

23. Taphoorn MJ, Stupp R, Coens C, et al. Health related quality of life in patients with glioblastoma: A randomized controlled trial. *Lancet Oncol.* 2005;6(12):937–944.

24. Bottomley A, Thomas R, Vanvoorden V, Ahmedzai S. Health related quality of life in non small cell lung cancer: methodological issues in randomised controlled trials. *J Clin Oncol.* 2003;21(15):2989–2992.

25. Bottomley A, Vanvoorden V, Flechtner H, Therasse P. EORTC Quality of Life Group and EORTC Data Center. The challenges and achievements involved in implementing quality of life research in cancer clinical trials. *Eur J Cancer.* 2003;39:275–85.

26. Efficace F, Bottomley A, van Andel G. Health related quality of life in prostate carcinoma patients. *Cancer.* 2003;97(2): 377–388.

27. Efficace F, Bottomley A, Osoba D, et al. Beyond the development of Health-Related Quality of Life (HRQOL) Measures: a checklist for evaluation HRQOL Outcomes in Cancer Clinical Trials- Does HRQOL evaluation in prostate cancer research inform clinical decision making. *J Clin Oncol.* 2003;21(18):3502–3511.

The Economics of Oncology Clinical Trials

Michaela A. Dinan and Shelby D. Reed

The cost of cancer care in the United States is increasing rapidly due to the aging of the population and the introduction, and increased use, of costly emerging medical technologies. Overall healthcare costs in the United States are approaching 20% of the U.S. gross domestic product (GDP) with nearly half of spending supported by governmental sources (1). As a result, demonstrating the economic value of new treatments is playing an increasingly large role in the development of any new medical technology. To generate early evidence on a treatment's value, economic analyses are frequently being conducted alongside prospective clinical trials. A consequence of this increasingly cost-aware environment is that researchers and physicians participating in clinical trial design and implementation will benefit from having a working understanding of the major principles of economic analyses.

In this chapter, we review the fundamental principles of economic analyses in the context of prospective clinical trials.

COSTS—A WORD OF CAUTION

This chapter begins with a word of caution. Many individuals who have not been formally trained in economic analyses are not aware of the nuances and depth of complexity that well-conducted economic analyses involve. As such, we start by describing some of the challenges relevant to any attempt to quantify healthcare costs in current U.S. practice before moving on to focus on how these studies are typically conducted within the context of a trial.

In most settings, there is a market value or transparent price that can be consistently assigned for goods and services. For example, the price of a product in Virginia is expected to be similar to the price of the same product in North Carolina. Even if there was some variation at the state level, one would not expect large differences between adjacent counties, and one certainly would not expect different people to pay different prices for the

same product at the same store. However, in healthcare, none of these assumptions are true. Payments for patients receiving the same treatments can vary a great deal between states, but can also substantially vary by city and between institutions (2). Even more surprising is that payments for patients undergoing the same treatment, at the same institution, for the same condition, may be vastly different due to different fee schedules negotiated between insurance companies and medical providers. Because of the nature of healthcare and the laws supporting it as a basic human right in the United States (i.e., Emergency Medical Treatment and Labor Act [EMTALA] for emergency care), "customers" cannot be turned away for certain services. The means by which hospitals and medical facilities balance the costs of those who can pay versus those who cannot set the stage for a widely variable, often obscure, pricing system in which physicians often do not know the cost of the tests and treatments they are prescribing. And, even when physicians learn the charges that appear on patients' bills for specific medical tests and treatments, they often bear little resemblance to the actual cost of supplies, personnel time, and other direct and overhead costs required to provide the services. This is in stark contrast to areas in which charges are known in advance and discussed up front by service providers, for example, as is the case for a mechanic or even veterinarian, as part of the consumer decision-making process.

Because of the opacity around medical costs, methods used to estimate costs in an economic evaluation must be carefully specified and can include payments made by the insurer, out-of-pocket payments by the patient, total payments, total charges, lost wages due to lost productivity, and the additional burden placed on family members or other caregivers. In addition, many interventions or treatments, in addition to their direct cost, may alter subsequent management strategies and patient outcomes, which can impact downstream costs. Of all these metrics, hospital listed charges vary the most widely, and are rarely used since most patients pay a lower price as negotiated by their insurance company.

Incremental costs are commonly used to indicate the additional cost of a change in treatment strategies or receipt of additional services and are often used in studies that examine the incremental impact of changes in treatment strategies. However cost is defined, it is important that costs incurred in different years are adjusted for inflation and that costs projected to be incurred in the future are discounted (typically at 3% per year in the United States) to represent their present value. Inflation rates are typically derived from the consumer price index for medical goods, and then reported with respect to the year for which costs were estimated (i.e., "$10,000 in 2015"). Because of the complexity of calculating healthcare costs, and the potential variation in the cost for a given service, close attention should be paid to the details and underlying assumptions of any cost estimate.

Costs can be described from multiple perspectives. In practice, cost estimates are often calculated from the payer's perspective, where costs represent payments made by the payer (often a health insurance company) to a healthcare provider. This approach allows for concrete figures that represent real-world costs to a specific stakeholder. However, details on payments for specific procedures or hospitalizations are often considered proprietary with the exception of public payers. Thus, Medicare fee schedules are one of the most widely used sources of cost weights used to value medical resources for economic evaluations. Alternatively, one can examine costs from the patient's perspective, which may include out-of-pocket payments, deductibles, lost wages, and expenses incurred for supportive care. The societal perspective is the most inclusive. In addition to all direct medical costs incurred, societal costs can include informal caregiving, nonmedical costs, and costs incurred in other sectors like social services or the judicial system.

When considering any of the aforementioned perspectives, one must also specify the time period over which costs are considered. This time period is sometimes referred to as the time horizon. A focus on short-term costs for acute episodes of care and the corresponding short time horizon is often appropriate. However, for patients with chronic diseases, a more appropriate horizon may be several months or years.

Bundled Episodes of Care

In assessing costs and how these might be interpreted, it is important to be aware that many payers no longer operate using the a la carte, fee-for-service system where each service or good is associated with a payment. For example, inpatient costs are increasingly "bundled" and rates of reimbursements set by a Diagnosis-Related Group (DRG) code, which consists of a single lump sum that is paid to hospitals to cover all care administered during a hospitalization. These DRG codes are based on estimates of how much an admission should reasonably cost given the reason for the admission and potential complicating factors. Similarly, surgical procedures are associated follow-up care, including complications within a predetermined time frame. Costs attributed to surgeries are often calculated as the sum of all costs accrued from the date of the surgery through 30 to 90 days following the surgery. These systems are designed to incentivize providers and hospitals to provide efficient care and minimize complications.

Additional Cost Considerations

Last, it should be noted that beyond the direct costs of treatment and associated toxicities and side effects, there are other costs such as overhead that may need to be considered in order to truly capture the full cost of a proposed intervention. For example, hospitals and medical facilities often incur fixed costs for building and maintaining their infrastructure, which does not result in direct payments or reimbursements. For example, hospitals are not directly reimbursed for the purchase of PET scanners, robotic surgery machines, or linear accelerators used to treat patients with radiation therapy. A single Da Vinci surgery system may cost $2 million, but only results in a 15% to 18% increase in direct charges for the surgery performed (3). New technologies are therefore often purchased to provide competitive market advantages, to increase patient volumes/revenues, or to recoup costs through reduction in operating room (OR) times, complications, or length of stay (3). Ensuring that all costs have been fully considered in analyses can help researchers provide the most complete perspective of healthcare and health system costs related to the proposed intervention.

GENERAL APPROACHES TO CLINICAL TRIAL ECONOMIC ANALYSIS: SINGLE- VERSUS MULTIPLE-ARM TRIALS

Trials contain either a single or multiple study arms, which essentially dictate the general goal of economic analyses.

In single-arm, nonrandomized trials, economic analyses can be used to characterize medical resource use and costs incurred by trial participants. Costs include the study intervention as well as associated tests and monitoring, medical services required to manage side effects or toxicities, and other downstream health outcomes. Because the cause of many healthcare costs cannot be readily or entirely disentangled, all-cause resource use and associated costs are commonly reported. For example, a patient with cancer may be hospitalized with a heart arrhythmia, but whether this was or was not related to cancer or treatment may not be discernable. Other metrics important to economic approaches may also be collected such as preference-based measures of health-related quality of life. In addition to collecting data to assess medical resource use, associated costs, and health-related quality of life, information on lost productivity, informal caregiving, and transportation for medical care can be used to provide a broader view of economic impact. Metrics estimated from these single-arm studies can then be used for later analyses or modeling approaches, discussed later in this chapter.

In multiarm trials, these same outcomes are examined with the goal of comparing costs in one arm versus another. Multiarm trials can either be randomized or nonrandomized. An example of a comparison of costs between randomized treatment arms can be seen during the initial adoption of PET imaging in the staging of non–small-cell lung cancer (NSCLC). In patients thought to have early-stage lung cancer, surgical resection is the standard of care. However, it was found that the use of PET scans in addition to conventional CT and bone imaging was able to detect occult metastatic disease in roughly 20% of these patients. As a result, the use of PET was able to decrease the rates of futile thoracotomy, as demonstrated in several randomized trials (4–6). An economic evaluation of one of these randomized trials demonstrated that PET improved care and saved money overall by reducing the rates of unnecessary surgery and hospitalization (7).

Nonrandomized, prospective trials, can either assign patients to arms based on patient, physician, or institution discretion or can occur in the context of phase I and II studies in which the assigned treatment changes over time (e.g., dose escalation studies or protocol amendments in which a certain treatment is added or withheld due to preliminary findings in the initial study cohort). An example of a study involving multiple nonrandomized treatment arms due to a mid-study protocol change was the RICOVER-60 trial of elderly patients with advanced diffuse large B-cell lymphoma. In this trial, radiation therapy was initially included after chemotherapy for all sites of bulky tumor. However, outcomes were so favorable using chemotherapy and radiation that an amendment was made partway through the study whereby radiation was no longer required, therefore providing a two-arm, nonrandomized opportunity to compare outcomes between these groups (8).

METHODS OF ANALYZING HEALTHCARE COSTS

Most researchers, clinicians, and policy makers are primarily interested in comparing the cost of two or more alternative treatment or management strategies. Economic analyses of healthcare costs take several forms, nicely reviewed by Preusller et al. (9). Sometimes the goal is simply to quantify the total cost of a specific treatment, which should include not only of "direct" cost of obtaining and administering treatment but also the costs of monitoring and treating associated toxicities or complications. In the situation where two approaches are proven to be equally effective, often the goal is to minimize costs. In many situations for new cancer therapies, however, there are small incremental gains in outcomes or reductions in toxicities with new treatments, and these gains are often expensive. In these settings, the gains in patient outcomes must be weighed against their costs. For the remainder of this chapter, we focus on these more common situations.

Cost Effectiveness Analyses (CEAs)

In recent years, the term "comparative effectiveness research" (CER) has been more commonly used to reflect the comparison of effectiveness between two or more management or treatment strategies. Many clinicians are familiar with the idea of efficacy, which indicates the *potential* benefit of an intervention when applied under a specific set of often ideal circumstances such as those encountered within the context of a clinical trial with a patient who completes treatment without any protocol violations. However, even more pertinent to policy is the idea of effectiveness, or the *actual realized* benefit that patients will receive on average in routine practice. For example, patients enrolled in clinical trials may have fewer comorbidities, and they may be younger and generally more fit than patients treated in routine practice. They may also be more likely to strictly adhere to the treatment regimen being evaluated. When the treatment is provided outside the context of a clinical trial in routine practice, the realized benefits of treatment may be a fair bit lower than observed in clinical trial populations. Nevertheless, most of the available evidence used in CEAs is either directly or indirectly based on clinical trials.

In CEAs, effectiveness can be measured in terms of overall survival, but can also be adjusted to take into account the quality of life during that survival. The use of "quality-adjusted life years" (QALYs) can accomplish this. The key outcome of CEAs is referred to as the incremental cost-effectiveness ratio (ICER), which indicates the additional cost of a new treatment divided by the number of years of life or QALYs gained. QALYs differ from overall survival in that they are adjusted for health-related quality of life, using numeric "utility weights," which are estimated on a scale from 0 to 1, where 0 is equivalent to dead and 1 indicates perfect health. Values between 0 and 1 represent the relative strength of preference or desirability of different health states. Health utilities can be estimated directly using standard gamble or time-trade-off techniques, but these can be challenging to implement in a clinical trial. In most trial settings, investigators use multiattribute health status instruments such as the EuroQol-5D (EQ-5D) or Health Utilities Index (HUI). These instruments are preference-weighted meaning that all possible responses to these instruments can be converted to utility weights derived from external studies.

At its core, formal CEA provides an objective and systematic way of quantifying the trade-off between the benefits and costs of alternative treatment options. The intent of CEAs is to assist decision makers in allocating limited resources to provide the greatest improvements in health outcomes for a population. Although CEAs are intended to be used only as a tool among other considerations in decision making, its application in practice poses many practical and political challenges. These challenges occur even in countries with a long history of using CEAs to inform treatment recommendations. For example, even though the United Kingdom has used CEAs to allow treatments within the National Health Service, public outcry led to the creation of the Cancer Drug Fund, which quickly overran its allocated budget and subsequently changed its processes. A review of the challenges and benefits of this system in the context of where CEA limits should be set was recently published by Drummond (10).

Over the past 20 years, there has been tremendous growth in the number of trials based on model-based CEAs (11). This growth has coincided with advances in methods and increased sophistication among individuals who review and use these studies to support decisions. An expert panel convened by the International Society for Pharmacoeconomics and Outcomes Research (ISPOR) has published good practice recommendations for implementing economic evaluations alongside clinical trials (12,13). Indeed, CEA is sufficiently specialized so that the typical trial investigator will not perform the CEA him or herself, but instead will engage an expert collaborator. This collaboration should begin during study design to guarantee that the study itself is designed to support a high-quality CEA and that the critical data elements needed for the CEA will be collected within the trial.

The ISPOR recommendations highlight the importance of evaluating effectiveness rather than efficacy and include clinical outcomes when possible. Because CEAs evaluate the incremental costs and benefits of one intervention versus another, the relevance of the comparators in the trial is crucial. In the event that QALYs are being assessed and utilities are needed, these guidelines recommend that such utilities are obtained directly from patients in these studies to obtain the most accurate estimates. The ISPOR panel further recommends that the collection of resource use, health utilities, and other related information be integrated into the trial protocol and that analyses of these data are conducted using the intention-to-treat principles. Drummond's book (14) provides a readable introduction on performing a CEA, and the U.S. Panel on Cost-Effectiveness in Health and Medicine provides an authoritative set of updated recommendations for conducting CEAs (15). Although journals such as *Value in Health and Pharmacoeconomics* publish numerous CEAs, these studies now commonly appear in mainstream and specialty medical journals such as *JAMA* and *Journal of Clinical Oncology*. A short list of key questions that can be used to help evaluate and develop a CEA is provided in Table 41.1.

TABLE 41.1 Key Questions to Help Evaluate CEA

Does the CEA model include the most relevant comparators?
Does the CEA include all the outcomes of interest to the relevant stakeholders? What is the perspective used to value costs?
Is the time horizon long enough to capture all downstream costs and health outcomes?
Are all medical resources valued appropriately?
How should outcomes be summarized?
How sensitive are the conclusions to changes in assumptions?

CEA, cost-effectiveness analysis.

Whether or not a specific intervention is considered "cost-effective" depends on the available resources and the target population's willingness to pay. The World Health Organization recommends considering cost-effectiveness in terms of GDP per capita (16). Using this schema, interventions are considered highly cost-effective (less than GDP per capita); cost-effective (between one and three times GDP per capita); and not cost-effective (more than three times GDP per capita). For the United States (2012 GDP per capita), this would equate to <$50,000, $50,000 to $150,000, and >$150,000, respectively. Others have cited larger willingness-to-pay thresholds in the United States (17), and the issue remains contentious (18).

Although a popular idea and often misquoted, exceedingly few medical technologies are cost-saving (decrease overall costs). Instead, most medical technologies or management strategies require CEAs to assess whether an approach is cost-effective. Ultimately, CEAs provide objective measures of the relative cost and benefit associated with a given treatment or management strategy. An informative example comes from CEAs that have been used to evaluate various screening colonoscopy strategies. A single screening colonoscopy costs approximately $3,000 to save 1 year of life, but screening every 10 years beginning at age 50 costs roughly $11,000 per year of life saved (19). However, screening every 10 years also saves 2 to 3 times more lives than a single screening colonoscopy, and is therefore recommended. Such analyses provide a detailed and objective framework with which patients, providers, and policy makers can make rational trade-offs in costs, care, and outcomes.

Important to any cost-effective analysis is the use of sensitivity analyses, which often demonstrate widely varying ICERs depending on the assumptions made in the model such as the cost of specific procedures and outcomes associated with various treatment strategies. Such sensitivity analyses can provide an indication of how reliable a given ICER might be with naturally occurring variation, under slightly different conditions, or applied to other populations.

Beyond Clinical Trials: Decision Modeling

There are many practical limitations of economic analyses conducted alongside clinical trials. The key limitation of clinical trial data is that a finite, specific population is being studied over an often limited time horizon. Modeling studies in health services research (HSR) refer to the creation of algorithms to describe complex associations and relationships between exposures, outcomes, and confounders (20). Modeling in CEA can be used to extend the time horizon beyond that observed in a clinical trial and to allow the analyst to bring in other relevant information from external studies. For example, modeling can be used to analyze the potential impact of a differential patient population, costs, time horizon, or any other factor that might impact the ultimate cost and/or effectiveness of an intervention.

Modeling can play a particularly important role in guiding the design of policies, guidelines, treatment approaches, or reimbursement that would otherwise be too time-consuming, costly, and complicated to analyze using direct interventional or conventional observational approaches. Modeling also provides a means of exploring relationships among data that cannot be directly observed or feasibly obtained in practice, such as those involving costs or long-term outcomes. Models used in HSR often examine the impact of various decision algorithms, new interventions, policies, or patient factors on associated outcomes or costs.

An example in the cancer literature comes from several analyses of the impact of Oncotype DX testing in breast cancer. Use of the Oncotype DX test, which predicts the benefit associated with receipt of chemotherapy, has been previously shown to change physician recommendations to prescribe less overall chemotherapy. Modeling studies of Oncotype DX testing have been used to perform CEAs and have predicted that the use of the assay has the potential to be cost-saving (21). The advantage of modeling is that various factors and their relative impact on outcomes of interest can be dissected. For example, predicted cost savings from Oncotype DX testing can vary when the analyst changes the utilization strategy, the age of the population, and the cost of chemotherapy. The obvious disadvantage of modeling is that many assumptions are left to the discretion of the analyst. Thus, the reader must carefully evaluate the assumptions used in the primary analysis and whether the analyst adequately varied uncertain assumptions and model parameters in sensitivity analyses.

GOING FORWARD: RATIONALE REIMBURSEMENT

As discussed previously in this chapter, overall healthcare costs have consistently increased over the past several decades and are projected to continue to grow in the future. Cancer costs comprise a substantial proportion of these costs and especially recent rises in costs. Because of the immense expense and often marginal benefit of emerging therapies in cancer, there have been increasing efforts to be more judicious about healthcare spending both within and outside the oncologic community. A detailed consideration of rational reimbursement models in healthcare is beyond the scope of this chapter and will undoubtedly continue to evolve long after the writing of this text. However, the reader should be generally aware of such efforts, since these rational models of reimbursement will provide yet another alternative metric or endpoint in which to calculate costs and may be of interest to clinical trialists.

Models of rational or incentive-based reimbursement for healthcare services include bundled payments, accountable care organizations (ACOs), self-insured large businesses, and other variations on capitated or episode-specific payments. Notable oncology-specific examples include those by the American Society of Clinical Oncology (ASCO), which has recently proposed potential methods of evaluating therapies using metrics of value to include quality of life, therapeutic value, toxicity, and palliation of symptoms (22). Other efforts by ASCO have included the Patient-Centered Oncology Payment (PCOP), in which providers may be reimbursed a set of standard, capitated payments for standard oncologic workflows such as first-line chemotherapy administration and supportive care. In 2012, the American Board of Internal Medicine (ABIM) launched the "Choosing Wisely" campaign, which was an effort across medical specialties to provide concrete examples of more cost-effective practices, with guidelines released by several oncology specialties including the American Society of Hematology and Oncology (ASH) and the American Society of Therapeutic Radiation Oncology (ASTRO).

SUMMARY

In this chapter, we hope to have provided a working knowledge needed by those participating in clinical design and implementation. Because the costs of cancer care in the United States have increased rapidly due to the adoption of expensive emerging medical technologies, they now play a significant role in the development and adoption of any new medical technology. The role of costs, methods to assess them, and their role in technology adoption will undoubtedly continue to evolve in the coming years. The increasing use of bundled payments, ACOs, and other rationally based reimbursement schemas will further contribute to their evolution. Expert health economists should be consulted early in the design of a clinical trial to consider design features that may impact an eventual CEA and to prepare for collection of appropriate data elements to accurately capture medical resource use, costs, and relevant health outcomes. Prospectively planned economic evaluations can provide high-quality information on a treatment's cost-effectiveness to be available when decision makers are making recommendations regarding its use and coverage. Collectively, these studies can help ensure that money spent on cancer care is used most efficiently to improving overall health outcomes.

REFERENCES

1. Keehan SP, Poisal JA, Cuckler GA, et al. National health expenditure projections, 2015-25: Economy, prices, and aging expected to shape spending and enrollment. *Health Aff (Millwood)*. 2016;35(8):1522–1531.
2. Newman D, Parente ST, Barrette E, Kennedy K. Prices for common medical services vary substantially among the commercially insured. *Health Aff (Millwood)*. 2016;35(5):923–927.
3. Link RE, Su LM, Bhayani SB, Pavlovich CP. Making ends meet: a cost comparison of laparoscopic and open radical retropubic prostatectomy. *J Urol*. 2004;172(1):269–274.
4. Fischer B, Lassen U, Mortensen J, et al. Preoperative staging of lung cancer with combined PET-CT. *N Engl J Med*. 2009;361(1):32–39.
5. Maziak DE, Darling GE, Inculet RI, et al. Positron emission tomography in staging early lung cancer: a randomized trial. *Ann Intern Med*. 2009;151(4):221–228, W-248.
6. van Tinteren H, Hoekstra OS, Smit EF, et al. Effectiveness of positron emission tomography in the preoperative assessment of patients with suspected non-small-cell lung cancer: the PLUS multicentre randomised trial. *Lancet*. 2002;359(9315):1388–1393.
7. Verboom P, van Tinteren H, Hoekstra OS, et al. Cost-effectiveness of FDG-PET in staging non-small cell lung cancer: the PLUS study. *Eur J Nucl Med Mol Imaging*. 2003;30(11):1444–1449.
8. Held G, Murawski N, Ziepert M, et al. Role of radiotherapy to bulky disease in elderly patients with aggressive B-cell lymphoma. *J Clin Oncol*. 2014;32(11):1112–1118.
9. Preussler JM, Denzen EM, Majhail NS. Costs and cost-effectiveness of hematopoietic cell transplantation. *Biol Blood Marrow Transplant*. 2012;18(11):1620–1628.
10. Drummond M. Clinical Guidelines: A NICE Way to Introduce Cost-Effectiveness Considerations? *Value Health*. 2016;19(5):525–530.
11. Neumann PJ, Thorat T, Shi J, et al. The changing face of the cost-utility literature, 1990-2012. *Value Health*. 2015;18(2):271–277.
12. Ramsey SD, Willke RJ, Glick H, et al. Cost-effectiveness analysis alongside clinical trials II-An ISPOR Good Research Practices Task Force report. *Value Health*. 2015;18(2):161–172.
13. Ramsey S, Willke R, Briggs A, et al. Good research practices for cost-effectiveness analysis alongside clinical trials: the ISPOR RCT-CEA Task Force report. *Value Health*. 2005;8(5):521–533.
14. Drummond MF, Schulpher MJ, Torrance GW, O'Brien BJ, Stoddart GL. *Methods for the Economic Evaluation of Health Care Programmes*. 3rd edn. New York, NY: Oxford University Press; 2005.
15. Neumann PJ, Sanders GD, Russell LB, eds, et al.*Cost-Effectiveness in Health and Medicine*. 2nd edn. New York, NY: Oxford University Press; 2016.
16. WHO. World Health Organization. Cost effectiveness and strategic planning (WHO-CHOICE) 2015; http://www.who.int/bulletin/volumes/93/2/14-138206/en/. Published 2015.
17. Ubel PA, Hirth RA, Chernew ME, Fendrick AM. What is the price of life and why doesn't it increase at the rate of inflation? *Arch Intern Med*. 2003;163(14):1637–1641.
18. Gafni A, Birch S. Incremental cost-effectiveness ratios (ICERs): the silence of the lambda. *Soc Sci Med*. 2006;62(9):2091–2100.
19. Sonnenberg A, Delco F. Cost-effectiveness of a single colonoscopy in screening for colorectal cancer. *Arch Intern Med*. 2002;162(2):163–168.
20. Ringel JS, Eibner C, Girosi F, et al. Modeling health care policy alternatives. *Health Serv Res*. 2010;45(5, Pt 2):1541–1558.
21. Vanderlaan BF, Broder MS, Chang EY, et al. Cost-effectiveness of 21-gene assay in node-positive, early-stage breast cancer. *Am J Manag Care*. 2011;17(7):455–464.
22. Schnipper LE, Davidson NE, Wollins DS, et al. American society of clinical oncology statement: a conceptual framework to assess the value of cancer treatment options. *J Clin Oncol*. 2015;33(23):2563–2577.

Special Considerations in Immunotherapy Trials

Claire F. Friedman, Katherine S. Panageas, and Jedd D. Wolchok

In 2013, *Science* magazine declared cancer immunotherapy to be the breakthrough of the year based on the positive results of clinical trials of antibodies that block negative regulators of T-cell function as well as the emergence of chimeric antigen receptor (CAR)-modified T cells. The antibody therapies include ipilimumab, which blocks anti-cytotoxic T-lymphocyte-associated protein 4 (CTLA-4), and pembrolizumab and nivolumab, which both block programmed death 1 (PD-1). While these agents initially demonstrated efficacy in advanced melanoma (1–3), the use of checkpoint inhibitors (CPIs) has subsequently expanded into other malignancies, including non–small-cell lung cancer (NSCLC) (4,5), renal cell cancer (6,7), bladder cancer(8), and Hodgkin's lymphoma (see Table 42.1) (15). Given the clinical efficacy of this class of drugs, a number of these antibodies received accelerated approval by the Food and Drug Administration (FDA) without phase III data. For example, pembrolizumab was FDA-approved for the treatment of melanoma in December 2014, three months after the phase I data was published (16).

As a result of these positive clinical trials, demonstrating proof of principle, the number of antibodies targeting immune checkpoints, as well as other immunologic approaches that are being tested in clinical trials, has dramatically expanded (17,18). The schema of drug development, including standards of clinical trial design, dose recommendation, patient selection, and efficacy assessments, implemented during the development of traditional chemotherapy will need to evolve to accommodate for the unique mechanisms of action and pharmacodynamics of immuno-oncology (IO). In this chapter, we discuss clinical trial design considerations for these agents.

PHASE I TRIAL DESIGN

The primary objectives of phase I trials have traditionally been to (a) establish the safety and tolerability of a novel agent and (b) determine the recommended phase II

dose (RP2D) for further investigation. Traditionally, the RP2D of cytotoxic drugs has been selected based on a dose-escalation schema and assumes there is a proportional increase between dose, efficacy, and toxicity for any given drug. This is based on the principle that the maximum tolerated dose (MTD) for cytotoxic chemotherapy agents that directly inhibit the growth of malignant cells will provide the greatest therapeutic effect. In contrast, CPIs and other IO agents, for the most part, have no direct effect on malignant cells. Instead, immune cells, such as T cells or natural killer cells, indirectly mediate the cytotoxic efficacy of this class of drugs. The traditional assumption of a linear relationship between efficacy and dose may not hold in this area of drug development. The objective of phase I trials may need to be modified to assess the minimum effective dose (MED) in phase I trials of immuno-oncologic agents.

Considering the Dose-Limiting Toxicity and MTD

Evaluation of an experimental treatment in a phase I trial may pertain to the evaluation of a dose of a single agent, the dose of combination agents (administered concurrently or sequentially), the schedule of administration, or a combination of dose and schedule. In phase I trials, the MTD is defined as the highest dose of a drug or treatment at which one or no dose-limiting toxicity (DLT) occurs in an expanded cohort of six patients (<33%), and it is usually the RP2D for further studies. For the determination of the MTD, whether or not a patient experiences a DLT is the endpoint of interest. The definition of the type and grade of toxicity considered to be dose limiting is determined at the trial design stage and is specific to the disease and drug under investigation. This has been commonly defined as any grade 3–4 non-hematological or grade 4 hematological toxicity, at least possibly related to the treatment, occurring during the first cycle of treatment (19). However, the definition of

TABLE 42.1 Checkpoint Inhibitors and Their FDA-Approved Indications

Compound	Disease	Indication	Dose
Ipilimumab (9)	Melanoma	Advanced unresectable melanoma	3 mg/kg q3 weeks x 4 doses
		Adjuvant treatment of patients with melanoma with involvement of regional lymph nodes after complete resection (total lymphadenectomy)	10 mg/kg q3 weeks
Nivolumab (10)	Melanoma	Advanced disease	240 mg q2 weeks
	NSCLC	Advanced disease	240 mg q2 weeks
	Renal cell carcinoma	Advanced disease relapsed or progressed after antiangiogenic therapy	240 mg q2 weeks
	Hodgkin's lymphoma	Disease relapsed or progressed after autologous HSCT and posttransplantation brentuximab vedotin	3 mg/kg q2 weeks
	Urothelial carcinoma	Locally advanced or metastatic disease that has progressed during a period of up to 1 year after first-line platinum-containing chemotherapy	240 mg q2 weeks
	SCC of the head and neck	Disease that has progressed during platinum chemotherapy or that has recurred or metastasized after platinum-based chemotherapy	3 mg/kg q2 weeks
Pembrolizumab (11)	Melanoma	Advanced disease	2 mg/kg q3 weeks
	NSCLC	First line in tumors with >50% PD-L1 expression	200 mg q3 weeks
	NSCLC	Disease with >1% PDL expression with disease progression on or after platinum chemotherapy	200 mg q3 weeks
	NSCLC	In combination with pemetrexed and carboplatin for first-line treatment	200 mg q3 weeks
	SCC of the head and neck	Recurrent or metastatic disease	200 mg q3 weeks
	Hodgkin's lymphoma	Refractory cHL, or those who have relapsed after three or more prior lines of therapy	200 mg q3 weeks
	Urothelial carcinoma	Upfront treatment for locally advanced or metastatic disease in patients who are not eligible for platinum chemotherapy OR disease that progressed during or following platinum chemotherapy within 12 months of neoadjuvant or adjuvant platinum chemotherapy	200 mg q3 weeks
	Microsatellite instability-high cancer	Solid tumors that have progressed following prior treatment and no other satisfactory alternatives	200 mg q3 weeks
Atezolizumab (12)	Urothelial carcinoma	Locally advanced or metastatic disease that has worsened during or following platinum-containing chemotherapy	1,200 mg q3 weeks
	NSCLC	Disease progression during or following platinum-containing chemotherapy	1,200 mg q3 weeks
Avelumab (13)	Merkel cell carcinoma	Metastatic disease	10 mg/kg q2 weeks

(continued)

TABLE 42.1 Checkpoint Inhibitors and Their FDA-Approved Indications (*continued*)

Compound	Disease	Indication	Dose
	Urothelial carcinoma	Locally advanced or metastatic disease that has worsened during or following platinum-containing chemotherapy or within 12 months of neoadjuvant or adjuvant platinum chemotherapy	10 mg/kg q2 weeks
Durvalumab (14)	Urothelial carcinoma	Locally advanced or metastatic disease that has worsened during or following platinum-containing chemotherapy or within 12 months of neoadjuvant or adjuvant platinum chemotherapy	10 mg/kg q2 weeks
Nivolumab + Ipilimumab (9,10)	Melanoma	Advanced disease	1 mg/kg + 3 mg/kg

cHL, classical Hodgkin's lymphoma; HSCT, hematopoietic stem cell transplantation; NSCLC, non–small-cell lung carcinoma; SCC, squamous cell carcinoma.

a DLT as well as limiting DLTs to the first cycle deserves reconsideration as IO agents have thus far had limited potential for causing acute or early onset toxicities. The majority of adverse events (AEs) from CPIs, known as immune-related adverse events (irAEs), occur after the first 30 days of exposure. For example, irAEs classically appear 8 to 10 weeks after starting ipilimumab (20). The median time to onset for irAEs in patients treated with pembrolizumab ranges from 1.3 months for hepatitis to 3.5 months for diarrhea (11), with similar data for nivolumab (10). Consequently, defining a DLT as a grade 3 or 4 event that occurs during the first cycle of treatment may not be sufficient to capture all AEs. There is a movement toward lengthening the DLT period to two cycles or up to 9 weeks, as has been done in a number of published IO trials (2,3,21,22). If a DLT period is not lengthened in order to allow rapid dose escalation, toxicities scoring as DLTs observed beyond cycle 1 should be thoroughly considered for the RP2D.

Dose-escalation designs can be generally classified into rule-based or model-based designs. Rule-based designs are simple to understand and implement, and do not require special software. These methods specify rules based on observed events to assign patients to specific dose levels and determine the MTD (most common rule-based design is the 3 + 3 design). Model-based designs assume a statistical model of the dose–toxicity relationship, patients are assigned dose levels, and determination of the MTD is based on the assumed model (most common model-based design is the continual reassessment method). Model-based designs may pose practical challenges with implementation if institutional resources are not in place.

The interplay between dose, efficacy, and toxicity has been examined for a number of CPIs. Toxicity and response appears to be dose-dependent for the anti-CTLA-4 antibody ipilimumab; patients treated with 10 mg/kg had a longer overall survival (OS) compared to those treated with 3 mg/kg (15.7 months [95% CI: 11.6–17.8] versus 11.5 months [95% CI: 9.9–13.3] [HR: 0.84,

p = .04]) (23). However, patients treated with 10 mg/kg also had a higher incidence of irAEs (24). On the other hand, anti-PD-1/PD-L1 antibodies have no clear correlation between dose, efficacy, and toxicities, as responses and AE rates seem equivalent beyond 1 to 2 mg/kg and up to 20 mg/kg either every 2 or 3 weeks (2,3,25). It remains to be seen whether antibodies that block or stimulate other checkpoint regulators have a dose-dependent effect. The agonist antibodies, which stimulate T-cell activation, may have a higher risk of toxicity even at low doses; in a phase 1 trial of TGN1412, an antibody against CD28, all six patients treated with the initial low dose of the experimental agent experienced life-threatening cytokine release syndrome (26).

The dose-finding data for CPIs were comprehensively examined by Postel-Vinay and colleagues who reviewed 13 phase 1 clinical trials of checkpoint blocking antibodies (27). In that series, only one trial identified per-protocol defined DLTs (28). In most of the other trials, the maximum administered dose (MAD), which is based on a prespecified dose range utilizing pharmacokinetic data, was used to guide the choice of the RP2D. In the limited number of studies that published pharmacokinetic data, it appears that CPIs have a relatively similar pharmacokinetic profile, including a dose-dependent Cmax and area under the curve, and a median half-life of 16 days (9–21 days) due to a common IgG backbone.

Given the uncertainty surrounding dosing and efficacy, both the anti-CTLA-4 and anti-PD-1 antibodies have been assessed at a number of doses and schedules. Ipilimumab was studied in four phase 1 trials at doses ranging from 3 mg/kg to 20 mg/kg; no MTD was established in any of the trials. Subsequently, three dose levels were compared in a phase II trial in metastatic melanoma (0.3, 3, and 10 mg/kg), which, together with a positive phase 3 experience at 3 mg/kg, led to the registration dose of 3 mg/kg for four cycles (1,24). Concurrently, patients with resected melanoma were enrolled on a study of the use of adjuvant ipilimumab at a higher dose (10 mg/kg) and with an alternative schedule (4 cycles q3 weeks with maintenance doses q3 months); this dose and schedule was FDA-approved in the adjuvant setting after it was shown to prolong progression-free survival (PFS) (29).

Pembrolizumab has been studied at different doses (2 mg/kg vs. 10 mg/kg) and different schedules (q2 weeks vs. q3 weeks) without a significant difference in efficacy or toxicity by dose or schedule (16,30). More recently, flat dosing of pembrolizumab at 200 mg q3 weeks has been FDA-approved for patients with squamous cell carcinoma of the head and neck and PD-L1 positive NSCLC (31,32). Adding additional uncertainty into dosing design is the use of alternative schedules when CPIs are used in combination. The combination of nivolumab 1 mg/kg and ipilimumab 3 mg/kg dosed q3 weeks for four doses is FDA-approved for the treatment of metastatic melanoma (33,34). Alternative dosing of the combination of ipilimumab and nivolumab was studied in a phase I trial of patients with metastatic NSCLC; patients were randomized to receive nivolumab 1 mg/kg every 2 weeks plus ipilimumab 1 mg/kg every 6 weeks, nivolumab 3 mg/kg every 2 weeks plus ipilimumab 1 mg/kg every 12 weeks, or nivolumab 3 mg/kg every 2 weeks plus ipilimumab 1 mg/kg every 6 weeks. Response rates and irAEs were similar in treatment groups who received nivolumab 3 mg/kg; both of these arms are considered promising for further study in the randomized phase 3 trial Checkmate 227 (35).

Treatment with combination immunotherapy is commonly used in melanoma, and phase I trials of combination therapies are increasingly being conducted in other diseases. Development of combination regimens is motivated by potentially synergistic effects thus leading to greater efficacy than either IO agent alone. The challenge is to increase overall efficacy without significantly increasing toxicity. Prioritization of potential drug combinations for clinical development can be overwhelming and toxicity data for a single agent may provide only limited information on the safety profile of the combination. In fact, the most effective and safest doses in the combination setting are rarely the same as those of the respective agents used in monotherapy (36). Dose-finding trials with combination treatments are complex and identification of the MTD of a combination regimen needs careful consideration (e.g., Are the toxicity profiles overlapping or additive? Is efficacy additive or synergistic?). In a dose-finding trial of combination regimens, a set of predetermined dose-level combinations are typically explored based on the MTD already known from monotherapy as well as any preclinical data demonstrating synergy. For simplicity, if a two-drug combination is being studied, the dose of one immunotherapy is escalated while the dose of the second agent is kept at a fixed dose until a tolerable combination dose level is achieved (37). In a more complex combination trial design the second drug may then be escalated or three

or more drug combinations may be evaluated. As with dose-finding trials of monotherapy, model-based or Bayesian adaptive designs have been proposed to escalate two agents simultaneously and may be superior to escalation algorithms in terms of maximizing safety and minimizing the number of patients required to reach the MTD (38,39).

Overlapping toxicities can limit escalation of the combination to active levels and it is recommended that combinations be derived with nonoverlapping toxicity profiles, if possible. In this scenario, the definition of DLT is specific to the IOs being studied. In practice, drug-combination phase I requires significant planning at the design preparation phase, to be sure the starting dose of each IO and the total number of combinations to be studied are set, as these studies can grow in sample size and cost very quickly (39). Typically, the entire space of possible combinations cannot be studied especially as more than two drug combinations are studied. It is plausible that combination immunotherapies can be evaluated in a phase II trial if there are no known or expected overlapping toxicities or pharmacokinetic/pharmacodynamic interaction. It is suggested in this scenario that an initial run-in phase is performed to evaluate the safety of the combination.

Novel Endpoints for Phase I Trials

Given these data, there has been discussion of altering the endpoint of phase I trials. Rather than looking for the MTD, the objective of a phase I could shift to identify a minimal immunologically active dose, for example by looking for a dose that achieves prespecified pharmacodynamic and/or pharmacokinetic parameters. Possibilities could include novel PET imaging endpoints that measure changes in PD-L1 expression (40) and/or T-cell infiltration (41) in tumors or PD-1 receptor occupancy on CD3+ peripheral blood mononuclear cells using flow cytometry (2,42,43). This approach could be especially instructive for compounds in which there is uncertainty about administration schedule (e.g., intermittent or continuous exposure) or therapy duration (predefined stopping point versus ongoing therapy regardless of response). However, pharmacodynamic evaluation remains an inexact science, as the relationship between the lab endpoint, that is, immunologic activity and clinical efficacy, is not always clear. For example, there may not be a linear relationship between increased tumor T-cell infiltration and tumor regression that translates into clinical benefit.

Expansion Cohorts

Phase I trials more frequently include a dose expansion phase after completion of a dose-escalation phase to further characterize toxicity, gain preliminary evidence on efficacy in a particular disease population, and determine the RP2D. It is well known that since conventional phase I sample sizes are too small to obtain reliable estimates, expansion cohorts are based on a prespecified number of patients (e.g., 5, 10, 15) to be treated at MTD in order to gain a more precise estimate of the probability of toxicity at that dose level. The RP2D may differ from the MTD as additional toxicity data are gathered through the expansion phase. If an expansion cohort is specified it must be clear how these data will be used. Oftentimes, multiple cohorts will be enrolled on trial during the dose expansion phase based on specific molecular characteristics, disease type, or both; however, justification of sample sizes can be difficult and can lead to a very large study without a clear rationale up front. This is illustrated by a single-center review of 522 phase I trials with expansion cohorts opened between 1988 and 2012. Sixty percent of trials with three or more cohorts provided no statistical justification of the sample size (44). These expansion cohorts are increasingly important for the safety assessment of CPIs given that irAEs are expected to occur beyond the first cycle and allow investigators to observe for delayed toxicities. In one systematic review among expansion cohorts with safety objectives, new toxicities were reported in 54% of trials and the RP2D was modified in 13% (45). Expansion cohorts also allow for early assessment of the efficacy of a compound as well as subpopulations for which that compound may be especially effective. These cohorts enable investigators to identify drugs that work best for specific patient populations in the context of a single trial, rather than using separate phase I trials and multiple phase II trials in specific patient populations. The costs and administrative burden associated with conducting separate trials can be greatly reduced.

One prime example of this was the phase I trial of nivolumab lead by Topalian and colleagues. Five expansion cohorts of patients were given the MAD of 10 mg/kg. Based on efficacy signal, three additional expansion cohorts of patients with melanoma, NSCLC, and renal cell carcinoma (RCC) were randomly assigned to receive drug at doses less than the MAD. Randomization enabled investigators to compare both safety and efficacy across multiple dose levels and disease types (2). However, the use of expansion cohorts in phase I trials has ballooned beyond expectations. For example, the anti-PD-L1 compound avelumab is being studied in a phase 1 trial with 16 expansion cohorts with a total projected enrollment of 1,706 people (NCT01772004, Clinicaltrials.gov). Study design of expansion cohorts should be structured more like phase II studies, which are designed to control for the possibility of false-positive or false-negative results, and have predefined stopping rules for futility to avoid exposing a high number of patients to the risk of ineffective or potentially dangerous treatment.

CONSIDERATIONS IN PHASE II AND PHASE III TRIAL DESIGN

Randomized Phase II Design

Typically, single-arm phase II trials are used in earlier drug development with the goal of establishing initial activity of a treatment. These trials tend to be single-institution studies and suffer from the confounding effects from accrual of patients with better risk profiles, trial eligibility definitions, and imaging and response assessments (46).

Given the pace at which immunotherapy drugs and combinations are being evaluated for efficacy, single-arm phase II trials may not be ideal for evaluating multiple experimental treatments. There has been increasing use of randomization in the phase II setting in order to evaluate multiple potential treatments and ensure better patient comparability. Randomized phase II trials fall into one of the following categories: randomization to parallel noncomparative arms; randomized selection; or randomized screening designs. A common strategy is to randomize patients to two parallel one-arm studies where each arm is compared to a null response rate and each arm will be assessed for promising activity compared to historical control response rates. Randomized selection or pick-the-winner designs are implemented when several regimens may be investigated at the end of the trial and one of the competing treatments will be selected to be studied further. The "winner" is selected based on the treatment with the highest response; however, criteria are specified in the design stage (e.g., 90% chance of selecting the better treatment when the response is 10% higher on one arm than the other). The goal is to have a high probability that you select the treatment that is not worse than the other. In these designs there is no intention to directly compare arms as in the definitive randomized phase III setting. Randomized screening designs are used when a treatment is compared against standard of care to obtain early evidence of increased efficacy (46).

In randomized discontinuation designs, all patients are treated in the first phase. Patients who respond and those who progress discontinue treatment. In the second phase, patients with stable disease are randomized to continue treatment or receive placebo and the proportion of patients who remain in stable disease are assessed in the two arms. Although this design limits the number of patients receiving placebo, if the expected number of patients with stable disease is small then this design may not be appropriate (47).

Patient Eligibility

Traditionally, phase II and III oncology trials have had strict eligibility criteria for patients to enter, including age greater than 18, excellent performance status

(Eastern Cooperative Oncology Group [ECOG] 0 or 1), preserved organ function, and no brain metastases. Appropriate eligibility criteria, which may require greater exclusions and a circumscribed patient population, are essential for the design of valid randomized controlled trials that aim to establish the efficacy of a new drug. However, many of the exclusion criteria commonly applied in randomized clinical trials are derived from cytotoxic chemotherapy and may not be relevant for IO agents. Overall, CPIs are well tolerated; the incidence of grade 3/4 irAEs from PD-1 blocking antibodies is less than 20% (4–7) and patient deaths are exceedingly rare, ≤2% (4,49). Exclusion criteria could therefore be expanded to include people with a lower performance status (ECOG 2). In addition, certain toxicities have little to no relevance for CPI treatment. For example, the rate of hematologic toxicity from immune-related agents is exceedingly low (33); this raises the question of why patients with abnormal blood counts are excluded from trials. In addition, activity and clinical benefit from CPIs have been observed in patients with brain metastases (49), a population of patients who are often excluded from clinical trials.

On the opposing side, clinical trials of IO agents have traditionally excluded patients with underlying autoimmune disease or patients on chronic immunosuppression out of fear that these novel treatments could worsen the underlying disease. Recent data published by Menzies and colleagues demonstrate that patients with underlying autoimmune disease do experience autoimmune disease flares when treated with anti-PD-1 therapy (38%) but only 4% of patients discontinued treatment due to the flare. Moreover, the response rate was only marginally lower than that published in large clinical trials (33%) (50).

Biomarkers

In the era of personalized medicine, where genetic sequencing is becoming increasingly inexpensive, there has been rapid advancement in targeted inhibition of oncogenic signaling pathways ("targeted therapy"). Drugs have been developed that are directed toward tumor-specific targets, including HER2 amplifications, EGFR mutations, ALK translocation, and BRAF mutations. There has been a simultaneous investment in finding biomarkers that may predict for response to CPI. Efficient development of new anticancer drugs may need to use clinical trial designs that are driven by predictive biomarkers to enable both evaluation of new treatments and identification of the patient subgroups in which these treatments are indicated (51). In this context, the clinical utility of a biomarker (in its role as the companion diagnostic for a specific new therapy) is defined by its ability to reliably identify a patient subgroup that benefits from the new therapy. The incorporation of biomarkers into clinical trial design has been

discussed extensively in reviews and elsewhere in this book (52).

Much of the initial effort toward defining a biomarker in IO has been directed toward the use of PD-L1 expression on tumor or infiltrating immune cells. PD-1, a CD28 receptor family member, is an inducible immune modulatory receptor. Upon interaction with its ligands B7 homolog 1 (PD-L1) and B7-DC (PD-L2), PD-1 plays important roles in negative regulation of T-cell responses to antigen stimulation and maintaining peripheral tolerance. In addition to the inducible expression pattern on conventional T cells, PD-1 is also found on regulatory T cells, follicular T and B cells, and antigen-presenting cells, including activated dendritic cells and monocytes. While PD-L1 expression has been associated with more favorable response rates to PD-1/PD-L1 agents, PD-L1 is not a static biomarker capable of binary discrimination of responsiveness. PD-L1 expression is inducible and can quickly vary over time in response to cytokines in the microenvironment. Moreover, there is disagreement about the antibody used, the threshold of positivity, and the cells on which this biomarker should be assessed (tumor versus tumor-infiltrating lymphocytes [TILs]).

In an initial study of nivolumab in patients with advanced solid tumors, zero of the 17 patients with PD-L1-negative tumors had an objective response compared to 36% of patients with PD-L1-positive tumors (2). Grosso and colleagues expanded on these findings by performing a retrospective review of patients with NSCLC and advanced melanoma who had received nivolumab. In the melanoma cohort, patients appeared to derive clinical benefit from nivolumab regardless of tumor PD-L1 expression, although patients with tumors higher in PD-L1 expression had more substantive clinical activity with a median OS of 21.1 versus 12.5 months (53). In patients treated with atezolizumab (MPDL3280A), a PD-L1 blocking antibody, PD-L1 expression on TILs was significantly associated with response to therapy in patients with NSCLC. This appeared to be a more important response correlate than tumor cell PD-L1 expression, but the relative impact of PD-L1 expression on tumor cells versus tumor-infiltrating immune cells may vary across tumor types (54). PD-L1 expression has been examined in a number of tumor types, including melanoma, bladder cancer, NSCLC, and gastric cancer; PD-L1 positivity seems to enrich for response to CPI in patients with melanoma (33), NSCLC (5), and bladder cancer (8) but does not appear to consistently predict likelihood of benefit to single-agent PD-1/PD-L1 blockade.

The significance of PD-L1 as a possible biomarker is also unclear in patients receiving the combination of ipilimumab and nivolumab. In most studies of this combination regimen, response rates to the combination have been similar, regardless of PD-L1 status (34,35,55,56). In a subset analysis of the phase III Checkmate 67 trial, a difference in PFS between combination immunotherapy and nivolumab monotherapy was most apparent for patients with PD-L1 negative (<5% expression) tumors (56). Nonetheless, patients with PD-L1 positive tumors also had a higher response rate with the combination compared to nivolumab monotherapy. At the present time, PD-L1 expression is considered an experimental biomarker with the exception of NSCLC, where PD-L1 positivity is required for administration of pembrolizumab.

Another potential biomarker is the presence of TILs. This was first examined by Hamid and colleagues, who obtained pre- and on-treatment biopsies from melanoma patients receiving ipilimumab. In comparing patients who derived clinical benefit from those who did not, 57.1% of those who benefited had a posttreatment increase in TILs and none had a decrease. In contrast, only 10% of those who did not benefit had an increase in TILs and 15% had a decrease ($p = .005$). In patients with melanoma treated with pembrolizumab, patients who derived clinical benefit from treatment had higher CD8+ T-cell densities at the invasive tumor edge compared to those who did not derive benefit. Moreover, serially sampled tumors exhibited an increase in CD8+ T-cell density in the response group but not in the progression group (Spearman's correlation $r = 0.71$, $p < .001$). Overall, the response group was associated with significantly higher numbers of CD8+, PD-1+, and PD-L1+ cells at both the invasive margin and the tumor center when compared to the progression group (57).

Melanoma and NSCLC have been shown to have the highest somatic mutation prevalence across human cancer subtypes, likely secondary to chronic mutagen exposure (i.e., ultraviolet [UV], cigarette smoke) (58). Given these data, it was then hypothesized that patient-mutated epitopes, known as neoantigens, may play an important role in the T-cell response driven by checkpoint blockade. This was first assessed by van Rooij and colleagues, who published a case report of a patient with stage IV melanoma who derived clinical benefit from ipilimumab treatment. They performed tumor whole-exome sequencing, which revealed 1,657 somatic mutations. Using a bioinformatics platform, the investigators derived 448 potential CD8 T-cell epitopes that were analyzed for reactivity against the patient's TILs. This demonstrated a dominant response against a mutated epitope in the ATR kinase. Mutated ATR-specific T cells were present before initiating ipilimumab therapy and expanded fivefold during therapy (59).

This hypothetical relationship between mutation load and clinical benefit from immunotherapy was explored further in two additional cohorts, one consisting of patients with melanoma and the other with metastatic NSCLC. In patients with melanoma, mutational load was associated with the degree of clinical benefit from ipilimumab but was not sufficient to predict benefit. Again, predicted neoantigens activated T cells in situ

from the patients treated with ipilimumab (60). In the lung discovery cohort ($n = 16$), a higher somatic non-synonymous mutation burden was associated with clinical efficacy of pembrolizumab (Mann–Whitney $p = .02$). In the entire set of sequenced tumors ($n = 34$), the PFS was higher in patients with a high nonsynonymous burden versus a low nonsynonymous burden (median PFS 14.5 vs. 3.7 months, log-rank $p= 0.01$, HR: 0.19, 95% CI: 0.05–0.70). Using a cut point of ≥178 nonsynonymous mutations, patients in the discovery cohort with a higher burden had a likelihood ratio for deriving clinical benefit of 3.0; the sensitivity was 100% (95% CI: 59–100) and the specificity was 67% (95% CI: 29–93). In the validation cohort, the sensitivity and specificity were 86% and 75%, respectively (61). These findings raise interesting hypotheses, but additional research is necessary to confirm these early associations.

Responses and Efficacy Assessment

Once an RP2D has been specified in the phase I setting, treatment efficacy is evaluated in phase II trials. Most phase II trials are based on a binary indicator such as tumor response that can be observed earlier than long-term events such as survival. A single-arm phase II design requires specification of desired improvement in response rates relative to historical control data, with the goal of making a decision to move on to a phase III definitive trial. Simon's two-stage single-arm design is commonly used, which includes an early stopping rule for futility after the first stage of enrollment and efficacy evaluation (62).

Determination of historical control benchmarks can be difficult when drug development is moving at a fast pace. Furthermore, definition of response rate as a measure of clinical efficacy is not straightforward for CPIs and may not be useful for drugs with a cytostatic mechanism of action.

The Response Evaluation Criteria in Solid Tumors (RECIST) are a unified set of criteria first implemented in 2000 and updated in 2009 to provide a simplified and uniform assessment of tumor response to therapy delivered under the auspices of a clinical trial. In brief, the radiologist selects up to five lesions (maximum of two lesions per organ) to designate as target lesions that are recorded and measured at baseline as well as each subsequent imaging scan. Progressive disease according to RECIST is defined as a 20% increase in the sum of the longest diameters of target lesions, unequivocal progression of nontarget lesions, and/or the development of new lesions. A complete response is disappearance of all target lesions, a partial response is at least a 30% decrease in the sum of the diameters of target lesions, and stable disease is anything that does not meet the aforementioned criteria.

While the RECIST criteria provide a reasonable framework when measuring the response to traditional therapies, such as cytotoxic therapy, tumor response to CPI is not always so linear. Atypical response patterns have been well-documented, initially in patients with advanced melanoma treated with ipilimumab. In some patients, a decrease in lesion size occurred after an initial increase, confirmed by biopsy as inflammatory cell infiltrates or necrosis. In others, a reduction in total tumor burden during or after the appearance of new lesions was observed. These atypical patterns of response have been labeled "pseudoprogression" and appear to reflect the unique dynamics of T-cell expansion and infiltration. The apparent increases in tumor burden that sometimes precede responses in patients receiving CPI may reflect either continued tumor growth until a sufficient immune response develops or transient immune-cell infiltrate associated with edema.

The incidence of pseudoprogression appears to vary based on the type of immunotherapy utilized. An initial report in patients who received ipilimumab for treatment of melanoma found that 9.7% of patients (22 of 227 patients) had clinical responses (partial response and stable disease) that would have been misclassified as disease progression by World Health Organization (WHO) criteria (63). The rate of pseudoprogression patients with advanced melanoma treated with anti-PD-1 antibodies appears to range from 6.7% to 12% (64,65). The incidence of pseudoprogression in other solid tumor types is unclear, although there are reports of atypical response patterns in bladder cancer, RCC, and NSCLC (66).

The primary concern regarding these atypical patterns of response is that patients who have progression of disease as determined by RECIST usually discontinue experimental treatment; however, patients with pseudoprogression ultimately derived clinical benefit from the therapy. This has raised questions about the use of RECIST and other standardized response assessment tools to study the activity of CPIs and resulted in the development of a set of alternative, immune-related response criteria (irRC) for the evaluation of immune therapy activity in solid tumors. In the irRC, in contrast, tumor burden is measured as a sum of target lesions with new lesions; new lesions do not necessarily count as progressive disease. In the irRC, an immune-related complete response (irCR) is the disappearance of all lesions, measured or unmeasured, and no new lesions; an immune-related partial response (irPR) is at least a 50% decrease in the total tumor burden from baseline as defined by the irRC; and immune-related progressive disease (irPD) is a 25% increase in tumor burden from the lowest level recorded. All other outcomes are considered immune-related stable disease (irSD) (63). These criteria have yet to be validated outside of clinical trials of melanoma and thus remain an exploratory endpoint.

In contrast to conventional chemotherapy, immunotherapies often demonstrate delayed clinical effects, which may not translate into a tumor response or even PFS. For example, sipuleucel-T immunotherapy for advanced prostate cancer prolongs OS without any effect on time to progression (TTP) or prostate-specific antigen (PSA) (67). OS remains the most important endpoint when evaluating effectiveness of a treatment. In a randomized phase III trial, patients who progress cross over to the experimental treatment or will receive alternative treatments off study, both of which can bias the OS comparison. Furthermore, if survival postprogression is long, it can be difficult to detect survival differences. For these reasons, there has been a shift away from OS to PFS (events are progression or death) or TTP (events are progression only) as the primary endpoint. Although PFS does not suffer from the same limitations as OS, measurement of progression with immunotherapy can be challenging and can affect estimation of PFS or TTP (68). Recent data suggests the hazard of favoring PFS as a primary endpoint over OS. The KEYNOTE-045 study compared second- or third-line pembrolizumab with investigator-choice chemotherapy as a treatment for patients with metastatic or locally advanced, unresectable urothelial carcinoma. The coprimary endpoints were OS and PFS. The median OS was 10.3 months with pembrolizumab versus 7.4 months with chemotherapy (HR: 0.73, $p = .0022$). The estimated 1-year OS rate was 43.9% with pembrolizumab compared with 30.7% in the chemotherapy arm. There was no significant difference in PFS (69). When there is late or delayed separation of the survival curves between two arms, intermediate endpoints such as milestone survival (survival probability at a specific time point) have been proposed for the evaluation of immunotherapies (70). Comparison of rates at a prespecified time point along the curve can be more powerful in this setting.

ASSESSING TOXICITY IN TRIALS—USING THE COMMON TERMINOLOGY CRITERIA FOR ADVERSE EVENTS (CTCAE)

In cancer clinical trials, AE are reported using the U.S. National Cancer Institute's (NCI's) Common Terminology Criteria for Adverse Events (CTCAE) (71). The original CTCAE were developed to document the adverse effects of chemotherapy but are also used in IO trials to document side effects termed "immune-related adverse events." Characterization of AEs by the CTCAE has implications for determining what constitutes a DLT and, consequently, the RP2D of investigational agents.

The majority of data documenting irAEs come from large published trials, mostly in patients with advanced melanoma, NSCLC, and RCC. Additionally, reports of large patient cohorts from expanded access programs and retrospective analyses have also provided information on the incidence of irAEs (72,73). In general, PD-1 inhibitors have a lower incidence of irAEs compared to those that block CTLA-4 such as ipilimumab, whereas the combination of nivolumab and ipilimumab has a higher rate of irAEs than either approach as monotherapy. For example, in a phase III trial in patients with advanced melanoma receiving nivolumab, ipilimumab, or the combination of both, grade 3/4 treatment-related AEs were observed in 16.3% of patients treated with nivolumab, 27.3% of patients treated with ipilimumab, and 55% of patients treated with the combination (33). Fortunately, despite this rate of grade 3/4 toxicity, irAEs leading to treatment-related patient death are exceedingly rare, ≤2% (4,48).

Investigators should think critically about classification of irAEs using the CTCAE, especially when considering DLTs. For example, in the phase I trial (CA209004) of nivolumab + ipilimumab, the dose cohort of ipilimumab 3 mg/kg + nivolumab 3 mg/kg was determined to have exceeded the acceptable levels of DLTs because of three patients having asymptomatic grade 3 or higher lipase elevations lasting for three or more weeks (22). This contributed to the determination of the 3 mg/kg of ipilimumab + 1 mg/kg of nivolumab dosing for subsequent studies in melanoma. However, it is unclear in the IO sphere what relationship isolated asymptomatic lab abnormalities may have with clinical events. In the case of lipase elevation, a subsequent retrospective review found that clinical pancreatitis was a rare event (1.7%) in patients receiving nivolumab + ipilimumab; these cases of pancreatitis represented 20% of patients with grade 3 or higher amylase, 6.3% of patients with grade 3 or higher lipase, and 20% of patients with grade 3 or higher elevations of both enzymes (74).

The NCI recently decided to modify the CTCAE criteria for amylase and lipase. In CTCAE v5.0, grade 4 amylase and lipase now require values exceeding five times the upper limit of normal (ULN) and must be associated with symptoms. Grade 3 amylase and lipase remain independent laboratory toxicities outside of a relevant clinical condition. Grade 3 AEs are considered DLTs in many clinical trials; this may have further ramifications for dictating the RP2D as novel IO agents are tested, potentially limiting access and exposure to effective new therapies. Investigators should reevaluate the criteria of the CTCAE in categorizing irAE and determining DLTs in the context of growing collective clinical experience.

CONCLUSIONS

The oncology clinical trial landscape is evolving rapidly with the incorporation of IO agents into the treatment algorithm of both solid and liquid tumors. Clinical investigators must be aware of the unique properties of these agents when designing trials, especially when considering toxicities and primary endpoints.

REFERENCES

1. Hodi FS, O'Day SJ, Mcdermott DF, et al. Improved survival with ipilimumab in patients with metastatic melanoma. *N Engl J Med.* 2010;363(8):711–723.
2. Topalian SL, Hodi FS, Brahmer JR, et al. Safety, activity, and immune correlates of anti-PD-1 antibody in cancer. *N Engl J Med.* 2012;366(26):2443–2454.
3. Brahmer JR, Tykodi SS, Chow LQ, et al. Safety and activity of anti-PD-L1 antibody in patients with advanced cancer. *N Engl J Med.* 2012;366(26):2455–2465.
4. Gettinger SN, Horn L, Gandhi L, et al. Overall survival and long-term safety of nivolumab (anti-programmed Death 1 antibody, BMS-936558, ONO-4538) in patients with previously treated advanced non-small-cell lung cancer. *J Clin Oncol.* 2015;33(18):2004–2012.
5. Garon EB, Rizvi NA, Hui R, et al. KEYNOTE-001 investigators. Pembrolizumab for the treatment of non-small-cell lung cancer. *N Engl J Med.* 2015;372(21):2018–2028.
6. Motzer RJ, Rini BI, Mcdermott DF, et al. Nivolumab for metastatic renal cell carcinoma: results of a randomized Phase II trial. *J Clin Oncol.* 2015;33(13):1430–1437.
7. Motzer RJ, Escudier B, Mcdermott DF, et al. CheckMate 025 investigators. Nivolumab versus Everolimus in advanced renal-cell carcinoma. *N Engl J Med.* 2015;373(19):1803–1813.
8. Rosenberg JE, Hoffman-Censits J, Powles T, et al. Atezolizumab in patients with locally advanced and metastatic urothelial carcinoma who have progressed following treatment with platinum-based chemotherapy: a single-arm, multicentre, Phase 2 trial. *Lancet.* 2016;387(10031):1909–1920.
9. Yervoy (R) [package insert]. Bristol-Myers Squibb; 2011. http://packageinserts.bms.com/pi/pi_yervoy.pdf
10. Opdivo (R) [package insert]. Bristol-Myers Squibb; 2014. https://packageinserts.bms.com/pi/pi_opdivo.pdf
11. Keytruda (R) [package insert]. Merck; 2017. https://www.merck.com/product/usa/pi_circulars/k/keytruda/keytruda_pi.pdf
12. Tecentriq (R) [package insert]. Genentech; 2016. https://www.accessdata.fda.gov/drugsatfda_docs/label/2016/761041lbl.pdf
13. Bavencio (R) [package insert]. EMD Serono; 2017. https://www.accessdata.fda.gov/drugsatfda_docs/label/2017/761049s000lbl.pdf
14. Imfinzi (R) [package insert]. AstraZeneca; 2017. https://www.accessdata.fda.gov/drugsatfda_docs/label/2017/761069s000lbl.pdf
15. Ansell SM, Lesokhin AM, Borrello I, et al. PD-1 blockade with nivolumab in relapsed or refractory Hodgkin's lymphoma. *N Engl J Med.* 2015;372(4):311–319.
16. Robert C, Ribas A, Wolchok JD, et al. Anti-programmed-death-receptor-1 treatment with pembrolizumab in ipilimumab-refractory advanced melanoma: a randomised dose-comparison cohort of a Phase 1 trial. *Lancet.* 2014;384(9948):1109–1117.
17. Vacchelli E, Bloy N, Aranda F, et al. Trial watch: immunotherapy plus radiation therapy for oncological indications. *Oncoimmunology.* 2016;5(9):e1214790
18. Buqué A, Bloy N, Aranda F, et al. Trial watch: immunomodulatory monoclonal antibodies for oncological indications. *Oncoimmunology.* 2015;4(4):e1008814
19. Paoletti X, Le Tourneau C, Verweij J, et al. Defining dose-limiting toxicity for Phase 1 trials of molecularly targeted agents: results of a DLT-TARGETT international survey. *Eur J Cancer.* 2014;50(12):2050–2056.
20. Weber JS, Dummer R, de Pril V, et al. MDX010-20 Investigators. Patterns of onset and resolution of immune-related adverse events of special interest with ipilimumab: detailed safety analysis from a Phase 3 trial in patients with advanced melanoma. *Cancer.* 2013;119(9):1675–1682.
21. Lutzky J, Antonia S, Blake-Haskins A, Segal NH. A Phase 1 study of MEDI4736, an anti–PD-L1 antibody, in patients with advanced solid tumors. *J Clin Oncol.* 2014;32(15, Suppl):3001.

22. Wolchok JD, Kluger H, Callahan MK, et al. Nivolumab plus Ipilimumab in advanced melanoma. *N Engl J Med Overseas Ed.* 2013;369(2):122–133.

23. Ascierto PA, del Vecchio M, Robert C, et al. Overall survival (OS) and safety results from a Phase 3 trial of ipilimumab (IPI) at 3 mg/kg vs 10 mg/kg in patients with metastatic melanoma (MEL). *Annals of Oncology.* 2016;27(Suppl 6). doi:10.1093/annonc/mdw379.01

24. Wolchok JD, Neyns B, Linette G, et al. Ipilimumab monotherapy in patients with pretreated advanced melanoma: a randomised, double-blind, multicentre, Phase 2, dose-ranging study. *Lancet Oncol.* 2010;11(2):155–164.

25. Patnaik A, Kang SP, Rasco D, et al. Phase I study of pembrolizumab (MK-3475; Anti-PD-1 Monoclonal Antibody) in patients with advanced solid tumors. *Clin Cancer Res.* 2015;21(19):4286–4293.

26. Hünig T. The storm has cleared: lessons from the CD28 superagonist TGN1412 trial. *Nat Rev Immunol.* 2012;12(5):317–318.

27. Postel-Vinay S, Aspeslagh S, Lanoy E, et al. Challenges of Phase 1 clinical trials evaluating immune checkpoint-targeted antibodies. *Ann Oncol.* 2016;27(2):214–224.

28. Ribas A, Camacho LH, Lopez-Berestein G, et al. Antitumor activity in melanoma and anti-self responses in a phase I trial with the anti-cytotoxic T lymphocyte-associated antigen 4 monoclonal antibody CP-675,206. *J Clin Oncol.* 2005;23(35):8968–8977.

29. Eggermont AM, Chiarion-Sileni V, Grob JJ, et al. Adjuvant ipilimumab versus placebo after complete resection of high-risk Stage III melanoma (EORTC 18071): a randomised, double-blind, Phase 3 trial. *Lancet Oncol.* 2015;16(5):522–530.

30. Robert C, Schachter J, Long GV, et al. KEYNOTE-006 investigators. Pembrolizumab versus Ipilimumab in advanced melanoma. *N Engl J Med.* 2015;372(26):2521–2532.

31. Reck M, Rodríguez-Abreu D, Robinson AG, et al. KEYNOTE-024 investigators. pembrolizumab versus chemotherapy for PD-L1-Positive non-small-cell lung cancer. *N Engl J Med.* 2016;375(19):1823–1833.

32. Seiwert TY, Burtness B, Mehra R, et al. Safety and clinical activity of pembrolizumab for treatment of recurrent or metastatic squamous cell carcinoma of the head and neck (KEYNOTE-012): an open-label, multicentre, Phase 1b trial. *Lancet Oncol.* 2016;17(7):956–965.

33. Larkin J, Chiarion-Sileni V, Gonzalez R, et al. Combined nivolumab and ipilimumab or monotherapy in untreated melanoma. *N Engl J Med.* 2015;373(1):23–34.

34. Postow MA, Chesney J, Pavlick AC, et al. Nivolumab and ipilimumab versus ipilimumab in untreated melanoma. *N Engl J Med.* 2015;372(21):2006–2017.

35. Hellmann MD, Rizvi NA, Goldman JW, et al. Nivolumab plus ipilimumab as first-line treatment for advanced non-small-cell lung cancer (CheckMate 012): results of an open-label, Phase 1, multicohort study. *Lancet Oncol.* 2017;18(1):31–41.

36. Wong KM, Capasso A, Eckhardt SG. The changing landscape of Phase I trials in oncology. *Nat Rev Clin Oncol.* 2016;13(2):106–117.

37. Mandrekar SJ. Dose-finding trial designs for combination therapies in oncology. *J Clin Oncol.* 2014;32(2):65–67.

38. Wages NA, Ivanova A, Marchenko O. Practical designs for Phase I combination studies in oncology. *J Biopharm Stat.* 2016;26(1):150–166.

39. Riviere MK, Le Tourneau C, Paoletti X, et al. Designs of drug-combination Phase I trials in oncology: a systematic review of the literature. *Ann Oncol.* 2015;26(4):669–674.

40. Hettich M, Braun F, Bartholomä MD, et al. High-resolution PET imaging with therapeutic antibody-based PD-1/PD-L1 checkpoint tracers. *Theranostics.* 2016;6(10):1629–1640.

41. Mccracken MN, Vatakis DN, Dixit D, et al. Noninvasive detection of tumor-infiltrating T cells by PET reporter imaging. *J Clin Invest.* 2015;125(5):1815–1826.

42. Liang M, Schwickart M, Schneider AK, et al. Receptor occupancy assessment by flow cytometry as a pharmacodynamic biomarker in biopharmaceutical development. *Cytometry B Clin Cytom.* 2016;90(2):117–127.

43. Brahmer JR, Drake CG, Wollner I, et al. Phase I study of single-agent anti-programmed death-1 (MDX-1106) in refractory solid tumors: safety, clinical activity, pharmacodynamics, and immunologic correlates. *J Clin Oncol.* 2010;28(19):3167–3175.

44. Dahlberg SE, Shapiro GI, Clark JW, Johnson BE. Evaluation of statistical designs in Phase I expansion cohorts: the Dana-Farber/Harvard Cancer Center experience. *J Natl Cancer Inst.* 2014;106(7). doi:10.1093/jnci/dju163

45. Manji A, Brana I, Amir E, et al. Evolution of clinical trial design in early drug development: systematic review of expansion cohort use in single-agent Phase I cancer trials. *J Clin Oncol.* 2013;31(33):4260–4267.

46. Mandrekar SJ, Sargent DJ. Randomized Phase II trials: time for a new era in clinical trial design. *J Thorac Oncol.* 2010;5(7):932–934.

47. Kopec JA, Abrahamowicz M, Esdaile JM. Randomized discontinuation trials: utility and efficiency. *J Clin Epidemiol.* 1993;46(9):959–971.

48. Weber JS, Antonia SJ, Topalian SL, et al. Safety profile of nivolumab (NIVO) in patients (pts) with advanced melanoma (MEL): a pooled analysis. *ASCO Meeting Abstracts.* 2015;33:9018.

49. Margolin K, Ernstoff MS, Hamid O, et al. Ipilimumab in patients with melanoma and brain metastases: an open-label, Phase 2 trial. *Lancet Oncol.* 2012;13(5):459–465.

50. Menzies AM, Johnson DB, Ramanujam S, et al. Anti-PD-1 therapy in patients with advanced melanoma and preexisting autoimmune disorders or major toxicity with ipilimumab. *Ann Oncol.* 2017;28(2):368–376.

51. U.S. Department of Health and Human Services. Enrichment strategies for clinical trials to support approval of human drugs and biological products. https://www.fda.gov/downloads/Drugs/GuidanceComplianceRegulatoryInformation/Guidances/UCM332181.pdf%20. Published 2012.

52. Freidlin B, Korn EL. Biomarker enrichment strategies: matching trial design to biomarker credentials. *Nat Rev Clin Oncol.* 2014;11(2):81–90.

53. Grosso J, Horak CE, Inzunza D, et al. Association of tumor PD-L1 expression and immune biomarkers with clinical activity in patients (pts) with advanced solid tumors treated with nivolumab (anti-PD-1; BMS-936558; ONO-4538). *ASCO Meeting Abstracts.* 2013;31:3016.

54. Herbst RS, Soria JC, Kowanetz M, et al. Predictive correlates of response to the anti-PD-L1 antibody MPDL3280A in cancer patients. *Nature.* 2014;515(7528):563–567.

55. Wolchok JD, Kluger H, Callahan MK, et al. Nivolumab plus ipilimumab in advanced melanoma. *N Engl J Med.* 2013;369(2):122–133.

56. Larkin J, Chiarion-Sileni V, Gonzalez R, et al. Combined nivolumab and ipilimumab or monotherapy in untreated melanoma. *N Engl J Med Overseas Ed.* 2015;373(1):23–34.

57. Tumeh PC, Harview CL, Yearley JH, et al. PD-1 blockade induces responses by inhibiting adaptive immune resistance. *Nature.* 2014;515(7528):568–571.

58. Alexandrov LB, Nik-Zainal S, Wedge DC, et al. Australian Pancreatic Cancer Genome InitiativeICGC Breast Cancer ConsortiumICGC MMML-Seq ConsortiumICGC PedBrain. Signatures of mutational processes in human cancer. *Nature.* 2013;500(7463):415–421.

59. van Rooij N, van Buuren MM, Philips D, et al. Tumor exome analysis reveals neoantigen-specific T-cell reactivity in an ipilimumab-responsive melanoma. *J Clin Oncol.* 2013;31(32):e439–e442.

60. Snyder A, Makarov V, Merghoub T, et al. Genetic basis for clinical response to CTLA-4 blockade in melanoma. *N Engl J Med.* 2014;371(23):2189–2199.

61. Rizvi NA, Hellmann MD, Snyder A, et al. Cancer immunology. Mutational landscape determines sensitivity to PD-1 blockade in non-small cell lung cancer. *Science.* 2015;348(6230):124–128.

62. Simon R. Optimal two-stage designs for Phase II clinical trials. *Control Clin Trials*. 1989;10(1):1–10.

63. Wolchok JD, Hoos A, O'Day S, et al. Guidelines for the evaluation of immune therapy activity in solid tumors: immune-related response criteria. *Clin Cancer Res*. 2009;15(23):7412–7420.

64. Hodi F, Ribas A, Daud A, et al. Patterns of response in patients with advanced melanoma treated with Pembrolizumab (MK-3475) and evaluation of immune-related response criteria (irRC). *J Immunother Cancer*. 2014;2(Suppl 3):P103.

65. Hodi FS, Sznol M, Kluger H, Sosman JA. Long term survival of ipilimumab-naive patients (pts) with advanced melanoma (MEL) treated with nivolumab (anti-PD-1, BMS-936558, ONO-4538) in a phase I trial. *J Clin Oncol*. 2014;32:9002.

66. Chiou VL, Burotto M. Pseudoprogression and immune-related response in solid tumors. *J Clin Oncol*. 2015;33(31):3541–3543.

67. Small EJ, Schellhammer PF, Higano CS, et al. Placebo-controlled Phase III trial of immunologic therapy with sipuleucel-T (APC8015) in patients with metastatic, asymptomatic hormone refractory prostate cancer. *J Clin Oncol*. 2006;24(19):3089–3094.

68. Dranitsaris G, Cohen RB, Acton G, et al. Statistical considerations in clinical trial design of immunotherapeutic cancer agents. *J Immunother*. 2015;38(7):259–266.

69. Bellmunt J, de Wit R, Vaughn D, et al. Keynote-045: open-label, Phase III study of pembrolizumab versus investigator's choice of paclitaxel, docetaxel, or vinflunine for previously treated advanced urothelial cancer. *J Immunother Can*. 2016;4(Suppl 2).

70. Chen TT. Milestone survival: a potential intermediate endpoint for immune checkpoint inhibitors. *J Natl Cancer Inst*. 2015;107(9). doi:10.1093/jnci/djv156

71. Callahan MK, Postow MA, Wolchok JD. CTLA-4 and PD-1 Pathway Blockade: combinations in the clinic. *Front Oncol*. 2014;4:385.

72. Horvat TZ, Adel NG, Dang TO, et al. Immune-related adverse events, need for systemic immunosuppression, and effects on survival and time to treatment failure in patients with melanoma treated with ipilimumab at memorial sloan kettering cancer center. *J Clin Oncol*. 2015;33(28):3193–3198.

73. Altomonte M, di Giacomo A, Queirolo P, et al. Clinical experience with ipilimumab 10 mg/kg in patients with melanoma treated at Italian centres as part of a European expanded access programme. *J Exp Clin Cancer Res*. 2013;32:82.

74. Friedman CF, Clark V, Raikhel AV, et al. Thinking critically about classifying adverse events: incidence of pancreatitis in patients treated with nivolumab + ipilimumab. *J Natl Cancer Inst*. 2017;109(4). doi:10.1093/jnci/djw260

43

Special Considerations in Radiation Therapy Trials

Amanda J. Walker, Hyun Kim, Paul G. Kluetz, Julia A. Beaver, Gideon Blumenthal, and Richard Pazdur

Radiation therapy is a prevalent treatment modality for malignancies and is indicated in the definitive management over half of patients with cancer. This is due to improved survival, local control, or toxicity profiles of radiation therapy compared to other treatment options (1). Despite these improvements, local and distant recurrences still occur and many survivors face complications regarding late radiation toxicities such as cardiovascular disease and soft-tissue fibrosis (2). Improvements in radiotherapy outcomes can provide enormous benefit to patients, both in terms of disease control and minimizing toxicities. This chapter is new to the 2017 Edition of *Oncology Clinical Trials* and highlights some important considerations regarding clinical trials with radiation therapy, with a focus on the clinical investigation of drugs in combination with external beam radiation therapy.

PRINCIPLES OF RADIATION THERAPY

While we cannot cover the expansive literature on the principles of radiation biology (3), we begin this chapter with a basic and simplified overview of the mechanism by which radiation exerts its therapeutic effect to facilitate the subsequent discussion on clinical trial considerations. The mechanism by which radiation therapy kills tumor cells, or renders them incapable of further cell division, includes direct DNA damage as well as indirect DNA damage caused by x-rays colliding with other molecules (e.g., water) in the target. Some of the main parameters that can be specified when prescribing radiation therapy are (a) the total dose of radiation (in Gy) over multiple treatments or fractions, (b) the dose per fraction, and (c) the frequency of treatment. Conventional radiation therapy when delivered with curative intent is typically delivered in 1.8 to 2.0 Gy daily fractions over a course of 6 to 8 weeks.

Therapeutic Index

Cell killing with radiation has a nonlinear relationship with fraction size such that a course of radiation therapy given in a smaller number of large fractions is more damaging to tissue than the same total dose given in larger number of smaller fractions. Moreover, there is a differential response between rapidly dividing cells (including tumor cells), compared with more slowly dividing cells (such as normal tissue cells), the latter being more prone to late radiation injury. The therapeutic index, or therapeutic ratio, defined as the ratio of tumor control probability to normal tissue complication probability, favors dividing the total dose into multiple small fractions when normal tissue is included in the treatment volume to minimize late radiation toxicity. Malignant tissue often has faulty DNA damage repair machinery and theoretically is unable to repair radiation-induced damage as well as normal tissue. In general, allowing at least 6 hours between treatment fractions and limiting treatment intervals to 24 hours allows for normal tissue repair while minimizing tumor repopulation, respectively. Therapeutic index is an important concept because, historically, the total doses and schedules used clinically have been determined more by what can be tolerated by the normal tissues rather than by what is sufficient to achieve high rates of tumor control. A number of strategies have been developed to optimize the therapeutic index, and the most common examples are described in the following.

Hypofractionation

The therapeutic ratio can be further improved by accounting for the intrinsic radiation susceptibility qualities of different tissues when determining the dose per fraction. Each tissue has an inherent radiosensitivity and ability to repair cells, often quantified as alpha (single hit or linear component of cell killing) and beta (quadratic component of cell killing) constants, respectively. The ratio alpha/beta is the dose at which the linear and quadratic components of cell death on an in vitro survival curve are equal. Tissues with low alpha/beta ratios are thought to be more resistant to low doses and there may be a therapeutic benefit in terms of disease control when using large fraction doses. While historically, most definitive daily treatment fraction sizes were 1.8 to 2.0 Gy, using fraction sizes larger than this over fewer total fractions is known as hypofractionation and had been demonstrated to be a successful approach thus far in breast and prostate cancer (4–7).

Stereotactic Body Radiation Therapy
The process of delivering high ablative doses of radiation using highly conformal treatment with image guidance is known as stereotactic ablative radiotherapy (SABR) or stereotactic body radiation therapy (SBRT). This treatment method allows for delivery of high doses of radiation in a small number of fractions (typically 1–5), and is used when radiation treatment is limited to small targets. Advantages of this treatment technique generally include higher rates of local disease control and minimal normal tissue irradiation.

Hyperfractionation
In contrast, hyperfractionation is the use of smaller fraction sizes given multiple times a day to complete the treatment course in a relatively similar overall calendar time. Hyperfractionation is often used to increase the treatment dose while maintaining a similar late toxicity incidence. For example, there is literature to suggest that delivering radiation therapy in twice daily fractions may reduce the risk of radiation-induced optic neuropathy in patients with head and neck cancer treated with curative intent (8).

Proton Therapy
While photon radiation is the most commonly prescribed radiation type, proton therapy is becoming more widely available and used. Protons and other heavy particles differ from photons in that particles travel to a certain depth and deposit all their energy, thus eliminating the exit dose that is intrinsic to photons passing completely through the body. This may potentially decrease normal tissue toxicity, and clinical trials in a number of disease sites are ongoing. Proton plans however are more sensitive to changes in the heterogeneity of the material through which the beam passes (tissue vs. air). Thus, protons prescribed to deposit their energy at the tumor edge may actually deposit the prescription dose in the normal organs at risk (OARs) located just distal to the tumor border (9).

Radiation in Combination With Systemic Therapy
The therapeutic index of radiation therapy can also be improved by combining radiation therapy with novel systemic agents intended to augment the biological effects of radiation therapy. Examples include radiosensitizers and drugs intended to prevent damage to normal tissue (i.e., radioprotectors). Furthermore, although perhaps not considered a *radiosensitizer* in the classic sense of the word, the addition of immunotherapy to radiation can afford additional synergistic local control benefits and potentially aid in the management of distant metastatic disease when given in combination with radiation therapy (10,11).

RADIATION CLINICAL TRIALS

In addition to exploring alternative doses and fractionations in clinical trials over the past two decades, a number of significant technical advances in the field of radiation oncology have been developed with efforts to improve outcomes via conformal techniques such as image guidance, intensity-modulated radiation therapy (IMRT), and charged particle irradiation. Although some benefits of these technologies may appear intuitive due to the fact that normal tissues may be spared from higher doses of radiation, often clinical trials are required to demonstrate the benefit of such techniques to justify their cost and the use of additional resources. Radiation clinical trials may evaluate clinical outcomes according to specific radiation technique, modality, fractionation, or dose. Examples include Radiation Therapy Oncology Group (RTOG) 0529, which investigated the difference in gastrointestinal and genitourinary toxicity in patients with anal cancer treated with IMRT compared to three-dimensional (3D) treatment planning (12). RTOG 1308 is an ongoing phase 3 randomized trial comparing the overall survival in inoperable non–small-cell lung cancer patients treated with proton versus photon chemoradiation therapy. Finally, RTOG 0617 compared overall survival in high-dose versus standard-dose radiation therapy with concurrent chemotherapy in inoperable stage III non–small-cell lung cancer (13). It is wise for investigators and cooperative groups to design trials that are able to demonstrate clinical benefit of one treatment technique/modality over another to provide relevance in clinical practice. Some of the trial design considerations discussed throughout the remainder of the chapter in the context of radiation–drug combinations also apply to trials investigating radiation therapy techniques or modalities.

DRUG DEVELOPMENT IN COMBINATION WITH RADIATION THERAPY

In addition to technological advances in radiation oncology described previously, medical oncology has also witnessed a concomitant increase in the development of novel molecularly targeted agents as our understanding of the molecular pathways driving tumorigenesis continues to improve and more druggable targets are identified. In fact, the therapeutic landscape has substantially changed in recent years for a number of cancer types due to drugs being developed based on improved understanding of tumor biology. For example, the standard of care for all patients with metastatic non–small-cell lung cancer is no longer a platinum doublet. Treatment options in the modern area include ALK inhibitors, EGFR inhibitors, and PD-1/PD-L1 inhibitors depending on the biology of the patient's disease (14).

Even though more targeted therapies are being used to treat metastatic disease, the systemic therapy that is used in combination with radiation therapy for a number of disease sites remains traditional cytotoxic chemotherapeutics, as demonstrated in Table 43.1 (15). Although the literature has reported improvements in disease control in a number of disease sites with the addition of chemotherapy to radiation compared to radiation alone, the addition of cytotoxic chemotherapy for radiosensitization often comes at the cost of increased toxicity due to lack of specificity for tumor cells. Thus, to further improve the outcomes of radiation therapy while minimizing normal tissue sensitization, a promising treatment approach is to combine novel targeted systemic agents with radiotherapy to improve the likelihood of durable control and minimize normal tissue toxicity. Furthermore, immunotherapy agents can also afford radiosensitization or synergistic benefits and potentially manage occult distant disease.

Clinical Trial Considerations With Radiation Therapy

Toxicity Evaluation

Radiation toxicity inherently has two components: acute (early) effects and chronic (late) effects, and any trial with radiation therapy should be designed to consider the entire spectrum of radiation toxicity. Acute effects are defined as occurring during or shortly after completion of radiation treatment and are generally not significantly influenced by fractionation. These early effects are usually temporary and gradually heal once the radiation therapy is completed. Late effects are defined as toxicity that is evident >90 days after treatment starts, may not occur until years after treatment completion, and may be permanent and progressive.

Investigators should consider prospectively evaluating for late toxicity in clinical trials involving radiation therapy to enhance the quality of toxicity data and to ensure that improvements in local control and survival do not occur at the expense of unacceptable late toxicities. Although it is often impractical to consider late toxicities in dose-escalation trials, any dose-escalation trial of a systemic agent used in combination with radiation therapy should incorporate a mechanism of capturing significant late effects of radiation therapy. Any such late toxicity should be ultimately considered in the determination of the dose and dose schedule to be taken forward in development. Published data indicate that only approximately 9% of early-phase combined modality trials prospectively identify late toxic effects as an endpoint and only approximately 12% of these trials report late effects in publication (16). Interestingly, the majority of these trials have a sufficient follow-up time (i.e., greater than 6 months) to evaluate for late effects.

Even when assessments for late effects of radiation therapy take place during clinical trials, the incidence of late effects may still be underreported due to the grading system used and the reporting methodology. In the Groupe d'Oncologie Radiothérapie Tête et Cou (GORTEC) 94–01, investigators reported an overall survival of 22% with concurrent chemoradiotherapy versus 16% with radiation alone (log-rank, $p = .05$) (17). The initial trial results showed high-grade late effects of 9% and 14% in the radiation and chemoradiotherapy arms, respectively. In the final report of the trial, the high-grade late effects at 5 years in the concurrent and radiation alone arms were 56% and 30%, respectively, when using the RTOG/European Organization for Research and Treatment of Cancer (EORTC) and National Cancer Institute/Common Terminology Criteria for Adverse Events (NCI/CTCAE)

TABLE 43.1 Drugs Used Concurrently With Radiation Therapy in the Definitive Management of Cancer

Malignancy	Drug(s) Used Concurrently With Radiation
Non–small-cell lung cancer	Cisplatin + etoposide Cisplatin + pemetrexed Paclitaxel + carboplatin
Small-cell lung cancer	Cisplatin + etoposide
Rectal cancer	Capecitabine 5-FU
Anal cancer	Mitomycin + 5-FU Mitomycin + capecitabine
Cervical cancer	Cisplatin Cisplatin + 5-FU
Head and neck cancer	Cisplatin
Esophageal cancer	Cisplatin + 5-FU Oxaliplatin + 5-FU Carboplatin + paclitaxel
Glioblastoma	Temozolomide
Bladder cancer	Cisplatin

5-FU, 5-fluorouracil.

Source: From National Comprehensive Cancer Network. NCCN clinical practice guidelines in oncology. https://www.nccn.org/professionals/physician_gls. Updated December 2016

grading systems. When toxicity assessment also included data from the Subjective, Objective, Management, Analytic (SOMA) system the rate of late effects was 47% in the radiation arm and 82% in the chemoradiotherapy arm ($p = .02$). Thus, the time points at which late effects are reported and the grading systems used can significantly affect the reporting of toxicity, which is an essential component in evaluating the clinical value of a treatment. Investigators may select the grading system(s) based on disease site, stage of disease, and patient population and multiple grading systems may be used for adverse events (AEs) of special interest. In addition to capturing toxicity information, it is also critical to document treatment parameters that are known to be associated with toxicities. For example, in a trial investigating definitive radiation therapy for lung cancer, investigators should not only describe the rates of pneumonitis, they should also describe the treatment parameters that are known to be associated with the risk of pneumonitis (e.g., the mean lung dose and other dose–volume histogram parameters for ipsilateral and total lung volume).

Patient-Reported Outcomes

Patient-reported outcome (PRO) measures are often assessed in trials to support a clinical benefit in safety or efficacy, complement our understanding of tolerability, or describe additional aspects of the patient's experience while receiving a cancer therapy. While health-related quality of life (HRQL) assesses many important aspects of a patient's life, when assessing the effect of a therapy it is important to discriminate the effect of the therapeutic intervention from other influences. Disease symptoms, symptomatic AEs, and physical function are important aspects of HRQL that are more "proximal" to the effect of the therapy under investigation, and may be more sensitive to the positive and negative effects of a cancer therapy on the patient and disease (18). When considering PRO measurement tools, generic fixed questionnaires measuring HRQL and their disease modules may lack the flexibility to adapt to different disease symptoms and drug/radiation toxicities encountered in contemporary drug development. One option is for investigators to employ a combination of questions selected from item libraries for relevant symptoms and use subsets or subscales of fixed questionnaires for more global domains (e.g., HRQL, social and emotional domains, etc.) that may be more agnostic to disease and treatment settings.

Like any other measure intending to provide evidence of treatment benefit, PRO endpoints should be clearly stated, generated from a well-defined and reliable PRO instrument, and appropriate statistical methods should be applied to generate substantial evidence of a meaningful treatment effect (19). Investigators should provide a prespecified plan for the analysis of PRO data including the threshold for an interpretation of a meaningful change in score(s). Procedures should be put in place to minimize missing data, and any concomitant medications that may affect the interpretation of the concept(s) being measured (e.g., use of concomitant pain medications when measuring pain) should be carefully recorded. While PRO efficacy endpoints can be challenging in cancer trials due to blinding and asymmetric loss of patients due to progression and death, there are successful examples of PRO endpoints supporting efficacy in the Food and Drug Administration (FDA) review of cancer therapies (20).

In addition to the use of PRO measures to support efficacy, PRO measures can play an important role in generating descriptive patient-centered data to further inform the safety and tolerability of each treatment arm in a trial, which is an important trial objective in any clinical investigation. One promising tool that can be used to assess symptomatic toxicities is the NCI's Patient-Reported Outcomes version of the Common Terminology for Adverse Events (PRO-CTCAE™) (21). Systematic assessment of important symptomatic toxicities at baseline and throughout treatment can provide a rich set of data on the patient's perception of the frequency, severity, and interference of treatment side effects, which can inform tolerability. There has been increased interest in longitudinal analysis of treatment side effects to understand the kinetics and impact of low grade but prolonged symptomatic toxicities (22). PRO measurement has the potential to provide important patient-centered longitudinal data on key symptomatic side effects that can be analyzed to complement existing clinician-based safety assessment.

In addition to the clinical trial setting, there is increasing interest in leveraging data from clinical practice electronic health record (EHR) systems, so called "real-world data." An area of active research is the use of electronic PRO assessment of symptomatic AEs and other aspects of a patient's health in the clinical setting to assist in patient communication and symptom control (23). PRO measures are particularly attractive when assessed electronically as they can provide a pipeline of structured clinical outcome data. The aggregation of this data can provide information on treatment effects in a more broad and representative population and exploration of PRO data from EHR systems may be a useful setting to explore late toxicities, a particular challenge in the controlled clinical trial setting due to the cost of prolonged follow-up.

Radiation Quality Assurance

The implementation of 3D planning, image-guided therapy, and sophisticated radiation delivery techniques such as IMRT and volumetric-modulated radiation therapy (VMAT) have resulted in more parameters to ensure the quality of treatment delivery (24). The quality of the radiation treatment plan and delivery ensures appropriate dosing to the tumor and sparing of normal tissues and is an important consideration in any clinical trial with radiation therapy.

RTOG 9704 and TROG 02.02 are examples of two clinical trials in which the data suggests that adherence to the radiation therapy protocols may have had an impact on patient outcomes. RTOG 9704 was a phase III, multi-institution trial evaluating the use of adjuvant gemcitabine versus *5-fluorouracil* (5-FU) chemotherapy prior to concurrent 5-FU and radiation therapy in resected pancreatic adenocarcinoma. The published data did not indicate a survival advantage for the use of gemcitabine as prescribed in the trial. Interestingly, the investigators demonstrated that adherence to the radiation therapy protocol requirements was associated with increased survival on multivariate analysis. The published data report that this survival benefit was even more strongly correlated than the assigned treatment arm (25). TROG 02.02 was an international, phase III trial evaluating radiotherapy with concurrent cisplatin plus tirapazamine for advanced head and neck cancer. Posttreatment review by the trial management committee revealed that 25.4% of patients had noncompliant radiation treatment plans. Of the protocol violations, 47% (12% overall) had deficiencies that would significantly impact tumor control. An unplanned retrospective analysis suggested that the 2-year overall survival for protocol compliant versus noncompliant plans was 70% versus 50%, respectively; hazard ratio (HR): 1.99, $p < .001$ (26).

A meta-analysis was performed of eight multi-institutional trials involving radiation therapy and evaluated the impact of radiation protocol compliance on cancer outcomes. The frequency of protocol deviations ranged from 8% to 71% (median = 32%). The investigators demonstrated that radiation deviations were associated with a decrease in overall survival (HR: 1.74, CI: 1.28–2.35, $p < .001$) and increased treatment failure (HR: 1.79, CI: 1.15–2.78, $p < .009$). Although the aforementioned secondary analyses are limited by the caveats of any retrospective analysis, they again suggest that higher quality radiation delivery is essential for improved cancer outcomes and therefore, should be considered in any clinical trial with radiation therapy.

Cooperative group investigators are now incorporating central radiation quality assurance into their trial designs. It is essential that protocol compliance and violations are catered to the specific radiation parameters of a study so as to not mislead the oncology community regarding the trial outcomes. For example, a large, phase III trial evaluating trimodality therapy for stage IIIA non–small-cell lung cancer randomized patients to concurrent chemoradiation therapy followed by surgery and adjuvant chemotherapy versus concurrent chemoradiation therapy followed by adjuvant therapy alone (27). The published results suggest there was no difference between the two treatment arms with respect to the primary endpoint of overall survival. The trimodality group was found to have a compliance rate with the protocol of 96% versus the nonsurgical arm radiation

compliance rate of 79%. At initial glance one may be led to attribute the inability to discern a benefit in the trimodality arm due to the poor radiation compliance. However, the trimodality arm was treated to a radiation dose of 45 Gy whereas the nonsurgical arm was treated to 61 Gy. As both arms had the same OARs but different dose levels, it is not surprising that the higher radiation arm had more protocol violations. In this scenario, the violations are inherent to the trial design and not a reflection of poor radiation quality assurance. Thus investigators should carefully consider the definitions of radiation protocol violations when designing clinical trials.

Trial Design Considerations

Patient Population. Selection of the optimal patient population is critical in conducting trials with drugs in combination with external beam radiation therapy. Early clinical trials with systemic anticancer agents alone typically enroll patients with metastatic and refractory cancer where the potential benefit of treatment outweighs the risks. Despite allowing for assessment of toxicity and response with relative ease, this patient population may not be relevant to improving outcomes with radiation therapy, where the patients are often treated with curative intent. The logical alternative for radiation–drug trials is to conduct trials in patients with potentially curable disease; however, this raises ethical considerations, especially when toxicities from the drug may lead to delay or interruption of curative radiation. One solution to overcome these ethical concerns is to enroll patients with an extremely high recurrence risk and therefore particularly poor prognosis, but for which definitive management may still be attempted. Examples include locally advanced or borderline resectable pancreatic cancer, *human papillomavirus* (HPV) negative locally advanced head and neck cancer, and unmethylated glioblastoma. As with any clinical investigation, patients must be fully informed that the experimental arm may lead to less favorable outcomes, including a higher risk of death, compared to the standard-of-care treatment.

Starting Dose. The primary objective of a phase I study of an oncology drug is usually to determine a recommended phase II dose (RP2D) that will subsequently be taken forward into further clinical development. When drugs are used concurrently with radiation therapy, particularly when synergy is expected with the combination, it is important to keep in mind that the maximum tolerated dose (MTD) or RP2D of a drug as a single agent may be much higher than the biologically active dose when used in combination with radiation. To efficiently develop radiation–drug combinations, one option is for investigators to conduct the radiation–drug combination studies shortly after the dose-escalation part of a phase I study, allowing for information regarding the drug's safety, tolerability, and pharmacokinetics/pharmacokinetics to be incorporated into the radiation trial(s).

Dose Escalation. Traditional dose-escalation designs, such as the classic "3 + 3," require each patient or cohort of patients to be fully evaluated for dose-limiting toxicities prior to enrolling additional patients. Cohort-of-three trials that include radiation therapy may be prohibitively long since subacute toxicities of radiation therapy can occur as late as 8 to 12 weeks following treatment, rather than within a few days or weeks of administration as is often the case with systemic agents alone. Spin-offs of the classic cohort-of-three trials that are aimed to reduce how often patient accrual is suspended include the rolling-six design and the continual reassessment method. A trial design that specifically addresses the late toxicity issues inherent in any radiation trial is the time-to-event continual reassessment method, which extends the cohort follow-up period and allows for staggered accrual without the need for complete dose-limiting toxicity follow-up of previously treated patients (28). Late effects of radiation therapy may manifest months to years after treatment and should be at least evaluated via posttrial monitoring. When subacute and late toxicities are not captured during dose escalation, this information should be considered in the determination of the final recommended dose to be used with radiation.

Regulatory Considerations

Despite the promise of combining drugs with radiation therapy, there has been a persistent lack of drug development using potential synergies between radiation and targeted systemic therapies. For example, since 2006 there have been more than 250 new drug and biological licensing applications approved by the Office of Hematology and Oncology Products at the FDA, and only one cancer therapy, cetuximab, was approved for use with radiation (29). The reasons for this discrepancy are complex and multifactorial, including limited regulatory precedent for drugs developed specifically for use with radiation therapy, as well as perceived challenges in trial design with radiation (30). In this section, we discuss the existing regulatory framework in which cancer drugs may be developed for use in combination with radiation therapy and describe the mechanisms in place for sponsors and investigators to obtain feedback from the FDA during the process of drug development.

Nonclinical Considerations. The development of a pharmaceutical is a stepwise process involving an evaluation of proof-of-concept and safety studies in animals before a first-in-human (FIH) study. In the case of drugs studied for use with radiation therapy, safety evaluation of the pharmaceutical alone in animal species is needed before initiating a FIH radiation combination study, assuming no previous human experience with the pharmaceutical is available. The more common scenario, however, is that the pharmaceutical has been already used as a single agent in patients, in which case nonclinical studies for the drug alone will have already been performed. For example, both temozolomide and cetuximab were initially approved for use as single agents in patients with recurrent glioblastoma and metastatic colorectal cancer, respectively (29,31). When a pharmaceutical is being specifically developed for use in combination with radiation therapy, in addition to the nonclinical safety assessment of the pharmaceutical alone, a study in animals comparing the toxicity in the presence and absence of radiation may provide useful information and assist in selecting the starting dose of drug in patients. Because each product development program is unique according to product characterizations and the oncology indication sought, discussion with the review division at the FDA/Office of Hematology and Oncology Products is encouraged during pre–investigational new drug (IND) application consultation and later during product development (32).

Clinical Considerations/Endpoints. For a drug to be marketed in the United States, it must demonstrate efficacy and an acceptable safety profile in adequate and well-controlled clinical trials. Efficacy can be demonstrated through clinical trials using a variety of measures. The appropriate primary efficacy endpoint(s) for a clinical trial will depend on the trial design and disease context, including specific disease site, organ of interest, and intent of therapy. Efficacy endpoints in cancer trials with a drug and radiation therapy include measurement of the disease, such as progression-free survival or clinical outcomes such as overall survival or measures of symptoms or function.

Demand for more rapid approval of drugs for patients with serious or life-threatening diseases has led to the establishment of expedited programs, including the accelerated approval pathway (21 CFR part 314, subpart H). To qualify for accelerated approval, the drug must provide a meaningful advantage over available therapies and demonstrate an effect on a surrogate endpoint or an intermediate clinical endpoint that is reasonably likely to predict clinical benefit. Given the uncertainty associated with an accelerated approval, sponsors must provide evidence to verify and describe clinical benefit in a subsequent clinical trial or trials (33). Although the FDA does not have a published guidance document that specifically addresses the development of radiation–drug combinations, the guidance on codevelopment of two or more INDs for use in combination may provide a helpful framework for investigators (34). Again, it is critical that the appropriate review division with relevant disease-specific expertise at the FDA is consulted on the specifics of a given clinical development program.

Opportunities to Obtain Feedback From the FDA. Given the limited regulatory precedent over the past decade for marketed products intended to be used specifically with radiation therapy, the FDA recommends obtaining feedback during the drug development process in the form of meetings (32,35). For example, a type B meeting, also known as a milestone meeting, is an opportunity for sponsors to meet with the FDA to discuss the development program at predefined milestones. Examples of type B meetings include pre-IND meetings, end-of-phase-I or end-of-phase-II meetings, and pre–New Drug Application or pre–Biologics License Application meetings. Sponsors or investigators may also submit special protocol assessments to confirm the acceptability of endpoints and statistical analysis plans before initiating trials anticipated to support drug marketing applications (36). A special protocol assessment agreement indicates concurrence by the FDA with the adequacy and acceptability of specific critical elements of overall protocol design, including entry criteria, trial design, endpoints, and planned analyses. These elements are critical to ensuring that the trial has the potential to meet regulatory requirements for approval.

Past FDA Approvals of Drugs in Combination With Radiation. Amifostine, temozolomide, and cetuximab are three drugs that have received supplemental indications for use specifically with radiation therapy. The data supporting each approval is discussed herein to provide examples of clinical trials and endpoints that successfully led to registration.

Amifostine is a free-radical scavenger and cytoprotective agent that was initially approved by the FDA in 1996 to reduce the cumulative renal toxicity associated with repeated administration of cisplatin in patients with advanced ovarian cancer. In 1999, it received a supplemental indication to reduce the incidence of moderate to severe xerostomia in patients undergoing postoperative radiation treatment for head and neck cancer, where the radiation port includes a substantial portion of the parotid glands (37). The latter approval was based on an open-label randomized control trial of 315 patients who received standard fractionated radiation of 50 to 70 Gy, with or without amifostine administered 15 to 30 minutes prior to each fraction (38). Patients were required to have at least 75% of both parotid glands within the radiation field to doses of at least 40 Gy. Primary endpoints included the incidence of grade 2 or higher acute xerostomia, grade 3 or higher acute mucositis, and grade 2 or higher late xerostomia. Acute toxicities were defined as occurring within 90 days or less from the start of radiation, and late toxicities were defined as occurring between 9 and 12 months following radiation. Locoregional control was the primary antitumor efficacy endpoint and included disease recurrence or persistence at the primary site or regional nodes. The incidence of grade 2 or higher acute

and late xerostomia, as assessed by the RTOG Acute and Late Morbidity Scoring Criteria, was significantly reduced in patients receiving amifostine. Acute grade 2 or higher xerostomia improved from 78% to 51%, and late grade 2 or higher xerostomia improved from 57% to 35% with the addition of amifostine. At 1 year following radiation, whole saliva collection following radiation showed that more patients given amifostine produced >0.1 gram of saliva (72% vs. 49%). In addition, the median saliva production at 1 year was higher in those patients who received amifostine. Stimulated saliva collections, however, did not show a difference between treatment arms. These improvements in saliva production were supported by the patients' subjective responses to a questionnaire regarding oral dryness. Although there were no differences between treatment arms in terms of locoregional failure at 18 months, due to concerns regarding tumor protection by the cytoprotectant, the proposed indication that included patients receiving both definitive and postoperative radiation therapy was amended to include only patients being treated with postoperative radiation therapy. The application was presented to an advisory committee, and it was felt that there were too few patients who received definitive radiotherapy and the follow-up time was too short to provide evidence that tumor protection would not be an issue in this setting.

Temozolomide is an alkylating agent that was initially approved by the FDA for the treatment of adult patients with refractory anaplastic astrocytoma. In 2005, it received a supplemental indication for the treatment of adult patients with newly diagnosed glioblastoma concomitantly with radiotherapy and then as maintenance treatment. The latter approval was based on an open-label randomized phase III trial with 573 patients who were randomized to receive either temozolomide + radiation therapy (n = 287) following by adjuvant temozolomide or radiation therapy alone (n = 286). In both arms focal radiation was delivered to a total of 60 Gy in 30 fractions. The addition of concomitant and maintenance temozolomide to radiotherapy showed a statistically significant improvement in overall survival compared to radiation alone. The HR for overall survival was 0.63 (95% CI: 0.52–0.75, p < .0001) in favor of the temozolomide arm. The median survival was increased by 2.5 months in the temozolomide arm.

Cetuximab is a monoclonal antibody that targets the human epidermal growth factor receptor that was initially approved by the FDA in 2004 for the treatment of metastatic colorectal cancer. In 2006, it received a supplemental indication for use in combination with radiation therapy for the treatment of locally or regionally advanced squamous cell carcinoma of the head and neck. The latter approval was based on an open-label randomized trial of 424 patients with locally or regionally advanced squamous cell carcinoma of the head and neck versus radiation therapy alone. Stratification factors were Karnofsky performance status (KPS; 60–80 vs. 90–100), nodal stage (N0 vs. N+), tumor stage (T1–3 vs. T4), and radiation therapy fractionation (concomitant boost vs. once daily vs. twice daily). Cetuximab was administered 1 week prior to starting radiation therapy and then weekly during treatment (1 hour prior to radiation). The primary outcome was duration of locoregional control and overall survival was also assessed. The addition of cetuximab to radiation therapy showed a statistically significant improvement in locoregional control compared to radiation alone. The HR for locoregional control was 0.68 (95% CI: 0.52–0.89, $p = .005$) and the median survival increased from 29.3 months to 49.0 months with the addition of cetuximab.

CONCLUSIONS

Radiation therapy continues to be a mainstay of both curative and palliative cancer therapies, and well-designed clinical trials are critical to demonstrating the clinical benefit of recent technologic advances and novel drug–radiation combinations. Unique considerations in clinical trials with radiation therapy include radiation toxicity assessment, PROs, and radiation quality assurance. As we have nearly exhausted our ability to improve radiation conformality and dose escalation, it is critical that investigators pursue biological methods of improving the therapeutic ratio through drugs that exploit inherent weaknesses within the tumor. Although novel drug–radiation combinations have the potential to significantly improve cancer outcomes, there is limited regulatory precedent for drugs approved specifically for the use with radiation therapy. Therefore, it is recommended that investigators engage with the FDA early and often in the process of drug development through meeting requests to obtain feedback regarding trial design and clinical endpoints that will ultimately support approval.

REFERENCES

1. Delaney G, Jacob S, Featherstone C, et al. The role of radiotherapy in cancer treatment: estimating optimal utilization from a review of evidence-based clinical guidelines. *Cancer*. 2005;104(6):1129–1137.
2. Darby SC, Mcgale P, Taylor CW, et al. Long-term mortality from heart disease and lung cancer after radiotherapy for early breast cancer: prospective cohort study of about 300,000 women in US SEER cancer registries. *Lancet Oncol*. 2005;6(8): 557–565.
3. Hall EJ, Giaccia AJ. Radiobiology for the Radiologist. 7th ed. Philadelphia, PA: Wolters Kluwer Health; 2011:556.
4. Whelan TJ, Pignol JP, Levine MN, et al. Long-term results of hypofractionated radiation therapy for breast cancer. *N Engl J Med*. 2010;362(6):513–520.
5. Bentzen SM, Agrawal RK, Aird EG, et al. START Trialists' Group. The UK Standardisation of Breast Radiotherapy (START) Trial B of radiotherapy hypofractionation for treatment of early breast cancer: a randomised trial. *Lancet*. 2008; 371(9618):1098–1107.
6. Bentzen SM, Agrawal RK, Aird EG, et al. START Trialists' Group. The UK Standardisation of Breast Radiotherapy (START) Trial A of radiotherapy hypofractionation for treatment of early breast cancer: a randomised trial. *Lancet Oncol*. 2008;9(4):331–341.
7. Dearnaley D, Syndikus I, Mossop H, et al. CHHiP Investigators. Conventional versus hypofractionated high-dose intensity-modulated radiotherapy for prostate cancer: 5-year outcomes of the randomised, non-inferiority, phase 3 CHHiP trial. *Lancet Oncol*. 2016;17(8):1047–1060.
8. Bhandare N, Monroe AT, Morris CG, et al. Does altered fractionation influence the risk of radiation-induced optic neuropathy? *Int J Radiat Oncol Biol Phys*. 2005;62(4):1070–1077.
9. Paganetti H. Range uncertainties in proton therapy and the role of Monte Carlo simulations. *Phys Med Biol*. 2012;57(11):R99–R117.
10. Golden EB, Chhabra A, Chachoua A, et al. Local radiotherapy and granulocyte-macrophage colony-stimulating factor to generate abscopal responses in patients with metastatic solid tumours: a proof-of-principle trial. *Lancet Oncol*. 2015; 16(7):795–803.
11. Postow MA, Callahan MK, Barker CA, et al. Immunologic correlates of the abscopal effect in a patient with melanoma. *N Engl J Med*. 2012;366(10):925–931.
12. Kachnic LA, Winter K, Myerson RJ, et al. RTOG 0529: a phase 2 evaluation of dose-painted intensity modulated radiation therapy in combination with 5-fluorouracil and mitomycin-C for the reduction of acute morbidity in carcinoma of the anal canal. *Int J Radiat Oncol Biol Phys*. 2013;86(1): 27–33.
13. Bradley JD, Paulus R, Komaki R, et al. Standard-dose versus high-dose conformal radiotherapy with concurrent and consolidation carboplatin plus paclitaxel with or without cetuximab for patients with stage IIIA or IIIB non-small-cell lung cancer (RTOG 0617): a randomised, two-by-two factorial phase 3 study. *Lancet Oncol*. 2015;16(2):187–199.
14. Blumenthal GM, Kluetz PG, Schneider J, et al. Oncology Drug Approvals: Evaluating Endpoints and Evidence in an Era of Breakthrough Therapies. *Oncologist*. 2017;22(7):762–767.
15. National Comprehensive Cancer Network. NCCN clinical practice guidelines in oncology. https://www.nccn.org/professionals/physician_gls. Updated December 2016.
16. Kim H, Dan TD, Palmer JD, et al. Quality and reporting accuracy of Phase 1 drug radiation clinical trials. *JAMA Oncol*. 2016;2(3):390–391.
17. Denis F, Garaud P, Bardet E, et al. Final results of the 94-01 French Head and Neck Oncology and Radiotherapy Group randomized trial comparing radiotherapy alone with concomitant radiochemotherapy in advanced-stage oropharynx carcinoma. *J Clin Oncol*. 2004;22(1):69–76.
18. Kluetz PG, Papadopoulos EJ, Johnson LL, et al. Focusing on core patient-reported outcomes in cancer clinical trials-response. *Clin Cancer Res*. 2016;22(22):5618.
19. Guidance for industry—Patient-reported outcome measures: use in medical product development to support labeling claims. http://www.fda.gov/downloads/Drugs/Guidances/UCM193282.pdf. Published 2009.
20. Deisseroth A, Kaminskas E, Grillo J, et al. U.S. Food and Drug Administration approval: ruxolitinib for the treatment of patients with intermediate and high-risk myelofibrosis. *Clin Cancer Res*. 2012;18(12):3212–3217.
21. Basch E, Reeve BB, Mitchell SA, et al. Development of the National Cancer Institute's patient-reported outcomes version of the common terminology criteria for adverse events (PRO-CTCAE). *J Natl Cancer Inst*. 2014;106(9):dju244.
22. Thanarajasingam G, Hubbard JM, Sloan JA, et al. The imperative for a new approach to toxicity analysis in oncology clinical trials. *J Natl Cancer Inst*. 2015;107(10):djv2161.
23. Basch E. Patient-reported outcomes—harnessing patients' voices to improve clinical care. *N Engl J Med*. 2017;376(2):105–108.

24. Williamson JF, et al. Quality assurance needs for modern image-based radiotherapy: recommendations from 2007 interorganizational symposium on "quality assurance of radiation therapy: challenges of advanced technology." *Int J Radiat Oncol Biol Phys*. 2008;7:1(1, Suppl): S2–S1.

25. Abrams RA, Winter KA, Regine WF, et al. Failure to adhere to protocol specified radiation therapy guidelines was associated with decreased survival in RTOG 9704—a Phase III trial of adjuvant chemotherapy and chemoradiotherapy for patients with resected adenocarcinoma of the pancreas. *Int J Radiat Oncol Biol Phys*. 2012;82(2):809–816.

26. Peters LJ, O'Sullivan B, Giralt J, et al. Critical impact of radiotherapy protocol compliance and quality in the treatment of advanced head and neck cancer: results from TROG 02.02. *J Clin Oncol*. 2010;28(18):2996–3001.

27. Albain KS, Swann RS, Rusch VW, et al. Radiotherapy plus chemotherapy with or without surgical resection for stage III non-small-cell lung cancer: a Phase III randomised controlled trial. *Lancet*. 2009;374(9687):379–386.

28. Cheung YK, Chappell R. Sequential designs for Phase I clinical trials with late-onset toxicities. *Biometrics*. 2000;56(4):1177–1182.

29. Erbitux Prescribing Information. http://www.accessdata.fda.gov/drugsatfda_docs/label/2015/125084s262lbl.pdf. Published 2015.

30. Ataman OU, Sambrook SJ, Wilks C, et al. The clinical development of molecularly targeted agents in combination with radiation therapy: a pharmaceutical perspective. *Int J Radiat Oncol Biol Phys*. 2012;84(4):e447–e454.

31. Temodar Prescribing Information. February 12th, 2016–October 19th, 2016. http://www.accessdata.fda.gov/drugsatfda_docs/label/2016/021029s031lbl.pdf

32. Guidance for industry: formal meetings between FDA and sponsors or applicants. http://www.fda.gov/downloads/Drugs/.../Guidances/ucm153222.pdf. Published 2009.

33. Guidance for industry: expedited programs for serious conditions—drugs and biologics. http://www.fda.gov/downloads/drugs/guidancecomplianceregulatoryinformation/guidances/ucm358301.pdf. Published 2014.

34. Guidance for industry: codevelopment of two or more new investigational drugs for use in combination. http://www.fda.gov/downloads/drugs/guidancecomplianceregulatoryinformation/guidances/ucm236669.pdf. Published 2013.

35. Walker AJ, Kim H, Saber H, et al. Clinical development of cancer drugs in combination with external beam radiation therapy: US Food and Drug Administration perspective. *Int J Radiat Oncol Biol Phys*. 2017;98(1):5–7.

36. Guidance for industry: special protocol assessment. http://www.fda.gov/downloads/Drugs/.../Guidances/ucm080571.pdf. Published 2002.

37. Ethyol Prescribing Information. https://www.accessdata.fda.gov/drugsatfda_docs/label/2017/020221s033lbl.pdf. Published 2017.

38. Brizel DM, Wasserman TH, Henke M, et al. Phase III randomized trial of amifostine as a radioprotector in head and neck cancer. *J Clin Oncol*. 2000;18(19):3339–3345.

Clinical Trials in Hematologic Malignancies

Neil Palmisiano, Bradley M. Haverkos, Sameh Gaballa, Joanne Filicko-O'Hara, Pierluigi Porcu, and Margaret Kasner

In 2016, there were an estimated 171,550 new diagnoses of hematologic malignancies in the United States (81,080 lymphomas, 60,140 leukemias, and 30,330 myelomas) (1). An estimated 1,237,824 patients are either living with, or in remission from, a hematologic malignancy in the United States (2). Unfortunately, approximately 58,320 individuals died from a hematologic malignancy in 2016 (1,2). As with other cancers, the key to improving outcomes across the hematologic malignancies is the rational development and prospective validation of new therapies through clinical trials. Progress, however, has been hampered by the fact that only an estimated 3% or less of U.S. cancer patients participate in clinical trials (3). After enrollment, a number of additional challenges threaten the successful and timely completion of a clinical trial. Progress can also be delayed due to a certain rate of attrition and some studies are interrupted and abandoned in the absence of robust early accrual (4). Thus, the timeline from the initial synthesis and screening of a new cancer drug to Food and Drug Administration (FDA) approval remains unacceptably long.

General barriers to clinical trial enrollment include lack of access, reluctance to enroll elderly patients (5), the challenge of obtaining informed consent for highly complex studies (a lengthy process if consent must be truly informed), the laborious procedure of verifying eligibility and starting a patient on the investigational treatment plan, patient misperceptions about risk, and unrealistic expectations (6–8). In addition, clinical trial participation in hematologic malignancies presents unique challenges and requires special considerations compared to studies involving solid tumors. These include: (a) the low incidence and extreme clinical and molecular heterogeneity of hematologic malignancies (responsible for only 9% of all cancer incidence, with hundreds of different clinicopathologic entities); (b) the use of distinct response criteria compared to solid tumors, often quite different among each disease type; (c) the presence of unique or distinct toxicities, such as tumor lysis syndrome (TLS), cytokine release syndrome (CRS), and acute infusion reactions; and (d) the fact that hematologic toxicity from drug-induced myelosuppression is often not considered a dose-limiting toxicity (DLT) and is not used to determine the maximum tolerated dose (MTD).

The choice of primary endpoints is also challenging. Often, clinical trials need to strike a balance between FDA-supported endpoints, cost, time, and sometimes biomarker assessment to meet regulatory stringency. A key understanding of the pathophysiology and clinical behavior of each malignancy, therefore, is a key element to trial success. Overall survival (OS) is, of course, the most important outcome, but earlier endpoints may also be valid. For example, for indolent lymphomas and multiple myeloma (MM), time to progression, time to next therapy, and OS are suitable endpoints, while for aggressive curable lymphomas and acute leukemia complete remission rate and progression-free survival (PFS) are very meaningful endpoints.

One additional important aspect when designing clinical trials for hematologic malignancies is to appropriately select the frequency and duration of the disease assessment time points, which will affect PFS. Routine imaging for the first two years can be appropriate for patients with aggressive curable lymphomas. In contrast, in patients with indolent lymphomas or MM the duration of follow-up and disease monitoring should be significantly longer as these diseases can relapse several years after primary therapy.

Recently, the identification of patient subgroups based on specific biomarkers has opened the door to clinical trials with "personalized therapy." Depending on the frequency of the biomarkers used as entry criteria, however, the potential population may be quite small. For example, if a trial accrues only leukemia patients with FLT3, IDH2, or TP53 mutations, the sample size will be significantly reduced, requiring large multicenter trials. A recent approach to overcome these challenges is the concept of "basket" trials. These trials would often include multiple disease subtypes or even completely different disease histologies, based on one or several biomarkers. One such example is the Molecular Analysis for Therapy Choice (MATCH) precision medicine clinical trial initiated by the National Cancer Institute (NCI), which tries to "match" patients with a certain genetic biomarker to the respective targeted agent (NCT02465060). Such trial designs incorporating biomarkers for inclusion (or exclusion) are likely to increase in the future as our understanding of the genetic basis of different lymphomas continues to evolve.

In this chapter, we provide a brief overview of the diagnostic and therapeutic challenges presented by the most common types of hematologic malignancies and offer a summary of the clinical research strategies informing the design and conduct of clinical trials in some of these neoplasms.

ACUTE MYELOID LEUKEMIA

The term acute myeloid leukemia (AML) encompasses a heterogeneous family of aggressive hematologic malignancies characterized by the clonal proliferation and compromised differentiation of immature myeloid precursors. Diagnosis is made primarily by obtaining a bone marrow biopsy and aspirate for review of morphology, immunophenotype by flow cytometry, cytogenetics analysis by conventional metaphase karyotype and fluorescence in situ hybridization (FISH), and targeted DNA next-generation sequencing (NGS) for commonly occurring mutations. Recently, updated World Health Organization (WHO) diagnostic criteria based more on recurrent cytogenetic and molecular

abnormalities than traditional morphologic analysis have been published (9). These criteria delineate different AML subtypes with unique clinical presentations and widely different outcomes (favorable risk vs. poor risk), thus informing treatment decisions and clinical trial eligibility (Table 44.1). For instance, the clinical course of acute promyelocytic leukemia (APL), with its hallmark t(15;17)(q22;q12) translocation affecting the retinoic acid receptor alpha (RARA) gene on chromosome 17 and the promyelocytic leukemia (PML) gene on chromosome 15, is characterized by severe disseminated intravascular coagulopathy (DIC) leading to life-threatening early bleeding complications, but the long-term outcome is favorable, with cure rates greater than 80% (10). This makes APL a favorable risk AML. Current therapy for APL consists of induction therapy with retinoic acid and arsenic trioxide or anthracycline based regimens, followed by consolidation strategies with similar drugs. Early mortality (during induction) for APL is now only ~10% and patients who enter molecular remission are unlikely to relapse. Most of the ongoing clinical trials for APL, therefore, target the small population of patients with relapsed or refractory disease or aim at further reducing early mortality by understanding and better treating severe coagulopathy. At the other end of the AML spectrum, a provisional entity characterized by intragenic mutations in the RUNX1 gene is characterized by inferior complete response (CR) rates to standard idarubicin and cytarabine (7 + 3) induction (48.4% vs. 68.1%) and poor OS at 5 years (22% vs. 36%), for RUNX1-mutated versus RUNX1 wild-type AML, respectively (11).

The different prognosis and treatment of these two diseases both called "AML" highlight several points

TABLE 44.1 AML Risk Categories

Favorable Risk		Poor Risk	
Cytogenetic Abnormalities	**Molecular Abnormalities**	**Cytogenetic Abnormalities**	**Molecular Abnormalities**
t(8;21)(q22;q22);RUN XI-RUNX1T1	Mut NPM and WT FLT3-ITD with NC	Complex (≥3 ChromosomalAbn)	FLT3-ITD with NC
Inv(16)(p13. q22) or t(16;16)(p13. 1q22); CBFB-MYH11	Mut CEPBα with NC	inv(3)(q21q26.2) or t(3;3)(q21;q26.2); RPN1-EVI1	TP53 Deletions
t(l.5:17);PML-RARα		−5 or del(5q)	
Intermediate Risk		−7 or del(7q)	
Cytogenetic Abnormalities	Molecular Abnormalities	Monosomal	
t(9;11)(p22;q23); MLLT3-MLL	NC without Molecular Abnormalities	t(6;9)(p22;q23);DEK- NUP214	
+8 Alone	Core-binding	t(v;11)(v;q23);MLL Rearrangement	

salient to clinical trial design in the cytogenetic and molecular diagnostic era. First, the underlying abnormalities that lead to malignancy define the disease better than morphologic appearance of the leukemic cells alone, and each subtype may have markedly different natural outcomes that will affect interventional responses. Because of these considerations, broad eligibility trials in AML must be designed to stratify based on risk profile and molecular classification. Second, diseases like APL, whose clinical course, treatment, and outcome is vastly better and different than other AML types should be treated on disease-specific protocols. Given that the cure rate for low- and even intermediate-risk APL with current therapy approaches 100%, trials that focus on reducing late complications, time on therapy, and cost, increasing patient satisfaction, and reducing early mortality are paramount to the development of new treatment strategies that offer similar outcomes.

Non-APL AML is conventionally treated in two phases: remission induction followed by consolidation. First developed in the 1970s, the combination of 3 days of an anthracycline and 7 days of infusional cytarabine (7 + 3) has remained the induction standard of care for fit individuals despite decades of trials. The exception to this dearth of new agents is midostaurin, a small molecule FLT3 inhibitor that has demonstrated significant efficacy on top of traditional induction chemotherapy in FLT3-mutated disease. The recent FDA approval of this medication demonstrates the first advance in upfront AML treatment in 30 years and the increasing importance of molecular diagnostics and targeted therapy for improving outcomes (12).

The morbidity and mortality of 7 + 3 chemotherapy is well-documented, limiting its use in those older, frail, or with significant concomitant medical issues. In one early series, more than a quarter of patients died during the 4 weeks after induction (13). Conversely, the therapy is quite effective at inducing remission in younger, fit patients with CR rates approaching 80%. Because of the wide disparities of effect and tolerability, clinical trials are commonly designed to enroll one but not both of these two groups.

Consolidation therapy in order to prevent relapse of disease follows induction. The decision to proceed with additional chemotherapy cycles with high-dose cytarabine (HiDAC) or an allogeneic hematopoietic stem cell transplantation (HSCT) in first remission for consolidation is largely guided by chance of relapse and fitness to undergo the rigors of the transplant process. Table 44.1 defines the recurrent cytogenetic and molecular abnormalities that help determine consolidation strategy. Studies demonstrate that any nonfavorable risk disease may benefit from transplantation after remission, while favorable risk disease does not (14).

When considering survival endpoints in leukemia clinical trials it is important to consider the effect of allogeneic HSCT as the proportion of patients offered transplant in CR may bias OS and relapse-free survival (RFS). In addition, it is worth looking at the percentage of patients able to proceed to allogeneic HSCT as a surrogate endpoint for early-phase trials, as OS and RFS data can take years to mature.

Consensus response criteria developed from working groups for acute leukemia are based on the fact that these malignancies are largely bone marrow based and recovery of normal hematopoiesis is important to confirm the elimination of the neoplastic clone in the bone marrow (15,16). Therefore, CR is defined by:

- A bone marrow biopsy with <5% blasts of normal phenotype
- Return of normal-appearing trilineage hematopoiesis
- Absolute neutrophil count >1,000/μL and platelet count >1,00,000/μL
- Resolution of any extramedullary sites of disease

Complete response with incomplete recovery (CRi) is indicative of disease that is responsive to therapy in the absence of recovery of adequate normal hematopoiesis in either platelets or neutrophils. The combined endpoint of CR/CRi is commonly used in early-phase trials (mostly phase II) to assess preliminary efficacy. Other responses include a partial response (PR), which is indicated by a greater than 50% reduction of marrow blasts from baseline, and stable disease (SD). Phase I trials may use a combined primary endpoint of CR/CRi/PR and sometimes include SD in order to pick up a signal of activity that would recommend further study. Complete cytogenetic response (CRc) is defined as the disappearance of previously seen cytogenetic abnormalities in the setting of CR and predicts outcome.

The advent of molecular diagnostics and highly sensitive flow cytometry has helped redefine the definition of response in AML. According to early studies, induction therapy is thought to reduce the number of malignant cells in the body from approximately 10^{12} to 10^9, below the limit of morphologic detection. However, induction chemotherapy alone rarely results in remissions lasting more than several weeks. Consolidation therapy is thought to reduce this burden even further in most cases, and to eliminate the leukemic burden in those who are cured. A significant proportion of patients who enter into a morphologic CR (<5% residual blasts) even after consolidation eventually relapse, implying that residual disease is present. Complicating this further, residual disease may not be uniformly spread throughout the marrow. Only until recently with the introduction of multiparameter flow cytometry (MFC) and real-time quantitative polymerase chain reaction (qRT-PCR) has this minimal residual disease (MRD) been more easily detectable (17). Each of these techniques has advantages and limitations. MFC relies on a leukemia-associated aberrant immunophenotype (LAIP) of leukemic blasts, and while more than 95% of AML have aberrant antigens, the presence of these antigens may shift from diagnosis to relapse in as many as 20% of cases. qRT-PCR has the potential to detect even lower concentrations of leukemic blasts (1/100,000) compared to MFC (1/1,000–1/10,0000), but only 80% of acute leukemias have an observable genetic lesion that can be detected by this method. Additionally, a subclone without the target genetic lesion may develop as a result of chemotherapy or clonal evolution, rendering this method unable to detect residual disease. More complicated still, no standardized definition of MRD currently exists, and the detection of MRD is not universally associated with relapse. Regardless, as these issues continued to be explored and their contribution to prognosis refined, even most earlier phase clinical trials incorporate some measurement of MRD as a secondary endpoint.

Several different types of treatment failure, including resistant disease, death in aplasia, and relapsed disease, have been defined. These designations are useful to differentiate the failure of a drug to effect the course of the disease from a death due to toxicity of a treatment in remission. Again, these designations are especially important in early-phase trials to determine preliminary efficacy and help determine if clinical development should move forward.

MYELODYSPLASTIC SYNDROMES

Myelodysplastic syndromes (MDSs) comprise a heterogeneous group of chronic myeloid neoplasms defined by clonal and ineffective hematopoiesis that leads to peripheral blood cytopenias. MDS is a malignancy primarily of elderly populations, with median age at time of diagnosis of 70 years. The clinical course of MDS can vary significantly, and a prognostic scoring system has been developed (Table 44.2) (18,19). Based on cytogenetic abnormalities, bone marrow blast percentage, and degree of cytopenias at diagnosis, a Revised International Prognostic Scoring System (IPSS-R) was devised that separates patients into gradients of risk categories corresponding with predicted OS (Table 44.2).

Given the older age of patients with MDS as well as the wide variation in prognosis and lack of curative

therapies, treatment for MDS is directed at restoring normal hematopoiesis as well as delaying transformation to AML. In higher risk disease, hypomethylating agents, such as azacitidine and decitabine, have become the standard-of-care benchmark for investigational therapies (20,21). Response criteria for MDS are similar to other blood-based malignancies but take into account the unique characteristics of the disease, including well-defined endpoints for hematologic improvement in neutrophil, platelet, and erythroid cell lines and definitions of transfusion independence of red cells. Given the advanced age of patients with MDS, quality of life (QOL) data are important and should be included among the clinical endpoints.

ACUTE LYMPHOBLASTIC LEUKEMIA

Much like AML, acute lymphoblastic leukemia (ALL) is diagnosed by bone marrow biopsy and flow cytometry, and is classified according to recurrent cytogenetic abnormalities. In general, ALL is treated with multiagent chemotherapy in induction, consolidation, intensification, and maintenance phases that can last for as long as several years. Prognosis, therapies, and therefore clinical trial design vary based on age, fitness, and genetic subgroups. For example, B-ALL with t(9:22) is treated by adding tyrosine kinase inhibitors (TKI), such as imatinib and dasatinib, to traditional induction and maintenance strategies with chemotherapies. Before the addition of TKIs, B-ALL with t(9:22) had very poor outcomes with median OS <1 year. However, in the post-TKI era along with allogeneic HSCT, long-term disease-free survival (DFS) rates >60% have been achieved. The comparison between the pre- and post-TKI area highlights the critical need for clinical trials to be designed to investigate drugs targeted to the molecular pathology that drives a particular malignancy. Another example of a recent change of strategy in adult ALL is the adoption of aggressive pediatric regimens in adolescents and young adults (AYA) under 30 years of age (22).

Clinical assessment and response criteria for ALL are largely similar to AML with several important points of difference. First, lymphoblasts have a marked

TABLE 44.2 MDS IPSS-R Risk Scores and Prognosis

	IPSS-R Risk Scores and Prognosis				
	Very Low	**Low**	**Intermediate**	**High**	**Very High**
Patients (%)	19%	38%	20%	13%	10%
Survival (y)	8.8	5.3	3	1.6	0.8
Time to t-AML (y)	NR	10.8	3.2	1.4	0.7

IPSS-R, Revised International Prognostic Scoring System; NR, not reached; t-AML, therapy-related acute myeloid leukemia.

predilection to cross the blood–brain barrier (BBB), and central nervous system (CNS) disease is significantly more common in ALL than AML. Clinical trials involving ALL should include cerebrospinal fluid (CSF) sampling prior to study entrance, and must make provisions to assess for CNS relapse during and after the course of therapy. In the relapsed setting, patients with prior history of CNS disease need not be excluded, as long as patients are free of symptoms at the time of enrollment, a complete course of CNS-directed therapy has been completed, and evidence of leukemia-free CSF is documented. Lymphoblasts also have a greater tendency to invade lymph nodes and form solid masses, and measurement of response should include an evaluation of nonmarrow disease (lymph nodes, spleen, and soft tissues). MRD measurement in ALL is also an import prognostic marker, and should be uniformly incorporated into clinical trial design though how to do this is still being refined.

LYMPHOMAS

Non-Hodgkin's lymphomas (NHLs) are a very large and heterogeneous family of hematologic malignancies that can be distinguished clinically into indolent and aggressive neoplasms and pathologically into B-cell and T/NK-cell lymphomas depending on their cell of origin (23). The most common aggressive B-cell lymphoma (BCL) is diffuse large B-cell lymphoma (DLBCL), which accounts for ~30% of all BCL. The most common indolent BCL is follicular lymphoma, which accounts for ~20%. Standard-of-care therapy options for these different lymphoma subtypes are drastically different. Thus, a good understanding of the clinical presentation and natural history of these neoplasms is crucial when designing clinical trials, as the appropriate clinical endpoints will be different for each subtype.

INDOLENT NON-HODGKIN'S LYMPHOMAS

Generally, indolent NHL (iNHL) are chronic, initially chemosensitive, but in the end incurable malignancies. During their life span, patients will require multiple lines of therapy, often with prolonged survivals. Moreover, iNHL due to their slow progression may not need to be treated immediately. Therefore, consensus criteria for initiation of therapy, usually based on symptoms and tumor burden, were developed early on. Thus, it is imperative, when designing a clinical trial for iNHL, that inclusion criteria account for clinical indications for initiation of therapy. The two most commonly used systems for initiation of therapy in iNHL are those proposed by the Groupe d-Etude des Lymphomes Folliculaires (GELF) and by the British National Lymphoma Investigation (BNLI) (24,25).

AGGRESSIVE NON-HODGKIN'S LYMPHOMAS

These lymphomas have a more aggressive clinical course, typically progress rapidly over weeks or a few months, and can be fatal if left untreated. The most common aggressive NHL of B-cell origin is DLBCL. Unlike iNHL, aggressive NHL can be cured with chemotherapy, but cure rates are very different depending on the biological subtype. For example, 'double-hit' lymphomas, a subset of DLBCL defined by the presence of genomic rearrangements involving the loci for the MYC and BCL2 genes, as detected by FISH, have a significantly worse prognosis compared to non-double-hit DLBCL and stratification based on these features at clinical trial enrollment is desirable (26). Clinical trials now routinely stratify patients with DLBCL according to cell of origin, defined by immunohistochemistry: germinal center (GC) type versus activated B-cell (ABC) or non-GC type. Prognosis is better for GC type DLBCL compared to non-GC type, and clinical trial design and outcome analysis need to consider these differences (27,28).

STAGING AND RESPONSE ASSESSMENT

The initial staging workup for lymphoma patients who are being screened for clinical trial enrollment requires imaging studies (often PET/CT scans), bone marrow biopsy, and occasionally CSF evaluation to exclude CNS involvement. The recent Lugano classification, based on the modified Ann Arbor staging system, is the current staging system for patients with NHL (Table 44.3) (29). Criteria for bulky disease vary by histology and no general cutoff has been validated (30). The 2014 Lugano classification, which provided updated response criteria for lymphoma clinical trials, has now been replaced by the International Working Group (IWG) Consensus Response Evaluation Criteria in Lymphoma (RECIL 2017) (31). The preferred imaging modality for patients with NHL depends upon the fluorodeoxyglucose (FDG) avidity of the histologic subtype. PET/CT is preferred for staging and assessment of response for FDG-avid lymphomas, while CT alone is preferred for FDG nonavid and variably avid histologies. Most lymphoma histologies are considered FDG-avid except for chronic lymphocytic leukemia/small lymphocytic lymphoma (CLL/SLL), lymphoplasmacytic lymphoma (LPL), mycosis fungoides (MF), and marginal zone lymphoma (MZL).

Responses are defined as complete or partial response and stable or progressive disease (PD). For FDG-avid histologies, a 5-point scale (Deauville score) is used to define PET responses according to FDG avidity, as follows:

1. No uptake
2. Uptake below blood pool
3. Uptake >mediastinal blood pool but below or equal to uptake in liver

TABLE 44.3 Revised Staging System for Primary Nodal NHL (Lugano classification)

Stage	Involvement	Extranodal (E) Status
Limited		
I	One node or a group of adjacent nodes	Single extranodal lesions without nodal involvement
II	Two or more nodal groups on the same side of the diaphragm	Stage I or II by nodal extent with limited contiguous extranodal involvement
II bulky	II as in the preceding with "bulky" disease	Not applicable
Advanced		
III	Nodes on both sides of the diaphragm; nodes above the diaphragm with spleen involvement	Not applicable
IV	Additional noncontiguous extralymphatic involvement	Not applicable

NHL, non-Hodgkin's lymphoma.

Extent of disease is determined by PET/CT for avid lymphomas and CT for nonavid histologies. Tonsils, Waldeyer's ring, and spleen are considered nodal tissue.

4. Uptake moderately more than liver uptake, at any site
5. Update markedly higher than liver (i.e., 2–3 x max standard uptake value [SUV] in the liver) and/or new lesions

Here x indicates new areas of uptake unlikely to be related to lymphoma.

Using this method, a Deauville score of 1 or 2 is consistent with a CR. Scores of 4 or 5 represent SD/PD. For most patients on clinical trials undergoing posttreatment PET/CT, a Deauville score of 3 usually is considered to represent a CR. For non-FDG avid lymphomas, the size of the lymph nodes found on CT scan is used to assess response.

Tumor Flares

Newer biologic agents with immune mechanisms of action (e.g., lenalidomide, rituximab, ibrutinib, brentuximab, checkpoint inhibitors, etc.) may lead to an initial "atypical response" or tumor flare in lymphoma and CLL that may mistakenly be interpreted as "progressive disease." This is usually seen within a first few weeks of initiation on treatment and represents an immune mediated response. This can be manifested by an increase in size of lymph nodes, lymphocytosis, bone pain, or increase in serum paraprotein. With time, these responses will convert to complete or partial responses and are important when designing clinical trials using immune agents to allow enough time (usually after 8 weeks) before assessing for response when using these agents.

Tools for Risk Stratification

In any study design, it is important to define the patient population and include or exclude patients according to their disease risk, when appropriate. Several clinical tools to assess lymphoma risk groups with different prognosis are available, which are routinely used to assess patient eligibility. The following are the most commonly used risk-stratification tools:

1. The original International Prognostic Index (IPI) and several variants are used in patients with DLBCL (32). The following factors were found to correlate significantly with shorter overall or relapse-free survival (age >60, elevated lactate dehydrogenase [LDH], Eastern Cooperative Oncology Group [ECOG] performance status ≥2, stage III or IV disease, number of involved extranodal disease sites >1). Patients are grouped in the following risk categories: low risk (0–1 score), low–intermediate risk (score of 2), high–intermediate (score of 3), or high risk (score above 4). The 3-year PFS among these risk groups is 87%, 75%, 59%, and 56%, respectively.
2. The original Follicular Lymphoma International Prognostic Index (FLIPI) (33) was devised based on an international study of long-term survival in patients with follicular lymphoma and identified five adverse prognostic factors (age >60, stage III or IV disease, hemoglobin <12, number of involved nodal areas >4, elevated LDH level). The corresponding risk groups are: low-risk (zero to one adverse factor), intermediate-risk (two adverse factors), and high-risk group (three or more adverse factors). The corresponding 5-year OSs were 91%, 78%, and 52%, among these groups respectively. The FLIPI2 (34) evaluates five parameters, some of which overlap with the original FLIPI score (age >60, bone marrow involvement, hemoglobin level <12, greatest diameter of the largest involved node more than 6 cm, and elevated serum beta-2 microglobulin level above the normal limit). The 3-year PFS rates of patients with low (no risk factors), intermediate (1–2 risk factors), or high (3–5 factors)

were 91%, 69%, and 51% respectively. The more recent M7-FLIPI (35) incorporates the FLIPI, ECOG performance status, and the mutational status of seven genes (EZH2, ARID1A, MEF2B, EP300, FOXO1, CREBBP, and CARD11). Patients are grouped into high-risk and low-risk groups with a 5-year event-free survival of 25% and 68%, respectively. This relatively new tool is currently limited to research studies and is not widely ready for routine clinical care.

3. The Mantle Cell Lymphoma International Prognostic Index (MIPI) (36) incorporates age, ECOG performance status, LDH, and white blood cell count and risk-stratifies patients with mantle cell lymphoma into three risk groups (low, intermediate, and high) with estimated 5-year survival of 60%, 35%, and 20%, respectively.

4. The Hodgkin's Lymphoma International Prognostic Score (IPS), also known as Hasenclever's score (37), is a score based on seven potential unfavorable features at diagnosis (serum albumin <4, hemoglobin <10.5, male gender, age >45, stage IV disease, white blood cell count >15,000/microL, absolute lymphocyte count <600/ microL and/or <8% of the total white blood cell count). The OS at 5 years correlates with the IPS score as follows: zero factors (98%), one factor (97%), two factors (91%), three factors (88%), four factors (85%), five or more factors (67%). The stratification of early-stage (IA–IIA) Hodgkin's disease into favorable and unfavorable varies by region. In the United States, most centers consider favorable disease as nonbulky (<10 cm) stage IA–IIA disease. In contrast, in Europe, other variables such as patient age and the erythrocyte sedimentation rate (ESR) are incorporated.

MULTIPLE MYELOMA

MM is characterized by the malignant proliferation of one or more clones of immunoglobulin-producing plasma cells. It is traditionally characterized by bone pain, lytic bone lesions, anemia, renal insufficiency, hypercalcemia, and an increased risk for infections. Most patients have increased production of a monoclonal immunoglobulin (M-protein) with decreased amounts of normal immunoglobulins (reciprocal hypogammaglobulinemia). MM currently accounts for about 15% of all hematologic malignancies and about 1.8% of all cancers (29,38). There are many presentations of MM, ranging from asymptomatic anemia to hypercalcemia, acute renal failure, and spinal cord compression. As patients are evaluated, it is important to be complete in the workup and to ensure the proper diagnosis to enroll patients on clinical trial.

The diagnostic criteria for MM have evolved substantially over the past two decades. Most recently, the International Myeloma Working Group (IMWG) (40) has defined MM as the presence of ≥10% clonal plasma cells in the bone marrow or biopsy proven bony or extramedullary plasmacytoma and one of the following: (a) serum calcium >0.25 mmol (1 mg/dL) higher than upper limit of normal (ULN) or 2.75 mmol/l (>11 mg/dL); (b) renal insufficiency (creatinine >2 mg/dL; 177 umol/L) or creatinine clearance <40 mL/min; (c) anemia (hemoglobin <10 g/dL or hemoglobin >2 g/dL below the lower limit of normal); (d) one or more osteolytic bone lesions on skeletal radiography, CT, or PET/CT; (e) clonal bone marrow plasma cells ≥60%; (f) abnormal serum free light chain (FLC) ratio ≥ (involved kappa) or ≤0.01 (involved lambda); (g) >1 focal lesions on MRI studies ≥1 mm.

The current International Staging System (41) is easy to use and has recently been refined to include chromosomal abnormalities detected by FISH, including del13, del17p13, t(4;14). t(11;14), and t(14;16) and the serum LDH. Response criteria in MM, as defined by the IMWG, have evolved recently as well (Table 44.4) (42,43). The current criteria incorporate marrow plasmacytosis, M-protein, FLC assays, as well as markers of MRD detected by next-generation flow (NGF) cytometry or NGS. Although more complex, use of the IMWG response criteria ensures that there is a consistent methodology and a consistent language to assess and follow patients on clinical trials in MM.

TABLE 44.4 International Staging System for Multiple Myeloma (International Myeloma Working Group)

	International Staging System		Revised ISS (R-ISS)
	B2M	Albumin	
Stage I	<3.5	≥3.5	ISS stage 1 and standard risk chromosomal abnormalities by iFISH and serum LDH ≤upper limit of normal
Stage II	3.5–5.5	<3.5	Not R-ISS stage 1 or III
Stage III			ISS stage III and either high-risk chromosomal abnormalities by iFISH or serum LDH >upper limit of normal

iFISH, immunofluorescence in situ hybridization; ISS, International Staging System; LDH, lactate dehydrogenase; R-ISS, Revised International Staging System.

Survival in MM has improved significantly in the past two decades, due to the introduction of multiple new therapies, including carfilzomib, daratumumab, elotuzumab, ixazomib, and pomalidomide. For many patients, progression of disease leads to a new line of therapy, which often extends survival, thereby making OS as a clinical trial endpoint difficult. Trials are generally designed to show improved response and improved PFS using the IMWG criteria.

FUTURE DIRECTIONS

Several new evolving technologies may influence clinical trial designs for hematologic malignancies in the near future. Currently, response is primarily defined by imaging studies, which do not account for the presence of MRD. Future lab tests for assessment of MRD, circulating tumor cells, or circulating tumor DNA (ctDNA) are likely to become integrated into clinical trial designs and eventually in routine clinical care. Finally, better understanding of the genetic blueprint and molecular complexity of the tumor may further refine our prognostic tools and the development of newer targeted therapies.

REFERENCES

1. American Cancer Society. www.cancer.org
2. National Cancer Institute. www.seer.cancer.gov
3. Murthy VH, Krumholz HM, Gross CP, et al. Participation in cancer clinical trials: race-, sex-, and age-based disparities. *JAMA.* 2004;291:2720–2726.
4. Cheng SK, Dietrich MS, Dilts DM. Predicting accrual achievement: monitoring accrual milestones of NCI-CTEP-sponsored clinical trials. *Clin Cancer Res.* 2011;17(7):1947–1955.
5. Townsley CA, Selby R, Siu LL. Systematic review of barriers to the recruitment of older patients with cancer onto clinical trials. *J Clin Oncol.* 2005;23(13):3112–3124.
6. Meropol NJ, Weinfurt KP, Burnett CB, et al. Perceptions of patients and physicians regarding phase I cancer clinical trials: implications for physician-patient communication. *J Clin Oncol.* 2003;21(13):2589–2596.
7. Agrawal M, Grady C, Fairclough DL, et al. Patients' decision-making process regarding participation in phase I oncology research. *J Clin Oncol.* 2006;24(27):4479–4484.
8. Manne S, Kashy D, Albrecht T, et al. Attitudinal barriers to participation in oncology clinical trials: factor analysis and correlates of barriers. *Eur J Cancer Care.* 2015;24(1):28–38.
9. Arber DA, Orazi A, Hasserjian R, et al. The 2016 revision to the World Health Organization classification of myeloid neoplasms and acute leukemia. *Blood.* 2016;127(20):2391.
10. Lo-Coco F, Avvisati G, Vignetti M, et al. Retinoic acid and arsenic trioxide for acute promyelocytic leukemia. *N Engl J Med.* 2013;369(2):111–121.
11. Gaidzik VI, Teleanu V, Papaemmanuil E, et al. RUNX1 mutations in acute myeloid leukemia are associated with distinct clinico-pathologic and genetic features. *Leukemia.* 2016;30(11):2160–2168.
12. Stone RM, Mandrekar S, Sanford BL, et al. The Multi-Kinase Inhibitor Midostaurin (M) Prolongs Survival Compared with Placebo (P) in Combination with Daunorubicin (D)/Cytarabine (C) Induction (ind), High-Dose C Consolidation (consol), and As Maintenance (maint) Therapy in Newly Diagnosed Acute Myeloid Leukemia (AML) Patients (pts) Age 18-60 with FLT3 Mutations (muts): An International Prospective Randomized (rand) P-Controlled Double-Blind Trial (CALGB 10603/RATIFY Alliance]). *Blood.* 2015;126(23):6.
13. Estey E, Smith TL, Keating MJ, et al. Prediction of survival during induction therapy in patients with newly diagnosed acute myeloblastic leukemia. *Leukemia.* 1989;3(4):257–263.
14. Mrozek K, Marcucci G, Nicolet D, et al. Prognostic significance of the European leukemiaNet standardized system for reporting cytogenetic and molecular alterations in adults with acute myeloid leukemia. *J Clin Oncol.* 2012;30(36):4515–4523.
15. Cheson BD, Bennett JM, Kopecky KJ, et al. Revised recommendations of the international working group for diagnosis, standardization of response criteria, treatment outcomes, and reporting standards for therapeutic trials in acute myeloid leukemia. *J Clin Oncol.* 2003;21(24):4642–4649.
16. Appelbaum FR, Rosenblum D, Arceci RJ, et al. End points to establish the efficacy of new agents in the treatment of acute leukemia. *Blood.* 2007;109(5):1810.
17. Grimwade D, Freeman SD. Defining minimal residual disease in acute myeloid leukemia: which platforms are ready for prime time? *Blood.* 2014;124(23):3345.
18. Greenberg PL, Tuechler H, Schanz J, et al. Revised international prognostic scoring system for myelodysplastic syndromes. *Blood.* 2012;120(12):2454–2465.
19. Della Porta MG, Tuechler H, Malcovati L, et al. Validation of WHO classification-based Prognostic Scoring System (WPSS) for myelodysplastic syndromes and comparison with the revised International Prognostic Scoring System (IPSS-R). A study of the International Working Group for Prognosis in Myelodysplasia (IWG-PM). *Leukemia.* 2015;29(7):1502–1513.
20. Fenaux P, Mufti GJ, Hellstrom-Lindberg E, et al. Azacitidine prolongs overall survival compared with conventional care regimens in elderly patients with low bone marrow blast count acute myeloid leukemia. *J Clin Oncol.* 2010;28(4):562–569.
21. Bhatt G, Blum W. Making the most of hypomethylating agents in myelodysplastic syndrome. *Curr Opin Hematol.* 2017;24(2):79–88.
22. Sanford B, Luger S, Devidas M, et al. Frontline-treatment of acute lymphoblastic leukemia (ALL) in older adolescents and young adults (AYA) using a pediatric regimen is feasible: toxicity results of the prospective US intergroup trial C10403 (Alliance). *Blood.* 2013;122(21):3903.
23. Swerdlow SH, Campo E, Pileri SA, et al. The 2016 revision of the World Health Organization classification of lymphoid neoplasms. *Blood.* 2016;127(20):2375–2390.
24. Ardeshna KM, Smith P, Norton A, et al. Long-term effect of a watch and wait policy versus immediate systemic treatment for asymptomatic advanced-stage non-Hodgkin lymphoma: a randomised controlled trial. *Lancet.* 2003;362(9383):516–522.
25. Brice P, Bastion Y, Lepage E, et al. Comparison in low-tumor-burden follicular lymphomas between an initial no-treatment policy, prednimustine, or interferon alfa: a randomized study from the Groupe d'Etude des Lymphomes Folliculaires. Groupe d'Etude des Lymphomes de l'Adulte. *J Clin Oncol.* 1997;15(3):1110–1117.
26. Dunleavy K. Double-hit lymphomas: current paradigms and novel treatment approaches. Hematology. *Am Soc Hematol Educ Program.* 2014;2014(1):107–112.
27. Thieblemont C, Briere J, Mounier N, et al. The germinal center/activated B-cell subclassification has a prognostic impact for response to salvage therapy in relapsed/refractory diffuse large B-cell lymphoma: a bio-CORAL study. *J Clin Oncol.* 2011;29(31):4079–4087.

28. Hans CP, Weisenburger DD, Greiner TC, et al. Confirmation of the molecular classification of diffuse large B-cell lymphoma by immunohistochemistry using a tissue microarray. *Blood*. 2004;103(1):275–282.

29. Cheson BD, Fisher RI, Barrington SF, et al. Recommendations for initial evaluation, staging, and response assessment of Hodgkin and non-Hodgkin lymphoma: the Lugano classification. *J Clin Oncol*. 2014;32(27):3059–3068.

30. Barrington SF, Mikhaeel NG, Kostakoglu L, et al. Role of imaging in the staging and response assessment of lymphoma: consensus of the International Conference on Malignant Lymphomas Imaging Working Group. *J Clin Oncol*. 2014;32(27):3048–3058.

31. Younes A, Hilden P, Coiffier B, et al. International Working Group consensus response evaluation criteria in lymphoma (RECIL 2017). *Ann Oncol*. 2017.

32. Ziepert M, Hasenclever D, Kuhnt E, et al. Standard international prognostic index remains a valid predictor of outcome for patients with aggressive CD20+ B-cell lymphoma in the rituximab era. *J Clin Oncol*. 2010;28(14):2373–2380.

33. Solal-Celigny P, Roy P, Colombat P, et al. Follicular lymphoma international prognostic index. *Blood*. 2004;104(5):1258–1265.

34. Federico M, Bellei M, Marcheselli L, et al. Follicular lymphoma international prognostic index 2: a new prognostic index for follicular lymphoma developed by the international follicular lymphoma prognostic factor project. *J Clin Oncol*. 2009;27(27):4555–4562.

35. Pastore A, Jurinovic V, Kridel R, et al. Integration of gene mutations in risk prognostication for patients receiving first-line immunochemotherapy for follicular lymphoma: a retrospective analysis of a prospective clinical trial and validation in a population-based registry. *Lancet Oncol*. 2015;16(9):1111–1122.

36. Hoster E, Dreyling M, Klapper W, et al. A new prognostic index (MIPI) for patients with advanced-stage mantle cell lymphoma. *Blood*. 2008;111(2):558–565.

37. Hasenclever D, Diehl V. A prognostic score for advanced Hodgkin's disease. International Prognostic Factors Project on Advanced Hodgkin's Disease. *N Engl J Med*. 1998;339(21):1506–1514.

38. Siegel RL, Miller KD, Jemal A. Cancer statistics, 2016. *CA Cancer J Clin*. 2016;66:7–30.

39. SEER Stat Fact Sheets: Myeloma. https://seer.cancer.gov/statfacts/html/mulmy.html

40. Rajkumr SV, Dimopoulos MA, Palumbo A, et al. International myeloma working group updated criteria for the diagnosis of multiple myeloma. *Lancet Oncol*. 2014;15:e538–e548.

41. Palumbo A, Avet-Loiseau H, Oliva S, et al. Revised international staging system for multiple myeloma: a report from the international myeloma working group. *J Clin Oncol*. 2015;33:2863–2869.

42. Durie BG, Harousseau JL, Miguel JS, et al. International uniform response criteria for multiple myeloma. *Leukemia*. 2006;20:1467–1473.

43. Kumar S, Paiva B, Anderson KC, et al. International myeloma working group consensus criteria for response and minimal residual disease management in multiple myeloma. *Lancet Oncol*. 2016;17:e328–e346.

45

Issues in Recruiting Elderly, Underserved, Minority, and Rural Populations (and Solutions)

Cecilia R. DeGraffinreid, Jill Oliveri, Chasity Washington, Cathy Tatum, and Electra D. Paskett

Clinical trials are often considered the gold standard of care for cancer treatment. However, the National Cancer Institute (NCI) reports less than 3% of adult cancer patients participate in clinical trials (1). Even more concerning is that participation rates among certain vulnerable populations are even lower (1). Underrepresentation of vulnerable populations in clinical trials greatly affects the generalizability of trial results and brings into question the therapeutic implication of the agent, device, or intervention being tested to be used as treatment options in all populations. Since less is known about treatment tolerance in these populations, treatment outcomes and overall survival are negatively impacted. The populations of concern include elderly (age 65 and older), minority (i.e., racial and ethnic), underserved (i.e., low socioeconomic level), and rural populations. Understanding these populations of interest, barriers to trial accrual, solutions to identified challenges, strategies for implementing solutions, and the importance of evaluation of implemented strategies is vital to enhancing accrual of vulnerable populations to clinical trials. This chapter focuses on understanding the cancer burden in these identified populations and describing barriers to accrual, followed by effective solutions to addressing barriers in these populations (Table 45.1).

This paper uses two frameworks to describe clinical trial accrual in vulnerable populations. First, the Accrual to Clinical Trials (ACT) framework, which posits that the majority of accrual barriers can be categorized as patient, system, and provider factors that influence or impact accrual to clinical trials (2). Patient-centered barriers include lack of awareness, distrust of the medical system, inadequate evidence of benefit, communication issues (e.g., language, literacy, style, etc.), cultural differences, and physical access to trials (Figure 45.1). Physician-related barriers include lack of awareness, belief that the standard therapy is best, desire not to lose control over the healthcare of the patient, lack of trial availability, and administrative burdens, while system barriers involve the research design, stringent eligibility criteria, lack of appropriate protocols, cost of trials, and navigational issues. The eight basic tenants of the ACT framework are: (a) adequately characterize the target population; (b) involvement of members of the target population in planning efforts; (c) take the message to the target population; (d) give back to the community; (e) enhance the credibility of a study by using a community spokesperson; (f) identify and remove barriers to participation; (g) improve staff sensitivity; and (h) provide education about importance of trial participation (2).

The second framework is the Multilevel Model of Health Disparities (3), which states that disparities are due to multilevel factors—from biology to policy—which interact synergistically to promote reduced access and increased risk of developing and dying from disease (Figure 45.2).

UNDERSTANDING POPULATIONS OF INTEREST

Elderly Patients

The growing number of cancer survivors can be credited both to improvements in cancer care and treatment, as well as an increasing number of older adults living significantly longer than previous generations. According to the U.S. Census Bureau, 14.1% of the population was 65 years or older in 2015, with the percentage increasing annually (4). With increasing age comes higher cancer incidence, and by 2020, about two thirds of all cancer survivors will be age 65 or older (5), and more than half will have completed treatment more than 5 years before (6). In 2013, the incidence rate of invasive cancer among older adults was 2,029/100,000 compared

TABLE 45.1 Barriers and Solutions to Clinical Trial Accrual by Underrepresented Population

Population	Barrier	Solutions
Elderly	Comorbidities Poor functional status Declining cognitive function Lower education/literacy Location of care Lack of transportation Lack of provider referral Provider's beliefs about clinical trials Provider–patient communication Clinical trial design (inclusion criteria) Time associated with presenting clinical trial	Utilize multilevel, multiple, and flexible strategies Patient education Physicians' recommendation Trial design; stratify on age or functional status; allowing patients with well-controlled comorbid conditions or conditions or organ systems of interest Obtaining a comprehensive geriatric assessment Addition of relevant endpoints Offering trials at local community hospitals Materials developed to accommodate low literacy patients
Racial and ethnic minorities	Implicit and explicit biases Fear and mistrust Lack or limited awareness of trials Economic/financial (lack of insurance, additional cost or copayments) Time away from work Transportation Lack of appropriate trials Not being offered a trial Provider's lack of knowledge about trials Provider–patient communication Provider's preference for standard treatment Language issues	Utilize multilevel, multiple, and flexible strategies Address biases Community engagement In-reach and outreach clinical trial education Offer extended/flexible hours Improve provider–patient communication Address trial design issues Address lack of trials for minority populations, especially advanced disease Utilize patient navigation to help address barriers
Rural	Lack or limited awareness of trials and how to access information about trials Economic/financial (lack of insurance, additional cost or copayments) Shortage of healthcare providers Time away from work Transportation Travel-/weather-related issues Social influences Provider–patient communication Mistrust of clinical trials Access to trials Provider's fear of losing patients Sponsor's requirements/paperwork	Utilize multilevel, multiple, and flexible strategies Offer extended/flexible hours Community, provider, patient, and hospital engagement Outreach education Use people in the community as outreach coordinators Utilize patient navigations to help address barriers Use community members for data collection and recruitment
Lower SES	Lack of financial resources Language barriers Lack of insurance Additional cost associated with trial participation Transportation Access to trials Time away from work	Utilize multilevel, multiple, and flexible strategies Use community health workers Utilize patient navigations to help address barriers Community engagement In-reach and outreach clinical trial education

SES, social economic status.

to 220/100,000 for those under age 65, and the age-adjusted mortality rate was 963/100,000 among those aged 65 and older compared to 54/100,000 for those under age 65 (7).

Elderly survivors (i.e., cancer survivors aged 65 and older) present unique perspectives and challenges in the cancer care delivery continuum. Compared to their younger counterparts, older survivors may adapt better

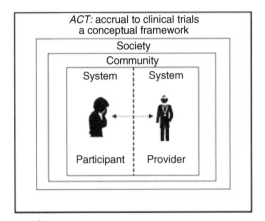

FIGURE 45.1 Accrual to clinical trial framework.

emotionally to their diagnosis; however, they are more likely to experience greater physical challenges, more comorbidities, and declining cognitive function (8). According to a study by Lewis et al. (2003), 32% of patients on phase II and phase III trials were aged 65 or older (9), and a similar proportion was reported by Unger et al. (10).

Despite their higher cancer incidence, older adults continue to be understudied, particularly within clinical trials. Specifically, vital information is lacking among elderly patient populations such as treatment risk and toxicity (9,11,12), interaction of comorbidities with treatment (13), or ability to tolerate treatment as part of the aging process. This lack of evidence may help explain physicians' less aggressive treatment plans for older patients (14). A study by Freedman et al. (15) found participation by elderly patients in adjuvant clinical trials has increased over time, although participation in neoadjuvant and metastatic trials has decreased. Elderly patients were also more likely to withdraw from protocol treatment early compared to their younger counterparts (i.e., <60 years old) (15); however, elderly clinical trial participants can benefit from longer overall survival compared to elderly cancer patients who do not participate (16).

A report by the Institute of Medicine (IOM) and the National Comprehensive Cancer Network (NCCN) encouraged cancer researchers to increase the scope of data collected on cancer treatments for older survivors, especially those with comorbidities (17,18) to enable treating physicians to deliver quality care that not only minimizes toxicity, but also improves quality of life, functional status and, ultimately, survival. Cost should not be a barrier to clinical trial participation since Medicare coverage expanded to include clinical trial treatments in 2000 (19).

Racial and Ethnic Minority Patients

As with other health conditions, cancer disparities persist among certain racial and ethnic minority groups. Historically, for example, African Americans have the highest cancer incidence and mortality rates while

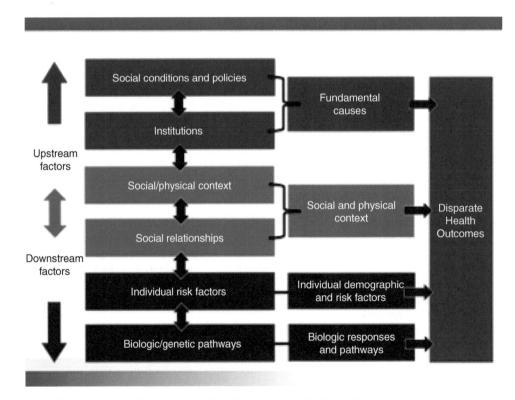

FIGURE 45.2 Model for analysis of population health and health disparities.

Source: From Warnecke RB, Oh P, Breen N, et al. Approaching health disparities from a population perspective: the National Institutes of Health Centers for Population Health and Health Disparities. *Am J Public Health.* 2008;98(9):1608–1615.

Asian/Pacific Islanders have the lowest rates (20). African Americans are more likely to be diagnosed with advanced disease and have lower specific-stage cancer mortality rates (20). African American women were historically diagnosed with invasive breast cancer at a lower rate than their Caucasian counterparts; however, the incidence rates among African American women have increased and are now similar to Caucasian women (21). Although the incidence and mortality rates for the four most common cancers are lower in some racial/ethnic groups (i.e., Hispanics, American Indians/Alaska Natives, Asian/Pacific Islanders) than for Caucasian, these groups have higher cancer incidence rates for infectious agent-associated cancers such as stomach and liver (20).

Over time the survival rates for African American and Caucasian women have increased; however, the survival rate remains 11% lower in African American women (20). In fact, the overall 5-year relative survival rate for all cancers has increased by 20% for Caucasians over the past 30 years and 24% for African Americans during this same time period, although African Americans still have a lower survival rate (Caucasian 68% and African Americans 61%) (21). The apparent difference between Caucasians and non-Caucasians relates to factors that limit the timeliness of patient-centered care (22).

Now, almost 25 years after the National Institutes of Health (NIH) 1993 Revitalization Act (23), which mandated that minorities be adequately represented in NIH-funded research studies, racial and ethnic minorities are still underrepresented in federally funded research (24) and in clinical trials (25–29). Also, a small proportion (<2%) of NCI-sponsored clinical trials have a racial or ethnic minority population as the focus of the trial (24). Although the percentage of racial and ethnic minority populations, especially Hispanic and African American, has increased over the past three decades, the percentage of members from these populations has not increased on clinical trials. Chen et al. noted that without a representative sample of racial or ethnic minorities in clinical trials, there will continue to be disparities in care, and the gap will likely continue to widen (24).

Differences associated with trial participation not only exist between Caucasians and racial and ethnic minorities, but also among the various minority groups (30). Chen et al. noted that between 2010 and 2030, a 99% increase in cancer incidence rates will occur for racial and ethnic minorities, and failure to include this population in clinical trials will result in a greater economic and social burden due to the increase of incidence and deaths from cancer (24). Underrepresentation of racial and ethnic minorities in clinical trials greatly affects the generalizability of the results and brings into question the therapeutic implication of the agent, device, or intervention being tested to be used as treatment options in all populations.

Rural Patients

Rural refers to a geographic area that is not urban or metropolitan and includes "all population, housing, and territory not included within an urban area. Whatever is not urban is considered rural" (31). The total population in rural counties in the United States is over 46 million, which represents 14% of the U.S. population and approximately 72% of its land mass (32). Rural populations are often underserved populations that experience desperate health outcomes and tend to have lower annual incomes when compared to urban areas (32). Rural areas have a shortage of physicians, nurses, and other healthcare providers, as well as poor access to specialty care (33). This contributes to health disparities in the population including higher cancer mortality. A study by Singh, et al. showed that those living in rural areas have a higher overall cancer mortality rate, with those in rural and nonmetropolitan urban areas experiencing 8% higher mortality than larger metropolitan or urbanized counties (34). This study also showed larger mortality disparities for rural residents in prostate, lung, cervical, and colorectal cancers.

Access to high-quality cancer care and cutting-edge treatments can positively impact cancer health disparities. Studies have shown that residents of rural areas are significantly less likely to be recruited to clinical trials (35). Rural residents are less likely to participate in a clinical trial than patients who live in urban areas (36).

Low Social Economic Status Patients

Social economic status (SES) is also a contributing factor in cancer disparities. Low SES is considered a risk factor for survival of cancer because it affects a person's ability to obtain cancer screenings, diagnostic testing, and treatment, thus leading to a higher likelihood of being diagnosed with advanced-stage cancers. Clegg et al. noted that individual-level SES patterns varied by cancer type; however, stage was consistent across cancers, with advanced stage being associated with lower SES (37,38). Other studies have shown that individuals living in low-SES areas (area-level SES) are more likely to present with advanced disease (39–41). In a study examining SES and tumor markers in ethnic populations and difference in tumor size and grade in breast cancer patients, results revealed many individual- and area-level SES factors accounted for ethnic differences in tumor size and stage of cancer (42).

Wong et al. noted that analysis of data for lung, esophageal, and pancreatic cancers from the SEER-Medicare database revealed that although there were differences in treatment across the SES groups, patients in the lower SES group were more likely not to receive cancer treatment (43). Survey data of cancer patients participating in a large national study also revealed that patients with low SES were less likely to participate in clinical trials and were more likely to cite cost as the reason for not participating in clinical trials (44,45). On the other hand, Unger et al. found that lower SES significantly predicted lower clinical trial participation in a population of elderly patients who were eligible for Medicare services, suggesting that SES may play a larger role in the disparity than cost of services (44).

BARRIERS TO ACCRUAL TO CLINICAL TRIALS

Elderly Patients

Patient Factors

Elderly patients, like other underserved populations, present certain characteristics that pose challenges in accruing to clinical trials. With increasing age comes increasing comorbidities. On average, elderly patients are diagnosed with 3.2 comorbidities compared with 1.9 for their younger counterparts (12), the most common being arthritis and hypertension (12,46). The elderly patient may have poorer functional status and is less likely to tolerate treatment well. Declining cognitive function may negatively affect survivorship care with respect to polypharmacy and care coordination across multiple providers (47). Most elderly survivors experience minimal cognitive decline while participating in clinical trials; however, one study found that those who received chemotherapy, received treatment for two or more comorbidities, were frail, or had limited function prediagnosis were more likely to experience cognitive decline during cancer treatment, which ultimately led to poorer physical function (47). Negative experiences such as these may lead clinicians to choose less aggressive treatment for their elderly patients (48).

Elderly patients may have less education, and therefore lower literacy, than younger patients, which can lead to fear and misunderstandings about clinical trials (12,49,50). In the not so distant past, older adults were more likely than younger adults to engage in passive decision making (51). On the other hand, many prefer to remain autonomous throughout the treatment process and refuse participation in a clinical trial if offered to remain in control of their treatment options (12). Other challenges such as location of care and transportation have been reported by elderly patients as reasons for not enrolling in clinical trials. In general, receipt of cancer care at a community hospital where relationships with primary oncologists are sustained is preferable to traveling to larger academic medical centers (52).

Provider Factors

Characteristics of cancer care providers also present challenges to clinical trial accrual of elderly patients. The strongest provider-level predictor of clinical trial participation is provider recommendation of and referral to clinical trials (53). Reasons for lack of recommendation or referral are varied. Oncologists may perceive

the available treatment as too toxic (12). In one study of patients with hematologic malignancies, elderly patients had greater odds of experiencing a grade 3 nonhematologic toxicity compared to younger patients (54); however, other studies have reported adequate treatment tolerance regardless of age (55–57). Other providers believe the best treatment is not available in active clinical trials, the patient is not eligible, or the patient's comorbidities would interfere with treatment response, even when the conditions did not render the patient ineligible. Sometimes clinicians are not even aware that a clinical trial was available (12).

Stage of disease and comorbidities (as they relate to age) may factor into a physician's decision to offer a clinical trial (58). Kemeny et al. examined the association among age, disease stage, comorbidity, and clinical trial recommendation and found that age was not a significant predictor of clinical trial recommendation for patients with stage I disease; however, older patients with stage II disease were less likely to be offered a clinical trial (12). In a study of older patients receiving adjuvant chemotherapy for breast cancer, Klepin et al. reported a median number of two comorbidities among patients, although the burden of these conditions was low. Four or more comorbid conditions and higher burden were associated with poorer overall survival, although neither showed a relationship with toxicity or time to relapse, suggesting that the mere presence of comorbid conditions may not be reason enough to exclude elderly patients from clinical trials (46).

Unfortunately, clinicians may not have the training or expertise needed to effectively communicate with or treat elderly cancer patients, particularly in more sensitive and potentially risky situations like clinical trials. A survey of hematology–oncology program directors revealed that only 32% of their training programs had a formal curriculum that addressed topics in geriatric oncology (59).

System Factors

System-level barriers relate mostly to clinical trial design and presentation to patients and where they are offered participation. While eligibility criteria rarely exclude patients based on chronologic age (i.e., patients must be under 65 years of age), the criteria routinely exclude patients based on their physiologic age as determined by comorbidities, functional status, and prior cancer diagnosis. Studies have shown that overall survival is associated with functional status and comorbidities (60,61). Furthermore, number, type, and burden of comorbidity are important to consider prior to enrollment in clinical trials since treatment options for different cancers affect different organ systems, making exclusion of patients of any age with a health history involving that organ warranted (46). Cardiac, renal, hepatic, and hematologic abnormalities commonly result in clinical trial exclusion due to anticipated effects of cancer treatment. Some studies exclude patients who are not ambulatory or cannot complete activities of daily living independently, while others exclude those with a prior cancer diagnosis (9). Considered independently or collectively, these exclusion criteria significantly decrease the number of elderly patients who may be eligible to participate in a clinical trial.

Another system-level barrier to clinical trial accrual among elderly patients is the presentation of clinical trials to patients, as well as location of the research. Older patients may require more time and resources to present a clinical trial in an understandable and informative manner. Frequently, clinical trial staff have time-sensitive schedules that do not allow the time needed to fully explain study involvement and allay patient fears (62). Furthermore, elderly patients are reluctant to travel to academic medical centers for treatment, preferring community hospitals instead (52). Regardless of location, few geriatric oncology clinics with staff trained in geriatric oncology exist in nonacademic centers (63), and comprehensive geriatric assessment is inconsistent and time-consuming.

Racial and Ethnic Minority Patients

Health systems, providers, and patients are contributors to racial and ethnic disparities in healthcare (64), and the same factors play a major role in racial and ethnic minority patients' accrual to clinical trials (2). These categorical barriers do not exist in isolation, rather they interact and intercept; there is almost a synergistic effect, thus impacting representation of racial and ethnic minorities at various stages and levels across the accrual continuum. In addition, biases on the part of the patient, providers, and systems influence all aspects of the accrual continuum.

These biases may be implicit or explicit in nature. Implicit biases are attitudes or stereotypes that affect an individual's or an institution's actions, understanding, and decisions in an unconscious manner (65,66). Individuals involved in the accrual process are unaware that they are acting upon a bias and, as a result of this automatic unintentional act, may undermine or damage the accrual process (65,66). Explicit biases are beliefs, attitudes, and/or stereotypes that an individual or institution consciously endorses (65). Both types of bias impact invitation and accrual to trials.

Patient Factors

Fear and mistrust of the medical system have widely been reported as barriers to trial participation among racial and ethnic minorities (2,67), including the concept of randomization, not wanting to be used as a "guinea pig" and loss of confidentiality and privacy (67). These fears and mistrust of the medical system are grounded in historical facts. The manner in which African American research participants' trust was abused during the

unethical conduct of the Tuskegee Syphilis Study (68) continues to fuel the mistrust and fear of research within many racial and ethnic minority communities. The Tuskegee study was conducted from 1932 to 1972 by the U.S. Public Health Services without obtaining informed consent from participants. The men in the study were told that they were being treated for "bad blood," not for syphilis, and treatment needed to cure syphilis was withheld so that researchers could better understand the natural history of the disease. This unethical research study is a major cause of mistrust and fear of the healthcare system and research that still has a profound impact on accrual to clinical trials.

Economic burden and financial issues are barriers to trial participation; lack of insurance, additional costs or copayments, time away from work, and time and expense to make additional trips to the hospital were significant barriers (67). However, being economically and financially sound is not a guarantee to equal access to quality care. Many minority patients report problems with patient–provider relationships. When they are afforded care, many minorities feel that they are left out of the decision-making process (67).

Provider Factors

Although economic and financial issues are pervasive barriers, not being offered a trial may be the barrier with the most impact associated with racial and ethnic minority underrepresentation in clinical trials. Failure to provide clinical trials as an option to patients is a barrier (67) and does not allow the patient to make an informed decision about treatment. The pros and cons of the various treatment options should be explained to the patient, thus allowing him or her to make an informed decision regarding the best course of care that may include all types of interventional clinical trials (therapeutic and nontherapeutic).

Some providers may not be aware of trials open at their institutions (67). New advances in treatments such as immunotherapy are being utilized as treatment options in clinical trials; however, this option is not always an option for or offered to minority patients (69); this is also true for lower SES, uninsured, and Medicaid patients (69). Provider bias may also play a role in patients not participating in trials (67); for example, providers may try to select the best participant for a trial or assume patients have logistical issues associated with participation, are unable to comprehend the trial requirements, or will be noncompliant (67). The IOM found similar findings in regard to providers, reporting: "Bias, stereotyping, prejudice, and clinical uncertainty on the part of healthcare providers may contribute to racial and ethnic disparities in healthcare" (64). Clearly, the provider's enthusiasm, provider–patient relationships, and the communication flow between the two parties are essential in enhancing accrual (67).

A study conducted with representatives/key stakeholders (i.e., cancer center directors, research staff, referring providers, and principal investigators) from five NCI-designated cancer centers yielded similar patient, provider, and system barriers as the reason for low accrual of racial and ethnic minorities (70). The stakeholders identified skepticism and distrust of clinical research, uncertainty of trial participation, lack of insurance, communication issues, and lack of awareness of clinical trials (70). Results of a study examining research professionals' perspectives regarding minority trial enrollment found that a majority of those surveyed agreed that the primary language and race of the patient and fear of unknown side effects were factors affecting trial enrollment (30).

System Factors

As with elderly patients, system-level factors also play a role in low accrual to clinical trials for racial and ethnic minority patients. In a study examining the reason for low accrual of Native Americans in community-based cancer centers, stringent inclusion criteria, lack of trials for the most common cancer sites, and lack of infrastructure to provide services were found to be reasons for low accrual of Native Americans to clinical trials (71). In addition to lack of trials for the most common cancer sites in various racial and ethnic populations, lack of trials for advanced disease is a challenge since underrepresented populations are more likely to be diagnosed at later stages (22,72).

Rural Patients

Rural populations experience similar barriers to other minority and or underserved groups when it comes to participation in cancer clinical trials. Rural populations have limited awareness or knowledge of clinical trials and are often not asked to participate and are thus often underrepresented in cancer clinical trials (73). However, due to geographic isolation and healthcare provider shortages, rural residents are more likely than those in urban settings to perceive limited access to locations in which to participate in a clinical trial (74).

Patient Factors

Patient-related barriers to clinical trial participation include transportation and work-related issues. Residents could not miss work in order to participate. Often rural residents desire or would need free transportation. They would prefer to drive less than 30 minutes in order to participate. Also depending on the season, bad weather or bad driving conditions could be a barrier (75). Social influences were also a barrier to rural residents who reported being discouraged by family members and friends who are often part of their decision-making process. Rural residents were more likely than urban residents to believe that clinical trials involved deception, and rural residents were less willing than urban residents to take part in a clinical trial in the future when asked (76).

Provider Factors

Providers play a very important role in a patient's decision to enroll in a clinical trial. As part of their decision-making process the influence of the family doctors/oncologists is strongly related to participation (77). Rural residents have reported lack of information from medical providers as a barrier. They are also more apprehensive regarding costs associated with trial participation (77). Also, if the researcher is unknown to the patient or speaks a different language, the rural patient may be less likely to participate in research (75). Rural healthcare providers may often fear losing patients to other providers. There is often mistrust of large academic medical institutions by community healthcare providers (78).

System Factors

The healthcare system itself plays an important role in the clinical trial recruitment and enrollment process. It is important for researchers to know that rural residents would be more likely to participate if a convenient site were chosen and season was taken into consideration when planning a trial. In some rural areas, there may be less information about how to access trials, a lack of basic trial design awareness and trial design requirements, and some misinformation about the role of clinical research to improving healthcare. There are also often study sponsor requirements and/or paperwork that influence participation by rural providers (78), limiting the ability to enroll patients on trials in their own communities.

Low-SES Patients

Patient Factors

Low SES is in itself a major barrier for all population groups, and lack of financial resources is cited as a primary reason for not participating in clinical trials. These patients may not have insurance to pay for care, let alone cover any additional cost associated with a clinical trial (44). Patients with low SES may have language or literacy barriers, may not have the time, or cannot afford to take leave from work to obtain necessary care, and may have transportation limitations that impede their ability to obtain care, especially if they do not live close to a facility offering clinical trials (38).

Provider Factors

As with other underrepresented populations, providers also contribute to poor accrual to clinical trials among lower SES patients. Unger and colleagues noted that patients with lower incomes were less likely than those with higher incomes to be offered a clinical trial even when one was available (44).

System Factors

Cancer patients may receive more comprehensive care at facilities where providers diagnose and treat high volumes of cancer patients, such as large cancer centers or academic research institutions (44,79), and patients with low SES may not have the means to get to these institutions. In addition, recruitment efforts focused on lower SES groups, among other underrepresented populations, are limited in most settings (35).

SOLUTIONS (WHAT WORKS) TO INCREASE ACCRUAL

Understanding the populations of interest and barriers to clinical trial accrual is essential to addressing the barriers. A multilevel approach that addresses barriers at the patient, provider, and system levels is important to finding solutions that address this problem. Solutions can be found across these levels but should be tailored to each population/group while also addressing individual barriers using strategies directed at all levels. Researchers have proposed multilevel approaches that also include interventions targeted at the individual level (patient and provider), system level, and interpersonal level (perceptions of organizational infrastructures, as well as attitudes and perceptions of each other [patient and provider], care received, and the doctor–patient relationship) (26).

Elderly Patients

Previous studies to improve elderly patient accrual to clinical trials have had limited success (15,80); however, there have been several trials in the recent past that focus solely on older cancer patients. Cancer and Leukemia Group B (CALGB) 369901 successfully recruited more than 1,200 breast cancer survivors aged 65 and older who had invasive, nonmetastatic breast cancer. They spoke either English or Spanish, demonstrated adequate cognitive function, and were ≤20 weeks from their definitive surgery. Using data collected from this elderly cohort, investigators examined the association of frailty with adherence to adjuvant hormonal therapy (81); the influence of patient and physician decision styles on chemotherapy use (82); the roles of personality, coping, and social support as predictors of long-term quality of life trajectories (83); and the associations among survivorship care plans, experiences of survivorship care, and functioning (84). Eligibility criteria were flexible enough to encourage participation while still providing cancer treatment and collecting valuable quality-of-life data.

Another CALGB trial (49907) recruited and enrolled more than 600 breast cancer patients (stage I–III) aged 65 and older to investigate an oral adjuvant chemotherapeutic agent (capecitabine) as an effective treatment option compared to standard chemotherapy (46).

Eligibility criteria included performance status of 0 to 2, adequate organ system function, and no comorbidities that would put the patient at increased risk for harm. Expected survival had to exceed 5 years, concurrent malignancy was prohibited, and previous cancer diagnoses must have had a risk of relapse ≤30%. A quality-of-life companion study was offered to these participants, and more than half (n = 350) were eligible. The valuable data provided by these elderly cancer patients allowed researchers to better understand the associations between comorbidity, chemotherapy toxicity, and outcomes (i.e., time to relapse, overall survival) (46), as well as other quality-of-life components of cancer treatment, particularly cognitive function (85) and social support (86). Unlike CALGB 369901, this study employed slightly more rigid eligibility criteria; however, in testing a chemotherapeutic agent, risk to organ systems was an important consideration that needed to be addressed.

After Medicare changed their policy to accommodate the costs of clinical trials in 2000, Southwest Oncology Group (SWOG) investigators analyzed trends in clinical trial accrual of elderly patients from 2001 to 2003 compared to previous years. This policy change alone accounted for a significant increase in trial participation among elderly patients, but only for those with supplemental private coverage of coinsurance costs (25% from 1993 to 1996; 31% from 1997 to 2000; 38% from 2001 to 2003) (10).

Although some studies focus exclusively on elderly patients, there are still numerous opportunities to move the science forward based on results of and lessons learned from previous studies. First, oncologists and clinical trial staff need to be better educated about the benefit of clinical trials to their elderly patients, as well as the availability of active clinical trials at their institutions. Several studies have noted that patients are likely to consider clinical trial participation if recommended by their physicians (12,49,53), and a clinical trial should be considered for every patient regardless of age (87). Relatedly, clinical trials need to be more widely offered for cancers other than breast cancer. While the population of breast cancer survivors is by far the largest, there is much to be learned from other cancer survivors as the experiences of breast cancer patients are not generalizable to the larger population.

Greater improvements to clinical trial accrual of elderly patients could be observed if clinical trials were redesigned to include, rather than exclude, this vulnerable population. One group, Eliminating Disparities in Clinical Trials (EDICT), works to address appropriate representation of underserved populations in clinical trials and has suggested that if mandates required inclusion of these vulnerable populations, accrual would naturally improve. Another strategy would be to stratify clinical trials on age or functional status to ensure adequate representation of older patients on every trial. An alternative may be that a certain proportion of participants for every trial be those aged 65 or older. Eligibility criteria could be modified to improve generalizability of results to the larger elderly population. Acknowledging that 80% of older adults have at least one chronic condition and almost 70% have at least two (88), allowing those whose comorbid conditions are well controlled and not involved in the organ system of interest to enroll in a clinical trial may not compromise treatment tolerance while still allowing valuable data to be collected on treatment effects in this subset (89). Lewis et al. predicted that if limitations on organ systems and functional status are removed from eligibility criteria, elderly patient participation would increase to 59.7% as these exclusions "almost fully explain the observed underrepresentation of the elderly in these trials relative to their burden of disease" (9). Subbiah et al. suggested considering risk factors strongly correlated with lack of clinical benefit (rather than age) when considering patients for clinical trials. Those who stand to benefit least from treatment have a performance status greater than 1 (on a scale of 0–5), have liver metastases, have had five or more prior treatments, or have had prior radiation therapy (55). Similarly, Balducci recommended a comprehensive geriatric assessment for all elderly patients prior to enrollment on a clinical trial, including functional status, comorbidity, mental status, emotional conditions, nutritional status, polypharmacy, and geriatric symptoms (90). Considering all of these factors collectively, rather than independently, may result in fewer adverse events (AEs) and more benefit from treatment (91). Finally, adding additional relevant endpoints for clinical trials, including quality of life, maintaining independence, and changes in general functioning could allow for monitoring treatment tolerance and trajectories (91,92).

Given that elderly patients are hesitant to seek and receive care at larger academic medical centers, more clinical trials should be offered at local community hospitals to allow patients to maintain their relationship with their primary oncologist and ease transportation barriers (93). Regardless of location, study materials (especially, informed consent forms and Health Insurance Portability and Accountability Act [HIPAA] authorizations) should be prepared to accommodate possible lower health literacy among older patients, and adequate staff should be employed and trained to foster clinical trial enrollment among this underserved population (62,92,94).

Racial and Ethnic Minority Patients

To improve accrual to clinical trials, it is important to take a multilevel approach and to develop flexible strategies that address barriers at the patient, provider, and system levels. It is also extremely important that there is a strong relationship between the patient, provider, and the system in order to ensure effective enrollment of minorities and other underserved populations to clinical trials. In a review of studies to identify successful community-engaged interventions to increase accrual of racial and ethnic minorities to clinical trials, Heller at al. noted that a multilevel approach that engaged the hospital, provider, and/or community was used by every study reviewed (95). There should be targeted recruitment efforts and utilization of these strategies directed at all levels as well as involvement of the community and patient families, as proposed in the ACT framework (2).

When deciding upon strategies it is important to understand and address biases, implicit or explicit, that are held by patients and providers within the system. Research has shown that implicit bias can be modified (65), and one method of addressing bias is through inreach and outreach educational activities. Engaging in community clinical trial education is a way to make members of various communities aware of clinical trials and to help eliminate or at least minimize the effect of the historically negative image of research. Outreach to the community and building strong community relationships and engagement is an effective means of enhancing trial enrollment (96). Providing training to all staff is vital to successful accrual; the receptionist as well as the clinical care team should be aware of trials and the importance of having representation of all populations in these studies. Changing the beliefs and norms of the community and organizations will foster better and open communication regarding healthcare.

Building a system infrastructure that encompasses the needs of the patient and the patient's family as well as the institution's need to meet accrual goals is essential. Having physicians understand that there are options other than standard treatment, integrating clinical trial recruitment within the patient care process (95), having a system in place to help patients with added cost such as parking and transportation (95), offering extended hours so that patients do not have to miss work (95), providing navigators to help the patient through the system by identifying barriers and helping to reduce those barriers (95,97), while fully engaging the patient in his or her care, are essential to having a patient-centered infrastructure. A strategy for enrolling patients to clinical trials is a good recruitment and retention plan that takes into consideration that recruitment strategies are not one size fits all; successful strategies utilized multiple and flexible approaches (95,96). There should be an understanding that some strategies may need to be tailored for different population groups being recruited to the trial. Also, inclusion and exclusion criteria that are necessary to maintain the integrity of the study but do not exclude patients for reasons that do not affect the safety of the patients or results of the study should be included in protocols. Ensuring that trials are available to the most common disease sites will help improve trial participation.

Fouad et al. conducted a 7-year study at an NCI-designated cancer center to investigate the impact of lay patient navigators on clinical trial participation and retention of African American patients (97). The study addressed patient- and system-level barriers; navigators were embedded into the clinical trial team (system) and worked directly with the patients to address individual barriers (97). Utilizing navigators increased enrollment and retention; referral of patients for clinical trials increased from 5.5.% to 16.6%, 80.4% of the patients referred who were eligible for a clinical trial enrolled in a clinical trial, and 74.5% of the participants working with a navigator completed the trial (97). The use of navigators has been found to be effective in helping patients through the hospital system (95).

Rural Patients

Strategies addressing barriers to awareness include targeting providers to explain the study and gain commitment to recruit and enroll their patients. The most successful programs used existing relationships and face-to-face meetings as cold calling, letters, or faxing information to providers were not successful (95). Strategies to address barriers to participation that proved successful were engaging hospitals, providers, and participants in underserved communities including rural areas. Pilot testing recruitment approaches and modifying methods as needed with input from community stakeholders also proved beneficial to recruitment (95). Some studies identified and provided incentives for community members to recruit participants from their social networks (98). In a review of effective recruitment strategies, Heller found that 70% of the studies used people from the community as outreach coordinators to educate and provide culturally relevant materials (95).

Public trust in research and the skills needed should be encouraged through training of researchers in health disparities. An understanding of culture and health disparities is essential to more diverse recruitment to clinical trials including from rural areas. Not doing so contributes to mistrust and inconsistent and inaccurate communication and literacy about research (78). Strategies to address barriers to participation have included the use of patient navigators to address financial, transportation, psychosocial, and other patient identified barriers. However, the most effective programs have used a combination of strategies to address the provider, participants, trust in the community, and the systems or locations in which the trials are being conducted (95).

The University of Maryland has developed a comprehensive multilevel approach to address community participation in clinical trials, which include infrastructure and personal barriers to clinical trial recruitment in rural as well as with other underserved populations (78). In a study conducted in rural Maryland, Baquet et al. found that reimbursement, insurance, more knowledge about the trial, follow-up, and providing additional healthcare played a role in the clinical trial participation decision of residents (35). Other things to consider include offering times of data collection outside of normal business hours; using local data collectors/recruiters from the community could also potentially improve response and participation rates (75). Living in a rural area may not alone be a cause or barrier for poor participation in clinical trials but combined with other factors or features of rural life, this impacts participation. Inclusion of rural people in healthcare research will ultimately have a positive influence on the quality of the healthcare they receive (75).

Low-SES Patients

Interventions utilized to enhance accrual of low SES to clinical trials have not been well studied, but should be delivered at the patient, provider, and system levels. Since low income is a factor that affects every population group, many of the multilevel interventions also apply to this population. Having a presence in low-SES communities is vital to enhancing accrual; this can be done by providing clinical trial education, providing resources for screenings, and utilizing the services of community health workers. Having a community health worker or patient navigator as part of the research team who is involved from the start of the accrual process will also hopefully enhance accrual. Training should be provided to all staff that includes sensitivity training, so that they are made aware that because someone is of a lower SES level they should not be treated differently than any other patient. Working within the system to help find transportation or provide transportation or parking vouchers will help elevate concerns about additional costs associated with trial participation (99). Covering the cost of copayments or coinsurance may be a means to improve trial participation (44), and provisions for time off from work or childcare needs should be important considerations (100). Providing translation services is also an important factor in engaging patients who do not speak English, as is creating research documents (e.g., informed consent form, HIPAA authorization) that are easily understandable by all patients. Ultimately, respecting every patient and providing them the service that everyone expects is the ultimate key to successful recruitment.

CONCLUSIONS

In spite of the many advances in cancer research over the past few decades, accrual of elderly, minority, rural, and underserved patients to clinical trials is still not consistent with their burden of disease, and evidence consistently demonstrates widespread disparities in clinical trial enrollment and participation. A clinical trial should be considered for every patient seen where clinical trials are available. Provider education can help correct misperceptions about clinical trial eligibility and availability. Clinicians and researchers need to better understand factors that influence a patient's decision to participate in clinical trials and ensure access, both from providers' and patients' points of view. New policies or initiatives, such as the Medicare policy change in 2000, may help ensure access to clinical trials for underrepresented populations (101). Without adequate representation, studies on new cancer treatments will be underpowered to answer important questions related to effectiveness, tolerance, and survival. Increasing accrual to clinical trials will improve surveillance and monitoring that will, in turn, identify other conditions (side effects and comorbidities) more quickly. Prompt treatment of these will lead to better symptom management, more frequent patient–provider communication, improved well-being, and better survival rates for all populations, and ultimately eliminate disparities in cancer outcomes (56).

REFERENCES

1. Colon-Otero G, Smallridge RC, Solberg LA Jr, et al. Disparities in participation in cancer clinical trials in the United States: a symptom of a healthcare system in crisis. *Cancer.* 2008;112(3):447–454.
2. Paskett ED, Katz ML, DeGraffinreid CR, Tatum CM. Participation in cancer trials: recruitment of underserved populations. *Clin Adv Hematol Oncol.* 2003;1(10):607–613.
3. Warnecke RB, Oh P, Breen N, et al. Approaching health disparities from a population perspective: the National Institutes of Health Centers for Population Health and Health Disparities. *Am J Public Health.* 2008;98(9):1608–1615.
4. US Census Bureau. *2011–2015 American Community Survey 5-Year estimates–age and sex.* 2016.
5. Parry C, Kent EE, Mariotto AB, et al. Cancer survivors: a booming population. *Cancer Epidemiol Biomarkers Prev.* 2011;20(10):1996–2005.
6. de Moor JS, Mariotto AB, Parry C, et al. Cancer survivors in the United States: prevalence across the survivorship trajectory and implications for care. *Cancer Epidemiol Biomarkers Prev.* 2013;22(4):561–570.
7. Howlader N, Noone AM, Krapcho M,et al., eds. *SEER cancer statistics review, 1975–2013,* Bethesda, MD: National Cancer Institute; 2016.
8. Rowland JH, Bellizzi KM. Cancer survivorship issues: life after treatment and implications for an aging population. *J Clin Oncol.* 2014;32(24):2662–2668.
9. Lewis JH, Kilgore ML, Goldman DP, et al. Participation of patients 65 years or older in cancer clinical trials. *J Clin Oncol.* 2003;21(7):1383–1389.
10. Unger JM, Coltman CA Jr, Crowley JJ, et al. Impact of the year 2000 Medicare policy change on older patient enrollment to cancer clinical trials. *J Clin Oncol.* 2006;24(1):141–144.
11. Mitka M. Too few older patients in cancer trials: experts say disparity affects research results and care. *JAMA.* 2003;290(1):27–28.
12. Kemeny MM, Peterson BL, Kornblith AB, et al. Barriers to clinical trial participation by older women with breast cancer. *J Clin Oncol.* 2003;21(12):2268–2275.
13. Yancik R, Wesley MN, Ries LA, et al. Effect of age and comorbidity in postmenopausal breast cancer patients aged 55 years and older. *JAMA.* 2001;285(7):885–892.
14. Foster JA, Salinas GD, Mansell D, et al. How does older age influence oncologists' cancer management? *Oncologist.* 2010;15(6):584–592.
15. Freedman RA, Foster JC, Seisler DK, et al. Accrual of older patients with breast cancer to Alliance systemic therapy trials over time: protocol A151527. *J Clin Oncol.* 2017;35(4):421–431.
16. Zafar SF, Heilbrun LK, Vishnu P, et al. Participation and survival of geriatric patients in Phase I clinical trials: the Karmanos Cancer Institute (KCI) experience. *J Geriatr Oncol.* 2011;2(1):18–24.
17. Institute of Medicine. *Delivering high-quality cancer care: charting a new course for a system in crisis.* Washington, DC: The National Academies Press; 2013.
18. Hutchins LF, Unger JM, Crowley JJ, et al. Underrepresentation of patients 65 years of age or older in cancer-treatment trials. *N Engl J Med.* 1999;341(27):2061–2067.
19. Centers for Medicare & Medicaid Services: Health Care Financing Administration. *Medicare coverage routine costs of beneficiaries in clinical trials.* September 19, 2000.
20. Siegel RL, Miller KD, Jemal A. Cancer statistics, 2017. *CA Cancer J Clin.* 2017;67(1):7–30.
21. American Cancer Society. *Cancer facts & figures 2017.* Atlanta, GA: American Cancer Society; 2017.
22. American Cancer Society. *Cancer facts & figures for African Americans.* Atlanta, GA: American Cancer Society; 2016.
23. National Institutes of Health, *The inclusion of women and minorities as subjects in clinical research—Amended October, 2001.* Washington, DC; 2001.
24. Chen MS, Jr, Lara PN, Dang JH, et al. Twenty years post-NIH Revitalization Act: enhancing minority participation in clinical trials (EMPaCT): laying the groundwork for improving minority clinical trial accrual: renewing the case for enhancing minority participation in cancer clinical trials. *Cancer.* 2014;120(Suppl 7):1091–1096.
25. Ford JG, Howerton MW, Lai GY, et al. Barriers to recruiting underrepresented populations to cancer clinical trials: a systematic review. *Cancer.* 2008;112(2):228–242.
26. Hamel LM, Penner LA, Albrecht TL, et al. Barriers to clinical trial enrollment in racial and ethnic minority patients with cancer. *Cancer Control.* 2016;23(4):327–337.
27. Tanner A, Kim SH, Friedman DB, et al. Promoting clinical research to medically underserved communities: current practices and perceptions about clinical trial recruiting strategies. *Contemp Clin Trials.* 2015;41:39–44.
28. Arevalo M, Heredia NI, Krasny S, et al. Mexican-American perspectives on participation in clinical trials: A qualitative study. *Contemp Clin Trials Commun.* 2016;4:52–57.
29. Salman A, Nguyen C, Lee YH, Cooksey-James T. A review of barriers to minorities' participation in cancer clinical trials: implications for future cancer research. *J Immigr Minor Health.* 2016;18(2):447–453.
30. Kurt A, Semler L, Jacoby JL, et al. Racial differences among factors associated with participation in clinical research trials. *J Racial Ethn Health Disparities*; 2016.
31. US Department of Health & Human Services. *Defining rural population.* 2017. https://www.hrsa.gov/ruralhealth/aboutus/definition.html
32. US Department of Agriculture Economic Research Service. *Rural America at a glance.* 2016.
33. The Council of State Governments, *Health care workforce shortages critical in rural America,* in *Capitol Facts & Figures.* 2011.
34. Singh GK, Jemal A. Socioeconomic, rural-urban, and racial inequalities in US cancer mortality: part I-all cancers and lung cancer and part II-colorectal, prostate, breast, and cervical cancers. *J Cancer Epidemiol.* 2011;2011:1–27.
35. Baquet CR, Commiskey P, Daniel Mullins C, Mishra SI. Recruitment and participation in clinical trials: socio-demographic, rural/urban, and health care access predictors. *Cancer Detect Prev.* 2006;30(1):24–33.

36. Geana M, Erba J, Krebill H, et al. Searching for cures: Inner-city and rural patients' awareness and perceptions of cancer clinical trial. *Contemp Clin Trials Commun.* 2017;5:72–79.

37. Clegg LX, Reichman ME, Miller BA, et al. Impact of socioeconomic status on cancer incidence and stage at diagnosis: selected findings from the surveillance, epidemiology, and end results: National Longitudinal Mortality Study. *Cancer Causes Control.* 2009;20(4):417–435.

38. Gross CP, Filardo G, Mayne ST, Krumholz HM. The impact of socioeconomic status and race on trial participation for older women with breast cancer. *Cancer.* 2005;103(3):483–491.

39. Mandelblatt J, Andrews H, Kao R, et al. The late-stage diagnosis of colorectal cancer: demographic and socioeconomic factors. *Am J Public Health.* 1996;86(12):1794–1797.

40. Mandelblatt J, Andrews H, Kerner J, et al. Determinants of late stage diagnosis of breast and cervical cancer: the impact of age, race, social class, and hospital type. *Am J Public Health.* 1991;81(5):646–649.

41. Merkin SS, Stevenson L, Powe N. Geographic socioeconomic status, race, and advanced-stage breast cancer in New York City. *Am J Public Health.* 2002;92(1):64–70.

42. Miller BA, Hankey BF, Thomas TL. Impact of sociodemographic factors, hormone receptor status, and tumor grade on ethnic differences in tumor stage and size for breast cancer in US women. *Am J Epidemiol.* 2002;155(6):534–545.

43. Wong SL, Gu N, Banerjee M, et al. The impact of socioeconomic status on cancer care and survival. in 2011 ASCO Annual Meeting. *Health Ser Res.* 2011 (suppl).

44. Unger JM, Hershman DL, Albain KS, et al. Patient income level and cancer clinical trial participation. *J Clin Oncol,* 2013;31(5):536–542.

45. Unger JM, Cook E, Tai E, Bleyer A. The role of clinical trial participation in cancer research: barriers, evidence, and strategies. *Am Soc Clin Oncol Educ Book.* 2016;35:185–198.

46. Klepin HD, Pitcher BN, Ballman KV, et al. Comorbidity, chemotherapy toxicity, and outcomes among older women receiving adjuvant chemotherapy for breast cancer on a clinical trial: CALGB 49907 and CALGB 361004 (alliance). *J Oncol Pract.* 2014;10(5):e285–e292.

47. Mandelblatt JS, Clapp JD, Luta G, et al. Long-term trajectories of self-reported cognitive function in a cohort of older survivors of breast cancer: CALGB 369901 (Alliance). *Cancer.* 2016;3555–3563.

48. Schonberg MA, Marcantonio ER, Li D, et al. Breast cancer among the oldest old: tumor characteristics, treatment choices, and survival. *J Clin Oncol.* 2010;28(12):2038–2045.

49. Townsley CA, Chan KK, Pond GR, et al. Understanding the attitudes of the elderly towards enrolment into cancer clinical trials. *BMC Cancer.* 2006;6:34.

50. Callahan EH, Thomas DC, Goldhirsch SL, et al. Geriatric hospital medicine. *Med Clin North Am.* 2002;86(4):707–729.

51. Davison BJ, Breckon E. Factors influencing treatment decision making and information preferences of prostate cancer patients on active surveillance. *Patient Educ Couns.* 2012;87(3):369–374.

52. Basche M, Barón AE, Eckhardt SG, et al. Barriers to enrollment of elderly adults in early-phase cancer clinical trials. *J Oncol Pract.* 2008;4(4):162–168.

53. Ayodele O, Akhtar M, Konenko A, et al. Comparing attitudes of younger and older patients towards cancer clinical trials. *J Geriatr Oncol.* 2016;7(3):162–168.

54. Tallarico M, Foster J, Seisler D, et al. Toxicities and related outcomes of elderly patients (pts) (≥65 Years) with hematologic malignancies in the contemporary era (Alliance A151611). *Blood.* 2016;128(22):536–536.

55. Subbiah IM, Wheler JJ, Hess KR, et al. Outcomes of patients ≥65 years old with advanced cancer treated on phase I trials at MD ANDERSON CANCER CENTER. *Int J Cancer.* 2017;140(1):208–215.

56. Mandelblatt JS, Makgoeng SB, Luta G, et al. A planned, prospective comparison of short-term quality of life outcomes among older patients with breast cancer treated with standard chemotherapy in a randomized clinical trial vs. an observational study: CALGB #49907 and #369901. *J Geriatr Oncol.* 2013;4(4):353–361.

57. Loconte NK, Smith M, Alberti D, et al. Amongst eligible patients, age and comorbidity do not predict for dose-limiting toxicity from phase I chemotherapy. *Cancer Chemother Pharmacol.* 2010;65(4):775–780.

58. Hurria A, Naeim A, Elkin E, et al. Adjuvant treatment recommendations in older women with breast cancer: a survey of oncologists. *Crit Rev Oncol Hematol.* 2007;61(3):255–260.

59. Naeim A, Hurria A, Rao A, et al. The need for an aging and cancer curriculum for. *J Geriat Oncol.* 2010;1(2):109–113.

60. Garrido-Laguna I, Janku F, Vaklavas C, et al. Validation of the Royal Marsden Hospital prognostic score in patients treated in the phase I clinical trials program at the MD Anderson Cancer Center. *Cancer.* 2012;118(5):1422–1428.

61. van Heeckeren WJ, Fu P, Barr PM, et al. Safety and tolerability of phase I/II clinical trials among older and younger patients with acute myelogenous leukemia. *J Geriatr Oncol.* 2011;2(3):215–221.

62. Hempenius L, Slaets JP, Boelens MA, et al. Inclusion of frail elderly patients in clinical trials: solutions to the problems. *J Geriatr Oncol.* 2013;4(1):26–31.

63. Mcneil C. Geriatric oncology clinics on the rise. *J Natl Cancer Inst.* 2013;105(9):585–586.

64. Institute of Medicine Committee on Understanding and Eliminating Racial and Ethnic Disparities in Health Care, Unequal Treatment. *Confronting Racial and Ethnic Disparities in Health Care.* Smedley BD, Stith AY, Nelson AR, ed. Washington, DC: National Academies Press; 2003.

65. Staats C, Capatosto K, Wright RA, Contractor D. *State of the science: implicit bias review 2016.* Columbus, OH: Kirwan Institute for the Study of Race and Ethnicity; 2016.

66. Brownstein M. Implicit bias. In Zalta EN, ed., *The Stanford encyclopedia of philosophy.* Metaphysics Research Lab: Stanford University; 2017.

67. Schmotzer GL. Barriers and facilitators to participation of minorities in clinical trials. *Ethn Dis.* 2012;22(2):226–230.

68. Centers for Disease Control and Prevention. US Public Health Service Syphilis Study at Tuskegee. 2013. https://www.cdc.gov/tuskegee/index.html

69. Flowers CR, Fedewa SA, Chen AY, et al. Disparities in the early adoption of chemoimmunotherapy for diffuse large B-cell lymphoma in the United States. *Cancer Epidemiol Biomarkers Prev.* 2012;21(9):1520–1530.

70. Durant RW, Wenzel JA, Scarinci IC, et al. Perspectives on barriers and facilitators to minority recruitment for clinical trials among cancer center leaders, investigators, research staff, and referring clinicians: enhancing minority participation in clinical trials (EMPaCT). *Cancer.* 2014;120(Suppl 7):1097–1105.

71. Guadagnolo BA, Petereit DG, Helbig P, et al. Involving American Indians and medically underserved rural populations in cancer clinical trials. *Clin Trials.* 2009;6(6):610–617.

72. American Cancer Society. *Cancer Facts & Figures for Hispanic/Latinos (2015–2016).* Atlanta: American Cancer Society; 2015.

73. Vanderpool RC, Kornfeld J, Mills L, et al. Rural-urban differences in discussions of cancer treatment clinical trials. *Patient Educ Couns.* 2011;85(2):e69–e74.

74. Kim SH, Tanner A, Friedman DB, et al. Barriers to clinical trial participation: a comparison of rural and urban communities in South Carolina. *J Community Health.* 2014;39(3):562–571.

75. Morgan LL, Fahs PS, Klesh J. Barriers to research participation identified by rural people. *J Agric Saf Health.* 2005;11(4):407–414.

76. Friedman DB, Bergeron CD, Foster C, et al. What do people really know and think about clinical trials? A comparison of rural and urban communities in the South. *J Community Health*. 2013;38(4):642–651.

77. Virani S, Burke L, Remick SC, et al. Barriers to recruitment of rural patients in cancer clinical trials. *J Oncol Pract*. 2011;7(3):172–177.

78. Baquet CR, Henderson K, Commiskey P, et al. Clinical trials: the art of enrollment. *Semin Oncol Nurs*. 2008;24(4):262–269.

79. National Cancer Institute. *Cancer Health Disparities Research*. 2017. https://www.cancer.gov/research/areas/disparities

80. Kimmick GG, Peterson BL, Kornblith AB, et al. Improving accrual of older persons to cancer treatment trials: a randomized trial comparing an educational intervention with standard information: CALGB 360001. *J Clin Oncol*. 2005;23(10):2201–2207.

81. Sheppard VB, Faul LA, Luta G, et al. Frailty and adherence to adjuvant hormonal therapy in older women with breast cancer: CALGB protocol 369901. *J Clin Oncol*. 2014;32(22):2318–2327.

82. Mandelblatt JS, Faul LA, Luta G, et al. Patient and physician decision styles and breast cancer chemotherapy use in older women: cancer and leukemia group B protocol 369901. *J Clin Oncol*. 2012;30(21):2609–2614.

83. Durá-Ferrandis E, Mandelblatt JS, Clapp J, et al. Personality, coping, and social support as predictors of long-term quality-of-life trajectories in older breast cancer survivors: CALGB protocol 369901 (Alliance). *Psychooncology*. 2017.

84. Faul LA, Luta G, Sheppard V, et al. Associations among survivorship care plans, experiences of survivorship care, and functioning in older breast cancer survivors: CALGB/Alliance 369901. *J Cancer Surviv*. 2014;8(4):627–637.

85. Freedman RA, Pitcher B, Keating NL, et al. Alliance for Clinical Trials in Oncology. Cognitive function in older women with breast cancer treated with standard chemotherapy and capecitabine on Cancer and Leukemia Group B 49907. *Breast Cancer Res Treat*. 2013;139(2):607–616.

86. Jatoi A, Muss H, Allred JB, et al. Social support and its implications in older, early-stage breast cancer patients in CALGB 49907 (Alliance A171301). *Psychooncology*. 2016;25(4):441–446.

87. Kimmick G. Clinical trial accrual in older cancer patients: the most important steps are the first ones. *J Geriatr Oncol*. 2016;7(3):158–161.

88. *National Council on Aging, Healthy Aging Fact Sheet*. Arlington, VA; 2016

89. Peairs KS, Barone BB, Snyder CF, et al. Diabetes mellitus and breast cancer outcomes: a systematic review and meta-analysis. *J Clin Oncol*. 2011;29(1):40–46.

90. Balducci L. Geriatric oncology. *Crit Rev Oncol Hematol*. 2003;46(3):211–220.

91. Lichtman SM. Geriatric oncology and clinical trials. *Am Soc Clin Oncol Educ Book*. 2015;e127–e131.

92. Townsley CA, Selby R, Siu LL. Systematic review of barriers to the recruitment of older patients with cancer onto clinical trials. *J Clin Oncol*. 2005;23(13):3112–3124.

93. Freedman RA, Seisler DK, Foster JC, et al. Risk of acute myeloid leukemia and myelodysplastic syndrome among older women receiving anthracycline-based adjuvant chemotherapy for breast cancer on Modern Cooperative Group Trials (Alliance A151511). *Breast Cancer Res Treat*. 2017;161(2):363–373.

94. Kornblith AB, Kemeny M, Peterson BL, et al. Cancer and leukemia group B. Survey of oncologists' perceptions of barriers to accrual of older patients with breast carcinoma to clinical trials. *Cancer*. 2002;95(5):989–996.

95. Heller C, Balls-Berry JE, Nery JD, et al. Strategies addressing barriers to clinical trial enrollment of underrepresented populations: a systematic review. *Contemp Clin Trials*. 2014;39(2):169–182.

96. Paskett ED, Reeves KW, Mclaughlin JM, et al. Recruitment of minority and underserved populations in the United States: the centers for population health and health disparities experience. *Contemp Clin Trials*. 2008;29(6):847–861.

97. Fouad MN, Acemgil A, Bae S, et al. Patient navigation as a model to increase participation of African Americans in cancer clinical trials. *J Oncol Pract*. 2016;12(6):556–563.

98. Vicini F, Nancarrow-Tull J, Shah C, et al. Increasing accrual in cancer clinical trials with a focus on minority enrollment: the William Beaumont Hospital community clinical oncology program experience. *Cancer*. 2011;117(20):4764–4771.

99. Nipp RD, Lee H, Powell E, et al. Financial Burden of cancer clinical trial participation and the impact of a cancer care equity program. *Oncologist*. 2016;21(4):467–474.

100. Unger JM, Gralow JR, Albain KS, et al. Patient income level and cancer clinical trial participation: a prospective survey study. *JAMA Oncol*. 2016;2(1):137–139.

101. Murthy VH, Krumholz HM, Gross CP. Participation in cancer clinical trials: race-, sex-, and age-based disparities. *JAMA*. 2004;291(22):2720–2726.

Telemedicine and Clinical Trials

Ana Maria Lopez

BACKGROUND

Oncology has led the way in evidence-based care due to its strong reliance on cancer clinical trials as the means by which new knowledge is translated into cancer care (1). This living bed-to-bedside and back again model has guided cancer clinical practice starting well into the past century. If clinical trials support progress in oncology care and less than 5% (2–4) of new cancer patients enroll in cancer clinical trials, would oncology science not be better served with improved access to cancer clinical trials and improved cancer clinical trial enrollment?

Although the answer to this question is a resounding yes and has been so for at least the past 50 years, the lament remains. In this chapter, we discuss what is known about the barriers and facilitators to cancer clinical trials and how technology may support solutions and innovations. Since facilitators and barriers generally have an obvious opposite partner, the discussion focuses on the facilitator. For example: the facilitator—enrollment in a clinical trial is positively associated with proximity to a cancer center—is partnered with the barrier—enrollment in a clinical trial is negatively associated with distance from a cancer center; the discussion focuses on the facilitator. Each discussion is followed by telemedicine solutions and innovations.

ENROLLMENT IN CANCER CLINICAL TRIALS

When asked, most cancer patients express awareness of, interest in, and value of cancer clinical trials (5,6). Maintaining and translating this interest of the majority of patients into a majority of cancer patients enrolling in cancer clinical trials would likely hasten clinical progress while improving clinical outcomes, including personalized outcomes, as enrollment would represent a broader segment of the population with cancer (7). This may also result in more equitable care as it has been suggested that disparities in access to cancer clinical trials contributes to inequities in cancer survivorship and cancer mortality (8–10).

TELEMEDICINE

Telemedicine is characterized by the use of telecommunications technology in the care of patients. Telemedicine technology has been developed to assist in the diagnosis, treatment, and follow-up care of patients (11). With the increasing recognition of team-based care, the term telehealth has been adopted as being more accurately reflective of team-based care. Telehealth is the term used for the remainder of this chapter and stands for a broad definition of telehealth, which includes mobile technologies, social media, and smartphone apps (12). Clinician is the general term used for the healthcare professional involved in the clinical care of the patient.

The technology that is available for telehealth use is increasingly accessible as it both improves and becomes less expensive with time. Although initially developed by National Aeronautics and Space Administration (NASA) to facilitate the clinical care of patients in space, that is, of the astronauts, the potential benefits of telehealth in bridging distance on Earth were quickly explored (13,14). Given the costs of the initial telehealth systems, general adoption of the technology was prohibitive for most. As the technology improved and costs decreased, adoption accelerated in the mid- to late-1990s (13) and has skyrocketed in this century (15). Telecommunication applications in healthcare have emerged as a boon market in the 21st century (16).

Telehealth consultations may take place in real-time (RT), store-forward (SF), or as a combination modality of the two (17). RT consultations are most like the in-person (IP) clinical encounter where the clinician and the patient are present and interact directly. The RT interaction requires patient and clinician to be available at the same time and necessitates high-resolution videoconferencing technology, training in its use, and access to technology support as needed. SF consultations are defined by those clinical interactions where direct patient–clinician interaction may not be necessary to answer the referral question. This consultation is most successful when the patient has a strong relationship with the clinician requesting the consultation. This referring clinician must be able to translate the teleclinical encounter for the patient and interpret the recommendations. For example, a patient with hepatitis C may work closely with the primary care physician and may intermittently have a virtual SF consultation with the hepatologist who reviews the patient's clinical findings—as reported by the primary care physician—the medications, treatment plan, and laboratory results. Although the assessment and recommendations would be provided by the telehepatologist, they would be relayed to the patient by the primary care physician who would be available to communicate with the patient and follow through on the treatment recommendations. SF, asynchronous telehealth consultations range from interpretation of laboratory results or radiology images to telepsychiatry consultations based on video recordings of structured behavioral health interviews (18–20).

Blending of the two modalities have also demonstrated success and most accurately mimic the IP clinical experience where the clinician may review clinical data (SF) and engage with the patient (RT). Telehealth efforts may also be used to facilitate interdisciplinary consultations by bringing together clinicians who are available locally with clinicians who are not present locally (21). Multiple examples of interprofessional telehealth consultations have been evaluated including physician based, nurse practitioner/physician assistant (PA/NP) based, nurse based, occupational or physical therapist based; including primary care, subspecialty, and home health teleconsultations (22–24); and may be conducted in RT,

SF, or blended modalities. The tele-clinical encounter can incorporate multiple attachments such as a tele-otoscope or electronic stethoscope to facilitate a complete physical exam with the limitation of virtual palpation; with Internet-based apps through which virtual house calls can be accessed; or with any of a wide-ranging blend of other available technology combinations through an individual's insurance company or on demand as direct-to-consumer care. Telehealth encounters are documented as part of the medical record as per standard of care. All telehealth encounters including the electronic transmission must meet Health Insurance Portability and Accountability Act (HIPAA) requirements (25). Reimbursement is variable and dependent on multiple factors outside of the scope of this chapter (26,27).

Broader dissemination of telecommunications technology such as the mobile applications of Skype and FaceTime and the prevalence of social media with potential video interaction open up new possibilities for telehealth communication and participant clinical trial engagement (28).

CANCER CLINICAL TRIAL FACILITATORS

Although much has been written outlining solutions to ameliorate enrollment in clinical trials, implementation of best practices has been difficult and improvement has been slow. Solutions can generally be categorized as community based, participant based, clinical team based, and research delivery system based (see Table 46.1).

TABLE 46.1 Factors That Impact Clinical Trial Enrollment and Measurable Outcome

Community	Participant	Clinical Team	Research Delivery System
Education Literacy* Health literacy (double-blind, randomization)* Numeracy* Language access* Cultural humility*	Education*	Education: • Lack of awareness and knowledge of cancer clinical trials • Importance of physician in clinical trial enrollment • Address bias	Identifying eligible participants
	Fear of unknown, side effects, time required, how care will be coordinated		Lack of partner engagement in clinical trial planning, outreach, recruitment, informed consent process, participant follow-up
	Desire to engage family	Lack of time	
Removed from researchers	Desire to engage caregivers	Community–academic partnerships	
Lack of trust in researchers	Distance and related factors		
Measurable Outcomes			
Increase participation in cancer clinical trials Fewer trials that close due to low accrual			

*Includes the factors outlined under the section Education (Community-Based Factors).

Community-Based Factors

Education

Outreach education to the community is essential to cancer clinical trial recruitment especially for prevention trials. Reaching the "at-risk well" cannot be accomplished effectively by waiting for potential participants to come to the cancer center but by going to where the potential participants are—to community centers, health fairs, and farmers' markets. Baseline education regarding cancer clinical trials—what they are, what they entail, and the potential benefits to the participant and the community—serves to "activate" the potential participant for both cancer prevention and therapeutic trials and to engage the family and community that supports him or her (29). This educational approach is not linked to a specific trial, is not taking place when a person is ill, and provides the potential participant baseline knowledge of cancer clinical trials that will better prepare him or her to consider the cancer clinical trial enrollment decision when a specific trial is offered during a time of illness.

Community-based education efforts may be enhanced by partnerships with patient advocacy groups (30) and with clinical trial participants and their families. The sharing of narratives may be very helpful to support understanding and address concerns regarding trust and safety (31). This may be especially important for the underrepresented potential participant whose historical experiences with clinical research may not have supported a trust relationship (32). Presenting the information with cultural humility (33) and with considerations of literacy, numeracy, health literacy, and language preference (34–37) is essential when engaging diverse populations that may include ethnically diverse, extremes of age, and rare disease communities (38–40).

As we move more effectively into patient- and community-centered work, these opportunities to engage the community regarding cancer clinical trials will not only improve community knowledge about cancer clinical trials but will enhance the cancer research agenda by allowing researchers to glean patient and community insights into research priorities, research design, and participant recruitment (41,42).

Telemedicine Innovations

Although most community-based educational interventions have often taken place in person and are reinforced by one-on-one engagement, the improved quality of videoconferencing technology can serve as a means to enhance community education and communication that well simulates the IP encounter (43). Distant synchronous or asynchronous community education can take place as a virtual classroom (44) with groups or individuals at the connecting sites thus expanding the reach of the clinical trial educator. The improvements and increased accessibility and use of similar technologies, that is, FaceTime or Skype, many of which are available on smartphones, have made videoconferencing

more familiar and thus more acceptable for populations including diverse populations (45,46).

Our definition of telehealth includes social media as a tool that may be effective to improve baseline community education about cancer clinical trials. With its broad reach, social media has the potential to reach a population widely, with limited effort, and via a modality that is already being regularly accessed by the community (47,48). Social media may be used for baseline education about cancer clinical trials or for education about a specific trial and/or recruitment for a specific trial. This medium may be especially effective in addressing the topics most difficult to grapple with regarding cancer clinical trials; these include the rationale for phase I trials, randomization, or why neither the participant nor the physician picks the treatment, and the meaning of double-blind studies (47,49–51).

Participant-Based Factors

Education

As noted earlier, the first step in facilitating participant enrollment in cancer clinical trials is community-based education. Community-based clinical trial education lays the groundwork for patient-centered cancer clinical trial decision-making and informed consent (52). Acknowledging the patient's decision-making preference creates an effective, respectful patient–clinician partnership that brings in caregivers, families, and clinical team members (53–55) as desired by the patient and allows the patient to express and reflect on the cancer clinical trial process (see Table 46.2). This approach recognizes the role of fear, enhances the participant's comfort level with his or her clinical trial decision, and promotes a spirit of reassurance and safety (56–58). Some common concerns expressed by potential participants include: clinical trial time commitment, access to clinical support at home to manage symptoms, and assistance in care, for example, addressing questions regarding intravenous line management (58,59).

Telemedicine Innovations

Education of the potential clinical trial participant can take place virtually with clinical/research team members that may include the physician, the clinical nurse, the research nurse, the study manager, and others. Considerations of literacy, health literacy, and numeracy are important for all clinical interactions. Telehealth solutions that address language access may utilize videoconferencing to increase access to language interpreters (60,61). As in the IP setting, the medical interpreter should receive instruction to paraphrase or translate directly, the clinician should allow time for the interpretation, and the line of vision between the patient and the clinician should be preserved. If an American Sign Language interpreter is needed, the interpreter should be in the view of the patient (62). Similarly, family members and clinical team members may be "beamed in" via

TABLE 46.2 Common Cancer Clinical Trial Questions

What does it mean to experiment on people?

How can I be sure research is ethical?

Who will have access to my information?

How will you ensure my privacy?

Will my family know that I'm on this trial?

What is double blind?

Is every study blinded?

Why can't I pick my treatment?

Why do I have to be randomized?

What will the benefit of the trial be to me?

What will you do with my tissue?

If I have the mutation, have I passed it on to my children?

How will I know the results of the trial?

Why does it take so long to know if the treatment will work?

What happens if you don't get enough participants?

What if I don't live long enough—will my family get the results?

What is the role of the placebo?

Why is only part of my care paid if I participate in the trial?

Why is part of my care paid if I'm on the trial and none if I'm not on the trial?

Why is only part of my care paid if I'm on the trial and all of my care covered if I go on hospice?

telecommunications technology as desired by the patient or needed for care or for the study, respectively (63). Smartphone or other mobile technology apps may be utilized to facilitate the recruitment–enrollment–retention process by assisting with symptom management, care coordination, line care, and scheduling (64–69).

Geography

Given that cancer clinical outcomes improve the closer the patient is to a cancer center (70,71), geography and access to transportation can be significant barriers both to care and to enrollment in cancer clinical trials. Distance is compounded by travel costs that may include the costs for the individual, for the caregiver and family, lost wages, childcare, and elder care. Participants may hesitate to access care for side effect management, care of indwelling lines, and for medical complications due to the requisite travel time and associated cost factors (72,73).

Telemedicine Innovations

Telemedicine was developed with the goal of bridging distance virtually (11,13,14). Although initially developed to address the distance faced by astronauts in space, telehealth applications have demonstrated efficacy in isolated populations, for example, incarcerated, rural, and frontier (74–76). More recently, acknowledgment of the maldistribution of healthcare resources and of the availability of a global market for healthcare delivery, has stimulated efforts to use telemedicine to improve access to care even in urban settings. In improving access to cancer clinical trials, telehealth applications can be effectively utilized to present the clinical protocol, assess eligibility, review the consent form, and arrange for follow-up discussions. Although the technology is generally thought of as bringing the patient to care virtually, it may also be helpful to bring others into the conversation as desired by the patient or as needed clinically. The patient's family member who is at a different location may be brought into the conversation as desired by the patient. The radiation oncologist who would be responsible for a portion of the trial may virtually engage the patient. Part of the interventional radiology preassessment for the indwelling line placement may be accomplished virtually—all to facilitate care and ease access to the trial. Geography as a barrier may dissolve as an illusion for most aspects of care and research access.

Clinical–Team-Based Factors

Lack of patient awareness of clinical trials is often cited as a significant factor for lack of participation in cancer clinical trials. Lack of *clinician awareness* is also a significant factor. Approximately two thirds of successful participants note the role of their physician (6), and often of their primary care physician as significant in their decision to enroll in the clinical trial (77). Although the academic center may be aware of trial availability, the local oncologist and/or the primary care physician and their respective clinical teams may be less aware not only of the availability of cancer clinical trials but also of the requirements, the clinical questions that are being addressed, and the interpretation of the outcomes (78,79). This has become increasingly complex as cancer studies include precision medicine trials and specialized biomarkers. With the rapidly changing landscape of actionable biomarkers, maintaining molecular biology literacy has become a full-time job for research oncologists. This specialization in cancer clinical trials makes it difficult for researchers to speak across different approaches and types of trials. The ability of academic research oncologists, clinical trialists, to bridge with the local clinicians, whether oncologists or primary care physicians, is essential to strengthen the referral networks necessary for cancer clinical trial engagement and proactively address the local clinician's concern of losing the care of the patient.

The clinicians in the referral network seek a better understanding of cancer clinical trials, of the specific trial in question (80), and of approaches to facilitate enrollment, for example, literacy, numeracy, health literacy, and language access. They also note lack of time and resources to recruit participants to trials (81). These efforts are intended to improve the clinician's cancer clinical trial presentation skills, broaden cancer clinical trial information dissemination, and thereby improve cancer clinical trial recruitment.

Telemedicine Innovations

Raising clinical trial awareness in the academic cancer center and in the referral community is a critical first step for participant entry into cancer clinical trials and may be facilitated through telecommunications technology. Whether synchronous or asynchronous, multiple examples of efficacy exist in the literature (82–86). Engaging interprofessional teams can broaden the referral network. Providing continuing education credit as part of the clinical trial effort that includes interprofessional team members not only serves as additional incentive but also adds value to the engagement.

Efforts to engage via social media have demonstrated varying effectiveness due to variable health professional engagement in the variety of tools available (87,88). Physician targeted platforms like Sermo and Doximity engage physicians in medical crowdsourcing and professional networking. Google+ Communities has multiple physician-related communities that may be specialty focused, international in focus, or have a targeted focus, that is, medical software information. Multiple professional social networks that include physicians but that are not limited to physicians exist such as LinkedIn. Which platform to engage depends on the goal of the outreach effort. An incentive for engagement and ease of use are necessary elements to ensure participation and maximize reach. To be successful, professional virtual engagement that is intended to support a clinical trial referral network needs to be accompanied by personal engagement (89,90).

Research Delivery System Based Factors

The prior discussion has focused on efforts to link the eligible potential clinical trial participant to the right cancer clinical trial. In addition to efforts facilitated by community-based, participant-based, and clinical–team-based factors, an analysis of the research delivery system may identify other opportunities. A solid research infrastructure is necessary to facilitate research processes including data management. When the effort is to include engagement of the community clinician, easing the burden of community cancer clinical recruitment and enrollment is important.

Telemedicine Innovations

These include efforts to identify potential participants via the electronic health record (EHR) (91), cancer registries (92), and other databases (93). If patients give permission and the EHR or other registry or database is set to search discrete fields related to cancer clinical trial enrollment, the EHR may alert the clinician or the clinical team of the patient's potential cancer clinical eligibility (94,95). Telehealth tools can streamline the recruitment process from engaging the referral network, disseminating clinical trial information, recruiting of participants, maintaining participant engagement to sharing results with the participants and the referral network (96). Examples include use of Twitter Chat to answer clinical trial inclusion questions, to engage participants, and to share results (97,98). Although this approach may not be a fit for all studies, this engagement of clinical trial participants and referral networks can be both successful and cost-effective.

Although referral practices may feel that due to time constraints the best that they can do is identify and refer potential participants as they come to clinic appointments, this approach misses participants because the study is not discussed at the time the patient is seen. With consent and adherence to privacy concerns, a tele-facilitated model may actively search the EHR or data registries for eligible participants prior to the clinical appointment. After the establishment of necessary institutional policies and agreements, trial eligibility may be confirmed at a distance or on site by a research team member at the academic center. This process provides the recruiting clinician with an actionable list of eligible patients based on preset criteria. Once referred to the study, the potential participant may meet with the research nurse through telehealth technology to begin the formal eligibility evaluation process. If eligible, the consent process may begin. Review of the consent form may take place virtually with the patient and his or her family members as desired by the patient. The technology allows for the patient's family to join whether they are in the same community as the patient or in another location. As discussed earlier, this approach is especially effective for patients who make decisions in consultation with others.

CONCLUSIONS

Cancer clinical trials from prevention to palliation are essential for progress in oncology (99). Limited enrollment in cancer clinical trials especially in the age of precision medicine may severely limit clinical progress. Telecommunications technology for healthcare has come a long way since initially conceptualized (see Figure 46.1) (100–102). Today, telehealth technology is better, faster, cheaper, and accessible as an app on a smartphone. Telehealth can be used to support academic and community partnerships that result in interprofessional cancer clinical trial networks. This collaborative

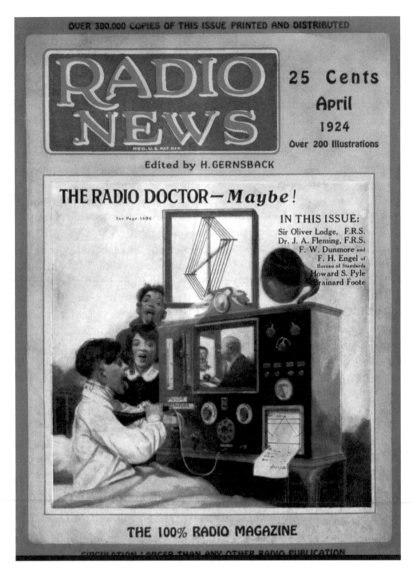

FIGURE 46.1 A prescient and early depiction of telecommunications technology use in healthcare.
Source: Radio News Cover Page. Reproduced with permission from Ziff Davis, LLC.

technology-enabled infrastructure can provide the elements needed to make for informed, patient-centered, value-congruent decisions. Professional and lay social networks can serve to reach patients with rare diseases for cancer clinical trials. Utilizing technology to educate patients and professionals about cancer clinical trials; facilitate trial planning; advertise, recruit, and walk participants through informed consent processes; and stay in touch with participants may not only improve cancer clinical trial recruitment and retention, it may also hasten progress.

REFERENCES

1. Ellis LM, Bernstein DS, Voest EE, et al. American Society of Clinical Oncology Perspective: raising the bar for clinical trials by defining clinically meaningful outcomes. *J Clin Oncol.* 2014;32(12):1277–1280.

2. Murthy VH, Krumholz HM, Gross CP. Participation in cancer clinical trials: race-, sex-, and age-based disparities. *JAMA* 2004; 291.291(22):2720–2726.

3. Lewis JH, Kilgore ML, Goldman DP, et al. Participation of patients 65 years of age or older in cancer clinical trials. *J Clin Oncol.* 2003;21(7):1383–1389.

4. Ford JG, Howerton MW, Lai GY, et al. Barriers to recruiting underrepresented populations to cancer clinical trials: a systematic review. *Cancer.* 2008;112(2):228–242.

5. Virani S, Burke L, Remick SC, et al. Barriers to recruitment of rural patients in cancer clinical trials. *J Oncol Pract.* 2011;7(3): 172–177.

6. Comis RL, Miller JD, Aldigé CR, et al. Public attitudes toward participation in cancer clinical trials. *J Clin Oncol.* 2003;21(5):830–835.

7. Siu, Lillian L, Tannock IF. Problems in interpreting clinical trials. In *Handbook of Statistics in Clinical Oncology. New York, NY, Marcel Dekker Inc;* 2001: 473–490.

8. Shavers VL, Brown ML. Racial and ethnic disparities in the receipt of cancer treatment. *J Natl Cancer Inst.* 2002; 94(5):334–357.

9. Deshazer C. Racial differences in the treatment of early-stage lung cancer. *N Engl J Med.* 2000;342(7):518–519.

10. Bach PB, et al. Survival of Blacks and Whites After a Cancer Diagnosis. *JAMA*. 2002;287(16):2106–2113.

11. Institute of Medicine and Committee on Evaluating Clinical Applications of Telemedicine. *Telemedicine: A Guide to Assessing Telecommunications in Health Care*. Institute of Medicine; 1996.

12. Darkins, AW, Cary MA. *Telemedicine and Telehealth: Principles, Policies, Performances and Pitfalls*. New York, NY: Springer publishing; 2000.

13. Simmons SC, Hamilton DR, McDonald PV. Telemedicine. In *Principles of Clinical Medicine for Space Flight*. New York, NY: Springer Publishing; 2008: 163–179.

14. Morrison DR, Hofmann GA. Cell separation and electrofusion in space. Space commercialization: Platforms and processing, *progress in Astronautics and Aeronautics, American Institute of Aeronautics and Astronautics, Washington, DC*. 1990:214–234.

15. Becker C, Frishman WH, Scurlock C. Telemedicine and Tele-ICU: the evolution and differentiation of a new medical field. *Am J Med*. 2016;129(12):e333–e334.

16. GoodenAM. Telemedicine a guide to online resources. *College & Research Libraries News*. 2016;77(3):135–139.

17. LocatisC, Ackerman M. Three principles for determining the relevancy of store-and-forward and live interactive telemedicine: Reinterpreting two telemedicine research reviews and other research. *Telemedicine e-Health*. 2013; 19(1):19–23.

18. Butler TN, Yellowlees P. Cost analysis of store-and-forward telepsychiatry as a consultation model for primary care. *Telemed J E Health*. 2012;18(1):74–77.

19. Maghazil A, Yellowlees P. Novel approaches to clinical care in mental health: from asynchronous telepsychiatry to virtual reality. In *Mental Health Informatics*. Springer Berlin Heidelberg; 2014: 57–78.

20. Yellowlees PM, Odor A, Iosif AM, et al. Transcultural psychiatry made simple—asynchronous telepsychiatry as an approach to providing culturally relevant care. *Telemed J E Health*. 2013;19(4):259–264.

21. Kucik, Corry J, Carmichael JJ. Telemedicine and Future Innovations. Trauma Team Dynamics. Springer International Publishing; 2016: 187–192.

22. Knight P, Bonney A, Teuss G, et al. Positive clinical outcomes are synergistic with positive educational outcomes when using telehealth consulting in general practice: a mixed-methods study. *J Med Internet Res*. 2016;18(2):e31.

23. Amadi-Obi A, Gilligan P, Owens N, et al. Telemedicine in pre-hospital care: a review of telemedicine applications in the pre-hospital environment. *Int J Emerg Med*. 2014;7:11.

24. Gilman M, Stensland J. Telehealth and medicare: payment policy, current use, and prospects for growth. *Medicare Medicaid Res Rev*. 2013;3(4):E1–E17.

25. Cole B, Stredler-Brown A, Cohill B, et al. The development of statewide policies and procedures to implement telehealth for part C service delivery. *Inter J Telerehabil*. 2016;8(2):77–82.

26. Lerouge C, Garfield MJ. Crossing the telemedicine chasm: have the U.S. barriers to widespread adoption of telemedicine been significantly reduced? *Int J Environ Res Public Health*. 2013;10(12):6472–6484.

27. Weinstein RS, Lopez AM, Joseph BA, et al. Telemedicine, telehealth, and mobile health applications that work: opportunities and barriers. *Am J Med*. 2014;127(3):183–187.

28. Drake TM, Ritchie JE. The Surgeon will skype tou now: advancements in E-clinic. *Ann Surgery*. 2016;263(4):636–637.

29. Wouda JC, Hbmvande W. Education in patient–physician communication: how to improve effectiveness? *Patient Educ Couns*. 2013;90(1):46–53.

30. Mahon E, Roberts J, Furlong P. Barriers to clinical trial recruitment and possible solutions: a stakeholder survey. *App Clin Trials*; 2015.

31. Ash JS, Cottrell E, Saxton L, et al. Patient narratives representing patient voices to inform research: a pilot qualitative study. *Stud Health Technol Inform*. 2015;208:55.

32. Banda DR, Libin AV, Wang H, et al. A pilot study of a culturally targeted video intervention to increase participation of African American patients in cancer clinical trials. *Oncologist*. 2012;17(5):708–714.

33. Erves JC, Mayo-Gamble TL, Malin-Fair A, et al. Needs, priorities, and recommendations for engaging underrepresented populations in clinical research: a community perspective. *J Community Health*. 2017;42(3):472–480.

34. Friedman DB, Kim SH, Tanner A, et al. How are we communicating about clinical trials? an assessment of the content and readability of recruitment resources. *Contemp Clin Trials*. 2014;38(2):275–283.

35. Utami D, Bickmore TW, Barry B, et al. Health literacy and usability of clinical trial search engines. *J Health Commun*. 2014;19(Suppl 2):190–204.

36. Kalichman SC, Cherry C, Kalichman MO, et al. Randomized clinical trial of HIV treatment adherence counseling interventions for people living with HIV and limited health literacy. *J Acquir Immune Defic Syndr*. 2013; 63(1):42–50.

37. Harris PA, Scott KW, Lebo L, et al. Research match: a national registry to recruit volunteers for clinical research. *Acad Med*. 2012;87(1):66–73.

38. Woolfall K, Shilling V, Hickey H, et al. Parents' agendas in paediatric clinical trial recruitment are different from researchers' and often remain unvoiced: a qualitative study. *PLoS One*. 2013;8(7):e67352.

39. Hurria A, Dale W, Mooney M, et al. Cancer and aging research group. Designing therapeutic clinical trials for older and frail adults with cancer: U13 conference recommendations. *J Clin Oncol*. 2014;32(24):2587–2594.

40. Anwuri VV, Hall LE, Mathews K, et al. An institutional strategy to increase minority recruitment to therapeutic trials. *Cancer Causes Control*. 2013;24(10):1797–1809.

41. Friedman DB, Tanner A, Kim S-H, et al. Improving our messages about research participation: a community-engaged approach to increasing clinical trial literacy. *Clin Investig* 2014;4(10):869–872.

42. Saliha A, D'Abundo ML. Improving the recruitment of minority populations in clinical trials: advocating for a strategic shift toward community-based recruitment. In *Encyclopedia of Strategic Leadership and Management*. IGI Global; 2017: 1354–1367.

43. Shi Y, Xie W, XU G, et al. The smart classroom: merging technologies for seamless tele-education. *IEEE Pervas Comput*. 2003;2:47–55.

44. Chipps J, Brysiewicz P, Mars M. A systematic review of the effectiveness of videoconference-based tele-education for medical and nursing education. *Worldviews Evid Based Nurs*. 2012;9(2):78–87.

45. Brooks NP. Telemedicine is here. *In World Neurosurgery*. Elsevier; 2016.

46. Angelica C. Wherever, whenever: health in the palm of your hand. *Looking Ahead The Cornell Roosevelt Institute Policy Journal*. 2014.

47. Chou W-Yings, Hunt YM, Beckjord EB, et al. Social media use in the united states: implications for health communication. *J Med Internet Res*. 2009;11(4):e48.

48. Ramo DE, Rodriguez TM, Chavez K, et al. Facebook recruitment of young adult smokers for a cessation trial: methods, metrics, and lessons learned. *Internet Interventions*. 2014;1(2):58–64.

49. Advani AS, Atkeson B, Brown CL, et al. Barriers to the participation of African-American patients with cancer in clinical trials: a pilot study. *Cancer*. 2003;97(6):1499–1506.

50. Bieniasz ME, Underwood D, Bailey J, et al. Women's feedback on a chemopreventive trial for cervical dysplasia. *Appl Nurs Res*. 2003;16(1):22–28.

51. Melisko ME, Hassin F, Metzroth L, et al. Patient and physician attitudes toward breast cancer clinical trials: developing interventions based on understanding barriers. *Clin Breast Cancer*. 2005;6(1):45–54.

52. Bensing J. Bridging the gap. The separate worlds of evidence-based medicine and patient-centered medicine. *Patient Educ Couns*. 2000;39(1):17–25.

53. Sepucha KR, Fowler FJ, Mulley AG. Policy support for patient-centered care: the need for measurable improvements in decision quality. *Health Aff*. 2004;Suppl Variation:VAR54–VAR62.

54. Arora NK, Mchorney CA. Patient preferences for medical decision making: who really wants to participate? *Medical Care*. 2000;38(3):335–341.

55. Barry MJ, Edgman-Levitan S. Shared decision making—the pinnacle of patient-centered care. *New Engl J Med*. 2012;366(9):780–781.

56. Townsley CA, Chan KK, Pond GR, et al. Understanding the attitudes of the elderly towards enrolment into cancer clinical trials. *BMC Cancer*. 2006;6(6):11.

57. Durant RW, Wenzel JA, Scarinci IC, et al. Perspectives on barriers and facilitators to minority recruitment for clinical trials among cancer center leaders, investigators, research staff, and referring clinicians: enhancing minority participation in clinical trials (EMPaCT). *Cancer*. 2014;120(Suppl 7):1097–1105.

58. Unger JM, Hershman DL, Albain KS, et al. Patient income level and cancer clinical trial participation. *J Clin Oncol*. 2013;31(5):536–542.

59. Piantadosi S. Clinical Trials: A Methodologic Perspective. John Wiley & Sons; 2013.

60. Jones D, Gill P, Harrison R, et al. An exploratory study of language interpretation services provided by videoconferencing. *J Telemed Telecare*. 2003;9(1):51–56.

61. Masland MC, Lou C, Snowden L. Use of communication technologies to cost-effectively increase the availability of interpretation services in healthcare settings. *Telemed J E Health*. 2010;16(6):739–745.

62. Lopez AM, Cruz M, Lazarus S, et al. Case report: use of American sign language in telepsychiatry consultation. *Telemed J E Health*. 2004;10(3):389–391.

63. Lindberg B, Nilsson C, Zotterman D, et al. Using information and communication technology in home care for communication between patients, family members, and healthcare professionals: a systematic review. *Int J Telemed Appl*. 2013;2013:1–31.

64. Luxton DD, Mishkind MC, Crumpton RM, et al. Usability and feasibility of smartphone video capabilities for telehealth care in the US military. *Telemed J E Health*. 2012;18(6):409–412.

65. Wang J, Wang Y, Wei C, et al. Smartphone interventions for long-term health management of chronic diseases: an integrative review. *Telemed J E Health*. 2014;20(6):570–583.

66. Girault A, Ferrua M, Lalloué B, et al. Internet-based technologies to improve cancer care coordination: current use and attitudes among cancer patients. *Eur J Cancer*. 2015;51(4):551–557.

67. Nasi G, Cucciniello M, Guerrazzi C. The role of mobile technologies in health care processes: the case of cancer supportive care. *J Med Internet Res*. 2015;17(2):e26.

68. Lopez AM. Telemedicine, telehealth, and e-health technologies in cancer prevention. In *Fundamentals of Cancer Prevention*. Springer Berlin Heidelberg; 2014: 259–277.

69. Ozdalga E, Ozdalga A, Ahuja N. The smartphone in medicine: a review of current and potential use among physicians and students. *J Med Internet Res*. 2012;14(5):e128.

70. Ambroggi M, Biasini C, del Giovane C, et al. Distance as a barrier to cancer diagnosis and treatment: review of the literature. *Oncologist*. 2015;20(12):1378–1385.

71. Lamont EB, Hayreh D, Pickett KE, et al. Is patient travel distance associated with survival on phase II clinical trials in oncology? *J Natl Cancer Inst*. 2003;95(18):1370–1375.

72. Barrington DA, Dilley SE, Landers EE, et al. Distance from a comprehensive cancer center: a proxy for poor cervical cancer outcomes? *Gynecol Oncol*. 2016;143(3):617–621.

73. Wolfson JA, Sun CL, Wyatt LP, et al. Impact of care at comprehensive cancer centers on outcome: Results from a population-based study. *Cancer*. 2015;121(21):3885–3893.

74. Starren JB, Nesbitt TS, Chiang MF. Telehealth. In Biomedical Informatics. London, UK: Springer Publishing. 2014;541–560.

75. Blotter JT, Fawson C. How has the Affordable Care Act impacted the implementation of telehealth programs in isolated rural areas? *UCUR 2016*. 2015.

76. Solomon A. Telehealth, Public Health, and Health Policy: Bridging the Geographic Divide for Rural Populations. 2015 APHA Annual Meeting & Expo. APHA, 2015.

77. Ford JG, Howerton MW, Lai GY, et al. Barriers to recruiting underrepresented populations to cancer clinical trials: a systematic review. *Cancer*. 2008;112(2):228–242.

78. Mccaskill-Stevens W, Pinto H, Marcus AC, et al. Recruiting minority cancer patients into cancer clinical trials: a pilot project involving the Eastern Cooperative Oncology Group and the National Medical Association. *J Clin Oncol*. 1999;17(3):1029–1029.

79. Brown JB. Abstract LB-142: Physician-engagement in cancer clinical trial recruitment: Leveraging partnerships among community-academic research institutions for direct accrual of racial/ethnic minorities and the medically underserved. *Cancer Res*. 2016;76(Supp 14):LB–142.

80. Siminoff LA, Zhang A, Colabianchi N, et al. Factors that predict the referral of breast cancer patients onto clinical trials by their surgeons and medical oncologists. *J Clin Oncol*. 2000;18(6):1203–1211.

81. Callahan EH, Thomas DC, Goldhirsch SL, et al. Geriatric hospital medicine. *Med Clin North Am*. 2002;86(4):707–729.

82. Arends R. Incorporating Telehealth in advanced practice registered nurse curriculum to impact rural and frontier population health. *Sigma Theta Tau International's 27th International Nursing Research Congress*. STTI 2016.

83. Marshall CL, Petersen NJ, Naik AD, et al. Implementation of a regional virtual tumor board: a prospective study evaluating feasibility and provider acceptance. *Telemed J E Health*. 2014;20(8):705–711.

84. Chelf JH, Agre P, Axelrod A, et al. Cancer-related patient education: an overview of the last decade of evaluation and research. *Oncol Nurs Forum*. 2001;28(7):1139–1147.

85. Augestad KM, Lindsetmo RO. Overcoming distance: video-conferencing as a clinical and educational tool among surgeons. *World J Surg*. 2009;33(7):1356–1365.

86. Dionne-Odom JN, Azuero A, Lyons KD, et al. Benefits of early versus delayed palliative care to informal family caregivers of patients with advanced cancer: outcomes from the ENABLE III randomized controlled trial. *J Clin Oncol*. 2015;33(13):1446–1452.

87. Burke MA, Fournier G, Prasad K. *Physician social networks and geographical variation in medical care*. Center on Social and Economic Dynamics; 2003.

88. Christakis NA, Fowler JH. *Connected: The Surprising Power of Our Social Networks and How They Shape Our Lives*. New York, NY: Little, Brown; 2009.

89. Denicoff AM, Mccaskill-Stevens W, Grubbs SS, et al. The National Cancer Institute-American Society of Clinical Oncology Cancer Trial Accrual Symposium: summary and recommendations. *J Oncol Pract*. 2013;9(6):267–276.

90. McAlearney AS, Reiter KL, Weiner BL, et al. Challenges and facilitators of community clinical oncology program participation: a qualitative study. *J Healthcare Manag*. 2013; 58(1):29.

91. Khan Y, Roth C, Payne P, et al. EHR-based clinical trial alert effects on recruitment to a neurology trial across Institutions: interim analysis of a randomized controlled study. *AMIA Jt Summits Transl Sci Proc*. 2013;2013:117.

92. Katapodi MC, Northouse LL, Schafenacker AM, et al. Using a state cancer registry to recruit young breast cancer survivors and high-risk relatives: protocol of a randomized trial testing the efficacy of a targeted versus a tailored intervention to increase breast cancer screening. *BMC Cancer*. 2013;13:11.

93. Simon R, Roychowdhury S. Implementing personalized cancer genomics in clinical trials. *Nat Rev Drug Discov.* 2013;12(5):358–369.
94. Grundmeier RW, Swietlik M, Bell LM. Research subject enrollment by primary care pediatricians using an electronic health record. *AMIA Annual Symposium proceedings.* Vol. 2007. American Medical Informatics Association; 2007.
95. Ferranti JM, Gilbert W, Mccall J, et al. The design and implementation of an open-source, data-driven cohort recruitment system: the Duke Integrated Subject Cohort and Enrollment Research Network (DISCERN). *J Am Med Inform Assoc.* 2012;19(e1):e68–e75.
96. Sabesan S, Zalcberg J. Telehealth models could be extended to conducting clinical trials-a teletrial approach. *Eur J Cancer Care.* 2016.
97. Attai DJ, Cowher MS, Al-Hamadani M, et al. Twitter social media is an effective tool for breast cancer patient education and support: patient-reported outcomes by survey. *J Med Internet Res.* 2015;17(7):e188.
98. Thompson MA. Social media in clinical trials. Am Society Clin Oncol. 2014; e101–e105.
99. Napoles A, Cook E, Ginossar T, et al. Applying a conceptual framework to maximize the participation of diverse populations in cancer clinical trials. *Adv Cancer Res.* 2017;133.
100. The Radio Doctor of the Future (Radio News 1924-04). http://www.magazineart.org/main.php?g2_view=core. DownloadItem&g2_itemId=25608&g2_serialNumber=2
101. Kinney AY, Boonyasiriwat W, Walters ST, et al. Telehealth personalized cancer risk communication to motivate colonoscopy in relatives of patients with colorectal cancer: the family CARE Randomized controlled trial. *J Clin Oncol.* 2014;32(7):654–662.
102. Breen S, Ritchie D, Schofield P, et al. The Patient Remote Intervention and Symptom Management System (PRISMS)–a Telehealth- mediated intervention enabling real-time monitoring of chemotherapy side-effects in patients with haematological malignancies: study protocol for a randomised controlled trial. *Trials.* 2015;16:472.

Cooperative Groups, Regulatory and Governing Bodies

Cooperative Groups and Global Clinical Trials in the Future

COOPERATIVE GROUPS: AN AMERICAN AND CANADIAN PERSPECTIVE

Joseph A. Sparano, Judith Manola, and Robert L. Comis†

The term "cooperative groups" is often used to denote federally funded research organizations that coordinate clinical trials carried out in multiple academic medical centers and community-based centers, typically accruing individuals with early- and advanced-stage cancer. For the most part, the groups focus on performing large, multicenter trials designed to test therapeutic strategies and potentially influence the standard of care, with the ultimate goal of reducing morbidity and mortality associated with cancer. This chapter focuses on past progress by the groups, and current adult cancer trials that will influence the standard of care in the future.

AN ABBREVIATED HISTORY OF THE COOPERATIVE GROUP SYSTEM

As described in greater detail in Chapter 2, the notion of using of systemic therapies to treat cancer dates back to the early 1900s (1). Cancer clinical trials date their history back to 1948, at which time Sidney Farber reported temporary remissions in five children with acute leukemia treated with intramuscular injections of aminopterin (2). Based in part on these results, the success observed in antibiotic and antimalarial therapy, including the first randomized clinical trial (of streptomycin for pulmonary tuberculosis [(3)]), the United States Senate Appropriations Committee instructed the National Cancer Institute (NCI) to establish a "cooperative system." Three groups were subsequently formed under the sponsorship of the NCI Cancer Chemotherapy National Service Center (4), including the Acute Leukemia Group A (led by Joseph Burchenal), Acute Leukemia Group B (led by Emil Frei, III), and the Eastern Solid Tumor

Group (led by Gordon Zubrod). The first publication of a randomized clinical trial in leukemia conducted by the cooperative groups was in 1958 by Emil Frei III on behalf of eight other coauthors and the "Acute Leukemia Group B" (5). The trial included 65 adult patients with acute leukemia randomized to receive 6-mercaptopurine plus methotrexate given either continuously or intermittently. Although the methods section of the publication stated: "The study followed the principles of a control clinical trial as advanced by Hill (6), and Marshall and Merrill (7)," the main focus was on the trial results indicating improved survival for those who achieved remission with the continuous schedule. The first publication of a clinical trial in pediatric cancer was in 1960 by Ruth Heyn by "Acute Leukemia Group A" in 168 children with acute leukemia randomized to 6-mercaptopurine alone or in combination with azaserine, which also mainly focused on the trial results indicating no benefit from addition of the second agent (8). The first publication of a clinical trial in solid tumors was in 1960 by Gordon Zubrod on behalf of 18 other coauthors and the "Eastern Cooperative Cancer Chemotherapy Group" (9). Although the publication included a description on the trial results, the report primarily focused on the methodology of performing the trial, including the use of a common clinical "protocol" by all collaborating investigators, randomized treatment assignment (nitrogen mustard vs. triethylene thiophosphoramide), target population (breast cancer, lung cancer, melanoma, and Hodgkin's disease), inclusion criteria (inoperable disease), standardized drug dosing and schedules, objective definitions and measurement of tumor response and trial endpoints (including survival), blinded outcome review, consistency of treatment parameters, prespecified statistical analysis plan, and specifics about "records to be kept" (e.g., screening logs, tumor measurement forms,

†deceased

and case report forms). By focusing mainly on the methodology of rigorously conducting a prospective clinical trial, the "Eastern Cooperative Cancer Chemotherapy Group," later known as the "Eastern Cooperative Oncology Group (ECOG)," provided a framework and foundation for cooperative group trials that exists to this day. This group was also the first to develop an internal auditing system, database management system, and electronic mail for communication, and also the first to develop standard response, performance status, and toxicity criteria (10), and to confirm the feasibility of engaging community practice sites in cancer clinical trials (11). In addition, statisticians involved in cooperative research have developed novel statistical methodologies for cancer clinical trials, including exponential methods for survival analysis (12), landmark analysis (13), and other novel analytical methods (14–16).

IMPACT OF COOPERATIVE GROUP TRIALS ON CANCER CARE

Clinical trials designed and coordinated by the cooperative groups have contributed to some of the most significant advances in cancer care in adults, some of which are summarized in Table 47.1. Multicenter trials coordinated by groups focused on pediatric cancer have also dramatically reduced cancer death rates from acute lymphocytic leukemia, Wilms tumor, medulloblastoma, neuroblastoma, and other pediatric cancers, as reviewed elsewhere (47). The advances in pediatric and adult cancer care made possible by the groups have contributed not only to declining cancer mortality rates in the United States and globally (48), but also to less cancer associated morbidity and an unprecedented number of cancer survivors (49).

REORGANIZATION OF THE NCI CLINICAL TRIAL SYSTEM

About 50 years after the initial reports from the cooperative groups, an Institute of Medicine (IOM) panel focused on the NCI-sponsored clinical trial system was convened at the request of the NCI director because the groups were at a ". . .critical juncture. . ." and faced ". . .numerous challenges. . ." (50). A report issued by the panel in 2010 acknowledged that: "The results of

TABLE 47.1 Selected Examples of Advances in Cancer Therapy Due to Cooperative Group Clinical Trials

Breast cancer
- Breast conserving surgery associated with comparable recurrence rates and survival compared with mastectomy (17–19)
- Sentinel lymph node biopsy produces comparable local–regional and systemic control as axillary dissection with less morbidity (20)
- Adjuvant polychemotherapy regimens reduce risk of recurrence and improve survival (21,22)
- Adjuvant endocrine therapy for up to 10 years reduces recurrence and improves survival in pre- and postmenopausal women with ER-positive breast cancer (23–27)
- Adjuvant trastuzumab reduces recurrence and improves survival when added to adjuvant chemotherapy in HER2-overexpressing breast cancer (28)
- Multiparameter gene expression assays identify subsets of patients with ER-positive disease who derive the greatest benefit from adjuvant chemotherapy (29–31)
- Chemoprevention with tamoxifen and raloxifene reduces breast cancer incidence in high-risk women (32,33)

Genitourinary cancer
- Adjuvant chemotherapy reduces recurrence and improves survival in testis cancer (20,34)
- Adjuvant antiandrogen therapy improves survival after surgery in high-risk prostate cancer (35)
- Chemotherapy improves survival when added to antiandrogen therapy as initial therapy for metastatic prostate cancer (36)

Colorectal cancer
- Adjuvant 5-fluorouracil containing therapy reduces recurrence and improves survival in colon cancer (37,38)
- Bevacizumab improves survival in metastatic colorectal cancer (39)

Thoracic cancer
- Screening with high-resolution CT reduces lung cancer mortality (40)
- Twice daily radiation improves survival in localized small-cell lung cancer (41)
- Bevacizumab improves survival in metastatic nonsquamous, non–small-cell lung cancer (42)

Hematologic cancers
- Pentostatin is effective for treatment of hairy cell leukemia (43)
- ATRA improves survival in acute promyelocytic leukemia (44)
- High-dose cytarabine more effective than autologous stem
- Addition of rituximab to CHOP chemotherapy improves survival in B-cell non-Hodgkin's lymphoma (45)
- Low-dose dexamethasone containing regimens associated with improved survival and less toxicity compared with high-dose regimens (46)

ATRA, all-trans retinoic acid.

Cooperative Group trials have steadily improved the care of patients with cancer in the United States and worldwide for more than 50 years," and provided recommendations for modernization of the system, including improving the speed and efficiency of the design and completion of clinical trials, incorporating innovative science and trial design, improving means to prioritize and complete trials, and incentivizing patients and physicians. Based on these recommendations, the NCI-sponsored clinical trial system was reorganized into National Clinical Trials Network (NCTN), including the research bases coordinating the trials, and the sites participating in the trials, including NCI-designed cancer centers, other medical centers, and community practices and academic medical centers, lead academic medical centers, and community-based practice sites and cancer centers. The reorganized group structures and network was launched on March 1, 2014, which included one pediatric and four adult cooperative groups with their associated operations and statistical and data management centers coordinating the research (Figure 47.1), and tissue banks collecting biospecimens, plus 30 sites funded as "lead academic participating sites" (LAPS) and 46 sites participating in the National Community Oncology Research Program (NCORP), including 12 sites specifically serving minority populations and 919 component/subcomponent sites (https://ncorp.cancer.gov/findasite/map.html) (51).

THE NATIONAL CLINICAL TRIALS NETWORK TRIALS PORTFOLIO

The NCTN research portfolio in adult cancers may be broadly classified as focused on integral biomarkers, precision medicine, immunotherapy, developmental therapeutics, local therapy, rare cancers, advanced imaging, and (via the NCORP program) cancer prevention/control, as described in the following and summarized in Table 47.2. This summary includes studies that are in progress or soon to be initiated as of December 2016, and selected pivotal studies performed by the NCI cooperative group legacy system that have completed accrual with results awaited.

Integral Biomarkers

Several studies have evaluated the role of integral biomarkers as a means to identify subpopulations most likely to benefit from standard chemotherapy or specific chemotherapy agents, and/or to refine the clinical utility of existing assays. For example, two trials in operable, estrogen receptor (ER) positive, HER2 negative breast cancer evaluated the role of the prognostic multiparameter gene expression assay (Onco*type* DX Recurrence Score [RS]) in patients with node-negative disease and an RS of 11 to 25 (TAILORx) (53), and 1 to 3 positive axillary nodes and an RS <25 (RxPonder)

(text continues on page 455)

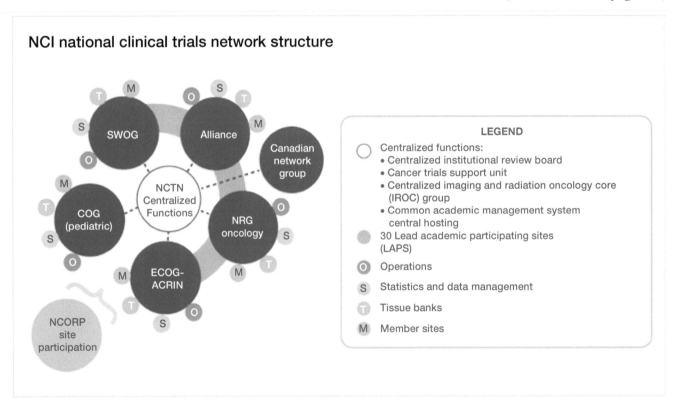

FIGURE 47.1 National Clinical Trials Network.

Source: Reproduced from National Clinical Trials Network. https://www.cancer.gov/PublishedContent/Images/research/areas/clinical-trials/nctn/nctn-clinical-trials-network.png.

TABLE 47.2 Selected Examples of Pivotal Completed and Current Cooperative Group Cancer Clinical Trials

NCI ID/ClinicalTrials.gov ID	Stage and Disease	Accrual	Trial Objective
Integral Biomarker Trials			
TAILORx (NCT00310180)	Resected stage I ER+, HER2- breast cancer	10,273	Biomarker: Onco*type* DX RS Objective: determine benefit of adjuvant chemotherapy if RS 11–25
RxPonder (NCT01272037)	Resected stage II–III ER+, HER2– breast cancer, 1–3+ nodes	4,639	Biomarker: Onco*type* DX RS Objective: Determine benefit of chemotherapy if RS ≤25
EA1131 (NCT02445391)	Resected triple negative breast cancer with residual disease after neoadjuvant chemotherapy	744	Biomarker: Prosigna (PAM50) assay Objective: Determine if platinum improves disease-free survival compared with capecitabine in the basal breast cancer subtype
E5202 (NCT00217737)	Resected stage II colon cancer	2,433	Biomarker: 18q and microsatellite stability Objective: Prospective validation of prognostic biomarkers and determine if benefit of adjuvant bevacizumab added to chemotherapy
B55 (NCT02032823)	Resected BRCA mutation associated operable breast cancer	330	Biomarker: germ-line BRCA mutation Objective: Determine benefit of 1 year of adjuvant olaparib in preventing recurrence
PRIMA (NCT02655016)	Stage III–IV ovarian cancer responding to first line platinum with HRD	305	Biomarker: HRD biomarker Objective: Determine benefit of PARP inhibitor niraparib in tumors with positive HRD biomarker
EA3132 (NCT02734537)	Resected stage III–IV squamous cell head/neck cancer	345	Biomarker: somatic p53 mutation Objective: Determine benefit of adding concurrent adjuvant platinum to radiation in p53 mutated tumors
EA3311 (NCT01898494)	Resected stage III–IV oropharyngeal cancer	377	Biomarker: p16 expression Objective: Determine if lower dose radiation as effective and less toxic
Precision Medicine			
MATCH (NCT02465060)	Advanced incurable cancer	6,000	Screening trial to identify new indications for targeted agents using targeted DNA sequencing assay
ALCHEMIST Trials Screening Trial (A151216)(NCT02194738)	Resected stage IB–IIIA non–small-cell lung cancer	Up to 8,300	Screen for molecular alterations in EGFR and ALK and PD-L1 expression
Treatment Trial EA4512 (NCT02201992)	ALKD alteration	378	Determine whether adjuvant crizotinib reduces recurrence risk in tumors with ALK alteration
A081105 (NCT02193282)	EGFR alteration	450	Determine whether adjuvant erlotinib reduces recurrence risk in tumors with EGFR alteration
EA5142 (NCT02595944)	No ALK or EGFR alteration	714	Determine whether adjuvant immunotherapy with nivolumab reduces recurrence

(continued)

TABLE 47.2 Selected Examples of Pivotal Completed and Current Cooperative Group Cancer Clinical Trials (*continued*)

NCI ID/ClinicalTrials.gov ID	Stage and Disease	Accrual	Trial Objective
LUNG-MAP S1400	Metastatic squamous cell lung carcinoma	Up to 10,000	Screening trial
S1400B (NCT02785913)	PI3K pathway alteration	59	Phase II: Determine efficacy of taselisib
S1400C (NCT02785939)	CDK alteration	59	Phase II: Determine efficacy of palbociclib
S1400D (NCT02154490)	FGFR pathway alteration	59	Phase II: Determine efficacy of AZD4557
S1400I (NCT02785952)	No alteration	350	Phase III: Compare efficacy of nivolumab vs. nivolumab plus ipilimumab
Immunotherapy			
EA5142 (NCT02595944)	Resected stage IB–IIIA non–small-cell lung cancer	714	Determine whether adjuvant nivolumab reduces recurrence risk
E1609 (NCT01274338)	Resected stage IIIB–IV melanoma	1,500	Determine whether adjuvant ipilimumab more effective than alpha-interferon in preventing recurrence
EA6141 (NCT02339571)	Unresectable stage IIIB–IV melanoma	400	Determine whether addition of GM-CSF to nivolumab/ipilimumab improves survival
EA3612 (NCT01950390)	Unresectable stage III–IV melanoma	168	Determine whether adding bevacizumab to ipilimumab improves progression-free survival
E1901 (NCT02003222)	BCR/ABL-negative B-cell acute lymphocytic leukemia	360	Determine whether adding blinatumomab to chemotherapy improves survival
Developmental Therapeutics			
S1207 (NCT01674140)	Resected stage II–III ER+, HER2– breast cancer	1,900	Determine whether 1 year of adjuvant everolimus improves disease-free survival
S0931 (NCT0112024)	Resected high-risk renal cell cancer	1,545	Determine whether 1 year of adjuvant everolimus improves recurrence-free survival
C-13 (NCT02664077)	Resected stage III colon cancer	1,118	Determine whether 2 years of adjuvant regorafenib improves disease-free survival
E2810 (NCT01575548)	Advanced renal cell cancer after metastasectomy	128	Determine whether adjuvant pazopanib improves disease-free survival after resection
E1A11 (NCT01863550)	Multiple myeloma	756	Determine whether adding carfilzomib improves survival compared with bortezomib
E3A06 (NCT01169337)	Smoldering myeloma	180	Determine whether lenalidomide delays progression to myeloma
S1403 (NCT02438722)	Metastatic non–small-cell lung cancer, EGFR mutant	605	Determine whether the afatinib/cetuximab combination improves progression-free survival and overall survival compared with afatinib alone
A031201 (NCT01949337)	Metastatic prostate cancer	1,311	Determine whether adding abiraterone to enzalutamide improves overall survival

(*continued*)

TABLE 47.2 Selected Examples of Pivotal Completed and Current Cooperative Group Cancer Clinical Trials (*continued*)

NCI ID/ClinicalTrials.gov ID	Stage and Disease	Accrual	Trial Objective
S1216 (NCT01809691)	Metastatic prostate cancer	1,204	Determine whether CYP17 inhibitor orteronel (TAK-700) improves survival compared with bicalutamide
E2112 (NCT02115282)	Metastatic ER+ breast cancer	600	Determine whether entinostat improves progression-free survival and/or overall survival when added to aromatase inhibitor therapy
A011106 (NCT01953588)	Resectable stage II–III ER+, HER2– breast cancer	2,820	Determine whether fulvestrant or fulvestrant plus anastrozole is more effective than anastrozole as neoadjuvant endocrine therapy
Local Therapy			
B51 (NCT01872975)	Resected clinical stage II–III breast cancer with pathologically negative nodes after neoadjuvant chemotherapy	1,636	Determine whether axillary radiation may be effectively spared
A011202 (NCT01901094)	Resected stage II–IIIA breast cancer with positive sentinel node biopsy	2,918	Determine whether axillary dissection may be effectively spared
S1101 (NCT01224665)	Muscle-invading bladder cancer	620	Determine whether extended pelvic lymphadenectomy improves disease-free survival after radical cystectomy
CC-003 (NCT02635009)	Small-cell lung cancer requiring PCI	304	Determine whether hippocampal avoidance during PCI results in less cognitive dysfunction and comparable intracranial recurrence
C140503 (NCT00499330)	Resectable stage IA non–small-cell lung cancer	1,258	Determine whether sublobar resection is as effective as lobectomy
R1308 (NCT01993810)	Unresectable stage II–IIIB non–small-cell lung cancer	560	Determine whether proton beam radiation improves overall survival compared with standard photon therapy
Advanced Imaging—Anatomic			
E4112 (NCT02352883)	DCIS	350	Determine mastectomy rate in patients with DCIS initially deemed candidates for breast conservation based on mammography and exam
ACRIN6694 (NCT01805076)	Resectable stage I–II breast cancer	536	Determine whether preoperative MRI reduces local recurrence rates
EA1141 (NCT02933489)	Female candidate for screening mammography	1,450	Compare cancer detection rates with abbreviated MRI and digital breast tomography
EA1151 (TMIST)	Female candidate for screening mammography	165,000	Compare cancer detection rates for clinically relevant cancers
ACRIN4703/DECAMP-1 (NCT01785342)	Smokers with indeterminate pulmonary nodules	500	Evaluate diagnostic performance of four previously established lung cancer biomarkers for a lung cancer diagnosis

(*continued*)

TABLE 47.2 Selected Examples of Pivotal Completed and Current Cooperative Group Cancer Clinical Trials (*continued*)

NCI ID/ClinicalTrials.gov ID	Stage and Disease	Accrual	Trial Objective
ACRIN4704/DECAMP-2 (NCT02504697)	Smokers with lung cancer or at high risk	880	Evaluate biomarkers in cross-sectional study of smokers with lung cancer, and longitudinal study of smokers at high risk for developing lung cancer
Advanced Imaging—Functional			
ACRIN 6685 (NCT00983697)	Potentially resectable T2–4, N0–3 squamous cell carcinoma of head/neck	292	Determine the negative predictive value for having pathologically negative nodes, and altering surgical treatment
C50801(NCT01118026)	Stage IA–IIB Hodgkin's disease	123	Evaluate response adapted approach to therapy
S1001 (NCT01359592)	Stage I–II B-cell non-Hodgkin's lymphoma	155	Evaluate FDG/PET directed approach to therapy
EA5123 (NCT02607423)	Potentially resectable T1-3N2 non–small-cell lung cancer	68	Evaluate FDG/PET to predict mediastinal node downstaging after preoperative chemotherapy
EAI141 (NCT02392429)	Acute myelogenous leukemia	57	Determine negative predictive value of posttreatment FLT PET/CT imaging for complete remission in comparison with bone marrow evaluation
EAI142 (NCT02398773)	Metastatic ER-positive breast cancer eligible for endocrine therapy	99	Determine negative predictive value of 18F FES uptake for clinical benefit from endocrine therapy
Cancer Control/Prevention			
A211102 (NCT01905046)	Women with ductal atypia on random periareolar fine needle aspiration	400	Determine whether a 1-year course of metformin reduces incidence of atypia on random periareolar fine needle aspiration
MA32 (NCT01101438)	Resected stage I–III breast cancer	3,649	Determine effect of metformin in improving disease-free survival
S0820 (NCT01349881)	Stage 0–III colorectal cancer with resection within 1 year	1,340	Determine the effect of eflornithine, sulindac, or combination in preventing a second primary high-risk adenoma or carcinoma
A221303 (NCT02349412)	Advanced lung and noncolorectal gastrointestinal cancers not being treated with curative intent	700	Determine whether early integration of palliative care services into standard oncology care in an outpatient setting improves quality of life
S1316 (NCT02270450)	Intra-abdominal cancer associated bowel obstruction	200	Determine number of days spent out of the hospital with surgery or nonsurgical management
E1Z11 (NCT01824836)	Postmenopausal women with breast cancer to receive adjuvant AI	1,000	Prospective validation of 10 specific single nucleotide polymorphisms and discontinuation of AIs due to musculoskeletal symptoms
S1200 (NCT01535066)	Breast cancer and AI-associated arthralgias	228	Determine effect of acupuncture in reducing severity of AI-induced arthralgias

(*continued*)

TABLE 47.2 Selected Examples of Pivotal Completed and Current Cooperative Group Cancer Clinical Trials (*continued*)

NCI ID/ClinicalTrials.gov ID	Stage and Disease	Accrual	Trial Objective
A221102 (NCT01573442)	Breast cancer and AI-associated arthralgias	224	Determine effect of testosterone in reducing severity of AI-induced arthralgias
GOG-0225 (NCT00719303)	Stage I–IV ovarian, fallopian tube, or primary peritoneal cancer	1,070	Determine effect of dietary intervention designed to promote increased levels of plasma carotenoids, control weight, and to ensure adequacy of micronutrient intake on progression-free survival
A011401 (NCT02750826)	Resected stage I–III breast cancer and body mass index 27 kg/m2 or higher	3,136	Determine effect of lifestyle weight loss intervention in improving disease-free survival
Rare Cancers			
EA2133 (NCT02560298)	Inoperable or metastatic anal carcinoma	80	Compare efficacy of cisplatin/5-FU with carboplatin/paclitaxel
EA8134 (NCT. . .)	Locally advanced squamous carcinoma of the penis	400	Role of neoadjuvant therapy, additional benefit from prophylactic pelvic lymph node dissection

5-FU, 5-fluorouracil; AI, aromatase inhibitor; ALCHEMIST, Adjuvant Lung Cancer Enrichment Marker Identification and Sequencing Trials; DCIS, ductal carcinoma in situ; DECAMP, Detection of Early lung Cancer Among Military Personnel consortium; FDG, fluorodeoxyglucose; GM-CSF, granulocyte–macrophage colony stimulating factor; HRD, homologous recombination deficiency; MATCH, Molecular Analysis for Therapy Choice; NCI, National Cancer Institute; PCI, prophylactic cranial irradiation; RS, Recurrence Score.

(54). Preliminary results from TAILORx indicate a 1% rate of recurrence at 5 years for patients with an RS <11 and negative axillary nodes treated with endocrine therapy alone (29). An ongoing trial (EA1131) is testing whether basal breast cancer subtype is more likely to benefit from adjuvant platinum than capecitabine therapy in high-risk populations with triple negative breast cancer and residual disease after neoadjuvant taxane/anthracycline containing therapy. Another trial in colon cancer (E5202) evaluated biomarkers to stratify patients; those with low-risk tumors (high levels of microsatellite instability [MSI-H] or absence of loss of heterozygosity of 18q/retention of 18q) were managed with observation alone after potentially curative surgery while those with high-risk tumors (microsatellite-stable or -low with 18q LOH) were assigned to adjuvant chemotherapy (55,56). Other studies are evaluating the role of poly(ADP-ribose) polymerase (PARP) inhibitors, including olaparib as adjuvant therapy for breast cancer associated with germ-line BRCA gene mutations (NSABP B55), or niraparib in patients with ovarian cancer associated with somatic BRCA-like DNA repair deficiency using a tissue-based homologous recombination deficiency (HRD) assay (PRIMA). In head and neck cancer, trials are using integral biomarkers to enrich for high-risk populations (p53 mutations) to add additional systemic therapy with cisplatin (E3132), or low-risk populations (p16+) to reduce radiation therapy (EA3311).

Precision Medicine

Initial plans for NCTN included a portfolio of "Precision Medicine" trials, including the Molecular Analysis for Therapy Choice (MATCH), Adjuvant Lung Cancer Enrichment Marker Identification and Sequencing Trials (ALCHEMIST), and LUNG-MAP suites of trials (57). The MATCH trial includes patients with advanced cancer, lymphoma, or myeloma with progressive disease following at least one line of standard systemic therapy and for whom there is no standard treatment known to prolong survival. Trial participants undergo analysis of a fresh or recent biopsy specimen of metastatic tumor using a multiplex assay including immunohistochemistry (PTEN, MHL1, MHL2) and targeted DNA sequencing including nearly 4,100 potentially deleterious variations in 143 genes of interest. A novel feature of the trial is that patients with targetable alterations (e.g., EGFR, HER2, MET, ALK, ROS1, BRAFV600E600K, PIK3CA, PTEN, NF1, GNAQ/GNA11, SMO/PTCH1, NF2, cKIT, FGFR, DDR, AKT, NRAS, CCND1-3) are matched to one of 24 arms with investigational agents or commercially available agents (e.g., afatinib, crizotinib, defactinib, dabrafenib, dasatinib, palbociclib, trametinib, vismodegib, and ado-trastuzumab emtansine) for nonapproved indications. It is anticipated that approximately 6,000 patients will be accrued, and that 20% of trial participants will be matched with an assigned treatment. The ALCHEMIST suite of trials includes patients with early-stage resectable non–small-cell lung cancer, about one half of whom are expected to recur. It is anticipated that up to about 8,000 patients will be enrolled on a screening trial (A151216) in which tumors are being characterized for EGFR or ALK alterations, of whom 10% with an EGFR alteration are enrolled on a trial testing adjuvant erlotinib (A081105) and 5% with an ALK alteration are enrolled on trial testing adjuvant crizotinib (E4512); the remainder are eligible for enrollment on a trial testing adjuvant immunotherapy with the PD1 inhibitor nivolumab (EA5142). In the LUNG-MAP suite of trials (S1400), patients with metastatic or inoperable squamous cell carcinoma of the lung undergo a tumor biopsy for biomarker analysis, and are assigned to biomarker-driven phase II treatment trials testing a PI3K pathway inhibitor (taselisib in S1400B), a CDK4/6 inhibitor (palbociclib in S1400C), or an FGFR inhibitor (AZD4557 in S1400D) if there is a targetable alteration, or a phase III immunotherapy trial (nivolumab vs. nivolumab plus ipilimumab) if there is no targetable alteration (S1400I).

Immunotherapy Trials

Agents blocking various immune checkpoint molecules, including CTLA4, PD-1, and PD-L1, are now approved based on improved survival in advanced melanoma and non–small-cell lung cancer, and on responses in bladder cancer (58). A number of clinical trials are in progress further evaluating the role of these agents for earlier stage of disease, including adjuvant therapy of non–small-lung cancer (E5142), melanoma (E1609, EA6141), and breast cancer (S1418), or in combination with other agents such as granulocyte–macrophage colony stimulating factor (GM-CSF; EA6141) or bevacizumab (EA3612) in advanced melanoma. Other approaches being tested include evaluation of the bispecific CD19-directed CD3 T-cell engager blinatumomab added to induction chemotherapy in BCR-ABL negative acute lymphocytic leukemia (E1910).

Developmental Therapeutics

A number of trials are focused on evaluating targeted therapeutic approaches in the management of operable high-risk cancers, including the mTOR inhibitor everolimus as adjuvant therapy of breast cancer (S1207) or renal cell cancer (S0931), and the multikinase inhibitor regorafenib as adjuvant therapy for high-risk colon cancer (NSABP C-13) and pazopanib for renal cancer after metastasectomy (E2810). In advanced disease, studies are evaluating the role of novel proteasome inhibitors such as carfilzomib in multiple myeloma (E1A11), lenalidomide in high-risk smoldering myeloma (E3A06), combination EGFR targeted therapy in non–small-cell lung cancer (S1403), combination antiandrogen therapy in metastatic prostate cancer (A031201, S1216), and the histone deacetylase inhibitor entinostat in metastatic ER-positive breast cancer (E2112). Neoadjuvant

endocrine therapy in ER+ breast cancer provides another therapeutic platform for testing novel treatment approaches; for example, fulvestrant and the combination of fulvestrant plus anastrozole are being compared with anastrozole alone (A011106).

Local Therapies

Several trials are addressing important questions in local disease control and minimizing adverse effects of local therapy, including extent of local–regional radiation therapy (NSABP B51) or axillary surgery (A011202) in breast cancer, extended pelvic lymphadenectomy in bladder cancer (S1011), hippocampal avoidance of prophylactic brain irradiation in small-cell lung cancer (CC-003), radiation therapy for primary small-cell lung cancer (C30610), surgery for primary non–small-cell lung cancer (C140503), and proton therapy in lung cancer (R1308).

Advanced Imaging

Several trials are focused on application of advanced imaging techniques in improving clinical outcomes, including use of MRI in ductal carcinoma in situ (E4112) and invasive breast cancer (ACRIN6694). Other trials are comparing screening modalities such as abbreviated MRI with digital tomosynthesis in women with radiographically dense breasts (EA1141), and digital tomosynthesis with standard digital mammography as a screening tool to detect clinically relevant cancers (EA1151). Other screening studies include surveillance of patients with solitary pulmonary nodules (ACRIN 4703) or early-stage lung cancer or high-risk populations (ACRIN 4704). Functional imaging studies involving PET are being evaluated in a number of trials, including tracers such as fluorodeoxyglucose (FDG; 2-deoxy-2-[fluorine-18]fluoro-D-glucose) in head/neck cancer (ACRIN 6685), Hodgkin's disease (C5080), B-cell lymphoma (S1001), lung cancer (EA5123), FLT (3'-deoxy-3'[(18)F]-fluorothymidine) in acute leukemia (EAI141), and FES (16a-18F-fluoroestradiol) in ER-positive metastatic breast cancer (EAI142).

Cancer Prevention/Control

This category includes the conduct of clinical trials focused on the behavioral, social, and population sciences to create or enhance interventions that, independently or in combination with biomedical approaches, reduce cancer risk, incidence, morbidity, and mortality, and improve quality of life. Examples of cancer prevention studies include evaluation of metformin as a chemopreventive agent in atypical ductal hyperplasia of the breast (A211102) and prevention of recurrence of invasive breast cancer (MA32), and eflornithine and sulindac to reduce risk of second colorectal cancers and adenomatous polyps (S0820). Several studies have focused on symptom control in advanced cancer (A221303) and bowel obstruction (S1316). Several studies have investigated aromatase inhibitor induced musculoskeletal toxicity by prospective validation of genetic predictors of this toxicity (E1Z11), or use of evaluation of supportive care measures such as acupuncture (S1200) or pharmacologic interventions (A221102). Other trials are evaluating whether diet and lifestyle factors in advanced ovarian cancer improve progression-free survival in advanced ovarian cancer (GOG-0225), or reduce recurrence in early breast cancer (A011401).

Rare Cancers

The cooperative groups collaborate with other members of the International Rare Cancers Initiative (IRCI) to plan prospective trials in cancers that are rare but associated with substantial morbidity and mortality. IRCI is a joint initiative between NCI and the National Institute for Health Research Cancer Research Network (NCRN), Cancer Research UK (CR-UK), and the European Organization for Research and Treatment of Cancer (EORTC) (59). Although there is no uniform definition of rare cancer, an incidence of less than 6/100,000/year has been proposed, which collectively account for about 20% of all cancers. One of the first trials to be developed by this initiative is a trial testing two standard chemotherapy regimens in advanced anal cancer (EA2133). Another is a multimodality study in advanced penile cancer (EA8134).

Cancer Care Delivery Research (CCDR)

CCDR is a new area of cancer research supported by NCI through the NCORP mechanism. CCDR is defined as the multidisciplinary field of scientific investigation that studies how social factors, financing systems, organizational structures and processes, health technologies, and provider and individual behaviors affect cancer. Although several CCDR projects have been launched, this area of research remains in its infancy.

SUMMARY AND CONCLUSIONS

Since the NCI Cooperative Group system was developed over 50 years ago, trials performed by the groups have contributed to some of the most important advances in cancer care. The next 50 years provide unprecedented opportunities because of the improved understanding of the biologic basis of cancer, the cancer microenvironment, and immune surveillance (60). The forthcoming years also provide unprecedented challenges because of increasing cancer burden due to aging of the population (61), the evolving molecular taxonomy and segmentation of common cancers into uncommon or rare subtypes, and the innumerable combinations of immunotherapeutic, targeted, and cytotoxic systemic and local therapies that may be studied. The cooperative group system is well positioned to address these challenges via the collaborative design and conduct of clinical trials that offer the greatest potential for impacting patient care, and that

would otherwise not be performed by the pharmaceutical industry. This is being accomplished through its network of participating investigators at academic and community sites, the collaborative nature of study design and conduct, its partnership with patients and advocate organizations, and its ability to collect and analyze clinically annotated biospecimens for correlative laboratory studies.

REFERENCES

1. DeVita VT Jr, Chu E. A history of cancer chemotherapy. *Cancer Res.* 2008;68:8643–8653.
2. Farber S, Diamond LK. Temporary remissions in acute leukemia in children produced by folic acid antagonist, 4-aminopteroylglutamic acid. *N Engl J Med.* 1948;238:787–793.
3. STREPTOMYCIN treatment of pulmonary tuberculosis. *Br Med J.* 1948;2:769–782.
4. Endicott KM. The national cancer chemotherapy program. *J Chronic Dis.* 1958;8:171–177.
5. Frei E 3rd, Holland JF, Schneiderman MA, et al. A comparative study of two regimens of combination chemotherapy in acute leukemia. *Blood.* 1958;13:1126–1148.
6. Hill AB. The clinical trial. *N Engl J Med.* 1952;247:113–119.
7. Marshall EK Jr, Merrell M. Clinical therapeutic trial of a new drug. *Bull Johns Hopkins Hosp.* 1949;85:221–230.
8. Heyn RM, Brubaker CA, Burchenal JH, et al. The comparison of 6-mercaptopurine with the combination of 6-mercaptopurine and azaserine in the treatment of acute leukemia in children: results of a cooperative study. *Blood.* 1960;15: 350–359.
9. Zubrod C, Schneiderman, M, Frei III E, et al. Appraisal of methods for the study of chemotherapy of cancer in man: comparative therapeutic trial of ntirogen mustard and triethylene thiophosphoramide. *J Chronic Dis.* 1960;11:7–33.
10. Oken MM, Creech RH, Tormey DC, et al. Toxicity and response criteria of the Eastern Cooperative Oncology Group. *Am J Clin Oncol.* 1982;5:649–655.
11. Begg CB, Carbone PP, Elson PJ, et al. Participation of community hospitals in clinical trials: analysis of five years of experience in the Eastern Cooperative Oncology Group. *N Engl J Med.* 1982;306:1076–1080.
12. Feigl P, Zelen M. Estimation of exponential survival probabilities with concomitant information. *Biometrics.* 1965;21:826–838.
13. Anderson JR, Cain KC, Gelber RD. Analysis of survival by tumor response. *J Clin Oncol.* 1983;1:710–719.
14. Gray RJ. Spline-based tests in survival analysis. *Biometrics.* 1994;50:640–652.
15. Gray RJ. A Bayesian analysis of institutional effects in a multicenter cancer clinical trial. *Biometrics.* 1994;50:244–253.
16. Gray RJ, Tsiatis AA. A linear rank test for use when the main interest is in differences in cure rates. *Biometrics.* 1989;45: 899–904.
17. Fisher B, Bauer M, Margolese R, et al. Five-year results of a randomized clinical trial comparing total mastectomy and segmental mastectomy with or without radiation in the treatment of breast cancer. *N Engl J Med.* 1985;312:665–673.
18. Fisher B, Anderson S, Bryant J, et al. Twenty-year follow-up of a randomized trial comparing total mastectomy, lumpectomy, and lumpectomy plus irradiation for the treatment of invasive breast cancer. *N Engl J Med.* 2002;347:1233–1241.
19. Fisher B, Jeong JH, Anderson S, et al. Twenty-five-year follow-up of a randomized trial comparing radical mastectomy, total mastectomy, and total mastectomy followed by irradiation. *N Engl J Med.* 2002;347:567–575.
20. Abdel-Wahab O, Mullally A, Hedvat C, et al. Genetic characterization of TET1, TET2, and TET3 alterations in myeloid malignancies. *Blood.* 2009;114:144–147.

21. Mansour EG, Gray R, Shatila AH, et al. Survival advantage of adjuvant chemotherapy in high-risk node-negative breast cancer: ten-year analysis–an intergroup study. *J Clin Oncol.* 1998;16:3486–3492.

22. Sparano JA, Wang M, Martino S, et al. Weekly paclitaxel in the adjuvant treatment of breast cancer. *N Engl J Med.* 2008;358:1663–1671.

23. Fisher B, Costantino J, Redmond C, et al. A randomized clinical trial evaluating tamoxifen in the treatment of patients with node-negative breast cancer who have estrogen-receptor-positive tumors. *N Engl J Med.* 1989;320:479–484.

24. Goss PE, Ingle JN, Martino S, et al. A randomized trial of letrozole in postmenopausal women after five years of tamoxifen therapy for early-stage breast cancer. *N Engl J Med.* 2003;349:1793–1802.

25. Davies C, Pan H, Godwin J, et al. Long-term effects of continuing adjuvant tamoxifen to 10 years versus stopping at 5 years after diagnosis of oestrogen receptor-positive breast cancer: ATLAS, a randomised trial. *Lancet.* 2013;381:805–816.

26. Pagani O, Regan MM, Walley BA, et al. Adjuvant exemestane with ovarian suppression in premenopausal breast cancer. *N Engl J Med.* 2014;371:107–118.

27. Pagani O, Regan MM, Francis PA, et al. Exemestane with ovarian suppression in premenopausal breast cancer. *N Engl J Med.* 2014;371:1358–1359.

28. Romond EH, Perez EA, Bryant J, et al. Trastuzumab plus adjuvant chemotherapy for operable HER2-positive breast cancer. *N Engl J Med.* 2005;353:1673–1684.

29. Sparano JA, Gray RJ, Makower DF, et al. Prospective Validation of a 21-Gene Expression Assay in Breast Cancer. *N Engl J Med.* 2015;373:2005–2014.

30. Paik S, Tang G, Shak S, et al. Gene expression and benefit of chemotherapy in women with node-negative, estrogen receptor-positive breast cancer. *J Clin Oncol.* 2006;24:3726–3734.

31. Albain KS, Barlow WE, Shak S, et al. Prognostic and predictive value of the 21-gene recurrence score assay in postmenopausal women with node-positive, oestrogen-receptor-positive breast cancer on chemotherapy: a retrospective analysis of a randomised trial. *Lancet Oncol.* 2010;11:55–65.

32. Fisher B, Costantino JP, Wickerham DL, et al. Tamoxifen for prevention of breast cancer: report of the National Surgical Adjuvant Breast and Bowel Project P-1 Study. *J Natl Cancer Inst.* 1998;90:1371–1388.

33. Vogel VG, Costantino JP, Wickerham DL, et al. Effects of tamoxifen vs raloxifene on the risk of developing invasive breast cancer and other disease outcomes: the NSABP Study of Tamoxifen and Raloxifene (STAR) P-2 trial. *JAMA.* 2006;295:2727–2741.

34. Williams SD, Stablein DM, Einhorn LH, et al. Immediate adjuvant chemotherapy versus observation with treatment at relapse in pathological stage II testicular cancer. *N Engl J Med.* 1987;317:1433–1438.

35. Messing EM, Manola J, Sarosdy M, et al. Immediate hormonal therapy compared with observation after radical prostatectomy and pelvic lymphadenectomy in men with node-positive prostate cancer. *N Engl J Med.* 1999;341:1781–1788.

36. Sweeney CJ, Chen YH, Carducci M, et al. Chemohormonal therapy in metastatic hormone-sensitive prostate cancer. *N Engl J Med.* 2015;373:737–746.

37. Moertel CG, Fleming TR, Macdonald JS, et al. Levamisole and fluorouracil for adjuvant therapy of resected colon carcinoma. *N Engl J Med.* 1990;322:352–358.

38. Wolmark N, Rockette H, Mamounas E, et al. Clinical trial to assess the relative efficacy of fluorouracil and leucovorin, fluorouracil and levamisole, and fluorouracil, leucovorin, and levamisole in patients with Dukes' B and C carcinoma of the colon: results from National Surgical Adjuvant Breast and Bowel Project C-04. *J Clin Oncol.* 1999;17:3553–3559.

39. Giantonio BJ, Catalano PJ, Meropol NJ, et al. Bevacizumab in combination with oxaliplatin, fluorouracil, and leucovorin (FOLFOX4) for previously treated metastatic colorectal cancer: results from the Eastern Cooperative Oncology Group Study E3200. *J Clin Oncol.* 2007;25:1539–1544.

40. National Lung Screening Trial Research T, Aberle DR, Adams AM, et al. Reduced lung-cancer mortality with low-dose computed tomographic screening. *N Engl J Med.* 2011;365:395–409.

41. Turrisi AT 3rd, Kim K, Blum R, et al. Twice-daily compared with once-daily thoracic radiotherapy in limited small-cell lung cancer treated concurrently with cisplatin and etoposide. *N Engl J Med.* 1999;340:265–271.

42. Sandler A, Gray R, Perry MC, et al. Paclitaxel-carboplatin alone or with bevacizumab for non-small-cell lung cancer. *N Engl J Med.* 2006;355:2542–2550.

43. Spiers AS, Moore D, Cassileth PA, et al. Remissions in hairy-cell leukemia with pentostatin (2'-deoxycoformycin). *N Engl J Med.* 1987;316:825–830.

44. Tallman MS, Andersen JW, Schiffer CA, et al. All-trans-retinoic acid in acute promyelocytic leukemia. *N Engl J Med.* 1997;337:1021–1028.

45. Habermann TM, Weller EA, Morrison VA, et al. Rituximab-CHOP versus CHOP alone or with maintenance rituximab in older patients with diffuse large B-cell lymphoma. *J Clin Oncol.* 2006;24:3121–3127.

46. Rajkumar SV, Jacobus S, Callander NS, et al. Lenalidomide plus high-dose dexamethasone versus lenalidomide plus low-dose dexamethasone as initial therapy for newly diagnosed multiple myeloma: an open-label randomised controlled trial. *Lancet Oncol.* 2010;11:29–37.

47. O'Leary M, Krailo M, Anderson JR, et al. Progress in childhood cancer: 50 years of research collaboration, a report from the Children's Oncology Group. *Semin Oncol.* 2008;35:484–493.

48. Jemal A, Center MM, DeSantis C, et al. Global patterns of cancer incidence and mortality rates and trends. *Cancer Epidemiol Biomarkers Prev.* 2010;19:1893–907.

49. DeSantis CE, Lin CC, Mariotto AB, et al. Cancer treatment and survivorship statistics, 2014. *CA Cancer J Clin.* 2014;64:252–271.

50. Nass S, Moses, HL, Mendelsohn J, Eds. A National Cancer Clinical Trials System for the 21st Century: Reinvigorating the NCI Cooperative Group Program. 2010;1–316.

51. Implementing a National Cancer Clinical Trials System for the 21st Century: Washington, DC:Second Workshop Summary; 2013.

52. National Clinical Trials Network. https://www.cancer.gov/PublishedContent/Images/research/areas/clinical-trials/nctn/nctn-clinical-trials-network.png

53. Sparano JA, Paik S. Development of the 21-gene assay and its application in clinical practice and clinical trials. *J Clin Oncol.* 2008;26:721–728.

54. Ramsey SD, Barlow WE, Gonzalez-Angulo AM, et al. Integrating comparative effectiveness design elements and endpoints into a phase III, randomized clinical trial (SWOG S1007) evaluating oncotypeDX-guided management for women with breast cancer involving lymph nodes. *Contemp Clin Trial.* 2013;34:1–9.

55. Watanabe T, Wu TT, Catalano PJ, et al. Molecular predictors of survival after adjuvant chemotherapy for colon cancer. *N Engl J Med.* 2001;344:1196–1206.

56. Ribic CM, Sargent DJ, Moore MJ, et al. Tumor microsatellite-instability status as a predictor of benefit from fluorouracil-based adjuvant chemotherapy for colon cancer. *N Engl J Med.* 2003;349:247–257.

57. Abrams J, Conley B, Mooney M, et al. National Cancer Institute's Precision Medicine Initiatives for the new National Clinical Trials Network. *Am Soc Clin Oncol Educ Book.* 2014;71–76.

58. Khalil DN, Smith EL, Brentjens RJ, et al. The future of cancer treatment: immunomodulation, CARs and combination immunotherapy. *Nat Rev Clin Oncol.* 2016;13:394.

59. Keat N, Law K, Seymour M, et al. International rare cancers initiative. *Lancet Oncol.* 2013;14:109–110.

60. Hanahan D, Weinberg RA. Hallmarks of cancer: the next generation. *Cell.* 2011;144:646–674.

61. Edwards BK, Howe HL, Ries LA, et al. Annual report to the nation on the status of cancer, 1973-1999, featuring implications of age and aging on U.S. cancer burden. *Cancer.* 2002;94:2766–2792.

COOPERATIVE GROUPS: A JAPANESE PERSPECTIVE

Kenichi Nakamura, Haruhiko Fukuda, and Yasuo Ohashi

A BRIEF HISTORY

Development of Japanese cooperative groups began in the 1980s, led by a number of researchers who began incorporating American cooperative group mechanisms (1). The history of cancer clinical trial groups in Japan resembles the earlier progress in the United States. Before the mid-1980s, although small groups in Japan engaged in clinical research, it was largely performed as observational studies without organized data coordinating centers. In the mid-1980s, several leaders introduced standard clinical trial methodology and cooperative group mechanisms that were initially developed in the United States. These researchers established clinical research groups with standing committees such as Data and Safety Monitoring Committees (DSMCs) and Protocol Review Committees (PRCs). In the early 1990s, the importance of data management and statistical methodology was recognized and several clinical trial groups formally organized data coordinating centers with full-time data managers and biostatisticians. From the late 1990s to the early 2000s, several groups gradually expanded the functions of their data coordinating centers and thus improved both the quality and quantity of their clinical trials. Since 2000, cooperative groups have formed corporate bodies, such as nonprofit organizations, or have been incorporated in academic institutions in order to stabilize their administrative or hiring structures. At the same time, they have introduced more sophisticated clinical trial methodologies from the United States or European countries and have developed an established cooperative group style to conduct large-scale phase III trials. They have begun performing site visit audits and quality control/assurance of radiotherapy or surgery. Because of these efforts, there are currently many established Japanese cooperative groups that can implement high-quality phase III trials.

REPRESENTATIVE CANCER COOPERATIVE GROUPS IN JAPAN

Table 47.3 shows six representative groups that belong to the Japanese Cancer Trial Network (JCTN) (2), a consortium of cancer cooperative groups involved in conducting nationwide large-scale clinical trials. As described later, JCTN has established guidelines to standardize trial implementation procedures. All six member groups, established before the mid-2000s, now operate a nationwide network to implement large-scale phase III trials with a standing data center. Funding sources are various. Some groups rely only on public funding sources from the Japan Agency for Medical Research and Development (AMED) or self-funding from academic institutions, whereas others receive donations or establish research contracts with pharmaceutical companies. Regarding their clinical trial portfolios, most trials have been conducted on approved commercial drugs. Combined treatment with approved drugs, surgery, radiotherapy, and/or endoscopy has been a main target, with only a few *Chiken* (trials to obtain approval directly for a drug indication) or Advanced Medical Care (AMC; *Senshin-Iryo*) trials (focusing on off-label drugs and aiming expanding indication indirectly). Although the primary goal of all groups is to establish better standard treatments, the proportion of phase III trials varies from 5% to 91%.

These cancer groups are discussed in the following sections. Examples of clinical trial contributions from these groups are listed in Table 47.4.

Japan Adult Leukemia Study Group

The Japan Adult Leukemia Study Group (JALSG) is a multi-institutional cooperative group for the development of treatments for adult leukemia and other hematologic malignancies. JALSG, one of the oldest Japanese cooperative groups, has established standard treatments for Japanese adult leukemia. Details can be found at www.jalsg.jp/english.

Japan Clinical Oncology Group

The Japan Adult Leukemia Study Group (JCOG) is the largest cooperative group in Japan, consisting of 16 disease- or modality-specific subgroups. The results of more than 50 JCOG clinical trials have been adopted in Japanese cancer treatment guidelines for various cancers, which are released by the disease-oriented academic societies. While the primary target of these trials is combination treatment with drugs, surgery, radiation, and/or endoscopy, the number of AMC trials aiming to expand drug indications for rare tumors is increasing. Structural details and clinical trial lists can be found at www.jcog.jp/en/index.html.

West Japan Oncology Group

The West Japan Oncology Group was originally established in 2000 (as The West Japan Thoracic Oncology Group; WJTOG) with the aim of improving the diagnosis and treatment of lung cancer. It has since expanded its scope to gastrointestinal and breast cancer. WJOG has published important evidence on lung and gastric cancers and has actively conducted correlative translational research. Details can be found at www.wjog.jp/index.html (in Japanese).

TABLE 47.3 Representative Cancer Cooperative Groups in Japan

Group	Year of Establishment	Target Disease	Number of Institutions	Annual Accrual (2015)	Funding Sources	Number of Clinical Trials (Interventional, Sept 2016)	Proportion of Phase III Trials
JALSG	1987	Adult leukemia	227	403	AMED, Pharmaceutical companies, donations	14 trials (*Chiken* 0, AMC 0) • Planning 4 • Accrual 6 • Follow-up 4	14%
JCOG	1990	Multidisease (16 disease or modality subgroups)	190	2295	NCC, AMED	94 trials (*Chiken* 0, AMC 7) • Planning 19 • Accrual 42 • Follow-up 33	88%
WJOG	2000	Lung, gastrointestinal, breast	256	464	AMED, industry, membership fees, donations	36 trials (*Chiken* 1, AMC 0) • Planning 7 • Accrual 10 • Follow-up 19	26%
CSPOR-BC (J-CRSU)	2001	Breast	133	470	Donations and contracts from pharmaceutical companies	6 trials (*Chiken* 0, AMC 0) • Planning 0 • Accrual 3 • Follow-up 3	83%
JGOG	2002	Gynecologic	191	1005	AMED	14 trials (*Chiken* 0, AMC 1) • Planning 3 • Accrual 5 • Follow-up 6	43%
JCCG	2014 (2003 for JPLSG, 2008 for JAPST)	Pediatric	176	1558	AMED	66 trials (*Chiken* 3, AMC 0) • Planning 15 • Accrual 30 • Follow-up 21	5%

AMC, Advanced Medical Care (system); AMED, (Japan) Agency for Medical Research and Development; CSFOR-BC, Comprehensive Support Project for Oncology Research of Breast Cancer; JALSG, Japan Adult Leukemia Study Group; JAPST, Japanese Association for Pediatric Solid Tumors; JCCG, Japan Children's Cancer Group; JCOG, Japan Clinical Oncology Group; JGOG, Japanese Gynecologic Oncology Group; JPLSG, Japanese Pediatric Leukemia/Lymphoma Study Group; J-CRSU, Japan Clinical Research Support Unit; NCC, National Cancer Center; WJOG, West Japan Oncology Group.

TABLE 47.4 Examples of Representative Clinical Trial Contributions of Japanese Cooperative Groups

Group	Examples of Clinical Trial Contributions
JALSG	• Equality of daunorubicin and idarubicin in induction chemotherapy for adult acute myeloid leukemia (AML) (JALSG-AML201) • Role of high-dose cytarabine (AraC) in consolidation chemotherapy for adult AML (JALSG-AML201) • Superiority of AM80 in maintenance therapy for adult acute promyelocytic leukemia (APL) (JALSG-APL204)
JCOG	• Role of lymph node dissection in gastric cancer (JCOG9501, JCOG9502, JCOG0110) • Role of irinotecan plus cisplatin in small-cell lung cancer (JCOG9511, JCOG0509) • Survival advantage of preoperative chemotherapy in esophageal cancer (JCOG9907)
WJOG	• Role of gefitinib in non–small-cell lung cancer with epidermal growth factor receptor (EGFR) mutation (WJTOG3405) • Role of carboplatin plus S-1 in advanced non–small-cell lung cancer (WJTOG 3605) • Role of irinotecan in advanced gastric cancer (WJOG 4007)
CSPOR	• Change of hormone therapy (from tamoxifen to aromatase inhibitor) as postoperative treatment for postmenopausal breast cancer (N-SAS BC 03) • A new standard therapy (S-1) as the first-line treatment for human epidermal growth factor receptor 2 (HER2)-negative metastatic breast cancer patients (SELECT-BC)
JGOG	• Survival advantage of dose-dense weekly paclitaxel and carboplatin in epithelial ovarian cancer (JGOG3016)
JCCG	• Efficacy of cisplatin plus pirarubicin in pediatric hepatic tumors (JPLT1, JPLT2) • Efficacy of early use of allogeneic hematopoietic stem cell transplantation for infants with acute lymphoblastic leukemia (MLL03) • Reduction of cumulative anthracycline doses for children with core-binding-factor AML (AML-05)

AML, acute myeloid leukemia; APL, acute promyelocytic leukemia; CSPOR-BC, Comprehensive Support Project for Oncology Research of Breast Cancer; JALSG, Japan Adult Leukemia Study Group; JCCG, Japan Children's Cancer Group; JCOG, Japan Clinical Oncology Group; JGOG, Japanese Gynecologic Oncology Group; WJOG, West Japan Oncology Group.

Comprehensive Support Project for Oncology Research of Breast Cancer

The Comprehensive Support Project for Oncology Research of Breast Cancer (CSPOR-BC) was established in 2001 as a project of the Public Health Research Foundation for supporting investigator-initiated clinical research. It has supported seven nationwide phase III breast cancer adjuvant trials and one phase III first-line trial for advanced disease with concomitant cohort studies. CSPOR-BC became an independent incorporated research association in 2013 and has started several studies, including a phase II study, and a first-line phase III study with quality of life (QOL) as a primary endpoint. Details can be found at www.csp.or.jp/cspor/en/ and cspor-bc.or.jp/study/index.html (in Japanese). The data management of CSPOR-BC has been conducted at the Japan Clinical Research Support Unit (J-CRSU.).

Japanese Gynecologic Oncology Group

The Japanese Gynecologic Oncology Group (JGOG) is a clinical research group that aims to establish optimal diagnostic and therapeutic methods for gynecologic malignancies. One of the strengths of JGOG is its international collaborative studies with the Gynecologic Oncology Group (GOG) of the United States and the Gynecologic Cancer Intergroup (GCIG), a global association of organizations. Details can be found at www.jgog.gr.jp/en/index.html.

Japan Children's Cancer Group

The Japan Children's Cancer Group (JCCG) is a nationwide clinical trial group for pediatric cancer. The JCCG was established in 2014 through the consolidation of a hematologic disease group (Japanese Pediatric Leukemia/Lymphoma Study Group [JPLSG]) and 6 pediatric solid tumor groups. It intends to study all types of pediatric cancer. Details can be found at jccg.jp/ (in Japanese).

ORGANIZATIONAL STRUCTURE

Most Japanese cooperative groups have basic organizational structures that are similar to those of their American counterparts. However, one important difference is that Japan does not have an oversight authority such as the National Cancer Institute Cancer Therapy Evaluation Program (NCI-CTEP). Therefore, each group has its own internal review system.

The structure of JCOG illustrates the typical organizational scheme of Japanese cooperative groups, because many other Japanese cooperative groups are modeled after JCOG. The three basic components are the headquarters (data center and operations office), study groups, and committees; an executive committee exists above them as a decision-making body (Figure 47.2). The JCOG headquarters, run by the National Cancer Center Hospital, consists of about 45 staff in the following 6 divisions: data management, biostatistics, information technology, general affairs, study coordination, and quality assurance. As a disease- or modality-specific investigators' group, JCOG comprises 16 study groups, and each of these groups has its own clinical trials and participating sites. Each group holds a 1-day group meeting 2 to 3 times a year where investigators discuss study concepts, study progress, report monitoring, and study results.

The roles of JCOG committees differ from those in the United States. For example, the PRC consists of active young investigators from the 16 study groups. Study concepts and full protocols are reviewed by investigators from other study groups (i.e., a peer-review system), and as such both should be understandable and compelling even for nonspecialists. The position of PRC reviewer is a stepping stone to that of study coordinator (physician responsible for day-to-day study management) and study chair (representative official of the study) of JCOG trials, so each group nominates young active investigators for educational purposes.

The DSMC takes on a wider range of roles such as protocol revision/amendment review, serious adverse event (SAE) review, regular monitoring report review, clinical study report review, and interim analysis review. In the United States, some of these responsibilities are managed by the NCI-CTEP. However, Japan does not have a similar authority, so the DSMC handles these various roles. The DSMC consists of senior-class active investigators (e.g., investigators with experience of study coordinators) from the 16 study groups, as well as other experts, including external statisticians. Thus, the functional mechanism of the DSMC is basically an internal peer-review system like the PRC. In addition to the PRC and DSMC, several other committees supervise or support the activity of the 16 study groups.

STUDY IMPLEMENTATION PROCESS

A JCOG case is described in this section to illustrate the typical study implementation process of a Japanese cooperative group (Figure 47.3).

Protocol Development

First, a new study idea is discussed at study group meetings that are held 2 to 3 times a year by each study

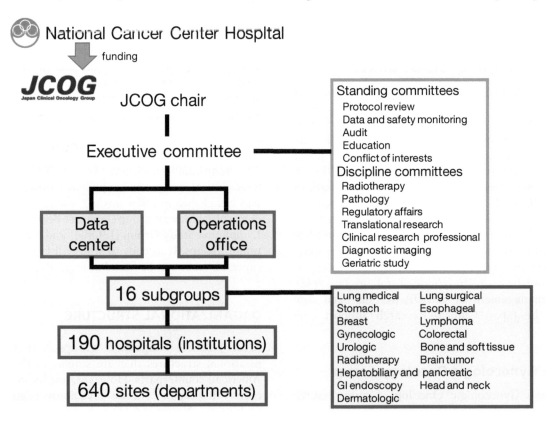

FIGURE 47.2 Typical Organizational Structure of Japanese Cooperative Groups from the Japan Clinical Oncology Group (JCOG).

Source: From JCOG, with permission.

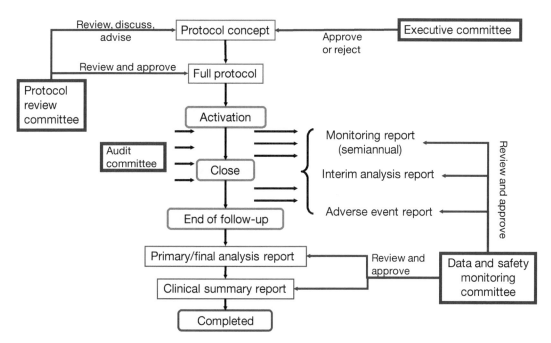

FIGURE 47.3 Study Process and Role of Committees.
GI, gastrointestinal.

group. From this step, attendees from the Data Center and Operations Office support planning and facilitate discussion of the study from methodologic points of view. Second, the study concept is reviewed by 8 to 10 PRC reviewers in a document review manner. Third, the reviewed study concept is discussed in a face-to-face PRC meeting. This meeting, which usually takes 3 hours, consists of intensive discussion focusing on the proposed study's social value, scientific validity, fair subject selection, and risk-benefit balance; as such, it plays an educational role for young investigators. Fourth, the study concept is taken up by the JCOG Executive Committee, which has the power to approve it. If approved, development of a full protocol occurs. Fifth, the full protocol is reviewed by the same PRC members who performed the concept review and approved by the PRC. The time from approval of the basic concept to approval of the full protocol varies from 3 months to 2 years, with an average of 15 months. The acceleration of the protocol development process has been an issue at JCOG, and several initiatives addressing this topic are ongoing in Data Center/Operations Office.

Although some Japanese cooperative groups have simpler protocol development processes, most of them have some internal review system consisting of concept review and full protocol review like JCOG. After the approval by each cooperative group's internal review, the study protocol is submitted to and reviewed by the institutional review board (IRB) at each participating institution and the study is activated for patient accrual at site by site.

Monitoring

Most Japanese cooperative groups have adopted a standardized central monitoring system, which is normal in American cooperative groups. In addition to day-to-day data monitoring, data managers issue a detailed monitoring report twice a year, and problems in the report are discussed at the study group meeting. Site visit monitoring is rarely performed except for investigator-initiated *Chiken*, because the risks of most trials are usually moderate and source data verification is performed during site visit audits. In 2015, Japanese ethical guidelines for clinical research were amended and renamed the "Ethical Guidelines for Medical and Health Research Involving Human Subjects" (from now on the "New Ethical Guidelines"). In these guidelines, study monitoring, either central or on-site, was mandated for invasive and interventional studies. Some small clinical trial groups and academic centers did not have formal monitoring systems before 2015, so they have initiated study monitoring by referring to materials such as the guidelines issued by JCTN.

Audits

Site visit audits are not mandated by the "New Ethical Guidelines." However, some Japanese cooperative groups have had their own internal auditing systems for quite a while because these groups are modeled after the NCI-sponsored cooperative group program. In Japan, site visit audits in investigator-initiated clinical trials were initially implemented by JCOG in 2000, and the other study groups were modeled after the JCOG audit system. Thus, central monitoring plus the site audit make up the basic quality control/assurance system in most Japanese groups. Because the number of institutions participating in Japanese cooperative groups is usually around 200, it is difficult to visit all institutions during a given cycle, usually 3 years. Although the frequency of site audits is relatively lower at Japanese cooperative groups than at American cooperative groups, the contents of monitoring reports are more detailed in Japan. JCTN has also issued guidelines regarding site audits.

Adverse Event Reporting

The definition of SAEs in the "New Ethical Guidelines" is the same as that of the International Council for Harmonisation Good Clinical Practice (ICH-GCP). Seriousness is defined by the Common Terminology Criteria for Adverse Events (CTCAE), and the translated Japanese version is widely used (translated by JCOG and available at the JCOG website). Usually, SAEs are reported to headquarters or the DSMC in each group. Then, SAEs are screened and reviewed internally. Suspected, unexpected, serious adverse reactions (SUSARs) are reported to the Pharmaceuticals and Medical Devices Agency (PMDA) in the case of *Chiken* and to the Ministry of Health, Labour and Welfare (MHLW) of Japan in the case of non-*Chiken*. JCTN has also issued guidelines for SAE reporting.

Biorepository

In past decades, many Japanese translational researchers have collected and analyzed blood and/or tissue specimens on a study-by-study basis, but only a few Japanese cooperative groups have their own permanent biorepository systems because the maintenance of such facilities is generally very costly. Beginning in 2013, JCOG initiated a biorepository in National Cancer Center Hospital East. Then, in a collaboration with BioBank Japan (BBJ), which is run by the Institute of Medical Science at the University of Tokyo, it was transferred to the JCOG-BBJ in 2015. BBJ is one of the largest biorepositories in Japan and is supported by AMED. In the context of this collaboration, JCOG has begun storing not only blood samples but also frozen tissue samples. In terms of JCOG clinical trials, the major benefit of this merged biorepository is high-quality, cleaned trial data. From now on, the publishing of many clinically relevant results are expected as a result of this collaboration. The pediatric group JCCG has also established the same scheme with BBJ and has started blood sample banking similar to JCOG.

ROLE OF COOPERATIVE GROUPS IN JAPAN

Until 2003, only pharmaceutical companies had been allowed to conduct a *Chiken*. In addition, off-label drug use has seldom been studied in clinical trials because it is rarely reimbursed by national health insurance. Consequently, the target of Japanese cooperative groups has been late-phase development combining approved drugs, radiotherapy, and/or surgery. The results of a number of such studies have been published and have contributed to improving the standard of care for various types of cancer. Such trials can be conducted even in nonspecialized community hospitals, and one of the strengths of Japanese cooperative groups is the large number of participating institutions and the high generalizability of trial results. Recently, some groups have focused more on translational research, but the primary goal of most cooperative groups is not drug development but rather late-phase clinical trials that seek to establish better standard therapies based on multimodal treatments.

Many drugs currently have been approved with very narrow indications (e.g., as second-line treatments for metastatic/unresectable disease). In addition, off-label drug use is rarely reimbursed by the national health insurance. Thus, clinical trials to expand indications to other subtypes or rare cancers have become more important because pharmaceutical companies are not always interested in such trials. The types of clinical trials listed in Table 47.5 would never be conducted by pharmaceutical companies because of a small market size or a potential decrease in their drug marketing.

However, this situation is gradually changing. Traditionally, *Chiken* trials were mainly conducted by the industry, and academic trials used only approved drugs. As is described later, investigator-initiated *Chiken* and AMC trials using off-label drugs have become possible. Today there are many innovative cancer drugs, but pharmaceutical companies usually conduct clinical trials only for major cancer types. In this setting, Japanese cooperative groups are required to perform new investigational drug studies introducing such new regulatory systems as investigator-initiated *Chiken* and AMC trials. Cooperative groups and pharmaceutical companies should share their responsibilities and collaboratively accelerate treatment development.

TABLE 47.5 Typical Clinical Trials in Japanese Cooperative Groups

- Preoperative chemotherapy compared with standard postoperative chemotherapy
- Comparison between continuous and intermittent administration
- Trials for rare cancers
- Direct comparison between a company's own product and that of a competitor
- Trials for elderly patients
- Trials combining surgery, radiotherapy, and/or endoscopy with drugs

ISSUES OF QUALITY

Over the past 30 years, Japan has established several cancer cooperative groups that can implement high-quality, large-scale phase III trials. However, several issues regarding quantity and/or quality still exist in terms of efficient treatment development.

The environment in which Japanese cooperative groups function has recently become more challenging. First, the regulations for academic trials have become stricter. The basic regulations for academic trials were previously specified by the "Ethical Guidelines for Clinical Research," issued by the MHLW, but they focused only on the protection of human subjects and did not mention quality control/assurance for the accuracy of the results in clinical research. However, in 2013 it was discovered that there was large-scale scientific misconduct in the cardiovascular field (3), with huge donations given to some related universities and suspicions of data manipulation by the industry's employees. In other words, the suspected studies were criticized due to lack of proper data quality control/assurance and appropriate management of conflicts of interest. Following this scientific misconduct, the MHLW amended the regulations and renamed them the "Ethical Guidelines for Medical and Health Research Involving Human Subjects" (the previously discussed "New Ethical Guidelines"). The new regulations mandate data monitoring, traceability of research data, and appropriate management of conflicts of interest. All of these procedures are essential for conducting high-quality clinical trials. The Japanese cooperative groups and academic centers that did not have the necessary systems to implement them are now struggling to adjust to these changes. Moreover, more rigorous laws are now being discussed in the Japanese Diet, one regarding clinical research using unapproved or off-label drugs and one pertaining to industry funding. If these bills focusing on clinical research are approved in the Diet, the activity of some Japanese cooperative groups and academic centers will temporarily diminish.

ISSUES OF QUANTITY

As Western cooperative groups published many pivotal study results, it became "fashionable" in the early 2000s, to establish cooperative groups in Japan and elsewhere. At that time, Japanese regulations made it relatively easy to perform academic trials without investigational new drugs (INDs; non-*Chiken*), requiring only patient protection and not study quality. In addition, as previously mentioned, there was no oversight authority for cooperative groups in Japan. These factors enabled Japanese investigators to easily organize clinical trial groups that conducted many postmarketing clinical trials. Pharmaceutical companies willingly gave them donations, partly to promote drug marketing. As a result, many local, small-sized clinical trial groups emerged and many postmarketing phase I, phase II, and small-size phase III trials were conducted. Figure 47.4 demonstrates Japanese cancer clinical trial groups that had registered a phase III trial as of July 2016 at the University Hospital Medical Information Network

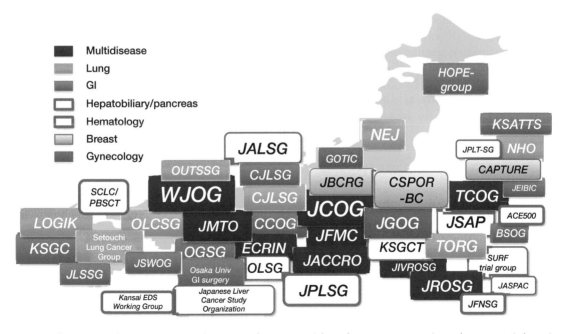

FIGURE 47.4 Multicenter Phase III groups in Japan (groups with at least one ongoing phase III trial registered in UMIN-CTR as of July 2016).

UMIN-CTR, University Hospital Medical Information Network Clinical Trial Registry.

Clinical Trial Registry (UMIN-CTR), a Japanese representative clinical trial registry. This chaotic situation has hampered efficient treatment development in Japan for three reasons: (1) similar trials using commercial drugs were conducted redundantly, (2) patients were dispersed over many clinical trial groups, and (3) operational procedures were not standardized. Because of the lack of a powerful oversight authority such as the NCI-CTEP, top-down control of Japanese clinical trial groups has been difficult. Therefore, some groups are engaged in a number of voluntary initiatives to improve this situation, as described later in the chapter.

JAPANESE REGULATION FOR CLINICAL TRIALS

Japanese academic clinical trials can generally be classified into three types: *Chiken*, AMC, and other investigator-initiated trials (IITs). The differences between these three types of IITs are summarized in Table 47.6.

Chiken is a clinical trial that aims to obtain drug approval corresponding to the Investigational New Drug (IND) trial in the United States. Investigators conducting *Chiken* must file a notification letter with the Pharmaceuticals and Medical Devices Agency (PMDA), the Japanese drug and device regulatory agency. *Chiken* is regulated by the Pharmaceutical Affairs Law and Japanese GCP. The latter is generally consistent with ICH-GCP but is more stringent than the "New Ethical Guidelines." Compared to the "New Ethical Guidelines," Japanese GCP is characterized, for example, by more comprehensive monitoring and auditing, validated data management systems, more rigorous data traceability, management of investigational drugs, detailed clinical study reports, and more rigorous record-keeping of various kinds of documents in each participating institution. Thus, *Chiken* is much more expensive than other clinical trial types. In addition, intensive support by clinical research coordinators (popularly known as CRCs in Japan; corresponding to research nurses or clinical research associates in the United States) is essential to conduct a *Chiken*, and most community hospitals do not have sufficient resources in this regard. Consequently, it is still difficult to conduct a large-scale, investigator-initiated *Chiken,* and the number of *Chiken* conducted by Japanese cooperative groups is quite low (see Table 47.3).

AMC is a health care–providing system based on the ministerial notification by the MHLW that enables the mixed use of the national health insurance system and nonreimbursed treatment. Generally, if a study includes an unapproved or off-label drug, the investigation is not reimbursed by the national health insurance system. However, in the case of *Chiken* and AMC, routine costs, but not the costs of unapproved or off-label drugs, are reimbursed. Approval as an AMC trial requires that the study protocol be reviewed and approved by a scientific committee under the MHLW, *Senshin-Iryo-Kaigi.* Basically, the clinical trial data of an AMC trial cannot be directly used for new, investigational drug applications to MHLW. However, if the published results of an AMC trial are accepted as "publicly well recognized (*kou-chi*)" in the investigators' community (e.g., adopted in a formal treatment guideline by regarding academic society for each cancer), the new drug indication can be approved by MHLW as a public knowledge-based application and be incorporated into the national health insurance system. Because most community hospitals prefer an AMC trial rather than a *Chiken* because of the less rigorous regulation, AMC has come to be used in several large-scale, multi-institutional trials of off-label drugs. In fact, JCOG has seven planned or ongoing AMC trials. Recently, newly developed drugs have been indicated for small disease subtypes, so the need for clinical trials examining off-label use is increasing. Expansion of drug indications is definitely best performed with *Chiken*, but AMC is sometimes chosen because of limited budgets. Also, most sites have difficulty participating in *Chiken* because of more rigorous regulations. Therefore, now *Chiken* tends to be conducted as small (<50 patients), single-arm trials for rare

TABLE 47.6 Regulatory Differences Among Japanese Investigator-initiated Trials

	Regulations	Indication	Application for Drug Approval	Mixed Use of National Health Insurance
Chiken	Pharmaceutical Affairs Law; Japanese GCP	Unapproved drug, off-label drug	Yes	Yes
Advanced Medical Care (AMC)	Notification of AMC by the MHLW; "New Ethical Guidelines"	Unapproved drug, off-label drug	No*	Yes
Other investigator-initiated trials	"New Ethical Guidelines"	Approved drug	No	No

AMC, Advanced Medical Care; GCP, Good Clinical Practice; MHLW, Ministry of Health, Labour, and Welfare of Japan.

*Potentially approved when the study result is publicly well recognized.

cancers, with a small number of participating hospitals (<10), and AMC trials tend to be a little larger (a few hundred), with more participating hospitals (several to a few dozen), and sometimes in a randomized trial setting (these tendencies are approximate). The difficulty in conducting investigator-initiated, large-scale *Chiken* trials is one of the current issues facing academic trials in Japan.

Clinical trials of approved drugs and/or devices are conducted under the "New Ethical Guidelines." This type of clinical trial accounts for more than 90% of trials by JCTN cooperative groups. Although the previous ethical guidelines subjected investigators to mild regulation, the recently activated "New Ethical Guidelines" are stringent, especially for invasive and interventional research. The changes from the former guidelines include (1) study monitoring (for invasive and interventional research), (2) assurance of study result traceability, (3) appropriate management of conflicts of interest, (4) registration of clinical trial results in addition to study design with a clinical trial registry (for interventional research), and (5) reinforcement of Institutional Review Board (IRB) function. Some clinical trial groups already had systems in place to manage such changes, but others did not. Thus, poor-quality clinical trials will no longer exist and the total number of clinical trials is anticipated to decrease for a while.

The "New Ethical Guidelines" were developed in response to recent scientific misconduct. In the same context, the Clinical Research Act is now being discussed in the Diet. The target of the new act is expected to be clinical research using unapproved or off-label drugs and research receiving industry funding. This new act is expected to be more stringent so as to increase the reliability and transparency of study results, and it will be the fourth approach to regulating clinical trials in Japan. Most Japanese IITs were conducted under liberal regulation, but this new act will require substantial changes, especially for Japanese clinical trial groups that rely mainly on industry funding.

FUNDING SOURCES

In response to the aforementioned large-scale scientific misconduct, pharmaceutical companies have developed transparency guidelines regarding their funding of academic trials. Previously, they gave donations to some groups without specifying the purpose for the money use, but the new guidelines require a documented contract between industry and clinical trial groups and mandate that funding be used for contracted research-related activity. As a result, the objectives of clinical trials conducted by Japanese cooperative groups are now restricted to those related to the funding provider. Therefore, it has become difficult to conduct a pure academic trial, such as direct comparison between competitive drugs, investigating an efficacy of shorter administration, or a surgery-radiation trial.

AMED, the national funding agency, was established in 2015. Before that, public funding for medical research was distributed independently by three ministries: the MHLW; the Ministry of Education, Culture, Sports, Science and Technology (MEXT); and the Ministry of Economy, Trade and Industry (METI). Because the funding from the three ministries was not necessarily well coordinated, AMED was established with the aim of distributing research funding more strategically and efficiently, with meticulous research progress management (4). The targets of AMED funding range from basic research to clinical trials. Support of clinical research is broad in scope, and includes drug development, clinical trials, and translational research.

Although AMED provides some competitive funding for clinical trials, it also funds clinical trial infrastructure for some academic centers but not for cooperative groups. One of the main initiatives of AMED in terms of clinical trial infrastructure involves Core Clinical Research Hospitals (CCRHs). CCRHs are required to have sufficient facilities for ICH-GCP–qualified clinical trials and to conduct a certain number of multi-institutional clinical trials. As of September 2016, there were eight certified CCRHs: Tohoku University Hospital, The University of Tokyo Hospital, Keio University Hospital, National Cancer Center Hospital, National Cancer Center Hospital East, Nagoya University Hospital, Osaka University Hospital, and Kyushu University Hospital. Most CCRHs are university hospitals, and their primary mission does not always focus on large-scale clinical trials. In addition, the headquarters of most Japanese clinical trial groups are unfortunately not involved with CCRHs except for that of JCOG, which is governed by the National Cancer Center Hospital. The minimal overlap between CCRHs and the headquarters of Japanese cooperative groups is a threat to late-phase treatment development for cancer.

On the other hand, the MHLW started funding the infrastructure of some Japanese cooperative groups beginning in 2012, but the funding is temporary (for 5 years), and the amount is much smaller than that in the CCRH program. Given this situation, some Japanese cooperative groups rely mainly on funding from pharmaceutical companies. However, because the goals of industry-funded academic trials are restricted to those related to the funding organization's interests, such groups lost their freedom to plan clinical trials focusing on their own clinical questions. Because nonindustry-related clinical trials are also important for the benefit of patients, it is desirable that AMED maintain a certain amount of competitive funding for academic trials as well as its funding for the infrastructure of qualified cooperative groups.

COOPERATION AMONG JAPANESE COOPERATIVE GROUPS

As shown in Figure 47.4, there are many cancer cooperative groups in Japan. Considering the country's population, the number of cooperative groups focusing on phase III trials may be too high. Moreover, study quality varies among groups. Although the "New Ethical Guidelines" require study monitoring and SAE reporting, there is no consensus about appropriate methods of monitoring, auditing, and SAE reporting. Against this background, several initiatives for cooperation among Japanese groups have been implemented.

Websites to Share New Study Ideas

One serious problem facing Japanese cooperative groups is duplication of clinical trials. When a new drug is approved, many groups start planning phase I or II trials of combination chemotherapy or preoperative/postoperative chemotherapy with the new drug. It is easy for small groups to conduct such small trials with approved drugs. Another problem in addition to that of duplication is that small groups conduct phase I or II trials without any plans for a subsequent phase III trial. This occurs because of lack of information about possible studies to be conducted by other groups and lack of communication with a large-scale cooperative group.

To resolve these problems, the National Cancer Center has launched a website (jctn.jp/english.html) to share information about study concepts being planned by participating clinical trial groups. After the start of patient enrollment, clinical trial information is basically open to the public and is presented in one of three certified Japanese clinical trial registries: the UMIN-CTR, Japan Pharmaceutical Information Center–Clinical Trials Information (JAPIC-CTI), and Japan Medical Association Center for Clinical Trials (JMACCT). (Note that clinicaltrials.gov is not a certified registry in Japan, so most Japanese trials are not listed there.) However, after accrual begins, it is too late to share such information, in which case groups cannot prevent duplication or facilitate collaboration; thus, sharing information during the planning phase is a key to success. As a result, each group periodically uploads its study idea to new websites, enabling them to check the study concepts of other groups and consider avoiding unnecessary duplication and/or opportunities for collaborations. The information is updated every 3 months. Currently, two disease-specific websites with limited access among the member groups have been launched; lung cancer sites with eight groups (CJLSG, JCOG, LOGIK, NEJSG, OLCSG, TCOG, TORG, WJOG), and gastrointestinal cancer sites with eight groups (CCOG, HGCSG, JACCRO, JCOG, KSCC, OGSG, TCOG, WJOG). The two groups behind each website have regular face-to-face meetings where collaboration is discussed. If the same ideas are

proposed by multiple groups, there is discussion about whether a collaborative study is possible or which group should take the initiative as the leading group. In fact, some collaborative studies have been realized in the fields of both lung and gastrointestinal cancer. An example is the JIPANG trial, which is a large-scale phase III trial evaluating the efficacy of postoperative chemotherapy with pemetrexed plus cisplatin in completely resected nonsquamous non–small-cell lung cancer compared to the standard treatment with vinorelbine plus cisplatin (UMIN-CTR number, UMIN000006737). The JIPANG trial is an all-Japan adjuvant trial that includes seven Japanese cooperative groups.

Moreover, these assemblies include both small groups focusing on exploratory studies and large groups focusing on confirmatory studies. By facilitating communication among them, a phase I or II result from a small group is expected to be adopted as a test treatment in a phase III trial conducted by a large group. In other words, this arrangement permits small groups to have an exit strategy and provides large groups with a source of promising treatment regimens.

Standardization of Study Implementation Methods

As shown in Figure 47.4, there are many cooperative groups and their study implementation methods are quite different. These differences are often a source of inconvenience and inefficiency for researchers in hospitals. Japanese site investigators usually participate in several clinical trial groups. If, for instance, the SAE reporting criteria or format differ among groups, investigators are required to learn each method every time they join a trial. In most cases, these differences involve long-standing practices developed in each group. Recently, the "New Ethical Guidelines" have required study monitoring and potential auditing for invasive and interventional studies, but concrete monitoring and auditing methods have not been described. Against this background, six representative Japanese cancer cooperative groups have shared their methods and discussed how these methods can be standardized. In 2015, the six groups organized JCTN and have published three JCTN guidelines: central monitoring, site visit audits, and SAE reporting.

These three guidelines have currently been adopted not only by JCTN groups but also by other Japanese clinical trial groups. This standardization will help improve study quality and facilitate collaborative studies between Japanese groups.

JCTN Central Monitoring Guidelines

The JCTN has adopted methods similar to those used by American cooperative groups. Thus, the central monitoring and site visit audit guidelines are the standard quality control/assurance system in JCTN. The

JCTN Central Monitoring Guidelines specify essential items to be listed in a regular monitoring report: general study information, patient accrual, progress of data submission, potential ineligible cases, distribution of background factors, reasons for off-protocol treatment, potential violations/deviations, safety information including SAEs, and secondary cancers. In general, a detailed monitoring report is to be issued twice a year. A template of a monitoring report with essential items (in Japanese) is available at the JCTN website (www.jctn.jp).

JCTN Site Audit Guidelines

The method of site visit audits is also similar to that of NCI-sponsored cooperative groups. These guidelines include a method to select sites or cases for site audits, concrete auditing procedures, items to be checked, assessment criteria, reporting procedures, and storage of audit records. Templates for the check sheet and audit report (in Japanese) are also available at the JCTN website.

JCTN SAE Reporting Guidelines

The definition of "seriousness" regarding adverse events is based on the CTCAE, but these guidelines allow groups to stipulate protocol-specific exceptions in SAE reporting. These exceptions are specified because some grade 4 adverse events in the CTCAE are not always considered life-threatening and are clinically manageable. These exceptions are listed and reviewed in the regular monitoring report. A template for the SAE reporting format is also available at the JCTN website.

Domestic Collaboration

As a result of this cooperation and standardization, the number of domestic collaborative studies has been increasing. In particular, JCOG and WJOG, both with established headquarters and a focus on multimodal treatment for adult solid cancer, have conducted six collaborative trials in lung cancer and gastric cancer since 2008. An example is the JCOG0802/WJOG4607L trial, which is a phase III randomized trial of lobectomy versus limited resection (segmentectomy) for small peripheral non–small-cell lung cancer (UMIN-CTR number, UMIN000002317) (5). Seventy-six sites participated in the trial, and the patient accrual was completed in 5 years with a total of 1,106 patients. Such a large-scale pivotal trial is a good example of the role of collaboration in facilitating patient accrual.

INTERNATIONAL COLLABORATION

Japanese cooperative groups have already participated in international collaborative trials, examples of which are listed in Table 47.7. From the Japanese perspective, international collaboration can be classified into four models.

Model 1: Participation in Overseas Groups

In this model, Japanese institutions join overseas cooperative groups and conduct a clinical trial under the governance of the overseas group. Data management is performed by the headquarters of the overseas group. An example is Japanese institutions from JGOG belonging to the NRG Oncology Group. Essentially all of the requirements for participating sites are imposed by NRG, but there is a coordinating center in Japan that serves as a liaison office between the NRG headquarters and the participating sites in Japan. Japanese institutions have been joining NRG trials continuously under this model.

Model 2: Collaboration With a Single Data Center

In this model, a Japanese cooperative group and an overseas cooperative group collaboratively conduct a clinical trial based on a unique protocol. Data management is performed by the leading group. While data quality is good, site management of the nonleading group can be challenging. An example is the collaboration between the European Organization for Research and Treatment of Cancer (EORTC) and JCOG, with EORTC as the leading group (6). Data management is performed by the EORTC, while site selection and site audits are performed by JCOG. The JCOG headquarters serve as a liaison office to support Japanese sites.

Model 3: Collaboration With Multiple Data Centers

In this model, Japanese cooperative groups and an overseas cooperative group conduct a collaborative trial with a unique protocol. Data management is performed separately at each data center. An advantage is that, in general, the trial is easy to conduct, but it is sometimes difficult to harmonize data management procedures and communication between data centers. An example is a collaborative study on gastric cancer between JCOG and the Korean Gastric Cancer Association (7). Data management is performed at the JCOG Data Center and Seoul National University using a common database format, and data management procedures were agreed on before the start of the trial. Intensive communication between data centers is required to smoothly implement this type of collaboration.

Model 4: Parallel Study With Multiple Data Centers

In this model, multiple cooperative groups independently conduct a clinical trial using the same study design and perform a combined analysis afterward. Study protocol and data management procedures are individually specified by each group, although the

TABLE 47.7   Examples of International Collaboration of Japanese Cooperative Groups

Group	Examples of International Collaboration
JCOG	• Phase III trial of reductive gastrectomy (with Korean Gastric Cancer Association) • Diagnostic validity study of the accuracy of magnetic resonance imaging after preoperative chemotherapy for hepatic metastases (with EORTC) • Collaborative phase III trial with International Rare Cancer Initiatives for small bowel carcinoma (with CR-UK et al.)
WJOG	• Phase III study of 3-weekly cisplatin plus S-1 versus 5-weekly cisplatin plus S-1 in advanced gastric cancer (with Korean group led by Asan Medical Center)
CSPOR	• Adjuvant tamoxifen and exemestane study in early breast cancer (TEAM study with 9 countries) • Adjuvant capecitabine after neoadjuvant chemotherapy (CREATE-X trial with Korean researchers)
JGOG	• Phase III trial of paclitaxel plus carboplatin versus irinotecan plus cisplatin for clear cell carcinoma of the ovary (JGOG3017) (with GCIG, Gynecologic Cancer Intergroup) • Phase II/III trial of weekly intravenous paclitaxel plus intraperitoneal carboplatin for epithelial ovarian, fallopian tube, or primary peritoneal cancer (JGOG3019) (with Korea Gynecologic Oncology Group, Singapore, New Zealand, Hong Kong, United States) • Phase II trial of temsirolimus for clear cell carcinoma of the ovary (as GOG-0268)
JCCG	• Randomized phase II trial of sodium thiosulfate in reducing ototoxicity for standard risk hepatoblastoma (with International Childhood Liver Tumour Strategy Group – SIOPEL) • Phase III trial for hepatoblastoma with temsirolimus added to high-risk stratum treatment (as an intergroup study with COG) • International randomized trial to evaluate the role of vinblastine for high-risk ALCL (as ALCL99) • International study for first relapsed acute lymphoblastic leukemia (as IntReALL SR 2010)

ALCL, anaplastic large cell lymphoma; COG, Children's Oncology Group; CR-UK, Cancer Research United Kingdom; CSPOR-BC, Comprehensive Support Project for Oncology Research of Breast Cancer; EORTC, European Organization for Research and Treatment of Cancer; JCCG, Japan Children's Cancer Group; JCOG, Japan Clinical Oncology Group; JGOG, Japanese Gynecologic Oncology Group; WJOG, West Japan Oncology Group.

groups share common eligibility criteria, protocol treatments, examination schedules, and study design. This type of collaboration is easy for most groups because they are allowed to adjust the study protocol or procedure in accordance with their preferred approach. However, it is sometimes difficult for multiple groups to stay in the same place and proceed at the same speed. JCOG once conducted a parallel study with an overseas group, but the overseas trial was terminated early due to slow accrual, and the study continues as a JCOG-only trial (JCOG1018).

Some examples of international collaborative trials by JCTN groups are shown in Table 47.7.

Global Clinical Trial Core Centers

International collaboration by Japanese cooperative groups has been supported by funding from the MHLW. In particular, the coordinating role of JGOG in its collaboration with the NRG Oncology Group was established by the Global Research Core Hospital program at Kitasato University. Taking over the MHLW program, AMED has newly selected two Global Clinical Trial Core Centers: the National Cancer Center Hospital and Osaka University Hospital. The National Cancer Center Hospital is planning to reinforce the collaboration between EORTC and JCOG through this program. This program is expected to cultivate core operational functions for international clinical research and facilitate greater collaboration with overseas groups.

CURRENT ENVIRONMENTAL ANALYSIS

Thanks to the great effort of visionary leaders, Japan has developed well-organized cooperative groups and generated a significant amount of evidence from large-scale phase III trials, especially involving combined treatments with surgery, radiotherapy, and/or approved drugs. These evidences have been adopted in Japanese treatment guidelines and have changed clinical practice in Japan. In contrast, Japanese cooperative groups lag behind Western groups in terms of incorporating innovations in cancer treatment.

A current strength, weakness, opportunity, and threat (SWOT) analysis of Japanese cooperative groups is shown in Table 47.8. It should be noted that this analysis was performed considering large-scale adult disease groups such as JCOG, WJOG, JALSG, and JGOG.

TABLE 47.8   Strength, Weakness, Opportunity, Threat (SWOT) Analysis of Japanese Cooperative Groups

Strengths	Weaknesses
• Capable of enrolling large numbers of patients with various cancer types and stages • Many motivated investigators • Clinical trials for rare tumors • High study quality and extensive experience of Japanese cooperative groups • Multimodal trials, including surgery, endoscopy, and radiotherapy • Strong relationship between Japanese cancer treatment guidelines and trial results by Japanese cooperative groups	• Few trials focused on drug approval (*Chiken*) • Few trials incorporating innovations in cancer treatment • Minimal translational research • Few international collaborative studies • Slow process of protocol development
Opportunities	**Threats**
• Establishment of national funding agency (AMED) • Funding opportunities for rare cancer, elderly patients, and intractable cancer • Funding opportunities for international collaborative studies	• More stringent regulations • Restricted use of industry funding • Minimal funding for cooperative group infrastructure • Complicated process for trials of off-label use (Advanced Medical Care: *Senshin-Iryo*)

AMED, Japan Agency for Medical Research and Development.

Cooperative group mechanisms are essential to develop better standard treatments for various cancer types. Closer communication will be needed to enable Japanese cooperative groups to adjust to rapidly changing circumstances with multiple stakeholders, including funding agencies, regulatory authorities, basic researchers, patient advocates, and international cooperative groups.

REFERENCES

1. Fukuda H. Development of Cancer Cooperative Groups in Japan. *Jpn J Clin Oncol*. 2010;40:881–890.

2. Japanese Cancer Trial Network (JCTN) website. http://www.jctn.jp

3. McCurry J. Former Novartis employee arrested over valsartan data. *Lancet*. 2014;383:2111.

4. Japan Agency for Medical Research and Development (AMED) website. http://www.amed.go.jp/en

5. Nakamura K, Saji H, Nakajima R, et al. A phase III randomized trial of lobectomy versus limited resection for small-sized peripheral non-small cell lung cancer (JCOG0802/WJOG4607L). *Jpn J Clin Oncol*. 2010;40:271–274.

6. Kataoka K, Nakamura K, Caballero C, et al. Collaboration between EORTC and JCOG—how to accelerate global clinical research partnership. *Jpn J Clin Oncol*. (in press).

7. Fujitani K, Yang HK, Mizusawa, et al. Gastrectomy plus chemotherapy versus chemotherapy alone for advanced gastric cancer with a single non-curable factor (REGATTA): a phase 3, randomised controlled trial. *Lancet Oncol*. 2016;17:309–318.

COOPERATIVE GROUPS: THE AUSTRALIAN PERSPECTIVE

Prudence A. Francis, Katrin Sjoquist, and Linda Mileshkin

The Australian healthcare system is underpinned by a universal government-funded public system, with private healthcare also available. A number of national clinical trial networks have been established in Australia, across a wide range of clinical disciplines and disease groups including oncology. Clinical trial networks (cooperative groups) are now recognized in Australia as an important component of both a high-quality healthcare system and a strong clinical trial enterprise that includes commercial and public good trials (1). The clinical trial groups in the Australian health system are considered particularly effective at conducting high-impact public good and investigator-initiated clinical trials. Australian clinical trial groups have developed extensive global partnerships to undertake multinational trials, although many trials have been designed and/or led by Australian researchers. Oncology cooperative clinical trial groups feature prominently among the Australian clinical trial networks as the earliest groups, and currently comprise approximately one third of all the national cooperative trial groups. In this chapter, three well-established

Australian oncology cooperative clinical trials groups are discussed with reference to past and current activities, along with consideration of future directions.

The first oncology cooperative clinical trial groups in Australia were founded in the 1970s, with hematologic malignancy and breast cancer clinical trials the focus of the earliest groups. Over subsequent decades, an expanding range of national oncology cooperative clinical trial groups developed (Table 47.9). Many of these groups are described as Australasian, due to participation of both Australia and New Zealand. Many of the clinicians involved in founding/leading Australian oncology cooperative clinical trial groups have undertaken additional oncology and research training overseas, and have obtained university postgraduate research degrees after completing oncology training.

In recent years, limited central infrastructure funding has been provided through a government-funded organization called Cancer Australia, to support the oncology cooperative groups' capacity to develop industry-independent cancer clinical trials. This is with the goal of increasing the number of cancer clinical trials and clinical trial sites in Australia, and increasing the participation in clinical trials of clinicians, researchers, and people affected by cancer. Clinical trials conducted by a cooperative group can potentially be funded through peer-reviewed grant funding from the Australian National Health and Medical Research

TABLE 47.9 Australian Oncology Cooperative Clinical Trial Groups

Established	Acronym	Cooperative Group Name
1973	ALLG	Australasian **Leukaemia and Lymphoma** Group
1978	ANZBCTG	Australia and New Zealand **Breast Cancer** Trials Group
1986	ANZCCSG ANZCHOG	Australian and New Zealand **Children's Cancer** Study Group (name change) Australian and New Zealand **Children's Haematology/Oncology** Group
1989	TROG	Trans-Tasman **Radiation** Oncology Group
1991	AGITG	Australasian **Gastro-Intestinal** Trials Group
1999	ANZMTG	Australia and New Zealand **Melanoma** Trials Group
2000	ANZGOG	Australia New Zealand **Gynaecological Oncology** Group
2004	ALTG	Australasian **Lung Cancer** Trials Group
2005	PoCOG	**Psycho-oncology** Co-operative Research Group
2007	COGNO	Cooperative Trials Group for **Neuro-Oncology**
2007	PaCCSC	**Palliative Care** Clinical Studies Collaborative
2008	ANZUP	Australia and New Zealand **Urogenital and Prostate Cancer** Trials Group
2008	ASSG	Australasian **Sarcoma** Study Group
2009	PC4	**Primary Care** Collaborative Cancer Clinical Trials Group

Council (NHMRC), Cancer Australia, or allied funding schemes, although such funding is increasingly highly competitive.

While all 14 oncology cooperative clinical trial groups operate under slightly different models, they are linked under the auspices of the Executive Officers Network. Established by the Clinical Oncology Society of Australia (COSA), this network exists to facilitate information exchange, support, and learning from common challenges. Several common challenges have been overcome through this network, including regulatory and administrative burdens, through establishment of a common clinical trial research agreement for cooperative group trials and an umbrella clinical trial insurance policy.

AUSTRALIA AND NEW ZEALAND BREAST CANCER TRIALS GROUP (ANZBCTG)

ANZBCTG was established in 1978 and is the largest independent oncology clinical trial research group in Australia and New Zealand. For almost 40 years, ANZBCTG has conducted a clinical trial research program for the treatment, prevention, and cure of breast cancer. The ANZBCTG research program involves multicenter national and international clinical trials and brings together more than 800 multidisciplinary

researchers across 90 institutions. More than 14,000 women have participated in the ANZBCTG breast cancer clinical trial research program and the group has contributed to approximately 1,000 publications to date. ANZBCTG clinicians' participation in and implementation of the results of the breast cancer research, has contributed to the significant improvement in breast cancer related mortality that has occurred over the last 30 years.

For large phase 3 adjuvant therapy, surgical, *ductal carcinoma in situ (*DCIS), or breast cancer prevention trials, ANZBCTG has traditionally contributed to international collaborative group trials coordinated by other groups. The group has contributed to numerous practice-changing international trials testing endocrine and HER2-targeted therapies, chemotherapy, and surgical trials (Table 47.10) (2–9). ANZBCTG participation has made an important contribution to the global clinical evidence base in breast cancer research. ANZBCTG has contributed to inform meta-analyses and overviews in breast cancer, including the Early Breast Cancer Trialists' Collaborative Group Oxford (EBCTCG) overviews, St. Gallen International Expert Consensus recommendations in primary breast cancer (10), and Cochrane systematic reviews.

While the ANZBCTG has not usually been the coordinating/lead group for phase 3 adjuvant breast cancer trials, ANZBCTG investigators have been involved in

TABLE 47.10   ANZBCTG Participation in International Collaborative Group Trials (Selected)

Trial (Activated)	Setting	Intervention	Outcome
IBCSG 9 (1988)	Adjuvant	CMF chemotherapy	Efficacy in postmenopausal node-negative ER-negative cancer
IBIS 1 (1992)	Prevention	Tamoxifen	Reduced risk of hormone receptor positive breast cancer
IBCSG 13 (1993)	Adjuvant	Tamoxifen	Efficacy in premenopausal hormone receptor positive breast cancer
IBCSG 10 (1993)	Surgical	No axillary dissection	Similar efficacy, better quality of life in women >60, clinically node-negative, planned for tamoxifen
ATLAS (1996)	Adjuvant	Tamoxifen	Efficacy of extended duration of therapy
ATAC (1998)	Adjuvant	Anastrozole	Superiority in postmenopausal hormone receptor positive breast cancer
BIG 1-98 (1999)	Adjuvant	Letrozole	Superiority in postmenopausal hormone receptor positive breast cancer
HERA (2001)	Adjuvant	Trastuzumab	Efficacy in HER2 positive early breast cancer

ANZBCTG, Australia and New Zealand Breast Cancer Trials Group.

designing international adjuvant breast cancer trials and chairing trials at an international level (11–14), with the adjuvant Suppression of Ovarian Function Trial (SOFT) conducted in premenopausal breast cancer, a recent example that contributed to updated American Society of Clinical Oncology treatment guidelines (15). The phase 3 LATER trial, conducted by ANZBCTG without international collaboration, tested the late reintroduction of adjuvant endocrine therapy, with results supporting reintroduction/longer duration of endocrine therapy (16). During the past decade, ANZBCTG has also been gaining experience in conducting neoadjuvant breast cancer trials. In 2017 ANZBCTG launched and is leading a multicenter international collaborative group trial (EXPERT) that is examining personalized radiation therapy for low-risk early breast cancer (NCT02889874).

ANZBCTG has conducted numerous independent phase 3 trials in metastatic breast cancer. Quality of life (QOL) assessments have been considered an important part of trials conducted at ANZBCTG centers. In the randomized ANZ 0001 first-line chemotherapy trial conducted in advanced breast cancer patients unsuited to more intensive regimens, quality-adjusted progression-free survival (PFS) was chosen as the primary endpoint (17), although capecitabine was found to result in an overall survival advantage compared with CMF chemotherapy. The most influential and highly cited phase 3 study in metastatic breast cancer conducted by the ANZBCTG was the ANZ 8101 trial, which was designed around a QOL endpoint. The trial initiated in 1982 compared continuous chemotherapy versus intermittent chemotherapy, in patients with advanced disease after an initial three cycles of chemotherapy, and found that QOL was better with a continuous chemotherapy strategy (18).

In 1994, ANZBCTG established a department dedicated to fund-raising and education/public awareness, which has successfully helped support the research programs and has resulted in the group having a sound financial position. As a consequence, ANZBCTG has the capacity to support Discretionary Funding research applications for pilot research projects that may subsequently lead to a group trial. ANZBCTG first invited a consumer to join its Scientific Advisory Committee in 1994, with an ANZBCTG Consumer Advisory Panel subsequently formed in 1999. Consumer Advisory Panel members are involved in the research process from the early planning stages, reviewing protocols, patient information, and consent forms, and provide an important consumer perspective in breast cancer clinical trial research.

AUSTRALASIAN GASTRO-INTESTINAL TRIALS GROUP (AGITG)

Established in 1991, the AGITG has grown substantially over the past 25 years, with over 800 current members. Both membership and international standing have expanded, with the group now leading international phase III trials and research that has defined new standards of care around the world. With the remit of conducting trials in different primary gastrointestinal (GI) cancers, successful trial conduct has necessitated strong collaborations with international trial groups, including the Canadian Cancer Trials Group (formerly NCIC-CTG), European Organization for Research and Treatment of Cancer (EORTC; Europe), and Oncology *Clinical Trials* Office (OCTO; United Kingdom). The group is truly multidisciplinary in nature, with representation from medical, radiation, and surgical subspecialties, as well as diverse allied health input and a strong Consumer Advisory Panel.

The AGITG's stated mission is to improve health outcomes through research in prevention, screening, and treatment in GI cancers. Key clinical trials and research exemplifying the group's success in achieving this goal include: major involvement in trials of imatinib for gastrointestinal stromal tumors (GIST), including pivotal phase 3 studies in advanced disease and adjuvant treatment in resected disease; and in collaboration with the NCIC-CTG, a pivotal phase 3 trial (NCIC-CTG/AGITG C0.17) that not only established cetuximab as an effective therapy for previously treated advanced colorectal cancer (19) but demonstrated that the benefit of such treatment was confined to patients without any mutations in the KRAS gene (20).

The role of imatinib (800 mg vs. 400 mg/day) in advanced GIST was established by the EORTC- ISG-AGITG 62005 phase III study, which found that PFS was improved at the higher dose level but there was no difference in overall survival (21). A subsequent AGITG led phase II REGISTER trial has closed to recruitment and is undergoing analysis. The REGISTER trial (ACTRN12608000392369) aims to evaluate a risk-modified dose-escalation strategy for patients with advanced GIST based on their underlying KIT mutation status (high risk: exon 9/wild type [WT] vs. low risk: exon 11). Now standard of care for intermediate- and high-risk resected GIST, the benefit of adjuvant imatinib, was established by another trial in which AGITG was a significant contributor (22). The 62024 randomized phase III international study demonstrated an improvement in failure-free survival and 3-year survival for participants receiving 2 years of imatinib versus placebo.

The NCIC-CTG/AGITG C0.17 trial is an example of practice-changing research, which has catalyzed further significant research advances. This randomized international phase III trial in advanced colorectal cancer, following failure of standard treatments, established both the benefit of cetuximab, the first approved epidermal growth factor receptor (EGFR) antibody in this setting (19), and the importance of *KRAS* mutations as predictive biomarkers for benefit from this treatment (20). Subsequent trials have sought to increase understanding of this class of agents and their role in therapy, with a recent randomized phase II AGITG trial exploring the benefit of cetuximab, with or without irinotecan, in tumors harboring *KRAS* G13D mutations (23). The ability to recruit 50 patients with a rare, molecularly defined subtype of colorectal cancer exemplifies the benefits of the collaborative group network of engaged investigators, where cross-referrals frequently occur to facilitate participation.

AUSTRALIA NEW ZEALAND GYNAECOLOGICAL ONCOLOGY GROUP (ANZGOG)

ANZGOG is the peak gynecological cooperative clinical trial group in Australasia, and has accrued over 1,000 women to gynecological cancer clinical trials since the group was established in 2001. ANZGOG has a multidisciplinary membership of over 700, which includes virtually all of the oncologists—medical, gynecological, and radiation, with a specific interest in gynecological cancer in Australia and New Zealand. The group has established collaborations with other cooperative groups involved in gynecological cancer research through its membership of the international Gynecologic Cancer InterGroup (GCIG). Because many gynecological cancers in fact are rare cancers, it is acknowledged that large phase 3 trials in these disease types usually require international collaboration. The GCIG (https://gciggroup.com) is an umbrella organization that encompasses all of the major cooperative groups working in gynecological cancer around the world. The GCIG has two face-to-face meetings per year and involves a number of disease-specific and research-type committees that discuss the development of new international clinical trials. ANZGOG representatives have chaired a number of these committees from Harmonisation to Symptom Benefit, and introduced a similar internal process of having disease-specific working groups (e.g., endometrial) to develop new clinical trial proposals. As consumers are critical stakeholders in health and medical research, ANZGOG embraces consumer and community participation in health and medical research, including a very active Consumer and Community Committee with a robust process for engaging consumers in clinical trial development.

ANZGOG has been a significant contributor to many large international trials, which have or will in the future change practice, and has contributed to or led more than 90 publications. These trials include GOG 182, which confirmed the optimum chemotherapy regimen for advanced ovarian cancer (24); GOG 199, which identified the role of prophylactic surgery in women with a high risk of ovarian cancer; CALYPSO (25), a trial leading to multiple high-impact publications about recurrent disease; and the preceding ICON6 and ICON7 trials, which determined the value of adding a biological agent to current standard chemotherapy treatment for ovarian cancer. ICON7 has already led to reimbursement of bevacizumab for ovarian cancer in the United Kingdom and Australia (26), and cediranib remains in development as an agent to treat ovarian cancer as a result of ICON6 (27).

As the lead international group, ANZGOG is responsible for three current trials with potentially practice-changing results in gynecologic cancers. The first of these, the Symptom Benefit trial (ACTRN12607000603415), has completed accrual and is undergoing analysis. Designed to develop better methods to evaluate clinical benefit in platinum-resistant/refractory ovarian cancer, it has resulted in the development and evaluation of a new instrument, the Measure of Ovarian cancer Symptoms and Treatment concerns (MOST) (28). With the importance of patient-reported outcomes (PROs) increasingly recognized as key clinical and trial endpoints, the MOST has the potential to become an important tool in both clinical practice and future trial design (29).

The OUTBACK trial (ACTRN12610000732088) is an adjuvant therapy trial in cervical cancer that completed the enrollment of 900 women with locally advanced cervical cancer planned to receive chemoradiation in mid 2017. This international phase III randomized trial led by ANZGOG seeks to determine whether the addition of adjuvant chemotherapy (carboplatin–paclitaxel), following standard chemoradiation to the pelvis, improves overall survival (30). The PARAGON trial (ACTRN12610000796088) also led by ANZGOG is one of the first examples of using a basket protocol to enable more efficient research into several rare cancer types at once. The aim is to investigate anastrozole, in patients with various estrogen-receptor/progesterone-receptor-positive metastatic gynecological cancers in a series of seven individual phase 2 studies embedded into a basket protocol (31,32). ANZGOG has also been successful in establishing substudies within several international trials. For example, within the recently completed PORTEC-3 trial examining the utility of adjuvant chemotherapy in high-risk endometrial cancer (33), ANZGOG has led substudies into radiation quality assurance (34) and patient preferences for chemotherapy (35).

NATIONAL HEALTH AND MEDICAL RESEARCH COUNCIL CLINICAL TRIALS CENTRE

The NHMRC Clinical Trials Centre in Sydney is the coordinating center for five of the Australasian Cancer Cooperative Trials Groups (CCTGs; AGITG, Australasian Lung Cancer Trials Group [ALTG], ANZGOG, Australia and New Zealand Urogenital and Prostate Cancer Trials Group [ANZUP], Cooperative Trials Group for Neuro-Oncology [COGNO]), and the statistical center for another group (ANZBCTG). The Clinical Trials Centre also conducts clinical trials in other cancers, as well as diabetes, neonatology, and cardiovascular diseases. As the only academic research organisation of its type in Australia, the NHMRC Clinical Trials Centre is nationally and internationally recognized for expertise in clinical trial methodology and conduct. As a founding member of Australian Clinical Trials Alliance (ACTA), the NHMRC Clinical Trials Centre seeks to design and deliver well-conducted, clinically relevant trials answering important questions for patients. One such example is the Sentinel Node biopsy versus Axillary Clearance (SNAC) breast cancer trial, conducted in collaboration with the Royal Australasian College of Surgeons (36). A randomized trial of 1,088 women, the SNAC trial established the benefits of sentinel node biopsy as compared to routine axillary clearance, for women with early breast cancer undergoing primary resection, with reduced upper limb morbidity in the sentinel node group at 1 and 3 years after surgery.

GENOMIC CANCER CLINICAL TRIALS INITIATIVE

In 2013, Cancer Australia established a Genomics Cancer Clinical Trials Initiative, which is led by the NHMRC Clinical Trials Centre at the University of Sydney in partnership with Zest Health Strategies. Not a clinical trial group itself, it is intended to build capacity to conduct genomic cancer clinical research activity across Australia, with the remit to support researchers to develop mutation-specific clinical trial concepts and grant applications involving cancers from more than one primary site and more than one of Australia's CCTGs. Recognizing that small, molecularly defined cohorts of tumors often exist across anatomically defined tumor types, this framework is designed to facilitate development of ideas that would be difficult to run within the established mechanisms of individual groups established around more traditional cancer type groupings. The most promising concept(s) each year are identified with input from the Scientific Steering group, and developed for submission to nationally competitive funding schemes. To date, three individual concepts have been submitted, and one has received funding.

FUTURE DIRECTIONS AND CHALLENGES

Despite their achievements, oncology cooperative clinical trial groups in Australia face a variety of challenges. The cumulative burden and lack of funding for long-term follow-up of breast trial participants is significant, although ANZBCTG were recently successful in obtaining 5 years of additional government funding for follow-up of the premenopausal women they randomized in the SOFT and TEXT trials. With progressively improving outcomes in early-stage breast cancer, it is increasingly difficult to demonstrate the types of improvements seen in previous generations of trials. As a consequence, there is a changing paradigm from large phase III breast cancer trials in which many sites could enroll a reasonable number of patients, to smaller niche trials with novel designs or molecularly defined cohorts. Sometimes only a finite number of Australian sites will be selected to participate by overseas collaborative partner groups in such trials, which may lead to disengagement of other sites or inability to retain trial support staff. With fewer large phase III trials, there is a move toward earlier phase, pilot, and neoadjuvant trials, which can require groups to adapt their skill sets and these types of trials may not be well-suited to the participation of all sites. Substantial administrative burdens result from small patient numbers in such trials. With the imperative to obtain trial results in a reasonable time frame, the shift toward use of surrogate endpoints as an alternative to overall survival or disease-free survival is increasingly explored, but may bring its own challenges. Australian investigators who collaborate internationally suffer the tyranny of distance, with the time and expense of traveling to meetings, in addition to different time zones producing unfavorable hours for teleconferencing.

Funding of investigator-initiated cooperative group clinical trials remains challenging. There is currently one main government-funded peer-reviewed grant cycle annually, with grant submissions due in March and outcomes not known till late in the year, with funding for successful grants initiated in January the following year. With the maximum duration of grant funding 3 to 5 years, this duration may still be insufficient to complete a clinical trial, requiring additional time-consuming submissions to obtain further funding. The maximum budget that can be obtained from this type of funding is generally insufficient to support the full cost of a large phase III oncology trial. Moreover, individual trials effectively compete against each other, as well as other types of research including basic scientific research, for a fixed pool of funding. Ideally, a dedicated pool of funding that represented a fixed proportion of the overall healthcare budget would be allocated for clinical trial research. For overseas group trial collaborations, fluctuating currencies can make trial budgets/payments less predictable. Competition with better funded industry trials also presents a challenge for cooperative groups and the need to provide site payments that reflect the actual costs of conducting research becomes increasingly important.

AUSTRALIAN CLINICAL TRIALS ALLIANCE TRIAL OF THE YEAR AWARD

In 2016, the ACTA introduced the "Trial of the Year Award" celebrating Australian leadership and excellence in clinical trials. Eligible trials are collaboratively developed, multicenter, investigator-driven, randomized controlled trials that were designed to improve patient-centered outcomes or healthcare delivery with primary results published in the previous year. The SOFT premenopausal early breast cancer trial was a finalist, with a randomized obstetric trial in preterm rupture of membranes winning the inaugural award. The ACTA Trial of the Year Award was presented on 20 May—International Clinical Trials Day—which commemorates the day in 1747 that naval surgeon James Lind began a clinical trial for scurvy. The award aims to acknowledge the major improvements in health outcomes that have resulted due to clinicians dedicated to finding answers to important clinical questions and members of the community who participate in clinical trials.

REFERENCES

1. Australian Clinical Trials Alliance: Report on the activities and achievement of clinical trials networks in Australia 2004–2014. 2015. www.clinicaltrialsalliance.org.au/publications
2. Cuzick J, Forbes JF, Sestak I, et al. Long-term results of tamoxifen prophylaxis for breast cancer – 96 months follow-up of the randomized IBIS 1 Trial. *J Natl Cancer Inst.* 2007;99:272–282.
3. International Breast Cancer Study Group. Tamoxifen after adjuvant chemotherapy for premenopausal women with lymph node-positive breast cancer: International Breast Cancer Study Group Trial 13-93. *J Clin Oncol.* 2006;24:1332–1341.
4. The ATAC (Arimidex, Tamoxifen Alone or in Combination) Trialists' Group. Anastrozole alone or in combination with tamoxifen versus tamoxifen alone for adjuvant treatment of postmenopausal women with early breast cancer: first result of the ATAC randomised trial. *Lancet.* 2002;359:2131–2139.
5. The Breast International Group (BOG) 1-98 Collaborative Group. A comparison of letrozole and tamoxifen in postmenopausal women with early breast cancer. *N Engl J Med.* 2005;353:2747–2757.
6. Davies C, Pan H, Godwin J, et al. Long term effects of continuing adjuvant tamoxifen to 10 years versus stopping at 5 years after diagnosis of oestrogen receptor-positive breast cancer. *Lancet.* 2013;381:805–816.
7. Piccart-Gebhart MJ, Procter M, Lleyland-Jones B, et al. Trastuzumab after adjuvant chemotherapy in HER2-positive breast cancer. *N Engl J Med.* 2005;353:1659–1672.
8. International Breast Cancer Study Group. Endocrine responsiveness and tailoring adjuvant therapy for postmenopausal lymph node-negative breast cancer: a randomized trial. *J Natl Cancer Inst.* 2002;94:1054–1065.
9. International Breast Cancer Study Group. Randomized trial comparing axillary clearance versus no axillary clearance in older patients with breast cancer: first results of International Breast Cancer Study Group Trial 10-93. *J Clin Oncol.* 2006;24:337–344.
10. Coates AS, Winder EP, Goldhirsch A, et al. Tailoring therapies-improving the management of early breast cancer: St Gallen International Expert Consensus on the Primary Therapy of Early Breast Cancer 2015. *Ann Oncol.* 2015;6:1533–1546.
11. International Breast Cancer Study Group. Multicycle dose-intensive chemotherapy for women with high-risk primary breast cancer: results of International Breast Cancer Study Group Trial 15-95. *J Clin Oncol.* 2006;24:370–378.
12. Francis P, Crown J, Di Leo A, et al on behalf of the BIG 02-98 Collaborative Group. Adjuvant chemotherapy with sequential or concurrent anthracycline and docetaxel: Breast International Group 02-98 randomized trial. *J Natl Cancer Inst.* 2008;100:121–133.
13. Pagani O, Regan MM, Walley BA, et al. Adjuvant exemestane with ovarian suppression in premenopausal breast cancer. *N Engl J Med.* 2014;371:101–118.
14. Francis PA, Regan MM, Fleming GF, et al. Adjuvant ovarian suppression in premenopausal breast cancer. *N Engl J Med.* 2015;372:436–446.
15. Burstein HJ, Lacchetti C, Anderson H, et al. Adjuvant endocrine therapy for women with hormone receptor-positive breast cancer: American Society of Clinical Oncology Clinical Practice Guideline Update on Ovarian Suppression. *J Clin Oncol.* 2016;34:1689–1701.
16. Zdenkowski N, Forbes JF, Boyle FM, et al. Observation versus late reintroduction of letrozole as adjuvant endocrine therapy for hormone receptor-positive breast cancer (ANZ 0501 LATER): an open label randomized controlled trial. *Ann Oncol.* 2016;27:806–812.
17. Stockler MR, Harvey V, Francis P, et al. Capecitabine versus classical CMF as first line chemotherapy for advanced breast cancer. *J Clin Oncol.* 2011;29:4498–4504.
18. Coates A, Gebski V, Bishop JF, et al. Improving the quality of life during chemotherapy for advanced breast cancer. *N Engl J Med.* 1987;317:1490–1495.
19. Jonker DJ, O'Callaghan CJ, Karapetis CS, et al. Cetuximab for the treatment of colorectal cancer. *New Engl J Med.* 2007;357:2040–2048.
20. Karapetis CS, Khambata-Ford S, Jonker DJ, et al. K-ras mutations and benefit from cetuximab in advanced colorectal cancer. *New Engl J Med.* 2008;359:1757–1765.
21. Verweij J, Casali PG, Zalcberg J, et al. Progression-free survival in gastrointestinal stromal tumours with high-dose imatinib: randomised trial. *Lancet.* 2004;364:1127–1134.
22. Casali PG, Le Cesne A, Velasco AP, et al. Time to definitive failure to the first tyrosine kinase inhibitor in localized GI stromal tumors treated with imatinib as an adjuvant: a European Organisation for Research and Treatment of Cancer Soft Tissue and Bone Sarcoma Group Intergroup Randomized Trial in collaboration with the Australasian Gastro-Intestinal Trials Group, UNICANCER, French Sarcoma Group, Italian Sarcoma Group, and Spanish Group for Research on Sarcomas. *J Clin Oncol.* 2015;33:4276–4283.
23. Segelov E, Thavaneswaran S, Waring PM, et al. Response to cetuximab with or without irinotecan in patients with refractory metastatic colorectal cancer harboring the KRAS G13D mutation: Australasian Gastro-Intestinal Trials Group ICECREAM Study. *J Clin Oncol.* 2016;34(19):2258–2264.
24. Bookman MA, Brady MF, McGuire WP, et al. Evaluation of new platinum-based treatment regimens in advanced-stage ovarian cancer: a Phase III Trial of the Gynecologic Cancer Intergroup. *J Clin Oncol.* 2009;27(9):1419–1425.
25. Wagner U, Marth C, Largillier R, et al. Final overall survival results of phase III GCIG CALYPSO trial of pegylated liposomal doxorubicin and carboplatin vs paclitaxel and carboplatin in platinum-sensitive ovarian cancer patients. *Br J Cancer.* 2012;107:588–591.
26. Oza AM, Cook AD, Pfisterer J, et al. ICON7 trial investigators. Standard chemotherapy with or without bevacizumab for women with newly diagnosed ovarian cancer (ICON7): Overall survival results of a phase 3 randomised trial. *Lancet Oncol.* 2015;16(8):928–936.
27. Ledermann JA, Embleton AC, Raja F, et al. ICON6 collaborators. Cediranib in patients with relapsed platinum-sensitive ovarian cancer (ICON6): a randomised, double-blind, placebo-controlled phase 3 trial. *Lancet.* 2016;387(10023):1066–1074.
28. King MT, Stockler MR, Butow P, et al. Development of the Measure of Ovarian Symptoms and Treatment concerns aiming for optimal measurement of patient-reported symptom benefit with chemotherapy for symptomatic ovarian cancer. *Int J Gyn Cancer.* 2014;24(5):865–873.

29. Friedlander M, Stockler MR, O'Connell R, et al. Is it time to change the primary endpoint in clinical trials in recurrent ovarian cancer (ROC)?: Symptom burden and outcomes in patients with platinum resistant/refractory (PRR) and potentially platinum sensitive ROC receiving ≥ 3 lines of chemotherapy (PPS ≥ 3)—The Gynecologic Cancer Intergroup (GCIG) Symptom Benefit Study (SBS). *J Clin Oncol* (ASCO Meeting Abstracts). 2015;33(15 suppl):5536.

30. Mileshkin LR, Narayan K, Moore KN, et al. A phase III trial of adjuvant chemotherapy following chemoradiation as primary treatment for locally advanced cervical cancer compared to chemoradiation alone: Outback (ANZGOG0902/GOG0274/RTOG1174). *J Clin Oncol* (Meeting Abstracts). 2014;32(15_suppl):TPS5632.

31. Mileshkin LR, Edmondson RJ, O'Connell R, et al. Phase II study of anastrozole in recurrent estrogen (ER)/progesterone (PR) positive endometrial cancer: the PARAGON trial—ANZGOG 0903. *J Clin Oncol* (Meeting Abstracts). 2016;34(15_suppl):5520.

32. Bonaventura A, O'Connell RL, Mapagu C, et al. Paragon (ANZGOG-0903): Phase 2 study of anastrozole in women with estrogen or progesterone receptor-positive platinum-resistant or -refractory recurrent ovarian cancer. *Int J Gynecol Cancer*. 2017;27(5):900–906.

33. de Boer SM, Powell ME, Mileshkin L, et al. Toxicity and quality of life after adjuvant chemotherapy and radiation therapy (RT) versus RT alone for women with high-risk endometrial cancer: first results of the randomised PORTEC-3 trial. *Lancet Oncol*. 2016;17(8):1114–1126.

34. Jameson MG, McNamara J, Bailey M, et al. Results of the Australasian (TROG) radiotherapy dummy run exercise in preparation for participation in the PORTEC-3 trial. *JMIRO*. 2016;60(4):554–559.

35. Blinman P, Mileshkin L, Khaw P, et al. Patients' and clinicians' preferences for adjuvant chemotherapy in endometrial cancer: an ANZGOG sub-study of the PORTEC-3 intergroup randomized trial. *Br J Cancer*. 2016;115:1179–1185.

36. Wetzig N, Gill PG, Zannino D, et al. Sentinel lymph node based management or routine axillary clearance? Three-year outcomes of the RACS sentinel node biopsy versus axillary clearance (SNAC) 1 trial. *Ann Sur Oncol*. 2015;22:17–23.

COOPERATIVE GROUPS: A LATIN AMERICAN PERSPECTIVE

Gustavo Werutsky

LATIN AMERICA DEMOGRAPHY AND SOCIOECONOMIC CHARACTERISTICS

Latin America is one of the biggest continents in the world, comprising 20 countries and an estimated population, as of 2015, of more than 626 million (1).

The predominant language is Spanish and Portuguese. Poverty continues to be one of the region's main challenges and according to the Economic Commission for Latin America and the Caribbean (ECLAC) it is the most unequal region in the world (2).

Latin American countries are characterized by sociocultural, economic, and political diversity, with wide socioeconomic and health disparities. Population is concentrated in large urban areas as well as most hospitals and cancer specialists working in tertiary cancer centers offering cutting-edge, complex, multimodality treatments. The geographical distribution imposes difficulties for cancer care for people living outside urban areas (3).

There are disparities in health-care spending across countries in Latin America. The average health expenditure is 7.7% of gross domestic product (GDP) compared to 9.5% in Japan or 9.6% in the United Kingdom. Several barriers to optimal treatment and lack of access to high-cost medications is a reality and therefore the total economic burden of cancer in Latin America, including medical and nonmedical costs, is estimated to be around US$4 billion (3,4).

In recent decades, economic growth, access to basic health care, and the increase in life expectancy have changed the morbidity and mortality profile of the population. In the context of this epidemiological transition, Latin American countries have focused their health investment on prevention and treatment of infectious diseases, whereas spending on noncommunicable diseases, such as cancer that represents the second most common cause of death in the region, has not been prioritized (5–9).

CANCER BURDEN IN LATIN AMERICA

Epidemiology

Cancer burden is a human and economic threat to low- and middle-income countries because 56% of the global new cases and 64% of deaths occur in developing countries. According to GLOBOCAN 2012, in Latin America and the Caribbean it is estimated that 1 million new cases and 603,000 deaths occur annually (10).

Although the overall incidence of cancer is lower in Latin America (age-standardized rate of 163 per 100,000) than in Europe (264 per 100,000) or the United States (300 per 100,000), the mortality burden is greater (11). The most common cancer types in Latin America are prostate, breast, and cervix uteri with the higher mortality being prostate, breast, and lung cancer respectively (10).

Cancer Registries

One of the pillars to cancer control is through investment in cancer registries to prioritize policies in prevention initiatives, effective interventions, and monitor results (12).

Latin America has a deficiency of high-quality cancer registries where only 6% of the population is covered by population-based cancer registries compared to 83% in North America and 32% in Europe. In Latin America, there are 48 cancer registries in 18 countries. A few centers in the region have produced quality statistics over a large period of time (13–15).

There are some initiatives to improve cancer registries in the region. The Union for International Cancer Control has a Global Initiative for Cancer Registry Development (GICR) in low- and middle-income countries, in collaboration with regional partners such as the Pan American Health Organization, Red de Institutos Nacionales de Cáncer, and Latin American excellence centers. GICR offers assistance to national authorities in planning and strengthening cancer registration through methodological, technical, educational support, and collaborative research (16,17).

Importantly, observational studies that are relatively inexpensive might contribute to better understanding the patterns of cancer care in the region and give some sort of experience for investigators and sites to run less complex studies. In Brazil, patients with breast cancer with public health coverage present with more advanced disease and worse survival when compared with those with private coverage (18).

CLINICAL TRIALS IN LATIN AMERICA

Clinical trials in the Latin American region are limited. In January 2017, only 5.9% of ongoing phase I to III cancer clinical trials registered in clinicaltrials.gov worldwide have been performed in Latin America (19). The majority of clinical trials ongoing in the region are phase II and III studies sponsored by pharmaceutical companies, wherein participating local investigators contribute in the recruitment. Trials funded by pharmaceutical companies have resulted in improved clinical trial infrastructure and investigators' experience. Enrolling patients from densely populated urban areas can be straightforward, whereas enrollment to trials that are of specific importance to rural and remote areas is much more challenging because of lack of infrastructure and investment (20).

The results of trials designed by developed countries may not necessarily attend overall to local Latin American patient needs and, more importantly, do not guarantee access to therapy. For example, a well-established therapy with 1-year adjuvant trastuzumab for early-stage HER2 positive breast cancer might not be cost effective in several Latin American countries (21). Besides that, adjuvant trastuzumab for breast cancer was only provided in the public health system in Brazil 8 years after its first regulatory approval in United States. Publications in peer-reviewed scientific journals from Latin American studies are also uncommon. A study shows that only 1% of abstracts in the American Society of Clinical Oncology (ASCO) annual meeting from 2001 to 2005 were from Brazilian investigators. Almost half of them were retrospective analyses. Several recently published major oncology studies have included a substantial number of patients from Brazil, thus ensuring co-authorship to Brazilian investigators (22).

The main challenges for clinical cancer research are described in Table 47.11. The limited funding for cancer research is a reality in Latin America, as they rely on public funding and are applied basically in postgraduation (e.g., PhD) grants. It is clear that the investment in research and development is lower in Latin America as Brazil invests 1.1% of GDP and Mexico 0.9%, which is two to three times less than developing countries (23). Also, the lack of financial support and specific regulation for academic clinical research have limited the possibility of local investigators to design and run clinical studies that are innovative or important to Latin American populations. Other barriers to clinical research in Latin America are lack of training and experience in developing and conducting clinical trials, site infrastructure to address specific research needs, delays in ethical and regulatory approval and, in some countries, the negative government perception about clinical research.

Latin American patient accrual rates are high and the data generated are generally of high quality, and most Latin American studies meet the high standards set by regulatory agencies in the United States and Europe for approval of new therapies (24).

Overcoming Barriers to Clinical Trials

Latin American countries have to take the opportunity to embark on incentive clinical research development in the era where large numbers of novel therapies that target specific tumor markers are creating an increasing need for international trial collaborations to enroll sufficient patients. Delays in initiating clinical trials have been a substantial challenge in the region, particularly in Brazil (25). Simplifying regulations and making regulatory agencies work more efficiently is a completely feasible measure that can boost countries' participation in clinical trials. Although challenged by the lack of public or alternative funding sources, academic studies can provide valuable information to Latin Americans in areas such as surgery, radiotherapy, and high prevalent cancers in the region. Lastly, patients and advocacy groups also have an increasing role in supporting clinical research. However, educational initiatives about clinical trials and access to information regarding where to find active studies are essential (26,27).

TABLE 47.11   Challenges for Cancer Research and Cooperative Groups in Latin America

Challenges	Description of Actual Situation
Cancer registry	Poor quality and little coverage population of cancer registries in Latin America.
Academic research organizations policy	No recognition and specific policies about academic research organizations.
Regulation for clinical research	Complex regulation and delay for clinical trial approval.
Funding	Lack of public and private funding for clinical research. Due to no specific regulations for academic research it is very costly for local investigators to run a clinical trial.
Observational studies	Continue and improve observational studies, which describe patterns of care in the region.
Information about clinical research for patients	Very limited information about clinical research is provided to patients. Health authorities and institutions have to make this educational communication available and easily accessible.
Education and training of investigators and other specialties	Lack of educational programs and workshops in clinical research.

Cooperative Groups in Latin America

The development of cooperative groups for cancer research in Latin America is recent and the majority have been established in the past 10 to 20 years. A list of cooperative research groups is described in Table 47.12. In general, the cooperative groups in Latin America were founded by a group of investigators, not institutions, with the aim to promote cancer research locally, address important questions from the regional population, and collaborate with studies internationally.

In general, these groups have limited personnel and infrastructure to manage clinical trials. Therefore they concentrate their work on translational or observational studies. There are several challenges faced by cooperative groups in Latin America to maintain their activities such as: financial constraints to support a minimum research structure, lack of funding to perform the studies, limited number of qualified cancer and clinical research specialists (physicians, statisticians, among others), inefficiency in the regulatory authority processes (delays in protocol approval), and a national and regional regulation,

which does not recognize academic research making the costs to run clinical trials prohibitive.

Therefore a few groups have the structure to run an entire clinical trial and it is attractive and beneficial to participate in international intergroup studies whereas a restricted number of activities are done by the local group at the same time gaining experience with study management. This model was used, for example, in intergroup breast cancer trials such as HERA and NeoALTTO with participation of groups in Peru (Grupo de Estudios Clínicos Oncológicos Peruano [GECOPERU]) and Brazil (**Grupo Brasileiro de Estudos em Cancer de Mama** [GBECAM]) (28,29).

Another type of interaction to support cancer clinical trials in the region is the Southwest Oncology Group (SWOG) Latin America Initiative, which offers many levels of collaboration with regional sites. SWOG statisticians serve as mentors, bringing years of experience running large-scale cancer trials to the table. Our expert clinicians and investigators provide advice on developing protocols. In turn, we get to be students and learn about cancer treatment and research in Latin America,

TABLE 47.12 Profile of Latin American Cooperative Cancer Research Groups

Name	Country	Tumor Types	Type of Studies
LACOG	Brazil and Latin America	All	Observational Clinical Trials Intergroup Studies
GBOT	Brazil	Thoracic	Observational
GBECAM	Brazil	Breast	Observational Intergroup Clinical Trials
EVA	Brazil	Gynecological	Observational
GOCCHI	Chile	All	Observational Clinical Trials Intergroup Studies
GECOPERU	Peru	All	Observational Clinical Trials Intergroup Studies
GOCUR	Uruguay	All	Observational Clinical Trials Intergroup Studies
GAICO	Argentina	All	Observational Clinical Trials Intergroup Studies
CLICaP	Mexico and Latin America	Lung	Observational Translational
ONCOLGroup	Colombia	All	Observational Translational

CLICaP, Latin American Consortium for Lung Cancer Research; EVA, Grupo Brasileiro de Tumores Ginecologicos; GAICO, Grupo Argentino de Investigación Clínica en Oncología; GBECAM, Grupo Brasileiro de Estudos em Cancer de Mama; GBOT, Grupo Brasileiro de Oncologia Torácica; GECOPERU, Grupo de Estudios Clínicos Oncológicos Peruano; GOCCHI, Grupo Oncologico Coopertivo Chileno de Investigacion; GOCUR, Grupo Oncológico Cooperativo Uruguayo; LACOG Latin American Cooperative Oncology Group; ONCOLGroup, Grupo Colombiano para la Investigación Clínica y Traslacional en Cáncer.

and the challenges and opportunities they face (30). Educational activities such as clinical trial workshops in Latin America were presented by local and international oncology societies such as the Sociedad Latinoamericana y del Caribe de Oncología Médica (SLACOM), GECOPERU, Sociedade Brasileira de Oncologia Clínica (SBOC), European Society of Medical Oncology (ESMO), and ASCO in order to teach the fundamental goals and organizational aspects of clinical trial design and conduct (31).

A description of the main activities and research contribution of each Latin American research group is presented in the following.

Latin American Cooperative Oncology Group (LACOG)

LACOG is a multinational group with its headquarters in Porto Alegre, Brazil. It is the most structured group in Latin America in terms of personnel and facilities to run clinical cancer studies. Investigators are from several countries, with the majority from Brazil, Argentina, Peru, Colombia, and Mexico. There are around 13 ongoing studies, observational and clinical trials, that are supported by pharmaceutical companies, the public, and government grants. LACOG also participates in intergroup studies. LACOG has published the results of its first international phase II trial (GLICO 0801) in breast cancer, and several abstracts of observational studies were presented in international conferences (32). Educational activities are organized by LACOG such as licensed Best of ASCO in Brazil, AACR International Conference on Translational Cancer Medicine, and Stat Course for nonstatisticians endorsed by the European Organization for Research and Treatment of Cancer (EORTC), among others (www.lacog.org.br).

Grupo Brasileiro de Estudos em Cancer de Mama (GBECAM)

GBECAM, dedicated to breast cancer research, was the first cooperative group launched in Brazil. The group has successfully conducted a retrospective study with more than 3,000 patients, which showed that patients treated in the public health system have worse breast cancer survival than those treated in the private sector (18). Also, GBECAM has participated in some international intergroup clinical trials such as ALTTO, NeoALTTO, and CIBOMA. The group faced financial constraints and merged its office activities with LACOG to form the LACOG breast cancer group (www.gbecam.org.br).

Grupo Brasileiro de Oncologia Torácica (GBOT)

GBOT has its headquarters in Porto Alegre, Brazil and shares the office facilities with LACOG. The group dedicates educational activities for patients and professionals as well as research in thoracic cancer, especially lung cancer. The group has a limited number of publications such as review articles or abstracts presenting retrospective studies of lung cancer in Brazil. Currently, there are no ongoing studies. GBOT is responsible for organizing the World Conference on Lung Cancer endorsed by the International Association for the Study of Lung Cancer (IASLC; www.gbot.med.br).

Grupo Brasileiro de Tumores Ginecologicos (EVA)

EVA is a dedicated gynecological oncology group from Brazil, which aims to develop observational and clinical trials in the country as well as international collaborations. EVA has a close collaboration with LACOG and a prospective registry (EVITA study) aiming to describe patterns of care of cervical cancer, the second most prevalent cancer in Brazil, was launched recently (www.eva.org.br).

Grupo Oncologico Coopertivo Chileno de Investigacion (GOCCHI)

GOCCHI is a Chilean group dedicated to studies of all cancer types. The group has launched their own observational studies, conducted few clinical trials, and participated in international intergroup trials. The group is a member of the Breast International Group (BIG) and International Breast Cancer Study Group (IBCSG). The group has made some local observational studies (i.e., PRECISO trial) and conducted translational research in the field of gastric cancer. In all studies, more than 2,500 patients were recruited in 20 studies to date. Recently, the group set up a biobank for translational research projects (www.gocchi.org).

Colombian Collaborative Group for Clinical and Molecular Research in Cancer (ONCOLGroup)

The group is a collaboration of investigators in Colombia. The group has published some observational and translational studies. A proper infrastructure to perform or collaborate in clinical trials has not been established (www.ficmac.org).

Peruvian Group of Oncological Cancer Research (GECOPERU)

GECOPERU is one of the most organized collaborative groups in Latin America with a coordinating office dedicated to study management. The group has done observational studies as well as participated in international intergroup phase II and III trials in breast cancer with BIG and IBCSG. The group conducts educational activities hosting the Best of World Conference on Lung Cancer and did a clinical trial workshop with SLACOM and ESMO (www.gecoperu.pe).

Grupo Oncológico Cooperativo Uruguayo (GOCUR)

GOCUR is a founded by the Uruguayan society of oncology and has a close relation with the ministry of health. The group has participated in pharmaceutical-sponsored trials and has been able to perform translational research projects. However, the country has very few clinical research sites, with regulation complexity and delays and lack of funding to support studies (www.sompu.org.uy).

Grupo Argentino de Investigación Clínica en Oncología (GAICO)

GAICO is a cooperative group, which has 16 member sites in Argentina. The group has participated in international intergroup trials performing some trial management activities. GAICO also organizes an annual conference on research and development in oncology. Recently the group created a website to inform about open cancer clinical trials, academic or pharma sponsored in Argentina (www.gaico.org.ar).

Latin American Consortium for Lung Cancer Research (CLICaP)

CLICaP was created in 2010 to develop collaborative studies on translational and clinical research in lung cancer. The group has published the most comprehensive translational study of the prevalent mutations EGFR, KRAS, and ALK/ROS1 in lung cancer including patients from several countries in Latin America (no website available).

CONCLUSIONS

Cancer clinical research today is promoted globally and despite the large population and economic importance in Latin America, it contributes a small proportion of clinical trials worldwide.

Drug development and science are crucial for social and health development; therefore, clinical research has to be considered a priority in the region. It is critical to identify and address the specific barriers for Latin America cancer research development. There is a lack of knowledge from governments and health authorities on the role and potential impact of academic research and cooperative groups. Despite the progress in cancer research in the past decades, the model cannot be based solely on the efforts of pharmaceutical companies but should include other stakeholders from institutions, governments, nongovernmental organizations, the private sector, and patient organizations. Latin America cooperative groups are strategic collaborators to provide information about local patient population and practice and to develop science in the region in the future.

In summary, there is great potential need for increasing clinical cancer trials in Latin America, However, a significant effort should be made to overcome barriers and change the clinical trial research scenario in Latin America so that such trials can be conducted.

REFERENCES

1. 2017 Revision of World Population Prospects. https://esa.un.org/unpd/wpp
2. Inclusive Social Protection in Latin America: a comprehensive, rights-based approach. http://www.cepal.org/en/publications/inclusive-social-protection-latin-america-comprehensive-rights-based-approach
3. Goss PE, Lee BL, Badovinac-Crnjevic T, et al. Planning cancer control in Latin America and the Caribbean. *Lancet Oncol.* 2013;14(5):391–436.
4. Atun R, de Andrade LO, Almeida G, et al. Health-system reform and universal health coverage in Latin America. *Lancet.* 2015;385(9974):1230–1247.
5. Ravishankar N, Gubbins P, Cooley RJ, et al. Financing of global health: tracking development assistance for health from 1990 to 2007. *Lancet.* 2009;373(9681):2113–2124.
6. Demographic Bulletin No. 72. Latin America and the Caribbean: Population Ageing. http://www.cepal.org/cgi-bin/getProd.asp?xml=/publicaciones/xml/1/13371/P13371.xml&xsl=/celade/tpl/p9f.xsl&base=/celade/tpl/top-bottom.xsl
7. Bloom DE, Cafiero ET, Jané-Llopis E, et al. The Global Economic Burden of Noncommunicable Diseases. Geneva: World Economic Forum; 2011. http://www3.weforum.org/docs/WEF_Harvard_HE_GlobalEconomicBurdenNonCommunicableDiseases_2011.pdf
8. Saad PM, Miller T., Martínez C. Impacto de los cambios demográficos en las demandas sectoriales en América Latina. *Rev Bras Est Pop.* 2009;26:237–261.
9. Balducci L, Ershler WB. Cancer and ageing: a nexus at several levels. *Nat Rev Cancer.* 2005;5(8):655–662.
10. Globocan. http://globocan.iarc.fr/Default.aspx
11. Ferlay J, Shin HR, Bray F, et al. Estimates of worldwide burden of cancer in 2008: GLOBOCAN 2008. *Int J Cancer.* 2010;127(12):2893–2917.
12. Curado MP, Bezerra de Souza DL. Cancer Burden in Latin America and the Caribbean. *Ann Glob Health.* 2014;80(5):370–377.
13. Curado MP, Edwards B, Shin HR, et al. Cancer Incidence in Five Continents Vol. IX. http://www.iarc.fr/en/publications/pdfs-online/epi/sp160/index.php
14. Strasser-Weippl K, Chavarri-Guerra Y, Villarreal-Garza C, et al. Progress and remaining challenges for cancer control in Latin America and the Caribbean. *Lancet Oncol.* 2015;16(14):1405–1438.
15. Banydeen R, Rose AM, Martin D, et al. Advancing Cancer Control Through Research and Cancer Registry Collaborations in the Caribbean. *Cancer Control.* 2015;22(4):520–530.
16. Cancer registries. Information for action in Latin America and the Caribbean. http://www.iccp-newstaging.uicctest.org/sites/default/files/resources/20120329-GICRCancerRegistriesInfoLatAmericaE.pdf
17. United Nations high-level meeting on noncommunicable disease prevention and control. http://www.who.int/nmh/events/un_ncd_summit2011/en
18. Liedke PE, Finkelstein DM, Szymonifka J, et al. Outcomes of breast cancer in Brazil related to health care coverage: a retrospective cohort study. *Cancer Epidemiol Biomarkers Prev.* 2014;23(1):126–133.
19. Clinicaltrials.gov. https://clinicaltrials.gov
20. Seruga B, Hertz PC, Le LW, et al. Global drug development in cancer: a cross-sectional study of clinical trial registries. *Ann Oncol.* 2010;21(4):895–900.
21. Buendía JA, Vallejos C, Pichón-Rivière A. An economic evaluation of trastuzumab as adjuvant treatment of early HER2-positive breast cancer patients in Colombia. *Biomedica.* 2013;33(3):411–417.
22. Saad ED, Pinheiro CM, Masson AL, et al. Increasing output and low publication rate of Brazilian studies presented at the American Society of Clinical Oncology Annual Meetings. *Clinics (Sao Paulo).* 2008;63(3):293–296.

23. Hermes-Lima M, Santos NC, Alencastro AC, et al. Whither Latin America? Trends and challenges of science in Latin America. *IUBMB Life*. 2007;59(4–5):199–210.

24. Latin America Office. https://www.fda.gov/AboutFDA/Centers Offices/OfficeofGlobalRegulatoryOperationsandPolicy/ OfficeofInternationalPrograms/ucm243682.htm

25. Metzger-Filho O, de Azambuja E, Bradbury I, et al. Analysis of regional timelines to set up a global phase III clinical trial in breast cancer: the adjuvant lapatinib and/or trastuzumab treatment optimization experience. *Oncologist*. 2013;18(2):134–140.

26. Lopes G. Cancer Control in Latin America and the Caribbean. http://am.asco.org/daily-news/cancer-control-latin-america-and-caribbean

27. Cazap E. A Vision of Independent Clinical Research in South America. http://www.ascopost.com/issues/may-15-2014/a-vision-of-independent-clinical-research-in-south-america

28. Piccart-Gebhart MJ, Procter M, Leyland-Jones B, et al. Trastuzumab after adjuvant chemotherapy in HER2-positive breast cancer. *N Engl J Med*. 2005;353(16):1659–1672.

29. de Azambuja E, Holmes AP, Piccart-Gebhart M, et al. Lapatinib with trastuzumab for HER2-positive early breast cancer (NeoALTTO): survival outcomes of a randomised, open-label, multicentre, phase 3 trial and their association with pathological complete response. *Lancet Oncol*. 2014;15(10):1137–1146.

30. Blanke CD. A Major Stride for our SWOG Latin America Initiative. http://www.swog.org/Media/frontline/2015/0311.asp

31. Advancing Clinical Cancer Research in Brazil and India. https://connection.asco.org/magazine/features/advancing-clinical-cancer-research-brazil-and-india

32. Gómez HL, Neciosup S, Tosello C, et al. A phase II randomized study of lapatinib combined with capecitabine, vinorelbine, or gemcitabine in patients with HER2-positive metastatic breast cancer with progression after a taxane (Latin American Cooperative Oncology Group 0801 Study). *Clin Breast Cancer*. 2016;16(1):38–44.

The Evolution of the Drug Evaluation Process in Oncology: Regulatory Perspective

THE EVOLUTION OF ONCOLOGY DRUG EVALUATION AT THE FDA

Steven J. Lemery, Gideon Blumenthal, Paul G. Kluetz, Patricia Keegan, Amy McKee, and Richard Pazdur

Since the release of the 2010 edition of the *Oncology Clinical Trials* textbook, the Food and Drug Administration (FDA) has embarked on multiple initiatives relevant to oncologists, patients, and the regulated industry. At its core, the FDA remains responsible for ensuring that drugs marketed in the United States are both safe and effective. The FDA also continues to regulate drug development, including the review of clinical trials conducted under an investigational new drug (IND) application. Since 2010, the FDA's role in cancer drug development has evolved, with new laws creating breakthrough therapy designation (BTD) based on preliminary clinical evidence of efficacy and allowing for approval of biosimilar products; new guidance documents (e.g., Co-development of Two or More New Investigational Drugs for Use in Combination and Pathological Complete Response Guidance in Breast Cancer); and numerous initiatives and workshops by the FDA Office of Hematology and Oncology Products (OHOP) to foster efficient and effective drug development regarding topics such as clinical trial designs, patient-reported outcomes (PROs), and dose finding. This chapter describes some of these initiatives while continuing to highlight important regulatory considerations from the prior version of this book.

The 2010 edition of *Oncology Clinical Trials* contained a section describing the structure of FDA centers, offices, and divisions pertaining to the review of products intended to treat or prevent cancer. This edition does not describe such structures other than to highlight that the FDA created an Oncology Center of Excellence to support an integrated approach to the clinical evaluation of drugs, biologics, and devices (1).

FDA DECISION MAKING

Laws passed by Congress provide the legal foundation for the FDA authorities. For example, the 1962 amendments to the Federal Food, Drug, and Cosmetic Act (FDCA) require FDA-approved drugs to be safe and effective. The statute authorizes the agency to write regulations that interpret the law. The regulations regarding the conduct of a clinical trial of an IND can be found in the Code of Federal Regulations (CFR), specifically in 21 CFR 312. Both statutes and regulations are legally binding for the regulated industry (e.g., pharmaceutical or device companies), clinical study investigators, and the FDA. The agency may publish guidance documents that describe its current thinking on how to comply with the regulations. Guidance documents are not legally binding except where the guidance cites the applicable statutes or regulations. Although not legally binding, the FDA recommends that sponsors seek advice from the agency prior to deviating from guidance.

Investigational New Drug

An IND is an exemption under the Interstate Commerce Act that allows for the interstate shipment of nonapproved drugs, also known as investigational drugs (2). There are certain legal requirements applicable to IND sponsors and clinical investigators when conducting a clinical investigation under an IND. These include informed consent requirements contained in 21 CFR 50, institutional review board (IRB) requirements contained in 21 CFR 56, and IND requirements contained in 21 CFR 312. The regulations under 21 CFR 312 describing the criteria for placing a clinical investigation or IND on hold, the IND exemption criteria for marketed drugs, and the responsibilities and obligations of sponsors and investigators have not been revised for more than a decade.

What Is An Investigational Drug?

A drug is defined as an article that is intended for use in the diagnosis, cure, mitigation, treatment, or prevention of disease *and* is an article (other than food) intended to affect the structure or any function of the body (3). Biological products (e.g., therapeutic cellular products, monoclonal antibodies, therapeutic cytokines) subject to licensure under section 351 of the Public Health Service Act may also be considered drugs within the scope of the FDCA (3). An IND is required in the United States to administer an unapproved drug to humans.

If an investigator intends to conduct a clinical trial using commercial supplies of a lawfully marketed drug product, an IND will not be required if the following conditions are met:

1. The clinical trial (investigation) is not intended to be reported to FDA as a well-controlled study that might support a new indication or support any significant change in the labeling (4).
2. The trial is not intended to support new promotional claims (advertising) for the drug (4).
3. The trial does not involve a route of administration, dosage level, or new patient population (or other factors) that significantly increase the risks associated with the drug (4).
4. The clinical trial is conducted in compliance with IRB and informed consent regulations (4).
5. The clinical trial is conducted in compliance with the requirements of 21 CFR 312.7 (this section of the regulations deals with the promotion and charging/commercialization of investigational drugs) (4).

In the past decade, the FDA issued guidance regarding IND exemptions. The guidance provides clarification regarding the types of manufacturing modifications that can be made to a lawfully marketed product (e.g., low-risk modifications including minor variations to solid dosage forms, such as changing color, scoring, or capsule size) and still be exempted from IND requirements, provided that the exemption criteria are otherwise satisfied (4). An earlier (2004) guidance provides examples of types of studies investigating the effects of lawfully marketed products in patients with cancer that are generally exempt from IND (e.g., small single-arm, noncommercial, dose-finding trials investigating the use of a drug in patients with a different tumor type) (5).

FDA Review of INDs

The FDA's major objectives during the review of an IND are to ensure the safety and rights of subjects, and to ensure that the quality of a scientific investigation (particularly in phase II and III trials) is adequate to permit an evaluation of safety and efficacy (6). Within 30 days of receipt of a new IND, the FDA will either allow the IND to proceed or will place the IND on hold. If an FDA reviewer discovers potential hold issues, a discussion between the clinical review division and the IND sponsor may occur prior to the 30-day deadline to resolve deficiencies in the IND.

When a study is placed on clinical hold, no patient may receive the investigational drug(s) under that IND until the FDA receives the necessary information to resolve the issues and states in writing that the clinical hold has been lifted. The FDA may also place a portion of the IND on hold (i.e., a partial hold). For example, the FDA may allow patients who have received the investigational drug without experiencing toxicity to continue to receive the drug while suspending accrual of treatment-naïve patients.

For phase I (first-in-human) studies, there are five reasons cited in the regulations (21 CFR 312.42) that allow the FDA to place a study on hold:

1. Unreasonable or significant risk of injury or illness to the subject
2. Investigators are not qualified by reason of their scientific training or experience
3. Misleading, erroneous, or incomplete Investigator's Brochure
4. Insufficient data submitted to assess the risk to subjects
5. Exclusion of men or women with reproductive potential from a study intended to treat a life-threatening disease that affects both sexes (this criterion does not apply to pregnant women or diseases that only affect one gender)

For phase II and III studies, a protocol can be placed on hold for the aforementioned five reasons and if the trial is clearly deficient in design to meet its stated objectives (7).

FDA Review Process for INDs

An IND must contain information pertaining to a drug's chemistry, manufacturing, and controls (CMC), and the drug's pharmacology and toxicology. A clinical protocol must also be submitted (8). The IND must contain an Investigator's Brochure, unless the IND is being submitted and conducted at a single clinical site by a sponsor–investigator (8). With the exception of certain single-patient INDs (see the section on expanded access), a sponsor must also complete and sign FDA Form 1571, in which the sponsor agrees to the following: (a) clinical investigations will not begin until 30 days after the date the IND is received by the FDA or notified by the FDA that the investigation will begin, (b) clinical investigations will not be initiated or will be discontinued if the FDA places the IND on hold, (c) an

IRB that complies with 21 CFR 56 will be responsible for initial and ongoing review of all studies under the IND, and (d) all clinical studies will be conducted in accordance with other applicable regulations (e.g., those pertaining to informed consent and those contained in the IND regulations under 21 CFR 312) (8).

When an IND is received, FDA Quality staff (e.g., chemists, biologists, or microbiologists as appropriate) review data regarding the drug substance, drug product, labeling information, microbial assessments, and environmental analyses to ensure the proper identification, quality, purity, and strength (or potency) of the product (8). Sponsor–investigators typically submit the required information through a letter of cross-reference obtained from the commercial sponsor of the investigational drug.

FDA toxicology reviewers assess animal studies and other toxicology data. They collaborate with the clinical reviewer to ensure the safety of the starting dose and to provide advice on monitoring for specific adverse events observed in nonhuman pharmacology and toxicology studies.

The FDA clinical reviewer assesses the adequacy of protocols and informed consent documents for risks to patients, as supported by animal or human data pertinent to establishing the safety of the proposed clinical trials. After initiation of the clinical investigation, the clinical reviewer evaluates amendments to the IND, which may include protocol amendments, new protocols, expedited safety reports, and annual reports. Clinical protocols submitted to OHOP are reviewed by healthcare practitioners with experience in the treatment of patients with cancer and management of adverse reactions of drugs that treat cancer. A statistician may be included as part of the IND review team, especially for phase 2 and 3 studies, to evaluate the appropriateness of the plans for data analysis and to confirm the results of data analyses submitted by the IND sponsor.

A clinical pharmacologist will review animal, and if available, human pharmacokinetic data and evaluate the scientific rigor of clinical plans for the characterization of the investigational drug's pharmacokinetic profile in the intended population and in special populations (e.g., in patients with hepatic or renal impairment). The clinical pharmacologist also evaluates plans for the characterization of the drug's effect on QTc prolongation and possible drug interactions, and determination of the incidence and clinical impact of immunogenicity, that is, antiproduct antibodies for biotechnology-derived products.

Sponsor and Investigator Responsibilities Regarding the IND

Sponsors and investigators must meet certain obligations when conducting studies under an IND. For example, IND sponsors are obligated to select qualified investigators, provide them with the information necessary to conduct an investigation properly, ensure proper monitoring of the investigation, ensure that the investigation is conducted in accordance with the general investigational plan and protocols contained in the IND, and ensure that the FDA and all participating investigators are promptly informed of significant new adverse effects or risks with respect to the drug (9). Investigators are obligated to conduct the study according to the signed investigator's statement, the investigational plan, and applicable regulations and for the protection of the rights, safety, and welfare of subjects under the investigator's care (e.g., obtaining informed consent) (10).

In 2010, the FDA amended the safety reporting rule (regulation) and subsequently issued new guidance in 2012 to decrease the number of expedited (i.e., 7 or 15 days) safety reports that are uninformative when reported as single events (11,12). The FDA requires sponsors to submit expedited safety reports for serious and unexpected *suspected* adverse reactions. Suspected means that there is evidence to suggest a causal relationship between the drug and the adverse event (12). Specifically, the guidance describes certain serious adverse events that should *not* be submitted as expedited serious adverse events including adverse events anticipated to occur in the study population independent of drug exposure (these other serious adverse events are submitted in IND annual reports). For example, a sponsor generally could not attribute a single case of myocardial infarction observed in an elderly individual with cancer who has received an investigational drug for multiple months (12). Similarly, single events such as "general health deterioration" cannot be attributable to a drug in a patient population with advanced cancer. Sponsors should evaluate such events in aggregate to make a determination that there was a causal relationship between the drug and the adverse event (12). The FDA issued an additional draft guidance in 2015 that describes how sponsors can conduct such aggregate analyses (13).

Evidence to date suggests that the goals of the amended safety reporting regulation have not been realized. The number of safety reports continues to increase and a random FDA-conducted audit of safety reports submitted to commercial INDs of investigational cancer drugs showed that most (86%) appeared to be uninformative, because they did not meet the criteria for expedited reporting (14). Based on these results, the FDA continues to engage with the industry to decrease the number of uninformative expedited safety reports submitted to the FDA and investigators (15). The agency hopes to foster a more comprehensive and thoughtful analysis of safety under an IND so that true safety signals can be identified and appropriately acted upon (13).

FDA EFFORTS TO FACILITATE DRUG DEVELOPMENT

The following paragraphs highlight areas where the FDA, and OHOP specifically, have taken steps to facilitate drug development or encourage novel approaches to clinical trials through new programs for expediting drug development. BTD was introduced legislatively; other items in the following are described in FDA guidance or other public forums (e.g., publications or workshops).

Breakthrough Therapy Designation

The Food and Drug Administration Safety and Innovation Act (FDASIA) was signed into law on July 9, 2012 (16). This Act allows the FDA to grant BTD for drugs that treat a serious or life-threatening condition and for which *preliminary* clinical evidence indicates that the drug may demonstrate substantial improvement over existing therapies on one or more clinically significant endpoints, observed early in clinical development (16–18). Unfortunately, confusion exists in the medical community regarding the level of evidence required to support a request for BTD. For example, 52% of responding physicians in a survey believed, incorrectly, that the FDA requires strong evidence (e.g., randomized trials) to grant BTD (19).

FDASIA stipulates that when a drug receives BTD, this will trigger closer interactions between the FDA and the sponsor covering all aspects of the development of the drug, and allows the FDA to take steps to ensure that the clinical trial designs are as efficient as practicable (16–18). The FDA can provide advice to sponsors regarding manufacturing to ensure that the drug will be available to the public following approval. A BTD also allows a new drug application (NDA) or biologic license application (BLA) to receive "rolling review," in which the FDA begins reviewing portions of an application before the application is complete. Finally, BTD facilitates an organizational commitment to expedite the development and review of the drug through early and intensive involvement of senior managers and other FDA review staff (18).

As of June 2016, the FDA approved 14 new drugs (i.e., new molecular entities) that received BTD for the treatment of patients with cancer: venetoclax, atezolizumab, alectinib, elotuzumab, daratumumab, osimertinib, palbociclib, nivolumab, blinatumomab, pembrolizumab, idelalisib, ceritinib, ibrutinib, and obinutuzumab (16). The FDA has also approved additional (supplemental) indications for approved drugs that were granted BTD for these new indications.

Breakthrough Designation Versus Fast-Track Designation

BTD is granted for drugs that treat a serious or life-threatening condition and for which preliminary *clinical* evidence *indicates* that the drug may demonstrate *substantial* improvement over existing therapies on one or more clinically significant endpoints. Fast-track designation (FTD) can be granted for the development program for drugs intended to treat a serious condition and for which nonclinical or clinical data demonstrate the *potential* to address an unmet medical need. FTD can be granted based on nonclinical data *and* a description of a development plan that addresses how a sponsor intends to address an unmet medical need for a specific population. Therefore, FTD should not imply that FDA has determined that clinical data exist to address that unmet need. Like BTD, FTD may allow a sponsor to request a rolling review of an NDA or BLA.

FDA Input on Trial Designs

Since 2010, the FDA has held meetings, released guidance, and published articles providing recommendations to sponsors and investigators to facilitate cancer drug development. The following describe a few of the FDA initiatives applicable to oncology clinical trials.

Dose Finding

In conjunction with the American Association for Cancer Research (AACR), the FDA cosponsored two dose-finding workshops (May 18–19, 2015 and June 13, 2016) attended by academia and industry. Following the first workshop, FDA staff coauthored several articles that encouraged a thoughtful approach to optimization of dose selection for drugs intended to treat patients with cancer (20–23). One of the messages of the meeting was that the "3 + 3" design used to determine a maximum tolerated dose (MTD) is not an efficient approach to identifying an optimal dose, and IND sponsors are encouraged to use integrated approaches to dose finding. For example, sponsors may use an adaptive/Bayesian model with continuous assessments of safety and efficacy data throughout the life cycle of drug development to provide a larger patient experience and more data supporting dose selection (22,23). Sponsors should also consider use of nonclinical and pharmacokinetic data when selecting a dose and carefully consider drug-related toxicities that occur beyond the first cycle when selecting a dosage regimen for further investigation (20–23). Dose optimization beyond phase 1 can also improve the safety and efficacy profile of a product, potentially leading to a more favorable outcome for a drug development program.

Seamless Oncology Drug Development

Increasingly in the clinical development of cancer drugs, the historical definitions for "phases" of clinical investigations (e.g., as described in 21 CFR 312.21) are meaningless, as sponsors conduct whole development programs within a single clinical trial (which have exceeded 1,500 patients). Such developmental approaches can be efficient and facilitate access to investigational drugs; however, concerns have been expressed regarding such protocols, including adequate oversight for drug-related toxicity. In fact, such approaches may be less efficient if they fail to ensure that the number of patients enrolled do not exceed that necessary to answer specific objectives, overinterpret interim data for future development, or fail to consider available data prior to initiation of new "stages" or "cohorts." To ensure that "seamless" development plans are efficient and scientifically driven, these protocols should have statistical plans that provide justification for the sample size for each discrete phase, stage, or cohort (24). Furthermore, an informed consent document appropriate for first-in-human use would not be appropriate in a study that subsequently enrolls hundreds of patients (24).

The FDA has held workshops regarding seamless development in oncology and has stated that these trial designs may be appropriate for certain drugs that appear highly active (i.e., drugs granted BTD) (24,25). Such designs are consistent with the FDA's goals to facilitate efficient development for these drugs (25). Nevertheless, trials should be carefully designed to ensure they are efficient and subject to external oversight of safety and more frequent real-time communication among sponsors, investigators, IRBs, regulators, and patients (24,25).

Biomarker-Directed Drug Development and "Master Protocols"

Master protocols offer another opportunity to increase the efficiency of drug development and bring promising new treatments to patients faster. A master protocol may include an evaluation of multiple drugs or may evaluate patients with multiple diseases, with or without a common control arm. Furthermore, a master protocol may be amended to add or drop new treatment arms or substudies. A common master protocol design allows for a patient's tumor to be tested for the presence of various biomarkers in order to assign the patient to treatment with drugs specifically targeted to treat that patient's particular tumor (26). Efficiency may be increased when such protocols use adaptive designs that, based on prespecified criteria, substitute a new investigational drug if one is not active or proceed to a randomized component (e.g., an adaptive trial) designed to formally evaluate the safety and effectiveness of the drug if promising activity is seen in a biomarker positive population.

The design and conduct of master protocols can be challenging and requires involvement from multiple stakeholders, including industry, patients, academia, and government (e.g., the National Cancer Institute [NCI] and the FDA). From a regulatory perspective, participation of both drug (or biologic) reviewers and device reviewers (Center for Devices and Radiological Health [CDRH]) may be necessary. CDRH review is often necessary to ensure that the companion diagnostic assay used to select patients for enrollment or specified treatment has acceptable performance characteristics and that the trial will also facilitate the development of the device to support approval of the device contemporaneously with the drug approval (27). Several master protocols have been successfully launched and are awaiting results (28–30).

Safety Collection

In addition to providing advice to sponsors regarding novel trial designs, FDA has published guidance about the extent of safety data collection necessary in late-stage premarket and postapproval clinical investigations (31). For example, it may be appropriate in certain settings to collect selective safety data in clinical trials for cancer drugs with well-established adverse event profiles. Such selective data collection (for example, collection limited to severe and serious adverse events or collection of complete safety data from a subset of patients) could decrease the costs of clinical trials and facilitate investigator and patient participation in clinical trials (31). Although the 2016 guidance describes situations where selective data collection may be appropriate, the guidance also recommends that sponsors obtain agreement with the agency prior to initiating a study with a selective data collection approach (31).

Patient Engagement and Patient-Reported Outcomes in Oncology

Recent legislation supports increased patient engagement and patient-centered data in drug development. FDASIA required that FDA host multiple patient-focused drug development (PFDD) meetings to gather the patient perspective across various disease areas; OHOP held PFDD meetings for breast cancer and lung cancer (32). As a result of these and other efforts, there is increased interest in the development of more robust clinical outcome assessments, including PRO data to assess symptom and functional outcomes in the research and clinical settings. OHOP cosponsored workshops with the Critical Path Institute's PRO Consortium to explore opportunities and challenges with measurement of PROs in cancer clinical trials (33). While the FDA reviews PRO data submitted in applications, inclusion of data in product labeling should be generated from well-defined and reliable assessments and should aim to distinguish the effect of the drug from other influences (34,35). To facilitate the inclusion of patient-centered data in product labeling, OHOP recommends that sponsors focus their analyses for FDA labeling on those symptom and functional areas most relevant to the drug and disease context under study. Three core areas include disease-specific symptoms (e.g., dyspnea, cough, and pain in patients with lung cancer or cognitive impairment in a patient with glioblastoma multiforme), physical function, and symptomatic adverse events. In addition to static health-related quality of life tools, flexible PRO item banks and libraries are available that can be adapted to different trial contexts such as the publicly available Patient-Reported Outcomes Measurement Information System (PROMIS) and the Patient-Reported Outcomes version of the Common Terminology Criteria for Adverse Events (PRO-CTCAE) (36,37). OHOP supports a thoughtful combination of static questionnaires and item banks or libraries to create a flexible and modular approach to

PRO assessment that provides a reasonably comprehensive picture of the patient experience most affected by therapy, to satisfy the needs of multiple drug development stakeholders (38,39).

Regardless of which PRO measures are employed, it is critical to maximize the rigor with which the data are collected and analyzed. For example, missing data can undermine the interpretation of PRO results. Sponsors should take care to mitigate missing data through adequate site training and monitoring. Sponsors also will need to carefully consider the schedule of assessments, which may differ based on trial objectives, disease context, and therapy under study (e.g., for an intermittently administered cytotoxic therapy versus a daily administered tyrosine kinase inhibitor). Although adverse event data can be presented descriptively in product labeling, for efficacy claims or other claims of treatment benefit, a PRO endpoint will need to be strictly defined with a pre-specified analysis plan addressing multiplicity. Sponsors should also provide data to support the threshold for and interpretation of a meaningful change in scores on each PRO instrument.

Other Initiatives

The FDA is working with various stakeholders to develop guidance on when it may be appropriate to expand eligibility criteria in cancer clinical trials. Rather than "copy and pasting" eligibility criteria from first-in-human trials through definitive, hypothesis-testing trials, sponsors should consider expanding eligibility to enroll patients who will likely receive the drug in the postmarketing setting. This might include patients with poor performance status, organ dysfunction, brain metastases, or HIV (40). Sponsors should also consider when there is sufficient safety in adults to support inclusion of children as young as 12 in adult protocols (41).

The FDA also encourages sponsors to enroll diverse patient populations that will be reflective of the U.S. patient population. Evaluation in diverse patient populations helps ensure that the drug is safe and effective across the spectrum of patients who will receive the drug in the postmarketing setting.

Real-World Evidence

Real-world data can be defined broadly as data generated or obtained outside of traditional clinical trials and collected for other purposes. Sources of real-world data include insurance claims, patient registries, electronic health records (EHRs), social media, and mobile applications and devices. The 21st Century Cures Act, signed into law by President Obama in 2016, defines evidence from clinical experience (real-world data) as "data regarding the usage, or the potential benefits or risks, of a drug derived from sources other than randomized clinical trials." While useful, this definition proposes a dichotomy that suggests randomization can only occur in a clinical trial. On the contrary, pragmatic clinical trials can employ randomization in the "real-world" setting (42).

Real-world evidence (RWE) can potentially complement conventional clinical trials to inform regulatory decision making. Potential applications for RWE in oncology include labeling expansion for efficacy, dose optimization, postmarketing safety surveillance, assessing the quality of Risk Evaluation and Mitigation Strategy (REMS) programs, assessing PRO and quality of life, and testing real-world performance of predictive biomarkers, to name a few. With the increased use of EHRs in oncology practices and new technologies to improve interoperability, curation, and analysis, RWE applications to inform regulatory decision making will likely increase in the next decade (43).

EXPANDED ACCESS FOR INVESTIGATIONAL DRUGS

Expanded access, also known as compassionate use, involves the administration of an unapproved investigational drug outside of a clinical trial. FDA regulations permit three categories of expanded access: expanded access for individual patients, including emergency use; expanded access for intermediate-size patient populations; and a treatment IND for larger populations (for example, for widespread treatment of patients following completion of clinical trials but prior to marketing authorization) (44). In June 2016, the FDA finalized a guidance that provides for a streamlined alternative to submitting an individual patient expanded access request (i.e., Form 3926) (45). This form requests only the pertinent information for individual patient submissions and will take an estimated 45 minutes to complete (46).

The following are the criteria for expanded access: (a) the patient has a serious or life-threatening disease or condition and there is no comparable or satisfactory alternative treatment; (b) the potential benefit justifies the potential risks; (c) the expanded access use will not interfere with the initiation, conduct, or completion of clinical investigations that could support marketing approval (44,45). The preferred mechanism for access to an investigational drug is a clinical trial to facilitate drug development, because the ultimate "access" for patients is drug approval (46). Nevertheless, the FDA recognizes that many patients will be ineligible for a specific clinical trial or live too far away from a clinical trial site, and therefore, expanded access is appropriate.

Although the FDA has long had a history of granting expanded access for investigational drugs, ultimately, the manufacturer of that drug (commercial sponsor) must first agree to provide access to the drug and supply a letter of cross-reference allowing the FDA to reference the necessary chemistry and manufacturing (CMC), toxicology, and clinical information in the commercial sponsor's IND to support the expanded access request. An IND or protocol for expanded access may begin 30 days after FDA receives the protocol or sooner than 30 days, upon notification by the FDA. In an analysis of over 1,332 INDs submitted to OHOP over a 3-year period (2012–2014), only two were not granted (i.e., placed on hold); and the median review time of all single-patient, investigator-initiated INDs in OHOP was 1 day (2 days in the analysis limited to single-patient, nonemergency INDs) (47).

Emergency use INDs may be granted in an imminently life-threatening situation, in which there is not sufficient time to formally submit an IND for review or to obtain IRB approval. In such instances, the FDA can review the information obtained by telephone conversation, facsimile transmissions, or email, with the formal IND submission to occur within 15 days of the FDA's authorization of use (44). Although initial treatment under an emergency IND can be administered prior to IRB approval, the IRB must be notified within 5 days posttreatment. Informed consent is still required under an emergency use IND except for very limited situations described in 21 CFR 50.23.

The Drug Approval Process

After passage of the 1962 Kefauver–Harris Amendments to the FDCA, marketing applications for approval of drugs (i.e., an NDA) required demonstration of substantial evidence of effectiveness obtained in adequate and well-controlled trials (48). Because of the plurality of the word "trials," applicants were generally expected to demonstrate evidence of effectiveness in more than one trial. In 1997, passage of the Food and Drug Administration Modernization Act (FDAMA) permitted the FDA to consider evidence from one adequate and well-controlled trial plus confirmatory evidence in certain circumstances (48). These circumstances include statistically persuasive findings in a large multicenter trial with consistent results across subsets on a serious outcome such as survival or irreversible morbidity, such that a second study would be considered unethical (48).

Accelerated Approval

FDA published the final rule for the accelerated approval regulations in 1992; these regulations were amended under FDASIA (18). Under these regulations, the FDA can grant accelerated approval to drugs that (a) treat a serious condition; (b) provide a meaningful advantage over available therapy; and (c) demonstrate an effect on a surrogate endpoint that is reasonably likely to predict clinical benefit or on a clinical endpoint that can be measured earlier than irreversible morbidity or mortality (IMM) that is reasonably likely to predict an effect on IMM or other clinical benefit (18). Under the provisions

of accelerated approval, applicants are required to study the drug further to verify and describe the clinical benefit if there is uncertainty as to the relation of the surrogate endpoint to clinical benefit, or of the observed clinical benefit to the ultimate outcome (18).

Accelerated approval requires substantial evidence of a treatment effect on a surrogate or intermediate endpoint (18). An application should provide evidence that the effect on the surrogate or intermediate endpoint is a real effect. Accelerated approval is not a mechanism for approval of drugs or a new indication for marketed drugs where the effect can be attributed to chance.

The European Medicines Agency (EMA) has a similar program called conditional marketing authorization (CMA) designed to expedite the approval of drugs for patients with seriously debilitating or life-threatening diseases and unmet need (49). The requirements differ for CMA in that EMA must determine that the benefit–risk profile is positive based on less than comprehensive clinical evidence (49). EMA must also determine that the confirmatory data will be provided in a reasonable time frame and the potential risk associated with the greater level of uncertainty about its benefit–risk is outweighed by the potential benefits to the public health (49). CMA is subject to yearly renewals and, in contrast to accelerated approval, can only be granted to initial marketing authorizations (49). The other important difference is that the FDA accelerated approval regulations specifically stipulate approval based on surrogate or intermediate endpoints rather than a preliminary assessment of risk–benefit.

Approval of Oncology Drugs—Endpoints

Improved understanding of the biology of cancer, coupled with unprecedented antitumor effects observed in clinical trials, has necessitated a reassessment of endpoints used to support the approval of drugs intended to treat patients with cancer (50).

Historically, an improvement in overall survival (OS) represented the highest level of efficacy for approval of new drugs for the treatment of cancer patients. In 1979, the U.S. Supreme Court (*United States vs. Rutherford*) concluded that a drug intended to treat terminally ill patients is effective if it prolongs life, improves physical condition, or reduces pain, and that a drug is safe if the potential to cause harm is offset by the potential therapeutic benefit (51). In multiple meetings held in the 1980s, the Oncologic Drugs Advisory Committee (ODAC) advised the FDA that a drug indicated for the treatment of cancer should improve mortality or relieve suffering to demonstrate clinical benefit (52).

Although approval based on OS is appropriate in certain diseases, OS may not be feasible in many situations, given that cancer in the genomic era is increasingly being subsegmented into smaller populations, and because clinical effects (e.g., on objective response rate [ORR]) may be of such a large magnitude that patients may be unwilling to participate in a randomized controlled trial (53). In some cases, the FDA has used effects on other endpoints such as progression-free survival (PFS) or durable ORR to support either accelerated approval or regular approval of drugs. When making approval decisions based on PFS or ORR, the FDA considers the context of the malignant neoplasm, whether there is an unmet medical need, the absolute magnitude of the treatment effect, the toxicity profile of the drug, and the overall risk–benefit profile (53).

For approvals based on ORR, the FDA has accepted single-arm, historically controlled trials, because (with rare exceptions) tumors do not shrink in the absence of therapy. For approval, the response rate and duration should be of sufficient magnitude to either be considered as a surrogate *reasonably likely* to predict benefit (for accelerated approval) or to be considered as a surrogate for clinical benefit (or considered as clinical benefit in and of itself). An illustrative example of how the FDA considered response rate to support regular approval was the approval of a new indication for crizotinib for the treatment of patients with ROS1-positive metastatic non–small-cell lung cancer (NSCLC) (54). The FDA granted regular approval based on an ORR of 66% with a median duration of response of 18.3 months as assessed by an independent radiology review committee. In granting regular approval, the FDA considered the magnitude of the treatment effect (both for response rate and response duration) *and* the favorable risk–benefit profile that crizotinib demonstrated in previous randomized trials in patients with ALK positive NSCLC. Given the rarity of ROS1-positive NSCLC, the large magnitude of treatment effects on ORR and duration of response, the modest treatment effects on ORR and duration of response observed with alternative therapies, and the benefit–risk established in previous randomized trials, the FDA agreed that a randomized clinical trial would be infeasible and unethical (equipoise would not exist).

Although regular approval was granted for crizotinib for ROS1-positive NSCLC, uncertainty may exist with respect to the relationship between an observed ORR and duration of response of a smaller magnitude (than seen with crizotinib) and the ultimate clinical benefit such that additional data may be necessary to support regular approval. In many cases, randomized trials may be necessary, because demonstration of clinical benefit requires assessment of an effect on PFS of large magnitude or an effect on OS. For regular approval based on PFS, the FDA considers many of the same factors discussed earlier in regard to ORR, including magnitude of effect, benefit–risk profile, natural history of the disease, and availability of alternative therapies. The FDA will also assess for any positive or negative trends on

OS when considering whether to approve a drug based on PFS. Furthermore, a well-thought-out, prospectively designed, and appropriately analyzed assessment of PROs could support FDA approval of a drug with PFS as the primary endpoint.

PFS as a study endpoint generally requires smaller sample sizes and shorter follow-up compared to OS (52). Furthermore, PFS will not be influenced by subsequent therapies, which could potentially confound assessments of effects on OS (52). Nevertheless, PFS can be subject to unintentional ascertainment bias by investigators with knowledge of the treatment administered; therefore, blinded independent assessments of radiographs are often required by the FDA to assess for and minimize the effects of such bias. Furthermore, attention to trial conduct is important in a study with a PFS endpoint, because missing data can complicate the analysis of PFS (52). When assessing the magnitude of an effect on PFS, FDA generally considers absolute magnitude of the treatment effects (e.g., absolute difference in median PFS) as well as the relative treatment effects as assessed by the hazard ratio. A clinically important plateau in the PFS curve limited to the treatment arm may provide additional support for a drug's clinical benefit. Finally, a modest PFS effect when a drug is directly compared to an active drug is ordinarily more clinically meaningful than a modest PFS effect when a drug is compared to placebo (or added to standard therapy).

In addition to the commonly used endpoints of ORR, PFS, and OS, the FDA has considered other endpoints for approval decisions when appropriate. For example, the FDA approved glucarpidase for the treatment of toxic plasma methotrexate concentrations in patients with delayed methotrexate clearance due to impaired renal function based on demonstration of rapid and sustained clinically important reductions in plasma methotrexate concentrations (55). Similarly, the FDA approved asparaginase Erwinia chrysanthemi for acute lymphoblastic leukemia in patients with hypersensitivity to *E. coli*-derived asparaginase based on the proportion of patients who achieved a serum trough asparaginase level greater than or equal to 0.1 International Units/mL, which has been shown to correlate with effective antitumor activity for asparaginase (56). In 2013, the FDA granted accelerated approval to pertuzumab in combination with trastuzumab and docetaxel as neoadjuvant treatment of patients with HER2 positive, locally advanced, inflammatory, or early-stage breast cancer (either greater than 2 cm in diameter or node positive) as part of a complete treatment regimen for early breast cancer based on demonstration of an improvement in pathological complete response rate and previous data in the metastatic setting demonstrating that pertuzumab improves OS of patients with HER2 positive breast cancer (57).

BIOSIMILARS

The Biologics Price Competition and Innovation Act (BPCI Act), enacted as part of the Affordable Care Act on March 23, 2010, created an abbreviated licensure pathway for biological products demonstrated to be biosimilar to or interchangeable with a U.S.-licensed reference product (58,59). The FDA approved the first biosimilar product, Zarxio, in March 2015 (60,61). The BPCI Act defined biosimilarity to mean "that the biological product is highly similar to the reference product notwithstanding minor differences in clinically inactive components" and that "there are no clinically meaningful differences between the biological product and the reference product in terms of the safety, purity, and potency of the product." (58,59). The act also requires (unless the FDA determines that an element is unnecessary) that a biosimilar application contain, among other things, information demonstrating that the biological product is biosimilar based on data derived from (a) analytical studies (demonstrating that the biological product is highly similar to the reference product notwithstanding minor differences in clinically inactive components); (b) animal studies, including an assessment of toxicity; and (c) a clinical study or studies, including an assessment of immunogenicity and pharmacokinetics or pharmacodynamics that are sufficient to demonstrate safety, purity, and potency in one or more appropriate conditions of use for which the reference product is licensed and intended to be used and for which licensure is sought for the biological product (58,59).

To demonstrate that a biological product is "highly similar" to the reference product, an IND sponsor will need to conduct an extensive analytical characterization of both products that will include structural and functional tests of multiple quality attributes including, among other things, primary structure, higher order structures, posttranslational modifications, oxidation or protein deamidation variants, and biological assays (59,62). The design and scope of clinical studies to assess for clinically meaningful differences will depend, in part, on the nature and extent of residual uncertainty about biosimilarity after conducting structural and functional characterization and, where relevant, animal studies (59,62).

As a scientific matter, in order to assess for clinically meaningful differences, the FDA expects biosimilar sponsors to conduct comparative assessments of pharmacokinetics and pharmacodynamics (if there are relevant pharmacodynamics markers) and a comparative assessment of immunogenicity in humans (59,63). Additional comparative clinical studies may also be necessary if residual uncertainty remains regarding whether clinically meaningful differences exist between the biosimilar product and the reference product (59).

The goal of such studies, if necessary, is to assess for clinically meaningful differences and not to reproduce the clinical trials that led to a determination that the reference product was safe and effective (59). As such, IND sponsors, with adequate justification, may conduct studies with different endpoints or populations than those that led to the approval of the reference product. One of the provisions of the BPCI Act specifically allows for extrapolation, which gives an applicant the ability to seek licensure, with adequate scientific justification, for one or more indications that were not studied in a clinical trial (59). Biosimilar sponsors should consider whether the clinical studies will be adequately sensitive to assess for clinically meaningful differences in order to support biosimilarity and to support, if appropriate, extrapolation of clinical data across indications (59).

Ultimately, the FDA will use a totality of the evidence approach when assessing whether a product is biosimilar to a reference product and whether the data support extrapolation. The provisions regarding extrapolation are fundamental to the abbreviated licensure pathway, which has the potential to increase treatment options for patients, reduce healthcare costs, and to reduce the need to conduct unnecessary trials (and divert resources) in patients with cancer and other diseases (64).

REFERENCES

1. Oncology Center of Excellence. 2016. http://www.fda.gov/AboutFDA/CentersOffices/OfficeofMedicalProductsandTobacco/ucm509057.htm
2. Chapter 21 Code of Federal Regulations (CFR) 312.
3. Guidance for Clinical Investigators, Sponsors, and IRBs, Investigational New Drug Applications (INDs) - Determining Whether Human Research Studies Can Be Conducted Without an IND. 2013.
4. 21 CFR 312.2.
5. Guidance for Industry, IND Exemptions for Studies of Lawfully Marketed Drug Products for the Treatment of Cancer. 2004.
6. 21 CFR 312.22(a).
7. 21 CFR 312.42.
8. 21 CFR 312.23.
9. 21 CFR 312.50.
10. 21 CFR 312.60.
11. 21 CFR 312.32.
12. Guidance for Industry and Investigators, Safety Reporting Requirements for INDs and BA/BE Studies. 2012.
13. Guidance for Industry, Safety Assessment for IND Safety Reporting. 2015.
14. Jarow JP, Casak S, Chuk M, et al. The majority of expedited investigational new drug safety reports are uninformative. *Clin Cancer Res*. 2016;22:2111–2113.
15. Archdeacon P, Grandinetti C, Vega JM, et al. Optimizing expedited safety reporting for drugs and biologics subject to an investigational new drug application. *Ther Innov Regul Sci*. 2014;48:200–207.
16. Frequently Asked Questions: Breakthrough Therapies. US Food and Drug Administration, 2016. http://www.fda.gov/RegulatoryInformation/Legislation/SignificantAmendmentstotheFDCAct/FDASIA/ucm341027.htm

17. Section 506(a) of the FD&C Act, as added by section 902 of FDASIA.
18. Guidance for Industry, Expedited Programs for Serious Conditions—Drugs and Biologics. 2014.
19. Kesselheim AS, Woloshin S, Eddings W, et al. Physicians' knowledge about FDA approval standards and perceptions of the "Breakthrough Therapy" designation. *JAMA*. 2016;315:1516–1518.
20. Bullock JM, Rahman A, Liu Q. Lessons learned: dose selection of small molecule-targeted oncology drugs. *Clin Cancer Res*. 2016;22:2630–2638.
21. Dambach DM, Simpson NE, Jones TW, et al. Nonclinical evaluations of small-molecule oncology drugs: integration into clinical dose optimization and toxicity management. *Clin Cancer Res*. 2016;22:2618–2622.
22. Janne PA, Kim G, Shaw AT, et al. Dose finding of small-molecule oncology drugs: optimization throughout the development life cycle. *Clin Cancer Res*. 2016;22:2613–2617.
23. Nie L, Rubin EH, Mehrotra N, et al. Rendering the 3 + 3 design to rest: more efficient approaches to oncology dose-finding trials in the era of targeted therapy. *Clin Cancer Res*. 2016;22:2623–2629.
24. Prowell TM, Theoret MR, Pazdur R. Seamless oncology-drug development. *New Engl J Med*. 2016;374:2001–2003.
25. Theoret MR, Pai-Scherf LH, Chuk MK, et al. Expansion cohorts in first-in-human solid tumor oncology trials. *Clin Cancer Res*. 2015;21:4545–4551.
26. Pazdur RBG, Blumenthal G. FDA innovation brings new therapies to lung cancer patients. FDA Voice. 2014.
27. Draft Guidance for Industry and Food and Drug Administration Staff. Principles for Codevelopment of an In Vitro Companion Diagnostic Device with a Therapeutic Product. 2016.
28. Malik SM, Pazdur R, Abrams JS, et al. Consensus report of a joint NCI thoracic malignancies steering committee: FDA workshop on strategies for integrating biomarkers into clinical development of new therapies for lung cancer leading to the inception of "master protocols" in lung cancer. *J Thorac Oncol*. 2014;9:1443–1448.
29. McNeil C. NCI-MATCH launch highlights new trial design in precision-medicine era. *J Natl Cancer Inst*. 2015;107.
30. Rugo HS, Olopade OI, DeMichele A, et al. Adaptive randomization of veliparib-carboplatin treatment in breast cancer. *New Engl J Med*. 2016;375:23–34.
31. Guidance for Industry. Determining the Extent of Safety Data Collection Needed in Late-Stage Premarket and Postapproval Clinical Investigations. 2016.
32. Patient-Focused Drug Development: Disease Area Meetings Planned for Fiscal Years 2013-2017. 2016. http://www.fda.gov/ForIndustry/UserFees/PrescriptionDrugUserFee/ucm347317.htm
33. Workshop on Clinical Outcome Assessments (COAs) in Cancer Clinical Trials. https://c-path.org/workshop-on-clinical-outcome-assessments-coas-in-cancer-clinical-trials/
34. 21 CFR 314.126.
35. 21 CFR 201.56(b)(1) and 201.57(c)(7).
36. Basch E. Toward patient-centered drug development in oncology. New Engl J Med. 2013;369:397–400.
37. Cella D, Riley W, Stone A, et al. The Patient-Reported Outcomes Measurement Information System (PROMIS) developed and tested its first wave of adult self-reported health outcome item banks: 2005–2008. *J Clin Epidemiol*. 2010;63:1179–1194.
38. Kluetz PG, Chingos DT, Basch EM, Mitchell SA. Patient-Reported Outcomes in Cancer Clinical Trials: Measuring Symptomatic Adverse Events With the National Cancer Institute's Patient-Reported Outcomes Version of the Common Terminology Criteria for Adverse Events (PRO-CTCAE). *Am Soc Clin Oncol Educ Book*. 2016;35:67–73.
39. Kluetz PG, Slagle A, Papadopoulos EJ, et al. Focusing on core patient-reported outcomes in cancer clinical trials: symptomatic adverse events, physical function, and disease-related symptoms. *Clin Cancer Res*. 2016;22:1553–1558.
40. Kim ES, Atlas J, Ison G, Ersek JL. Transforming clinical trial eligibility criteria to reflect practical clinical application. *Am Soc Clin Oncol Educ Book*. 2016;35:83–90.
41. Chuk MK, Mulugeta Y, Roth-Cline M, et al. Enrolling adolescents in disease/target-appropriate adult oncology clinical trials of investigational agents. *Clin Cancer Res*. 2017;23:9–12.
42. Vestbo J, Leather D, Diar Bakerly N, et al. Effectiveness of fluticasone furoate-vilanterol for COPD in clinical practice. *New Engl J Med*. 2016;375:1253–1260.
43. Sherman RE, Anderson SA, Dal Pan GJ, et al. Real-World evidence–what is it and what can it tell us? *New Engl J Med*. 2016;375:2293–2297.
44. 21 CFR 312 Subpart I.
45. Guidance for Industry, Individual Patient Expanded Access Applications: Form FDA 3926. 2016.
46. Kim T, Lurie P, Pazdur R. US Food and drug administration efforts to facilitate the use of expanded access programs. *J Clin Oncol*. 2015;33:3979–3980.
47. Lemery S, Mailankody S, Kazandjian D, et al. Food and drug administration analysis of 1332 single patient and emergency use expanded access (Compassionate Use) requests for patients with cancer over a duration of three years (2012–2014). *J Clin Oncol*. 2016;34(suppl):abstr 6523.
48. Guidance for Industry. Providing Clinical Evidence of Effectiveness for Human Drug and Biological Products. 1998.
49. Martinalbo J, Bowen D, Camarero J, et al. Early market access of cancer drugs in the EU. *Ann Oncol*. 2016;27:96–105.
50. Kluetz PG, Pazdur R. Looking to the future in an unprecedented time for cancer drug development. *Semin Oncol*. 2016;43:2–3.
51. US v Rutherford, 442 US 544. 1979.
52. Guidance for Industry. Clinical Trial Endpoints for the Approval of Cancer Drugs and Biologics (Services UDoHaH, ed). 2007.
53. Blumenthal GM, Pazdur R. Response rate as an approval end point in oncology: back to the future. *JAMA Oncol*. 2016;2:780–781.
54. Kazandjian D, Blumenthal GM, Luo L, et al. Benefit-risk summary of crizotinib for the treatment of patients with ROS1 alteration-positive, metastatic non-small cell lung cancer. *Oncologist*. 2016;21:974–980.
55. Glucarpidase. 2012. http://www.fda.gov/Drugs/InformationOnDrugs/ApprovedDrugs/ucm288016.htm
56. Asparaginase Erwinia chrysanthemi. 2011. http://www.fda.gov/AboutFDA/CentersOffices/OfficeofMedicalProductsandTobacco/CDER/ucm280543.htm
57. Amiri-Kordestani L, Wedam S, Zhang L, et al. First FDA approval of neoadjuvant therapy for breast cancer: pertuzumab for the treatment of patients with HER2-positive breast cancer. *Clin Cancer Res*. 2014;20:5359–5364.
58. Sections 7002(a)(2) and (b)(3) of the Affordable Care Act, adding sections 351(k), 351(i)(2), and 351(i)(4) of the PHS Act.
59. Guidance for Industry. Scientific Considerations in Demonstrating Biosimilarity to a Reference Product. 2015.
60. FDA BLA Approval Letter. 2015. http://www.accessdata.fda.gov/drugsatfda_docs/appletter/2015/125553Orig1s000ltr.pdf
61. FDA News Release, FDA approves first biosimilar product Zarxio. 2015. http://www.fda.gov/NewsEvents/Newsroom/PressAnnouncements/ucm436648.htm
62. FDA Guidance for Industry. Quality Considerations in Demonstrating Biosimilarity of a Therapeutic Protein Product to a Reference Product. 2015.
63. FDA Draft Guidance. Clinical Pharmacology Data to Support a Demonstration of Biosimilarity to a Reference Product. 2014.
64. Cavallo J. Is this the dawn of cancer biosimilars? a conversation with Gary H. Lyman, MD, MPH, FASCO; Andrew D. Zelenetz, MD, PhD; Leah Christl, PhD; and Steven Lemery, MD, MHS. ASCO POST. 2016.

THE EVOLUTION OF THE DRUG EVALUATION PROCESS IN THE EU

Francesco Pignatti, Emmanuelle Kempf, and Pierre Demolis

Disclaimer: The views expressed in this article are the personal views of the authors and may not be understood or quoted as being made on behalf of or reflecting the position of the agencies or organizations with which the authors are affiliated.

INTRODUCTION

Drug regulation has evolved rapidly in the European Union (EU) since the 1960s when requirements for quality efficacy and safety for pharmaceuticals in the common EU market have been harmonized among member states. Over the years, a number of legislative changes have introduced new tools for cancer drug regulation, including incentives for orphan drugs, requirements on pediatric plans, and mechanisms for early approval.

Standards of cancer drug development and evaluation have continued to evolve over the years, as researchers and drug regulators have aimed to optimize clinical trial designs, particularly in terms of patient selection and shorter trial durations. Such approaches aim to offer "early access" to drugs for patients with high unmet medical needs, while dealing with challenges such as small populations, and also managing uncertainties while confirmatory data are being collected.

The following sections of this chapter describe:

- The EU regulatory system from a historical perspective, explain the role of the European Medicines Agency (EMA), and how drug evaluation is performed
- Different types of approvals that are available in the EU and how these have been used in recent years
- Existing EMA guidelines on the conduct of clinical trials for marketing authorization and key aspects such as choice of endpoint and use of external controls
- Clinical trials and interaction with academia and good clinical practices
- Perspectives on future developments in cancer drug evaluation

THE DRUG REGULATORY SYSTEM IN THE EUROPEAN UNION

Harmonization of Pharmaceutical Legislation

Cooperation between the countries of the EU has initially focused on establishing a common European market, to allow the free movement of goods, services, and people across national borders, and bringing the different economic policies of the member states closer together. Gradually the EU has become actively involved in issues such as environmental protection, health, consumer rights, competition and safety in the transport industry, education, and culture. In the early 1960s, the determination to prevent reoccurrence of the thalidomide disaster led to European law requiring that every medicinal product for human use that is to be placed on the market must first be granted a marketing authorization delivered by a competent authority (1). While aiming to safeguard public health, this law also reflected other important objectives for Europe, such as encouraging the development of the pharmaceutical industry and the achievement of a single market for pharmaceuticals.

The harmonization process moved on in 1975 with a directive detailing which tests and trials had to be carried out by companies seeking a marketing authorization (2). A second directive defined the criteria for the examination of applications and introduced a procedure to facilitate the adoption of a common position by the member states (3). A Committee for Medicinal Products for Human Use (CHMP) was set up, ensuring adequate scientific expertise at the regulatory level. Further procedures were introduced in 1986, targeting high-technology medicinal products, with a view of arriving to identical decisions throughout the EU.

A major step was achieved in 1995 with the coming into operation of the EMA and the establishment of a "centralized procedure" (4). The EMA has been primarily responsible for the scientific evaluation of marketing authorization applications via this procedure. The EMA coordinates the works of its scientific committees, which are based on the scientific resources made available by the national competent authorities. The EMA also coordinates the supervision of medicinal products that have been authorized within the EU. The scientific committee responsible for preparing the opinions on questions relating to the evaluation of medicinal products for human use is the CHMP.

An application through centralized procedure can lead to a single marketing authorization that is valid across the EU. Initially, this new procedure did not supersede the existing process based on national authorizations, except for certain "biotech" products. However, since 2006, it became mandatory also for other types of products, including new oncology drugs and drugs for orphan diseases.

In almost 60 years of legislation, EU law has enforced uniform rules governing aspects of the authorization, production, distribution, and proper use of medicines in the EU. Member states have maintained autonomy on matters such as clinical trial authorization, pricing, and reimbursement.

The Role of the European Medicines Agency

The CHMP is responsible for conducting an evaluation of the quality, safety, and efficacy of medicinal products submitted through a centralized procedure to the highest possible standards; this follows a strict timetable. The CHMP includes one member and one alternate nominated by each member state and up to five co-opted members, chosen by reason of their role and experience in the evaluation of medicinal products. In addition, a wide network of experts has been established over the years to serve on working parties or expert groups of the CHMP. A number of other committees, such as the Pharmacovigilance Risk Assessment Committee and the Committee for Advanced Therapies, complete the system.

The scientific review of a marketing authorization application is coordinated by the EMA and consists of an alternation of periods of active evaluation (scientific assessment, drafting of reports, discussion and adoption of opinion and accompanying documents at the level of the CHMP), with periods where the clock is stopped and where the applicant is asked to resolve certain deficiencies or objections. The total duration of the process is a maximum of 210 days of active time, plus the stop clock (which should generally not exceed 8 months, according to a CHMP policy; Figure 48.1 [5]).

Once the evaluation is completed, the CHMP gives a favorable or unfavorable opinion as to whether to grant the authorization. The applicant is given the opportunity to withdraw the application prior to opinion or to appeal to the CHMP against its opinion. Once a final opinion is adopted, it is forwarded together with all necessary translations to the European Commission. (The European Commission is an EU institution that holds executive powers over the EU and is responsible for

implementing decisions). This is the start of the decision-making process leading to a legally binding decision.

Within 15 days of receipt of the opinion from the CHMP, the European Commission prepares a draft decision. The draft decision is forwarded to a regulatory committee called the "Standing Committee on Medicinal Products for Human Use," where representatives of the member states can raise objections. If objections are raised, the CHMP may be asked to formulate a reply, and a fresh procedure can be started based on the CHMP answer. If the Standing Committee's opinion is favorable, the European Commission can proceed with the decision making process. If the European Commission does not receive a favorable opinion from the Standing Committee, the matter is referred to the Council of the European Union. (Together with the European Parliament, the Council is the main decision-making body of the EU).

Scientific Advice

The EMA, particularly acting through its committees, advises about undertakings on the conduct of the various tests and trials necessary to demonstrate the quality, safety, and efficacy of medicinal products. To this end, the field of activity of the scientific committees of the EMA has been enlarged, and their operating methods and composition have been modernized. Over the years, scientific advice for future applicants seeking marketing authorization has been provided more generally and in greater depth. Similarly, structures allowing the development of advice for companies, in particular small- and medium-sized enterprises, have been put in place. The scientific committees consult standing working parties open to experts from the scientific world appointed for this purpose, while retaining total responsibility for the

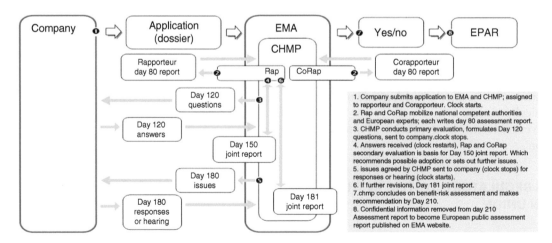

FIGURE 48.1 Submission and evaluation of a drug application through the centralized procedure.

CHMP, Committee for Proprietary Medicinal Products; CoRap, Corapporteur; EMA, European Medicines Agency; EPAR, European Public Assessment Report; Rap, Rapporteur.

Source: From Phillips LD, Fasolo B, Zafiropoulos N, Beyer A. Is quantitative benefit-risk modelling of drugs desirable or possible? Drug Discovery Today: Technologies; 2011.

scientific opinions issued. There exist fee waivers for scientific advice provided to designated orphan medicinal products (so-called "protocol assistance").

TYPES OF APPROVAL

Standard Approval

Applicant companies are required to submit the results of pharmaceutical and nonclinical tests and clinical trials to enable a sufficiently well founded and scientifically valid judgment as to whether the potential risks are outweighed by the therapeutic efficacy of the product. The risks relate to patients' health or public health (6).

If there are comprehensive data and the benefit-risk balance is positive, a standard approval is granted and is valid for 5 years. During this period, the CHMP assesses periodic safety update reports and the results from any outstanding post-authorization measures (e.g., results of stability studies, long-term follow-up of clinical trials) on a regular basis. After 5 years, the benefit-risk balance is reevaluated and the marketing authorization can be renewed indefinitely or for another 5 years. The marketing authorization will be refused if the benefit-risk balance is not favorable or if the therapeutic efficacy is insufficiently substantiated (Figure 48.2).

What constitutes comprehensive data for standard approval is a matter of scientific judgment, and EMA guidelines address specific requirements for marketing authorization for different therapeutic areas, including oncology (7). Randomized controlled trials (RCTs) are generally required using time-related endpoints such as overall survival (OS) or progression-free survival (PFS). RCTs are mostly active-controlled, with a minority of trials using placebo or best care. Masking is often not feasible because of the distinct toxicity profiles of the different drugs except for the less toxic targeted agents, for which double-blind placebo-controlled RCTs have been possible. Nonrandomized studies using historical controls have been accepted in some cases as a basis for standard approval if a "dramatic effect" in terms of objective tumor response was shown in a homogenous population with predictable outcome and no alternative treatment.

Conditional Approval

Conditional approval is reserved for drugs that treat, prevent, or diagnose (a) seriously debilitating or life-threatening diseases, (b) rare diseases (orphan drugs) or drugs to be used in emergency situations in response to threats recognized either by the World Health Organization or by the EU (8). With this approval, which differs from standard approval in that the clinical data submitted are not yet comprehensive, the applicant company is obliged to submit further data from ongoing or new trials or further pharmacovigilance data to confirm that the benefit-risk balance is positive.

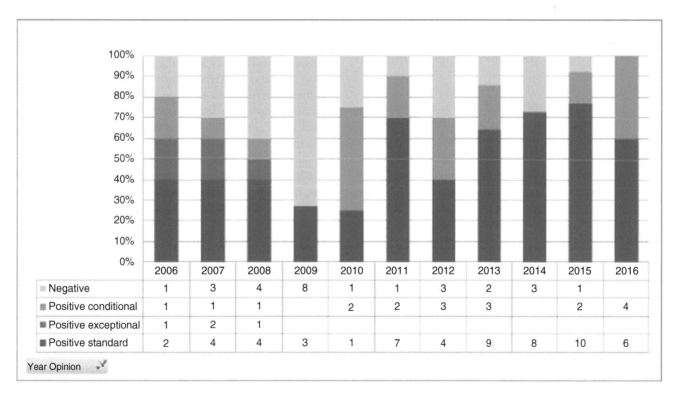

Year Opinion	2006	2007	2008	2009	2010	2011	2012	2013	2014	2015	2016
Negative	1	3	4	8	1	1	3	2	3	1	
Positive conditional	1	1	1		2	2	3	3		2	4
Positive exceptional	1	2	1								
Positive standard	2	4	4	3	1	7	4	9	8	10	6

FIGURE 48.2 Outcome for initial cancer drug applications (2006–2016) by type of outcome. "Negative" outcome includes withdrawn applications.

Several criteria have to be fulfilled for granting of a conditional marketing authorization:

- The benefit-risk balance must be positive.
- It must be likely that the applicant company will provide comprehensive data postapproval.
- Available methods to prevent, diagnose, or treat the condition must be unsatisfactory or, even if satisfactory methods exist, the drug must offer a major therapeutic advantage.
- The benefits to public health deriving from the immediate availability of the product must outweigh the risks due to the fact that the data are not yet comprehensive.

A conditional approval is only valid for 1 year but can be renewed. The renewal is given on the basis of the confirmation of the benefit-risk balance, taking into account the specific obligations and the time frame for their fulfillment. For conditional approval, prior to expiry of the authorization the applicant company submits a report on the fulfillment of the obligations, and the CHMP assesses the benefit-risk balance. Once it is judged that remaining data have been provided or are no longer required, the marketing authorization can be converted to a "standard" authorization. If at any time the benefit-risk is considered to be negative, the marketing authorization can be suspended or revoked.

Patients and health care professionals are given clear information about the conditional nature of such approvals, including details about the renewal of the approval in the summary of product characteristics. For instance, the initially approved summary of product characteristics for sunitinib informed prescribers that sunitinib

(. . .) has been authorized under a 'conditional approval' scheme. This means that further evidence on this medicinal product is awaited, in particular about the effect of SUTENT in terms of progression-free survival in patients with MRCC [metastatic renal cell carcinoma]. A study is being conducted to investigate this. The European Medicines Agency (EMEA) will review new information on the product every year (. . .). (9)

It has been recognized that conditional marketing authorization (MA) is an important tool for ensuring timely access to medicines in areas of unmet medical need (Figure 48.3) (10). However, delays have been observed in the timelines for reaching reimbursement decisions nationally, compared to standard approvals (11). EMA has been encouraging early dialogue with companies on conditional MAs and involving other stakeholders (in particular, health technology assessment organizations) in this process, aiming at facilitating timely completion

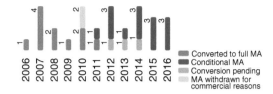

FIGURE 48.3 Conditional marketing authorizations (MA) granted by year. The CHMP reviews all data collected annually to decide about a further renewal of the authorization or its conversion into a standard marketing authorization. On average, a conditional MA is converted into a standard MA within 4 years. From 2006 to 2016, 17/30 (57%) conditional MAs were granted for oncology drugs.

EMA, European Medicines Agency; MA, marketing authorization.

Source: Courtesy of Z. Sebris, EMA.

of studies required for health economic evaluation and access to medicines for patients.

Approval Under "Exceptional Circumstances"

Exceptional circumstances status is reserved for situations where it is impossible to provide comprehensive data because (a) the disease is too rare, (b) the current state of scientific knowledge does not allow comprehensive data to be collected, or (c) it would be contrary to medical ethics to collect such data. For the remaining situations, approval under exceptional circumstances is similar to conditional approval in that there are requirements for postapproval studies that form the basis for a yearly reassessment of the benefit-risk balance. However, postapproval studies normally do not lead to comprehensive data and standard approval because of the intrinsic difficulty of doing so. Also for approval under exceptional circumstances, the legislation requires that the package leaflet and any medical information draw the attention of the medical practitioner to the fact that the data available concerning the medicinal product in question are as yet inadequate in certain specified respects. Trabectedin for the treatment of patients with advanced soft tissue sarcoma was an example of an approval under "exceptional circumstances." The CHMP concluded that the benefit-risk balance was positive but that adequate exploratory data should be made available to identify patients who are most likely to respond. Individual subgroups based on histology were considered too rare for adequately powered RCTs to be conducted against best supportive care to explore factors associated with response to treatment within reasonable time. Thus, because of the rarity of the disease, the CHMP considered that the marketing authorization could be granted under exceptional circumstances. The applicant committed to explore further the population that might benefit most from the treatment as a specific obligation.

THE EMA GUIDELINE ON ANTICANCER MEDICINAL PRODUCTS

The EMA has issued guidance on the clinical development of new anticancer drugs. The first EMA guideline on the clinical development of new anticancer agents was issued in 1996. This was based on a previous text from 1990 adopted by the CHMP (12). Since its first publication, this regulatory clinical guideline has reflected the experience of EMA and the focus was on confirmatory (phase III) studies for conventional cytotoxic compounds. Two revisions followed in 2001 and 2003, including a number of improvements and updates (e.g., use of the Response Evaluation Criteria In Solid Tumors [RECIST] for response evaluation). The third revision was published in 2006 and provides additional guidance for new oncology drugs that behave variably as cytostatic or cytotoxic agents (7).

The current version of the main guideline (revision 4, published in 2013) includes new guidance on the development of noncytotoxic (i.e., cytostatic) agents and immunotherapy. For noncytotoxic drugs, the early stages of clinical drug development are more complex and must be tailored according to the assumed pharmacology of the individual compound as defined in nonclinical studies. The integration of information from exploratory (phase I/II) and confirmatory (phase III) studies is of primary importance for a successful development and authorization for these types of agents.

In terms of evidentiary standards for approval, two related issues are often debated between regulators and applicant companies—namely the design of the study and the choice of endpoint. Regardless of the type of agent, phase III trials should be designed with the aim of establishing the benefit-risk balance of the drug in a well-characterized target population. These studies should be RCTs and, where possible blinded or include blinded evaluation. Acceptable primary endpoints include OS and PFS or disease-free survival (DFS). If PFS or DFS is the selected primary endpoint, OS should be reported as a secondary and vice versa. When OS is reported as a secondary endpoint, the required number of events and duration of follow-up will depend on the results with regard to the primary endpoint, availability and activity of next-line therapies, expected survival after progression, and safety results comparing test with reference. However, the estimated treatment effect on OS should be sufficiently precise to ensure that there are no relevant detrimental effects on this endpoint. In situations where there is a large effect on PFS, a long expected survival after progression, or a clearly favorable safety profile, precise estimates of OS may not be needed for approval. When PFS is reported as secondary endpoint, consistency is expected with regard to the treatment effect on OS.

In patients with tumor-related symptoms at baseline, symptom control, if related to antitumor effects, is a valid measure of therapeutic activity and may serve as primary endpoint in studies investigating late-line therapy, provided that the study can be conducted under proper double-blind conditions and that other sources of possible bias can be minimized. In certain cases, time to symptomatic tumor progression may also be an adequate primary measure of patient benefit.

There are also examples where tumor response-related activities (e.g., limb-saving surgery) may be reasonable primary measures of patient benefit. However, analyses of location- or cause-specific events should in general be avoided because the focus may be drawn away from the main objective, namely the overall success of the treatment strategy in question.

In double-blind studies and especially in the palliative setting, health-related quality of life using generally accepted instruments might be a valuable secondary endpoint.

It is acknowledged that at the time of first submission for marketing authorization, there may be unresolved issues (e.g., identification of important pharmacological factors to explain the outcome of the confirmatory studies). Nevertheless, to the extent that this is possible throughout the clinical development, the study of biomarkers is highly recommended, in particular for noncytotoxic agents. This will form the basis for exploring ways to select responders and guide further studies to be conducted postmarketing.

The use of external control (including historical control) is discussed in International Council for Harmonisation of Technical Requirements for Pharmaceuticals for Human Use (ICH) E10 and it concluded that "the inability to control bias restricts use of the external control design to situations where the treatment effect is dramatic and the usual course of the disease highly predictable" (13). Dramatic effects are uncommonly documented in the treatment of malignancies, but it is acknowledged that such effects, obvious to any qualified observer, are seen occasionally. In these cases, prospective confirmation in randomized, reference-controlled studies is not only unacceptable to investigators, patients, and ethics committees, but also unnecessary.

Four appendices complement the guideline. The first is an appendix on methodological aspects related to measuring PFS as primary endpoint in phase III trials. The second deals with the use of patient-reported outcome measures. The third provides condition-specific appendix guidance for non–small cell lung cancer, prostate cancer, chronic myeloid leukemia, myelodysplastic syndromes, hematopoietic stem cell transplantation, breast cancer, and chronic lymphocytic leukemia. The fourth provides recommendations relevant to childhood malignancies and pediatric drug development. (The full text of the guidelines is available on the EMA website: www.ema.europa.eu).

CLINICAL TRIALS AND INTERACTION WITH ACADEMIA

Role of Academia in Cancer Research

Academic researchers achieved the first successes in cancer care starting mostly after World War II. Thanks to significant achievements in chemistry and biology, highlighted in 1953 by the full description of the DNA double helix in Cambridge by James Watson and Francis Crick, the knowledge of carcinogenesis improved—and therefore the biological rationales related to anticancer drug development. At that time, medical oncology as a full specialty did not exist. Hematologists had quite an easy access to tumor biology thanks to bone marrow biopsies, which led to the first clinical successes in immunotherapy, like the first worldwide allograft in acute myeloid leukemia in 1963 by Georges Mathé in France. On the other hand, surgeons to whom all the patients with breast cancer were referred developed the concept of hormonal therapies, based on the positive effects of surgical castration in the United Kingdom.

Before the 1980s, the academic world led anticancer drug development, while the pharmaceutical industries started to invest in this new field, mostly with a compassionate purpose. Researchers were in charge of the screening and the synthesis of new compounds. Influenced by the program launched in the United States by the National Institutes of Health (NIH), a few European early oncologists created in 1962 the Groupe Européen de Chimiothérapie Anticancéreuse (GECA). This became the European Organization for Research and Treatment of Cancer (EORTC), once English became the consensual language of international scientific communication. The European collaboration of some of the first-generation oncologists aimed at developing anticancer drugs from bench to bedside. This comprehensive drug development process split in two parts in the late 1980s when pharmaceutical industries hired academic researchers to develop cancer-specific drugs. The financial investment required to build drug pipelines became unsustainable for the academic world, which has since focused on basic science and late-stage clinical trials.

Academic trials have contributed important advances in establishing new treatment standards and have played a particularly important and innovative role, often in neglected or orphan diseases, and generally in therapeutic areas where the clinical development is difficult, such as oncology and pediatrics. The recent extension of the marketing authorization for arsenic trioxide in the EU for induction of remission and consolidation in adult patients with newly diagnosed low-to-intermediate risk acute promyelocytic leukemia is a good example.

High-quality clinical trials (whether academic or not) are necessary to provide the main evidence of efficacy and safety in a marketing authorization application. Academic sponsors of investigational drugs or drugs in new indications must keep in mind that a marketing authorization may be a necessary subsequent step. In these situations, it is advisable to seek agreement with the regulatory and other decision makers about the evidentiary standards. In 1964, the Declaration of Helsinki merged the ten principles of the 1947 Nuremberg Code, regarding ethical issues in the conduct of clinical research, with the 1948 Declaration of Geneva, which was supposed to refresh the Oath of Hippocrates after WWII. In 2008, the Good Clinical Practices (GCP) guideline from the ICH was added. The GCP guideline focuses more on procedural aspects than on ethical issues related to the conduct of clinical research.

There is only one standard of GCP, but the implementation in the context of each trial may be proportional to the risks and complexity of the trial and prior knowledge of the product. GCP inspections may take place as part of the verification of applications for marketing authorization.

Interaction With Academia

Academia play an important role in helping the EU medicine's regulatory network to keep abreast of the opportunities and challenges brought by science and to have access to the right expertise to evaluate these innovative medicines. Academia is a recognized source of scientific knowledge and excellence that provides the EMA regulatory network with expert input to ensure that medicines are evaluated and monitored to the highest scientific standards. As regulatory approaches continue to evolve the collaboration between the regulatory network and academia is necessary to ensure preparedness for future challenges and opportunities offered by advances in science and technology. In 2017, the EMA has introduced a framework for collaboration with academia (14). (Formal frameworks for interacting with patients, health care professionals, and the pharmaceutical industry were adopted by the EMA's Management Board in 2005, 2011, and 2015.) The framework's overall objectives are:

1. To raise awareness of the mandate and work of the EMA regulatory network as a means to increase academia's engagement and trust in the regulatory system that addresses society's needs
2. To promote and further develop the regulatory support to foster the translation of academic research into novel methodologies and medicinal products that meet the regulatory standards required to address patients' and public and animal health's needs
3. To ensure that the best scientific expertise and academic research are available to support timely and effective evidence generation, regulatory advice and guidance, and decision making in regulatory processes

4. To work in collaboration with the regulatory network in developing regulatory science that addresses novel approaches, novel endpoints, and methodologies, adapting to scientific progress while affording appropriate patient safety

In order to achieve its overall objectives, the framework will rely on the following elements: mapping of academic entities with an interest in the regulatory activities, evolution of available expertise to keep pace with advances in scientific knowledge, identifying opportunities to promote research and knowledge generation, promoting and reinforcing dialogue through effective communication, and monitoring progress and output of the cooperation with academia.

PERSPECTIVES ON FUTURE DEVELOPMENTS

The year 2015 marked the 50th anniversary of the adoption of the first law concerning the authorization of pharmaceuticals at the EU level, which set the basis for some of the key principles that are still valid today. Over the past 50 years, a large body of legislation has been developed around the principle that to safeguard public health, no medicinal product can be marketed without prior authorization, with the progressive harmonization of requirements for the granting of marketing authorizations and postmarketing monitoring implemented across the entire EU. The most significant achievement has been providing Europe with centralized pharmaceutical assessment and authorization. A host of experts from agencies of member states and other stakeholders now work together to provide European citizens and the health care sector access to quality medicinal products that are safe and effective. The EU's assessment and authorization system for medicines is a major achievement in itself (15).

Despite the many achievements there are still many challenges ahead. Some of the most pressing challenges are related to budgetary constraints of health systems and access to innovative treatments. While the regulators focus on the benefit-risk balance of a drug, the payers base their decisions on its comparative effectiveness and cost-effectiveness. If cancer patients are to get access to innovations more quickly, the medical evidence on which the marketing authorization has been approved might lack clinically relevant data regarding long-term effects on survival as required by certain health economic evaluations. Also, some endpoints such as PFS, used to approve the drugs, might not correlate with OS assessed in further postapproval analysis. In Europe, each EU member state follows national and independent public health policies in order to reimburse the cost of approved drugs. According to distinct budget priorities, some countries might not be able to afford the increasing price of innovations such as checkpoint inhibitors or combination therapy with innovative drugs. For example, in the past decade, France reimbursed its people for more drugs than Scotland or Poland, increasing the discrepancy related to patient access to innovations across Europe (16). Collaboration is intrinsic to the values of the EU and its organizations and may help address some of these challenges. A successful example of such collaboration in terms of efficient transfer of information and joint advice to companies is an EMA's collaboration with the health technology assessment organizations from the European Network for Health Technology Assessment (EUNetHTA). However, pricing and reimbursement are likely to remain at the heart of debates in the years to come.

Cancer drug regulators will continue to face challenges in a number of areas such as orphan and pediatric medicines, which are a growing feature of the drug therapy world. The trend toward personalized medicine will add to these challenges. Targeted therapies explore and introduce new indications that may sometimes describe very small populations. This may bring into question the use of classical designs (large comparative trials) and usual endpoints, making the development of some anticancer drugs always closer to what is applied for orphan conditions. Dealing with new, more complex therapeutic options and new medicine delivery systems will undoubtedly create new challenges for regulators. There is also growing interest to explore new types and levels of evidence for testing new medical products, going beyond the traditional RCTs. Despite growing complexities, regulators will have to retain the capacity to step back and engage with patients and other stakeholders in a language they understand, keeping them informed of regulatory, technical, and medical developments (15). The EMA has developed a framework for more patient involvement in the benefit-risk assessment and is exploring the role of patient preference studies in the regulatory context (17,18).

Building a pipeline of promising anticancer drugs represents a financial burden that the academic world cannot afford anymore. Yet, their biological rationale and the further assessment of their clinical relevance and optimization of treatment may be part of the scope of academic research. Specifically, the evidence gap between EMA approvals and the evidence required for cost-effectiveness evaluations might be filled by academic medical evidence, such as clinical trials but also real-life/real-world data from cancer registries, patients' long-term follow-up and perspectives, comparative effectiveness studies, and so on. It is also possible that "payers" will take a more active role in supporting such studies in a cooperative manner across the EU.

REFERENCES

1. Council Directive 65/65/EEC of 26 January 1965 on the approximation of provisions laid down by Law, Regulation or Administrative Action relating to proprietary medicinal products. *Official J EurCommun P*. 1965;22:0369–0373.
2. Council Directive 75/318/EEC of 20 May 1975 on the approximation of the laws of Member States relating to analytical, pharmaco-toxicological and clinical standards and protocols in respect of the testing of proprietary medicinal products. *Official Journal L*. 1975;147:0001–0012.
3. Second Council Directive 75/319/EEC of 20 May 1975 on the approximation of provisions laid down by Law, Regulation or Administrative Action relating to proprietary medicinal products. *Official Journal L*. 1975;147:0013–0022.
4. Council Regulation (EEC) No 2309/93 of 22 July 1993 laying down Community procedures for the authorization and supervision of medicinal products for human and veterinary use and establishing a European Agency for the Evaluation of Medicinal Products. *Official Journal L*. 1993;214:1–21.
5. Phillips LD, Fasolo B, Zafiropoulos N, Beyer A. Is quantitative benefit-risk modelling of drugs desirable or possible? *Drug Discov Today Technol*. 2011;8:e3–e10.
6. Commission Directive of 25 June 2003 amending Directive 2001/83/EC of the European Parliament and of the Council on the Community code relating to medicinal products for human use. 2003.
7. CPMP/EWP/205/95/Rev.3. Guideline on the Evaluation of Anticancer Medicinal Products in Man. 2005. http://www.ema.europa.eu/ema/index.jsp?curl=pages/regulation/general/general_content_001122.jsp&mid=WC0b01ac0580034cf3
8. Commission Regulation (EC) No 507/2006 of 29 March 2006 on the conditional marketing authorisation fro medicinal products for human use falling within the scope of Regulation (EC) No 726/2004 of the European Parliament and of the Council. 2006.
9. European Medicines Agency. Sutent (sunitinib): summary of product characteristics. http://www.ema.europa.eu/docs/en_GB/document_library/EPAR_-_Product_Information/human/000687/WC500057737.pdf. Published 2018.
10. EMA report. Conditional marketing authorisation. http://www.ema.europa.eu/docs/en_GB/document_library/Report/2017/01/WC500219991.pdf
11. Martinalbo J, Bowen D, Camarero J, et al. Early market access of cancer drugs in the EU. *Ann Oncol*. 2016;27(1):96–105.
12. Evaluation of anticancer medicinal products in man. CPMP Working Party on Efficacy of Medicinal Products. *Pharmacol Toxicol*. 1990;67(5):454–458.
13. Choice of Control Group and Related Issues in Clinical Trials (E10). International conference on harmonisation of technical requirements for registration of pharmaceuticals for human use. http://www.ich.org/fileadmin/Public_Web_Site/ICH_Products/Guidelines/Efficacy/E10/Step4/E10_Guideline.pdf. Published 2000.
14. REF2 European Medicines Agency. Framework of collaboration between the European Medicines Agency and academia. http://www.ema.europa.eu/docs/en_GB/document_library/Regulatory_and_procedural_guideline/2017/03/WC500224896.pdf. Published 2017.
15. 50 Years of EU Pharma Legislation: Achievements and Future Perspectives. https://ec.europa.eu/health/sites/health/files/human-use/50years/docs/50years_conf_report.pdf
16. Pujolras LM, Cairns J. Why do some countries approve a cancer drug and others don't? *J Can Policy*. 2015;4:21–25. doi:10.1016/j.jcpo.2015.05.004
17. Postmus D, Mavris M, Hillege HL, et al. Incorporating patient preferences into drug development and regulatory decision making: results from a quantitative pilot study with cancer patients, carers, and regulators. *Clin Pharmacol Ther*. 2016;99(5):548–554.
18. Postmus D, Richard S, Bere N, et al. Individual trade-offs between possible benefits and risks of cancer treatments: results from a stated preference study with patients with multiple myeloma. *Oncologist*. 2018;23(1):44–51.

THE EVOLUTION OF THE DRUG EVALUATION PROCESS IN JAPAN

Hiroyuki Sato, Tomohiro Yamaguchi, Yuki Ando, and Takahiro Nonaka

NEW DRUG REVIEW PROCESS IN JAPAN

Establishment of a Review Agency

To respond to events involving health damage caused by drugs, the Fund for Adverse Drug Reactions Suffering Relief was established in October 1979. Its function was to provide quick relief to patients with adverse drug reactions (ADRs). This fund began to implement research and development (R&D)–type activities in 1987, and it later became the Organization for Pharmaceutical Safety and Research (OPSR) in 1994. OPSR began giving advice for clinical trials planning and performing good clinical practice (GCP)/good laboratory practice (GLP) inspections as part of the review process for new drug applications in 1997. In the same year, the Pharmaceuticals and Medical Devices Evaluation Center (PMDEC) was established at the National Institute of Health Sciences in order to develop a complete regulatory review system, increasing the complexity of review activities. The Japan Association for the Advancement of Medical Equipment (JAAME) was established in 1995 to improve the review processes of medical devices.

The Pharmaceuticals and Medical Devices Agency (PMDA) was established on April 1, 2004, in accordance with the Act on the Pharmaceuticals and Medical Devices Agency (Act No. 192 of 2002). The PMDA, the agency for reviewing new drugs, consolidated the operations allocated to PMDEC, OPSR, and JAAME in order to further evaluate reviews and postmarketing safety. Its mission is to contribute to improved public health by giving prompt relief to people who have suffered ADRs or infections from biological products; provide advice and reviews regarding the quality, efficacy, and safety of drugs and medical devices using a system that integrates the entire process from preclinical research to approval; and collect, analyze, and deliver postmarketing safety information.

New Drug Review

In the PMDA, five new drug offices (Office of New Drug I to V), the Office of Cellular and Tissue-based Products, and Office of Vaccines and Blood Products evaluate the efficacy, safety, and quality of drugs for which applications have been submitted for regulatory approval; these offices base their work on current scientific and technologic standards. Activities involve clinical trial consultation meetings that give advice to sponsors of clinical

trial–related design and evaluation. Each review office has review teams for each therapeutic area. Under the guidance of an office director and a review director, a review team conducts new drug review and consultation. As a general rule, each review team is made up of experts from the pharmaceutical sciences, medical sciences, toxicology, biostatistics, and other related fields. There is a team leader and deputy team leader.

Once an applicant has submitted the materials to the PMDA in Common Technical Document format, reviewers begin their review based on the materials. After discussion by the review team, questions about drug efficacy, safety, and dosage regimen are sent to the applicant, and the applicant addresses the queries. The review team sometimes asks the applicant to conduct additional analysis of the data based on suggestions by reviewers. The review team and the applicant repeat this procedure in order to complete the review report of the product. The report by the PMDA review team consists of descriptions related to the efficacy and safety of the product in specialized fields such as Chemistry, Manufacturing and Control (CMC), toxicology, pharmacology, pharmacokinetics, medical sciences including biostatistics, in addition to the background of the disease and the drug. The review report also includes the results of the on-site and document-based inspections for evaluating whether application data comply with GCP as conducted by the Office of Nonclinical and Clinical Compliance. After completion of the review report, the review team has scientific discussion with the external experts about the results of the review. The review team adds descriptions based on the discussion to the review report to complete the review and sends it to the Ministry of Health, Labour, and Welfare (MHLW). The MHLW consults the Pharmaceutical Affairs and Food Sanitation Council for advice about the approval of the drug. Then finally the MHLW may give approval of the drug.

CURRENT TOPICS IN DRUG DEVELOPMENT AND REVIEW IN JAPAN

Clinical Development Strategy for New Drug Applications in Japan

The guideline for the clinical evaluation methods of anticancer drugs, termed the first guideline, was issued in February 1991 (1). This guideline stipulated that the results of the phase III clinical trial were allowed to be submitted after drug approval, although the plan for that trial needed to be submitted by the time of drug approval. More than 10 years had passed since the first guideline was issued, and the situation concerning the development and review of new drugs had improved. However, the Japanese "drug-lag" issue, a several years' delay in new drug approval in Japan,

---

The views expressed here are the result of an independent study and do not represent the viewpoints or findings of the PMDA.

became apparent. Considering this situation, the first guideline for anticancer drugs was revised and issued in November 2005 (2). The revised guideline dictated that the results from phase III studies must be submitted at the time of application, at least for drugs indicated for major cancers, such as non–small cell lung cancer, gastric cancer, colorectal cancer, and breast cancer. In addition, based on the International Council on Harmonisation (ICH) E5 Guideline "Ethnic Factors in the Acceptability of Foreign Clinical Data," (3) the revised guideline stated that the clinical development strategies using foreign confirmatory clinical trial data were encouraged to promote efficient and rapid development of new oncology drugs in Japan. It should be noted that this may imply that drug development in Japan is delayed compared with that in other regions. Thus, these strategies can contribute to decreasing drug lag, but cannot remove drug lag entirely.

Multiregional clinical trials (MRCTs) potentially lead to simultaneous new drug applications and approval worldwide. When MRCTs are conducted, the differences in intrinsic and extrinsic ethnic factors that can cause differences in drug efficacy and safety among participating regions should be thoroughly considered through trial design, conduct, analysis, and interpretation of the results. In Japan, we have had substantial experience discussing development strategies using foreign clinical data in the PMDA consultation meetings with sponsors held in the planning stage of the clinical trials. Of particular interest, based on the accumulated experience of the consultations for MRCTs, "Basic Principles on Global Clinical Trials" was issued as a guidance document for MRCT planning in September 2007 (4). Several topics frequently discussed in consultation meetings were covered in the guidance document, such as the necessity for pharmacokinetic and dose-response information in Japanese prior to the MRCTs; management of potential differences in efficacy variables, controls, or concomitant drugs; and the appropriate sample size of Japanese subjects.

Since the issuance of "Basic Principles on Global Clinical Trials," Japan's participation in global clinical trials has been steadily increasing. The methods of cooperation between Japan and foreign countries have also been diversified. In global drug development, well-conducted global clinical trials are important not only for industries but also for regulatory authorities that evaluate study results. In order to react to the progress and changes, "Basic Principles on Global Clinical Trials (Reference Cases)" was developed in September 2012 (5). Furthermore, considering the cases that safety data in a foreign population has already been obtained to some extent at a beginning of Japanese drug developments, in order to prevent Japan from missing an opportunity to participate in MRCTs, the "Basic Principles for Conducting Phase I Trials in the Japanese Population Prior to Global Clinical Trials" was issued in October 2014 (6).

Since we have many approved cases using MRCTs including Japanese patients as the pivotal trials in clinical data packages, experience evaluating MRCT results is growing in Japan. The major target diseases of the MRCTs have been cancer and cardiovascular disease, but the conditions under study have recently expanded and now include neurologic/psychiatric, inflammatory, and metabolic diseases. Based on the publication data (7), we investigated the number of approved anticancer drugs/applications that were submitted in Japan between November 2005 and March 2015. This survey covered 100 applications (excluding the application based on evidence in the public domain) in that period. Figure 48.4 shows the trends of the number of drugs approved in Japan with MRCTs compared with those with the other strategy (e.g., local trial, foreign trial), along with percentages of the total number of approved drugs. From 2005 to 2008, the percentage of approved cases using

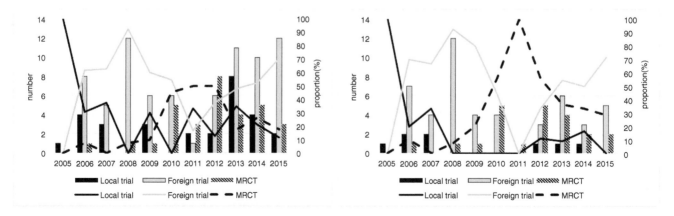

FIGURE 48.4 Trends of the number of approved drugs shown by the columns and the percentages of the total number of approved drugs shown by the line (left side, all applications; right side, orphan drug).

MRCT, multiregional clinical trials.

foreign clinical trial data was larger than that of the other strategies. However, from 2009, the percentage of the approved drugs using MRCTs increased by 20% to 30%.

Recently, a study investigated the relationship between the clinical development strategies and the lag in drug development (difference between the submission dates of new drug applications [NDAs] in the United States and Japan) to identify an appropriate strategy for NDA submission in Japan (8). This research demonstrated that the lag in drug development was markedly shorter in the clinical development strategies with MRCTs. Based on these results, although we should not draw a conclusion, the percentage of the approved drugs using MRCTs seems to be surpassing that using the other strategy in the clinical development of oncology drugs.

Oncology Phase I Clinical Trials in Japan

The process of developing pharmaceuticals involves several stages of evaluation. Following satisfactory preclinical evaluations in animal models, phase I trials are conducted in humans to determine the optimal dose and schedule of administration based on tolerability. Phase I trials also play an important role in understanding toxicity.

Despite groundbreaking research being done in Japanese laboratories involving the discovery of various molecular targets for cancer treatment including BRCA1, EML4-ALK, RET, and PD-1 (9–12), clinical development of many promising molecular-targeted agents and immune-checkpoint inhibitors have been launched in Western countries, with most of the first-in-human (FIH) trials conducted outside Japan. Practically speaking, the primary purpose of phase I trials in Japan has been to confirm tolerability in Japanese patients.

Between 2013 and 2015, 24 new oncology products received approval in Japan, including three products (nivolumab, alectinib hydrochloride and tipiracil hydrochloride, and trifluridine) that were first approved in Japan before any other countries. Alectinib hydrochloride, however, was the only drug with an FIH trial conducted in Japan.

In addition, the median research and development (R&D) lag, which is defined as the length of time from initiation of an FIH trial abroad until the start of a phase I trial here in Japan, is 77 months (range, 6–515 months). In comparison, the median drug lag, which is defined as the length of time from drug approval in the United States until approval here in Japan is 31 months (range, 1–388 months). It appears the R&D lag is one of the contributing reasons for our drug lag (13).

Increasing the number of FIH trials in Japan is advisable not only to shorten the drug lag that prevents Japanese patients from accessing new and effective drugs, but also to further Japan's valuable contributions to the development of such drugs.

What are the reasons for the scarcity of FIH trials in Japan? In terms of regulatory issues, pharmaceutical regulations in Japan are based on the ICH guidelines, which do not appear to be a major barrier to conducting FIH trials in Japan. As for infrastructure issues, however, there are only a limited number of Japanese institutions that can conduct FIH trials, which is most certainly one of the principle obstacles to initiating such trials in Japan.

In an effort to address the infrastructure problem, the Japanese government has annually awarded $1 million since 2006 to 10 centers of excellence, including the National Cancer Center Hospital in Tokyo (14–15). As a result, the facilities and resources necessary for early drug development in those institutions has improved with a corresponding increase in the number of FIH trials as well as translational research being conducted in Japan (e.g., mogamulizumab, alectinib hydrochloride, and TAS-115) (16–18). Although such financial assistance has contributed to a modest increase in the number of FIH trials being conducted in Japan, additional governmental support is necessary.

Foreign pharmaceutical companies are conducting their drug discovery research outside Japan; therefore, the rationale for not conducting FIH trials in Japan is quite understandable. As for domestic pharmaceutical companies (e.g., Eisai, Takeda, Chugai, and Ono), which are contributing to the development of innovative oncology products by discovering promising seeds in Japan, even they sometimes conduct their FIH trials outside Japan (e.g., CH5183284) (19).

Reflecting the recent globalization of drug development, global phase I trials are now being conducted more often with Japanese institutions participating in some of these global phase I trials (e.g., ASP8273, ABL001, EGF816, HDM201, FGF401) (20–24). Japanese regulatory concerns with respect to global phase I trials presently are (a) that competitive enrollment in every dose-escalation cohort may cause dose escalation without confirming tolerability in Japanese patients and (b) whether important information such as safety issues, including occurrence of severe adverse events or dose-limiting toxicities, will be shared among all participating institutions in each country without delay. Despite these concerns, increased active participation of Japanese institutions in global phase I trials is one of the important options for boosting the number of FIH trials in Japan.

Personalized Medicine in Oncology and Regulation of Companion Diagnostics in Japan

In order to respond to all the recent medical innovations in recent years and to address scientific issues in advanced science and technology, the PMDA established a Science Board in May 2012. The Board consisted of experts in areas such as medicine, dentistry, pharmaceutical science, and engineering. The PMDA uses the Science

Board to communicate with universities, research institutions, and health care professionals to discuss the evaluation of innovative drugs, medical devices, and cellular and tissue-based products. Furthermore, the PMDA attempts to deal with state-of-the-art technology through its review and safety procedures as well as its Pharmaceutical Affairs Consultation on R&D Strategy. The Science Board has produced a document titled "Summary of Discussion on the Assessment of the Current Status of Personalized Medicine related to Development and Regulatory Review."

Rapid advances in technology, together with a deeper cancer biology, have transformed the field of oncology and raised hopes for implementation of more personalized medicine. A key component to achievement of personalized medicine in oncology is the development of biomarkers for treatment selection. Biomarkers that are particularly important for personalized medicine can be broadly categorized as prognostic or predictive biomarkers. Predictive biomarkers are baseline measurements that provide information about which patients are likely or unlikely to benefit from a specific treatment. A predictive biomarker is often designated for use of a particular new treatment using a companion biomarker (a companion diagnostic) in the development of the new treatment. For example, a biomarker that captures overexpression of the human epidermal growth factor receptor 2 (HER2), which transmits growth signals to breast cancer cells, can be a companion biomarker in developing a molecularly targeted drug for breast cancer patients, trastuzumab, which blocks the effect of HER2.

In Japan, in vitro diagnostics (IVDs) have been categorized into class I products (self-certified), class II products (subject to third-party certification), and class III products (subject to PMDA review under marketing authorization applications [MAAs] and approved by the MHLW), mainly depending on risk profile. Companion diagnostics generally fall under class III and usually require review not only by PMDA officers but also by outside advisory experts.

The Japanese regulatory view on companion diagnostics and selection of patients based on biomarker status is mostly in agreement with the concept papers in the United States and the European Union. The Companion Diagnostics Working Group, founded in April 2012, summarized this view. In July 2013, the MHLW/PMDA published its "Notification on approval applications for in vitro companion diagnostics and corresponding therapeutics products" document (25–27), which defines companion diagnostics as IVDs for use in tandem with a specific drug. In the notification, the companion diagnostics are defined as products designed to do one of the following:

- To identify patients who are expected to respond better to a specific therapeutic product

- To identify patients who are likely to be at high risk for developing adverse events associated with a particular therapeutic product
- To be necessary for optimizing the treatment, including dose, schedule, and discontinuation of a particular therapeutic product

On the other hand, the Questions and Answers (Q&As) of the notification excludes the following "in vitro diagnostic agents or medical devices intended simply for disease diagnosis" products from the companion diagnostics.

- Tests used to identify the disease, check the treatment effect, assist in follow-up observation, or evaluate the severity in routine clinical practice
- Biochemical assays related to organ functions such as serum creatinine, transaminases, and blood glucose level
- Hematological assays such as prothrombin time
- Bacterial or viral identification and susceptibility tests for infections

The notification specifies that MAAs of therapeutic products and corresponding companion diagnostics should be submitted at the same time. This encourages sponsors planning to develop drugs and their corresponding companion diagnostics to cooperate with each other from the early stages of the product development stage.

In December 2013, the MHLW/PMDA published a report titled "Technical guidance on development of in vitro companion diagnostics and corresponding therapeutic products." (28). The MHLW/PMDA recommended in principle that both biomarker-positive and biomarker-negative patients be included in clinical trials, preferably at the early development phase because the exclusion of biomarker-negative patients from early development phases would preclude examination of the clinical cutoff value and the difference in benefit-risk balance between biomarker-positive and biomarker-negative patients. In the report, the MHLW/PMDA did not mention statistical requirements regarding clinical data on biomarker-negative patients in early-phase trials because statistical standards concerning biomarker-negative patients had not been established.

In addition, the MHLW/PMDA mentioned that it is necessary, in principle, to conduct prospective randomized controlled trials for the development of drugs and their corresponding companion diagnostics. However, it is difficult to conduct prospective randomized controlled trials in some instances, such as:

- Cases where it is difficult or inappropriate to verify qualification by prospective randomized controlled trials, such as cases where limiting the patient population to be treated based on the status of the efficacy biomarker would make it extremely difficult to conduct a randomized controlled trial from the viewpoint of sample size

- Cases where it is difficult to verify its qualification by prospective randomized controlled trials from an ethical point of view, such as when the safety biomarker may be associated with extremely serious adverse events

In the report, the MHLW/PMDA also mentioned that evaluation of the biomarker based primarily on the results of retrospective analyses is acceptable if the analyses meet all of the following five conditions:

1. The retrospective analysis uses measurement methods that have undergone certain analytical test validation.
2. An appropriate hypothesis has been defined, and statistical analysis on the biomarker has been planned, before data are analyzed.
3. Statistically appropriate analysis in terms of multiplicity adjustment, and so on, has been planned and conducted.
4. The retrospective analysis derives from randomized controlled trials that were appropriately planned and conducted and in which data were obtained, from all registered participants, wherever possible.
5. Consistent analytical results have been obtained from results of two or more independent clinical trials, each of which meets all of the previous four conditions.

EXAMPLE OF THE ISSUES IN NEW DRUG EVALUATION IN JAPAN

The Evaluation of the Treatment Effect for the Japanese Population in Multiregional Clinical Trials

As described previously, Japan's participation in global clinical trials has been steadily increasing. One of the important issues in MRCTs is the evaluation of the treatment effect for local region population. The Q&A No. 11 document for the ICH E5 guideline suggests an approximate strategy, which is based on demonstrating a significant effect in the entire study together with *consistent trends* in treatment comparisons across the regions (29). However, the term *consistent trends* is not explicitly defined and could be interpreted arbitrarily. In addition, this guideline also mentions that it is difficult to generalize what study results would be judged persuasive, as this is clearly a regional determination.

In Japan, "Basic Principles on Global Clinical Trials" describes a sufficient statistical power to detect statistically significant difference, which should not necessarily

be secured within the Japanese subpopulation. However, if results from a Japanese subgroup are markedly different from those in the entire study population, the reasons for it should be examined and an additional clinical trial may be needed where necessary (4). In "Basic Principles on Global Clinical Trials (Reference Cases)," when evaluating the data, the precision of the point estimate (e.g., standard deviation) should be taken into account as well as the point estimate itself based on the sample size (5). Furthermore, the results of the secondary endpoints in a Japanese subgroup should be evaluated to ensure that the results are consistent with those on primary endpoints in the Japanese subgroup. Similarly, any clear safety differences between the Japanese subgroup and the overall study population warrant investigation. If any differences are apparent, whether the data from the global trial can corroborate the efficacy and safety of the drug in Japanese patients should be carefully evaluated. Systematic consideration of reasons for the difference should be made using relevant data such as results of subgroup analysis of individual factors.

An example of the evaluation of the treatment effect for Japanese population in oncology drug development is described in the following discussion. In May 2012, the application for pertuzumab was submitted based on the results of a phase III study (30). The purpose of this study was to demonstrate the superiority of the pertuzumab combination therapy group over the placebo combination therapy group. This study was conducted in 204 centers in 25 countries, including Japan. Participating patients with distant metastatic or recurrent HER2-positive breast cancer had not received chemotherapy to investigate the efficacy and safety of concomitant use of pertuzumab or placebo added to trastuzumab/docetaxel combination therapy.

All 808 patients enrolled in the study (402 patients in the pertuzumab combination therapy group, 406 patients in the placebo combination therapy group) were included in the intent-to-treat (ITT) population for efficacy analysis. The primary endpoint of the study was progression-free survival (PFS) based on the assessment of the independent review facility (IRF). Results of the final analysis of PFS (IRF assessment) in each group are shown in Table 48.1.

In this study, it was speculated that, assuming that the efficacy (hazard ratio) expected for the Japanese population is similar to that of the total population, consistent results would be obtained with conditional probability of 80% provided that 30 events are observed in Japan. Thus, the study was continued under blinded conditions until 30 events for PFS (IRF assessment) occurred in Japanese patients.

Of the 53 Japanese patients included in the ITT population, 26 were in the pertuzumab combination therapy group and 27 were in the placebo combination therapy group. As a result, the hazard ratio (95% confidence interval [CI]) in Japanese patients was 1.92 [0.91,

TABLE 48.1 Final Results of Progression-Free Survival (ITT population, IRF assessment)

	Pertuzumab Combination Therapy Group	Placebo Combination Therapy Group
Number of patients	402	406
Number of deaths or progression (%)	191 (47.5)	242 (59.6)
Median [95% CI] (months)	18.5 [14.6, 22.8]	12.4 [10.4, 13.2]
Hazard ratio* [95%CI]	0.62 [0.51, 0.75]	
p value (two-sided)[†]	< .0001	

CI, confidence interval; IRF, independent review facility; ITT, intent-to-treat.

*Cox proportional hazard model adjusted for stratification factors (prior treatment status and region).

[†]Stratified log-rank test (stratified by prior treatment status and region).

4.04], and the PFS analysis results in the Japanese population are not consistent with those of the overall study population.

The PMDA and the drug manufacturer considered this result. The discrepancy in the distribution of the following background factors between the treatment groups in the Japanese population was observed in the following parameters: visceral disease status (visceral or nonvisceral disease), HER2 expression level assessed by immunohistochemistry, Eastern Cooperative Oncology Group (ECOG) performance status, and hormone receptor (estrogen/progesterone) expression level. Table 48.2 shows simultaneous distribution of above prognostic factors in the Japanese population.

Results of Cox regression analysis of the total population suggested that visceral disease status, HER2 expression assessed by immunohistochemistry, and ECOG performance status all affected PFS (i.e., prognostic factors). The hazard ratio [95% CI] in the Japanese population adjusted by these prognostic factors using the Cox proportional hazard models was 1.91 [0.69, 5.27]. Any differences in efficacy between Japanese and non-Japanese patients were investigated using a multivariate analysis model with "Japanese/non-Japanese patients" and "interactions between treatment group and Japanese/non-Japanese patients" added to the model. The result suggested the existence of interactions between the efficacy in the Japanese population and the non-Japanese population.

It is suggested that the inconsistency was possibly caused by the small sample size in the Japanese population and the nonuniformity in the distribution of the prognostic factors between the treatment groups. The explanation was considered to be acceptable, but it is practically difficult to conclude, based on the results of this study, that pertuzumab is expected to be effective in Japanese patients, for the following reasons:

1. Analytical results suggest the presence of interactions of treatment effect (PFS) and ethnicity (Japanese population vs. non-Japanese population).
2. Estimates of the treatment effect in the Japanese population based on the multivariate analysis models taking account prognostic factors failed to clearly show the efficacy of pertuzumab.

TABLE 48.2 Simultaneous Distribution of Prognostic Factors in the Japanese Intent-to-Treat Population

Visceral Disease	HER2 Expression Level	ECOG PS	Pertuzumab Combination Therapy Group (N = 26)*	Placebo Combination Therapy Group (N = 27)*
Yes	2+	0	6 (23.1)	0
Yes	2+	1	1 (3.8)	0
Yes	3+	0	15 (57.7)	9 (33.3)
Yes	3+	1	0	5 (18.5)
No	2+	0	2 (7.7)	1 (3.7)
No	2+	1	0	0
No	3+	0	2 (7.7)	11 (40.7)
No	3+	1	0	1 (3.7)

ECOG PS, Eastern Cooperative Oncology Group performance status; HER2, human epidermal growth factor receptor 2.

*Number of patients (%).

Many other case examples have showed different outcomes for the Japanese population and the entire study population. One cause of these differences could be the sample size of the Japanese population. Although no generally recommended method of calculating the Japanese sample size currently exists (see articles by Kawai et al. [(31)], Uesaka [(32)], and Quan et al. [(33)]), the Japanese sample size is significantly affected by the power and the number of regions in the entire study population. In some cases, the proportion of the Japanese subjects for the entire study population is sufficient at approximately 20%, but in other cases it is more than 40%. However, different results between the Japanese population and the study population may occur by chance with a probability of 20% to 30%. Furthermore, in actual clinical trials, inclusion could be insufficient in terms of balance between Japan and the other regions or feasibility of the study.

In this section, we presented an example of the evaluation of the treatment effect for Japanese population. For actual review or consultation, the issues of an MRCT are considered on a case-by-case basis. We believe that it is important to understand these issues, to perform continuous research concerning them, and to have frequent discussions among industry, academia, and regulatory groups.

NEW INITIATIVES OF REGULATORY REVIEW

Advanced Review With Electronic Data

The Japan Revitalization Strategy (adopted by the Cabinet on June 14, 2013) indicated that it is essential to strengthen the system of the PMDA with respect to both quality and quantity. The Healthcare and Medical Strategy (an agreement among relevant ministers, June 14, 2013) further states that PMDA shall take the initiative in using clinical data for its reviews. After the 3-year preparation period and conducting several pilot projects, the PMDA formally started to accept patient level clinical study data with new drug submission in October 2016 (34,35). This change has had a major impact on the new drug review process in Japan. The PMDA will take the initiative to conduct its analysis and investigation, using clinical trial data submitted electronically. In an application review for individual new drugs, reviewers can conduct various analyses that will provide direct answers to their scientific questions that arise in the review, without asking sponsors to reanalyze data. The analyses will allow the reviewers to make more objective and scientific decisions and further contribute to the quality of the review. The clinical study data are submitted in the standardized format using international data standards developed by the Clinical Data Interchange Standards Consortium (CDISC). Collecting data in a standardized format will allow reviewers cross-product analysis of accumulated clinical study data in the near future. Such investigation will lead to further understanding of course of a disease and its prognosis, as well as the efficacy and safety of similar drugs. It is expected that more guideline documents for clinical evaluation of drugs and guidelines for evaluation methodologies will be published based on the investigation of accumulated study data. In addition, it is anticipated that more informative advice will be provided in clinical trial consultation meetings based on the more scientifically analyzed information. The promotion of such activities is critical to contribute to the increased efficiency of the developments of drugs, including oncology drugs, for life-threatening diseases.

Initiatives to Utilize Real-World Evidence for Regulatory Decision Making

According to the Bipartisan Policy Report, the level of research and development (R&D) efficiency (number of drugs approved per billion dollars of R&D spending) has actually declined in the United States despite an investment of more than $1.5 trillion in R&D over the past 2 decades (36). The extraordinarily high cost of drug development has led to a proportionate increase in drug prices, which in turn causes serious economic problems for patients, medical facilities, and government health-support programs.

In Japan, expenditures on imported medical and drug patents are inordinately high because there are so few Japanese pharmaceutical mega-firms that can develop innovative drugs by themselves. One of the direct consequences is that Japanese universal health care is facing a crisis in cancer treatment (37). It is essential for all stakeholders including the PMDA, therefore, to achieve efficient drug development in order to continue our innovative efforts in the life sciences with the goal of improving overall public health. One of the anticipated solutions in realizing this objective is the utilization of real-world evidence (RWE).

According to draft guidance issued in the United States by the Food and Drug Administration (FDA), RWE is derived from real-world data sources, including electronic health records used within provider settings, laboratory information systems, pharmacy and radiology systems, and administrative claims systems and registries. Other sources include patient-generated data captured on home-based and portable monitoring devices as well as patient information-sharing networks and social media. Real-world data are gathered from sources outside of randomized controlled trials, and reflect the actual experiences of patients during routine patient care (38). The FDA has undertaken several proactive initiatives to promote the use of RWE in regulatory decision making.

At the present time, there are few reliable clinical databases in Japan that can be used for regulatory decision making. The Cabinet Office has proposed a plan, however, to develop a platform incorporating the world's most advanced medical information and communication technology capabilities with the Japanese universal health care system. Using vast amounts of medical examination and treatment data in such a reliable and effective manner should contribute significantly to the development of cutting-edge drugs, therapies, and medical devices in Japan. The use of artificial intelligence in combination with this enormous amount of data also could lead to the development of a system to provide more efficient medical treatment in the health care field (39).

The PMDA and its partners have recently undertaken several initiatives to generate RWE including MID-NET, a large-scale electronic health record database; the MIHARI project, designed to develop a new safety assessment system for postmarketing drugs using Japanese electronic health care data; and a clinical innovation network with a patient registry–based infrastructure aimed at facilitating Japanese clinical trials (40,41). A number of barriers are still to be overcome, however, such as ensuring the transparency and accuracy of the health care data, which will be essential if we are to rely on such information to take appropriate regulatory action. In order to achieve our overall objective of improving public health, therefore, collaborative interaction among academia, the pharmaceutical industry, and the PMDA will be of critical importance.

REFERENCES

1. Japan antibiotics research association. Guideline for evaluation methods of anticancer drugs in Japan. 1991 (in Japanese).
2. Ministry of Health, Labour and Welfare. The revision of the guideline for clinical evaluation methods of anticancer drugs in Japan. 2005 (in Japanese). https://www.pmda.go.jp/files/000206740.pdf
3. International Conference on Harmonization. E5 Guideline: Ethnic Factors in the Acceptability of Foreign Clinical Data (R1). 1998. https://www.pmda.go.jp/files/000156836.pdf
4. Ministry of Health, Labour and Welfare. Basic Principles on Global Clinical Trials. 2007. https://www.pmda.go.jp/files/000157900.pdf
5. Ministry of Health, Labour and Welfare. Basic Principles on Global Clinical Trials (Reference Cases). 2012. https://www.pmda.go.jp/files/000208185.pdf
6. Ministry of Health, Labour and Welfare. Basic Principles for Conducting Phase I Trials in the Japanese Population Prior to Global Clinical Trials. 2014. https://www.pmda.go.jp/files/000157777.pdf
7. Pharmaceutical and Medical Devices Agency. Information search for ethical drug. https://www.pmda.go.jp/PmdaSearch/iyakuSearch
8. Ueno T, Asahina Y, Tanaka A, et al. Significant differences in drug lag in clinical development among various strategies used for regulatory submissions in Japan. Clin Pharm Therap. 2014;95:533–541.
9. Miki Y, Swensen J, Shattuck-Eidens D, et al. A strong candidate for the breast and ovarian cancer susceptibility gene BRCA1. Science. 1994;266:66–71.
10. Soda M, Choi YL, Enomoto M, et al. Identification of the transforming EML4-ALK fusion gene in non-small-cell lung cancer. Nature. 2007;448:561–566.
11. Takahashi M, Ritz J, Cooper GM. Activation of a novel human transforming gene, ret, by DNA rearrangement. Cell. 1985;42:581–588.
12. Ishida Y, Agata Y, Shibahara K, Honjo T. Induced expression of PD-1, a novel member of the immunoglobulin gene superfamily, upon programmed cell death. EMBO J. 1992;11:3887–3895.
13. Unpublished data based on Pharmaceuticals and Medical Devices Agency. Review report (in Japanese). Accessed October 28, 2016.
14. Sinha G. Japan works to shorten "drug lag"; boost trials of new drugs. J Natl Cancer Inst. 2010;102:148–151.
15. McCurry J. Japan unveils 5-year plan to boost clinical research. Lancet. 2007;369:1333–1336.
16. Yamamoto K, Utsunomiya A, Tobinai K, et al. Phase I study of KW-0761, a defucosylated humanized anti-CCR4 antibody, in relapsed patients with adult T-cell leukemia-lymphoma and peripheral T-cell lymphoma. J Clin Oncol. 2010;28:1591–1598.
17. Seto T, Kiura K, Nishio M, et al. CH5424802 (RO5424802) for patients with ALK-rearranged advanced non-small-cell lung cancer (AF-001JP study): a single-arm, open-label, phase 1–2 study. Lancet Oncol. 2013;14:590–598.
18. Matsubara N, Shitara K, Naito Y, et al. First-in-human study of TAS-115, a novel oral MET/VEGFR inhibitor, in patients with advanced solid tumors. J Clin Oncol. 2015; 33(Suppl):Abstr 2532.
19. Zanna C, Vaslin A, Voss MH, et al. Preliminary clinical pharmacokinetics and pharmacodynamics of Debio 1347 (CH5183284), a novel FGFR inhibitor. J Clin Oncol. 2015; 33(Suppl):Abstr 2540.
20. Yu HA, Oxnard GR, Spira AI, et al. Phase I dose escalation study of ASP8273, a mutant-selective irreversible EGFR inhibitor, in subjects with EGFR mutation positive NSCLC. J Clin Oncol. 2015;33(Suppl):Abstr 8083.
21. Ottmann OG, Alimena G, DeAngelo DJ, et al. ABL001, a Potent, Allosteric Inhibitor of BCR-ABL, Exhibits Safety and Promising Single- Agent Activity in a Phase I Study of Patients with CML with Failure of Prior TKI Therapy. Blood 2015; 126: 138
22. A Phase I/II, Multicenter, Open-label Study of EGFRmut-TKI EGF816, Administered Orally in Adult Patients With EGFRmut Solid Malignancies. ClinicalTrials.gov. https://clinicaltrials.gov/ct2/show/NCT02108964
23. Study to Determine and Evaluate a Safe and Tolerated Dose of HDM201 in Patients With Selected Advanced Tumors That Are TP53wt. ClinicalTrials.gov. https://clinicaltrials.gov/ct2/show/NCT02143635
24. FGF401 in HCC and Solid Tumors Characterized by Positive FGFR4 and KLB Expression. ClinicalTrials.gov. https://clinicaltrials.gov/ct2/show/NCT02325739
25. Ministry of Health, Labour and Welfare. Notification on approval application for in vitro companion diagnostics and corresponding therapeutic products (PFSB/ELD Notification No. 0701-10, English). https://www.pmda.go.jp/english/rs-sb-std/standards-development/cross-sectional-project/0005.html
26. Ministry of Health, Labour and Welfare. Questions and answers on companion diagnostics and corresponding therapeutic products (Administrative Notice). https://www.pmda.go.jp/english/rs-sb-std/standards-development/cross-sectional-project/0005.html
27. Nagai S, Urata M, Sato H, et al. Evolving Japanese regulation. Nat Biotechnol. 2016;34:141–144.
28. Ministry of Health, Labour and Welfare. Technical guidance on development of in vitro companion diagnostics and corresponding therapeutic products (Administrative Notice, English). https://www.pmda.go.jp/english/rs-sb-std/standards-development/cross-sectional-project/0005.html

29. International Conference on Harmonization. E5 Guideline: E5 Implementation Working Group Questions & Answers (R1). 2006. https://www.pmda.go.jp/files/000156278.pdf

30. Pharmaceutical and Medical Devices Agency. Review report for pertuzumab. https://www.pmda.go.jp/files/000153631.pdf

31. Kawai N, Chuang-Stein C, Komiyama O, Ii Y. An approach to rationalize partitioning sample size into individual regions in a multiregional trial. *Drug Inform J.* 2008;42:139–147.

32. Uesaka H. Sample size allocation to regions in a multiregional trial. *J Biopharm Stat.* 2009;19:580–594.

33. Quan H, Zhao PL, Zhang J, et al. Sample size considerations for Japanese patients in a multi-regional trial based on MHLW guidance. *Pharm Stat.* 2010;9:100–112.

34. Ministry of Health, Labour and Welfare, Basic Principles on Electronic Submission of Study Data for New Drug Applications. 2014.

35. Ministry of Health, Labour and Welfare, Notification on Practical Operations of Electronic Study Data Submissions. 2015.

36. Bipartisan Policy Center, Using Real-World Evidence to Accelerate Safe and Effective Cures. http://cdn.bipartisanpolicy.org/wp-content/uploads/2016/06/BPC-Health-Innovation-Safe-Effective-Cures.pdf

37. Fujiwara Y, Yonemori K, Shibata T, et al. Japanese universal health care faces a crisis in cancer treatment. *Lancet Oncol.* 2015; 6:251–252.

38. Draft Guidance for Industry and Food and Drug Administration Staff, Use of Real-World Evidence to Support Regulatory Decision-Making for Medical Devices. http://www.fda.gov/ucm/groups/fdagov-public/@fdagov-meddev-gen/documents/document/ucm513027.pdf

39. Cabinet Office, Government of Japan, Japan Revitalization Strategy 2016. http://www.kantei.go.jp/jp/singi/keizaisaisei/pdf/2016_hombun1_e.pdf

40. Takahashi F. Current Situation and Challenges of Medical Information Database Network (MID-NET) Project. *Regul Sci Med Product.* 2015;5:235–243 (article in Japanese).

41. Ishiguro C, Takeuchi Y, Uyama Y, et al. The MIHARI project: establishing a new framework for pharmacoepidemiological drug safety assessments by the Pharmaceuticals and Medical Devices Agency of Japan. *Pharmacoepidemiol Drug Saf* 2016;25:854–859.

49

Clinical Trials in the Year 2025

Apostolia M. Tsimberidou, Peter Müller, and Richard L. Schilsky

Over the past decade, unprecedented treatment breakthroughs have occurred in oncology. New technologies have improved our understanding of genomic, transcriptional, proteomic, epigenetic, and immune mechanisms and aberrations in carcinogenesis. This knowledge, in turn, has stimulated translational research and the discovery of drugs that have improved the outcomes of patients with cancer. Functional genomics and nonclinical model systems have enabled the validation of novel therapeutic strategies, and exciting new data have been reported in preclinical and clinical studies. Ongoing research aims to discover the molecular mechanisms associated with resistance to novel therapies and tumor heterogeneity. The basic strategies of anticancer therapy now include immunotherapy and targeting cancer stem cells, the microenvironment, angiogenesis, and epigenetic mechanisms. Further advances in technology and the use of bioinformatic analyses of complex data to fully characterize tumor biology and function, as well as highly dynamic tumoral changes in time and space, will continue to improve cancer diagnosis and prognosis.

Efficient and carefully designed clinical trials hold the promise of expediting the development of novel anticancer drugs with the potential of curing cancer. For some time, biomarkers have been integrated into early-phase clinical trials of targeted agents and immunotherapy for optimal patient selection. The rapid evolution of cancer in patients who are undergoing therapy requires repeated testing of tumor characteristics and optimization of treatment by selecting a strategy or drug that will inhibit the function of the emerging tumor drivers of disease progression. Cancer clinical trials in the coming years will need to take into consideration the changing landscape of the patients' tumor profiles at the molecular level, as well as the patients' comorbidities. The trials' adaptive designs should allow for changes in therapeutic management (e.g., the addition of investigational drugs) while the trial is ongoing, while preserving the integrity of the trial design and the quality of the trial data. Furthermore, to optimize enrollment of patients with rare tumor subtypes, clinical trials will need to be available immediately when a patient needs treatment. To accomplish this goal, we need to change the paradigm of trial enrollment from the traditional approach of having the patient seek out the trial to an approach of delivering the trial to the patient at the point of care.

Clinical trial data sharing will be essential to prevent redundancy, improve efficiency, and enhance sample size for the analysis of small populations. A standardized database that contains all ongoing clinical trials, eligibility criteria, and up-to-date response, response duration, overall survival (OS), and toxicity data will be a vital tool. More importantly, real world "N of 1" databases such as American Society of Clinical Oncology's CancerLinQ will provide an invaluable learning resource to optimize the treatment of patients with cancer.

Historically, randomized clinical trials have been the gold standard for proof of clinical evidence. These trials typically involve a large number of patients, often require protracted recruitment periods, and are generally very expensive. The eligibility criteria limit the use of the drug or strategy under investigation to highly selected patient populations that are often not representative of patients seen in community practice. In the current era of precision medicine, the notion of one treatment being effective for a large homogeneous patient population is becoming increasingly hard to sustain. Many clinical trials are therefore now designed to address the heterogeneity of patient populations by using adaptive treatment allocation, population enrichment, and sequential stopping. Indeed, in some studies the discovery of relevant subpopulations for adaptive treatment assignment is part of the trial design. The factors that lead investigators to consider such novel study designs are the increasing use of targeted therapies and immunotherapy, stricter standards for efficient and ethical study design, and advances in statistical methods to support such designs.

A typical example is Investigation of Serial Studies to Predict Your Therapeutic Response With Imaging And moLecular Analysis 2 (ISPY-2) (1), an adaptive phase II trial designed to identify effective treatment regimens for patient subsets on the basis of molecular characteristics (biomarker signatures). The design includes the facility to recommend specific treatments and subpopulations for a confirmatory phase III study if preliminary efficacy thresholds are met. Berry et al. (2) developed ISPY-2 as a special case of a larger class of designs known as platform trials, that is, studies that simultaneously evaluate many therapies in a particular disease area. Several recent studies have been designed to identify subgroups likely to benefit from treatment (2), and an important common theme of many novel trial designs is the use of adaptive features.

Finally, the process of selecting clinical trials should be patient-centered, that is, the patient should have access to the available data and participate in the treatment decision-making process with the guidance of the oncologist. Evolving technological advancements are expected to expedite complete tumor characterization (genomics, proteomics, immune markers, other evolving biologic markers), which can be used in treatment selection at the time of diagnosis. This patient-centric model will be enabled by easily accessible databases that contain meaningful data from completed and ongoing clinical trials. Innovative clinical trials will be designed using data from "N of 1" databases (the accuracy of which is invaluable) and will empower continued optimization of treatment selection based on what is learned from previously treated patients.

In this chapter, we review novel elements of clinical trial design that we expect to be commonly used by the year 2025. We expect that clinical trials will be more patient-centered, exploit patient tumor biology (genomics, proteomics, immunomarkers), rely on rapid and comprehensive tumor profiling, and be recorded in databases that patients may search themselves. The role of patients will be one of active participants in the trial rather than as study subjects.

UPDATING CONTINUOUS INFORMATION

In an ideal world, clinical studies would adjust treatment assignments, continuation decisions, and reports in real time as information accrues, while ensuring the integrity of the trial design and the quality of the data. While one can argue that decisions should be based on all available information, such continuous information updating is usually not considered in clinical trials because of the difficulty in maintaining control over "type I" error rates. However, such purely computational and analytical constraints are less of a concern with early-phase studies where simulation-based error rates are acceptable.

There are many ways in which continuous information updating can be achieved. At the highest level, standardized databases should accurately list all clinical trials, eligibility criteria, up-to-date response data, response duration, and OS and toxicity. At the other

end of the spectrum, clinical studies should at least allow for continuous information updating for individual patients across repeat observations and multiple cycles or stages of treatment. Such updating would be implemented in interim analyses, which would require revised methods to be available to investigators. There is some progress toward this goal in the recent literature on clinical trial design. For example, Lee et al. (3) have proposed a design for dose-finding studies with multiple treatment cycles. The design uses information from earlier cycles to optimize later cycle responses, allowing within-patient adaptation.

The implementation of continuous updating requires careful consideration of the design criteria. Among the recorded toxicity and efficacy outcomes for each patient in each treatment cycle, it is convenient to introduce a formal utility function to summarize the relative preferences for different outcomes. "Preferences" refers to an aggregate criterion, taking into account the goals of all stakeholders. Practically, the investigators who develop the study protocol would elicit a specific set of the investigators' preferences.

Averaging with respect to estimated probabilities of unknown quantities, including in particular future outcomes, under a considered dose assignment, we get expected utilities. These expected utilities are then used to assign an optimal dose for each patient.

Figure 49.1 shows expected second cycle utilities for a study with five dose levels. The plots mark the optimal second cycle dose (optimal dose, indicated by star). The different color lines show utilities for different assumed first cycle responses, making dose allocation a patient-specific decision. (The dose allocation is patient-specific, based on a patient's first cycle responses, but not chosen by the patient.) All probabilities are evaluated under hierarchical two-cycle toxicity and efficacy outcomes as a regression on dose. The model is flexible, allows for nonmonotonic dose–response relationships, and learns about the degree of dependence at all levels of the model. This brief example illustrates how future trials can make increasingly more efficient use of available data. In this scenario, future clinical trials provide a framework and the information to allow for more active patient participation, by providing more patient-specific information (i.e., in this scenario patient-specific information is available, but is not used). Current clinical practice and available databases do not readily allow sharing of information across studies, institutions, and organizations. However, the basic tools, methods, and computational engines are already available.

NONRANDOMIZED DATA SOURCES

An important and largely unused source of information is observational data that are routinely collected in registries, as claims data, in electronic medical records, and

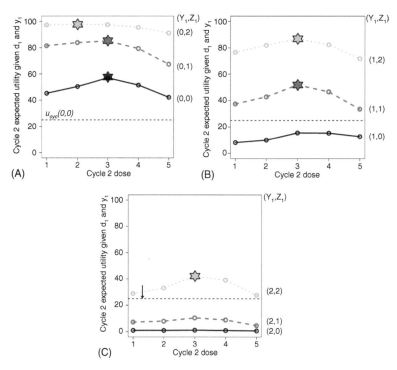

FIGURE 49.1 Two-cycle dose escalation. Panels (A) through (C) plot second cycle expected utilities as a function of first cycle outcomes for an ordinal response for patients with first cycle mild toxicity (B), moderate toxicity (C), and severe toxicity (A), respectively. A conventional dose–response curve would plot probability of toxicity against dose. Instead of probability of toxicity we plot expected utility, which combines relative clinical preferences for toxicity and efficacy outcomes. Instead of a single curve for all patients we show different curves, arranged by first cycle toxicity and efficacy outcome. A star marks the patient-specific optimal cycle 2 dose for patients with different cycle 1 outcomes. The dashed horizontal line shows for comparison the relative utility of no toxicity and no efficacy. The star on each of the different color lines indicates the optimal dose.

from other data sources. The use of this wealth of data to inform clinical studies is limited by the lack of randomization. Current research in clinical trial design is developing methods that use mathematical postprocessing to remove the severe biases that may arise from lack of randomization. Such tools are of critical importance and may eventually enable investigators to make full use of all available data.

A specific example of postprocessing adjustment for lack of randomization is inference for dynamic treatment regimens (DTRs), where a multistage treatment regimen follows a set policy based on earlier stage responses and possibly other baseline covariates. In cancer, later stage therapies are salvage therapies and can often not be randomized, even when frontline therapy is randomized. The patient outcome data are often obtained from postmarketing registries or other observational data sets. The lack of randomization for subsequent lines of therapy may limit the interpretability of the randomized treatment results, particularly OS, the endpoint that most clinicians, patients, and regulators consider to be the most important. Although many stakeholders in a clinical trial still prefer OS data, such data are increasingly difficult to obtain due to multiple lines of therapy being applied in a nonrandomized fashion. Mathematical postprocessing provides a potential

solution. As an example of the nature of the required adjustments, we briefly describe one method that was recently developed by Xu et al. (4).

Figure 49.2 shows an example of a DTR with induction therapy A and salvage therapies in the case of resistance and progression, respectively. In Xu et al. (5), one of the choices for A is fludarabine plus cytosine arabinoside (ara-C) plus idarubicin and one of the choices for salvage therapy is treatment with high-dose ara-C. There are in all 12 possible DTRs, that is, 12 possible paths through the diagram. The aim is to compare these 12 regimens on the basis of expected OS. But the comparison is complicated by the lack of randomization, which is typical for DTRs, and it is impossible to compare regimens on the basis of the observed data only. Xu et al. (5) introduce statistical inference to adjust for this lack of randomization in the assignment of salvage treatments, which are the two later stage treatment decisions (flow diagram, lower half). Popular methods in the literature that allow such adjustments include double robust methods (6) that model the probability of treatment assignment and a regression of outcome on treatment. The strength of these methods is that inference remains consistent (i.e., correct in the hypothetical case of enrolling an unlimited number of patients) even if one of the two models is wrong. However, inference could

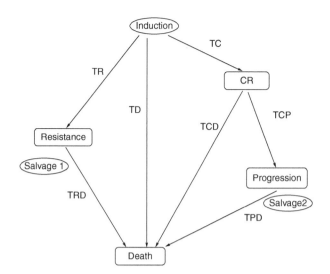

FIGURE 49.2 Dynamic treatment regimen with randomized frontline therapy (induction) and nonrandomized salvage treatments. Model-based inference is used to adjust for the lack of randomization.

CR, complete response; TC, time to complete response; TCD, time from CR to death; TCP, time from CR to progression; TD, time to death; TPD, time from progression to death; TR, time to resistance; TRD, time from resistance to death.

be misleading when both models are wrong, as is unfortunately the case in many applications.

Alternatively, Xu et al. (5) introduced an approach based on flexible modeling of possible transition times under all treatment options. It is critical here that the model has full support, i.e., it is allowed to represent essentially any true survival distribution. This is achieved with flexible models for random distributions known as nonparametric Bayesian inference (7). For details, we refer to the discussion in Xu et al. (5). Figure 49.3 summarizes results in a massive simulation study.

For each simulated data set we estimated the treatment effect using different methods. The different colors in the figure show the distribution of estimated treatment effects over these 1,000 simulations for each of the different methods. The purple curve, on the furthest to the right, corresponds to inference that ignores the lack of randomization. We see a substantial bias, with estimated treatment effects between four and five units. The blue and the green curves correspond to two methods for calculating the inverse probability of treatment weighting. Both methods correctly adjust for the lack of randomization on average, but still show substantial variation. The red curve corresponds to inference under the proposed nonparametric Bayesian model. In summary, with careful consideration of the experimental setup and statistical postprocessing it is possible to obtain meaningful inference about treatment effects even without randomized treatment assignment. This enables investigators to exploit the available information in nonrandomized data. The goal of the different approaches is to infer treatment effect with minimal bias, and this is depicted as the narrowest histogram in the figure.

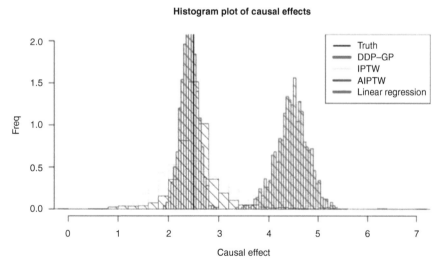

Histogram plot of causal effects

FIGURE 49.3 Dynamic treatment regimen. The figure shows estimated treatment effects under massive repeat simulation. The estimated treatment effects are plotted on the x-axis. The y-axis shows the frequency of the respective estimates as a histogram. Different color histograms correspond to different methods. The simulation study is set up to have a true treatment effect of 2.5 units (marked as a vertical line in the plot). That is, the closer a histogram is to 2.5 (on the horizontal axis), the better the corresponding method. Overall, 1,000 repeat simulations of possible trial realizations were then carried out under this assumed truth. The red histogram (labeled DDP-GP) uses a flexible nonparametric Bayesian model; the green and the cyan histograms are methods that adjust for the lack of randomization with an approach known as inverse probability weighting; the pink histogram is without adjustment for the lack of randomization.

SUBGROUP ANALYSIS: DISCOVERY AND TREATMENT ALLOCATION

In recent years, the treatment of cancer has been transformed by targeted therapies that inhibit specific enzymes, growth factor receptors, signal transducers and immuno-therapeutic strategies, thereby interfere with a variety of cellular processes that are essential for cancer progression and survival. Characterization of genomic, transcriptional, proteomic, immune and epigenetic changes has led to the development of targeted therapies and immunotherapies which have increased response, progression-free survival, and/or OS in patients with certain cancer types. The development of such treatments results in challenging demands on innovation in clinical trial design. Designs need to enable discovery of the patient subpopulation that will benefit the most from specific treatments. Subgroups are characterized by baseline markers, including in particular genomic alterations, and are typically restricted to minimum size to allow for reliable inference about treatment effects and optimal choices. Innovative designs should continue to take into consideration the increasing number of new tests and the complexity of treatment selection, as each patient's tumor has a unique constellation of molecular aberrations. This unique patient molecular profile makes it challenging to test and identify the optimal drug or drug combination for each individual patient.

The recent literature describes many innovative designs for subgroup analysis. For example, in a model-based study designed to find the optimal treatment allocation for different subpopulations of patients, the subpopulations were identified by biomarkers, and the subgroup-based adaptive design included multiple rounds of splitting the patient population into subpopulations defined by dichotomizing biomarker values (8). Figure 49.4 illustrates the formation and inference of the subpopulations, and Figure 49.5 shows how estimated subpopulations are used in the protocol.

A practical implementation would limit the number of recursive splits to, for example, three rounds. For a total sample size of approximately 300 patients, this leads to a design with favorable operating characteristics. After an initial testing phase the design calls for adaptive treatment allocation. Adaptation is determined by the discovered subgroups of patients (Table 49.1).

The subgroup-based adaptation is useful whenever a treatment is expected to be of most benefit for only a small patient subpopulation and when the endpoint is binary. Implementing such inference for subgroups in the process of a clinical trial will, in the future, allow investigators to study combination treatments in small and unique subsets of patients.

PLATFORM AND BASKET TRIALS: MULTIDRUG AND MULTIDISEASE TRIALS

Targeted therapies are likely to benefit patients across different diseases, giving rise to another important challenge for clinical trial design. In cancer, recent developments in genomic profiling technologies have led to the

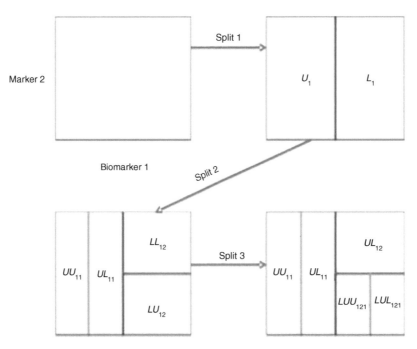

FIGURE 49.4 Subgroup-based adaptive design. The model includes partitioning the patient population by repeated splits with respect to thresholds of biomarkers. The design implements interpatient adaptation by allowing for different treatment allocations in each subpopulation. In the figure, the letters "L" and "U" mark subpopulations characterized by biomarker values below ("lower") and above ("upper") the respective thresholds.

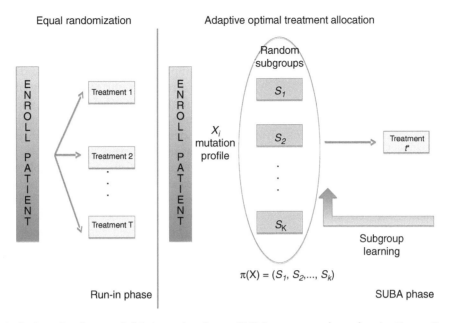

FIGURE 49.5 SUBA design. During an initial run-in phase, SUBA uses equal randomizations. Once adaptive allocation starts, subgroup-based adaptive estimates subgroups (see Figure 49.4) and allows for subgroup-specific allocation probabilities.

SUBA, subgroup-based adaptive.

TABLE 49.1 The Average Numbers of Patients Assigned to Three Treatments After the Run-In Phase in up to Three Different Subsets Under Four Alternative Methods: ER, outcome AR, Reg, and the Proposed SUBA Design i in 1,000 Simulated Trials Under Six Different Scenarios for a Hypothetical Truth. The Average Is With Respect to (Hypothetical) Repeat Simulation. The Simulation Setup Includes Three Treatment Arms. In Simulation Scenarios 2 Through 5, the Simulation Truth Includes a Patient Subpopulation That Benefits Most From Some of the Treatments (Such Subpopulation Is Indicated by Boldface in the Results for SUBA). In Scenario 1, Treatment 1 Is Best for All Patients, and in Scenario 6 All Treatments Are Equal (Null Scenario).

Scenario		ER			AR			Reg			SUBA		
	Subset	1	2	3	1	2	3	1	2	3	1	2	3
1	/	66.8	66.6	66.6	83.0	65.4	51.6	119.5	70.1	10.4	**177**	18.7	4.2
2	S1	33.5	33.1	33.2	33.4	33.2	33.3	35.2	32.9	31.7	**72.6**	18.47	8.9
	S2	33.3	33.5	33.4	33.4	33.3	33.5	35.4	33.0	31.8	8.6	17.8	**73.8**
3	S1	19.5	19.1	19.3	22.2	17.6	18.0	18.7	16.4	22.8	**41.1**	8.9	7.8
	S2	25.2	25.2	25.4	21.1	26.8	27.8	24.1	21.9	29.8	13.7	**35.9**	26.2
	S3	22.1	22.3	22.0	24.6	20.5	21.3	21.3	19.0	26.1	11.3	11.5	**43.5**
4	S1	33.3	33.1	33.4	43.0	42.3	14.5	51.8	48.0	0.0	**52.8**	47.0	0.1
	S2	33.5	33.5	33.2	42.3	43.5	14.4	51.8	48.4	0.0	50.8	**49.3**	0.1
5	S1	33.3	33.1	33.4	39.1	38.5	22.2	51.5	48.3	0.1	**51.1**	47.1	1.6
	S2	33.5	33.5	33.2	38.3	39.3	22.6	51.2	48.9	0.1	47.1	**51.5**	1.6
6	/	66.8	66.6	66.6	66.7	66.9	66.5	65.0	67.8	67.1	66.9	64.2	68.9

AR, adaptive randomization; ER, equal randomization; Reg, regression; SUBA, subgroup-based adaptive.

development of therapies designed to target specific biomarkers and molecular pathways. Examples are the use of trastuzumab for HER2 positive breast cancer (9) and the recommendation against using epidermal growth factor receptor antibodies for *RAS*-mutated colorectal cancer. Some studies investigate the matching of tumor molecular alterations regardless of the patients' cancer types. That is, the study enrolls patients across different diseases. Such trials are known as basket trials and give rise to challenging design questions (2). By the year 2025 we expect to see many such trials, with many treatments successfully graduating from such basket trials to more confirmatory studies. A recent example is Park et al. who recommend neratinib for neoadjuvant therapy in high-risk clinical stage II or III breast cancer among patients with HER2 positive, hormone receptor negative cancer (12). The study showed a high probability that a future study will confirm a benefit.

A fully adaptive design to select disease, treatment, and patient subpopulations for a clinical trial (IMPACT 2) is being conducted at The University of Texas MD Anderson Cancer Center. In this trial, patients with various tumor types undergo tumor biopsy followed by genomic profiling (next-generation sequencing). Patients with U.S. Food and Drug Administration (FDA)-approved drugs for their indication are excluded from randomization. Patients with a targetable molecular alteration are eligible for randomization to targeted therapy (clinical trial or off-label FDA-approved targeted therapy for a different indication) or nontargeted therapy. At the time of disease progression or serious toxicity, patients can cross over to the other arm. The primary endpoint is progression-free survival.

One goal of the study is to identify the subpopulations of patients who benefit most from each of the included targeted therapies. In other words, to identify a subpopulation that could best define eligibility criteria for a future confirmatory study of a particular targeted therapy for specific tumor types. Genomic analysis of tumor samples is performed at the time of enrollment to identify tumor molecular aberrations and to assign treatment for every patient.

Figure 49.6 shows the eligible patient population, by disease and molecular aberrations, and a set of matched targeted therapies. Figure 49.7 illustrates the nature of the inference under this design.

The proposed design includes the use of a criterion that scores all possible subsets of patients for use in the adaptive treatment allocation and reporting as a benefiting subgroup. The criterion includes the difference in average log hazard ratio. The difference is relative to the overall population and identifies a threshold at a minimum clinically meaningful difference. The criterion also includes the estimated size of the subpopulation. Subpopulations with fewer patients are clinically less interesting than large subpopulations that correspond to potentially large benefits if a future confirmatory trial can validate a significant treatment effect. The underlying probability model is a flexible nonparametric Bayesian survival regression. An important feature of the design is that the criterion for selecting subpopulations for adaptive allocation and reporting on one hand, and the probability model on the other hand, are separated. For the probability model, the most possible flexibility is desirable for the best prediction. Finally, the subsets with the best outcomes are selected.

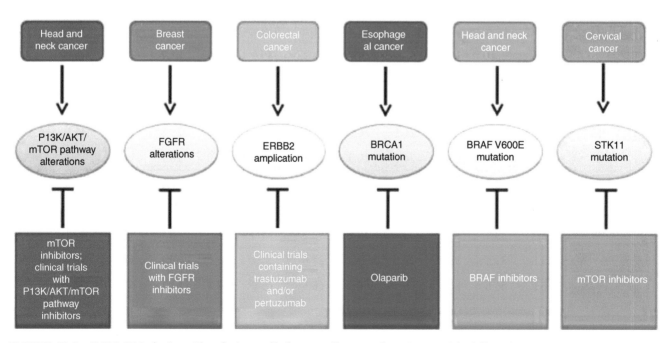

FIGURE 49.6 IMPACT 2 design. The design calls for enrollment of patients with different tumor types. On the basis of their molecular alterations, patients are eligible for certain targeted therapies.

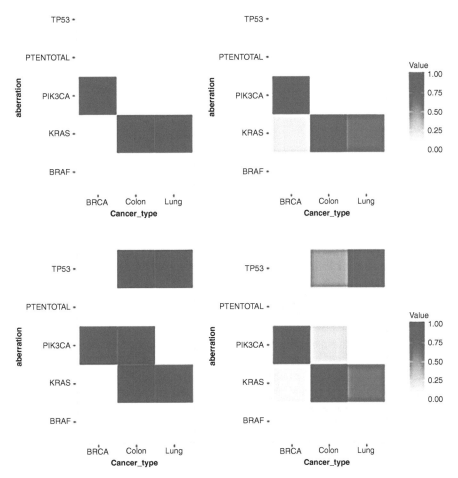

FIGURE 49.7 IMPACT 2 design. The figure shows two hypothetical scenarios. The two left side panels show the assumed truth in two hypothetical scenarios. The figures show the probabilities, under the assumed truth in these simulations, of patients benefiting from targeted therapy. The probabilities are shown by tumor type and molecular aberration. The two right side panels show the final inference under the proposed study design. That is, simulating patient responses under the assumed truth and proceeding with the proposed study design and inference, the right side panels show how often the particular subset was identified in a massive repeat simulation. Blue cells represent mutation-tumor pairs with treatment effect different from the overall population under simulation truth; the two right panels show how often (in massive repeat simulation) each subpopulation was recommended. Dark blue (white) indicates that the corresponding subgroup was recommended in 100% (0%) of the repeat simulations, and lighter blue shades correspond to in-between frequencies.

NOVEL EFFICACY ENDPOINTS

In recent years, there has been a move toward increased engagement of patients in the clinical trial process. A natural consequence will likely be the development and validation of new study endpoints that better reflect outcomes of importance to patients. Conventional indicators of toxicity and clinical benefit will increasingly be replaced by more study- and patient-centric outcome measures. These goals interface well with ongoing research into the more efficient and real-time use of available data and the corresponding development of novel methods. We briefly discuss a typical example of an unusual design criterion and how it relates to the use of more sophisticated methods.

A clinical trial for patients who experience air leaks after pulmonary resection compares the standard procedure versus the use of a novel hydrogel sealant (Progel), which was developed to reduce the probability of air leaks and/or accelerate time until leak resolution (4). Figure 49.8 shows historical control data (black and white histogram) versus hypothetical data of Progel use (red shaded histogram). Progel is expected to shift the distribution toward shorter resolution times and may prevent air leaks from developing at all. Common study designs to compare the two treatments would be based on a comparison of the averages of time to resolution. However, this is clinically inappropriate and practically infeasible in this trial. It is clinically inappropriate because a short resolution period is clinically far more

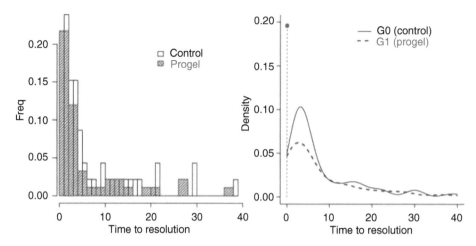

FIGURE 49.8 The left panel shows hypothetical times to resolution of the air leak for patients assigned to control (black histogram) and Progel (red shaded histogram). Based on these data we built a model for the distribution of resolution times under the two treatments (right panel). Note the substantial probability point mass at zero for one of the distributions.

preferable than a period longer than 10 days. As a consequence, a reduction of 1 day is far more important for short resolution times than the same reduction starting from a much longer resolution time. It is practically infeasible because available sample sizes under realistic accrual rates would not allow sufficient statistical power for a comparison of mean resolution times.

A novel trial design was therefore implemented to allow the study to proceed. First, Xu et al. recognized that for patients, reduction in resolution times is more important for early days than for late days. This was formalized by introducing a formal utility as a function of time to resolution and building a design criterion on such utility as an efficacy endpoint. For such novel efficacy endpoints, the use of flexible probability models is important. For example, in the case of this study, meaningful use of the proposed utility function requires a flexible survival regression that goes beyond the usual parametric families and allows for the estimation of small but possibly important changes, especially in the

early days after surgery. An alternative is the use of flexible models for random distributions known as nonparametric Bayesian inference (7). For details, we refer to the discussion in Xu et al. (4). The important feature is that inference allows learning about particular changes in probabilities for resolution within the first few days.

Figure 49.9 summarizes inference. Under the proposed design we are able to carry out the study, which would have been impossible under a traditional study design due to sample size requirements beyond realistic accrual targets.

IMMUNOTHERAPY

Designing innovative clinical trials for novel drug classes can be challenging. During the past decade, breakthroughs in the development of cancer immunotherapies have revolutionized the treatment of patients with cancer. Some, including checkpoint blockade

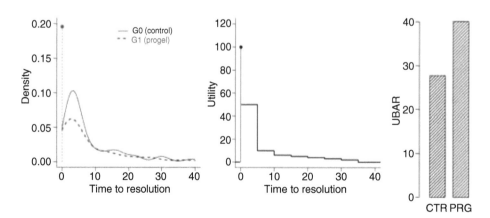

FIGURE 49.9 Weighting the random resolution times under each treatment (left panel) with elicited utilities (center panel), we get weighted average utilities (right panel) for the two treatments.

inhibitors, specifically anti-PD-1 and anti-PD-L1 agents (i.e., pembrolizumab [Keytruda], nivolumab [Opdivo], and atezolizumab [Tecentriq]), are already approved by the FDA to treat particular cancer types based on their significant antitumor activity and favorable safety profile. Other immunotherapeutic strategies that are being developed in current studies include therapies that employ T-cell expansion and dendritic cells.

An example of a challenging issue is the choice of criteria for optimal selection of treatment. Based on the current state of our knowledge, patient selection criteria could include various tumor biomarkers such as mutational burden, POLE or POLD mutations, PD1 or PD-L1 expression, microsatellite-instability status, and new immunotherapy markers now in development; comorbidities; and the toxicity profile of the anticancer therapy and risk factors for toxicity associated with the use of immunotherapy. Some recently published clinical trial designs like subgroup-based adaptive design or its extension proposed in Guo et al. (10) and the IMPACT 2 design allow such adaptive treatment allocation. Additionally, they allow for the discovery of relevant subgroups as part of the same study, at varying levels of generality.

Other issues are the need to allow for nonmonotonic dose/response functions and the opportunity to design seamless phase I/II studies. The lack of monotonicity implies the use of an optimal biologic dose instead of the maximum tolerated dose usually used for cytotoxic agents. In contrast to studies of cytotoxic agents, recently completed immunotherapy studies have used the same patient population for phases I and II. This allows for more efficient study designs and a seamless phase I to II transition. This is implemented in several recently proposed designs. For example: Guo et al. (11) explicitly allow for dose insertion, i.e., the addition of a new dose level that was not originally prespecified in the trial design. This feature becomes more important with nonmonotonic dose/response curves.

Currently, many patients on clinical trials with immunotherapeutic agents are treated for 1 month after the time of disease progression. Although only 5% to 10% of patients are known to have "pseudoprogression," the proportion of patients who continue treatment is often much higher. Biomarkers for early identification of patients with real progression should be developed. More importantly, progression-free survival should be calculated from the time of true disease progression for accurate reporting of clinical outcomes. The existing gap in understanding markers of response and resistance, particularly in immunotherapy-treated patients, combined with the serious toxicity of these treatments (particularly irreversible endocrinopathies) emphasizes the need for coordinated efforts among academic centers, community healthcare providers, basic scientists, pharmaceutical companies, and oncology organizations to better define informative biomarkers and clinical endpoints.

CONCLUSIONS

We are on the threshold of translating discoveries in cancer biology into improved clinical outcomes for a greater number of cancer patients than ever before. This requires innovative clinical trials that account for tumor heterogeneity and clinical evolution in their design and execution. Clinical trials in 2025 are expected to be patient-centric, with patients being informed about their tumor profiles and available treatments and having a central role in the selection of their therapeutic approaches with the guidance of their oncologists. Advances in technology are expected to enable complete tumor characterization (genomics, proteomics, immune markers, other evolving biologic markers), which can be used in treatment selection at the time of diagnosis and subsequent lines of treatment. This patient-centric model will be enabled by easily accessible databases with meaningful data from completed and ongoing clinical trials. The design of innovative clinical trials will be informed by "N of 1" databases (the accuracy of which is invaluable) and will enable continued optimization of treatment selection based on learning from previously treated patients on the same study. In this unique time in history, optimization of the design of clinical trials and discovery of novel therapeutic approaches that target the molecular basis of cancer will accelerate the translation of discoveries in basic sciences into efficient clinical trials that hold the promise to expedite the cure of cancer by offering a precision medicine approach to every patient with cancer.

ACKNOWLEDGMENTS

The authors would like to thank Elangovan Krishnan, MBBS, PhD, Investigational Cancer Therapeutics, University of Texas, MD Anderson for assistance with the references; and Juhee Lee, Applied Mathematics & Statistics, University of California at Santa Cruz, and Yanxun Xu, Department of Applied Mathematics and Statistics, Johns Hopkins University, for assistance with some of the figures.

REFERENCES

1. Barker AD, Sigman CC, Kelloff GJ, et al. I-SPY 2: an adaptive breast cancer trial design in the setting of neoadjuvant chemotherapy. *Clin Pharmacol Ther*. 2009;86(1):97–100.
2. Berry DA. The brave new world of clinical cancer research: adaptive biomarker-driven trials integrating clinical practice with clinical research. *Mol Oncol*. 2015;9(5):951–959.
3. Lee J, Thall PF, Ji Y, Muller P. Bayesian dose-finding in two treatment cycles based on the joint utility of efficacy and toxicity. *J Am Stat Assoc*. 2015;110(510):711–722.
4. Xu Y, Thall P, Mueller P, and Mehran R. A Bayesian nonparametric utility-based design for comparing treatments to resolve air leaks after lung surgery. *Bayesian Analysis*. 2017;12:639–652.
5. Xu Y, Müller P, Wahed AS, Thall PF. Bayesian Nonparametric Estimation for Dynamic Treatment Regimes With Sequential Transition Times. *J Am Stat Assoc*. 2016;111(515):921–950.

6. Bang H, Robins JM. Doubly robust estimation in missing data and causal inference models. *Biometrics*. 2005;61(4):962–973.

7. Johnson WO, de Carvalho M. Nonparametric Bayesian methods in biostatistics and bioinformatics. In: Mitra R, Müller P. *Bayesian Nonparametric Biostatistics*. Springer-Verlag; 2015: 15–23.

8. Xu Y, Trippa L, Muller P, Ji Y. Subgroup-based adaptive (SUBA) designs for multi-arm biomarker trials. *Stat Biosci*. 2016;8(1):159–180.

9. Hudis CA. Trastuzumab–mechanism of action and use in clinical practice. *New Engl J Med*. 2007;357(1):39–51.

10. Guo W, Ji Y, Catenacci DV. A subgroup cluster-based Bayesian adaptive design for precision medicine. *Biometrics*. 2016.

11. Guo W, Ni Y, Ji Y. TEAMS: Toxicity- and Efficacy-based dose insertion design with adaptive model selection for phase I/II dose-escalation trials in oncology. *Stat Biosci*. 2015;7(2):432–459.

12. Park JW, Liu MC, Yee D, et al. Adaptive randomization of neratinib in early breast cancer. *N Engl J Med*. 2016;375(1):11–22.

RECOMMENDED READING

Berry DA. Adaptive clinical trials in oncology. *Nat Rev Clin Oncol*. 2011;9(4):199–207.

Baladandayuthapani V, Ji Y, Talluri R, et al. Bayesian random segmentation models to identify shared copy number aberrations for array CGH data. *J Am Stat Assoc*. 2010;105(492):1358–1375.

Barski A, Zhao K. Genomic location analysis by ChIP-Seq. *J Cell Biochem*. 2009;107(1):11–18.

Lai TS. Adaptive design. In Halbi S, ed. *Oncology Clinical Trials: Successful Design, Conduct and Analysis*. 2016.

Misale S, Yaeger R, Hobor S, et al. Emergence of KRAS mutations and acquired resistance to anti-EGFR therapy in colorectal cancer. *Nature*. 2012;486(7404):532–536.

Pan H, Xie F, Liu P, et al. A phase I/II seamless dose escalation/expansion with adaptive randomization scheme (SEARS). *Clinical Trials (London, England)*. 2014;11(1):49–59.

Wages NA, Slingluff CL, Jr., Petroni GR. A Phase I/II adaptive design to determine the optimal treatment regimen from a set of combination immunotherapies in high-risk melanoma. *Contemporary Clin Trials*. 2015;41:172–179.

Xu Y, Lee J, Yuan Y, et al. Nonparametric Bayesian bi-clustering for next generation sequencing count data. *Bayes Anal*. 2013;8(4):759–780.

Xu Y, Müller P, Tsimberidou A, Berry DA population-finding design with covariate-dependent random partitions. *Technical report, Johns Hopkins University*. 2016.

Zang Y, Lee JJ. Adaptive clinical trial designs in oncology. *Chin Clin Oncol*. 2014;3(4):49.

Index

AACR. *See* American Association for Cancer Research
ABIM. *See* American Board of Internal Medicine
ACA. *See* Affordable Care Act
accrual to clinical trials (ACT) framework
  barriers and solutions, 429
  elderly patients
    CALGB trial, 435
    comprehensive geriatric assessment, 436
    EDICT, 435
    eligibility criteria, 436
    patient factors, 432
    provider factors, 432
    SWOG investigators, 435
    system-level barriers, 432–433
  low-SES patients
    low income, 437
    patient factors, 434
    provider factors, 434
    system factors, 435
    translation services, 437
    transportation, 437
  racial and ethnic minority patients
    implicit bias, 436
    multilevel approach, 436
    NCI-designated cancer center, 437
    patient factors, 433
    provider factors, 433–434
    system factors, 434
    system infrastructure, 436
  rural patients, 434, 437
ACHRE. *See* Advisory Committee on Human Radiation Experiments
ACT. *See* adoptive cell therapy
ACTA. *See* Australian Clinical Trials Alliance
ACT framework. *See* accrual to clinical trials (ACT) framework
acute lymphoblastic leukemia (ALL), 422–423
acute myeloid leukemia (AML)
  acute prolymphocytic leukemia, 420
  allogeneic HSCT, 421
  consolidation therapy, 421
  CR/CRi, 421
  diagnosis, 420

induction therapy, 420
molecular diagnostics, 421–422
mortality, 420
non-APL AML, 421
nonrandomized phase II trial
  confidence intervals, 75
  design and hypothesis test, 74–75
  testing and estimation, 75
randomized phase III trial
  deaths and associated times, 80–82
  design and hypothesis test, 79–80
  Kaplan–Meier survival function estimates, 82–84
  standard errors, 82
treatment failure, 422
adaptive clinical trial designs
  Bayesian design, 132–133
  biomarkers, 126
  interim data monitoring, 293–295
  Lai-Lavori-Liao test, 183
  phase I/II designs, 179–180
  phase II/III designs, 182–183
  phase I studies
    approximate dynamic programming, 177–178
    Beta prior distribution, 178
    cohort-by-cohort up-and-down scheme, 176
    cytostatic therapies, 178–179
    cytoxic treatments, 176
    maximum tolerated dose, 176
    relatively benign drugs, 176
    up-and-down designs, 176
  phase II study, 179
  phase III (survival-endpoint) trials
    information time, 180
    Kaplan-Meier estimator, 180
    logrank statistic, 181
    modified Haybittle-Peto test, 181
    overall survival, 180
    studentized cumulative hazard difference, 181
    time-sequential test statistics, 181–182
adaptive least absolute shrinkage and selection operator (ALASSO), 318
ADC toxicity. *See* antibody–drug conjugates (ADC) toxicity

AdEERS. *See* Adverse Event Expedited Reporting System
adoptive cell therapy (ACT), 146
Advanced Medical Care (AMC) trials, 470–471
Adverse Event Expedited Reporting System (AdEERS), 216
adverse events (AEs)
  attribution of, 212
  collection of, 211
  documentation, 212
  elements used, 202
  IND sponsor reporting to FDA, 214, 215
  NCI/CTEP reporting guidelines
    Adverse Event Reporting System, 215
    CAEPR list, 218, 219
    expedited AE reporting, 216–218
    funding and infrastructure, 214–215
    routine AE reporting, 215
    SAE review and processing, 215–216, 218
  PI reporting to IND sponsor
    CRF, 212–213
    expedited reporting, 213–214
    SAE/AESI report, 213
  requirements, 202
  routine, 201
  serious adverse events, 201–202
  term and grade selection, 211–212
  terminology
    comparison, 207–209
    MedDRA®, 207, 209–210
    NCI CTEP, 210
  treatment-related toxicities, 222
adverse events of special interest (AESI), 213
advisory board, 28
Advisory Committee on Human Radiation Experiments (ACHRE), 13
AEs. *See* adverse events
AESI. *See* adverse events of special interest
Affordable Care Act (ACA), 256
aggressive non-Hodgkin's lymphomas, 423
AGITG. *See* Australasian Gastro-intestinal Trials Group
AJCC. *See* American Joint Committee on Cancer

ALASSO. *See* adaptive least absolute shrinkage and selection operator

alemtuzumab, dose-related neutropenia, 226

alkylating agents, 11

ALL. *See* acute lymphoblastic leukemia

allopurinol, 225

AMC trials. *See* Advanced Medical Care trials

American Association for Cancer Research (AACR), 492

American Board of Internal Medicine (ABIM), 397

American Joint Committee on Cancer (AJCC), 304, 313

American Society of Clinical Oncology (ASCO), 5, 337, 397, 484

amifostine, 416

AML. *See* acute myeloid leukemia

analgesia, 146

anchor-based methods, QOL score, 173

angiogenesis, 259

angiotensin-converting enzyme inhibitors, 226

antibody–drug conjugates (ADC) toxicity, 227

antineoplastic agents, 221

ANZBCTG. *See* Australia And New Zealand Breast Cancer Trials Group

ANZGOG. *See* Australia New Zealand Gynaecological Oncology Group

ASCO. *See* American Society of Clinical Oncology

atezolizumab, toxicities, 228

attitudinal barriers, clinical trial enrollment, 251–252

attribution of adverse events, 212

Australasian Gastro-intestinal Trials Group (AGITG), 478–479

Australia And New Zealand Breast Cancer Trials Group (ANZBCTG)
 breast cancer research, 477
 fund-raising and education/public awareness, 478
 phase 3 LATER trial, 478
 quality of life assessments, 478
 Suppression of Ovarian Function Trial, 478

Australian Clinical Trials Alliance (ACTA), 480

Australia New Zealand Gynaecological Oncology Group (ANZGOG), 479

Australian healthcare system
 ACTA Trial of the Year Award, 480–481
 AGITG, 478–479
 ANZBCTG, 477–478
 ANZGOG, 479
 future directions and challenges, 480
 Genomics Cancer Clinical Trials Initiative, 480
 NHMRC Clinical Trials Centre, 479–480
 oncology cooperative clinical trial groups, 476

balanced randomization, 191

barriers to clinical trial
 ethnic and racial minorities, 253
 non-English speakers, 253–254
 older adults, 254
 organizational barriers, 255–256
 patient factors, 251–253
 provider factors, 254–255

baseline data, 200, 201

basket trials, 125

BATTLE trial. *See* Biomarker-integrated Approaches of Targeted Therapy for Lung Cancer Elimination trial

Bayesian designs
 adaptive clinical trial designs, 178
 adaptive randomization, 132–133, 138–139
 advantages, 140
 binary endpoint, 139
 "calibrated Bayes" designs, 132
 clinical study designs, 131–132
 coherent probability model, 132
 correlated ordinal toxicity monitoring, 137–138
 decision-theoretic approach, 133
 elicitation of priors, 136–137
 extracorporeal membrane oxygenation, 140
 frequentist stopping rules, 132
 historical priors, 135–136
 issues, 139
 likelihood principle, 132
 modeling toxicity and biomarker expression, 138
 operating characteristics, 132, 137
 precision medicine, 133
 real-time updating
  early stopping rules, 133
  fully sequential design, 135
  multiarm trial, 134
  phase II adaptive randomization designs, 135
  phase I oncology dose-finding study, 134–135
  seamless phase II–III design, 135
  single-arm phase II study, 133
  statistical software, 133
 review-and-revise process, 132
 subgroup-based Bayesian adaptive trial, 139

Bayesian single-arm phase II designs, 117

Bayesian statistics, 131

Bayesian two-stage design, 116

Bayes rule, 131

Bayh–Dole Act, 22

BBJ. *See* BioBank Japan

B-cell lymphoma (BCL), 423

BCL. *See* B-cell lymphoma

Belmont Report, 13

beneficence, 15–16

Bernard, C., 9

bevacizumab, randomized trial, 67

bias, 188–189

biased coin randomization, 193

BICR approach. *See* blinded independent central review approach

binary endpoints, 144, 327

BioBank Japan (BBJ), 468

biologic license application (BLA), 214, 492

Biologics Price Competition and Innovation Act (BPCI Act), 497

biomarker, 323

Biomarker, Imaging and Quality of Life Studies Funding Program (BIQSFP), 270

Biomarker-integrated Approaches of Targeted Therapy for Lung Cancer Elimination (BATTLE) trial, 126, 157, 183

biomarkers
 adaptive designs, 126
 categories, 122
 endpoint biomarkers, 369
 enrichment design, 124
 FISH assay, 126–127
 ICH assays, 126
 immunotherapy trials
  atezolizumab, 404
  melanoma, 405
  nivolumab, 404
  PD-L1 expression, 404–405
  phase III Checkmate 67 trial, 404–405
  tumor-infiltrating lymphocytes, 405
 negative predictive value, 127
 pharmacodynamic, 369
 positive predictive value, 127, 128
 predictive, 122–123 (*see also* predictive biomarker)
 prevalence biomarker, 128
 prognostic, 123–124 (*see also* prognostic biomarker)
 regulatory approval, 124
 treatment interaction design, 124–125
 tumor heterogeneity, 271–272
 umbrella trials, 125–126

Biomarkers Qualification program, 243

Biospecimen Reporting for Improved Study Quality (BRISQ) guidelines, 305

BIQSFP. *See* Biomarker, Imaging and Quality of Life Studies Funding Program

BLA. *See* biologic license application

blinded independent central review (BICR) approach
 objective response rate, 377
 progression-free survival, 376

bootstrapping, prognostic model, 321

BPCI Act. *See* Biologics Price Competition and Innovation Act

break-through therapy designation (BTD), 26, 489, 492

breast cancer, HER2 overexpression, 123

BreastQ, 235

brentuximab vedotin, 227

BRISQ. *See* Biospecimen Reporting for Improved Study Quality (BRISQ) guidelines

BTD. *See* break-through therapy designation
budget, 36

CAEPR list. *See* Comprehensive Adverse Events and Potential Risks list
CALGB. *See* Cancer and Leukemia Group B
CALIBER, 51
CALYPSO trial, 479
Cancer and Leukemia Group B (CALGB), 305
  HAI/systemic therapy, 308–309
  multivariable analyses, 310
  patient accrual, 309
  stratified randomization, 309–310
  40502 trial, 292
Cancer Care Delivery Research (CCDR), 461
cancer clinical trial facilitators
  clinical-team–based factors, 444–445
  community-based factors, 443
  geography, 444
  participant-based factors, 443–444
  research delivery system, 445
Cancer Research UK (CR-UK), 461
cancer symptoms, 233
Cancer Therapy Evaluation Program (CTEP), 3, 201
capillary leak syndrome, 228
case report form (CRF)
  data collection (*see* data collection, CRF)
  design and layout, 204
  edit checks and queries, 204–205
  review and testing, 205
  templates, 204
  timeline, 198
cause-specific hazard regression, 351, 353
CBER. *See* Center for Biologics Evaluation and Research
CCDR. *See* Cancer Care Delivery Research
CCOP. *See* Community Clinical Oncology Program
CCRHs. *See* Core Clinical Research Hospitals
CDISC. *See* Clinical Data Interchange Standards Consortium
CDE Browser. *See* Common Data Element Browser
CDF. *See* cumulative distribution functions
CDP. *See* clinical development plan
CDRH. *See* Center for Devices and Radiological Health
CDx testing. *See* companion diagnostic testing
CEAs. *See* cost effectiveness analyses
cell theory, 8
censored data
  Kaplan-Meier estimates, 382
  time-to-event analyses, 375–376
censoring, 316
Center for Biologics Evaluation and Research (CBER), 20
Center for Devices and Radiological Health (CDRH), 493

Certificate of Confidentiality (COC), 21–22
cetuximab, 416–417
CFR. *See* Code of Federal Regulations
CHARMS. *See* Critical Appraisal and Data Extraction for Systematic Reviews of Prediction Modelling Studies
charter, data monitoring committees, 297
checkpoint inhibitors (CPIs), 399, 400
chemotherapy-induced diarrhea (CID), 224
chemotherapy-induced nausea and vomiting (CINV), 224
chemotherapy-induced peripheral neuropathy (CIPN), 224
Chiken clinical trial, 470
CID. *See* chemotherapy-induced diarrhea
CINV. *See* chemotherapy-induced nausea and vomiting
CIPN. *See* chemotherapy-induced peripheral neuropathy
classification trees, 317–318
CLIA. *See* Clinical Laboratory Improvement Amendments
CLICaP. *See* Latin American Consortium for Lung Cancer Research
Clinical Data Interchange Standards Consortium (CDISC), 37, 513
clinical data management, 37
clinical development plan (CDP)
  academia–industry relationship
    academic discoveries, 29
    advisory board, 28
    contract and budget negotiations, 29–30
    contract research organizations, 29
    correlative studies, 27–28
    financial conflict, 31
    ICH-GCP guidelines, 27
    ICMJE policy, 30
    independent data monitoring committees, 28–29
    investigator-initiated study, 29
    medical science liaison teams, 30
    open communication, 27
    pharmaceutical trade associations, 30
    safety evaluation team, 29
    steering committee, 28
    venture investments, 29
  clinical planning, 26
  companion diagnostic test, 26
  first-in-human study, 24
  Gantt charts, 26
  indication selection, 25
  molecular selection assay, 25–26
  new molecular entity declaration, 24
  pembrolizumab drug approval, 26
  preclinical toxicology and pharmacology experiments, 26
  primary elements, 24–25
  standard of care regimen, 26
  target product profile, 24–25
  three-phase drug development paradigm, 26
clinical endpoint, 64, 323
clinical equipoise, 190

Clinical Laboratory Improvement Amendments (CLIA), 281
clinical outcome assessments (COAs), 165
  clinician-reported outcomes, 234
  factors influencing, 233
  observer-reported outcomes, 234
  performance outcomes, 234
clinical research associates (CRAs), 251
clinical trials
  definition, 2
  methodology, 2
  motivation, 3
  phase I, 2
  phase II, 2
  phase III, 2, 3
  resources, 5
  scope, 3–5
  in 2025
    continuous information updating, 517, 518
    discovery and treatment allocation, 520
    immunotherapy, 524–525
    ISPY-2, 516–517
    multidrug and multidisease trials, 520, 522
    nonrandomized data sources, 517–519
    novel efficacy endpoints, 523–524
Clinical Trials Transformative Initiative (CTTI), 295
clinician-reported outcomes (ClinRO), 234
ClinRO. *See* clinician-reported outcomes
clustered regularly interspaced short palindromic repeats (CRISPR), 20
cluster randomization, 194–195
CMA. *See* conditional marketing authorization
COAs. *See* clinical outcome assessments
COC. *See* Certificate of Confidentiality
Code of Federal Regulations (CFR), 13, 33, 489
coherent probability model, 132
COI. *See* conflict of interest
Colombian Collaborative Group for Clinical and Molecular Research in Cancer (ONCOLGroup), 486
colorectal adenocarcinoma
  companion diagnostic assay, 280–281
colorectal cancer
  AGITG, 478–479
Common Data Element (CDE) Browser, 204
Common Rule, 13, 45, 46
Common Terminology Criteria For Adverse Events (CTCAE), 202, 210, 211, 222, 406–407
Community Clinical Oncology Program (CCOP), 255
companion diagnostic (CDx) testing
  biomarker identification, 278
  challenges, 284
  clinical trial designs, 284
  clinical trials and drug development
    crizotinib clinical trials, 283
    erlotinib, 282

companion diagnostic (CDx) testing (*cont.*)
gefitinib, 282
IDEAL-1 and IDEAL-2, 282
INTACT trials, 282
colorectal adenocarcinoma, 280–281
definition, 277
gastrointestinal cancer, 286
guidelines, 282
laboratory assay, 281–282
laboratory developed tests, 284–285
lung cancer, 285–286
mammary carcinoma, 279
non–small-cell lung cancer, 279–280
prototypic laboratory test, 281
statistical analysis, 282
targeted agents codevelopment, 283–284
targeted therapy validation, 277, 278
competing risk survival analysis
breast cancer trial, 346
definition, 346
disease-site–specific endpoints, 346
resources for, 353
statistical methods
cause-specific hazard regression, 351, 353
cumulative incidence function, 347–350
cumulative incidence regression, 350, 352
hazard function, 346–347
notations, 347
overall survival function, 347
subdensity function, 347
time-to-event endpoints, 346, 347
complete cytogenetic response (CRc), 421
completely randomized design, 192–193
complete response (CR), 66, 421
component selection and smoothing operator (COSSO), 318
Comprehensive Adverse Events and Potential Risks (CAEPR) list, 218, 219
Comprehensive Support Project for Oncology Research of Breast Cancer (CSPOR-BC), 465
concept development, IIT
components, 33
concept sheet, 33
innovative and forward-thinking trial design, 34
institutional requirements, 34
new drug combination strategy, 34
risks associated with, 33
conceptual model development, PROs, 235–236
concordance index, 320
conditional marketing authorization (CMA), 495
confidence interval, 114
conflict of interest (COI), 22
consent language, 16, 17
CONSORT statement. *See* Consolidated Standards of Reporting Clinical Trials statement
continual reassessment method (CRM), 87

Bayesian designs, 134–135
dose–toxicity model, 111
for POCRM, 111
single cytotoxic agent
dose allocation method, 109
dose-limiting toxicity, 108
"empiric" model, 108
maximum tolerated dose, 108
model-based toxicity probabilities, 109
one-parameter power model, 109–110
pseudodata prior, 108
rule-based design, 109
skeleton values, 108, 109
two-parameter model, 110
two-stage continual reassessment method, 109, 110
time-to-event toxicity outcomes, 110–111
continuous outcome, meta-analysis, 360
contract research organizations (CROs), 29, 38, 297
contracts, 37
cooperative group clinical trials
Acute Leukemia Group A, 452
Acute Leukemia Group B, 452
advances in cancer therapy, 453
antibiotic and antimalarial therapy, 452
Eastern Solid Tumor Group, 452, 453
NCI Cancer Chemotherapy National Service Center, 452
NCI clinical trial system, 453–454
NCTN research portfolio
advanced imaging, 457–458, 460
Cancer Care Delivery Research, 461
cancer prevention/control, 458–461
developmental therapeutics, 456–457, 460
immunotherapy trials, 456, 460
integral biomarkers, 454, 455, 459
International Rare Cancers Initiative, 461
local therapies, 457, 460
precision medicine, 455–456, 459–460
Core Clinical Research Hospitals (CCRHs), 471
correlative studies
assay reproducibility and robustness, 274–275
formalin-fixed, paraffin-embedded tissues, 272–274
tumor heterogeneity, 270–272
uneven quality of clinical annotation, 275
COSSO. *See* component selection and smoothing operator
cost effectiveness analyses (CEAs)
decision making, 395–396
decision modeling, 397
GDP per capita, 396
incremental cost-effectiveness ratio, 395
ISPOR recommendations, 396
multiattribute health status instruments, 395
quality-adjusted life years, 395

screening colonoscopy costs, 396
cost of cancer care
cost effectiveness analyses, 395–397
fee-for-service system, 394
healthcare and health system costs, 394
incremental costs, 394
inflation rates, 394
market value, 393
medical costs, 393
medicare fee schedules, 394
patient's perspective, 394
payments for patients, 393
short-term costs, 394
societal costs, 394
surgical costs, 394
Cox proportional hazard model, 346, 351
CPIs. *See* checkpoint inhibitors
CR. *See* complete response
CRAs. *See* clinical research associates
CRc. *See* complete cytogenetic response
CRF. *See* case report form
CRi. *See* incomplete recovery
CRISPR. *See* clustered regularly interspaced short palindromic repeats
Critical Appraisal and Data Extraction for Systematic Reviews of Prediction Modelling Studies (CHARMS), 313
crizotinib clinical trials, 283
CRM. *See* continual reassessment method
CROs. *See* contract research organizations
cross-validation, prognostic model, 321
CR-UK. *See* Cancer Research UK
cryotherapy
oropharyngeal mucositis, 224
CSPOR-BC. *See* Comprehensive Support Project for Oncology Research of Breast Cancer
CTCAE. *See* Common Terminology Criteria For Adverse Events
CTEP. *See* Cancer Therapy Evaluation Program
CTLA-4. *See* cytotoxic T-lymphocyte-associated protein 4
CT scans
contrast media, 258
hepatocellular carcinoma, 259
multidetector CT, 258
multiphase imaging protocols, 258
target lesion determination, 262
tumor change detection, 260, 261
tumor size variations measurement, 266
CTTI. *See* Clinical Trials Transformative Initiative
cumulative distribution functions (CDF), 171
cumulative incidence function
of cancer and noncancer, 349
definition, 348
Gray's test, 349–350
NSABP B-04 breast cancer trial, 349, 350
1–Kaplan-Meier estimates, 349, 350
cumulative incidence regression, 350, 352
cytochrome P450 isoenzymes, 229–230

cytokine therapy, 228
cytostatic therapies, 65
cytotoxic therapy
  cytotoxic agents, 223–224
  hematologic toxicities, 224
  nonhematologic toxicities, 224–225
cytotoxic T-lymphocyte-associated protein
    4 (CTLA-4), 228

data analysis and interpretation
  CONSORT statement, 303
  harmonization of regulatory
      requirements, 303
  manuscripts reporting
    abstract, 304
    adverse events, 308
    CALGB trial, 308–310
    efficacy, 308
    elements, 303
    introduction, 304
    patient characteristics, 306–308
    REMARK, 310–311
    statistical methods, 305–306
    study conduct, 305
    study population, 304
    title and authorship, 304
    treatment and administration, 304–305
    tumor biomarker studies, 305
  standardization, 303
  statistical considerations, 303
Data and Safety Monitoring Board
    (DSMB), 309
Data and Safety Monitoring Committee
    (DSMC), 221
data-capture strategy, PROMs, 238
data collection, CRF
  amount and frequency, 203
  baseline data, 201
  eligibility data, 201
  follow-up and survival data, 203
  treatment data, 200
    adverse events reporting, 201–202
    cycle number, 201
    dose modifications, 201
    dose received, 201
    off-treatment reason and date, 201
    response and disease assessment data,
        202
    treatment continuation, 201
    treatment received date, 201
    tumor measurement data, 202–203
data missing at random (MAR), 375
data monitoring committees (DMCs)
  charter, 297, 298
  Clinical Trials Transformative Initiative,
      295
  communication and recommendations,
      299–301
  composition, 295
  contract research organizations, 297
  data monitoring plan, 297
  independent statistician model, 297
  meetings, 297
  modern industry model, 296
  organizational flow for, 296

report preparation
  data freeze, 299
  endpoint summaries, 299
  open reports, 299
  poor report preparation, 299, 300
  scheduled data transfer, 297–298
  sweeping, 298–299
responsibilities, 296
roles, 295–296
statistical and data analysis center, 296
data monitoring plan (DMP), 297
DCE-MRI. See dynamic contrast-enhanced
    MRI
decision-theoretic approach, 133
Declaration of Helsinki, 13, 14
developmental therapeutics, 460
DFS. See disease-free survival
Diagnosis-Related Group (DRG) code, 394
dichotomous outcome, meta-analysis, 360
diffuse large B-cell lymphoma (DLBCL),
    423
discordant-risk randomized design, 340
disease-free survival (DFS), 306
  adjuvant setting, 68
  practical and methodological challenges,
      68–69
  surrogate endpoint, gastric cancer,
      329–331
  time-to-event endpoints, 68
distribution-based methods, QOL score, 173
DLBCL. See diffuse large B-cell lymphoma
DLT. See dose-limiting toxicity
DMCs. See data monitoring committees
DMP. See data monitoring plan
dose-finding algorithm, 88
dose-limiting toxicity (DLT), 85, 108
DRG code. See Diagnosis-Related Group
    code
drug absorption
  food effect, 100
  pH-dependent absorption, 100–101
drug development
  immunotherapy trials, 399
  radiation therapy
    clinical considerations/endpoints, 415
    cytotoxic chemotherapeutics, 412
    dose-escalation designs, 415
    FDA approvals of drugs, 416–417
    nonclinical considerations, 415
    patient population, 414
    patient-reported outcome measures,
        413
    radiation quality assurance, 413–414
    starting dose, 414–415
    toxicity evaluation, 412–413
  surrogate endpoint, 324
drug evaluation process
  European Medicines Agency
    anticancer medicinal products, 503
    conditional approval of drugs,
        501–502
    exceptional circumstances status, 502
    future perspectives, 505
    harmonization process, 499
    role of, 500

role of academia, 504–505
scientific advice, 500–501
standard approval of drugs, 501
Food and Drug Administration
  biomarker-directed drug development,
      493
  BIOSIMILARS, 497
  breakthrough therapy designation, 492
  Code of Federal Regulations, 489
  dose finding, 492
  Federal Food, Drug, and Cosmetic
      Act, 489
  investigational new drug, 490–491,
      495
  PRO measures, 493
  real-world data, 494
  safety collection, 493
  seamless oncology drug development,
      492–493
in Japan
  advanced review with electronic data,
      513
  Basic Principles on Global Clinical
      Trials, 508
  companion diagnostics, 509–511
  ICH E5 Guideline, 508
  JAAME, 507
  multiregional clinical trials, 508,
      511–513
  new drug applications, 509
  new drug review, 507
  OPSR, 507
  personalized medicine, 509–511
  phase I clinical trials, 509
  PMDA, 507
  PMDEC, 507
  real-world evidence, 513–514
DSMB. See Data and Safety Monitoring
    Board
DSMC. See Data and Safety Monitoring
    Committee
dynamic contrast-enhanced MRI
    (DCE-MRI)
  antiangiogenics, 259–260
  response criteria, 265–266
  semiquantitative and quantitative
      methods, 260, 262
  tumor perfusion interpretation, 266

early breast cancer, genomic signatures
  clinical and pathological characteristics,
      336
  magnitude of chemotherapy benefit, 342
  MammaPrint, 336–337
  Oncotype DX, 336–337
  predicted risk categories, 336
Early Breast Cancer Trialists' Collaborative
    Group Oxford (EBCTCG), 477
Eastern Cooperative Oncology Group
    (ECOG), 453
EBCTCG. See Early Breast Cancer
    Trialists' Collaborative Group
    Oxford
ECMO. See extracorporeal membrane
    oxygenation

ECOG. *See* Eastern Cooperative Oncology Group
economic analysis
  cost of cancer care (*see* cost of cancer care)
  multiarm trials, 395
  single-arm, nonrandomized trials, 394–395
eCRFs. *See* electronic CRFs
EDC technology. *See* electronic data capture technology
EDICT. *See* Eliminating Disparities in Clinical Trials
EFPIA. *See* European Federation of Pharmaceutical Industries and Associations
EGAPP panel. *See* Evaluation of Genomic Applications in Practice and Prevention panel
EGFR inhibitor therapy. *See* epidermal growth factor receptor inhibitor therapy
EHR. *See* electronic health record
elderly patients
  ACT framework
    CALGB trial, 435
    comprehensive geriatric assessment, 436
    EDICT, 435
    eligibility criteria, 436
    patient factors, 432
    provider factors, 432
    SWOG investigators, 435
    system-level barriers, 432–433
  age-adjusted mortality rate, 429
  cancer incidence, 430
electrolyte abnormalities, tumor lysis syndrome, 225
electronic CRFs (eCRFs)
  benefits of, 199
  design and layout, 204
  edit checks and queries, 205
  template development, 204
electronic data capture (eDC) systems, 198, 199
electronic data capture (EDC) technology, 37
electronic health record (EHR)
  patient-reported outcome measures, 413
  telehealth, 445
electronic signatures, 42
eligibility data, 200, 201
Eliminating Disparities in Clinical Trials (EDICT), 435
EMA. *See* European Medicines Agency
empiric medicine, 7
endpoint model development, PROs, 237–238
endpoints
  clinical endpoint, 64
  definition, 64
  novel measurements, 70
  phase II and phase III clinical trials
    disease-free survival, 65, 68–69

overall survival, 69–70
  patient PFS, 65, 68–69
  quality of life, 70
  response rate, 66–68
phase I trials, 64–65
primary, 64
secondary, 64
surrogate endpoint, 64
enrichment design, biomarker, 124
environmental-related factors, 314
EORTC trial. *See* European Organization for Research and Treatment of Cancer trial
epidemiology, 9
epidermal growth factor receptor (EGFR) inhibitor therapy
  diarrhea, 225
  mAbs, 225
  rash with, 225
  small molecule TKIs, 225
  standard dose modifications, 225
EQ-5D. *See* EuroQol-5D
esophageal cancer, response endpoint, 146
ethical justification, randomization, 190
ethical principles
  ACHRE, 13
  Belmont Report, 13
  beneficence, 15–16
  Certificate of Confidentiality, 21–22
  COI regulations, 22
  data and tissue banking, 20
  ethical violations, 13
  gene therapy/transfer studies, 20
  informed consent, 16–19
  IRB submissions, 20–21
  justice, 14
  National Bioethics Advisory Committee, 13
  phase I clinical trials, 19
  respect for persons, 14, 16
  state and federal regulations, 14
  violations and deviations, 21
European Federation of Pharmaceutical Industries and Associations (EFPIA), 30
European Medicines Agency (EMA), 243–244, 495
  anticancer medicinal products, 503
  conditional approval of drugs, 501–502
  exceptional circumstances status, 502
  future perspectives, 505
  harmonization process, 499
  role of, 500
  role of academia, 504–505
  scientific advice and guidelines, 500–501
  standard approval of drugs, 501
European Organization for Research and Treatment of Cancer (EORTC) trial, 50
  core questionnaire, 234–235
  QLQ-C30
    instruments, 387
    scoring, 388
    time schedule, 388

EuroQol-5D (EQ-5D), 171–172, 395
EVA. *See* Grupo Brasileiro de Tumores Ginecologicos
Evaluation of Genomic Applications in Practice and Prevention (EGAPP) panel, 337
Ewing, J., 8, 9
experimental bias, 189
external validation, prognostic model, 320
extracorporeal membrane oxygenation (ECMO), 140

FACIT. *See* Functional Assessment of Chronic Illness Therapy
FACT-G. *See* Functional Assessment of Cancer Therapy-General
fast-track designation (FTD), 492
FDA. *See* Food and Drug Administration
FDAAA. *See* Food and Drug Administration Amendments Act of 2007
FDAMA. *See* Food and Drug Administration Modernization Act
FDASIA. *See* Food and Drug Administration Safety and Innovation Act
FDCA. *See* Federal Food, Drug, and Cosmetic Act
febrile neutropenia, treatment-related, 223
Federal Food, Drug, and Cosmetic Act (FDCA), 489
federal regulatory requirements, 35
Federalwide Assurance (FWA), 16
fee-for-service system, 394
^{18}F-FDG PET/CT
  response criteria, 264–265
  standard uptake value, 260
  tumor size and metabolic changes, 260, 261
FFPE tissues. *See* formalin-fixed, paraffin-embedded tissues
FIH study. *See* first-in-human study
Finkelstein's likelihood-based score test, 379
first-in-human (FIH) study, 24, 221
FISH assays. *See* fluorescence in situ hybridization (FISH) assays
Fisher's exact test, 119
fixed-effects models, meta-analysis, 362
Fleming's K-stage designs, 115
FLIPI. *See* Follicular Lymphoma International Prognostic Index
fluorescence in situ hybridization (FISH) assays, 126–127
Follicular Lymphoma International Prognostic Index (FLIPI), 304, 424–425
Food and Drug Administration (FDA), 207–209
  biomarker-directed drug development, 493
  BIOSIMILARS, 497
  breakthrough therapy designation, 492
  Code of Federal Regulations, 489

dose finding, 492
Federal Food, Drug, and Cosmetic Act, 489
investigational new drug (*see* investigational new drug)
PRO measures, 493
real-world data, 494
safety collection, 493
seamless oncology drug development, 492–493
Food and Drug Administration Amendments Act of 2007 (FDAAA), 30
Food and Drug Administration Modernization Act (FDAMA), 495
Food and Drug Administration Safety and Innovation Act (FDASIA), 492
formalin-fixed, paraffin-embedded (FFPE) tissues, 270
biomarker quantification, 272
DNA exome sequencing studies, 272
feasibility studies, 272
fixation and storage conditions, 273–274
flash-frozen studies, 272
NanoString platform, 273
pathological assessments, 272
RNA expression data, 273
RNA quality, 273
tissue gene expression patterns, 274
FTD. *See* fast-track designation
Functional Assessment of Cancer Therapy-General (FACT-G), 234–235
Functional Assessment of Chronic Illness Therapy (FACIT), 234
FWA. *See* Federalwide Assurance

GAICO. *See* Grupo Argentino de Investigación Clínica en Oncología
Gantt charts, 26
gastric cancer, surrogate endpoint
disease-free-survival, 329–331
meta-analysis, 328–329
progression-free survival, 330–332
gastroesophageal adenocarcinoma (GEC), 139
gastrointestinal cancer, EGFR overexpression, 286
gastrointestinal stromal tumors, AGITG, 478
gastrointestinal (GI) toxicities, 224
GBECAM. *See* Grupo Brasileiro de Estudos em Cancer de Mama
GBOT. *See* Grupo Brasileiro de Oncologia Torácica
GCIG. *See* Gynecologic Cancer InterGroup
GCP guidelines. *See* Good Clinical Practice guidelines
GEC. *See* gastroesophageal adenocarcinoma
GECOPERU. *See* Peruvian Group of Oncological Cancer Research
Gehan's two-stage designs, 114–115
Genetic Information Nondiscrimination Act (GINA), 20

Genomics Cancer Clinical Trials Initiative, 480
genomic signatures
clinical trial designs for
discordant-risk randomized design, 340–341
fine-tuned modeling, 341
intermediate-signature-risk randomized design, 341
issues, 340
operating characteristics, 340
cost-effectiveness, 341
development, 337
early breast cancer, 336–337
K-fold cross-validation process, 342, 343
permutation scheme, 342
randomized controlled trials, 336
signature values, 336
as treatment-effect modifiers, 341–343
geriatrics, pharmacokinetics, 105
GICR. *See* Global Initiative for Cancer Registry Development
GINA. *See* Genetic Information Nondiscrimination Act
ginseng root, 230
Global Initiative for Cancer Registry Development (GICR), 483
GOCCHI. *See* Grupo Oncologico Coopertivo Chileno de Investigacion
GOCUR. *See* Grupo Oncológico Cooperativo Uruguayo
Good Clinical Practice (GCP) guidelines, 35
GORTEC. *See* Groupe d'Oncologie Radiothérapie Tête et Cou
grapefruit juice, 230
Gray's test, 349–350
Groupe d'Oncologie Radiothérapie Tête et Cou (GORTEC), 412
Grupo Argentino de Investigación Clínica en Oncología (GAICO), 487
Grupo Brasileiro de Estudos em Cancer de Mama (GBECAM), 486
Grupo Brasileiro de Oncologia Torácica (GBOT), 486
Grupo Brasileiro de Tumores Ginecologicos (EVA), 486
Grupo Oncológico Cooperativo Uruguayo (GOCUR), 486–487
Grupo Oncologico Coopertivo Chileno de Investigacion (GOCCHI), 486
Gynecologic Cancer InterGroup (GCIG), 479

Harvey, W., 9
Hasenclever's score, 425
hazard function, 346–347
hazard ratio, noninferiority trial, 161
healthcare costs. *See* cost effectiveness analyses
Health Insurance Portability and Accountability Act (HIPAA), 13–14
health-related quality of life (HRQoL)
compliance, 388–389
cross-sectional analysis, 389
interpretation of results, 389

longitudinal modeling, 389
missing data, 388
randomized controlled trial
advanced breast cancer, 390
glioblastoma, 390
glioblastoma patients, 390
instruments, 387–388
objectives, 387
sample size, 388
scoring, 388
time schedule, 388
reporting and evaluating, 391
SISAQOL initiative, 389
time-to-event based summaries, 389
health services research (HSR), 397
Health Utilities Index (HUI), 395
hematologic malignancies
acute lymphoblastic leukemia, 422–423
acute myeloid leukemia, 420–422
lymphoma, 423–425
multiple myeloma, 425–426
myelodysplastic syndromes, 422
overall survival, 419
primary endpoints, 419
trial designs, 420
hematologic toxicities
cytotoxic therapy, 224
targeted therapy, 226
hepatic impairment, pharmacokinetics, 104
HER2. *See* human epidermal growth factor receptor 2
heterogeneity, meta-analysis
fixed-effects models, 362
individual trial variability, 362
patient-level treatment effect modifiers, 363
random-effects model, 362
sensitivity analyses, 363
trial-level effect modifiers, 362
hierarchical two-level model, 327
HIPAA. *See* Health Insurance Portability and Accountability Act
Hippocratic physicians, 7
histology-stage-based approach, 133
Hodgkin, T., 8
hormone replacement therapy (HRT), 304
host-related factors, 314
HRQoL. *See* health-related quality of life
HRT. *See* hormone replacement therapy
HSR. *See* health services research
HUI. *See* Health Utilities Index
human epidermal growth factor receptor 2 (HER2), 58, 123
hyperfractionation, 411
hypofractionation, 410–411

iAUROC. *See* integrated area under the ROC curve
ICER. *See* incremental cost-effectiveness ratio
ICH. *See* International Council for Harmonisation
ICH-GCP guidelines. *See* International Council for Harmonisation Good Clinical Practice guidelines

ICMJE policy. *See* International Committee of Medical Journal Editors policy
ICON7 trial, 479
IDE. *See* investigational device exemption
IDMC. *See* Independent Data Monitoring Committee
IIT. *See* investigator initiated trial
image-guided stereotactic body radiotherapy (IG-SBRT), 51
imaging techniques
  computer-aided response assessment, 266–267
  CT scans
    contrast media, 258
    hepatocellular carcinoma, 259
    multidetector CT, 258
    multiphase imaging protocols, 258
    target lesion determination, 262
    tumor change detection, 260, 261
    tumor size variations measurement, 266
  image acquisition techniques, 268
  MRI, 258–260
  objective response rate, 262
  PET scanners, 259
  radiomics, 266
  response assessment criteria, 263–266
  sources of variability, 266
  time to progression assessment, 263
IMM. *See* irreversible morbidity or mortality
immune-checkpoint inhibitors, 24
immune-related adverse events (irAEs), 227
immune-related partial response (irPR), 406
Immune-Related Response Criteria (irRC), 67, 377, 406
Immune-Related Response Evaluation Criteria in Solid Tumors (irRECIST), 67–68
immune-related stable disease (irSD), 406
immunohistochemical (IHC) assays, 126
immunotherapy
  antibody therapies, 399
  cancer vaccine, 89
  checkpoint blockade agents, 89
  checkpoint blockade inhibitors, 525–526
  checkpoint inhibitors, 399, 400
  drug development, 399
  immune checkpoint molecules, 460
  Mel 63 trial
    immunologic endpoints, 91
    protocol-specific dose-limiting adverse events, 90–91
    treatment combinations, 90
  minimal toxicity, 90
  model-based allocation, 91–92
  nonmonotonic dose/response curves, 526
  patient selection criteria, 526
  phase II and phase III trial design
    biomarkers, 404–405
    patient eligibility, 403–404
    randomized phase, 403
    responses and efficacy assessment, 405–406
  phase I trial design
    expansion cohorts, 402–403

maximum tolerated dose, 399, 401–402
  novel endpoints for, 402
  objectives, 399
  protocol-specific immunological endpoints, 90
  pseudoprogression, 525
  sample size and accrual, 92
  single-agent immunotherapy, 90
  statistical modeling framework, 90
  toxicities
    cytokine therapy, 228
    immune checkpoint inhibitors, 228
    immune overactivation, 227
    immune-related adverse events, 227
    oncolytic viruses, 227–228
    vaccine therapy, 227
  toxicity assessment, 406–407
Immunotherapy for Prostate Adenocarcinoma Treatment (IMPACT) trial, 58, 300, 522–523
IMPACT trial. *See* Immunotherapy for Prostate Adenocarcinoma Treatment trial
IMRT. *See* intensity-modulated radiation therapy
IMWG. *See* International Myeloma Working Group
incomplete recovery (CRi), 421
incremental cost-effectiveness ratio (ICER), 395
incremental costs, 394
IND. *See* investigational new drug
Independent Data Monitoring Committee (IDMC), 28–29, 56
individual–level association, 327
individual participant data (IPD), 354–355
indolent non-Hodgkin's lymphomas (iNHL), 423
inducers, 101, 102
industry-sponsored clinical trials, 33
  patient-reported outcomes (*see* patient-reported outcomes)
informative censoring, 161, 379–380
informed consent
  children, 18
  in clinical research, 40
  cognitively impaired individuals, 18–19
  consent language, 16, 17
  elements, 16, 17
  emergency use protocol, 19
  investigator initiated trial, 36
  NCI informed consent templates, 43–45
  non-English speaking individuals, 18
  oral consent, 17
  physician investigators, 18
  planning for, 40
  principal investigator, 16
  principle, 40
  requirements for, 40
  research participants, 40–41
  therapeutic misconception, 18
  written consent document (*see* written consent document)
inhibitors, 101, 102

iNHL. *See* indolent non-Hodgkin's lymphomas
Inoue-Thall-Berry model, 182
institutional review board (IRB), 35–36, 41
insurance, clinical trial enrollment
  Affordable Care Act, 256
  commercial insurance, 255
  IND application, 256
  policy changes, 255
  retrospective study, 255
  state laws, 255–256
integral biomarkers, 454, 455
integrated area under the ROC curve (iAUROC), 320
intensity-modulated radiation therapy (IMRT), 411
intent-to-treat (ITT) analysis, 151, 155–156, 191, 306
interferon (IFN) a-2b toxicities, 228
interim data monitoring
  adaptive designs, 293–295, 301
  data monitoring committees, 295–301
  formal analysis plans, 290
  group-sequential tests, 290–291
  monitoring activities, 290
  one-sample designs, 293
  statistical methods, 290
  trial-wide error risk, 290
interleukin 2 (IL-2) toxicities, 228
intermediate-signature-risk randomized design, 341
internal validation, prognostic model, 320
International Committee of Medical Journal Editors (ICMJE) policy, 30
International Council for Harmonisation (ICH), 35, 303
International Council for Harmonisation Good Clinical Practice (ICH-GCP) guidelines, 27, 43, 44, 207–209
International Myeloma Working Group (IMWG), 425
International Rare Cancers Initiative (IRCI), 461
International Society for Pharmacoeconomics and Outcomes Research (ISPOR) recommendations, 396
interval censoring, 376
investigational device exemption (IDE), 38
investigational new drug (IND), 45, 256
  accelerated approval, 495
  clinical trial, 490
  definition, 490
  drug approval process, 495
  endpoints, 495–496
  FDA review, 490–491
  legal requirements, 489
  safety reporting, 214
  sponsor and investigator responsibilities, 491
Investigation of Serial Studies to Predict Your Therapeutic Response With Imaging And moLecular Analysis 2 (ISPY-2), 516–517

investigator, 33
investigator initiated trial (IIT)
    clinical data management, 37
    concept development, 33–34
    consent development, 36
    contracts, 37
    monitoring and oversight, 37–38
    multicenter trial, 38–39
    pharmacovigilance, 38
    protocol budget, 36
    protocol development, 34–36
    sponsor–investigator role, 33
    study activation, 37
IPD. See individual participant data
ipilimumab, 67, 228, 399
IPSS-R. See Revised International
        Prognostic Scoring System
irAEs. See immune-related adverse events
IRB. See institutional review board
irinotecan, 146
irPR. See immune-related partial response
irRC. See Immune-Related Response
        Criteria
irRECIST. See Immune-Related Response
        Evaluation Criteria in Solid Tumors
irreversible morbidity or mortality (IMM),
        495
ISPOR recommendations. See International
        Society for Pharmacoeconomics
        and Outcomes Research
        recommendations
irSD. See immune-related stable disease
ISPY-2. See Investigation of Serial Studies
        to Predict Your Therapeutic
        Response With Imaging And
        moLecular Analysis 2
ITT analysis. See intent-to-treat analysis
ixabepilone, 292

JAAME. See Japan Association for
        the Advancement of Medical
        Equipment
JALSG. See Japan Adult Leukemia Study
        Group
Japan Adult Leukemia Study Group
        (JALSG), 463
Japan Adult Leukemia Study Group
        (JCOG), 463
Japan Agency for Medical Research and
        Development (AMED), 471
Japan Association for the Advancement of
        Medical Equipment (JAAME), 507
Japan Children's Cancer Group (JCCG),
        465
Japanese Cancer Trial Network (JCTN),
        463
    central monitoring guidelines, 472–473
    SAE reporting guidelines, 473
    site audit guidelines, 473
Japanese cooperative groups
    AMC trials, 470–471
    Chiken clinical trial, 470
    CSPOR, 465
    domestic collaboration, 473
    funding sources, 471

history, 463
international collaboration, 473–474
issues of quality, 469
issues of quantity, 469–470
Japan Adult Leukemia Study Group, 463
Japan Children's Cancer Group, 465
Japanese Cancer Trial Network, 463,
        472–473
Japanese Gynecologic Oncology Group,
        465–468
New Ethical Guidelines, 471
organizational structure, 465–466
role of, 468
SWOT analysis, 474–475
websites, 472
West Japan Oncology Group, 463
Japanese Gynecologic Oncology Group
        (JGOG), 465
    adverse event reporting, 468
    biorepository, 468
    monitoring, 467
    organizational structure, 466
    protocol development, 466–467
    roles of, 466
    site visit audits, 467–468
JCCG. See Japan Children's Cancer Group
JCTN. See Japanese Cancer Trial Network
JGOG. See Japanese Gynecologic
        Oncology Group
JIPANG trial, 472
justice, 14

Kaplan-Meier method, 346
knowledge barriers, clinical trial
        enrollment, 251–252

laboratory developed tests (LDT), 284–285
LACOG. See Latin American Cooperative
        Oncology Group
Lai-Lavori-Liao test, 183
LAIP. See leukemia-associated aberrant
        immunophenotype
Lan–DeMets error-spending functions, 292
LAR. See legally authorized representative
LASSO. See least absolute shrinkage and
        selection operator
Latin America
    cancer burden, 483
    clinical trials, 483–484
    cooperative groups
        breast cancer trials, 485
        CLICaP, 487
        EVA, 486
        GAICO, 487
        GBECAM, 486
        GBOT, 486
        GECOPERU, 486
        GOCCHI, 486
        GOCUR, 486–487
        LACOG, 486
        ONCOLGroup, 486
        profile of, 485
        SWOG Latin America Initiative, 485
    demography and socioeconomic
        characteristics, 483

Latin American Consortium for Lung
        Cancer Research (CLICaP), 487
Latin American Cooperative Oncology
        Group (LACOG), 486
LCSS-Meso. See Lung Cancer Symptom
        Scale adapted for patients with
        mesothelioma
LDT. See laboratory developed tests
least absolute shrinkage and selection
        operator (LASSO), 318
left censoring, 376
legally authorized representative (LAR),
        18–19, 40, 44
leukemia-associated aberrant
        immunophenotype (LAIP), 421
licorice root, 230
logistic regression model, 316
log-rank test, 181, 346
longitudinal modeling, HRQoL, 389
low social economic status (SES) patients,
        431–432
    low income, 437
    patient factors, 434
    provider factors, 434
    system factors, 435
    translation services, 437
    transportation, 437
Lugano classification, 423, 424
Lung Cancer Symptom Scale adapted for
        patients with mesothelioma (LCSS-
        Meso), 235
LUNG-MAP protocol, 126, 157
lymphoma
    aggressive non-Hodgkin's lymphoma, 423
    indolent non-Hodgkin's lymphoma, 423
    Lugano criteria, 264
    risk-stratification tools, 424–425
    staging and response assessment,
        423–424
    tumor flare, 424
Lyric criteria for lymphoma, 264

MAA. See marketing authorization
        application
magnetic resonanace imaging (MRI)
    anatomical information, 258
    dynamic contrast-enhanced MRI
        antiangiogenics, 259–260
        response criteria, 265–266
        semiquantitative and quantitative
            methods, 260, 262
        tumor perfusion interpretation, 266
    multiple sequences, 259
MammaPrint signature, 336–337
mammary carcinoma, companion
        diagnostic assay, 279
Mantle Cell Lymphoma International
        Prognostic Index (MIPI), 425
MAR. See data missing at random
marketing authorization application
        (MAA), 26
maximum tolerated dose (MTD), 59–60,
        65, 85, 108, 399, 401–402
MB-CCOP. See Minority-Based Community
        Clinical Oncology Program

MCAR. *See* missing completely at random
MCID. *See* minimal clinical important difference
MD Anderson Cancer Center's Symptom Index (MDASI), 235
MDASI. *See* MD Anderson Cancer Center's Symptom Index
MDSs. *See* myelodysplastic syndromes
Measure of Ovarian cancer Symptoms and Treatment concerns (MOST), 479
MedDRA. *See* Medical Dictionary for Regulatory Activities
mediation analysis, 326
Medical Dictionary for Regulatory Activities (MedDRA), 207, 209–210
medical science liaison (MSL) teams, 30
Medicare fee schedules, 394
meetings, data monitoring committees, 297
melanoma, treatment response endpoint, 146
meta-analysis
    heterogeneity, 362–363
    impact of, 365–366
    multivariate, 364
    network, 364
    one-stage approach, 361
    outcomes and effect measures, 360–361
    planning, 360
    results interpretation, 363
    two-stage approach, 361–362
methotrexate, 11
MFC. *See* multiparameter flow cytometry
MHLW. *See* Ministry of Health, Labour and Welfare
minimal clinical important difference (MCID), 387
minimal residual disease (MRD), 421–422
minimization randomization
    cumulative imbalance, 195–196
    Pocock–Simon approach, 197
    stratification variable, 196–197
    Taves method, 196
Ministry of Health, Labour and Welfare (MHLW), 468, 471, 507, 510–511
Minority-Based Community Clinical Oncology Program (MB-CCOP), 253
MIPI. *See* Mantle Cell Lymphoma International Prognostic Index
missing at random (MAR), 173
missing completely at random (MCAR), 173, 375
missing data
    censored data, 375–376
    clinical trials, 380–382
    data missing at random, 375
    EMA guideline, 375
    health-related quality of life, 388
    immune-related response criteria, 377
    missing completely at random, 375
    missing not at random, 375
    objective response rate, 377
    progression-free survival, 376–377
    statistical analysis, 378–380
    study designs and strategies, 377–378

missing not at random (MNAR), 173, 375
missing QOL data, 172–173
mitomycin C (MMC), 146
MM. *See* multiple myeloma
MMC. *See* mitomycin C
MNAR. *See* missing not at random
modified Haybittle-Peto test (modHP test), 181
molecular selection assay, 25–26
monoclonal antibody therapy, infusion reactions, 226–227
MOST. *See* Measure of Ovarian cancer Symptoms and Treatment concerns
MPN-SAF. *See* Myeloproliferative Neoplasm Symptom Assessment Form
MRCTs. *See* multiregional clinical trials
MRD. *See* minimal residual disease
MRI. *See* magnetic resonanace imaging
MSL teams. *See* medical science liaison teams
MTD. *See* maximum tolerated dose
multiagent dose-finding trials
    DLT probability, 85–86
    dose–toxicity relationship, 86
    maximum tolerated dose combination, 85
    neratinib and temsirolimus combination, 85
    possible escalation combinations, 86
    tolerable dose diagram, 86
    toxicity order, 86
multiattribute health status instruments, 395
multicenter trial, IIT
    definition, 38
    maintaining communication in, 39
    pharmaceutical sponsored studies, 38
    site/investigator selection, 38
    sponsor obligations in, 38
    subsite clinical trial agreements, 38
multiparameter flow cytometry (MFC), 421–422
multiple myeloma (MM)
    diagnostic criteria for, 425
    international staging system, 425
    survival, 426
multiregional clinical trials (MRCTs), 508, 511–513
multistage phase II trial
    Bayesian two-stage design, 116
    Fleming's K-stage designs, 115
    Gehan's two-stage designs, 114–115
    optimal adaptive two-stage designs, 116
    Simon's optimal two-stage designs, 116
multivariate meta-analysis, 364
multivariate prognostic classifiers
    complete cross-validation, 373–374
    gene expression profiling, 373
    high-dimensional genomic assays, 373
    predictive index, 373
    for preoperative chemoradiotherapy, 373
    resubstitution estimate, 373
    split-sample method, 373
myeloablative therapy, randomization, 191

myelodysplastic syndromes (MDSs), 422
Myeloproliferative Neoplasm Symptom Assessment Form (MPN-SAF), 165–166
myelosuppression, 224

nab-paclitaxel, 292
NanoString platform, 273
narrow therapeutic range (NTR), 101
National Bioethics Advisory Committee, 13
National Cancer Institute (NCI)
    clinical trial system, 453–454
    Common Terminology Criteria for Adverse Events, 210
    informed consent templates, 43–45
National Cancer Institute Community Cancer Centers Program (NCCCP), 255
National Cancer Institute Community Oncology Research Program (NCORP), 255
National Clinical Trials Network (NCTN)
    trials, 270
    advanced imaging, 457–458, 460
    Cancer Care Delivery Research, 461
    cancer prevention/control, 458–461
    developmental therapeutics, 456–457, 460
    immunotherapy trials, 456, 460
    integral biomarkers, 454, 455, 459
    International Rare Cancers Initiative, 461
    local therapies, 457, 460
    precision medicine, 455–456, 459–460
National Community Oncology Research Program (NCORP), 454
National Institute for Health Research Cancer Research Network (NCRN), 461
National Institutes of Health (NIH)
    Recombinant DNA Advisory Committee, 20, 35
    1993 Revitalization Act, 431
National Surgical Adjuvant Breast and Bowel Project (NSABP), 349
NCCCP. *See* National Cancer Institute Community Cancer Centers Program
NCCTG trial. *See* North Central Cancer Treatment Group trial
NCI. *See* National Cancer Institute
NCORP. *See* National Community Oncology Research Program
NCRN. *See* National Institute for Health Research Cancer Research Network
NCTN trials. *See* National Clinical Trials Network trials
NDAs. *See* new drug applications
network meta-analysis, 364
neuropathic pain, 145
neutropenia, treatment-related, 224
neu vaccine Neuvax (E75), 58
new drug applications (NDAs), 98, 214

new drug combination strategy, 34
new molecular entity (NME) declaration, 24
NHL. *See* non-Hodgkin's lymphoma
NIH. *See* National Institutes of Health
nivolumab, 399
NME declaration. *See* new molecular entity declaration
nonhematologic toxicities, 224–225
  chemotherapy-induced peripheral neuropathy, 224
  cytopenias, 224–225
  dose modification guidelines, 223
  gastrointestinal (GI) toxicities, 224
  oropharyngeal mucositis, 224
  targeted therapy, 225–227
  tumor lysis syndrome (TLS), 225
non-Hodgkin's lymphoma (NHL)
  aggressive, 423
  indolent, 423
  phase II trial of thalidomide
    confidence interval, 77
    design and hypothesis test, 75–76
    testing and estimation, 76–77
noninferiority trial design
  endpoints and metrics, 160–161
  experimental product, 159
  interval, 160
  noninferiority margin
    constancy assumption, 162, 163
    control effect, 162
    goals of, 161–162
    limited historical data, 162
    time-to-event endpoints, 162–163
  outcomes of, 160
  placebo effect, 159
  practical considerations, 163
noninformative censoring, 161
non-small-cell lung cancer (NSCLC)
  ALK gene rearrangement, 128
  basket trials, 125
  companion diagnostic assay, 279–280
    ALK gene rearrangements, 283
    crizotinib therapy, 283
    EGFR overexpression, 282
    erlotinib therapy, 282
    gefitinib therapy, 282
    TKI therapy, 283
  pemetrexed diosodium treatment, 122–123
  randomized phase II trial
    Bayesian estimator, 73
    confidence interval, 74
    design and hypothesis test, 72–73
non-toxicity endpoints, 65
normally distributed endpoints, 327
North Central Cancer Treatment Group (NCCTG) trial, 305
NSABP. *See* National Surgical Adjuvant Breast and Bowel Project
NSCLC. *See* non-small-cell lung cancer
NTR. *See* narrow therapeutic range
Nuremberg Code, 13, 14

obesity-based changes, pharmacokinetics, 105
objective response rate (ORR), 262
  missing data
    BICR evaluation, 377
    metastatic disease setting, 377
    postbaseline tumor assessment data, 380
  noninferiority trial, 160
O'Brien–Fleming method, 292
observer-reported outcomes (ObsRO), 234
ObsRO. *See* observer-reported outcomes
ODAC. *See* Oncologic Drugs Advisory Committee
Office for Human Research Protections (OHRP), 13, 207–209
Office of Hematology and Oncology Products (OHOP), 493
OHOP. *See* Office of Hematology and Oncology Products
OHRP. *See* Office for Human Research Protections
ONCOLGroup. *See* Colombian Collaborative Group for Clinical and Molecular Research in Cancer
Oncologic Drugs Advisory Committee (ODAC), 69, 375
oncolytic viruses, 227–228
Oncotype DX testing, 336–337, 342, 397
one-size-fits-all approach, 133
OPSR. *See* Organization for Pharmaceutical Safety and Research
organizational barriers, clinical trial enrollment
  geography/location, 255
  insurance, 255–256
  trial availability, 255
Organization for Pharmaceutical Safety and Research (OPSR), 507
origins of oncology
  cancer medicine, 7–8
  cancer recognition, 7
  cancer science, 8
  clinical trials
    anecdotal reports, 9
    chemicals, 10
    epidemiology, 9
    experimental medicine, 9
    landmark study, 9
    modern chemotherapy, 10–11
    smoking and lung cancer correlation, 10
    streptomycin trial, 9–10
  empiric medicine, 7
  Hippocratic physicians, 7
  human evidence of neoplasia, 7
  modern era, 8–9
oropharyngeal mucositis, 224
ORR. *See* objective response rate
OS. *See* overall survival
OUTBACK trial, 479
outcome-adaptive randomization, 194
ovarian cancer, sunitinib monotherapy, 146–147
overall survival (OS), 69–70, 160

overfitting, prognostic model, 320

Paget, S., 8
pancreatic cancer, randomized phase II trial
  confidence intervals, 79
  design and hypothesis test, 77–78
  testing and estimation, 78–79
PANGEA protocol, 139
paper case report form
  advantages and disadvantages, 199
  design and layout, 204
  template development, 204
PARAGON trial, 479
PARP. *See* poly-ADP ribose polymerase
partial order continual reassessment method (POCRM), 111
  dose-finding algorithm, 88
  dose–toxicity orders, 87
  estimation procedure, 87–88
  single trial illustration, 88–89
  two-stage, 87
partial response (PR), 66
Patient-Centered Oncology Payment (PCOP), 397
patient-focused drug development (PFDD), 493
patient recruitment delay, 51, 53
patient-related barriers, clinical trial enrollment
  communication, 252
  decision aids, 252–253
  knowledge and attitudinal barriers, 251–252
  logistical issues, 251
patient-reported outcomes (PROs), 413
  cancer studies, 241–243
  conceptual model development, 236–237
  endpoint model development, 237
  HRQOL, 234
  prognostic indicator, 234
  PROMs (*see* patient-reported outcomes measures)
  and regulators, 243–244
  selection of, 237
  Skindex and BreastQ, 235
  strategic purposes, 235
  value messages, 237, 244
Patient-Reported Outcomes Measurement Information System (PROMIS), 174, 235
patient-reported outcomes measures (PROMs)
  analysis and reporting, 239–240
  challenges, 241
  criteria for, 241
  data-capture strategy, 238–239
  EORTC core questionnaire, 234–235
  FACT-G, 234–235
  investigator meetings, 241
  MD Anderson Cancer Center's Symptom Index, 234
  measurement strategy, 237–238
  PRO-CTCAE, 234–235
  PROMIS, 235

patient-reported outcomes measures
(PROMs) (*cont.*)
protocol specifications, 241
QLQ-C30, 234–235
selection of, 237
site training, 242–243
study site preparation, 242–243
translations, 237, 241–242
validity and reliability, 234, 235
vendor management, 241
Patient-Reported Outcomes version of the
Common Terminology Criteria for
Adverse Events (PRO-CTCAE),
172–173, 235, 413
PBPK models. *See* physiologically based
pharmacokinetics models
PCOP. *See* Patient-Centered Oncology
Payment
PD. *See* pharmacodynamics; progressive
disease
pediatrics, pharmacokinetics, 105
pembrolizumab, 26, 399
PERCIST. *See* Positron Emission
tomography Response Criteria In
Solid Tumors
PerfO. *See* performance outcomes
performance outcomes (PerfO), 234
permuted block design randomization
advantage, 193
block size selection, 193
features, 194
randomization list construction, 193
personalized medicine trials, 60
Peruvian Group of Oncological Cancer
Research (GECOPERU), 486
PET scanners. *See* positron emission
tomography scanners
PFDD. *See* patient-focused drug
development
PFS. *See* progression-free survival
Pharmaceutical Research and
Manufacturers of America
(PhRMA), 30
Pharmaceuticals and Medical Devices
Agency (PMDA), 510–511
Pharmaceuticals and Medical Devices
Evaluation Center (PMDEC), 507
pharmacodynamic biomarkers, 369
pharmacodynamics (PD), 106
pharmacokinetics
concentration vs. time curve, 99, 100
drug absorption, 100–101
drug administration routes, 100
drug distribution, 101
drug metabolism
drug–drug interaction, 101–102
phase II reactions, 101
phase I reactions, 101
excretion, 102
geriatrics, 105
hepatic impairment, 104
new drug applications, 98
obesity-based changes, 105
parameters, 98–100
pediatrics, 105

phase I clinical trials, 103
phase II clinical trials, 103
phase III clinical trials, 103–104
pregnancy/lactation, 104
renal impairment, 104
pharmacovigilance, 38
phase I clinical trials
adaptive designs
approximate dynamic programming,
177–178
Beta prior distribution, 178
cohort-by-cohort up-and-down
scheme, 176
cytostatic therapies, 178–179
cytoxic treatments, 176
maximum tolerated dose, 176
relatively benign drugs, 176
up-and-down designs, 176
dose-limiting toxicity, 85
immunotherapy, 89–92
maximum tolerated dose, 85
multiagent dose-finding trials, 85–86
partial order continual reassessment
method, 87–89
patient heterogeneity, 93–96
phase II clinical trials
bivariate designs, 118
extended-dose temozolomide, 113
fully sequential designs, 117
goal of, 113
multistage designs, 114–116
randomized designs, 119
single-stage designs, 113–114
time-to-event endpoints, 118–119
phase III clinical trials
adaptive designs
information time, 180
Kaplan-Meier estimator, 180
logrank statistic, 181
modified Haybittle-Peto test, 181
overall survival, 180
studentized cumulative hazard
difference, 181
time-sequential test statistics, 181–182
biomarkers, 157
endpoint considerations, 148
monitoring, 156–157
multiarm trials, 156
patient population, 148
randomization, 148–149
sample size and study duration, 149
time-to-event data
intent-to-treat principle, 151, 155–156
log-rank test, 149
notation, 149
product limit estimator, 149
random censorship model, 149
sample size and power calculations,
150–156
subset analyses, 156
PHI. *See* protected health information
PH model. *See* proportional hazards model
PhRMA. *See* Pharmaceutical Research and
Manufacturers of America
Physician Payments Sunshine Act, 31

physiologically based pharmacokinetics
(PBPK) models, 104
platinum compounds, 11
PMC. *See* Precision Medicine Core
PMDA. *See* Pharmaceuticals and Medical
Devices Agency
PMDEC. *See* Pharmaceuticals and Medical
Devices Evaluation Center
Pocock–Simon approach, 197
POCRM. *See* partial order continual
reassessment method
poly-ADP ribose polymerase (PARP), 58
Pool Adjacent Violators Algorithm, 178
population pharmacokinetics, 103–104
PORTEC-3 trial, 479
Positron Emission tomography Response
Criteria In Solid Tumors
(PERCIST), 265
positron emission tomography (PET)
scanners
3`-deoxy-3`-18 fluorothymidine, 259
^{18}F-FDG signals, 259
response criteria, 265
shortcomings, 259
tumor glucose metabolism
quantification, 259
PR. *See* partial response
PRE-ACT. *See* Preparatory Education
About Clinical Trials
Precision Medicine Core (PMC), 313
prediction error, 328
predictive biomarker
BRAF, 369
disease-free survival, 369
drug effectiveness, 369
HER2 gene, 369
phase II designs, 371
phase III pivotal clinical trial
candidate biomarker, 372
enrichment design, 371–372
interim analysis, 372
test positive and negative patients, 372
umbrella designs, 372
predictive index, 373
Preferred Reporting Items for Systematic
review and Meta-Analysis
(PRISMA) guidelines, 358, 359
pregabalin, 145
Preparatory Education About Clinical
Trials (PRE-ACT), 252
prevalence biomarker, 128
primary endpoint, 64
principal investigator (PI), 16
PRISMA guidelines. *See* Preferred
Reporting Items for Systematic
review and Meta-Analysis
prognostic biomarker
multivariate analysis, 370
multivariate prognostic classifiers,
372–373
Oncotype DX breast cancer, 370
prognostic classifiers, 370
therapeutic decision making, 370
prognostic model
classification trees, 317–318

criteria for, 313
environmental-related factors, 314
host-related factors, 314
importance, 313–314
logistic regression model, 316
overall survival, 314
proportional hazards model, 316–317
regression models, 313
risk models, 313
"small n, large p" problem, 318–319
stratified randomized trials, 314
study design, 315–316
tumor-related factors, 314
validation, 320–321
variable selection methods, 318
programmed death 1 (PD-1) inhibitors, 221
progression-free survival (PFS), 306
advantage, 68
clinical relevance, 69
missing data
blinded independent central review, 376–377
censoring rules, 379
definition, 376
disease progression timing, 379
double-blinded studies, 377
E2100 trial, breast cancer, 381
informative censoring, 379–380
ITT principle, 379
Kaplan-Meier analysis, 380
lost to follow-up, 380
primary PFS analysis, 380, 381
progressive disease, 376
noninferiority trial, 160–161
practical and methodological challenges, 68–69
surrogate endpoint, gastric cancer, 330–332
time-to-event endpoints, 68
progressive disease (PD), 66
PROMIS. See Patient-Reported Outcomes Measurement Information System
PROMs. See patient-reported outcomes measures
proportional hazards (PH) model, 316–317
PROs. See patient-reported outcomes
prostate-specific antigen (PSA), 57
protected health information (PHI), 21
protein programmed cell death-ligand 1 (PD-L1), 228
protocol development, IIT
protocol template, 34
regulatory requirements, 35–36
software platforms, 35
supporting company requirements, 36
version control, 34
proton therapy, 411
PSA. See prostate-specific antigen

QLQ-C30, 234–235
QOL. See quality of life
quality of life (QOL), 70
CONSORT statement, 173–174

design considerations
assessment timing, 168
clinic visits, 169
conceptual framework, 167
constructs/concepts, 167–168
eligibility criteria, 167
open-label and nonrandomized trials, 169
patient burden, 168
PRO integration, 169
questionnaire administration mode, 168
target patient population, 167
interpretation, 173
minimum standards, 167
missing data, 380
MPN-SAF, 165–166
multistep development process, 166
patient-reported outcome, 165
patient self-report, 165
resources for assessment, 165
SISAQOL, 174
statistical analysis strategies, 169–173
racial and ethnic minority patients
ACT framework
implicit bias, 436
multilevel approach, 436
NCI-designated cancer center, 437
patient factors, 433
provider factors, 433–434
system factors, 434
system infrastructure, 436
African Americans, 430–431
NCI-sponsored clinical trials, 431
radiation quality assurance, 413–414
radiation therapy
clinical trials, 411
drug development
clinical considerations/endpoints, 415
cytotoxic chemotherapeutics, 412
dose-escalation designs, 415
FDA approvals of drugs, 416–417
nonclinical considerations, 415
patient population, 414
patient-reported outcome measures, 413
radiation quality assurance, 413–414
starting dose, 414–415
toxicity evaluation, 412–413
mechanism, 410
parameters, 410
principles, 410–411
Therapeutic Index, 410
Radiation Therapy Oncology Group (RTOG), 411
radiosensitizer, 411
random-effects model, 362
randomization
balanced vs. unbalanced, 191
bias, 188–189
biased coin, 193
cluster, 194–195

disadvantages and logistic difficulties, 190
ethical justification, 190
goals of, 189
historical controls, 190
intention-to-treat analysis, 191
issues of control, 188
minimization, 195–197
outcome-adaptive, 194
permuted block design, 193–194
phase III trials, 148–149
randomized consent design, 190
replacement, 193
replication, 188
scientific justification, 190
simple, 192–193
and stratification, 195
timing of, 190–191
randomized controlled trials (RCTs), 355
health-related quality of life, 386–387
non–small-cell lung cancer
Bayesian estimator, 73
confidence interval, 74
design and hypothesis test, 72–73
pancreatic cancer
confidence intervals, 79
design and hypothesis test, 77–78
testing and estimation, 78–79
rasburicase, 225
RCTs. See randomized controlled trials
real-time (RT) consultations, 441
real-time quantitative polymerase chain reaction (qRT-PCR), 421–422
real-world evidence (RWE), 494
RECIST. See Response Evaluation Criteria in Solid Tumors
Recommendations for the Development of Informed Consent Documents for Cancer Clinical Trials, 43
REDCap, 199
REGISTER trial, 478
replacement randomization, 193
reportable payment, 31
Reporting Recommendations for Tumor Marker Prognostic Studies (REMARK), 310–311
research participants recruitment
barriers
clinical study location, 247
communication plan, 247
feasibility planning discussions, 248
participant registries, 248
recruitment materials and outreach activities, 247
unrecognized study participants, 248–249
community outreach, 249
rapid response to inquiries, 249
social media plan, 249–250
study letters/emails, 249
Response Assessment in Neuro-Oncology (RANO) Criteria, 144
response endpoint
esophageal cancer, 146
melanoma, 146

Response Evaluation Criteria in Solid
    Tumors (RECIST), 144, 171, 405,
    406
    complete response, 66
    cytotoxic agents, 66–67
    false-positive and false-negative
        responses, 67
    Immune-Related Response
        Criteria, 67
    irRECIST criteria, 67–68
    partial response, 66
    patient overall response, 66
    progressive disease, 66
    response criteria, 263–264
    stable disease, 66
    time to progression of disease, 67
    version 1.1, 66, 202
Revised International Prognostic Scoring
    System (IPSS-R), 422
RICOVER-60 trial, 395
right censoring, 376
risk–benefit ratio, 221
rituximab, 226
RTOG. See Radiation Therapy Oncology
    Group
rural patients
    cancer mortality rate, 431
    solutions to clinical trial accruals, 437
    U.S. population, 431
RWE. See real-world evidence

SAEs. See serious adverse events
SBRT. See stereotactic body radiation
    therapy
safety evaluation team (SET), 29
scientific justification, randomization,
    190
SCUBA design. See Subgroup ClUsterbased
    Bayesian Adaptive design
SD. See stable disease
SDAC. See statistical and data analysis
    center
secondary endpoint, 64
selection bias, 189
selection designs
    binary endpoints, 144
    ovarian cancer, sunitinib monotherapy,
        146–147
    overall survival endpoint, lung cancer,
        145
    randomization, 143–144
    response endpoint, 146
    sample size calculations, 145
    schema for, 143
    single-protocol infrastructure, 143
    standard-of-care control arms, 143
    statistical principles, 143
    time-to-event outcomes, 144–145
    toxicity endpoint, 145–146
Sentinel Node biopsy versus Axillary
    Clearance (SNAC) breast cancer
    trial, 480
serious adverse events (SAEs), 38,
    201–202, 213
SET. See safety evaluation team

Setting International Standards in
    Analyzing Patient-Reported
    Outcomes and Quality of Life
    Endpoints Data (SISAQOL)
    initiative, 389
SHIVA trial, 60
Simon's optimal two-stage designs, 116
simple randomization, 192–193
simple stratification, 195
single-agent toxicity profiles, 86
single-cell whole-exome DNA, 271
single-stage phase II trial
    confidence interval, 114
    hypothesis testing framework
        probability density function, 113
        response variable, 113
        statistical test, 113
        TMZ example, 114
sipuleucel-T (Provenge) vaccine, 227
SISAQOL initiative. See Setting
    International Standards in
    Analyzing Patient-Reported
    Outcomes and Quality of Life
    Endpoints Data initiative
site initiation visit (SIV), 37
SIV. See site initiation visit
Skindex, 235
small molecule inhibitors, 225
SNAC breast cancer trial. See Sentinel
    Node biopsy versus Axillary
    Clearance breast cancer trial
Social Security Death Index, 203
societal costs, 394
SOFT. See Suppression of Ovarian
    Function Trial
SOMA system. See Subjective, Objective,
    Management, Analytic system
Southwest Oncology Group (SWOG) Latin
    America Initiative, 485
Specific Protocol Exceptions to
    Expedited Reporting (SPEER),
    218
SPEER. See Specific Protocol Exceptions to
    Expedited Reporting
split-sample validation, prognostic model,
    320
sponsor, 33
stable disease (SD), 66
Standard Terms of Agreement for Research
    Trial (START), 30
START. See Standard Terms of Agreement
    for Research Trial
statistical analysis strategies
    quality of life
        arm-level QALYs, 172
        cross-sectional analyses, 170
        endpoints, 169–170
        EuroQoL's EQ-5D, 171–172
        ITT approach, 169
        longitudinal analyses, 171
        MFSAF v2.0, 171
        missing QOL data, 172–173
        multiplicity, 172
        summary measures and summary,
            170–171

statistical and data analysis center (SDAC),
    296
STE. See surrogate threshold effect
steering committee, 28
stereotactic body radiation therapy (SBRT),
    411
    design considerations, 94
    phase I/II trial, 93–94
    trial conduct, 94–96
St. John's Wort, 230
store-forward (SF) consultations, 441
stratification, 195
stratified randomization, 195
stromal cells, 271
subgroup-based Bayesian adaptive trial, 139
Subgroup ClUsterbased Bayesian Adaptive
    (SCUBA) design, 139
Subjective, Objective, Management,
    Analytic (SOMA) system, 413
subsite clinical trial agreements, 38
substrates, 101, 102
Sunshine Act, 31
Suppression of Ovarian Function Trial
    (SOFT), 478
surrogate endpoint, 64
    biological plausibility, 323
    in cancer, 324–325
    definition, 323–324
    drug development, 324
    failures with, 324
    gastric cancer
        disease-free survival, 329–331
        meta-analysis, 328–329
        progression free survival, 330–332
    individual-level association, 323
    meta-analytic approach
        binary endpoints, 327
        examples, 328, 329
        longitudinal measures, 327–328
        normally distributed endpoints, 327
        surrogacy criteria, 328
        time-to-event endpoints, 327
        two-stage modeling strategy, 327
        unit of analysis, 328
    need for, 324
    single trial
        examples, 326
        Prentice's definition and criteria,
            325–326
        statistical approaches, 326
    treatment effect prediction, 328
surrogate imaging biomarkers
    phase II trials, 259
    tumor size changes, 259
surrogate threshold effect (STE), 323, 328
survival analysis
    competing risk survival analysis (see
        competing risk survival analysis)
    Cox proportional hazard model, 346
    events of interest, 346
    Kaplan-Meier method, 346
    log-rank test, 346
    time-to-event data, 346
SUSAR. See suspected, unexpected, serious
    adverse reaction

suspected, unexpected, serious adverse reaction (SUSAR), 214, 468
SWOG Latin America Initiative. *See* Southwest Oncology Group Latin America Initiative
systematic error, 188, 189
systematic reviews
　cancer conferences, 358
　Cochrane systematic reviews, 357
　consistent data collection, 358–359
　data availability bias, 356–357
　impact of, 365–366
　IPD approach, 354–355
　meta-analysis (*see* meta-analysis)
　objective and eligibility criteria, 355–356
　PRISMA flow diagram, 358, 359
　publication bias, 357
　quantitative synthesis, 354
　randomized controlled trials, 355
　search strategies, 355
　study selection bias, 356
　vs. traditional reviews, 354, 355
　validity and reliability, 359–360

TAILORx trial, 341
TALENT clinical trials, 282
talimogene laherparepvec (Imylgic), 227
targeted therapies, 65
targeted therapy toxicities
　adverse reactions, 225
　antibody–drug conjugates toxicity, 227
　EGFR inhibitors, 225
　hematologic toxicities, 226
　monoclonal antibody therapy, 226–227
　off-target toxicities, 225
　on-target toxicity, 225
　small molecule inhibitors, 225
　VEGF inhibitors, 225–226
target product profile (TPP), 24–25
taxanes, 11
telecommunications technology
　prescient and early depiction, 446
　telemedicine (*see* telemedicine)
telemedicine
　clinical-team–based factors, 444–445
　community-based factors, 443
　geography, 444
　participant-based factors, 443–444
　research delivery system, 445
　telehealth, 441
　　consultations, 441–442
　　costs, 441
　　encounters, 442
　　interdisciplinary consultations, 442
　　technology, 441
temozolomide, 416
　null response rate, 114
　phase II trials
　　confidence interval, 114
　　Fleming two-stage design, 115
　　fully sequential designs, 117
　　Gehan's approach, 115
　　Simon minimax design, 116
TH. *See* tumor heterogeneity

Therapeutic Index, 410
therapeutic misconception, 18
three-phase drug development paradigm, 26
thrombocytopenia, 224
TILs. *See* tumor-infiltrating lymphocytes
time-dependent area under the receiver operating characteristic (tAUROC) curve, 320
time-to-event continual reassessment method (TITE-CRM), 110–111
time-to-event endpoints, 68, 327, 346, 347
　censoring, 376
　meta-analysis, 360
　noninferiority margin, 162–163
　selection designs, 144–145
time to progression (TTP), 67, 263
tissue banking, 20
TITE-CRM. *See* time-to-event continual reassessment method
TLS. *See* tumor lysis syndrome
toxicity endpoints, 64–65
toxicity order, 86
TPP. *See* target product profile
Transparent Reporting of a Multivariable Prediction Model for Individual Prognosis Or Diagnosis (TRIPOD), 313
trastuzumab
　prognostic marker, 123
　regulatory approval, 124
treatment data, 200
　adverse events reporting, 201–202
　cycle number, 201
　dose modifications, 201
　dose received, 201
　off-treatment reason and date, 201
　response and disease assessment data, 202
　treatment continuation, 201
　treatment received date, 201
　tumor measurement data, 202–203
treatment interaction design, biomarkers, 124–125
treatment-related toxicities
　adverse events, 222
　class-specific toxicities, 221–222
　cytochrome P450 isoenzymes, 229–230
　cytotoxic therapy, 223–225
　dose modification rules, 222, 223
　"first-in-human" trials, 221
　hematologic toxicities, 223, 224
　immunotherapy, 227–228
　preclinical animal studies, 221
　risk–benefit ratio, 221
　targeted therapy toxicities, 225–227
trial failure
　examples, 48
　excess of complexity
　　diffusion of innovation, 53–54
　　feasibility assessment, 54–57
　　formal comparative testing failure, 53
　　IG-SBRT, 51

patient recruitment delay, 51, 53
slow recruitment, 53
Trial 22113 LungTech study scheme, 51, 52
features, 48
lack of recruitment
　clinician conflicting interests, 50–51
　insufficient coordination across departments, 51
　randomization, 48, 50
personalized medicine, 60
phase I clinical trials, 59–60
phase II-to-phase III transition
　drug mechanism of action, 57–58
　excess of optimism, 58–59
taxonomy, 49–50
window-of-opportunity trials, 60
trial–level association, 327, 330, 331
Trial 22113 LungTech study scheme, 51, 52
TRIBUTE clinical trial, 282
TRIPOD. *See* Transparent Reporting of a Multivariable Prediction Model for Individual Prognosis Or Diagnosis
TTP. *See* time to progression
tumor heterogeneity (TH), 139
　biomarker studies, 271–272
　DNA sequencing approaches, 270
　immunohistochemistry, 271
　immunotherapies, 271
　longitudinal studies, 271
　RNA in situ hybridization, 271
　single-cell whole-exome DNA, 271
　stromal cells, 271
tumor-infiltrating lymphocytes (TILs), 146, 405
tumor lysis syndrome (TLS), 225
tumor-related factors, 314
tumor response rate
　definition, 66
　phase II endpoint, 68
　phase III trials, 68
　as a primary endpoint, 66
　RECIST, 66–68
two-stage continual reassessment method, 109, 110
two-stage meta-analysis models, 361–362

UA. *See* unit of analysis
UI. *See* unit of interest
umbrella trials, 125–126
UMIN-CTR. *See* University Hospital Medical Information Network Clinical Trial Registry
unbalanced randomization, 191
unit of analysis (UA), 194–195
unit of interest (UI), 194–195
University Hospital Medical Information Network Clinical Trial Registry (UMIN-CTR), 469–470
U.S. National Research Act, 13

vaccine-based immunotherapy, 89
vaccine therapy, toxicities, 227

value messages, PROs, 237
variable importance (VIMP) score, 318
variable selection approach
    prognostic factor, 320
variance–covariance matrix, 327
vascular endothelial growth factor (VEGF)
        inhibitors, 221–222
    bleeding events, 226
    diarrhea, 225–226
    hypertension, 226
VEGF inhibitors. *See* vascular endothelial
        growth factor inhibitors

vemurafenib therapy, 125
vendor management, PROMs, 241
von Waldeyer-Hartz, W., 8

WCLC. *See* World Conference on Lung
    Cancer
West Japan Oncology Group (WJOG), 463
WHO response assessment criteria, 263
window-of-opportunity trials, 60
World Conference on Lung Cancer
        (WCLC), 358
WJOG. *See* West Japan Oncology Group

written consent document
    electronic signatures, 42
    exceptions, 44–46
    headings, 42–43
    informational elements, 41
    institutional review board, 40
    online readability programs, 41
    participants, 41
    plain language guidelines, 41
    readability and understandability,
        41–42
    valid informed consent, 43